GOTH'S

MEDICAL PHARMACOLOGY

GOTH'S MEDICAL PHARMACOLOGY

Wesley G. Clark, Ph.D.
Associate Professor
Department of Pharmacology
Southwestern Medical School
The University of Texas Southwestern Medical Center at Dallas
Dallas, Texas

D. Craig Brater, M.D.
Professor of Medicine and Pharmacology
Chairman
Department of Medicine
Director of Clinical Pharmacology
Indiana University School of Medicine
Indianapolis, Indiana

Alice R. Johnson, Ph.D.
Professor
Department of Biochemistry
The University of Texas Health Center at Tyler
Tyler, Texas

Thirteenth Edition
with 421 illustrations

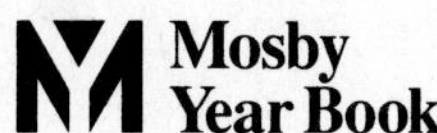

St. Louis Baltimore Boston Chicago London Philadelphia Sydney Toronto

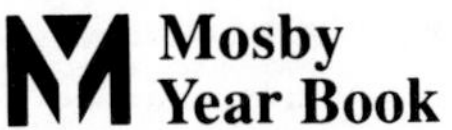

Dedicated to Publishing Excellence

Editor: Kimberly Kist
Assistant Editor: Penny Rudolph
Project Manager: Gayle May Morris
Designer: Jeanne Wolfgeher

Thirteenth Edition

A Mosby imprint of Mosby—Year Book, Inc.

Printed in the United States of America

Mosby–Year Book, Inc.
11830 Westline Industrial Drive, St. Louis, Missouri 63146

Library of Congress Cataloging-in-Publication Data

Clark, Wesley G.
Goth's medical pharmacology.—13th ed./Wesley G. Clark, D. Craig Brater, Alice R. Johnson.
p. cm.
Includes bibliographical references and index.
ISBN 0-8016-0953-4
1. Pharmacology. I. Brater, D. Craig. II. Johnson, Alice R. III. Title. IV. Title: Medical pharmacology.
[DNLM: 1. Pharmacology. QV 4 C596g]
RM300.C513 1991
615′.1—dc20
DNLM/DLC
for Library of Congress 91-25666
CIP

95 96 GW/DC 9 8 7 6 5 4

Contributors

Burnell R. Brown, Jr., M.D., Ph.D., F.F.A.R.C.S.
Professor and Head
Department of Anesthesiology
Professor, Department of Pharmacology
Associate Dean for Phoenix Programs
University of Arizona Health Sciences Center
Tucson, Arizona

William B. Campbell, Ph.D.
Professor
Department of Pharmacology
The University of Texas Southwestern Medical Center at Dallas
Dallas, Texas

Barton A. Kamen, M.D., Ph.D.
Professor
Departments of Pediatrics and Pharmacology
The University of Texas Southwestern Medical Center at Dallas
Dallas, Texas

Bill H. McAnalley, Ph.D.
Research Director
Carrington Laboratories, Inc.
Irving, Texas

James W. Smith, M.D.
Chief
Infectious Diseases Section
Dallas Veterans Affairs Medical Center
Professor
Department of Internal Medicine
The University of Texas Southwestern Medical Center at Dallas
Dallas, Texas

Alvin Taurog, Ph.D.
Professor
Department of Pharmacology
The University of Texas Southwestern Medical Center at Dallas
Dallas, Texas

Michael R. Vasko, Ph.D.
Associate Professor
Departments of Pharmacology and Toxicology, Anesthesia, and Internal Medicine
Indiana University School of Medicine
Indianapolis, Indiana

This edition is dedicated to the memory of
Dr. Andres Goth.

Preface

Dr. Andres Goth, who wrote and edited this textbook from the first edition in 1961 through the eleventh edition in 1984, died on October 1, 1990. He had served for over 30 years as Chairman of the Department of Pharmacology at what is now the University of Texas Southwestern Medical Center at Dallas. Dr. Goth's editions of this text were used in medical schools by many thousands of physicians who are currently in practice, and those editions served the present editors as the model for both the twelfth edition and for the present one, which we dedicate to his memory. We continue the original intention of Dr. Goth, expressed in his preface to the first edition, "to present current pharmacologic knowledge with particular reference to principles and concepts . . . . written primarily for students and practitioners."

This edition contains two new chapters, one on second-messenger systems and the other on treatment of motor disorders. Histamine and antihistamines are now considered together in a single chapter; antidepressants and antimanic drugs are likewise grouped together as are antianxiety drugs, hypnotic drugs, and alcohol. In contrast, several topics are now discussed separately; these include serotonin and its antagonists, kinins and other peptides, hypothalamic releasing factors and growth hormone, drugs used to treat mycobacterial and fungal infections, antimalarials, and anthelmintics. The extensive topic of antibiotics is now covered in two chapters. Although we have limited the overall length of this textbook, coverage is provided of virtually all the important drugs that have become available since the previous edition. In addition, Appendix B, which provides extensive pharmacokinetic data, has been enlarged about 25%.

Wesley G. Clark
D. Craig Brater
Alice R. Johnson

Contents

Section fourteen Prescription writing and drug compendia

Appendixes

Chapter 1

Introduction

Chemical agents not only provide the structural basis and energy supply of living organisms but also regulate their functional activities. Interactions between potent chemicals and living systems contribute to our knowledge of biologic processes and provide effective methods for treatment, prevention, and diagnosis of many diseases. Compounds used for these purposes are called *drugs*, and their actions on living systems lead to *drug effects*.

Pharmacology deals with the properties and effects of drugs and, in a more general sense, with interactions between chemical compounds and living systems. It is a discipline of biology that is closely related to physiology and biochemistry. Nevertheless, pharmacology is unique in that it deals especially with mechanisms of action of biologically active substances.

Although the specific aim of many pharmacologists is to define the biologic activity of chemical compounds, the use of such agents can also contribute greatly to knowledge of living systems. In other words, drugs are frequently used as probes to help dissect fundamental aspects of physiology and pharmacology. This contribution to understanding of life processes is valuable to biologic sciences in general and to medicine in particular. However, some aspects of pharmacology are of less relevance to the study of medicine. To emphasize this distinction, the title *Medical Pharmacology* was chosen for this book.

SUBDIVISIONS OF PHARMACOLOGY AND RELATED DISCIPLINES

Several fields of study may be considered subdivisions of pharmacology or disciplines related to it.

Pharmacodynamics is the study of drug actions and effects, whereas *pharmacokinetics* deals with the disposition of drugs and their elimination from the body.

Emphasis on mode of action of chemical compounds distinguishes pharmacology from other basic medical sciences. As used in medicine, the term *pharmacology* is essentially synonymous with pharmacodynamics.

Chemotherapy is the subdivision of pharmacology that, according to the definition first proposed by Paul Ehrlich, deals with drugs that can destroy invading organisms without destroying the host. This term is used when referring to use of antimicrobial agents and also to drug treatment of malignancy.

Pharmacy is concerned with the preparation and dispensing of drugs. Today the pharmacist has little to do with preparation of drugs, most of which are manufactured by pharmaceutical companies. Dispensing of drugs by the pharmacist now provides additional services, such as counselling of patients about their medications, screening of prescription records for potential drug interactions, and assessment of appropriate dosage.

Therapeutics refers to the treatment of disease.

Pharmacotherapeutics is the application of drugs for treatment of disease.

Toxicology is the science of poisons. Although toxicology may be viewed as a special extension of pharmacology, it has developed into a separate discipline for a variety of reasons. Forensic and environmental medicine requires the services and knowledge of toxicologists with special training in drug identification and poison control.

HISTORICAL DEVELOPMENT OF PHARMACOLOGY

Although a detailed discussion is beyond the scope of this textbook, the history of pharmacology can be divided into two periods. The early period began in antiquity with empiric observations regarding the use of crude medicinal preparations. It is interesting that even primitive cultures discovered relationships between drugs and disease. The use of drugs has been so prevalent throughout history that Sir William Osler stated (1894) with some justification that "man has an inborn craving for medicine."

In contrast to this ancient period, modern pharmacology is based on experimental investigations concerning the site and mode of action of drugs. Application of the scientific method to the study of drugs was initiated in France by François Magendie and was expanded by Claude Bernard (1813-1878). The name of Oswald Schmiedeberg (1838-1921) is commonly associated with the development of experimental pharmacology in Germany, and John Jacob Abel (1857-1938) played a similar role in the United States.

The growth of pharmacology was greatly stimulated by the rise of synthetic organic chemistry, which provided new tools and new therapeutic agents. More recently, pharmacology has benefited from developments in other basic sciences, such as molecular biology, and in turn contributes to their growth.

One of the most dynamic areas of pharmacologic research deals with drug receptors and related topics; for example, discovery of the endorphins occurred shortly after identification of receptors for exogenous opioid compounds. One of the basic functions of pharmacology is to characterize receptors and map out their distribution in the body.

Some of the greatest changes in medicine during recent decades are directly attributable to the discovery of new drugs. Progress in this field is not without its problems, however. Sometimes newly marketed medications are found to be unsafe and must be withdrawn. Studies during development of new drugs do not generally include enough patients (perhaps several thousand would be needed) to identify rare but serious adverse effects. Such effects occur so infrequently during the developmental process that they are likely to avoid detection. As a consequence, it is inevitable that some new drugs are found lacking when used in sufficient numbers of patients to identify all their effects. Furthermore, it is difficult for the practicing physician to stay abreast of rapid developments in the field of pharmacology. Hence all physicians must have a solid understanding of basic principles. These shortcomings notwithstanding, the successes have more than made up for problems that occur with drugs.

PLACE OF PHARMACOLOGY IN MEDICINE

There are several reasons for considering pharmacology an increasingly important basic science in medicine. Some of these are obvious; others are not yet generally recognized.

Large numbers of drugs (approximately 1000) are used in the practice of medicine. They cannot be administered intelligently or safely without an understanding of their mode of action, side effects, toxicity, and kinetics. As powerful new drugs are introduced, adequate pharmacologic knowledge on the part of the physician is mandatory. Pharmacologic terms and concepts are used so commonly in clinical journals that a physician without a good grounding in the subject will find it difficult to read and evaluate the current medical literature.

Pharmacology is taught in medical schools for other reasons. As a basic science it contributes important concepts to the understanding of health and disease. Drugs are used widely in research as chemical tools for elucidating basic mechanisms, and they are also used for diagnostic purposes.

Pharmacology is also important in medicine because of the commercial influences exerted on the physician in the selection of drugs. Knowledge of the principles of pharmacology provides the physician with the ability to evaluate critically and rationally the claims made for new drug preparations.

Finally, numerous functions in the body are regulated by endogenous compounds that interact with specific receptors. Many commonly used drugs mimic or oppose the action of these endogenous compounds or alter their metabolism. When viewed in this light, pharmacology forms not only the scientific basis of drug therapy but also contributes to our understanding of bodily functions.

CLINICAL PHARMACOLOGY

Although pharmacology is concerned with drug effects in all species of animals, medicine is directly concerned with clinical pharmacology, which deals with drug actions in human beings. One reason for this more specific interest is that results of studies on animals cannot always be applied to humans because of species differences in the response to a drug or in its kinetics.

Clinical pharmacology provides scientific methods for the determination of usefulness, potency, and toxicity of new drugs in humans, necessary requirements for their development. In addition, their use in patients after marketing entails continued evaluation of drug disposition and effect. Clinical pharmacologists play a major role in the design, conduct, and interpretation of such studies.

section one

General aspects of pharmacology

Chapter 2

Drug-receptor interactions

Most drugs exert potent and specific actions in the body by forming a bond, which is generally reversible, with a cellular constituent termed a *receptor*. Drugs that interact with receptors to elicit a response are termed *agonists*; compounds that interact with receptors to prevent the action of agonists are referred to as *specific pharmacologic antagonists*. Those that can act either as an agonist or an antagonist, depending on circumstances, are called partial agonists or antagonists.

The existence of cellular receptors for a drug can be deduced from (1) relationships between structure and activity in a homologous series of compounds, (2) quantitative studies on agonist-antagonist pairs, and (3) selective binding of radioactive drugs to cells, membranes, or the isolated receptor itself.

The function of a receptor is to recognize a specific chemical signal and to discriminate between this appropriate structural signal and other molecules. The drug-receptor interaction is then coupled, usually through a second messenger such as cyclic AMP or the phosphoinositide system (see Chapter 3), to an effector mechanism that evokes a cellular response.[1,2,6,9] The presence of receptors at an anatomic site is one determinant of the selective nature of many drug actions because a receptor-specific drug will not affect tissues that lack that receptor. For example, acetylcholine applied directly to a motor end-plate elicits an action potential. Since only the end-plate region contains the receptors, application of acetylcholine a short distance away has no effect.

Not all drug actions are mediated by receptors. For example, volatile anesthetics, metal-chelating agents, and osmotic diuretics exert effects that are not mediated by specific receptors. On the other hand, drugs of the autonomic nervous system, opioid analgesics, most antipsychotics, and many other drugs act on specific receptors.

RECEPTOR THEORY

The *receptor concept* was first proposed by Langley in 1878 and was used extensively by Paul Ehrlich in his studies on chemotherapy. While investigating the opposing actions of pilocarpine and atropine on salivary secretion, Langley suspected the presence of some substance in the nerve endings or glands with which the drugs combine. As conceived by Ehrlich, receptors are groups of protoplasmic macromolecules with which drugs combine *reversibly* or *irreversibly*.

According to current concepts, there are several types of drug receptors.[1,8,9,11] Some are on the external surface of the plasma membrane of target cells. Examples are receptors that interact with peptide hormones and releasing factors or with drugs that mimic or block the actions of autonomic mediators such as the catecholamines.[8,11]

These receptors are, for the most part, coupled to second messengers (see Chapter 3). Other receptors are located in the cytoplasm of target cells, for example, those that combine with drugs that mimic or block the actions of steroid hormones.[1] With these the drug-receptor combination is translocated to the nucleus where it may regulate expression of a gene and thereby the concentration of a specific messenger ribonucleic acid (mRNA) and, ultimately, protein synthesis. Still other receptors, such as those for thyroid hormone, are in the nucleus.

The binding forces in drug-receptor interactions consist of covalent, ionic, and hydrogen bonds as well as van der Waals forces. Covalent binding, because of its high energy, causes essentially irreversible effects. If a drug is an antagonist such as phenoxybenzamine, formation of a covalent bond results in *noncompetitive* antagonism, termed noncompetitive because adding higher concentrations of agonist cannot displace the antagonist to cause an effect. In contrast, *competitive* antagonism involves formation of a variety of weaker, reversible bonds. *Ionic bonds* are interactions between cationic and anionic groups; pH, which affects the number of negatively and positively charged groups, may influence this type of binding. *Hydrogen bonds* result from attractions between hydrogen atoms and pairs of free electrons on nearby oxygen or nitrogen atoms. The *van der Waals bond* is a weak interaction between dipoles. Although the bond energy is only about 0.5 kcal per mole—compared with 100 kcal per mole for the covalent bond—van der Waals bonds are very important in drug-receptor interactions for several reasons. First, the binding forces are summed over a large number of interacting atoms. Second, because drugs and receptors "fit" in three-dimensional space, a better fit allows more bonds to form; this permits the receptor to discriminate between a highly specific drug and another compound with a conformation that fits less well. Finally, the relatively weak van der Waals bond allows for drug effects of short duration. Ionic, hydrogen, and van der Waals bonds also permit competition for binding.

DRUG-RECEPTOR INTERACTIONS

The basic function of a receptor is to discriminate a true signal from noise.[1] To receive the signal, the receptor must have an affinity for the drug, as determined by the binding forces discussed above. At the same time, receptors must have specificity, in other words, an appropriately low affinity for less active drugs; this allows discrimination among various potential signals.

Affinity is quantified by study of the dose-response relationship between a drug and a receptor. One of several methods may be used. In systems in which only dose and response can be determined, the log of the dose is plotted against the response (Fig. 2-1). In such studies, the dose of a drug that produces a response that is 50% of the maximum is referred to as the "ED_{50}" (effective $dose_{50}$).

Newer methods that usually require a radioactive drug can quantify the relationship between the concentration of free drug and that which is specifically bound.

The binding of a drug (D) and a receptor (R) can be represented as follows:

$$[D] + [R] \xrightarrow{k_1} [DR]$$

The rate at which they combine is described by the rate constant k_1. Since most drug-receptor interactions are reversible, it is also true that

$$[DR] \xrightarrow{k_2} [D]+[R]$$

At equilibrium the rates of the forward and backward reactions are equal, and

$$k_1[D][R]=k_2[DR]$$

The concept of K_d emerges if the above equation is rewritten:

$$DR;DR=\frac{k_2}{k_1}=K_d$$

K_d is the equilibrium dissociation constant; its magnitude indicates the affinity of the receptor for the drug. In the above equation, if half of the receptors are bound to a drug, the concentrations of R and DR are equal; thus they cancel. Under such conditions K_d = [D]. This means that the concentration of drug necessary to bind 50% of the receptors equals the K_d. If this concentration is low, affinity is high. For example, a K_d of 10^{-10} indicates a hundredfold greater affinity than a K_d of 10^{-8}.

Affinity and intrinsic activity

Affinity then represents the tenacity with which a compound combines with the receptor. A drug with a lower K_d has greater affinity for the receptor, stimulates the receptor at a lower concentration, and thus elicits a response at lower concentrations than does a drug with a higher K_d. This concept is illustrated in Fig. 2-1, A, where drug A has a greater affinity and therefore greater *potency* than drug B. In many systems the magnitude of response is a direct function of the number of receptors occupied, that is, the maximal response develops when all of the receptors are occupied. Receptors for catecholamines are examples. In other systems only a fraction of

FIG. 2-1 *Log dose-response curves illustrating the difference between potency and efficacy.* ***A,*** *Drug A is much more potent than drug B, but both cause the same maximal effect.* ***B,*** *Drug A is not only more potent but also has greater efficacy; it produces a greater peak effect than drug B.*

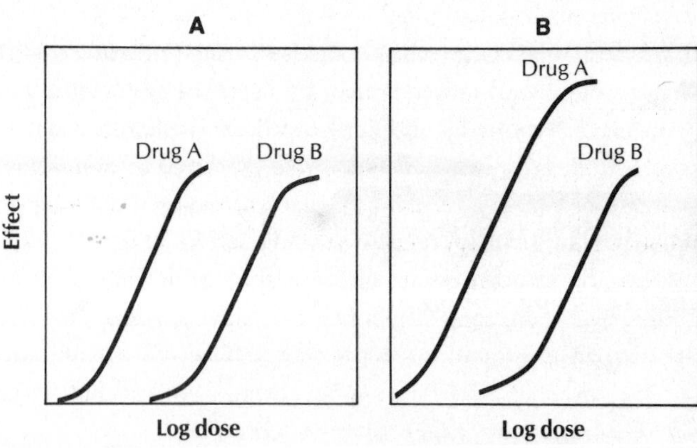

the available receptors need be bound to agonist to elicit a maximal response; such systems are said to have *spare receptors*. Receptors for insulin are an example of this type, because occupancy of only about 20% of available insulin receptors elicits a maximal response.

One drug may not only have a higher affinity than another compound but may also produce a greater maximal effect, as illustrated in Fig. 2-1, *B*. Because drug A causes a greater peak effect than drug B, it is said to have greater *intrinsic activity* or *efficacy*. Drug B might be a *partial agonist*, that is, one that acts on the same receptor as the full agonist (it might even have similar or greater affinity), but it cannot produce the same maximal effect, regardless of concentration, because its efficacy is less. Therefore the response is a function not only of the concentration of the drug-receptor complex but also of efficacy, which may be defined as the capacity to stimulate relative to a given receptor occupancy.

In summary, an agonist is a drug that has both affinity for a receptor and intrinsic activity. An antagonist has affinity for the receptor but lacks intrinsic activity. An antagonist may in turn be either competitive or noncompetitive.

Drugs that do not act on specific receptors

The biologic activity of anesthetics and some other agents is believed to depend not on drug-receptor interactions but on the *relative saturation* at some cellular phase (Ferguson's principle).[4] Whenever chemically unrelated drugs produce the same effect at the same relative saturation, they are unlikely to act on specific receptors. Probably by reaching a certain level of saturation at some cellular site (the so-called biophase), they hinder some metabolic function or disrupt membrane organization.

Receptor regulation

The response to a drug depends partially on the number of available receptors, and this number may be affected by the continued presence of the drug. Many receptors, including those that activate adenylyl cyclase (for example β-adrenergic receptors) and insulin receptors, decrease in number or undergo *downregulation* with continued drug administration. This phenomenon is sometimes referred to as *desensitization, tachyphylaxis*, or *tolerance*.[8,10] Although there is great interest in downregulation, it should be pointed out that most drugs can be administered repeatedly or continuously without development of significant desensitization. In the case of insulin this is accounted for by the availability of spare receptors. With other drugs recovery of responsiveness occurs rapidly between doses, perhaps due to the fluctuating concentration of drug, so that downregulation associated with peak concentrations has time to reverse during trough concentrations. Tachyphylaxis to some drugs (for example, nitrates or diuretics) occurs through mechanisms unrelated to receptors.

There are a few examples of increased receptor numbers. Thyroid hormone increases the number of β-adrenergic receptors in the myocardium, consistent with the clinical impression that hyperthyroid persons are more sensitive to catecholamines. When skeletal muscle is denervated, receptors for acetylcholine, which are normally localized in the end-plate region, spread over the surface of the muscle fibers. Tardive dyskinesia, a motor disorder associated with chronic antipsychotic medication, has been attributed to upregulation of dopamine receptors.

Receptor-related diseases

There is great interest in the role of receptor changes in certain diseases.[7] Practically all patients with myasthenia gravis have antibodies to acetylcholine receptors. In some forms of insulin-resistant diabetes, there are antibodies to insulin receptors.[5] Other interesting examples of receptor-related diseases are testicular feminization (androgen insensitivity), familial hypercholesterolemia (decrease in receptors for low-density lipoproteins),[3] and several endocrine diseases that may represent receptor insensitivity rather than hormonal deficiencies.

QUANTITATIVE ASPECTS OF DRUG POTENCY AND EFFICACY

A drug is said to be "potent" when it has great biologic activity per unit weight. Plotting the dose of a drug on a logarithmic scale against a measured effect generates a sigmoid curve, usually referred to as a *log dose-response* curve. Any point on such a curve could indicate the potency of a drug, but for comparative purposes the ED_{50} is most often selected. In Fig. 2-1, *A*, drugs A and B produced parallel dose-response curves. The ED_{50} of drug B may be 10 times greater than that of drug A. As a consequence, it may be said that drug A is 10 times more potent than drug B. *It is essential to remember that potencies are compared on the basis of doses that produce the same effect and not by comparison of the magnitudes of effects elicited by the same dose.*

A clinically relevant example of a potency relationship, typical of that illustrated in Fig. 2-1, *A*, is that of the diuretic drugs chlorothiazide and hydrochlorothiazide. It takes about 1 g of chlorothiazide to achieve the same effect as 100 mg of hydrochlorothiazide; hydrochlorothiazide is 10 times more potent than chlorothiazide.

Fig. 2-1, *B*, illustrates another property of a drug that should not be confused with potency. Drug A is not only 10 times more potent than drug B, but it also has a higher maximum or "ceiling" of activity; it exhibits greater *efficacy,* or *power,* an expression of intrinsic activity. Diuretics can be used to illustrate this phenomenon. Chlorothiazide and hydrochlorothiazide have equal ceilings of activity. Furosemide, however, has not only greater potency than these two drugs but also a higher ceiling, that is, it promotes excretion of a larger amount of sodium chloride. Consequently, furosemide is not only more potent than chlorothiazide but also has greater efficacy.

Potency and efficacy are often confused in medical terminology. Potency alone is an overrated advantage in therapeutics. If drug A is 10 times more potent than drug B but has no other virtues, this may mean only that the patient will take tablets containing fewer milligrams of drug A. Pharmaceutical companies often emphasize that a drug is more potent than some other drug. This in itself is of little importance to the physician. On the other hand, if the drug has greater efficacy, it may accomplish results that are unattainable with a less powerful compound.

AGONIST, ANTAGONIST, AND PARTIAL AGONIST

An agonist is a drug that has affinity and efficacy. It interacts with receptors and elicits a response. Acetylcholine is a good example of an agonist. However, if a log dose-response curve to acetylcholine (at muscarinic receptors) is obtained in the presence of the antagonist atropine, it will be found that atropine shifts the log

FIG. 2-2

Log dose-response curves illustrating differences between a competitive antagonist and a noncompetitive antagonist. ***A,*** *A competitive antagonist decreases potency but not efficacy; there is a parallel shift of the log dose-response curve to the right.* ***B,*** *A noncompetitive antagonist decreases both efficacy and potency; the log dose-response curve is not only shifted to the right but the maximal effect is also reduced.*

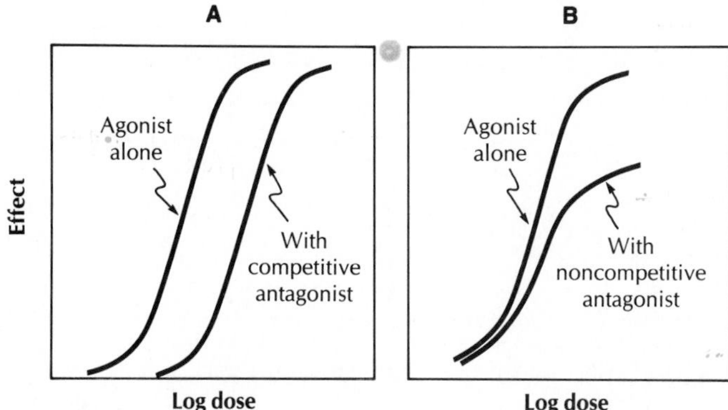

dose-response curve of acetylcholine to the right, although atropine given alone causes no effect.

Atropine competes with acetylcholine for muscarinic receptors; in other words, the antagonist has affinity but lacks efficacy. Because administration of greater amounts of acetylcholine to a patient or tissue exposed to atropine can eventually replace the atropine and elicit a response, this is an example of *competitive* or *surmountable* antagonism, in contrast to noncompetitive antagonism described in the next section. The key feature of competitive antagonism is *parallel displacement of the log dose-response curve to the right without a shift in the maximum* (Fig. 2-2, *A*).

Somewhere between pure agonists and pure antagonists are the drugs termed *partial agonists*. They have affinity and some (but not complete) intrinsic activity. Given alone they act like an agonist; given in combination, they may antagonize the action of a full agonist by interfering with binding of the latter to their receptors.

NONCOMPETITIVE ANTAGONISM

In the case of atropine and acetylcholine the antagonist and agonist compete for the same receptor, as evidenced by the parallel shift in the log dose-response curve without a shift in the maximum. In some instances the antagonist may combine irreversibly with the receptor, and increasing the concentration of the agonist can never fully overcome the inhibition. The net effect will be a decrease in the maximum height of the log dose-response curve, which is believed to reflect a decrease in the number of drug-receptor complexes (Fig. 2-2, *B*). There is no change in the K_d of the drug; the affinity of the drug for the available receptors is unaltered.

PROBLEM 2-1. The graph below depicts the linear segment of a typical log dose-response curve. What is the dose (X) *that induces* Y *units of response? How many units is* Y*?*

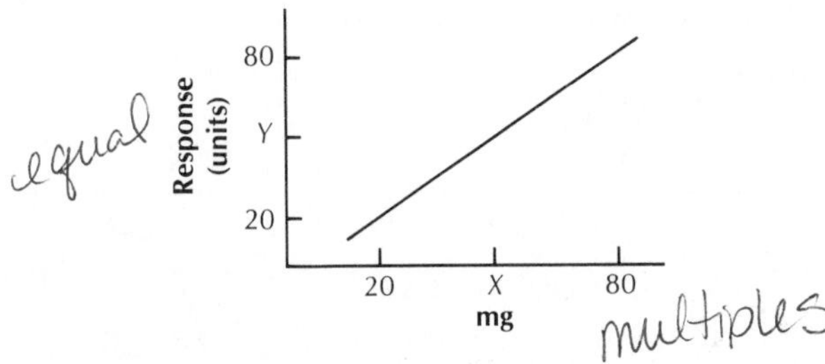

Since dosage is plotted on a log *scale, equal increments on the abscissa represent equal* multiples *so that X = 40 mg. In contrast, the magnitude of the response is plotted on a* linear *scale, so that equal increments on the ordinate represent* equal *changes in response; Y therefore equals 50 units.*

REFERENCES

1. Baxter JD, Funder JW: Hormone receptors, *N Engl J Med* 301:1149, 1979.
2. Berridge MJ, Irvine RF: Inositol trisphosphate, a novel second messenger in cellular signal transduction, *Nature* 312:315, 1984.
3. Brown MS, Goldstein JL: A receptor-mediated pathway for cholesterol homeostasis, *Science* 232:34, 1986.
4. Ferguson J: Use of chemical potentials as indices of toxicity, *Proc R Soc Lond [Biol]* 127:387, 1939.
5. Flier JS, Kahn CR, Roth J: Receptors, antireceptor antibodies and mechanisms of insulin resistance, *N Engl J Med* 300:413, 1979.
6. Hurwitz L, Suria A: The link between agonist action and response in smooth muscle, *Annu Rev Pharmacol* 11:303, 1971.
7. Jacobs S, Cuatrecasas P: Cell receptors in disease, *N Engl J Med* 297:1383, 1977.
8. Lefkowitz RJ: Direct binding studies of adrenergic receptors: biochemical, physiologic, and clinical implications, *Ann Intern Med* 91:450, 1979.
9. Motulsky HJ, Insel PA: Adrenergic receptors in man: direct identification, physiologic regulation, and clinical alterations, *N Engl J Med* 307:18, 1982.
10. Overstreet DH, Yamamura HI: Receptor alterations and drug tolerance, *Life Sci* 25:1865, 1979.
11. Snyder SH: Drug and neurotransmitter receptors in the brain, *Science* 224:22, 1984.

Chapter 3

Second-messenger systems

Stimulation of a receptor typically initiates a series of events that lead to the final response of the tissue, whether this response is secretion, contraction, relaxation, change in rate, or something else. The link is often provided by so-called *second messengers*, a term originally coined with reference to the role of cyclic AMP (cyclic adenosine 3′,5′-monophosphate) in glycogenolysis.[16] Three such systems are described below to illustrate current knowledge of the complexities inherent in conversion of receptor stimulation to response. Table 3-1 indicates many of the receptors that have been linked to these systems.

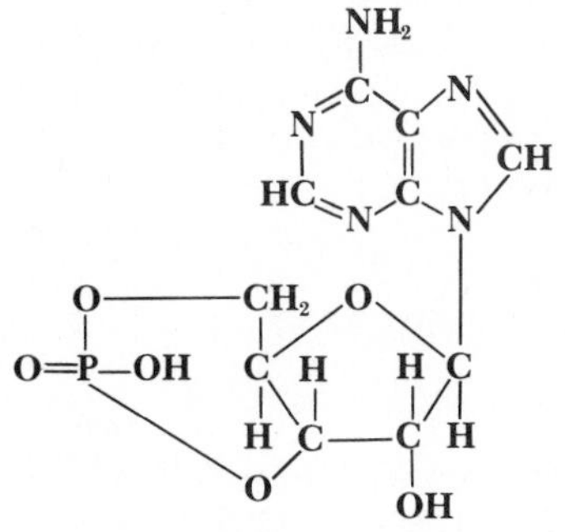

Cyclic adenosine 3′,5′-monophosphate

G PROTEINS, ADENYLYL CYCLASE, AND CYCLIC AMP

Stimulation of a β-adrenergic receptor by norepinephrine, epinephrine, or other β-receptor agonists (see Chapter 18) activates a membrane-bound protein, one of a family of guanine nucleotide-binding regulatory proteins called *G proteins*,[2,8] that requires GTP for activity (Fig. 3-1). This particular protein is designated G_s because the end result of its activation is stimulatory, that is, activation of adenylyl cyclase (also called adenyl or adenylate cyclase). In its inactive state G_s is composed of three different subunits: α to which GDP is attached, β, and γ . Binding of the agonist to its receptor alters G_s to favor replacement of GDP by GTP. When GTP binds to G_s, the βγ component splits off, freeing the α(GTP) subunit. This α subunit can then activate adenylyl cyclase, which catalyzes formation of cyclic AMP from ATP (Fig. 3-2). Cyclic AMP in turn activates a cytoplasmic cyclic AMP–dependent protein kinase by attaching to two regulatory subunits of the kinase and releasing two catalytic subunits[10] that promote phosphorylation of serine residues on proteins. This phosphorylation step controls a variety of activities, depending on the particular tissue involved. The α(GTP)

TABLE 3–1 Second-messenger systems and related receptors[2,5,12,15]

Receptor type or agonist	Second-messenger system		
	G_s	G_i, G_o	PIP_2
ACTH	Yes		
Adenosine	A_2	A_1	
Adrenergic	β_1, β_2	α_2	α_1
Angiotensin II		Yes	Yes
Bradykinin			B_2
Calcitonin, CGRP	Yes		
Cholecystokinin			CCK_A
Dopamine	D_1	D_2	
FSH	Yes		
GABA		$GABA_B$	
Glucagon	G_2		G_1
Histamine	H_2		H_1
Leukotriene			LTB_4, LTD_4
LH	Yes		
Muscarinic		M_2	M_1, M_3
Neurotensin		Yes	Yes
Opioid		δ, μ	
Oxytocin			OT
Prostacyclin	IP		
Prostaglandin D	DP		
Prostaglandin E_2	EP_2	EP_3	EP_1, EP_3
Prostaglandin $F_{2\alpha}$			FP
Purinergic		P_{2T}	P_{2Y}
Serotonin (5-HT)		$5\text{-}HT_{1A}$, $5\text{-}HT_{1B}$, $5\text{-}HT_{1D}$	$5\text{-}HT_{1C}$, $5\text{-}HT_2$
Somatostatin		Yes	
Substance P			NK_1, NK_2, NK_3
Thromboxane A_2			TP
Vasopressin	V_2		V_{1A}, V_{1B}

subunit has GTPase activity; as it converts to α(GDP), $\beta\gamma$ subunits reattach and the protein is restored to its inactive conformation. Amplification occurs in this system because repeated stimulation of one receptor can cause overlapping activation of several molecules of G protein and because inactivation of the α subunit is relatively slow. The membrane may also contain a similar G protein called G_i because its activation inhibits adenylyl cyclase. It is not clear if G_i inhibits the cyclase directly or if it acts as a source of $\beta\gamma$ subunits that inhibit dissociation of G_s.

There are several other G proteins.[2,8] G_o, like G_i, is inhibitory for adenylyl cyclase and is the most abundant G protein in the brain. Both G_i and G_o often elicit effects through pathways involving activation of K^+ channels, inhibition of Ca^{++} channels, or Na^+/H^+ exchange.[2,3,11,13] G_k refers to a G_i-type protein that activates K^+ channels.[17] G_t (transducin) in the rods of the retina is activated when rhodopsin is exposed to light.

Turnover cycle of a G protein. Squares *represent inactive conformations as they relate to modulation of effector functions.* Circular *and* semi-circular shapes *represent activated forms of the G protein. Activation is both GTP and Mg^{++} dependent and is stabilized by subunit dissociation to give an activated α-GTP complex plus the $\beta\gamma$ dimer. Hydrolysis of GTP by the α subunit deactivates the complex, increases its affinity for $\beta\gamma$, and leads to reassociation to give an inactive G protein with GDP bound to it. Re-initiation of the activation cycle requires release of GDP and renewed binding of GTP.* ***FIG. 3-1***

From Birnbaumer L, Abramowitz J, Brown AM: Biochim Biophys Acta 1031:163, 1990.

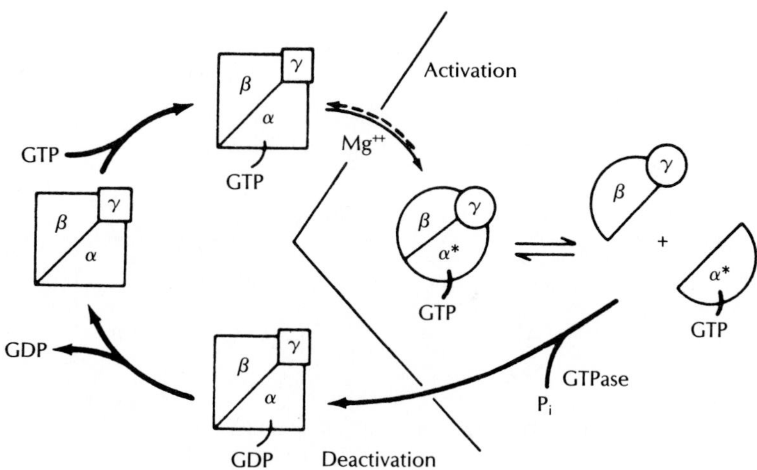

Role of the cyclic AMP-dependent protein kinase in signal transduction. ***FIG. 3-2***

From Krebs EG: JAMA October 6, 262:1815-1818, Copyright 1989, American Medical Association.

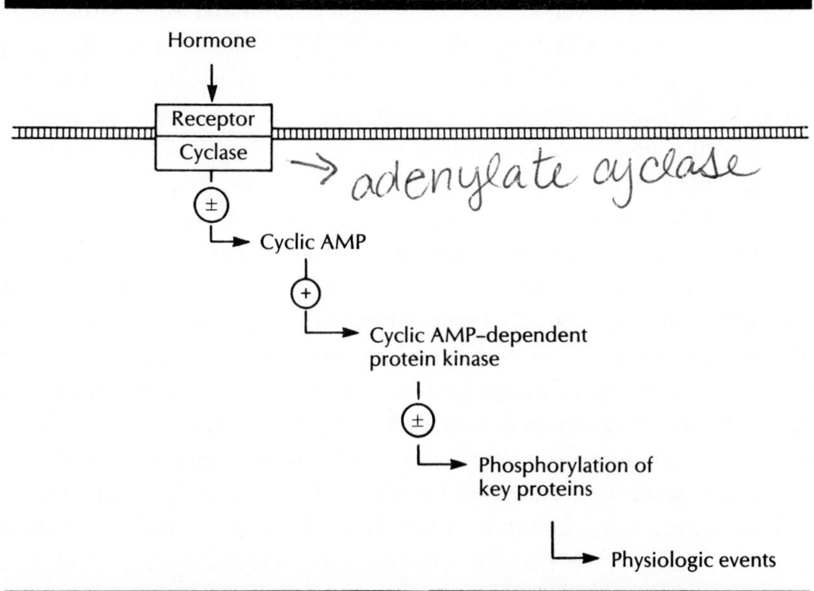

FIG. 3-3 *Schematic representation of the metabolism of inositol phosphates released from phosphoinositides. Activation of the receptor* (R), *which is coupled to phospholipase C* (PLC) *through a G protein* (G), *leads to hydrolysis of* PIP_2*; two key metabolites, diacylglycerol* (DG) *and inositol 1,4,5-trisphosphate* [Ins(1,4,5)P_3], *are formed. Under certain conditions, hydrolysis of PIP and PI may also release diacylglycerol after receptor stimulation. Diacylglycerol stays in the plasma membrane to activate protein kinase C (PKC), which is translocated to the membrane after stimulation. Ins(1,4,5)*P_3 *mobilizes intracellular calcium (*$Ca^{++}{}_i$*) from the store in the endoplasmic reticulum* (ER). *Ins(1,3,4,5)*P_4 *has a role in entry of extracellular* Ca^{++}*, which also appears to depend on an action of Ins(1,4,5)*P_3.

From Chuang D-M: Reproduced, with permission, from the Annual Review of Pharmacology and Toxicology, Vol 29, © 1989 by Annual Reviews Inc, p 71.

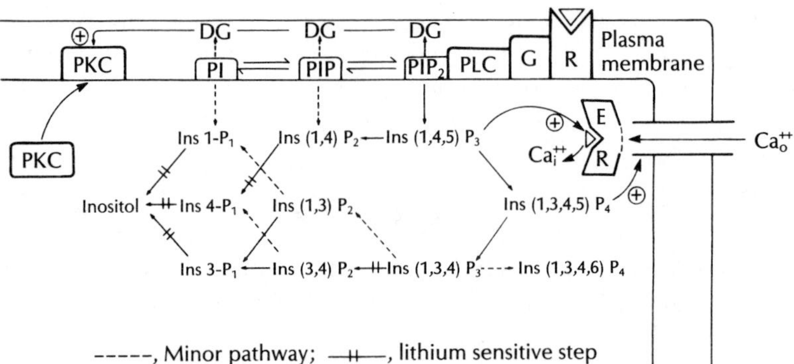

The designation G_p (or more specifically G_{plc}) has been used for the G protein, apparently neither G_s nor G_i, that is an integral link between receptor stimulation and activation of the phosphoinositide system discussed next.

THE PHOSPHOINOSITIDE SYSTEM

Inositol (hexahydroxycyclohexane) consists of a saturated ring with a hydroxyl group on each of the six carbons. The enzyme PI synthetase converts inositol to phosphatidylinositol (PI) in the endoplasmic reticulum.[5] A small portion of the PI is transported to the plasma membrane where it undergoes repeated phosphorylation to form phosphatidylinositol 4-phosphate (PIP) and then phosphatidylinositol 4,5-bisphosphate (PIP_2), an important component of this second-messenger system (Fig. 3-3). In this case interaction of an agonist with its receptor activates a G protein (G_p) that activates phospholipase C. This enzyme splits PIP_2 into inositol 1,4,5-trisphosphate (IP_3) and 1,2-diacylglycerol (DAG). Each of these products in turn activates other systems.[5,14] IP_3 leaves the plasma membrane to stimulate intracellular receptors and release Ca^{++} from the endoplasmic reticulum; this free Ca^{++} may bind to calmodulin (see next section) or modulate the state of various ion channels.[7,12] IP_3 also promotes translocation of protein kinase C from the cytosol to the plasma membrane. The DAG remains in the plasma membrane and acts with Ca^{++} to activate protein kinase C; furthermore, DAG sensitizes the enzyme to activation by Ca^{++}. Once activated the kinase can phosphorylate serine residues in a variety of proteins.

IP_3 is converted to a number of products, some active such as inositol 1,3,4,5-

tetrakisphosphate (IP_4), which may promote entry of extracellular Ca^{++},[5] perhaps via Ca^{++} movement from one intracellular pool to another.[1] Other products are less active or inactive, such as the dephosphorylated metabolites that eventually release free inositol. Fig. 3-3 indicates how Li^+, which is used in management of affective disorders (see Chapters 26 and 28), inhibits regeneration of free inositol. Lack of sufficient inositol in the brain for conversion to PIP_2 would tend to limit the activity of this second-messenger system and may contribute to the therapeutic effect of the ion.

CALCIUM ION AND CALMODULIN

An increase in unbound cytosolic Ca^{++} concentration can serve as a second messenger, although it may simply be a further step in a series initiated by activation of a G protein or release of IP_3.[7,9] Certain Ca^{++} channels are influenced directly or indirectly by G proteins.[2,6] The roles of IP_3 and IP_4 in increasing intracellular Ca^{++} are discussed above. Regardless of the source or initiating stimulus, the free Ca^{++} can bind to calmodulin or some other calcium-binding protein.[4] Calcium-calmodulin activates a variety of enzymes, such as myosin light-chain kinase (important for smooth muscle contraction) and cyclic nucleotide phosphodiesterase (important for hydrolysis and inactivation of cyclic AMP).[9] Although not a second messenger in the usual context, Ca^{++} that enters a neuron through voltage-gated channels during passage of an action potential is an essential factor for neurotransmitter release.

REFERENCES

1. Berridge MJ, Irvine RF: Inositol phosphates and cell signalling, *Nature (Lond)* 341:197, 1989.
2. Birnbaumer L, Abramowitz J, Brown AM: Receptor-effector coupling by G proteins, *Biochim Biophys Acta* 1031:163, 1990.
3. Brown DA: G-proteins and potassium currents in neurons, *Annu Rev Physiol* 52:215, 1990.
4. Carafoli E: Intracellular calcium homeostasis, *Annu Rev Biochem* 56:395, 1987.
5. Chuang D-M: Neurotransmitter receptors and phosphoinositide turnover, *Annu Rev Pharmacol Toxicol* 29:71, 1989.
6. Dolphin AC: G protein modulation of calcium currents in neurons, *Annu Rev Physiol* 52:243, 1990.
7. Exton JH: Mechanisms of action of calcium-mobilizing agonists: some variations on a young theme, *FASEB J* 2:2670, 1988.
8. Gilman AG: G proteins and regulation of adenylyl cyclase, *JAMA* 262:1819, 1989.
9. Hanley RM, Steiner AL: The second-messenger system for peptide hormones, *Hosp Pract* 24(8):59, 1989.
10. Krebs EG: Role of the cyclic AMP-dependent protein kinase in signal transduction, *JAMA* 262:1815, 1989.
11. Limbird LE: Receptors linked to inhibition of adenylate cyclase: additional signaling mechanisms, *FASEB J* 2:2686, 1988.
12. Neher E: The use of the patch clamp technique to study second messenger-mediated cellular events, *Neuroscience* 26:727, 1988.
13. Nicoll RA, Malenka RC, Kauer JA: Functional comparison of neurotransmitter receptor subtypes in mammalian central nervous system, *Physiol Rev* 70:513, 1990.
14. Rana RS, Hokin LE: Role of phosphoinositides in transmembrane signaling, *Physiol Rev* 70:115, 1990.
15. Receptor nomenclature supplement, *Trends Pharmacol Sci* January, 1991.
16. Sutherland EW, Øye I, Butcher RW: The action of epinephrine and the role of the adenyl cyclase system in hormone action, *Recent Prog Horm Res* 21:623, 1965.
17. Szabo G, Otero AS: G protein mediated regulation of K^+ channels in heart, *Annu Rev Physiol* 52:293, 1990.

Chapter 4

Determinants of response to drugs

The previous two chapters discussed the response to drugs at the level of the receptor and subsequent second messengers. Response in this context can be measured as binding to a receptor or as the end effect on the second messenger, such as an increase in intracellular cyclic AMP or Ca^{++} concentration. At the tissue level, these events culminate in a response, such as contraction of a muscle or release of a hormone, that can be quantified more readily.

DOSE-RESPONSE IN MAN

Extrapolation still further to the whole animal or to human beings involves quantitation of response by measurement of clinical endpoints such as change in blood pressure caused by a catecholamine or by an antihypertensive drug, change in Na^+ excretion caused by a diuretic, or change in glucose concentration elicited by a hypoglycemic agent. These global endpoints, which represent a summation of the effects of a drug and of homeostatic mechanisms as well, are the focus of the clinician. For example, assume one assesses the response to a vasodilating antihypertensive agent by measuring blood pressure; the decrease in pressure will be a function of not only the magnitude of vasodilatation caused by the drug but also of the dampening of overall pressure change by reflex tachycardia, by baroreceptor-mediated release of catecholamines, and so forth. The latter factors might cause underestimation of the drug's efficacy as a vasodilator. Nevertheless, the change in blood pressure would provide a good assessment of the clinical effect of the drug.

THERAPEUTIC DOSAGE

When one assesses the relationship between the dose or concentration of a drug and in vivo endpoints of response, the relationship is a sigmoid-shaped curve, as was shown in Chapter 2 (Fig. 2-1) when the effect of a drug at its receptor was described. Response to a drug is often thought of mainly in terms of benefit; it should not be forgotten that the response may just as well be toxic. The relationship between doses (or concentrations) that cause a beneficial effect and those that are toxic defines the *therapeutic margin* or *margin of safety* of a drug. This concept is illustrated schematically in Fig. 4-1 where sigmoid relationships are shown for both therapeutic and toxic effects. In the upper panel of the figure, the distance between the curves representing toxicity and benefit of a drug is great. Such an agent is said to have a wide therapeutic margin; a dose large enough to assure maximal benefit can be given with little risk of toxicity. In contrast, the lower panel of Fig. 4-1 represents a drug with a narrow margin of safety. In a dose that causes maximal benefit, this drug entails considerable risk of toxicity. There is little margin for error in chosing the proper dose for such agents.

FIG. 4-1 *Relationship between drug dose or concentration and both beneficial and toxic effects. The box in each panel represents the range of therapeutic doses or concentrations.*

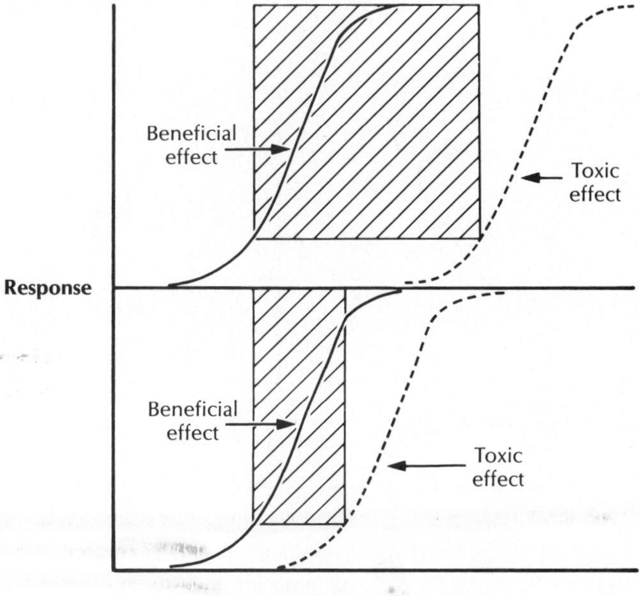

VARIABILITY IN RESPONSE TO DRUGS

Experimental studies show that the dose or concentration of a drug that will give a fixed response varies considerably. Fig. 4-2 illustrates the gaussian distribution of drug effect. Biologic variation in drug effect is an important reason to individualize dosage and adjust treatment to the requirements of a given patient. Some of the numerous factors that contribute to variability of response are discussed below.

Hypersusceptibility

Because of biologic variation, disease, or the presence of another medication, some persons may develop a much greater than normal response to an ordinary dose of a drug. For example, a thyrotoxic patient may have an exaggerated cardiovascular response to injected epinephrine. Similarly, a patient with subclinical asthma may experience symptoms of bronchial constriction from doses of histamine or β-adrenergic antagonists that are innocuous in normal persons. Such patients are at the sensitive end of a gaussian frequency distribution curve (Fig. 4-2). Hypersusceptibility is sometimes referred to as *drug intolerance*.

Drug idiosyncrasy

The term *idiosyncrasy* has been used rather vaguely in medicine to apply to drug reactions that are *qualitatively* different from the effects obtained in the majority of patients and cannot be attributed to drug allergy. Occasionally extreme susceptibility of an individual to an expected pharmacologic action has also been called an idiosyncrasy. As discussed in Chapter 8, some of these responses can be attributed to an inability to metabolize a drug.

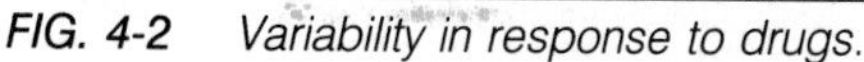

FIG. 4-2 *Variability in response to drugs.*

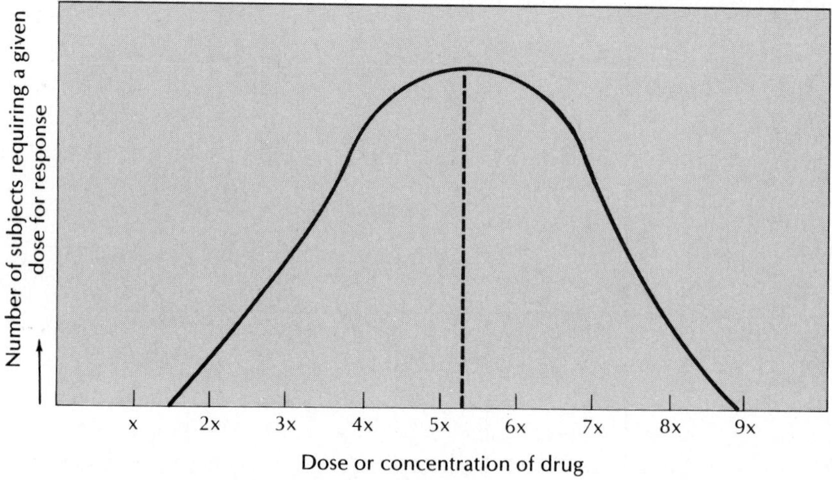

Drug allergy

Drug allergy is a response that results from a previous sensitizing exposure to a drug; it is mediated by an immunologic mechanism. Drug allergy differs from drug toxicity in a number of respects: (1) The reaction occurs in only a fraction of the population. (2) Dose is irrelevant in that a minute amount of an otherwise safe drug can elicit a severe reaction. (3) The manifestations of the reaction are different from the usual pharmacologic effects of the drug. (4) There is a primary sensitizing period before the individual responds with the unusual reaction. (5) When the sensitizing agent is a protein or a hapten, which forms covalent bonds with proteins, circulating antibodies may be demonstrated in sensitized individuals, and skin tests, though hazardous, may show a positive reaction to the offending drug.

In most drug allergies, the complete antigen is not known nor is the form in which the drug acts as a hapten. For example, a patient may develop a skin rash after ingestion of a sulfonamide, yet show no reaction to the same drug injected intracutaneously. This is generally true for drugs of small molecular weight and the *immediate* type of allergies elicited by them. In *contact dermatitis*, on the other hand, skin tests are often positive.

Immediate and delayed drug allergies

The terms *immediate* and *delayed reactions* originated from observations of the rapidity with which the positive skin test to allergens becomes manifest. Thus in anaphylactic hypersensitivity, skin-test results are immediate; in delayed reactions, such as tuberculin hypersensitivity, it is many hours before there is a visible change in the skin where the antigen was injected. In addition, there are profound differences in the immunologic bases of the two types of hypersensitivity. Circulating antibodies mediate immediate but not delayed hypersensitivity. The latter is mediated by sensitized cells.

Among the many types of drug allergy, some are considered immediate, others are delayed, and still others can not be accurately classified. *Anaphylaxis*, *urticaria*, *angio-*

neurotic edema, *drug fever*, and *asthma* are clearly immediate reactions. *Serum sickness* reactions are characterized by a delay in their appearance. This same delay is observed after the first administration of a foreign serum. Once sensitized, however, an individual often reacts rapidly to the same agent. For example, methyldopa may be taken daily by an individual for 1 to 2 weeks before fever and joint pain develop. Subsequent administration of a small dose of the drug will produce the same reaction in a matter of hours. *Contact dermatitis* is undoubtedly a delayed allergy. Many other cutaneous reactions and some severe hematologic disturbances elicited by drugs probably also belong in the delayed category.

Disease processes that influence response

Pathologic processes may also influence the response to drugs. In some, but not all, instances this can be explained by disease-induced changes in drug elimination (see Chapter 10). It is obvious that in severe renal disease one must cautiously use drugs that depend on the kidney for excretion.[3] If the dose of digoxin is not adjusted in patients with renal insufficiency, fatal toxicity can occur. In severe liver disease, similar care must be exercised in the use of drugs that are normally inactivated by hepatic processes.[2,4,6,7]

Presence of other drugs

When more than one drug is given to the same patient, their actions may be completely independent of one another. Alternatively, the effect of a combination may be greater or less than that which could have been obtained with either drug alone.

ADDITIVE EFFECT, SYNERGISM, AND POTENTIATION

When the combined effect of two drugs is the algebraic sum of their individual responses, it is sometimes referred to as an *additive effect* or as an example of *summation*. However, the correct way to consider additivity is in terms of doses rather than effects. If a certain dose of drug A and a certain dose of drug B produce the same effect quantitatively (that is, are *equieffective*), the drugs are additive if half of each of these doses used simultaneously elicits the same effect as the full dose of either drug alone. If the response is appreciably greater than that of the full dose of either drug alone, the drugs are said to be synergistic; *synergism* refers to a greater than additive effect.

Potentiation is the best term for the case in which a drug that appears to have no action when given alone increases the potency (not the efficacy) of a second drug. This occurs, for example, when one drug interfers with the destruction or disposition of a second drug, thus increasing the response to a given dose of the latter.

Unfortunately, many people interpret these terms differently; one should ask for clarification if the meaning is not obvious.

ANTAGONISM

Drug antagonism may be of several types: chemical, physiologic, pharmacologic, and pharmacokinetic.

Chemical antagonism. A drug may combine with another in the body, just as it would in a test tube. This is the basis of action of chemical antidotes. For example, dimercaprol (British antilewisite, BAL) can combine with mercury, lead, or arsenic.

Physiologic antagonism. Two drugs may influence a physiologic system in opposite directions, one drug canceling the effect of another. The simultaneous injection of properly adjusted doses of vasodilator and vasoconstrictor drugs may not change blood pressure. Similarly, stimulants and depressants of the central nervous system can antagonize each other.

Pharmacologic antagonism. Two drugs may bind reversibly or irreversibly to the same receptor site; the inactive or weaker member of the pair inhibits access of the potent drug (see Chapter 2). Examples of pharmacologic antagonism are the antihistaminic-histamine and atropine-acetylcholine relationships.

Pharmacokinetic antagonism is briefly discussed below.

Drug Interactions in Clinical Pharmacology

In addition to the large variety of pharmacodynamic interactions that can occur as noted above, one drug may also interact with another by several pharmacokinetic mechanisms. Both pharmacodynamic and pharmacokinetic interactions influence the variability among patients in response to a drug. Pharmacokinetic interactions are discussed in detail in Chapter 70; they include (1) altered absorption from the gastrointestinal tract,[1,5] (2) reduced binding to plasma proteins, (3) altered renal excretion,[3] (4) inhibition of metabolic degradation, and (5) induction of metabolic degradation. Potentiation or antagonism can result from such interactions. Examples of pharmacokinetic antagonism include the binding of tetracycline to milk products or antacids precluding absorption,[1,5] enhanced metabolism of a number of drugs by phenobarbital or rifampin, and increased renal excretion of weakly acidic compounds in an alkaline urine.

Cumulation, tolerance, and tachyphylaxis

Response to a certain dosage of a drug can be greatly influenced by special features of drug metabolism such as cumulation, tolerance, and tachyphylaxis.

Cumulation

Most drugs are eliminated from the body by first-order reactions, that is, a constant fraction of a drug is eliminated per unit of time (see Chapter 5). Within 4 half-lives 94% of the drug is eliminated. If a drug is administered frequently in relation to its half-life, it will accumulate in the body. Eventually, however, a *plateau* or *steady-state* is reached when elimination equals the amount of drug being administered. A good example is the drug digitoxin, which has a half-life of 7 days; because it is administered on a daily basis, it gradually accumulates in plasma. After 4 half-lives of dosing (28 days), digitoxin will have accumulated to 94% of its final steady-state level.

Tolerance

Tolerance is an interesting phenomenon characterized by the need for increasing amounts of a drug to obtain the same quantitative effect. Drugs vary greatly in their tendency to induce tolerance; perhaps the best-known examples are the opium alkaloids. The adult therapeutic dose of morphine is ordinarily about 10 mg, but if the drug is administered repeatedly, increasing doses are necessary to obtain the same analgesic effect. Finally, enormous doses (perhaps 5 g daily) are used by an addict who has developed pronounced tolerance. With some agents, like the β-adrenergic agonists, tolerance appears to involve uncoupling of receptors from their second messenger or, over a longer period, removal of the receptors from the cell surface and eventually their destruction. A moderate degree of tolerance to several drugs is the result of liver metabolic enzyme induction (see Chapter 7). The actual mechanisms of tolerance to many drugs remain poorly characterized.

TACHYPHYLAXIS

The term tachyphylaxis refers to rapidly developing tolerance. This occurs with vasopressin, nitrates, and indirectly acting sympathomimetic amines such as amphetamine. The first injection of vasopressin or amphetamine produces a much greater elevation of blood pressure than does a second injection after only a brief interval.

Although mechanisms of tachyphylaxis are often poorly understood, there are exceptions. Amphetamine releases norepinephrine from adrenergic nerve endings; tachyphylaxis is probably a consequence of depletion of a pool of releasable norepinephrine. The same mechanism plays a role in tachyphylaxis to histamine releasers. In other instances the action of a drug may persist at the receptor site, but its overt manifestations are concealed by compensatory reflexes or by desensitization of the receptor.

REFERENCES

1. Azarnoff DL, Huffman DH: Therapeutic implications of bioavailability, *Annu Rev Pharmacol Toxicol* 16:53, 1976.
2. Bass NM, Williams RL: Guide to drug dosage in hepatic disease, *Clin Pharmacokinet* 15:396, 1988.
3. Fabre J, Fox HM, Dayer P, Balant L: Differences in kinetic properties of drugs: implications as to the selection of a particular drug for use in patients with renal failure with special emphasis on antibiotics and β-adrenoceptor blocking agents, *Clin Pharmacokinet* 5:441, 1980.
4. Howden CW, Birnie GG, Brodie MJ: Drug metabolism in liver disease, *Pharmacol Ther* 40:439, 1989.
5. Koch-Weser J: Bioavailability of drugs, *N Engl J Med* 291:233 and 503, 1974.
6. Williams RL: Drug administration in hepatic disease, *N Engl J Med* 309:1616, 1983
7. Williams RL, Mamelok RD: Hepatic disease and drug pharmacokinetics, *Clin Pharmacokinet* 5:528, 1980.

Chapter 5

Pharmacokinetic principles in the use of drugs

Pharmacokinetics is the study of the time course of absorption, distribution, metabolism, and excretion of drugs and their metabolites in the intact organism. A schema of pharmacokinetics is shown below:

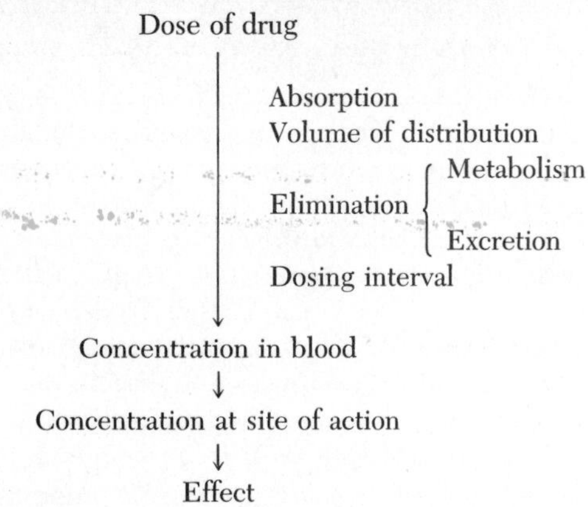

Understanding and quantification of pharmacokinetic parameters allows better selection of a dose and dosing interval to achieve the desired effect (while avoiding toxicity) in an individual patient.

PRINCIPLES OF PHARMACOKINETICS

Pharmacokinetic parameters

BIOAVAILABILITY

For use of drugs in patients, the important pharmacokinetic parameters are bioavailability, half-life, volume of distribution, and clearance.[1-5] Bioavailability is the proportion of a dose that enters the body.[6] This parameter is designated F, the fraction of drug absorbed. With intravenous administration, bioavailability is 100% ($F = 1.0$). Drugs given by other routes may exhibit incomplete bioavailability ($F = <1.0$). The clinician must have a quantitative estimate of bioavailability to select an appropriate dose, particularly for oral administration.

HALF-LIFE

Half-life is not an independent parameter that describes drug kinetics; instead it is a hybrid function of the fundamental parameters clearance and volume of distribution (see Table 5-1). An alteration in half-life attributable to clearance has therapeutic implications different from those of a change secondary to volume of distribution. Historically, half-life has been used uncritically without realizing its limitations.

Half-life is important primarily as an indication of the time required for a dosing regimen to achieve *steady-state* concentrations of drug in blood. Steady-state is the condition in which the concentration of a drug in blood has leveled out; the concentration fluctuates between a consistent maximum (peak) and a consistent minimum (trough); for an example see Fig. 5-4. If a loading dose is not administered, 4 to 5 half-lives elapse before the drug reaches steady-state concentrations in the patient. To be more precise, after 4 half-lives the drug will have reached 94% of its steady-state concentration. For a drug such as digoxin then, which has a half-life of about 36 hours in patients with normal renal function, approximately 1 week must elapse before steady-state is achieved. Likewise, if the dose of a drug is changed, whether increased or decreased, 4 to 5 times the half-life must elapse to reattain steady-state. Similarly, if drug half-life changes, as is common with a change in the patient's disease state, a new steady-state will be reached after 4 to 5 times the *new* half-life.

It is important to interpret drug concentrations and clinical end points of response in relation to whether the patient is at steady-state. Changing dosage of a drug before the patient has reached steady-state with one regimen can be a confusing and potentially hazardous exercise.

VOLUME OF DISTRIBUTION

The volume of distribution (V_d) of a drug describes the relationship between the blood concentration attained with initial dosing and the dose of drug given; that is,

$$\text{Concentration initially achieved} = \text{Dose}/V_d$$

This volume should *not* be ascribed physiologic meaning or interpretation; it is a derived parameter. Clinically, the volume of distribution is used to calculate the loading dose of a drug required to reach an initial target blood concentration. For example, if a concentration of 10 μg/ml is needed and if the volume of distribution is 100 L, the loading dose would be 1000 mg:

$$\text{Concentration initially achieved} = \frac{\text{Dose}}{V_d}$$

$$10\ \mu\text{g/ml} = \frac{\text{Dose}}{100{,}000\ \text{ml}}$$

This calculation is independent of clearance. Importantly, diseases can affect the volume of distribution and thereby alter the loading dose needed. In this example, if a disease had decreased the volume of distribution of the drug from 100 L to 50 L, and the patient was given the same 1000 mg loading dose, the circulating concentration would predictably be 1000/50, or 20 μg/ml, and toxicity could result.

To reemphasize, a loading dose is administered to achieve a therapeutic concentration of a drug quickly. Otherwise, one must wait 4 to 5 times the half-life to reach steady-state. In turn, volume of distribution determines the loading dose.

PROBLEM 5-1. What loading dose of phenytoin, an antiepileptic drug, would you give intravenously to achieve rapidly a therapeutic concentration for control of generalized tonic-clonic seizures in a 70 kg man? Use Appendixes A and B for additional information. Try to derive your answer by small, but logical, steps rather than with an equation as presented above. Then use the equation to check your answer. You may find that you don't need to memorize an equation to solve such problems.

To determine a loading dose of the drug you will also need to know its V_d and the desired plasma concentration. From Appendix B you find that the V_d of phenytoin is 0.6 L/kg; from Appendix A (Table A1) you find that the therapeutic concentration range is 10-20 μg/ml. Let's assume you are cautious and choose 10 μg/ml (or 10 mg/L) as the desired concentration. The V_d of this patient will equal 70 kg (his weight) times 0.6 L/kg (the V_d per kilogram) or 42 L. If you want 10 mg of drug in each liter you will give a loading dose of 420 mg.

CLEARANCE

Clearance is usually referred to as blood, plasma, or serum clearance, depending on the particular fluid assayed. Clearance is equivalent to an amount of body fluid sufficient to account for all drug removed per unit of time. Therefore a serum clearance of 100 ml/min means that in 1 minute all of the drug could have been eliminated from 100 ml of serum (keeping in mind, of course, that serum does not actually exist within the body). This removal can occur through distribution to tissues, metabolism, or excretion.

Clinically, clearance is important for determination of the amount of drug needed to *maintain* a steady-state concentration. By definition, at steady-state:

$$\text{Rate in} = \text{Rate out}$$

The rate of drug entering is a function of the dose administered, the fraction, F, of that dose absorbed if administered orally, and the time interval over which it is administered:

$$\text{Rate in} = F \times \text{Dose/Dosing interval}$$

The rate of drug leaving the body is a function of its steady-state concentration (Cp_{ave}) and its clearance (Cl):

$$\text{Rate out} = Cp_{ave} \times \text{Cl}$$

Therefore, at steady-state:

$$F \times \text{Dose/Dosing interval} = Cp_{ave} \times \text{Cl}$$

or with the equation rearranged:

$$Cp_{ave} = \frac{F \times \text{Dose}}{\text{Dosing interval} \times \text{Cl}}$$

It is obvious from this relationship that changes or individual differences in bioavailability, in dosing regimen (dose and dosing interval), and in clearance can influence the steady-state concentration of a drug. Disease effects on drug clearance must be compensated for by the maintenance regimen; by a change in the dose or the frequency with which it is administered, or both. The method selected for adjusting the dosage regimen influences the magnitude of difference between peak and trough concentrations of drug, that is, the fluctuation above and below the average drug concentration. The more frequently a drug is administered, the less fluctuation and vice versa.

No best method can be promulgated for adjustment of the maintenance regimen of a drug.[1-5] The general relationship between dosing frequency and fluctuation of drug concentrations must be coupled with knowledge of the influence of specific disease

TABLE 5–1 Pharmacokinetic principles

$$\text{Initial concentration achieved} = \frac{\text{Loading dose}}{\text{Volume of distribution}}$$

$$\text{Steady-state concentration maintained} = \frac{\text{Fraction absorbed} \times \text{Maintenance dose}}{\text{Dosing interval} \times \text{Clearance}}$$

$$\text{Half-life} = \frac{0.693 \times \text{Volume of distribution}}{\text{Clearance}}$$

states on the pharmacokinetics and dynamics of specific drugs. This allows selection of an initial dosage regimen that can then be adjusted to the individual patient by assessment of clinical end points of response and by measurement of serum concentration of the drug.

PROBLEM 5-2. What oral dose of desipramine, a drug used to alleviate psychologic depression, would you give every 12 hours to maintain a therapeutic concentration in a 50 kg woman? As in Problem 5-1, use Appendixes A and B for additional information, and try to derive your answer by logical steps. Then use the equation above to check your answer.

To determine a maintenance dose you need to know the clearance of the drug, the desired plasma concentration and, because oral administration is used, the drug's bioavailability. From Appendix B you find that the clearance of desipramine is 10-30 ml/min/kg and that its bioavailability is 40% to 50%; according to Appendix A (Table A1) the therapeutic concentration range is 0.1-0.25 μg/ml. Assume that you are trying to maintain a concentration of 0.2 μg/ml (or 0.2 mg/L) and that clearance and bioavailability in this patient are at the high end of the ranges listed. The clearance of desipramine in this patient will equal 50 kg (her weight) times 30 ml/min/kg (the clearance per kilogram) or 1.5 L/min (1500 ml/min), which (at a serum concentration of 0.2 μg/L) is equivalent to removal of 0.3 mg/min. In 1 hr 18 mg of drug will be inactivated, and over 12 hr 216 mg will be inactivated. Because the bioavailability of desipramine is only 50%, twice this amount or 432 mg should be taken every 12 hr.

Clinical use of pharmacokinetic parameters

Table 5-1 summarizes the clinically most important pharmacokinetic principles. To reiterate, volume of distribution is important for loading dose, clearance for maintenance dose, and half-life for determining the time required to reach steady-state. It is important to note that half-life can be affected by changes in volume of distribution or clearance. Therefore, knowing only that the half-life of a drug is altered in a particular disease state does not allow one to decide on the appropriate adjustment of therapy. One must dissect this parameter into its component terms of volume of distribution and clearance and alter therapy accordingly.

Table 5-2 illustrates these points with the drugs digoxin and lidocaine and shows how changes in volume of distribution or clearance affect therapeutic decisions. As shown by the table, the actual quantitative effect on half-life is a function of the relative magnitude of change of each of its determinants. For example, assessing the effect of congestive heart failure only on the half-life of lidocaine would indicate no need to adjust dose, whereas clearly both loading and maintenance doses of this drug should be reduced in this therapeutic setting.

MODELS OF DRUG DISPOSITION

Studies on drug distribution, absorption, and excretion have led to the concept that the body may be considered to consist of different compartments.[1-5] In the simplest

FIG. 5-1 *Schematic representation of drug disappearance curves and biologic half-life. The y axis is on the linear scale in* **A** *and on the logarithmic scale in* **B.** *Drug A has a biologic half-life of 1 hour. The biologic half-life of drug B is 2 hours.*

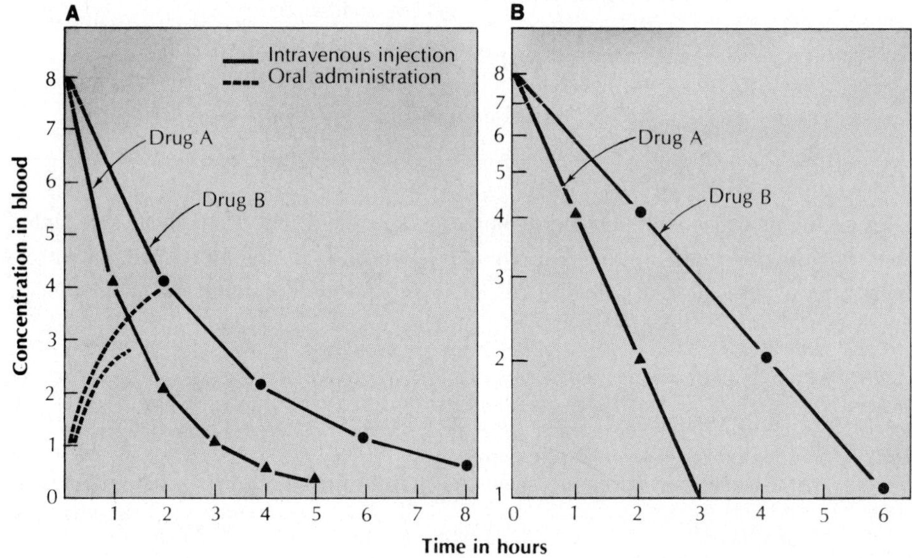

TABLE 5–2 Clinical illustration of pharmacokinetic principles

Clinical setting	Kinetic parameter V_d	Cl	$T_{1/2}$	Dosing Load	Maintenance
Digoxin in mild to moderate renal failure	—*	↓	↑	—	↓
Digoxin in end-stage renal failure	↓	↓↓	↑	↓	↓↓
Lidocaine in liver disease	—	↓	↑	—	↓
Lidocaine in congestive heart failure	↓	↓	—	↓	↓

*No change.

form, a drug passes from one compartment to another in direct proportion to its concentration gradient. In other words, a *constant fraction* (rather than a constant amount) of drug moves between compartments. Drugs with this characteristic are said to obey *first-order* kinetics as opposed to zero-order, saturable, or Michaelis-Menten kinetics. In a *one-compartment model*, it is assumed that drugs are homogeneously distributed throughout tissues and fluids of the body.

One-compartment model

In most instances a graphic representation of the time course of both absorption and elimination of drugs describes an exponential decay curve (Fig. 5-1, A). If the same data are graphed on semilogarithmic paper, the result is a straight line (Fig. 5-1,

Diagram of a two-compartment open model of drug disposition. *FIG. 5-2*

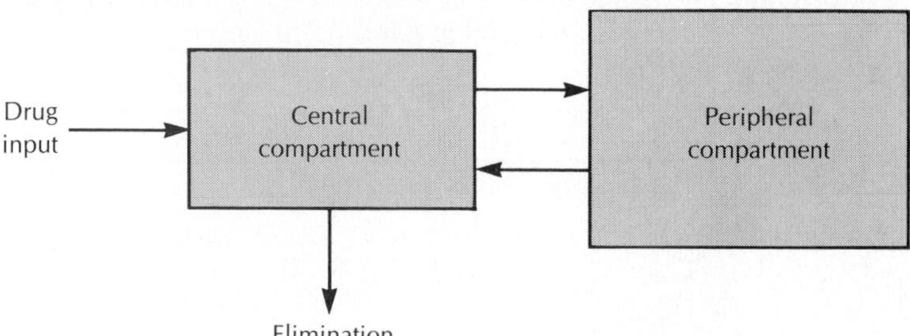

B). The intercept of the extrapolated line on the ordinate indicates the initial concentration that would be achieved when the drug is administered intravenously and it distributes instantaneously throughout the body. This hypothetical concentration is used experimentally to calculate volume of distribution (see equation on p. 25). Clearance is calculated from the dose administered divided by the *a*rea *u*nder the *c*urve (AUC) of the graph shown. Lastly, half-life, the time required for a 50% decrease in concentration of the drug, can also be derived from the graph. It is apparent from Fig. 5-1, *B*, that, in this model, half-life is independent of the concentration of the drug.

Two-compartment open model

The single-compartment model assumes an instantaneous and homogeneous distribution of drug throughout the body. This is obviously an oversimplification. A two-compartment open model more adequately describes the distribution of many drugs (Fig. 5-2). The plasma concentration profile that occurs with this type of model is shown in Fig. 5-3 where the curve has two distinct components; the first is related to distribution and the second to elimination. Transforming the curve as shown in the figure allows derivation of values for A, B, α, and β, from which relevant pharmacokinetic parameters can be calculated.

The two-compartment model incorporates a small central compartment and a larger peripheral compartment. Although no specific anatomic spaces are implied, the central compartment usually corresponds to the blood and extracellular fluid of highly perfused organs. The peripheral compartment consists of less well perfused tissues such as skin, fat, and muscle. It is further assumed that drugs initially enter and are eventually eliminated from the central compartment, though there is also reversible transfer to the peripheral compartment, which can act as a reservoir.[1-5]

These different models allow calculation of volume of distribution, clearance, and half-life, which can then be used to derive dosage regimens to achieve the desired concentration of drug in individual patients.

Zero-order elimination

For some drugs elimination is a zero-order process; that is, a *fixed quantity* of drug is eliminated per unit of time. The best example is alcohol. It is assumed that saturation of the metabolizing enzymes is responsible for the deviation from first-order kinetics. For a few drugs, such as aspirin and phenytoin, the type of elimination is dose

FIG. 5-3 *Logarithm of drug concentration in blood plotted against time* (solid line) *after intravenous administration of a drug whose disposition can be described by a two-compartment model. Broken line (– – –) represents extrapolation of terminal (B) phase. The · - · - · - line was obtained by method of residuals.*

From Dvorchik BH, Vesell ES: Clin Chem 22:868, 1976.

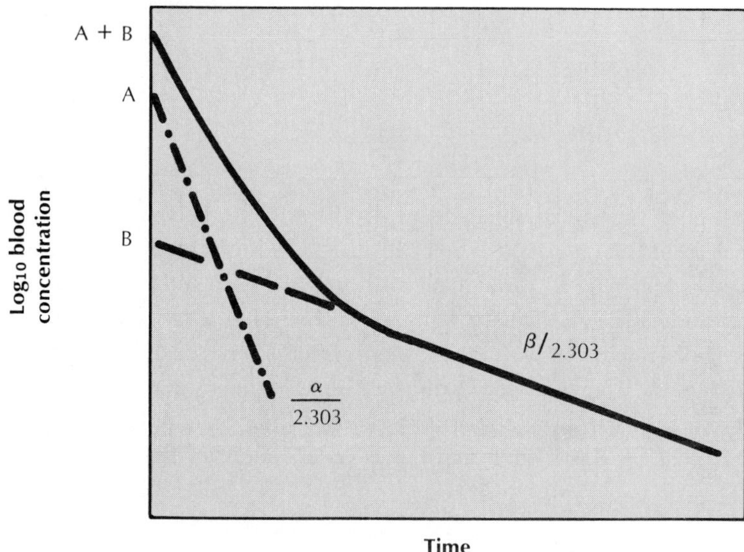

related. At low concentrations first-order kinetics prevail; saturation of elimination processes by higher concentrations results in zero-order elimination. For such drugs (assuming that volume of distribution remains constant) half-life is increased at higher concentrations because clearance is reduced.

With first-order drugs, doubling dosage doubles steady-state plasma concentration. With zero-order drugs, this does not occur. At low doses phenytoin follows first-order kinetics; therefore, doubling the dosage from 100 mg/day to 200 mg/day would increase its plasma concentration from 5 μg/ml to 10 μg/ml. If dosage is doubled again to 400 mg/day, zero-order kinetics may be reached so that the plasma concentration does not simply double again, to 20 μg/ml, but instead increases disproportionately to 30 or 40 μg/ml, concentrations that are usually toxic. Dosage of drugs that follow zero-order kinetics should be increased by small increments because the plasma concentration that will ensue is less predictable than that for drugs following first-order kinetics.

DOSAGE SCHEDULES AND PHARMACOKINETICS

Drugs may be administered in a single dose or in a repetitive fashion. Fig. 5-1, *A*, shows two drug-concentration curves, to which a one-compartment model applies, after administration of a single intravenous dose. If the drug is administered orally in a single dose, the curve will have an ascending limb (shown in dashes), a peak, and a descending limb. Variations in absorption and elimination may greatly influence the concentration curve, as reflected by changes in magnitude of the peak effect, the time required to achieve peak effect, and the duration of action of the drug.

Plot of concentration of a drug in blood after repetitive oral administration of equal doses at equal time intervals. *FIG. 5-4*

From Dvorchik BH, Vesell ES: Clin Chem 22:868, 1976.

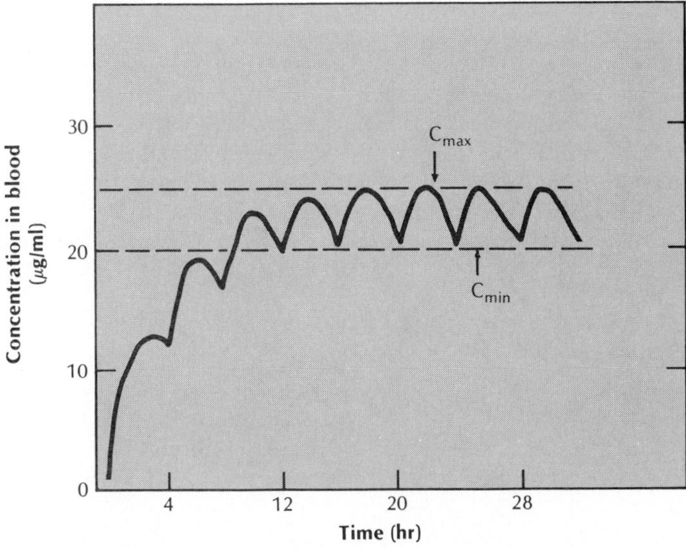

Repetitive dosing

If a drug is given repeatedly at intervals shorter than the time necessary for its complete elimination (which is roughly 4 to 5 times the half-life), it will accumulate in the body. A typical plot is depicted in Fig. 5-4. It can be seen that the drug concentration rises until it reaches a *plateau*, namely steady-state. The curve also shows fluctuations, the extent of which is determined by the individual maintenance dose, the dosage interval, and the elimination half-life. Frequent administration of a drug tends to minimize these fluctuations, whereas administration of the same total dose over more widely spaced intervals exaggerates them. The importance of fluctuations depends on the drug and the clinical setting. With some drugs, such as penicillin, large fluctuations are acceptable, whereas with drugs used to treat abnormal cardiac rhythms relatively constant blood concentrations are necessary to achieve the therapeutic objective while avoiding toxicity.

In general, if a drug has a short duration of action, the following methods are available for prolonging its action:

1. *Frequent administration*. Most sulfonamides are administered every 4 hours.
2. *Slowing absorption*. Enteric coating and other pharmaceutic maneuvers may accomplish this.
3. *Slowing elimination*, for example, by (a) interfering with renal secretion (probenecid blocks the excretion of penicillin) or (b) inhibiting drug metabolism. Allopurinol (now used to treat gout) was originally developed to block the metabolic degradation of mercaptopurine.

PROBLEM 5-3. *A sleeping medication has a half-life of 1 hour. It is administered in a dose of 100 mg, and the patient wakes up when only 12.5 mg remain in the body. How many hours will the patient sleep? If 200 mg of the same drug is administered, how much longer will the patient sleep? The answer can be found by comparison with Fig. 5-1. Doubling the dose simply adds one half-life to the duration of sleep.*

REFERENCES

1. Fenster PE: Clinical uses of pharmacokinetic principles in prescribing cardiac drugs, *Med Clin North Am* 68:1281, 1984.
2. Fleishaker JC, Smith RB: Compartmental model analysis in pharmacokinetics, *J Clin Pharmacol* 27:922, 1987.
3. Gibaldi M, Levy G: Pharmacokinetics in clinical practice. 1. Concepts, *JAMA* 235:1864, 1976.
4. Gibaldi M, Levy G: Pharmacokinetics in clinical practice. 2. Applications, *JAMA* 235:1987, 1976.
5. Greenblatt DJ, Koch-Weser J: Clinical pharmacokinetics, *N Engl J Med* 293:702 and 964, 1975.
6. Ther L, Winne D: Drug absorption, *Annu Rev Pharmacol* 11:57, 1971.

Chapter 6

Drug absorption and distribution

Absorption of drugs entails their passage across membranes. After oral administration they must cross the intestinal epithelium, and after subcutaneous or intramuscular injection they must cross capillary walls to reach the circulation. As a drug circulates, a portion will traverse additional cellular boundaries to distribute to various body tissues.

PASSAGE OF DRUGS ACROSS BODY MEMBRANES

For a drug to reach its site of action it must pass through various membranes. Fig. 6-1 depicts the general course of a drug in the body. Absorption, capillary transfer, penetration into cells, and excretion are basic examples of the movement of drugs across membranes.

Because of its lipoid nature, the cell membrane is highly permeable to lipid-soluble substances. Since water and other small lipid-insoluble compounds such as urea also readily enter cells, it is believed that the lipid membrane has pores or channels that allow passage of small lipid-insoluble molecules.

In addition to passive movement of many substances across body membranes, it is necessary to postulate more complex processes for the passage of glucose, amino acids,

FIG. 6-1 *Movement of drug in the body. After absorption, drug in the plasma* (shaded) *can be bound to protein; only unbound drug is accessible to the site of action and to routes of metabolism and excretion. Metabolized products or excreted drug in renal tubular fluid or intestinal tract may reenter the plasma space before final elimination.*

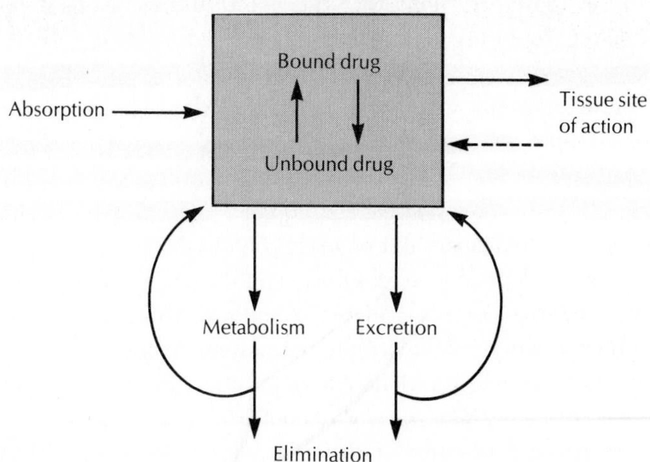

and some inorganic ions and drugs. A simplified summary of the various mechanisms follows:

1. Passive transfer
   a. Simple diffusion
   b. Filtration
2. Specialized transport
   a. Active transport
   b. Facilitated diffusion
   c. Pinocytosis

The essential features of these transfer mechanisms will be described briefly.

Passive transfer

Simple *diffusion* of a substance across a membrane is characterized by a rate of transfer that is directly proportional to the concentration gradient across the membrane. Both lipid-soluble substances and lipid-insoluble molecules of small size may cross membranes by this process. *Filtration* through a porous membrane refers to bulk flow of a solvent along with substances dissolved in it, except for molecules that are larger than the pores. The glomerular membrane of the kidney is a good example of a filtering membrane.

A special situation exists in the case of weak electrolytes, including most drugs. Cell membranes are more permeable to the nonionized, and therefore more lipid-soluble (lipophilic), form of a given drug than to its ionized and more water-soluble (hydrophilic) form. As a consequence, the passage of many drugs across membranes and into cells is a function of the pH of the environment and the pK_a of the drug.

The concept of pK_a is derived from the Henderson-Hasselbalch equation. For an acid:

$$pK_a = pH + Log \frac{\text{Molecular concentration of nonionized acid}}{\text{Molecular concentration of ionized acid}}$$

For a base:

$$pK_a = pH + Log \frac{\text{Molecular concentration of ionized base}}{\text{Molecular concentration of nonionized base}}$$

It follows from these equations that the pH resulting in equal portions of the ionized and nonionized forms of a drug is the same as its pK_a. In other words, a substance is half-ionized in an environment in which the pH is equal to its pK_a.

Although these concepts may seem academic, they explain several important principles. For example, weak acids are well absorbed from the stomach because the acidic pH causes most of the drug to be in the nonionized, more absorbable form. In contrast, weak bases are not appreciably absorbed until they reach the less acidic intestine. The influence of urinary pH on excretion of salicylic acid or phenobarbital is another example of the dependence of diffusion on the pK_a of drugs. Once these drugs enter the urine, a more alkaline pH increases the proportion of drug that is ionized. This decreases the tendency for the drug to be passively reabsorbed across the tubular epithelium and enhances its excretion. This property is the rationale for inducing an alkaline urine when treating salicylate or phenobarbital intoxication.

The pK_a values for a number of drugs are listed in Table 6-1. It should be

TABLE 6–1 pK_a Values for some weak acids and bases (at 25° C)

Weak acids	pK_a	Weak bases	pK_a
Salicyclic acid	3.00	Reserpine	6.6
Aspirin	3.49	Codeine	7.9
Sulfadiazine	6.48	Quinine	8.4
Barbital	7.91	Procaine	8.8
Boric acid	9.24	Ephedrine	9.36
		Atropine	9.65

TABLE 6–2 Effect of pH on the ionization of salicyclic acid (pK_a = 3)

pH	Percent nonionized
1	99.0
2	90.9
3	50.0
4	9.1
5	1.0
6	0.1

remembered that for acidic drugs the lower the pK_a, the stronger the acid, whereas for basic drugs the higher the pK_a, the stronger the base.

Relationships between pH, pK_a, and ionization of an acidic drug are exemplified with salicylic acid in Table 6-2.

Specialized transport

The passage of many substances into cells and across body membranes cannot be explained simply on the basis of diffusion or filtration. For example, compounds may be taken up against a concentration gradient, selectivity of transport can be shown for compounds of the same size, competitive inhibition can occur among substances transported by the same mechanism, and in some instances metabolic inhibitors can block transport processes.

Some of these phenomena are explained by the existence of specific *carriers* in membranes. *Active transport* refers to transport of substances against a concentration or electrochemical gradient. For example, many drugs are actively secreted into the urine. *Facilitated diffusion* is a special form of carrier transport that has many characteristics of active transport, except that the substrate does not move against a concentration gradient. The uptake of glucose by cells is an example of facilitated diffusion. *Pinocytosis* refers to the ability of cells to engulf small droplets. Aminoglycoside antibiotics enter the proximal tubule of the kidney by this mechanism.

ABSORPTION

The process whereby a drug initially enters body fluids is referred to as *absorption*. The rate of this process depends on the route of administration, solubility and other physical properties of the drug, disease states affecting absorptive processes, and so on.

Absorption from the gastrointestinal tract

Drugs are administrated by the oral route in many different forms—solutions, suspensions, capsules, and tablets with various coatings.[1,2,5] For absorption a drug must be in solution in molecular form. When a drug is not given in solution, its rate of absorption will be slowed by the time necessary for the tablet or capsule to release the drug (dissolution) and for the drug to dissolve in the gastrointestinal fluid. For example, ketoconazole, an antifungal drug, requires an acidic pH to dissolve. If gastric acidification is impaired, the drug does not dissolve and none is absorbed. The rate of dissolution is determined by the pharmaceutic formulation, which thus influences absorption. Once a drug is in solution, absorption is a function of the membrane of the gastrointestinal tract and can be accounted for by simple diffusion across a membrane having the characteristics of a lipoid structure with water-filled pores.

As discussed previously, the gastrointestinal membrane is permeable to nonionized lipid-soluble forms of drugs and is virtually impermeable to the ionized form. Weak acids, such as salicylates and barbiturates, are largely nonionized in the acidic gastric fluid and are therefore well absorbed from the stomach. Despite this, factors such as gastric emptying time and surface area may result in absorption of a greater fraction of weak acids from the intestine than from the stomach. In contrast, weak bases, such as quinine or ephedrine, are poorly absorbed from the stomach.

In the small intestine the surface area is much greater than that of the stomach, and the pH of intestinal contents is more alkaline. The mucosal membrane of the small intestine is also more permissive or porous than that of the stomach. Hence, many drugs, whether they are acids or bases, are absorbed primarily in the proximal small intestine. Therefore how soon the stomach empties its contents into the intestine will influence how quickly drugs are absorbed.[4] For example, if quinine is retained in the stomach, its absorption may be considerably delayed. Several drugs that affect gastric emptying greatly influence absorption; opioid analgesics slow emptying whereas metoclopramide hastens it.

Passive intestinal absorption does not account for uptake of all substances. Special mechanisms exist for the absorption of sugars, amino acids, and compounds related to normal nutrients. Similarly, some inorganic ions, such as sodium and chloride, are well absorbed despite the fact that they are charged.

In the oral cavity the mucosa also behaves as a lipid-pore membrane, and drugs may be absorbed after sublingual administration. Nitroglycerin is administered in this manner.

FIRST-PASS EFFECT

When administered orally, drugs that pass through the intestinal wall enter the liver before reaching systemic sites. Even with complete gastrointestinal absorption a fraction of the dose may not traverse the liver because of metabolism within it or, in some cases, within the gut. This concept is referred to as the "first-pass effect" or "presystemic elimination." This process is important for many drugs, one of the best studied being propranolol. Occasionally, it is important clinically to circumvent this first-pass effect. For example, swallowed nitroglycerin does not readily reach the systemic circulation because the first-pass effect is so great. Consequently, this drug is frequently administered under the tongue where it is absorbed into vessels that do not drain into the liver.

For drugs that exhibit an important first-pass effect, a decrease in the metabolic capability of the liver can augment absorption. For example, in patients with severe cirrhosis the bioavailability of propranolol is twice that in patients with normal hepatic function.

Absorption with parenteral administration

The rate of absorption from subcutaneous or intramuscular sites depends largely on two factors: the solubility of the preparation and the blood flow through the region.[3] Suspensions or colloidal preparations are absorbed more slowly than aqueous solutions. Advantage can be taken of this fact when prolonged absorption is desirable. For example, protamine is added to insulin to form a suspension and thereby slow absorption from the subcutaneous depot. Various penicillin suspensions also prolong therapeutic action by slowing absorption.

The importance of local blood flow is illustrated by very slow absorption of drug from a subcutaneous site in the presence of peripheral circulatory failure. This has been observed after administration of morphine to patients in shock. In contrast, the greater flow per unit weight of muscle is responsible for more rapid absorption of drugs from this tissue than from subcutaneous fat. Furthermore, the rate of blood flow to different muscle groups differs, and absorption rate can depend on the particular muscle chosen for the injection site.

Certain consequences of these facts are of clinical importance. Cooling an area of subcutaneous injection will slow absorption, a desirable effect if an excessive dose has been inadvertently injected or if an untoward reaction begins to develop. In contrast, massage of the site will increase blood flow and hasten absorption.

Rate-controlled drug delivery

There is increasing interest in methods of administration that maintain a fairly uniform drug concentration in the blood and thereby at its site of action. Examples are constant-infusion pumps, sustained-release gastrointestinal delivery systems, and transdermal devices.[2] Pumps can be worn externally or implanted under the skin. Insulin-infusion pumps are being used in diabetics. When pilocarpine is used in eyedrops to treat glaucoma, frequent administration is necessary because of rapid clearance. A device that releases the drug uniformly can now be placed under the lower eyelid. Patches applied to the skin are used increasingly for transdermal administration of scopolamine, nitroglycerin, estrogen, and clonidine. Whether such an approach is feasible depends greatly on the physicochemical characteristics of the drug itself and the structure (for example, the skin) through which the drug is absorbed. Enteric-coated tablets are commonly used to provide a sustained level of drug in the body, but, despite its popularity, this dosage form cannot generally be considered a predictable method of administering drugs. There is great variation in rates of gastric emptying and of dissolution of such preparations. They may even be eliminated unchanged in the feces. This uncertainty has led to development of other methods for sustaining intestinal release of drug. For example, one system uses osmotic force to pump drug out of a permeable tablet at a constant rate. Such systems reliably attain stable drug concentrations in plasma throughout a dosing interval.

DISTRIBUTION OF DRUGS IN THE BODY

Once a drug reaches the plasma, it must cross various barriers to reach its site of action. The first of these barriers is the capillary wall. Through diffusion and filtration most drugs rapidly cross the capillary wall, which has the usual characteristics of biologic membranes. Lipid-soluble substances diffuse through the endothelium, whereas lipid-insoluble drugs pass through pores that represent an important fraction of the total surface area. The capillary transfer of lipid-insoluble substances is inversely related to molecular size. Large molecules are transferred so slowly that, for example, dextran solutions can be used as plasma substitutes to retain fluid within the vascular compartment.

Factors affecting distribution of drugs

Factors that affect distribution of drugs in the body include (1) binding to plasma proteins, (2) the rate of blood flow to various organs, (3) cellular binding, (4) concentration in fatty tissues, and (5) the blood-brain barrier.

Binding of drugs to plasma proteins increases the concentration of drug in blood relative to that in extracellular fluid.[8] It also provides a depot, since the bound portion of the drug is in equilibrium with the free form. As the unbound fraction is excreted or metabolized, additional drug dissociates from the protein. Protein binding can prolong the half-life of a drug, because the bound fraction is not filtered through renal glomeruli and is also protected from biotransformation. The protein-bound fraction of a drug also is restricted from reaching its site of action and is inactive. The protein responsible for binding of acidic drugs is usually albumin. Basic drugs are bound to α_1-acid glycoprotein.[6] Many hormonal agents are bound to other types of proteins; for example, transcortin binds glucocorticoids.[8]

The binding capacity of proteins is limited. Once binding becomes saturated, a small increment in dose can cause a large increase in unbound drug with a concomitant increase in effect, including toxicity. In hypoalbuminemia, toxic manifestations of drugs may develop with customary doses due to the deficiency of binding protein.

Drugs may influence protein binding of other substances or drugs.[7] Thus salicylates decrease the binding of thyroxin to proteins. The binding of bilirubin to albumin may be inhibited by a variety of drugs, such as sulfisoxazole and salicylates. This can be particularly hazardous in neonates when this mechanism increases the accessibility of bilirubin to the brain; fatal kernicterus has occurred in premature infants who were given sulfisoxazole. Other examples of drug interactions based on displacement from protein binding are discussed in Chapter 70.

The *rate of blood flow* affects delivery of drug to various organs. After intravenous administration, the concentration of a highly lipophilic compound in a well perfused tissue such as the brain rapidly reaches equilibrium with unbound drug in plasma. Muscle, which is less well perfused, takes up the drug more slowly. Despite the ability of fat to concentrate the drug if exposed to it for a prolonged period, fat, because of its limited blood flow, absorbs the drug most slowly. The almost immediate anesthetic action of thiopental is due to its rapid uptake by the brain. Recovery of consciousness then occurs within minutes as less well perfused tissues continue to absorb the drug, the concentration of drug in blood decreases, and the anesthetic rapidly distributes out of the brain.

The *cellular binding* of drugs is usually a result of affinity for some cellular constituent. The high concentration of the antimalarial drug quinacrine in liver or muscle is probably caused by its affinity for nucleoproteins.

The *concentration of drug in fatty tissues* also affects distribution. Highly lipid-soluble drugs like glutethimide distribute into fat, which then serves as a depot. Extraction of such drugs from plasma by metabolism or excretion results in egress from fat into blood with restoration of the circulating concentration.

The *blood-brain barrier* provides a unique example of unequal distribution of drugs. Even if injected intravenously, many drugs fail to reach the central nervous system, the cerebrospinal fluid, or the aqueous humor, or they enter much less rapidly than they enter other tissues. There are, however, some brain regions with a weak blood-brain barrier; these include the neurohypophysis and the area postrema.

The capillaries in the central nervous system are enveloped by glial cells, which present a barrier to many water-soluble compounds, although they are permeable to lipid-soluble substances. Thus quaternary amines penetrate the central nervous system poorly, whereas general anesthetics do so with ease.

Of great importance in clinical medicine is the increase in barrier permeability produced by inflammation. For example, administration of large doses of penicillin to normal persons fails to produce detectable concentrations of the antibiotic in cerebrospinal fluid. From such data alone, one might conclude a lack of potential efficacy of the drug in meningitis. However, penicillin can penetrate readily into the spinal fluid of patients with inflamed meninges and is commonly used in some forms of meningitis.

Although many drugs do not reach the cerebrospinal fluid well, they can move efficiently in the reverse direction by filtration across the arachnoid villi and by secretion across the choroid plexus. The peritoneal membrane exhibits similar parallels in which transport from the peritoneum into blood is much greater than the reverse. For example, patients treated by peritoneal dialysis frequently develop peritoneal infections. Instillation of many antibiotics into the peritoneum results in substantial absorption into the systemic circulation. The converse is not true; very little of these antibiotics enters the peritoneal space after systemic injection.

The passage of drugs from blood into *milk* may be explained by diffusion of the nonionized, non–protein-bound fraction. Sufficient amounts may reach the milk to cause adverse effects in the breast-fed infant. On the other hand, many drugs appear in milk only in small quantities and are generally of no clinical significance for the infant. In general, large doses of drugs should not be administered to a mother who is breast-feeding her child without considering the potential danger to the infant.

REFERENCES

1. Azarnoff DL, Huffman DH: Therapeutic implications of bioavailability, *Annu Rev Pharmacol Toxicol* 16:53, 1976.
2. Goldman P: Rate-controlled drug delivery, *N Engl J Med* 307:286, 1982.
3. Greenblatt DJ, Koch-Weser J: Intramuscular injection of drugs, *N Engl J Med* 295:542, 1976.
4. Heading RC: Gastric emptying: a clinical perspective, *Clin Sci* 63:231, 1982.
5. Koch-Weser J: Bioavailability of drugs, *N Engl J Med* 291:233 and 503, 1974.
6. Kremer JMH, Wilting J, Janssen LHM: Drug binding to human alpha-1-acid glycoprotein in health and disease, *Pharmacol Rev* 40:1, 1988.
7. MacKichan JJ: Protein binding drug displacement interactions: fact or fiction? *Clin Pharmacokinet* 16:65,1989.
8. Øie S: Drug distribution and binding, *J Clin Pharmacol* 26:583, 1986.

Chapter 7

Drug elimination by metabolism and excretion

Drug elimination (clearance) occurs by metabolism and excretion. The former takes place predominately in the liver where drugs are converted from less polar, more lipid-soluble compounds to more polar, hydrophilic compounds that are more readily excreted, predominately via the kidney.

DRUG METABOLISM

Chemical reactions in drug metabolism

The chemical reactions involved in drug metabolism or *biotransformation* are classified as microsomal oxidations, nonmicrosomal oxidations, reductions, hydrolyses, and conjugations (Table 7-1).[5] These pathways of metabolism will each be discussed, with specific examples. Since microsomal enzymes play a predominant role in biotransformation, their functions are summarized first.

TABLE 7–1 Types of drug metabolism and responsible enzymes

Drug metabolism	Enzymes
Oxidations of aliphatic and aromatic groups	Cytochrome P-450
Hydroxylation	
N-dealkylation	
0-dealkylation	
S-dealkylation	
Deamination	
Desulfuration	
Sulfoxidation	
N-oxidation	
Nonmicrosomal oxidation	Alcohol dehydrogenase
Reductions of azo and nitro groups	Flavin enzymes
Hydrolyses of esters and amides	Esterases
Conjugations	Transferases
Glucuronidation	
Glycine conjugation	
Sulfation	
Acetylation	
Mercapturic acid synthesis	
Methylation	

Microsomal Enzymes

The microsomal enzymes of the liver, which are part of the smooth endoplasmic reticulum, convert many lipid-soluble drugs and foreign compounds into more water-soluble metabolites.[5] These enzymes constitute a mixed-function oxidase system. As an example, consider the oxidation reaction that occurs in the presence of nicotinamide adenine dinucleotide phosphate (NADPH) and oxygen. The enzyme system transfers one atom of oxygen to the drug while another atom of oxygen is reduced to form water. The general scheme is as follows:

$$NADPH + A + H_2 \rightarrow AH_2 + NADP^+$$

$$AH_2 + O_2 \rightarrow \text{"Active oxygen"}$$

$$\text{"Active oxygen"} + \text{Drug} \rightarrow \text{Oxidized drug} + A + H_2O$$

$$\text{Result:} \quad NADPH + O_2 + \text{Drug} = NADP^+ + H_2O + \text{Oxidized drug}$$

In this scheme, *A* is cytochrome P-450, the terminal oxidase for a variety of drug oxidations. Cytochrome P-450 is so named because this hemoprotein in its reduced state combines with carbon monoxide to form a product with an absorption peak at 450 nm. There are numerous isoenzymes of cytochrome P-450, discussed in more detail in Chapter 8, with specificity for different drugs and different reactions. Another essential enzyme in the reaction is NADPH cytochrome P-450 reductase, which reduces the oxidized P-450.

Microsomal Oxidations

Hydroxylation of aromatic rings. Phenytoin is changed to *p*-hydroxyphenytoin. Phenobarbital is converted to *p*-hydroxyphenobarbital.

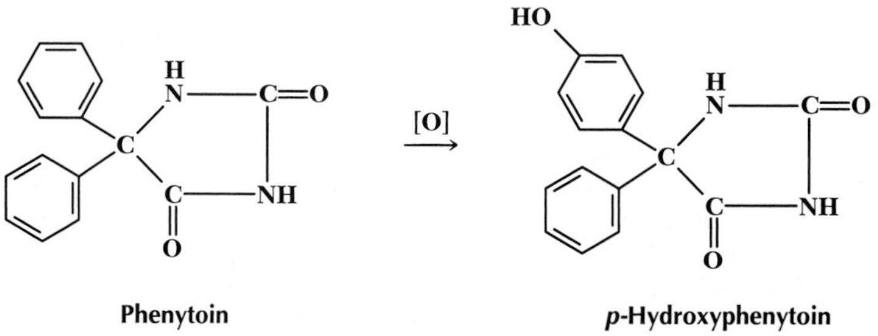

Phenytoin $\xrightarrow{[O]}$ ***p*-Hydroxyphenytoin**

Side-chain oxidation (aliphatic hydroxylation). Tolbutamide is metabolized to hydroxytolbutamide. Pentobarbital is metabolized to pentobarbital alcohol.

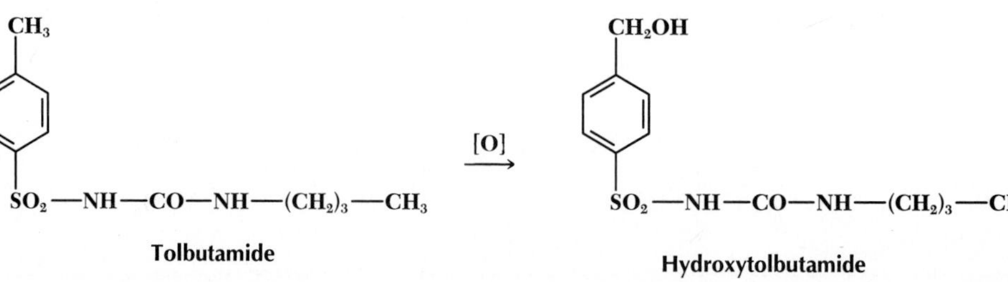

Tolbutamide $\xrightarrow{[O]}$ **Hydroxytolbutamide**

N-dealkylation. Imipramineis demethylated to desipramine. A clinically important caveat with this pathway is that it appears to be less subject to induction and inhibition by other drugs as compared with hydroxylation reactions.

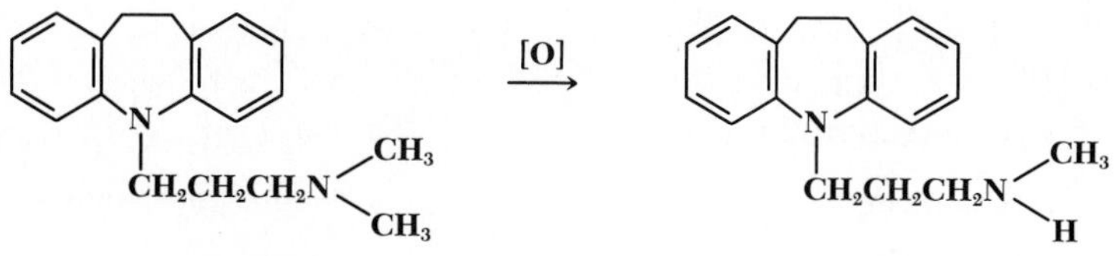

$CH_2CH_2CH_2N(CH_3)_2$ $\xrightarrow{[O]}$ $CH_2CH_2CH_2N(CH_3)H$

Imipramine **Desipramine**

O-dealkylation. Encainide is changed to *O*-demethylencainide.

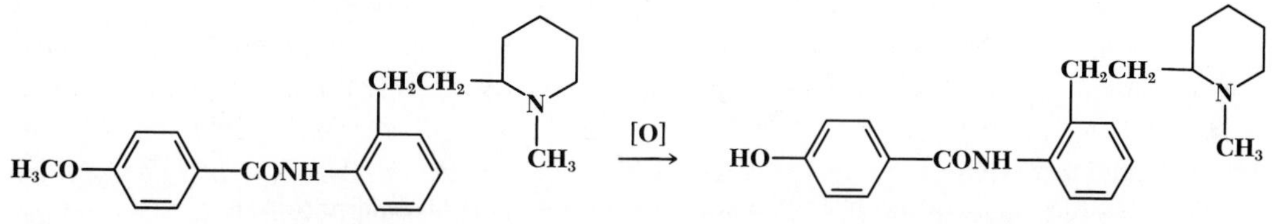

H_3CO—CONH— CH_2CH_2 N CH_3 $\xrightarrow{[O]}$ HO—CONH— CH_2CH_2 N CH_3

Encainide ***O*–Demethylencainide**

S-dealkylation. 6-Methylthiopurine is demethylated to 6-mercaptopurine.

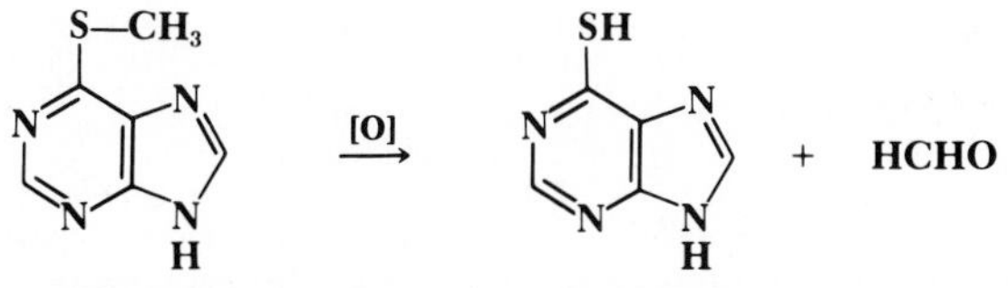

S—CH_3 $\xrightarrow{[O]}$ SH + HCHO

6-Methylthiopurine **6-Mercaptopurine**

Deamination. Amphetamine is oxidized to phenylacetone.

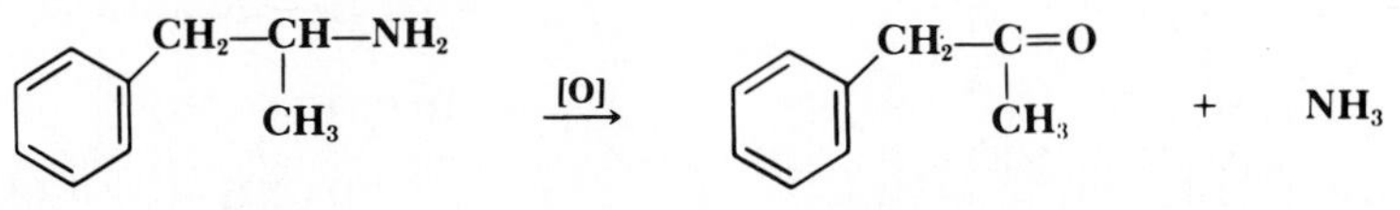

CH_2—CH—NH_2 (CH$_3$) $\xrightarrow{[O]}$ CH_2—C=O (CH$_3$) + NH_3

Amphetamine **Phenylacetone**

Desulfuration. Parathion becomes an active cholinesterase inhibitor after oxidation to paraoxon.

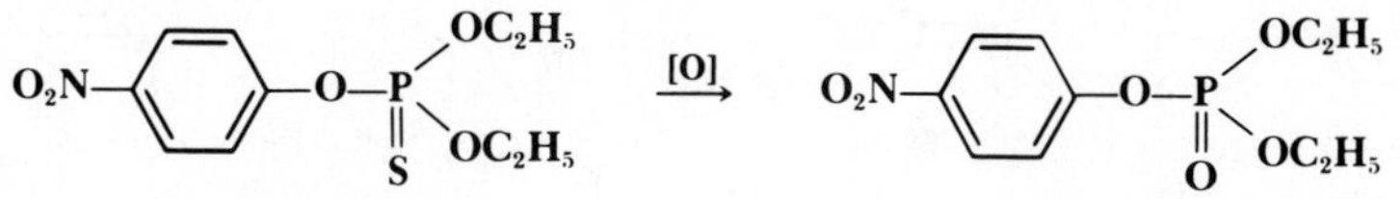

O_2N—O—P(=S)(OC_2H_5)$_2$ $\xrightarrow{[O]}$ O_2N—O—P(=O)(OC_2H_5)$_2$

Parathion **Paraoxon**

Sulfoxidation. Chlorpromazine is converted to chlorpromazine sulfoxide.

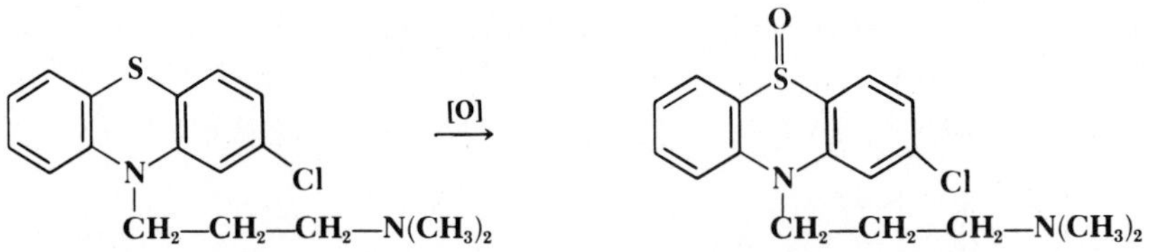

Chlorpromazine **Chlorpromazine sulfoxide**

N-oxidation. Meperidine is oxidized to meperidine *N*-oxide.

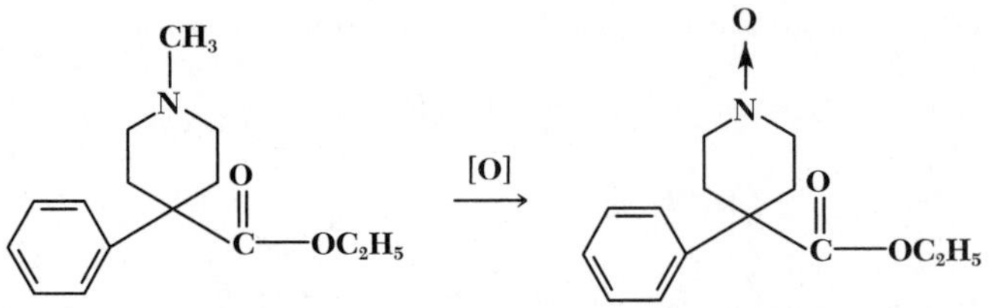

Meperidine **Meperidine *N*–oxide**

NONMICROSOMAL (ALCOHOL) OXIDATION

Ethyl alcohol is changed to acetaldehyde primarily in the cytoplasm by alcohol dehydrogenase. However, oxidation to the same product also takes place within microsomes.

$$\underset{\text{Ethyl alcohol}}{CH_3CH_2OH} + NAD^+ \xrightarrow{[0]} \underset{\text{Acetaldehyde}}{CH_3CHO} + NADH + H^+$$

REDUCTIONS

Nitroreduction. Chloramphenicol is reduced to the arylamine.

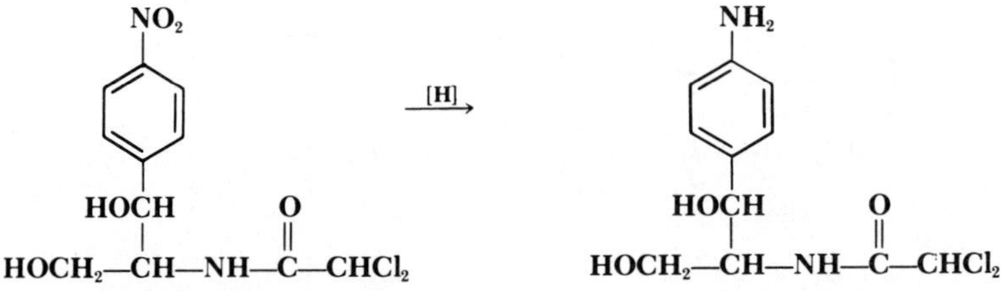

Chloramphenicol **"Arylamine"**

Azoreduction. Prontosil is reduced to sulfanilamide.

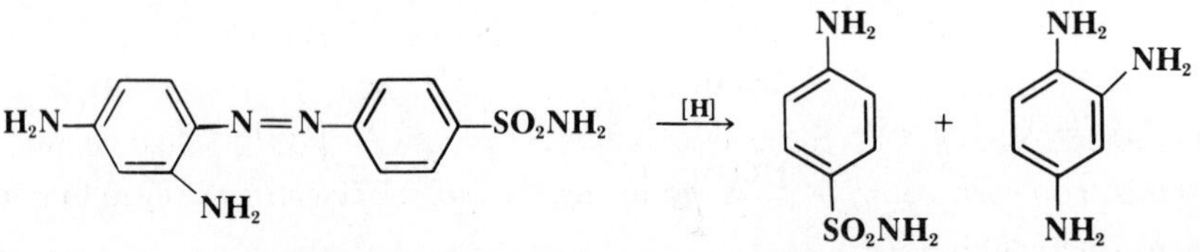

Prontosil **Sulfanilamide**

Alcohol dehydrogenation. Chloral hydrate is changed to trichloroethanol, the active moiety.

$$Cl_3C{-}CH(OH){-}OH + NADH + H^+ \longrightarrow Cl_3C{-}CH_2{-}OH + NAD^+ + H_2O$$

Chloral hydrate   Trichloroethanol

HYDROLYSIS

Enalapril. Enalapril is hydrolyzed to active enalaprilat.

$$C_6H_5CH_2CH_2{-}CH(COOC_2H_5){-}NH{-}CH(CH_3){-}C(=O){-}N(\text{pyrrolidine-COOH}) \xrightarrow{[+\ H_2O]} C_6H_5CH_2CH_2{-}CH(COOH){-}NH{-}CH(CH_3){-}C(=O){-}N(\text{pyrrolidine-COOH}) + C_2H_5OH$$

Enalapril   Enalapril   Ethyl alcohol

CONJUGATIONS

The most important conjugation reactions are glucuronide synthesis, glycine conjugation, sulfate conjugation, acetylation, mercapturic acid synthesis, and methylation.

Glucuronide synthesis. Phenols, alcohols, carboxylic acids, and compounds containing amino or sulfhydryl groups may undergo glucuronide conjugation. Glucuronide formation is one of the most common routes of drug metabolism. Not only does this process occur with parent compounds, but many metabolites formed by microsomal oxidation are in turn conjugated to a glucuronide before excretion. The mechanism of the reaction is as follows:

$$\text{Uridine diphosphoglucuronate} + \text{ROH} \xrightarrow[\text{transferase}]{\text{Glucuronyl}} \text{RO glucuronide} + \text{Uridine diphosphate}$$

Morphine is an example of a drug excreted almost entirely as glucuronides. Morphine-3-glucuronide, the major metabolite, is inactive; active morphine-6-glucuronide is also formed.

$$\text{Morphine (3-HO, 6-OH; } CH_3N\text{)} \longrightarrow \text{Morphine-3-glucuronide (3-O-}C_6H_9O_6\text{, 6-OH; } CH_3N\text{)}$$

Morphine   Morphine-3-glucuronide

Glucuronide bonds form either an ester or an ether linkage. That shown for morphine is the latter. The former is labile and the conjugate can hydrolyze to reform the parent compound.

Glycine conjugation. Glycine conjugation is characteristic for certain aromatic acids. It depends on the availability of coenzyme A, glycine, and glycine-*N*-acylase. A typical reaction is as follows:

COOH, OH —(ATP + CoA)→ C(=O)—CoA, OH —(Glycine)→ C(=O)—NH—CH_2—COOH, OH

Salicyclic acid　　Salicyl—CoA　　Salicycluric acid

Drugs conjugated with glycine in humans include salicylic acid, isonicotinic acid, and *p*-aminosalicylic acid. These drugs are also metabolized by other pathways, which may be more important quantitatively than glycine conjugation.

Sulfate conjugation. Phenols, alcohols, and aromatic amines may undergo sulfate conjugation. The sulfate donor is 3′-phosphoadenosine-5-phosphosulfate (PAPS). The major metabolite of acetaminophen in children is the sulfate; in adults its major metabolite is a glucuronide.

NHC(=O)—CH_3, OH —(PAPS)→ NHC(=O)—CH_3, O-sulfate

Acetaminophen　　Acetaminophen sulfate

Acetylation. Derivatives of aniline are acetylated in the body. In addition to sulfanilamide and related compounds, drugs such as *p*-aminosalicylic acid, isoniazid, and procainamide are transformed by this mechanism. The general reaction involving an amine, acetyl coenzyme A, and a specific acetylating enzyme may be depicted as follows:

$$RNH_2 + CoASCOCH_3 \xrightarrow{\text{Acetyltransferase}} RNHCOCH_3 + CoASH$$

The acetylating ability of individuals may differ considerably and shows a bimodal distribution; patients can be grouped as slow acetylators as opposed to rapid acetylators (see also Chapter 8). In the case of isoniazid, a low degree of acetylation shows some correlation with the incidence of toxic reactions such as peripheral neuritis.

$CONHNH_2$ → $CONHNHCOCH_3$

Isoniazid　　Acetylated isoniazid

Mercapturic acid synthesis. Mercapturic acid synthesis is not a common pathway in humans. Some drugs containing an active halogen or a nitro group may be changed to mercapturates. In fact, the thiol derivative of nitrates is thought by some to be the active intermediate that causes vasodilatation.

Methylation. Norepinephrine and epinephrine are metabolized in part to normetanephrine and metanephrine by O-methylation, whereas nicotinic acid is metabolized to *N*-methylnicotinic acid, an example of N-methylation. The source of methyl groups is *S*-adenosylmethionine.

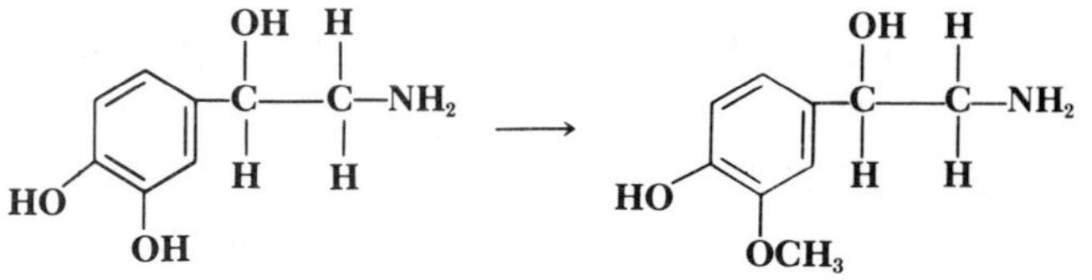

OH H — C—C—NH_2 (H, H); HO, OH → OH H — C—C—NH_2 (H, H); HO, OCH_3

Norepinephrine Normetanephrine

Drug metabolism and detoxification

Drug metabolism, for the most part, changes a drug to more water-soluble metabolites that are usually, but not necessarily, inactive. The term *detoxification* is not accurate, since the body can also form a toxic metabolite from a less toxic drug. For example, a normally minor intermediate step in acetaminophen metabolism is formation of a reactive compound that can damage hepatocytes. With usual doses the liver is protected because this metabolite is neutralized by a thiol (sulfhydryl) group. If the sulfhydryl groups are exhausted by an overdose, exposure of hepatocytes to the toxic metabolite causes cell necrosis. Hence the morbidity and mortality of acetaminophen intoxication are attributable to hepatic failure. Treatment is logically aimed at replenishing thiol donors by administering *N*-acetylcysteine.

Factors that affect the metabolism of drugs

Most drugs are metabolized at rates proportional to their plasma concentrations (first-order or linear kinetics, see Chapter 5) because therapeutic concentrations are not high enough to saturate drug-metabolizing enzymes. If saturation does occur, metabolism becomes zero order and obeys saturable or Michaelis-Menten kinetics. A number of conditions can affect access of drug to metabolizing enzymes or change the amount or activity of the enzymes; all would be expected to affect clearance of the drug and thereby its plasma concentration during maintenance dosing.

FLOW-LIMITED AND CAPACITY-LIMITED METABOLISM

Drugs metabolized by the liver are conveniently separated into those that are flow limited and those that are capacity limited.[7,8] Examples are listed in Table 7-2. Simplistically, hepatic metabolic capacity is very high for drugs that are flow limited, and the liver's only limitation to metabolism is the amount of drug that reaches it. Such drugs exhibit a high *hepatic extraction ratio*; in other words, the liver metabolizes a large fraction of the drug (as much as it "sees"), which, in turn, is determined by blood flow to the liver. For such drugs, the first-pass effect is substantial, though not always complete; a decrease in hepatic metabolism can diminish first-pass elimination and

TABLE 7–2 Examples of flow-limited and capacity-limited drugs in terms of their hepatic metabolism

Flow-limited	Capacity-limited
Lidocaine	Chlordiazepoxide
Meperidine	Cimetidine
Metoprolol	Diazepam
Propranolol	Lorazepam
	Naproxen
	Theophylline
	Tolbutamide
	Warfarin

thereby increase drug bioavailability. Changes in plasma protein binding have no effect on clearance of flow-limited drugs because free drug is metabolized rapidly enough to allow dissociation of bound drug from plasma protein, followed by metabolism of newly free drug until all the drug that enters the liver, whether initially free or bound, is metabolized.

For drugs that are less readily metabolized, so-called capacity-limited agents that have a low hepatic extraction ratio, plasma protein binding is an important determinant of clearance. A high degree of binding, an inherent characteristic of many drugs, limits clearance. Conversely, a decrease in binding, as when another drug competes for the same site, presents more unbound drug to the liver for metabolism; there is a subsequent increase in the amount metabolized and a reduction in total plasma concentration. However, because the reduction in binding also increases the proportion of free, pharmacologically active drug, effects are typically unchanged or only transiently enhanced. In other words, a lower total concentration of drug is now sufficient to maintain a concentration of unbound drug comparable to that before binding was inhibited.

Enzyme induction and inhibition

Phenobarbital, rifampin, and many other lipid-soluble drugs may increase the amount of microsomal hydroxylase. Clinically this increases clearance of the drug itself and of some other drugs, which may be sufficient to require an increase in dose. Because enzyme induction requires synthesis of new protein, it occurs gradually over a course of several days and may take 1 or 2 weeks to attain its maximal effect (see also Chapter 70 on drug interactions).

Premature infants, persons with liver disease, and elderly patients may have a deficiency of microsomal enzymes and thereby a diminished metabolic capacity for many drugs. Some drugs inhibit drug-metabolizing enzymes; drug clearance is then decreased, often necessitating a decrease in dose to avoid toxic concentrations. For example, cimetidine, omeprazole, and ciprofloxacin diminish the metabolic clearance of theophylline to one-half of normal, mandating a comparable dosage reduction. In contrast to induction of drug metabolism, inhibition occurs quickly, with the first dose of the interacting drug.

Schematic of a chiral compound. The two configurations are not superimposable but are mirror images of one another. *FIG. 7-1*

$$\mathrm{COOH{-}\overset{\overset{\displaystyle CH_3}{|}}{\underset{\underset{\displaystyle R}{|}}{C}}{-}H} \quad \Bigg| \quad \mathrm{H{-}\overset{\overset{\displaystyle CH_3}{|}}{\underset{\underset{\displaystyle R}{|}}{C}}{-}COOH}$$

Mirror

Stereoselective drug metabolism

Many compounds, both exogenous and endogenous, can exist in three-dimensional space in two different configurations, which are mirror images of one another (Fig. 7-1). These asymmetric or *chiral* three-dimensional structures are called *stereoisomers* or *enantiomers*. They have identical chemical characteristics such as melting point but, when in solution, rotate light in opposite directions. Of primary importance to therapy, enantiomers may differ in terms of disposition and biologic effects.[1-6] For example, (S)-warfarin is more potent than (R)-warfarin in inhibiting synthesis of vitamin K–dependent clotting factors. Furthermore, these isomers are bound to different extents by plasma proteins and are metabolized differently by the liver. Moreover, the metabolic pathway for (R)-warfarin is inhibited by cimetidine, whereas the pathway for the (S)-isomer is not.

As another example, the ability of ibuprofen and related agents (see Chapter 35) to inhibit prostaglandin synthesis resides in the (S)-enantiomer; the (R)-configuration lacks this activity. Like warfarin, the stereoisomers vary in degree of protein binding and extent of metabolism.

Numerous drugs are administered as *racemic* mixtures, namely, as equal portions of each stereoisomer, primarily because such mixtures are the natural product of pharmaceutical synthesis. Some drugs for which important pharmacokinetic and/or pharmacodynamic differences between stereoisomers are known are listed in Table 7-3. For many other drugs, unfortunately, isomers have not been adequately compared, leaving clinicians with uncertainty concerning possible differences. Scientists are currently urging that future development of drugs focus on pure stereoisomers, as now occurs with marketed products such as levodopa, naproxen, and propoxyphene. This should improve the therapeutic margin of drugs with asymmetric conformations.[1-3]

EXCRETION OF DRUGS

The most important route of excretion for most drugs is the kidney. Many drugs are also excreted into bile, but some can then be reabsorbed from the intestine (so-called enterohepatic circulation), making this route quantitatively less important. Elimination of drugs in the feces or through the lungs and the salivary and sweat glands is important only in special cases to be discussed under individual drugs.

Three major processes are involved in the renal handling of drugs: glomerular filtration, tubular reabsorption, and tubular secretion. A common course of a drug is filtration through the glomeruli, with or without secretion into the proximal tubule,

TABLE 7–3 Examples of drugs administered as racemic mixtures, with known, important differences between enantiomers

Disopyramide	Pentobarbital
Flecainide	Pindolol
Ibuprofen	Propafenone
Ketamine	Sotalol
Labetalol	Tocainide
Mephenytoin	Verapamil
Mexiletine	Warfarin

followed by partial reabsorption from more distal tubular segments. Because water is reabsorbed to a much greater extent than most drugs are, the concentration of a drug in urine is usually greater than that in plasma and is never less.

Filtration of a drug at the glomerulus is mainly a function of molecular size. Most drugs are smaller than the glomerular fenestrations (about 40 angstroms), and so unbound drug in plasma is filtered freely. An exception is large molecular weight (70,000) dextran, all of which is free in plasma but none of which is filtered due to the size constraint.

Just as in the gastrointestinal tract, the fraction of drug in tubular fluid that is uncharged will be a function of the urinary pH and the pK_a of the drug. Drugs that are bases are excreted to a greater extent if the urine is acidic, whereas acidic compounds are excreted more readily if the urine is alkaline. A practical application of this principle is in treatment of poisoning by the weak acids phenobarbital and salicylic acid; an alkaline urine increases the proportion of ionized drug, thereby decreasing reabsorption and enhancing excretion. Administration of sodium bicarbonate is a therapeutically useful strategy for management of either type of poisoning.

Since urine is normally acidic, the elimination of weakly acidic drugs by excretion alone would require a very long time. Fortunately, metabolism tends to transform these drugs into stronger electrolytes, thereby increasing the percentage in the ionic form and limiting tubular reabsorption.

In addition to glomerular filtration with passive tubular reabsorption, the renal tubule can actively secrete organic anions and cations. Classic examples of such organic anions are penicillin and probenecid; examples of organic cations are cimetidine and procainamide. These active transport pathways also secrete other agents, and competition for active tubular secretion occurs among the various anions and cations (see also Chapter 70).

Some drugs, such as penicillins secreted by the tubules, have very short half-lives. To slow elimination, tubular secretion can be inhibited by a drug like probenecid, a compound specifically developed for this purpose. Usually, however, it is simpler to maintain a drug in the body for longer periods of time by prolonging its absorption rather than by impairing elimination. This is the reason for the development of penicillin preparations that are absorbed slowly after intramuscular injection.

Many disease processes, including primary renal disease, diminish renal excretion of drugs and mandate dose adjustment to compensate for decreased renal clearance. This is discussed in greater detail in Chapter 10.

REFERENCES

1. Ariëns EJ: Implications of the neglect of stereochemistry in pharmacokinetics and clinical pharmacology, *Drug Intell Clin Pharm* 21:827, 1987.
2. Ariëns EJ, Wuis EW, Veringa EJ: Stereoselectivity of bioactive xenobiotics: a pre-Pasteur attitude in medicinal chemistry, pharmacokinetics and clinical pharmacology, *Biochem Pharmacol* 37:9, 1988.
3. Drayer DE: Pharmacodynamic and pharmacokinetic differences between drug enantiomers in humans: an overview, *Clin Pharmacol Ther* 40:125, 1986.
4. Jamali F, Mehvar R, Pasutto FM: Enantioselective aspects of drug action and disposition: therapeutic pitfalls, *J Pharm Sci* 78:695, 1989.
5. La Du BN, Mandel HG, Way EL: *Fundamentals of drug metabolism and drug disposition*, Baltimore, 1971, Williams & Wilkins.
6. Lam YWF: Stereoselectivity: an issue of significant importance in clinical pharmacology, *Pharmacotherapy* 8:147, 1988.
7. Wilkinson GR: Clearance approaches in pharmacology, *Pharmacol Rev* 39:1, 1987.
8. Williams RL: Drug administration in hepatic disease, *N Engl J Med* 309:1616, 1983.

Chapter 8

Pharmacogenetics: genetic differences in drug metabolism and response

VARIABILITY IN DRUG RESPONSE

A perplexing problem for both pharmacologists and physicians is the variation in response to a particular drug that occurs among normal subjects, as well as among patients. This interindividual variability necessitates a correspondingly wide range of doses among patients. Differences in clearance of a drug among individuals can range from fourfold to fortyfold, the extremely wide range occurring more typically with drugs metabolized in the liver. The clinical consequences of differences in dose requirement mandated by such variability cannot be overemphasized.

Variability of drug metabolism or response

When a fixed dose of drug is given to a large population of normal subjects and an index of metabolism of the drug or a specific quantitative response to the drug is measured and plotted, several types of curve can be generated. The most common shapes of this distribution curve are *unimodal* and *bimodal* (Fig. 8-1). For most drugs, when a population is tested, a unimodal, gaussian distribution curve of drug response is obtained. This curve can arise from purely environmental differences, such as a dose-related effect of smoking on the metabolism of a certain drug. In addition, genetic differences in which genes at multiple loci contribute to the variation may be responsible. This latter type of control is called *polygenic*. Polygenic control is at least partially involved in regulation of such traits as blood pressure, intelligence, and intensity of skin color.

Bimodal curves of drug metabolism or response are usually produced by monogenically controlled conditions, such as those listed in Table 8-1, but can also arise from environmental differences; for example, one mode representing metabolism of theophylline by normal persons and another mode representing subjects receiving an inhibitor of theophylline metabolism such as cimetidine.

When metabolism or response to a drug exhibits bimodal distribution, an additional step in exploring pharmacogenetics is to perform family studies on individuals located at the extremes of the distribution curve. Individuals at the extremes are most likely to exhibit a sufficiently distinctive metabolism or response to drugs to permit clear-cut identification of its transmission through several generations. By determining whether a particular type of drug metabolism or response conforms to a pattern of Mendelian laws for inheritance of dominant and recessive traits, investigators can tell whether a genetic mechanism controls the variation in drug metabolism or response observed in the population.[2,6,14,15] Moreover, the specific kind of genetic control

FIG. 8-1

Schematic illustration of unimodal versus bimodal distribution of drug metabolism or response. When a standard dose of a drug is given to a large number of persons and a drug effect or metabolism is measured, the usual finding is a normal frequency distribution as in ***A.*** *On the other hand, a discontinuous variation, as exemplified by the bimodal distribution shown in* ***B,*** *often indicates a genetically determined abnormality in drug action or metabolism.*

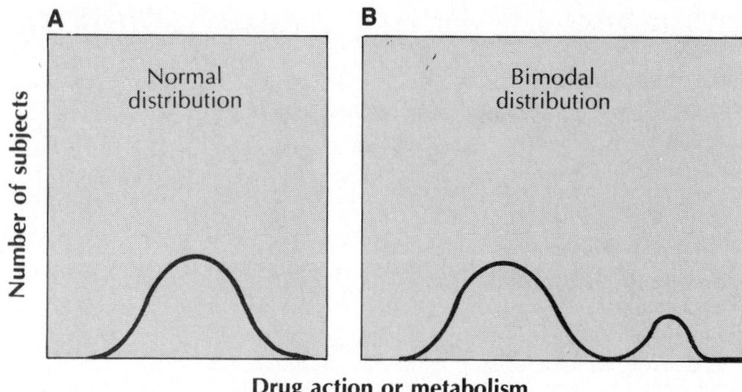

(autosomal dominant or recessive; X-linked dominant or recessive) can be discovered. Further studies utilizing techniques of molecular biology can determine the genetic defect at the level of the gene, messenger RNA, and the protein itself.[6]

PHARMACOGENETICS

Pharmacogenetics deals with genetically caused variations in drug response or metabolism. Some pharmacogenetic conditions in humans that affect either drug metabolism or the response to a drug are listed in Table 8-1.

In pharmacogenetics the ultimate goal is the ability to screen populations by a simple, rapid, safe test to ascertain how a particular trait is inherited, its incidence in a given group, and differences in frequency among various patient populations.

In pharmacogenetic studies the plasma half-life or clearance of a drug was traditionally used as the principal test of gene structure and function. For many polymorphisms of drug metabolism, current methods simply entail administration at bedtime of an innocuous test substance (for example, caffeine to assess acetylation or dextromethorphan to assess cytochrome P-450 II D6) and collection of an overnight urine sample. The ratio in the urine of parent drug to metabolite can discriminate slow from normal metabolizers; the former have predominately parent drug with little metabolite, whereas normal metabolizers have the converse.

PHARMACOGENETIC DIFFERENCES IN DRUG METABOLISM

An enzyme that controls metabolism of a drug has been identified in several pharmacogenetic conditions. Mutations decrease metabolic activity so that the parent drug accumulates, often causing toxicity. Thus one can identify the condition by documenting decreased clearance of the parent compound, decreased appearance of a metabolite, or a greatly increased concentration of parent drug relative to metabolite.[2] If persons possessing such genetic abnormalities can be identified *before* they receive a drug, one can avoid toxicity by giving a much reduced dose or by choosing another agent. For these reasons, familiarity with pharmacogenetic conditions can help physicians administer drugs more safely.

TABLE 8–1 Genetic conditions that alter drug metabolism or response

Defect	Typical substance(s)	Chromosome location	Incidence*
Altered drug metabolism			
Acatalasia	Hydrogen peroxide		1% O
Atypical cholinesterase	Succinylcholine		0.04%
Slow acetylation (Arylamine *N*-acetyltransferase deficiency)	Sulfamethazine, caffeine, procainamide, dapsone, hydralazine, isoniazid		50% W 10% O 33% H
Deficiency of cytochrome P-450 isoenzymes			
P-450 IA2	Phenacetin, theophylline	15	
P-450 IIC9	Mephenytoin, hexobarbital, diazepam, tolbutamide (?)	10	2%-5% W 20% O
P-450 IID6	Debrisoquin, sparteine, tricyclic antidepressants, encainide, flecainide, propafenone, metoprolol, propranolol, timolol, dextromethorphan, codeine	22	5%-10% W 0% O
P-450 IIIA4	Cyclosporine, erythromycin, ethinylestradiol, lidocaine, midazolam, nifedipine, quinidine	7	
Methyltransferase deficiency	Azathioprine		0.3%
Sulfotransferase deficiency	Acetaminophen, methyldopa		
Altered drug response			
Warfarin resistance	Warfarin		
Inability to taste phenylthiourea or phenylthiocarbamide	Drugs containing N—C—S functional group		
Glucose-6-phosphate dehydrogenase deficiency	Various analgesics, various sulfonamides, antimalarials		10% B†

**B*, Black; *H*, Hispanic; *O*, Oriental; *W*, White.
†In the United States.

Acatalasia

The condition acatalasia was discovered in a patient during application of hydrogen peroxide to the gums to sterilize a wound after surgery.[12] Instead of bubbles of oxygen forming by the action of the enzyme catalase as occurs in normal persons, the peroxide remained unchanged and caused toxicity by denaturing tissue proteins. The patient lacked catalase in her oral mucosa and erythrocytes, as did three of her five siblings. The parents were second cousins—consanguinity is a risk factor for autosomal recessive inheritance, the mode of transmission of acatalasia. The incidence of this condition reaches 1% in certain regions of Japan, and the deficiency also occurs in Switzerland. Only sporadic cases have been reported in the United States. An impressive lesson from the discovery of acatalasia is that an observant clinician, the Japanese oral surgeon Takahara, made an important contribution by being alert to the possibility that genetic differences can cause unusual reactions to drugs. Takahara postulated that his patient responded inappropriately to the peroxide because she lacked the normal form of the enzyme required to eliminate the drug. He proved his theory to be correct by gathering similar cases from 27 Japanese families.

Atypical plasma cholinesterase

Another example of a pharmacogenetic lesion that can produce toxicity is that of atypical plasma cholinesterase. Individuals homozygous for the mutant gene cannot adequately hydrolyze succinylcholine, a compound administered during anesthesia to produce muscle relaxation. Normally, succinylcholine is rapidly metabolized by plasma cholinesterase. However, in homozygous patients the drug remains active in the body for much longer periods than usual. Succinylcholine can then produce prolonged paralysis of respiratory musculature and, if mechanical respiration is not available, death. When succinylcholine was introduced in 1952 and administered widely in England as a preanesthetic agent, several deaths occurred in persons who had inherited from each parent a mutant gene at the cholinesterase locus. One in 25 persons is a heterozygote; homozygotes occur once among 2500 persons.

Arylamine N-acetyltransferase (NAT)

Acetylation of a number of drugs occurs via NAT. Isoniazid is used to treat tuberculosis. Persons with the genetically transmitted trait of fast acetylation of isoniazid may not be adequately treated on a fixed low dose because of rapid biotransformation. In contrast, slow acetylators receiving a normal dose may develop toxic effects. Isoniazid-induced polyneuritis—pain, tingling, and muscular weakness in the upper and lower extremities—occurs more frequently in slow than in rapid acetylators of isoniazid.[4] Fortunately, the neuritis can be effectively treated with vitamin B_6 (pyridoxine).

Approximately 50% of the population in the United States are slow acetylators, being homozygous for a recessive form of the gene for NAT.[7] Fast acetylators are either heterozygous or homozygous for the dominant allele. Like several other genetically controlled variations in humans, this hereditary variation in acetylation exhibits pronounced geographic differences in gene frequency. For example, slow inactivation is uncommon in Eskimos, 95% of whom are rapid acetylators, and only slightly more common in Japanese, 90% of whom are rapid acetylators. In Latin America, approximately 67% of the population are rapid acetylators.

Isoniazid is also an example of how toxicity can develop not only from drug accumulation but also from metabolites. Rapid acetylators of isoniazid are more liable than slow acetylators to develop hepatitis after chronic isoniazid administration; presumably a metabolite is the offending agent.

Fast and slow acetylation also occurs for several other drugs, including certain sulfonamides, the antihypertensive drug hydralazine, and the antiarrhythmic procainamide. Continued administration of high doses of hydralazine in slow, but not fast, acetylators can lead to severe toxicity in the form of a lupus erythematosus–like syndrome. Procainamide can cause the same syndrome, particularly in slow acetylators. That this condition is due to procainamide itself was proved by studies showing that the acetylated metabolite, *N*-acetylprocainamide, can be administered safely to patients who had previously developed procainamide-induced lupus.

Isoenzymes of cytochrome P-450

The antihypertensive drug debrisoquin is used in England but not in the United States. Patients receiving debrisoquin vary widely in their hypotensive responses to the adrenergic-blocking action of the drug, but there is a close correlation between debrisoquin plasma concentration and the resultant decline in blood pressure.[11] In 94 unrelated volunteers the urinary ratio of the parent drug to the primary metabolite, 4-hydroxydebrisoquin, was measured after a single oral dose of 10 mg of debrisoquin.[10] In three of these subjects the ratio was very high, suggestive of a deficiency of the hepatic cytochrome P-450–dependent monooxygenase that 4-hydroxylates debrisoquin. Furthermore, family studies of these three volunteers suggested transmission of the metabolic deficiency as an autosomal recessive trait.[10] Most side effects, as well as the most pronounced antihypertensive activity of debrisoquin, occurred in these slow metabolizers.

Virtually simultaneously with the report of a genetic basis for poor metabolism of debrisoquin, a report appeared from Germany of an exaggerated response to sparteine associated with diminished metabolism and autosomal recessive genetic transmission.[5] These observations stimulated an explosion of information concerning different isoenzymes of cytochrome P-450 and genetic defects thereof.[1-3] It is now known that many drugs depend on the isoenzyme that metabolizes debrisoquin and sparteine (Table 8-1).[3,6,16] In the 8% to 10% of Caucasian patients who are poor metabolizers of these drugs a variety of responses can occur, for example, exaggerated responses to debrisoquin and sparteine. In contrast, no change in effect occurs with flecainide because it is mainly eliminated by the kidney; metabolism is only a minor clearance pathway. On the other hand, codeine must be metabolized to morphine to cause its effects, and poor metabolizers have a diminished response to this opiate.

The genetic defect in poor metabolizers of debrisoquin and sparteine is a mutation(s) that results in a splicing defect in the messenger RNA for the enzyme; none of the cytochrome P-450 isoenzyme is synthesized.[2,6] Heterozygotes have a normal metabolic capacity, and only homozygotes express the poor metabolizer phenotype. Because the incidence of poor metabolism is relatively high in the white population, and because the implications of this phenotype are considerable in terms of numbers of drugs, an argument could be made for prospective screening of white patients who are to receive drugs metabolized by this isoenzyme.[3] At present such screening is possible only in specialized laboratories.

Work in this area has also identified isoenzymes of cytochrome P-450 that are specific for metabolism of other drugs (Table 8-1).[2,6,8,13,17] It is highly likely that additional isoenzymes will be characterized in the future, particularly because it is estimated that there may be up to 200 different isoenzymes of cytochrome P-450.[2,6] Clinicians must stay alert to developments in this area.

Methyltransferase deficiency

Deficiency of methyltransferase has been identified in only about 1 of 300 patients.[9,14] However, this defect is of particular importance because of its potentially devastating consequences. Patients with autoimmune disorders and those receiving organ transplants are commonly treated with azathioprine, a drug metabolized by methyltransferase. In patients deficient in this enzyme, small doses of azathioprine can cause profound bone marrow depression.[9]

PHARMACOGENETIC CONDITIONS THAT AFFECT DRUG ACTIONS

WARFARIN RESISTANCE

Resistance to warfarin in humans is one of several mutations that modify the response to a drug by altering the receptor (Table 8-1). In subjects with the mutant gene, anticoagulation occurs only after many times the normal dose of warfarin.

Warfarin inhibits production of several blood components necessary for clotting, probably by competing with vitamin K for a receptor. In cases of warfarin resistance the mutant receptor may be envisioned as a structurally altered molecule that fails to bind warfarin as strongly as the normal one and therefore does not readily produce anticoagulation; this alteration also results in a stronger than normal binding of vitamin K.

Differences in the capacity to taste phenylthiocarbamide

Most persons are able to taste dilute solutions of phenylthiocarbamide (PTC, phenylthiourea) and chemically related compounds containing the thiocyanate group, whereas a few individuals cannot. Because metabolism of some thiocyanate compounds appears to be no different in tasters and nontasters, this difference in ability to taste PTC suggests that a receptor mutation may exist in nontasters. Interestingly, this difference in taste threshold may influence food preferences and thus consumption of potential goitrogenic compounds. Enlargement of the thyroid gland, called *goiter*, can be produced in rats by PTC. Several vegetables, including turnips, brussels sprouts, and kale, contain a goiter-producing chemical, and nodular goiters are more common among nontasters than among tasters of PTC.

Control of glucose-6-phosphate dehydrogenase (G-6-PD) deficiency

A more complicated condition is G-6-PD deficiency, which affects about 100 million people in the world, primarily in areas where malaria is endemic. In the United States one in 10 black males is affected. Individuals with any one of 80 different mutations that occur at a specific site on the X chromosome develop hemolytic anemia after exposure to a large number of drugs, including analgesics, sulfonamides, and antimalarials. Some dietary constituents, such as fava beans (of the plant *Vicia fava*), can also cause hemolysis in susceptible subjects.

The mechanism believed responsible for hemolysis is complex but probably initially involves a shortage of NADPH. NADPH is produced by G-6-PD. NADPH itself then serves as a cofactor for glutathione reductase. Thus G-6-PD deficiency ultimately leads to a deficiency of reduced glutathione. In normal persons, the red cell membrane is maintained in a functional state by a supply of reduced glutathione adequate to keep membrane proteins in a reduced and operative condition. Highly reactive drug metabolites oxidize membrane proteins; if these oxidized metabolites are not rapidly reduced by glutathione, hemolysis ensues. Thus a genetically induced enzyme deficiency results in decreased usable glutathione, thereby allowing reactive drug metabolites to produce hemolysis.

REFERENCES

1. Balant LP, Gundert-Remy U, Boobis AR, von Bahr Ch: Relevance of genetic polymorphism in drug metabolism in the development of new drugs, *Eur J Clin Pharmacol* 36:551, 1989.
2. Brøsen K: Recent developments in hepatic drug oxidation: implications for clinical pharmacokinetics, *Clin Pharmacokinet* 18:220, 1990.
3. Brøsen K, Gram LF: Clinical significance

of the sparteine/debrisoquine oxidation polymorphism, *Eur J Clin Pharmacol* 36:537, 1989.

4. Drayer DE, Reidenberg MM: Clinical consequences of polymorphic acetylation of basic drugs, *Clin Pharmacol Ther* 22:251, 1977.
5. Eichelbaum M, Spannbrucker N, Steincke B, Dengler HJ: Defective N-oxidation of sparteine in man: a new pharmacogenetic defect, *Eur J Clin Pharmacol* 16:183, 1979.
6. Gonzalez FJ: The molecular biology of cytochrome P450s, *Pharmacol Rev* 40:243, 1989.
7. Grant DM, Mörike K, Eichelbaum M, Meyer UA: Acetylation pharmacogenetics: the slow acetylator phenotype is caused by decreased or absent arylamine *N*-acetyltransferase in human liver, *J Clin Invest* 85:968, 1990.
8. Jacqz E, Hall SD, Branch RA, Wilkinson GR: Polymorphic metabolism of mephenytoin in man: pharmacokinetic interaction with a co-regulated substrate, mephobarbital, *Clin Pharmacol Ther* 39:646, 1986.
9. Lennard L, Van Loon JA, Weinshilboum RM: Pharmacogenetics of acute azathioprine toxicity: relationship to thiopurine methyltransferase genetic polymorphism, *Clin Pharmacol Ther* 46:149, 1989.
10. Mahgoub A, Idle JR, Dring LG, et al: Polymorphic hydroxylation of debrisoquine in man, *Lancet* 2:584, 1977.
11. Silas JH, Lennard MS, Tucker GT, et al: Why hypertensive patients vary in their response to oral debrisoquine, *Br Med J* 1:422, 1977.
12. Takahara S, Sato H, Doi M, Mihara S: Acatalasemia. III. On the heredity of acatalasemia, *Proc Jpn Acad* 28:585, 1952.
13. Veronese ME, Miners JO, Randles D, et al: Validation of the tolbutamide metabolic ratio for population screening with use of sulfaphenazole to produce model phenotypic poor metabolizers, *Clin Pharmacol Ther* 47:403, 1990.
14. Weinshilboum R: Methyltransferase pharmacogenetics, *Pharmacol Ther* 43:77, 1989.
15. Weinshilboum R: Sulfotransferase pharmacogenetics, *Pharmacol Ther* 45: 93-107, 1990.
16. Woosley RL, Roden DM, Dai G, et al: Co-inheritance of the polymorphic metabolism of encainide and debrisoquin, *Clin Pharmacol Ther* 39:282, 1986.
17. Yasumori T, Murayama N, Yamazoe Y, Kato R: Polymorphism in hydroxylation of mephenytoin and hexobarbital stereoisomers in relation to hepatic P-450 human-2, *Clin Pharmacol Ther* 47:313, 1990.

Chapter 9

Effects of age on drug disposition

BARRIERS TO INVESTIGATION

For many years physicians have recognized that infants, particularly neonates, and elderly patients receiving drugs with low therapeutic indices frequently need lower doses to avoid toxicity. Only recently have some mechanisms responsible for changed dosage requirements of such patients been firmly established. For almost every drug investigated, rates of absorption, distribution, metabolism, or excretion differ in very young or in elderly subjects compared with young adults.[6,8,10,13,17-19] Unfortunately, many earlier studies assessed kinetics only by measuring half-life. Hence the changes noted could not be ascribed clearly to changes either in volume of distribution or in clearance. For example, early studies of some benzodiazepines showed an increase in half-life with aging, assumed to represent a decrease in metabolic capacity, that is, clearance.[12,16] Subsequent studies have shown that this half-life change represents primarily an increase in volume of distribution with some benzodiazepines, such as diazepam and chlordiazepoxide, and a decrease in clearance with others. Physicians should be aware of the limitations of much of the data in this area.

Patients at the extremes of age present special problems to the clinician. To identify how drugs are handled in "normal" neonates or geriatric persons, such subjects must be carefully examined to exclude concomitant pathologic conditions.

In young subjects, disposition of drugs changes as their livers and kidneys mature and grow and increase their eliminating capabilities. Similarly, body composition is altered during this period of rapid growth and development. Changes in drug disposition in geriatric subjects are largely the consequence of degenerative alterations in structure and function of the heart, liver, and kidney (Table 9-1). Cardiac output declines approximately 1% per year from age 19 onward, and with age a decreased proportion of this output is distributed to the liver and kidneys. The liver's metabolic capacity and the kidney's excretory capacity both decrease with age. Moreover, the concentration of circulating albumin (to which many drugs bind) declines with age,[3,9,11,24] the proportion of body fat to muscle increases, and total body water decreases, all of which can influence the distribution of drugs (Table 9-1). Age-related changes in the structure and function of critical organs undoubtedly occur at different rates in different subjects. Accordingly, patients of the same chronologic age exhibit varied degrees of cardiovascular, hepatic, or renal function. This variability is even more pronounced when disease-induced changes in organ function are superimposed on those due to age.

TABLE 9–1 Physiologic changes in elderly patients that may influence drug disposition

Physiologic change	Potential effect on drug disposition
Changes in gastrointestinal function	
↑ Gastric pH; ↑ prevalence of achlorhydria	↓ Absorption of acid-soluble drugs (example: ketoconazole)
Delayed gastric emptying	Delay in absorption and/or ↓ rate of absorption
↓ Absorptive surface	?
↓ Splanchnic blood flow	?
Changes in body composition	
↓ Lean body mass; ↑ adipose mass	↑ V_d of lipid-soluble drugs (example: diazepam)
↓ Total body water	↓ V_d of water-soluble drugs (example: ethanol)
Changes in plasma protein binding	
↓ Plasma albumin concentration	↑ V_d and clearance of total drug; no change in unbound drug
Changes in hepatic function	
↓ Liver size	?
↓ Hepatic blood flow	↓ Clearance and first-pass metabolism of highly extracted (flow-dependent) drugs (example: propranolol)
↓ Hepatic metabolism	↓ Clearance of capacity-limited drugs
Changes in renal function	
↓ Glomerular filtration rate and blood flow	↓ Clearance of drugs and metabolites excreted by the kidney

V_d, Volume of distribution.

DRUG DOSING IN CHILDREN

In experimental investigations, drugs are administered on the basis of a certain number of milligrams per kilogram of body weight, since the disposition of a drug often is roughly a function of body mass. For the same reason the weight of the patient should be considered when a dose is calculated. Certain formulas allow adjustment of dose according to weight. For example, Clark's rule is as follows:

$$\text{Dose for child} = \text{Adult dose} \times \frac{\text{Weight of child in pounds}}{150}$$

The assumption is that children need a smaller dose because their weight is less, but this is only an approximation. It has been pointed out that a child is not simply a "small adult" and that a child's reaction to drugs can be influenced by factors of growth and development, not just size.[20] The dose of a drug for children is more appropriately proportional to weight to the 0.7 power.[5] Since body surface is similarly related to body weight, it has been suggested that pediatric doses should be calculated on the basis of surface area in square meters (m^2). Tables are available that relate the weight of a child in pounds to surface area and to the approximate percentage of adult dose. The calculations are based on a surface area in adults of 1.73 m^2. Thus a 22-pound child having a surface area of 0.46 m^2 should receive 27% of the adult dose. A child weighing 121 pounds with a surface area of 1.58 m^2 would receive 91% of the adult dose.

DRUG ABSORPTION

For most compounds there are no data on the effects of age on gastrointestinal absorption. However, certain documented changes in gastrointestinal function that occur with age should, from a purely theoretic point of view, alter drug absorption. For example, gastric emptying time is reduced in elderly patients, probably as a result of increased stomach pH (see below). Shortened retention of drugs in the stomach would accelerate their delivery to absorptive sites in the small intestine and hasten overall absorption.

Another critical factor that affects drug absorption is intestinal blood perfusion, which decreases by 40% to 50% in elderly patients as compared with rates in young adults. This reduction could slow absorption by decreasing transfer of compounds across the serosal membrane. For example, passive absorption of xylose in the gut declines by 40% from ages 18 to 40 years to ages 70 to 80 years.[8] Despite these theoretic considerations suggestive of reduced rates of gastrointestinal drug absorption with age, no effect has been observed on either the rate or amount of gastrointestinal absorption of a variety of agents.

About 20% of elderly patients have a diminished ability to acidify their gastric contents and are either hypo- or achlorhydric.[2,7,14] Because absorption from some pharmaceutic formulations requires acid-induced dissolution in the stomach, patients with acidification defects will exhibit malabsorption of such drugs; an example is ketoconazole, an antifungal agent.

DRUG DISTRIBUTION

The aging process entails changes in body composition that can influence the distribution of drugs (Table 9-1). Lean body mass diminishes while that of adipose tissue increases with age. As age exceeds 65 years the portion of body weight that is fat increases from 18% to 36% in elderly men and from 33% to 45% in women.[15] In addition, total body water decreases 10% to 15% between ages 20 and 80.[13] These changes can affect the distribution of drugs among tissues. Thus drugs, such as ethanol, that are restricted to total body water have a smaller volume in which to distribute; relative to dose, they attain a higher blood concentration in elderly patients.[23] Conversely, highly lipid-soluble drugs, such as diazepam, have relatively more adipose tissue in which to distribute and hence exhibit larger volumes of distribution in elderly patients.[12,16]

The albumin concentration in plasma declines with age (Fig. 9-1).[9] Whether this decrease is a consequence of reduced albumin synthesis, increased catabolism, or a combination of both is uncertain. Reduced albumin concentration per se should exert no pharmacokinetic or pharmacodynamic effect on drugs not highly bound to this protein. In contrast, one would predict that the unbound (free) fraction of a highly bound drug would increase, thereby increasing its distribution into tissues and its volume of distribution. Furthermore, the greater fraction of free drug at metabolic and excretory sites may favor elimination. In this scenario the elderly should eliminate highly bound drugs more quickly. However, the opposite may occur if the activity of

FIG. 9-1 *Change in mean (±SE) serum albumin concentrations according to age in 11,090 hospitalized medical patients.*

From Greenblatt DJ: Am Geriatr Soc 27:20, 1979.

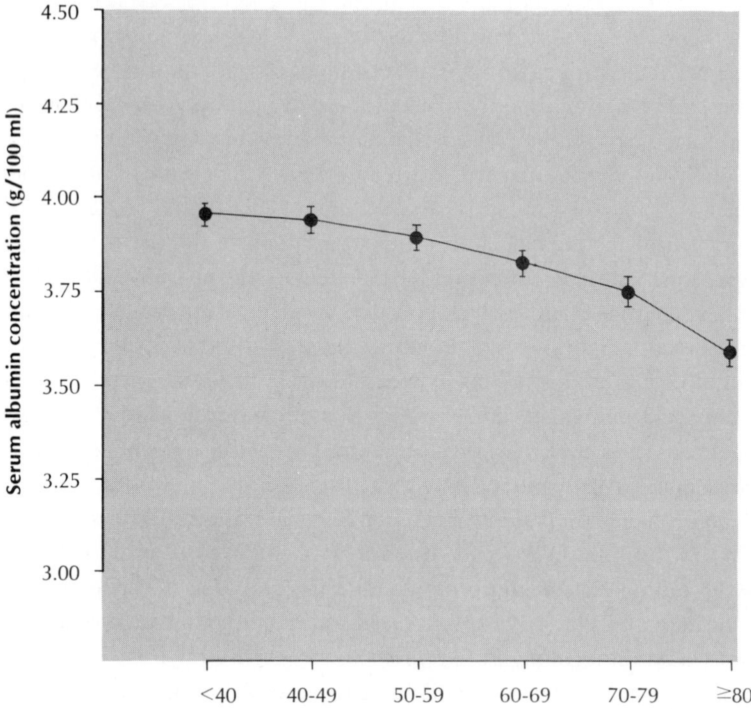

the eliminating organs is sufficiently impaired with age (see below); in this case, an increase in unbound, active drug will cause an exaggerated response.[21] A lower dose would then be needed to avoid toxicity. When the percent binding of specific drugs to albumin was compared in geriatric subjects and normal, middle-aged adults, a wide range of results was obtained. The implication of these data is that it is difficult to predict whether an individual elderly patient will manifest a change in drug binding. The physician should be alert to this possibility and monitor all elderly patients accordingly.

A number of basic drugs, for example propranolol, are highly bound to α_1-acid glycoprotein, an acute phase reactant. Although the concentration of this protein may be altered in disease states, age per se does not affect its concentration.[22] Consequently, there is little need for concern, based on patient age, about protein binding of basic drugs.

DRUG METABOLISM

A number of changes in hepatic physiology occur with aging (Table 9-1). Hepatic conjugating and metabolizing capacity increases throughout infancy. In elderly patients absolute liver size and its weight as a proportion of body weight decrease with age. Whereas in younger patients liver weight is about 2.5% of total body weight, in elderly patients this value declines to about 1.6%.[13,17] Because liver size per se is probably not a limiting factor in drug metabolism, it is doubtful that this change is an important determinant of altered drug metabolism in elderly patients.

On the other hand, aging-related reductions in hepatic blood flow and in the intrinsic capacity of the liver to metabolize drugs are major factors. At age 65 hepatic blood flow is reduced 40% to 45% compared with that in younger patients.[10,13,17] Such decrements can theoretically diminish the elimination of drugs that have a high extraction rate, the so-called flow-limited agents, elimination of which is dependent on hepatic blood flow. Verification of this postulate has occurred through studies of propranolol and lidocaine. Thus clinicians should realize that dosage of any such drug may need modification in elderly patients.

Flow-limited drugs are also subject to enhanced bioavailability if taken by mouth because first-pass elimination is diminished. Thus for drugs such as labetalol, metoprolol, and propranolol two changes in disposition occur with decreased hepatic blood flow, and their effects are additive. The net result is that dosage reduction must correct for both decreased clearance and increased bioavailability. If a drug is administered intravenously dosage adjustment need correct only for diminished clearance; if given by mouth changes in both clearance and bioavailability mandate an even greater dosage reduction.

Elderly patients also seem to have a diminished ability to metabolize drugs over and above any change in hepatic blood flow.[1,6,10,13,17,19] This effect is usually restricted to so-called phase I reactions, that is, hydroxylation, N-dealkylation, sulfoxidation, reduction, and hydrolysis. In contrast, conjugation or phase II reactions are unimpaired. These pathways include glucuronidation, acetylation, and sulfation. As a consequence, a priori prediction of whether a capacity-limited drug may be cleared slowly in an elderly patient requires knowledge of its metabolic pathways. In general, clinicians should anticipate decreased clearance in elderly patients and should consider administration of lower doses.

DRUG EXCRETION

Many drugs and their metabolites are eliminated from the body by renal excretion. If the extent to which renal mechanisms contribute to elimination of a particular drug is 40% or more, it is likely that doses will need to be reduced in elderly patients and in premature infants. Examples include digoxin and aminoglycoside antibiotics. Estimates of the degree of renal impairment are derived from creatinine clearance. Importantly, in elderly patients serum creatinine concentrations yield a poor estimate of renal function unless adjusted for age as in the following, commonly used, algorithm[4]:

$$\text{Creatinine clearance corrected to a 72 kg body weight} = \frac{140 - \text{age}}{\text{Serum creatinine (in mg/dl)}} \quad \text{(Women} = 85\% \text{ of this value)}$$

From an estimate of creatinine clearance, various nomograms permit selection of appropriately lower doses of drugs in patients with renal insufficiency, including the elderly.

TABLE 9–2 Drug-dosing changes for elderly patients

Drug	Dosing adjustment
Analgesics	
Meperidine	Avoid: active metabolite (normeperidine) accumulates, toxic to central nervous system
Morphine	Active metabolite (morphine 6-glucuronide) may accumulate if renal function impaired
Nalbuphine	F quadruples, ¼ usual dose
Propoxyphene	Cl ↓, ½ usual dose
Antianxiety agents, sedatives, and hypnotics	
Bromazepam	Cl and V_d ↓, ½ usual dose
Brotizolam	Cl ↓, ½ usual dose
Quazepam	Avoid: active metabolite accumulates
Hydroxyzine	Cl ↓, ½ usual dose
Antibiotics	
Amantadine	Cl ↓, ½ usual dose
Aminoglycosides	Cl ↓, ½ usual dose
Roxithromycin	Cl ↓, ½ usual dose
Anticholinergic and cholinergic drug	
Cisapride	Elimination ↓, quantitative guidelines not available, use cautiously or avoid
Anticonvulsants	
Primidone	½ Usual dose to adjust for accumulation of active metabolite
Valproic acid	Cl ↓, ⅓ usual dose
Vigabatrin	Cl of active S-enantiomer ↓, ⅓ usual dose
Antidepressant	
Trazodone	Cl ↓, ½ to ⅔ usual dose
Antihistamine	
Famotidine	Cl ↓, ½ usual dose
Anti-inflammatory agents (nonsteroidal)	
Diflunisal	Cl ↓, ½ usual dose
Ketorolac	Cl ↓, ½ usual dose
Naproxen	Cl ↓, ½ usual dose
Bronchodilator	
Theophylline	Cl ↓, ½ to ¾ usual dose
Cardiovascular agents	
Antianginal agents	
Amlodipine	Cl ↓, ½ usual dose
Felodipine	Cl ↓, ½ usual dose
Isrodipine	Cl ↓, ⅓ to ½ usual dose
Verapamil	Cl ↓, ¾ usual dose
Antiarrhythymic agents	
Cifenline	Cl and V_d ↓, ½ usual dose
Quinidine	Cl ↓, ½ usual dose

Cl, Clearance; *F*, fractional absorption or oral bioavailability; V_d, volume of distribution.

TABLE 9–2 Drug dosing changes for elderly patients—cont'd

Drug	Dosing adjustment
Antihypertensives	
α_1-Adrenergic antagonists	
Doxazosin	Cl ↓, ½ usual dose
Indoramin	Cl ↓, ½ usual dose
Terazosin	Cl ↓, ½ usual dose
Urapidil	Cl ↓, ½ usual dose
β-Adrenergic antagonists	
Acebutolol	½ Usual dose to account for accumulation of active metabolite
Betaxolol	Cl ↓, ½ usual dose
Labetalol	Cl ↓, F ↑, ½ usual dose
α_2-Adrenergic agonist	
Rilmenidine	Cl ↓, ½ usual dose
Converting enzyme inhibitors	
Cilazapril	Cl ↓, ½ usual dose
Perindopril	Cl ↓, F ↑, ½ usual dose
Vasodilator	
Nitroprusside	Toxic metabolite (thiocyanate) may accumulate
Hypoglycemic agent	
Acetohexamide	Avoid: active metabolite (hydroxyhexamide) accumulates
Hypouricemic agent	
Allopurinol	⅓ to ½ Usual dose to account for accumulation of active metabolite (oxipurinol)
Miscellaneous agents	
Buflomedil	Cl ↓, ⅔ usual dose
Levodopa	Cl ↓, ½ usual dose
Terodiline	Cl ↓, ⅓ usual dose

CONCLUSIONS

Effects of age on drug absorption, distribution, metabolism, elimination, and various combinations of these have been the subject of recent reviews.[1,6,10,13,17-19] The magnitude of such age-related changes depends on both the pharmacologic profile of the particular drug and clinical characteristics of each patient. Because so many diverse factors that can influence drug disposition change concomitantly in such subjects, it is often difficult to determine specific mechanisms responsible for the pharmacokinetic characteristics of a given drug in a particular patient. For these reasons and because our present knowledge is limited, physicians need to exercise special care to avoid toxicity when drugs are administered singly or in combination to very young or old patients. In general the best approach is to start with lower doses and to increase dosage slowly and in small increments.

Table 9-2 offers changes in dosing recommendations for elderly patients. In addition, for any drug in Appendix B for which reduced renal function mandates a change in dose, the decrement in renal function with age must be taken into account. These suggestions derive from published data. Many drugs are absent from Table 9-2 only because they have not been studied. Thus cautious use of any drug is urged.

REFERENCES

1. Beers MH, Ouslander JG: Risk factors in geriatric drug prescribing: a practical guide to avoiding problems, *Drugs* 37:105, 1989.
2. Bender AD: Effect of age on intestinal absorption: implications for drug absorption in the elderly, *J Am Geriatr Soc* 16:1331, 1968.
3. Bender AD, Post A, Meier JP, et al: Plasma protein binding of drugs as a function of age in adult human subjects, *J Pharm Sci* 64:1711, 1975.
4. Cockcroft DW, Gault MH: Prediction of creatinine clearance from serum creatinine, *Nephron* 16:31, 1976.
5. Done AK: Drugs for children. In Modell W, editor: *Drugs of choice 1972-1973,* St Louis, 1972, Mosby–Year Book.
6. Everitt DE, Avorn J: Drug prescribing for the elderly, *Arch Intern Med* 146:2393, 1986.
7. Geokas MC, Haverback BJ: The aging gastrointestinal tract, *Am J Surg* 117:881, 1969.
8. Gorrod JW: Absorption, metabolism and excretion of drugs in geriatric subjects, *Gerontol Clin* 16:30, 1974.
9. Greenblatt DJ: Reduced serum albumin concentration in the elderly: a report from the Boston Collaborative Drug Surveillance Program, *J Am Geriatr Soc* 27:20, 1979.
10. Greenblatt DJ, Sellers EM, Shader RI: Drug disposition in old age, *N Engl J Med* 306:1081, 1982.
11. Hayes MJ, Langman MJS, Short AH: Changes in drug metabolism with increasing age. I. Warfarin binding and plasma protein, *Br J Clin Pharmacol* 2:69, 1975.
12. Macklon AF, Barton M, James O, Rawlins MD: The effect of age on the pharmacokinetics of diazepam, *Clin Sci* 59: 479, 1980.
13. Montamat SC, Cusack BJ, Vestal RE: Management of drug therapy in the elderly, *N Engl J Med* 321:303, 1989.
14. Montgomery RD, Haeney MR, Ross IN, et al: The aging gut: a study of intestinal absorption in relation to nutrition in the elderly, *Q J Med* 47:197, 1978.
15. Novak LP: Aging, total body potassium, fat-free mass, and cell mass in males and females between ages 18 and 85 years, *J Gerontol* 27:438, 1972.
16. Ochs HR, Greenblatt DJ, Divoll M, et al: Diazepam kinetics in relation to age and sex, *Pharmacology* 23:24, 1981.
17. Ouslander JG: Drug therapy in the elderly, *Ann Intern Med* 95:711, 1981.
18. Richey DP, Bender AD: Pharmacokinetic consequences of aging, *Annu Rev Pharmacol Toxicol* 17:49, 1977.
19. Schmucker DL: Age-related changes in drug disposition, *Pharmacol Rev* 30:445, 1979.
20. Shirkey HC, Ericson AJ: Adverse reactions to drugs—their relation to growth and development. In Shirkey HC, editor: *Pediatric therapy,* ed 6, St Louis, 1980, Mosby–Year Book.
21. Upton RA, Williams RL, Kelly J, Jones RM: Naproxen pharmacokinetics in the elderly, *Br J Clin Pharmacol* 18:207, 1984.
22. Veering BT, Burm AGL, Souverijn JHM, et al: The effect of age on serum concentrations of albumin and α_1-acid glycoprotein, *Br J Clin Pharmacol* 29:201, 1990.
23. Vestal RE, McGuire EA, Tobin JD, et al: Aging and ethanol metabolism, *Clin Pharmacol Ther* 21:343, 1977.
24. Wallace S, Whiting B, Runcie J: Factors affecting drug binding in plasma of elderly patients, *Br J Clin Pharmacol* 3:327, 1976.

Chapter 10

Effects of occupation and disease on drug disposition

FACTORS THAT ALTER RESPONSE OF DRUG-METABOLIZING ENZYMES

As discussed in Chapter 8, genetic factors contribute appreciably to interindividual variations in drug pharmacokinetics. In addition, we are chronically exposed to numerous environmental compounds and conditions that can induce or inhibit the activity of hepatic mixed-function oxidases. There is a dynamic interaction between the genes that control these oxidases and environmental factors. Chemicals such as DDT, polychlorinated biphenyls, and polycyclic hydrocarbons can induce hepatic drug-metabolizing enzyme activity. As shown later in this chapter, disease states can also greatly change a subject's ability to eliminate drugs. Overall, then, a host of factors can influence drug handling in an individual patient.

OCCUPATIONAL CHEMICALS THAT ALTER DRUG-METABOLIZING CAPACITY

The field of occupational medicine has expanded greatly with the recognition that various human diseases develop from chronic exposure to certain chemicals. This association was first documented in the eighteenth century by Percival Potts. He reported that English chimney sweeps were at high risk of developing cancer of the scrotum. Today we know that exposure at work to asbestos, benzene, phenol, vinyl chloride, radium, and x rays also increases the risk of developing certain forms of cancer. Thus there are numerous examples of occupationally induced diseases. An additional new aspect of occupational medicine is the influence of chemicals encountered at work on a subject's capacity to metabolize drugs. Overall, the physician must be aware of myriad possible influences on drug handling and response in an individual patient.

EFFECTS OF DISEASE ON DRUG DISPOSITION

A single disease may cause multiple changes in the separate processes of drug absorption, distribution, metabolism, excretion, and effect. When each of the individual effects is measured and all effects are summated, the net change in "drug response" may be substantial or, alternatively, it can be negligible as a result of the balancing of one action by another in an opposite direction.

Alterations in drug half-life are often reported, but it is important to reemphasize that such data do not provide sufficient information for adjustment of dosage. Either a change in volume of distribution (important for loading dose) or a change in clearance (important for maintenance dose), or both can alter a drug's half-life. Furthermore, if large parallel changes occur in both clearance and volume of distribution of a drug, there may be no effect on half-life, yet dosing will need to be altered.

An important point is that a disease may affect the disposition of different drugs in different ways. Each drug has a distinct pharmacologic profile, and the way a disease alters the disposition of a particular drug depends on the drug's specific characteristics. In hypoalbuminemia the disposition of drugs that are extensively bound to albumin, such as warfarin and naproxen, will be changed, whereas the disposition of isoniazid and gentamicin, which bind negligibly to albumin, will not be altered. As another example, hepatocellular disease affects the disposition of propranolol but does not affect some other pharmacologically similar drugs like nadolol.

The clinical consequences of an alteration in drug disposition produced by disease will also be determined by the drug's margin of safety. For example, a change of 200% in the clearance of penicillin will probably have little or no clinical consequence, whereas a change of 20% in the clearance of digoxin, procainamide, or lidocaine may prove critical. By the same token, a decrease in albumin binding of warfarin from 99% to 98% may, at first, seem trivial. However, it may have a profound toxicologic consequence because the pharmacologically active free concentration has doubled (from 1% to 2%). In contrast, a decrease of 1% in albumin binding of methotrexate, from the normal of about 50%, has negligible clinical consequences even though the drug has a narrow therapeutic margin.

To illustrate how diseases can influence handling of and response to drugs, it is useful to consider the effects of several prototypic disease states on each of the pharmacokinetic processes. The extent to which a disease affects these processes will depend on the particular drug, and one should not presume that drugs in the same class are affected to the same degree by a certain disease. Among the drugs listed in Appendix B are many whose elimination is altered by diseases of the liver or kidney.

Drug absorption

Effects of disease states on absorption depend on many factors, including the site of drug administration. Until recently little was known about how disease alters oral absorption of drugs.[5] Large variability in rates of absorption of many orally administered drugs, in both patients and normal volunteers, make it difficult to identify specific disease- or drug-induced changes. Because most drugs are absorbed in the proximal small intestine, they must pass through the stomach before absorption can occur. Gastric emptying, in turn, is subject to effects of numerous physiologic and pathologic conditions plus pharmacologic effects of other drugs. For example, impaired absorption of acetaminophen occurs in patients with delayed gastric emptying and pyloric stenosis.[8] In patients with slow gastric emptying, levodopa may be ineffective.[2]

Changes in gastric pH can also affect absorption. Achlorhydria decreases the solubility of ketoconazole and impairs its absorption. In contrast, aspirin is absorbed significantly faster and peak plasma salicylate concentration is higher in patients with achlorhydria than in control subjects.[9]

In jejunal disease folic acid absorption is diminished.[4] In ileal disease the transport of bile acids may be impaired. This can reduce enterohepatic transport of many lipid-soluble drugs because bile acids promote absorption of fat and certain fat-soluble compounds, including many drugs and vitamins A, D, K, and E. By similar mechanisms, in steatorrhea fat-soluble drugs and vitamins may be lost in the feces. Ileal disease may also impair vitamin B_{12} absorption, since this vitamin is absorbed from the ileum after it forms a complex with intrinsic factor produced by the gastric parietal cell. Surgical removal or defective function of the ileum attributable to processes such as inflammatory bowel disease and tropical sprue can cause vitamin B_{12} malabsorption and pernicious anemia. Vitamin B_{12} absorption can also be impaired when intrinsic factor is deficient, as in patients with disease-induced parietal cell dysfunction or with precipitating or blocking antibodies to intrinsic factor.

Some inactive drugs are converted to an active form by gut bacteria, the best example being cleavage of sulfasalazine, a drug used to treat chronic ulcerative colitis. Diseases or drugs that change the nature of the intestinal flora can affect the disposition of drugs metabolized by gut bacteria. Approximately 10% of patients have an intestinal flora that inactivates digoxin, thereby decreasing its bioavailability. Eradication of these bacteria with broad-spectrum antibiotics can decrease digoxin inactivation, increase absorption (bioavailability), and result in a higher plasma concentration.[7] In contrast, absorption of digoxin in some patients is reduced by the antibiotic neomycin; the mechanism is not understood, but it is postulated that disruption of the intestinal mucosa by the antibiotic somehow impairs digoxin absorption.[6]

Drug distribution

Binding of many drugs to albumin can be altered, particularly in diseases of the liver and kidney associated with a decreased concentration of plasma albumin. In cirrhosis and nephrosis the unbound fraction of many drugs is elevated, compared with conditions of normal protein and albumin concentrations.

In uremia accumulation of endogenous compounds that compete for albumin-binding sites can reduce drug binding. For example, phenytoin binding is decreased,[10] and the percent unbound correlates with blood urea nitrogen and serum creatinine concentrations. Binding of other organic acids, including clofibrate, sulfonamides, thyroxin, and tryptophan, is also impaired. In addition to disease-associated *quantitative* changes in binding to albumin, *qualitative* changes occur; the avidity of phenytoin binding to albumin is reduced in uremia.[11]

Many basic drugs bind to α_1-acid glycoprotein, an acute-phase reactant. The concentration of this protein decreases in patients with cirrhosis but can increase substantially in acute clinical syndromes such as myocardial infarction. Lidocaine, for example, is bound to this protein; binding increases and the free fraction decreases in patients with acute myocardial infarction.[12]

These situations illustrate the danger of selecting a dose solely on the basis of total drug concentration in plasma rather than on the free concentration; only the latter reflects pharmacologic activity. Because it is usually not clinically practical to determine free drug concentrations, clinicians must assiduously assess clinical endpoints of pharmacologic response in their patients.

Hepatic drug metabolism

There are drugs that are avidly removed by the liver (flow-limited, high hepatic extraction ratio) and those with slower rates of removal (capacity-limited, low extraction ratio), even though both types are eliminated by hepatic metabolism.[16-18] An extraction ratio greater than 0.8, for agents such as propranolol and lidocaine, indicates that the liver removes nearly all of the drug that reaches it. Therefore alterations in blood flow accompanying liver disease can greatly change hepatic clearance of such compounds. For these drugs, liver disease can also diminish first-pass metabolism and enhance bioavailability. In contrast, for drugs with a low hepatic extraction ratio (less than 0.2), such as antipyrine and aminopyrine, the metabolic capacity of the liver is the determinant of removal; blood flow has little influence. For these drugs, disease-induced hepatocyte dysfunction primarily affects metabolic capacity.

The most common form of liver disease in the United States, alcoholic cirrhosis, is characterized by remissions and exacerbations and by variable progression over time. During the early stage of the disease, metabolism of many drugs may actually be faster than that in normal subjects because multiple doses of ethanol induce the cytochrome P-450–dependent monooxygenases.[15] However, with time the disease converts functional hepatocytes into fibrous bands incapable of metabolizing drugs. Since it is difficult to predict precisely how a particular patient with cirrhosis will eliminate a drug that is dependent on hepatic metabolism, the best course is to give these patients lower than normal doses initially and to observe them closely to make certain that toxicity does not occur.

Fig. 10-1 illustrates how well aminopyrine, a relatively safe test drug, is metabolized by patients with different forms of liver disease, compared with patients with normal cardiovascular, hepatic, and renal function. Hepatic metabolizing capacity is not impaired in patients with fatty liver and cholestasis; it is reduced, however, in patients with hepatocellular diseases, such as cirrhosis, infectious hepatitis, and certain metastatic cancers or hepatomas.

In contrast to aminopyrine metabolism, warfarin disposition during acute viral hepatitis is unchanged[19]; oxazepam metabolism is normal during acute viral hepatitis and cirrhosis.[13] Between these extremes, a group of drugs of which clindamycin is an example exhibits intermediate or moderate changes in disposition in liver disease.[1] Thus a wide range of alterations may occur in liver disease, depending on the drug studied and its particular dispositional characteristics.

In addition to primary diseases of the liver, disorders of other organs may secondarily affect hepatic metabolism of drugs. For example, hepatic function may be impaired in congestive heart failure, if pooling of blood in the liver reduces hepatic perfusion. Reduced hepatic blood flow should decrease uptake of drugs with a high extraction ratio. Hence congestive heart failure reduces elimination of lidocaine.[14] However, for drugs with low hepatic extraction it is unlikely that heart failure will affect elimination unless hepatic congestion is sufficient to impair metabolic functions. Fig. 10-2 shows that patients admitted to the hospital with acute congestive failure were unable to eliminate aminopyrine as rapidly as they could after treatment. This documents that the hemodynamic changes associated with congestive heart failure can be sufficient to impair hepatic drug metabolism.

Renal excretion of drugs

Some drugs are eliminated primarily by renal excretion; renal disease slows their removal. Therefore the dose of these drugs must be reduced, the extent of reduction

Metabolism of aminopyrine measured as excretion of $^{14}CO_2$ in breath of patients with various forms of liver disease compared with control patients. *FIG. 10-1*

Modified from Hepner GW, Vesell ES: Ann Intern Med 83:632, 1975.

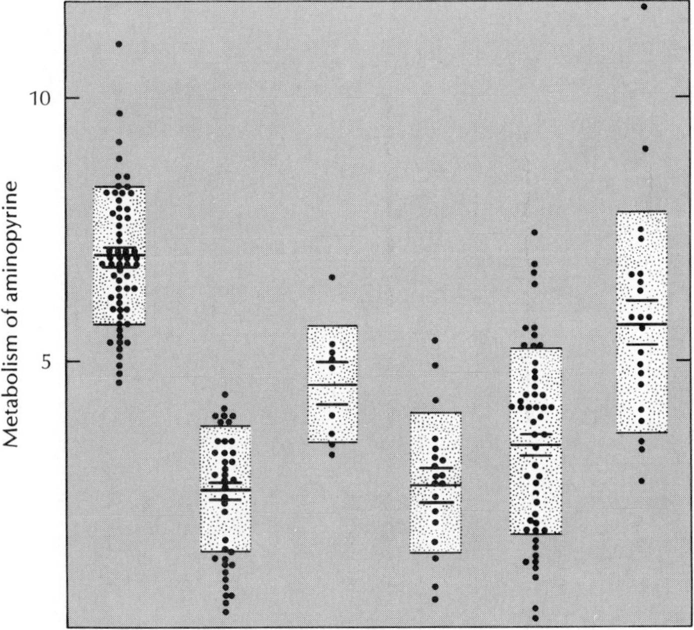

depending on the severity of the renal disease. Methods for dose adjustment in such patients have been promulgated by several investigators. In a simple version, a linear relationship exists between the overall elimination rate constant (k_e) and the endogenous creatinine clearance (Cl_{cr}):

$$k_e = k_{nr} + \delta \cdot Cl_{cr}$$

In this equation, k_{nr} is the mean extrarenal elimination rate constant in anuric patients (which is assumed to remain constant) and δ is a constant relating Cl_{cr} to the renal elimination rate constant (k_r) of the drug. This equation can be used for numerous drugs; simple nomograms have been devised to allow estimation, from the value of Cl_{cr}, of the rate of drug elimination in a patient with kidney disease.[3]

Appendix B provides data, from which dosage adjustments can be calculated, on the change in excretion of drugs in patients with renal disease.

PERSPECTIVE

The information provided in this and preceding chapters emphasizes the extreme plasticity and sensitivity of human pharmacokinetic processes to perturbation by numerous factors. A physician who is aware of the principles illustrated will succeed in selecting a dosage regimen that is therapeutic rather than toxic or ineffective. Several steps are available to help the physician optimize the patient's therapeutic regimen: (1)

FIG. 10-2 *Metabolism of aminopyrine measured by excretion of $^{14}CO_2$ in eight patients before and after treatment of congestive heart failure. Notice improvement in hepatic capacity to metabolize aminopyrine with treatment of congestive heart failure as indicated by markedly increased $^{14}CO_2$ output after treatment.*

Modified from Hepner GW, Vesell ES, Tatum KR: Am J Med 65:271, 1978.

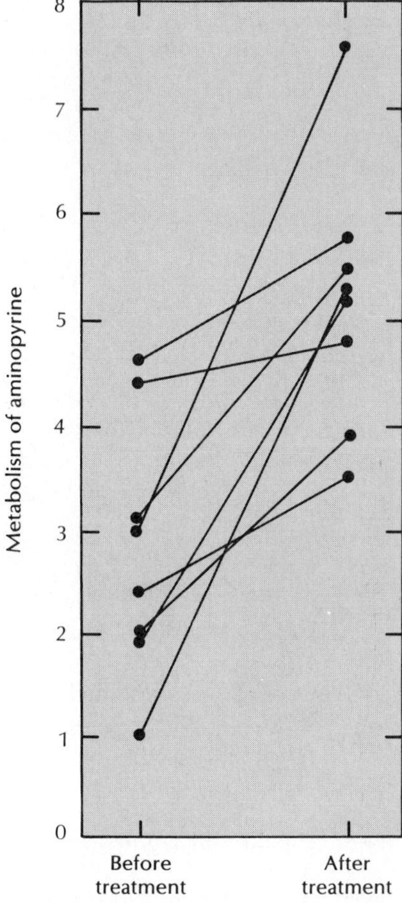

quantitative (rather than qualitative) prospective dose adjustment based on patient-derived data, such as presented in Appendix B; (2) close clinical observation of the patient for qualitative therapeutic, as well as toxic, signs of drug action; (3) assessment of quantitative clinical end points for certain drugs (such as anticoagulants or antihypertensive agents) against which the dose can be titrated; (4) measurement of drug concentrations in biologic fluids (see Appendix A). Thus, despite the fact that many factors influence rates of drug elimination in individual patients and render dosage selection difficult, the physician can proceed in a rational, deliberate manner to approximate the best dosage and to derive the maximal therapeutic benefit from available drugs, while minimizing risks of toxicity.

REFERENCES

1. Avant GR, Schenker S, Alford RH: The effect of cirrhosis on the disposition and elimination of clindamycin, *Am J Dig Dis* 20:223, 1975.
2. Bianchine JR, Calimlim LR, Morgan JP, et al: Metabolism and absorption of L-3,4-dihydroxyphenylalanine in patients with Parkinson's disease, *Ann NY Acad Sci* 179:126, 1971.
3. Dettli L: Individualization of drug dosage in patients with renal disease, *Med Clin North Am* 58:977, 1974.
4. Hepner GW, Booth CC, Cowan J, et al: Absorption of crystalline folic acid in man, *Lancet* 2:302, 1968.
5. Levine RR: Factors affecting gastrointestinal absorption of drugs, *Am J Dig Dis* 15:171, 1970.
6. Lindenbaum J, Maulitz RM, Butler VP, Jr: Inhibition of digoxin absorption by neomycin, *Gastroenterology* 71:399, 1976.
7. Lindenbaum J, Rund DG, Butler VP, Jr, et al: Inactivation of digoxin by the gut flora: reversal by antibiotic therapy, *N Engl J Med* 305:789, 1981.
8. Nimmo J, Heading RC, Tothill P, Prescott LF: Pharmacological modification of gastric emptying: effects of propantheline and metoclopramide on paracetamol absorption, *Br Med J* 1:587, 1973.
9. Prescott LF: Gastrointestinal absorption of drugs, *Med Clin North Am* 58:907, 1974.
10. Reidenberg MM: Kidney disease and drug metabolism, *Med Clin North Am* 58:1059, 1974.
11. Reidenberg MM, Odar-Cederlöf I, von Bahr C, et al: Protein binding of diphenylhydantoin and desmethylimipramine in plasma from patients with poor renal function, *N Engl J Med* 285:264, 1971.
12. Routledge PA, Stargel WW, Wagner GS, Shand DG: Increased alpha-1-acid glycoprotein and lidocaine disposition in myocardial infarction, *Ann Intern Med* 93:701, 1980.
13. Shull HJ, Wilkinson GR, Johnson R, Schenker S: Normal disposition of oxazepam in acute viral hepatitis and cirrhosis, *Ann Intern Med* 84:420, 1976.
14. Thomson PD, Melmon KL, Richardson JA, et al: Lidocaine pharmacokinetics in advanced heart failure, liver disease, and renal failure in humans, *Ann Intern Med* 78:499, 1973.
15. Vesell ES, Page JG, Passananti GT: Genetic and environmental factors affecting ethanol metabolism in man, *Clin Pharmacol Ther* 12:192, 1971.
16. Williams RL: Drug administration in hepatic disease, *N Engl J Med* 309:1616, 1983.
17. Williams RL, Benet LZ: Drug pharmacokinetics in cardiac and hepatic disease, *Annu Rev Pharmacol Toxicol* 20:389, 1980.
18. Williams RL, Mamelok RD: Hepatic disease and drug pharmacokinetics, *Clin Pharmacokinet* 5:528, 1980.
19. Williams RL, Schary WL, Blaschke TF, et al: Influence of acute viral hepatitis on disposition and pharmacologic effect of warfarin, *Clin Pharmacol Ther* 20:90, 1976.

Chapter 11

Effects of diet on drug disposition

Relationships between diet and drug disposition in human subjects were not even suspected until carefully designed studies clearly established such interactions and indicated the need for future investigations.[1] Dietary factors can not only affect drug absorption, as one would expect, but also influence drug metabolism.

EFFECTS OF STARVATION ON DRUG DISPOSITION

Because starvation is such an extreme, one would expect it to cause pronounced pharmacokinetic alterations. In support of this notion is the observation that in fasting rodents the rate of hepatic metabolism of some drugs is greatly reduced.[3,8] In contrast, there were no major changes in rates of drug metabolism in obese, otherwise healthy, human subjects after 7 to 10 consecutive days on a diet in which the total daily carbohydrate intake was less than 15 g.[13] This diet was sufficient to cause ketosis, as well as weight loss that ranged from 3.6 to 15 kg. When uncorrected for body weight, the volume of distribution of both antipyrine and tolbutamide was significantly lower after fasting than before, presumably because the early loss of weight during fasting is mainly due to loss of body water rather than reduced fat or muscle mass. The extent of decrease in volume of distribution was proportional in each subject to the weight lost so that, when correction was made for body weight, fasting had no effect on the volume of distribution of either drug. Other drugs metabolized by hepatic microsomal oxidations, including sulfisoxazole, isoniazid, and procaine, were also studied.[12] When allowance was made for body weight, neither half-life nor clearance of the five above drugs was changed in obese subjects. Although fasting decreased sulfisoxazole excretion, this was probably secondary to a decline in urine flow and in urinary pH, both of which favor nonionic diffusion of the drug back into the circulation. General conclusions regarding the failure of acute fasting to alter hepatic metabolism have been further documented in female patients with anorexia nervosa.[2]

In contrast to acute fasting, malnutrition has been shown to affect drug metabolism. If malnutrition is sufficiently severe to cause hypoalbuminemia, binding of acidic drugs decreases. In addition, microsomal oxidation of test substrates has been shown to decrease. This appears to be particularly true in patients who have both protein and energy substrate deficiencies, rather than the latter alone.[1]

EFFECTS OF DIET ON DRUG ABSORPTION

Food can have considerable effects on drug absorption. In general, ingestion of food delays gastric emptying. This in turn delays delivery of ingested drugs to absorption sites in the small intestine and delays the appearance of drug in the plasma.

Usually, ingestion of drugs with food also prolongs their absorption so that a lower peak concentration is reached. Lastly, some foodstuffs decrease the bioavailability of specific drugs if they are coingested. The classic example of this phenomenon is the chelation of tetracycline by milk products, which prevents absorption of the antibiotic. It should be clear that food can affect drug absorption in many ways. If there is concern about this possibility, patients should be instructed to take their medications 1 hour before or 2 or more hours after a meal.

An interesting additional effect of food on absorption has been the recent description of "dose-dumping" of a sustained-release theophylline product caused by a high-fat meal.[5] Ingestion of this formulation with a high-fat meal resulted in loss of the sustained-release characteristics, by unknown mechanisms.

EFFECTS OF DIET ON DRUG EXCRETION

Renal elimination of certain compounds can be altered by fasting or starvation as in the case of sulfisoxazole; renal excretion of this drug decreases during fasting, probably due to changes in urinary pH secondary to starvation ketosis. Renal excretion of drugs eliminated by glomerular filtration might also be affected by nutrition. Protein loads increase the filtration rate. In settings of parenteral or enteral nutrition, this increase may be sufficient to enhance renal elimination of drugs such as aminoglycosides to a clinically important degree, thereby requiring larger than usual doses.

ALTERATIONS IN DRUG METABOLISM CAUSED BY DIETARY MANIPULATION

A dramatic change in drug metabolism caused by dietary manipulation was described by Kappas and associates,[7] who showed that on an isocaloric diet the rate of antipyrine and theophylline metabolism was halved as the percentage of total calories as carbohydrate doubled from 35% to 70% and the percentage of protein decreased from 44% to 10%, the remainder being fat. The switch from high to low protein with a reverse change in carbohydrate content affected antipyrine and theophylline half-life (Fig. 11-1) by decreasing clearance, with no effect on the volume of distribution. The mechanism of this effect is unknown.

Many patients who receive drugs are debilitated and chronically ill. They may have inadequate nutrition, and the proportion of their diet that is carbohydrate, protein, or fat may change. For such patients drug elimination may be affected. Furthermore, some of the normal population use various weight-loss diets; these persons could also be susceptible to changes in drug-metabolizing capacity.

EFFECTS OF CHARCOAL BROILING ON DRUG DISPOSITION

The way in which food is prepared can also affect drug disposition. Isolated intestinal preparations from rats fed charcoal-broiled beef (rather than beef cooked while covered with foil, which prevents formation of polycyclic hydrocarbons) exhibited an elevenfold increase in intestinal metabolism of phenacetin.[9] Similarly, in eight healthy volunteers, eating charcoal-broiled beef shortened plasma antipyrine and theophylline half-lives by 22%.[6] This observation was attributable to an increase in metabolism, since no change occurred in the volume of distribution of either drug while clearance of both increased.

FIG. 11-1 *Theophylline half-lives in six normal subjects maintained on their usual home diets and on two test-diet periods. Each bar represents mean ±SE for the six subjects.* P, *Protein;* C, *carbohydrate;* F, *fat. Values for diets* 1, 3, *and* 4, *are not significantly different from each other. Value for diet* 2 *is significantly different from that of diet* 1 *(p = 0.05) and diet* 3 *(p = 0.01).*

From Kappas A, Anderson KE, Conney HA, Alvares AP: Clin Pharmacol Ther 20:643, 1976.

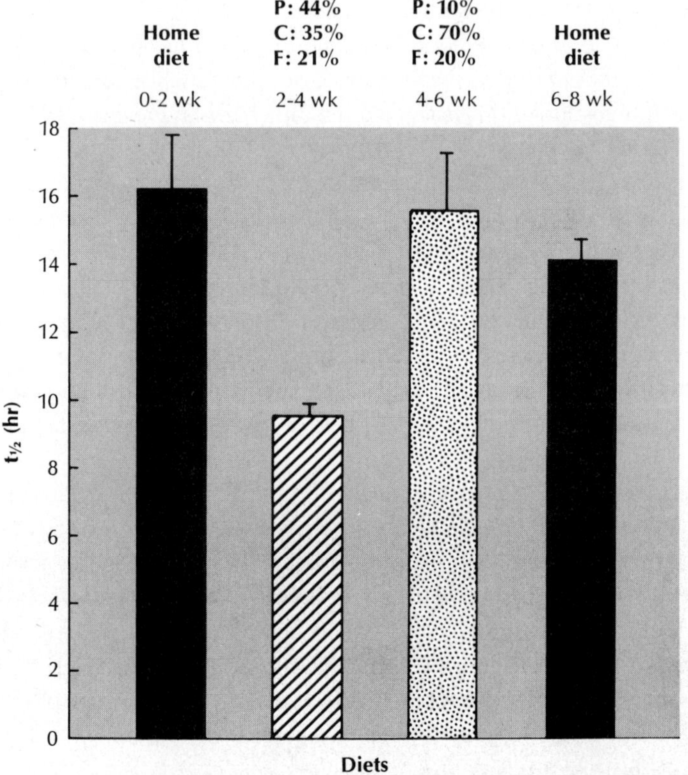

INDUCTION OF METABOLISM BY BRUSSELS SPROUTS AND CABBAGE

In rats a diet containing certain cruciferous vegetables, such as brussels sprouts, cabbage, turnips, broccoli, cauliflower, or spinach, induced intestinal benzo[*a*]pyrene hydroxylase activity and the intestinal enzymes that metabolize 7-ethoxycoumarin, hexobarbital, and phenacetin.[10,14] Certain indoles in these vegetables are potent inducers of these enzymes. A similar study in 10 healthy volunteers showed that on a 7-day diet rich in brussels sprouts and cabbage antipyrine clearance increased by 11% and mean plasma phenacetin concentrations decreased by 34% to 67%.[11] Although such an effect is not clinically important for antipyrine, dosage modification could conceivably be necessary for some drugs.

THEOBROMINE AS A METABOLIC INHIBITOR

Studies with the methylxanthine theobromine, a nutritional constituent of such dietary staples as chocolate and cocoa, revealed that daily theobromine intake decreases the capacity to eliminate theobromine itself.[4] After 2 weeks on a

Decay of a single oral dose of theobromine (6 mg/kg) before and after 2-week dietary abstention from methylxanthines. *FIG. 11-2*

From Drouillard DD, Vesell ES, Dvorchik BH: Clin Pharmacol Ther 23:296, 1978.

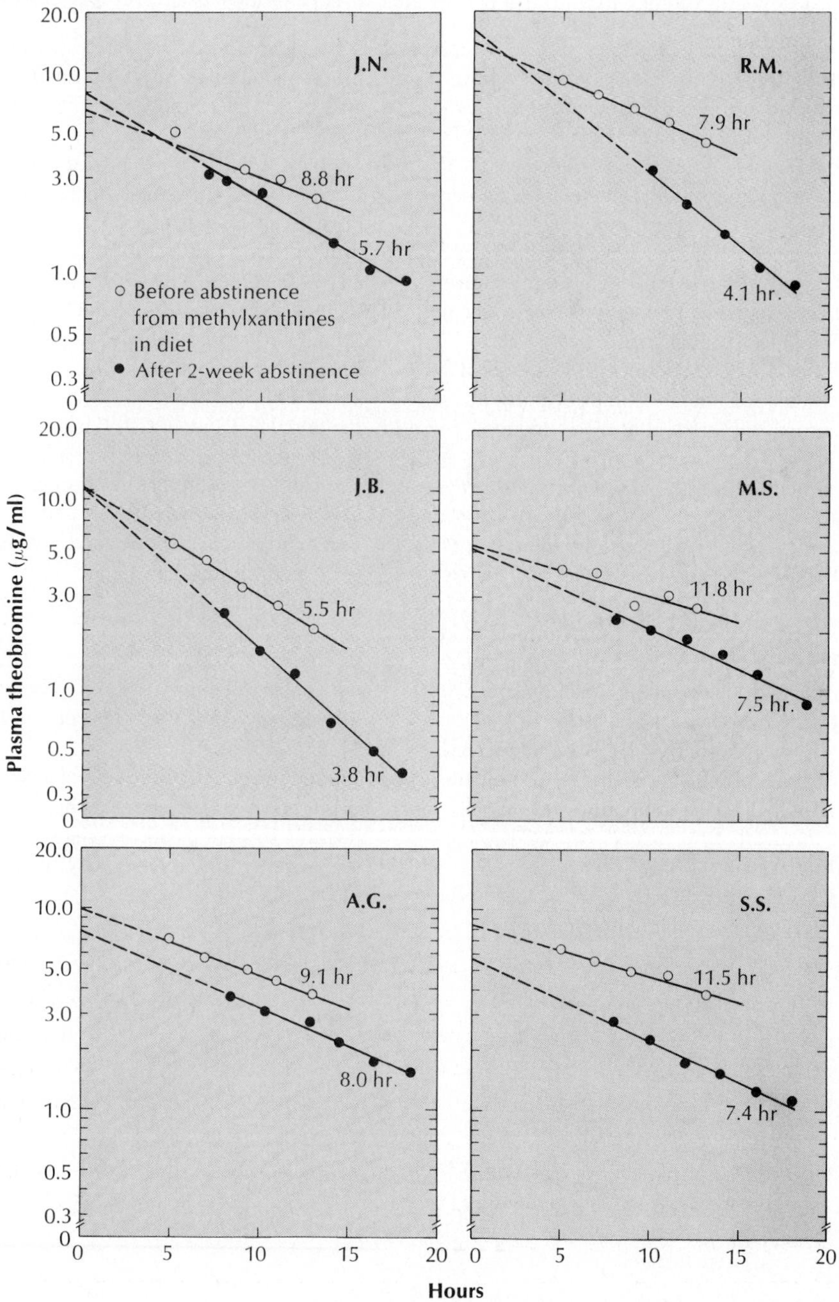

methylxanthine-free diet, each of six healthy male subjects had increased his capacity to eliminate a test dose of theobromine (Fig. 11-2).

A clinical study showing that theobromine also inhibits theophylline elimination suggests that its dietary intake might influence theophylline dosage requirements.

REFERENCES

1. Anderson KE: Influences of diet and nutrition on clinical pharmacokinetics, *Clin Pharmacokinet* 14:325, 1988.
2. Bakke OM, Aanderud S, Syversen G, et al: Antipyrine metabolism in anorexia nervosa, *Br J Clin Pharmacol* 5:341, 1978.
3. Dixon RL, Shultice RW, Fouts JR: Factors affecting drug metabolism by liver microsomes. IV. Starvation, *Proc Soc Exp Biol Med* 103:333, 1960.
4. Drouillard DD, Vesell ES, Dvorchik BH: Studies on theobromine disposition in normal subjects: alterations induced by dietary abstention from or exposure to methylxanthines, *Clin Pharmacol Ther* 23:296, 1978.
5. Hendeles L, Thakker K, Weinberger M: Food-induced dose dumping of Theo-24, *Am Pharm* NS25:592, 1985.
6. Kappas A, Alvares AP, Anderson KE, et al: Effect of charcoal-broiled beef on antipyrine and theophylline metabolism, *Clin Pharmacol Ther* 23:445, 1978.
7. Kappas A, Anderson KE, Conney AH, Alvares AP: Influence of dietary protein and carbohydrate on antipyrine and theophylline metabolism in man, *Clin Pharmacol Ther* 20:643, 1976.
8. Kato R, Gillette JR: Sex differences in the effects of abnormal physiological states on the metabolism of drugs by rat liver microsomes, *J Pharmacol Exp Ther* 150:285, 1965.
9. Pantuck EJ, Hsiao K-C, Kuntzman R, Conney AH: Intestinal metabolism of phenacetin in the rat: effect of charcoal-broiled beef and rat chow, *Science* 187:744, 1975.
10. Pantuck EJ, Hsiao K-C, Loub WD, et al: Stimulatory effect of vegetables on intestinal drug metabolism in the rat, *J Pharmacol Exp Ther* 198:278, 1976.
11. Pantuck EJ, Pantuck CB, Garland WA, et al: Stimulatory effect of brussels sprouts and cabbage on human drug metabolism, *Clin Pharmacol Ther* 25:88, 1979.
12. Reidenberg MM: Obesity and fasting: effects on drug metabolism and drug action in man, *Clin Pharmacol Ther* 22:729, 1977.
13. Reidenberg MM, Vesell ES: Unaltered metabolism of antipyrine and tolbutamide in fasting man, *Clin Pharmacol Ther* 17:650, 1975.
14. Wattenberg LW: Studies of polycyclic hydrocarbon hydroxylases of the intestine possibly related to cancer: effect of diet on benzpyrene hydroxylase activity, *Cancer* 28:99, 1971.

Chapter 12

Drug development

New drugs originate from many different sources. Fortuitous observations with natural products, unexpected clinical observations with the use of known compounds, physiologic or biochemical investigations, and basic pharmacologic experiments provide leads for therapeutic discoveries.

Until recently, most new drugs were discovered by testing (screening) large numbers of natural products or synthetic compounds for a variety of biologic activities. Once a compound is found to have an effect, numerous chemical modifications are made and tested until one is found to be suitable for further evaluation. Current drug development increasingly focuses on prospective designing for a specific chemical effect. For example, if studies of pathophysiology indicate a potential beneficial effect of inhibiting a specific enzyme, further development in the past required screening of thousands of compounds for inhibitory activity. In contrast, current strategies entail research to define the active site of the enzyme, including its structural conformation. A drug might then be synthesized to interact specifically with this active site.

A promising drug that seems safe enough in preliminary testing is then carried through the following series of steps:

1. Animal studies
   a. Acute, subacute, and chronic toxicity
   b. Therapeutic index
   c. Pharmacokinetics and metabolic pathways
2. Human studies[1,2]
   a. Phase 1: preliminary pharmacologic evaluation
   b. Phase 2: controlled clinical evaluation
   c. Phase 3: extended clinical evaluation
   d. Phase 4: postmarketing surveillance for some drugs

ANIMAL STUDIES

ACUTE, SUBACUTE, AND CHRONIC TOXICITY

The most common measure of acute toxicity is the median lethal dose (LD_{50}), that is, the dose that is lethal to 50% of the animals tested. The LD_{50} is determined by administering various doses of a drug to groups of animals. Ordinarily only a single dose is given to each animal. The percentage of animals dying in each group is plotted against the dose, and the dose that kills 50% of the animals is estimated. It should be obvious that the LD_{50} of any drug is of interest only to experimental pharmacologists and not to clinicians.

Historically, at least three different species were used to determine acute toxicity;

observations were made not only on the LD_{50} but also on the types of symptoms that developed. Currently, studies of lethality are done as infrequently as possible to minimize the toll on animals.

In subacute toxicity studies the mode of administration and the dosage depend on the proposed clinical trial. Usually the drug is administered orally. Several doses are used, some within the range of the estimated human dose and others that are considerably greater, in order to characterize toxic manifestations. Observations include a variety of laboratory studies, such as hematologic examinations and renal and hepatic function tests.

Chronic toxicity studies last many months and might extend through several generations to detect possible teratogenic effects of a drug. Several species are used because some species are more suitable than others for the demonstration of specific adverse effects. At various intervals selected animals are killed, and thorough pathologic examinations are performed.

Therapeutic index

The LD_{50} of a drug is not nearly so important as the difference between the dose required for toxicity and the therapeutic dose. Nevertheless, in *animal experiments* the therapeutic index, defined as the ratio of the LD_{50} to the median effective dose (ED_{50}), has been widely used as an initial approximation of drug toxicity.

$$\text{Therapeutic index} = \frac{LD_{50}}{ED_{50}}$$

Clinically, of course, the concept of effectiveness in relation to nonlethal toxicity (margin of safety) is more important than any specific ratio. A physician is most interested in knowing how far the usual therapeutic dose can be exceeded before adverse effects are encountered.

HUMAN STUDIES: CLINICAL PHARMACOLOGY

Animal studies provide a general profile of the toxicity, pharmacologic activity, and pharmacokinetics of a new drug. Even with this information, the initiation of clinical studies is risky. There are numerous examples of drugs that passed all the preclinical criteria for safety but caused serious adverse effects in humans. Not only is there great species variation in toxicity; there are also many adverse effects that simply cannot be ascertained in animals. These effects include drowsiness, nausea, dizziness, nervousness, epigastric distress, headache, weakness, insomnia, fatigue, tinnitus, heartburn, skin rash, depression, increased energy, vertigo, nocturia, abdominal distention, flatulence, stiffness, and urticaria.

Because of such discrepancies between animal data and human responses, initial clinical studies on any drug must be undertaken with great care, with the methodology meticulously planned, and with special attention to *relevance* (pertinence of data), *representativeness* (selection of material to eliminate bias), and *reliability* (repeatability of results). An *Investigational New Drug* (IND) application must be filed with the Food and Drug Administration (FDA) before any clinical evaluation is initiated.

Phase 1: preliminary pharmacologic evaluation

Very small doses of the drug are first administered to healthy human volunteers. The objectives of phase 1 studies are to assess toxicity and to determine the best route of administration and the safe dosage range.[1,2] In most instances it is also essential to characterize the absorption, metabolism, and excretion of the new drug. Otherwise the investigator cannot tell whether ineffectiveness is a consequence of lack of absorption or of rapid elimination. About 20 to 100 subjects are studied in phase 1, and approximately 50% of all compounds tested are abandoned because of toxicity, lack of efficacy, or both.

Ethical aspects of human experimentation have been the subject of much discussion and will not be considered in detail here. The important points, however, are that the subject must truly volunteer for testing (that is, be able to give informed consent and not be subjected to coercion) and that the investigator must be competent.

Phase 2: controlled clinical evaluation

Whereas phase 1 studies are usually performed in healthy individuals, in the second phase studies are conducted in patients in whom the drug is projected for use.[1,2] Up to 100 to 200 patients are studied to assess the safety and efficacy of the new drug in blind or double-blind studies employing comparisons to placebo, another active drug, or both. Adverse effects must be reported promptly to the sponsoring company and to the FDA, and specific studies are sometimes initiated to ascertain the significance of any unexpected findings.

Phase 3: extended clinical evaluation

Phase 3 evaluations of a new drug comprise large-scale clinical trials that may last for prolonged periods (sometimes a year or more) and involve a thousand or more patients. These trials are designed to determine whether chronic use provides a favorable benefit to risk ratio.[1,2] The investigators for such trials must not only be competent clinicians but must also have experience and training in the field of drug evaluation.

Data from all phases are compiled into a New Drug Application (NDA), which is submitted to the FDA in support of an application for marketing approval. Assuming that the studies demonstrate to the satisfaction of the FDA that the drug is safe and effective, the investigational drug may be approved for distribution and use. In making decisions concerning such matters, the FDA often utilizes independent advisory groups composed of experts in the clinical area in which the new drug is proposed for use.

Phase 4: postmarketing surveillance

It would seem that with all these safeguards, approval of a drug by the FDA would be free of hazard. Unfortunately, many unusual side effects, idiosyncrasies, and allergies may be observed only after extensive use by large numbers of patients. Even though an NDA contains data on several thousand patients, serious adverse effects that occur at frequencies of one in 5,000 or even less may remain undetected. As a result, some drugs now undergo postmarketing surveillance in which data concerning efficacy and toxicity are systematically gathered after the drug has been marketed. In this manner effects can be assessed from a much larger data base in terms of patient exposure. It is hoped that this approach will allow early detection of adverse effects that were not detected in initial trials with fewer patients over shorter periods of time.

The treatment IND

The AIDS epidemic has led to development of the treatment IND or "parallel track," the goal of which is to provide earlier access to drugs for patients with devastating diseases. This program allows desperately ill patients to take drugs that have not yet been approved by the FDA for marketing.[1] A physician can prescribe an investigational drug to patients with "immediate life-threatening disease" if no comparable or satisfactory alternative drug is available. In turn, the FDA has defined "immediate life-threatening disease" as one with a reasonable likelihood of death within months or of premature death unless immediately treated. Clinical conditions that fit this definition include AIDS, advanced heart failure, and metastatic cancers. The drug must be under active investigation toward an NDA, and it must be unique in its therapeutic potential. This program has made new antiviral drugs available to patients with AIDS. There is concern, however, that such access may impede recruitment of sufficient numbers of patients into controlled trials.

REFERENCES

1. Kessler DA: The regulation of investigational drugs, *N Engl J Med* 320:281, 1989.
2. Miller HI, Young FE: The drug approval process at the Food and Drug Administration: new biotechnology as a paradigm of a science-based activist approach, *Arch Intern Med* 149:655, 1989.

section two

Drug effects on the nervous system and neuroeffectors

Chapter 13

General aspects of neuropharmacology

The more than 10 billion neurons that constitute the human nervous system communicate with each other through chemical mediators. They also exert their effects on peripheral structures by release of neurotransmitters and not by electrical impulses.

Acetylcholine and norepinephrine are the predominant mediators in the autonomic nervous system. They act on effector organs through second-messenger systems. In autonomic ganglia and at the skeletal neuromuscular junction, acetylcholine opens ion channels. The role of presynaptic *autoreceptors*, which influence release of neurotransmitters, is of current interest and will likely be important for development of new drugs.

Amines, acetylcholine, certain amino acids and peptides, and adenosine serve as neurotransmitters and modulators within the central nervous system. Among the amines, norepinephrine, dopamine, serotonin (5-hydroxytryptamine), and probably histamine and epinephrine are important. Amino acids such as glutamic and aspartic acids excite postsynaptic membranes of many neurons, whereas γ-aminobutyric acid (GABA) and glycine are inhibitory transmitters. Substance P, the endorphins, and the enkephalins are examples of peptidergic neurotransmitters. As techniques have improved for assessing ligand binding to membrane recognition sites (putative receptors), the number of known and postulated receptor types and subtypes has proliferated. The discovery that neurons may release more than one active compound (so-called *co-transmitters*), for example an amine and a peptide, adds another level of complexity to be unraveled when one is trying to understand drug actions.[13]

Numerous drugs mimic or influence the action of chemical mediators. Those that act by less well understood mechanisms are classified according to their clinical usage.

THE CHEMICAL NEUROTRANSMISSION CONCEPT

Similarities between responses to certain drugs and responses to nerve stimulation were noted before this century. For example, muscarine, obtained from mushrooms, slowed heart rate, just like vagal stimulation. Similarly, adrenal extracts caused effects similar to those after stimulation of sympathetic nerves (Oliver and Shafer, 1895).

Definitive proof of chemical neurotransmission was provided in 1921 by experiments of Loewi and of Cannon and Uridil. In his classic experiment Loewi demonstrated that when the vagus nerve of a perfused frog heart was stimulated, a substance was released that slowed a second heart with no neural connections to the first.[18] Cannon and Uridil[6] found that stimulation of sympathetic input to the liver released a substance that was similar to epinephrine in many respects. This mediator, at first named "sympathin," is now known to be norepinephrine. Identification of the neurotransmitter in adrenergic axons as norepinephrine was provided by von Euler.[27]

Acetylcholine was first studied systematically by Dale.[7] The "quantum hypothesis" of acetylcholine release and of the role of synaptic vesicles in neuromuscular and synaptic transmission is a contribution of Katz and co-workers.[8,15] The discovery by Brodie and Shore[5] of monoamine release by reserpine led to great expansion of knowledge of the metabolism and functions of catecholamines in the nervous system. Axelrod[3] developed the concept of uptake of catecholamines by sympathetic nerves. The importance of these discoveries is attested to by the Nobel prizes awarded to many of the early investigators.

These discoveries showed that nerves release compounds that in turn influence the effectors. Instead of classifying drugs as sympathomimetic and parasympathomimetic, it was often more useful to classify nerves on the basis of the mediator released from them. This led to the concept of *cholinergic* and *adrenergic* nerve fibers.

SITES OF ACTION OF CHEMICAL MEDIATORS

The role of neurotransmitters at various anatomic sites is well established in some cases and is surmised in others. The generally accepted information on the site of action of these compounds may be summarized as follows:

1. Postganglionic parasympathetic nerve endings on smooth muscle, cardiac muscle, and exocrine glands: acetylcholine
2. Postganglionic sympathetic nerve endings on smooth muscle, cardiac muscle, and exocrine glands: norepinephrine (except for sweat glands)
3. All autonomic ganglionic synapses: acetylcholine
4. Motor fiber terminals at skeletal neuromuscular junctions: acetylcholine
5. Central nervous system synapses: acetylcholine, norepinephrine, dopamine, serotonin, histamine, glutamic and aspartic acids, GABA, glycine, adenosine, and numerous peptides

Postjunctional actions are emphasized in the following discussion, but there is growing evidence for presynaptic actions as well (see p. 142).

Sites of action of mediators in the autonomic nervous system are relatively well established, compared with the more complex central nervous system. Selective localization of active compounds in the brain with the use of immunocytochemical staining and biochemical identification of their binding sites are used to establish transmitter roles.

Regulation of sweat glands, adrenal medulla, and vascular smooth muscle

Sweat glands are an important exception to the generalization that norepinephrine is the chemical mediator to sympathetically innervated structures. These glands are activated by cholinergic drugs and inhibited by anticholinergic drugs. Thus postganglionic fibers innervating sweat glands are cholinergic rather than adrenergic.

The adrenal medulla secretes primarily epinephrine in response to cholinergic stimulation, a response inhibited by ganglionic blocking agents. On an embryologic basis, the adrenal medulla is a modified sympathetic ganglion. It is therefore not surprising that it responds to acetylcholine, the mediator that activates both sympathetic and parasympathetic postganglionic neurons.

Most vascular regions do not receive parasympathetic innervation; instead neural control of vascular tone is mediated by variation in sympathetic activity. Nevertheless, circulating muscarinic agonists, as well as a large number of unrelated agents, dilate blood vessels by releasing from endothelial cells a very short-acting substance called endothelium-derived relaxing factor (EDRF).[2] Relaxation has been attributed to subsequent formation of cyclic GMP in vascular smooth muscle. EDRF is thought by many investigators to be nitric oxide (NO) or another compound that releases NO.

RECEPTOR CONCEPT IN NEURO-PHARMACOLOGY

Neurotransmitters affect membranes by interacting with specific receptors. The existence of these receptors may be deduced from structure-activity studies on a series of chemically similar compounds or from shifts of dose-response curves in the presence of specific antagonists. The following receptors may be postulated for some of the neurotransmitters:

1. Acetylcholine acts on muscarinic and nicotinic receptors. Cholinergic receptors in smooth muscles, cardiac muscle, and exocrine glands are termed *muscarinic* because muscarine, a quaternary amine alkaloid, has an action similar to that of acetylcholine at these sites. Several muscarinic receptor subtypes exist,[10] but there is some disagreement as to their location and designation. M_1-receptors are selectively blocked by pirenzepine; one subtype (M_{1a}) is found in the hippocampus and another (M_{1b}) in autonomic ganglia. The heart contains $M_2(M_{2a})$-receptors, whereas $M_3(M_{2b})$-receptors have been located in smooth muscles, exocrine glands, and presynaptically on cholinergic neurons. Atropine and most related drugs are nonspecific antagonists at muscarinic receptors.

Acetylcholine, as well as nicotine, acts on *nicotinic* receptors in autonomic ganglia and at skeletal neuromuscular junctions. However, the receptors at these two sites are not identical. The action of acetylcholine at end-plate regions of skeletal muscle is antagonized by tubocurarine, whereas receptors in ganglia are blocked by hexamethonium. At nicotinic sites, unlike muscarinic sites, an excess of agonist causes persisting depolarization and blockade of transmission. There are also muscarinic and nicotinic receptors in the central nervous system.

2. Norepinephrine acts on adrenergic receptors that are classified as *alpha* (α) and *beta* (β). Drugs that block these receptors are known as α- and β-*adrenergic blocking agents*. In addition, α-receptors are divided into α_1- and α_2-receptors, and β-receptors are divided into β_1- and β_2-receptors (see p. 142).

3. Dopamine acts on dopaminergic receptors in the central nervous system, in ganglia, and in the kidney. Dopaminergic receptors are blocked by antipsychotic drugs. Dopamine also acts on β_1-receptors in the heart and in higher doses on α-receptors.

4. Serotonin acts on serotonergic receptors in the central nervous system and in some peripheral organs. Its action is blocked by antagonists such as methysergide.

5. Histamine acts on histaminergic receptors classified as H_1 and H_2. The antihistamines commonly used to treat hay fever are H_1-receptor antagonists, for example, diphenhydramine. H_2-receptor antagonists are relatively newer; a typical example is cimetidine.

In general, less is known about receptors for amino acid and peptide transmitters, although a great many have been studied (see Table 3-1).

Newer concepts of receptor structure

The nicotinic end-plate receptor and the β-adrenergic receptor are examples of two quite distinct types (sometimes termed superfamilies) of receptor, the former being an ion channel and the latter coupled to a G protein second-messenger system (see Chapter 3). Understanding of the structure and function of the nicotinic receptor derives to a large extent from studies on eels and rays that have electric organs with an extremely high density of receptors. Binding sites for acetylcholine reside on components of a funnel-shaped ion channel (Fig. 13-1) that extends beyond both sides of the cell membrane and is composed of five subunits designated α, α, β, γ, and δ. Binding of acetylcholine to both α subunits maximally opens the channel. The arrangement of the subunits is controversial, but the α subunits are not adjacent. Although the details are uncertain, each of the subunits is thought to be composed of a protein with four hydrophobic segments embedded within the plasma membrane, connected by hydrophilic loops extending into the cytoplasm or into the extracellular space.[19] Other members of this family are $GABA_A$, glycine, $5\text{-}HT_3$, and NMDA receptors.

The β-adrenergic receptor is thought to consist of a single protein with seven hydrophobic transmembrane regions, again linked by cytoplasmic and extracellular segments of various lengths (Fig. 13-2). There is evidence that other G protein–related receptors, such as muscarinic receptors, α_2-adrenergic receptors, some serotonin receptors, and rhodopsin, share this general configuration.

PROBLEM 13-1. *What accounts for the muscarinic or nicotinic nature of a cholinergic agent? Crystallographic analysis indicates that acetylcholine is a flexible molecule; rotation is possible at two different bonds. Muscarinic and nicotinic drugs differ from acetylcholine in the degree of rotation at sites*

FIG. 13-1

Three-dimensional model of the funnel-shaped acetylcholine receptor from Torpedo californica. Left, *Side view;* right, *view of extracellular surface with tentative assignment of subunit types.*

From McCarthy MP, Earnest JP, Young EF, Choe S, Stroud RM. Reproduced, with permission, from Annu Rev Neurosci *9:387, copyright 1986, by Annual Reviews Inc.*

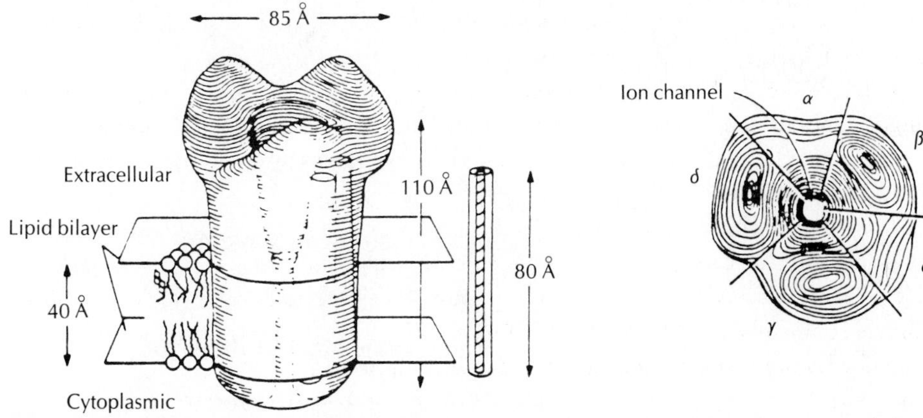

of torsion. Thus acetylcholine has both muscarinic and nicotinic activities, whereas purely muscarinic or nicotinic congeners have constraints imposed by conformational factors.

SEQUENCE OF CHEMICAL EVENTS AT SYNAPSES AND NEUROEFFECTOR JUNCTIONS

The following steps occur in junctional transmission: (1) synthesis of the mediator, (2) binding (storage) of the mediator in a potentially active form, (3) neuronal depolarization, entry of Ca^{++}, and release of the mediator, (4) binding of the mediator to a postjunctional receptor, (5) change in postjunctional ion conductance or second-messenger function, (6) removal or inactivation of the mediator, and (7) recovery of the postjunctional membrane. Theoretically, drugs could influence any of these steps, and, indeed, there are examples of many such interactions, as shown in Table 13-1.

A synapse is the site of transmission of the nerve impulse between two neurons. The axonal terminal is separated from the postsynaptic membrane by a cleft that is about 20 nm in width. Electron micrographs show that the presynaptic element contains numerous vesicles in which the transmitter is stored.

Transmission of the nerve impulse across a synapse is quite different from axonal conduction. First, transmission is unidirectional. Second, when the axon is stimulated

FIG. 13-2 *Structure of the human β_2-adrenergic receptor, as it may be organized within the cell membrane.*

From Dohlman HG, Caron MG, Lefkowitz RJ: Reprinted in part with permission from Biochemistry 26:2657, 1987. Copyright 1987 American Chemical Society.

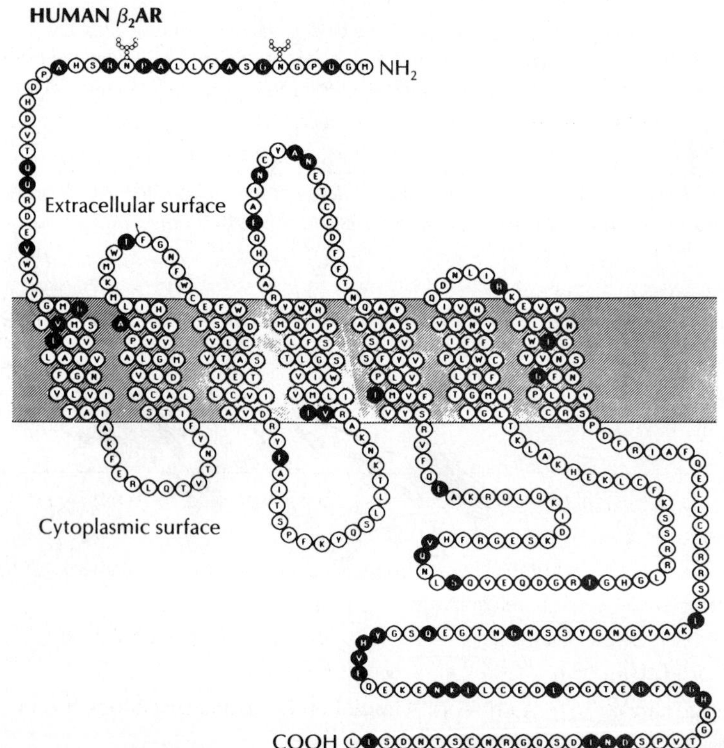

TABLE 13–1 Sites of drug action in relation to junctional transmission

Site of drug action	Mediator involved: Acetylcholine	Mediator involved: Norepinephrine
Synthesis of mediator inhibited by	Hemicholinium	Metyrosine
Transport of mediator into granules inhibited by	Vesamicol	Reserpine
Release of mediator enhanced by	Carbachol	Tyramine, amphetamine
Release of mediator inhibited by	Botulinum toxin	Bretylium
Depolarization of postsynaptic membrane promoted by	A. Muscarine Choline esters Pilocarpine B. Nicotine Choline esters C. Nicotine Choline esters	Catecholamine and related amines
Depolarization of postsynaptic membrane inhibited by	A. Atropine B. Hexamethonium C. *d*-Tubocurarine	α-Receptor blocking agents: e.g., phenoxybenzamine β-Receptor blocking agents: e.g., propranolol
Removal or inactivation of mediator inhibited by	Anticholinesterases	Cocaine, tricyclic antidepressants

A, Cholinergic neuroeffector site; *B,* Ganglionic site; *C,* Skeletal neuromuscular site.

electrically, there is a delay of about 0.2 second before the postsynaptic element is depolarized.

At a skeletal neuromuscular junction an axon terminal of the somatic motoneuron lies within the gutters of the end-plate region (Fig. 13-3). A neuronal action potential causes Ca^{++} influx, which releases acetylcholine from vesicles in the axon terminal.[22,26] Acetylcholine diffuses across the gap and changes the permeability of the postjunctional membrane to cations. The release process is inhibited by Mg^{++}.

At the termination of autonomic nerve fibers at neuroeffector junctions in smooth muscles, cardiac muscle, and exocrine glands, there are no specialized structures analogous to the motor end-plate. Transmitters are discharged from varicosities along the terminal plexuses into the extracellular space where they reach receptors by diffusion. See Figs. 13-4 and 13-5 for a display of organs innervated by the autonomic nervous system and a schema of parasympathetic and sympathetic outflows to neuroeffector cells.

EVIDENCE FOR CHOLINERGIC AND ADRENERGIC NEUROTRANSMISSION

The role of a mediator in neurotransmission is suggested or established by some or all of the following:

1. Presence of the transmitter in the axon along with enzymes responsible for its production and destruction
2. Similarity of the mediator's effect to that of nerve stimulation
3. Release of the transmitter by nerve stimulation
4. Blockade of the effect of nerve stimulation by drugs that block the transmitter's action

FIG. 13-3 *Cholinergic nerve terminal depicting the synthesis, storage, and release of acetylcholine (ACh), its hydrolysis by acetylcholinesterase, and its action on cholinergic receptors on the effector cell and presynaptic membrane.*

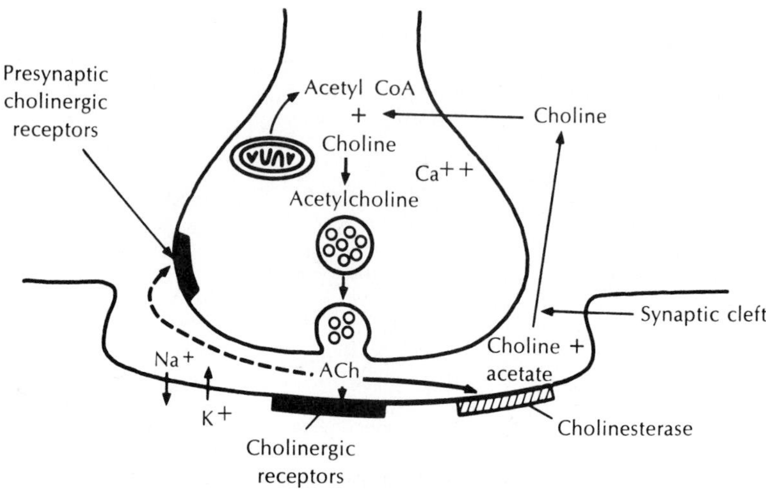

FIG. 13-4 *Autonomic innervation of various organs.*
Redrawn from a Sandoz Pharmaceuticals publication.

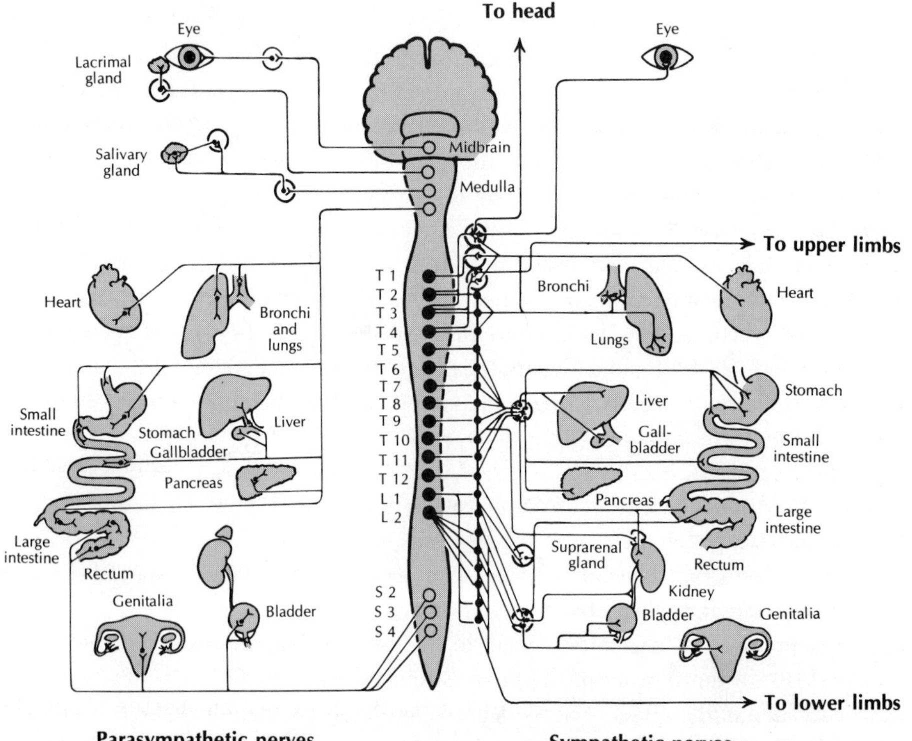

FIG. 13-5 *Schematic representation of autonomic innervation of neuroeffector cells.* ACh, *Acetylcholine;* NE, *norepinephrine.*

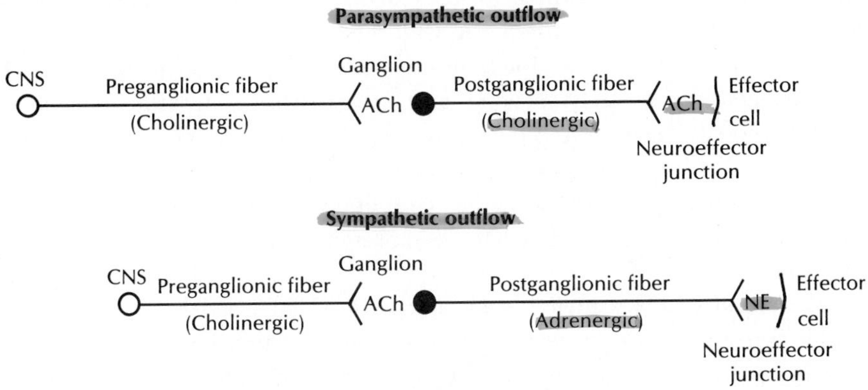

Most of these criteria can be met in studies of neuromuscular and ganglionic transmission, but there are formidable difficulties in proving the transmitter role of a substance in the central nervous system.[21] A chemical is often, at least tentatively, accepted as a central transmitter if it occurs in relatively high concentrations in brain regions that exhibit the capacity for high affinity, preferably stereospecific, binding of the substance. Further evidence is provided if local electrical stimulation and micro-injection of the compound elicit similar responses. Agents that selectively deplete the brain of a particular compound can be very useful for assessing physiologic roles of probable neurotransmitters.

FACTORS INFLUENCING RESPONSE OF EFFECTORS TO CHEMICAL MEDIATORS

The response of effector cells may be altered dramatically under certain circumstances.[14] Direct radioligand studies indicate that the number of receptors may change. An increase in receptor number is referred to as *upregulation*; a decrease in receptor number is *downregulation*. Prolonged exposure to high concentrations of an adrenergic agonist reduces the number of receptors. In the case of β-adrenergic receptors coupled to adenylyl cyclase, a brief exposure to agonist can cause a less drastic, readily reversible *desensitization* in which the receptor is phosphorylated and uncoupled from its second-messenger system.[12] Desensitization can be specific for the stimulating agonist (homologous) or may extend to agonists that act on other receptor types (heterologous). Receptors can also become sequestered at a site inaccessible to agonist or second messenger, perhaps preceding their destruction.

In contrast, a reduction in tissue catecholamines has a different effect; sustained depletion of norepinephrine by chronic administration of reserpine, can cause *supersensitivity* to catecholamines. Similarly, chronic administration of a ganglionic blocking agent to a guinea pig can increase the sensitivity of its isolated ileum to histamine, K^+, and serotonin, as well as to the normal postganglionic mediator acetylcholine. Such effects may explain changes in sensitivity to drugs in certain disease states. For example, the propranolol withdrawal syndrome (see p. 165) has been attributed to an increase in receptor number and enhanced responsiveness to endogenous catecholamines.

Cocaine and tricyclic antidepressants enhance the effects of endogenous and exogenous catecholamines by interfering with their prejunctional reuptake by adrenergic terminals (see p. 95). Thus the transmitter persists in the neuroeffector junction for a longer period at greater concentrations. *Denervation supersensitivity* after surgical postganglionic denervation of the nictitating membrane, which is correlated with degeneration of adrenergic nerve terminals, is explained on a similar basis. It is specific for catecholamines and related amines, develops within 48 hours after denervation, and is undoubtedly related to disappearance of the catecholamine uptake mechanism.

A specialized supersensitivity develops in denervated skeletal muscle. A week or two after denervation, the surface of the entire muscle fiber becomes responsive to externally applied acetylcholine, whereas only the end-plate region was sensitive before denervation. This observation is explained by the spread of new acetylcholine receptors across the muscle surface.

In contrast to supersensitivity induced by denervation or prolonged inactivity, more rapid sensitization to neurotransmitters and related drugs can also occur. Inhibitors of acetylcholinesterase immediately potentiate the actions of acetylcholine. Similarly, drugs that interfere with reflex mechanisms may allow greater fluctuation in a physiologic parameter such as blood pressure when another agent is administered. For example, ganglionic blocking agents increase the effectiveness of injected vasopressor drugs by interfering with buffering reflexes.

NEUROTRANSMITTER KINETICS AND THE NERVOUS SYSTEM

Aside from acetylcholine, the best studied neurotransmitters are nitrogenous bases synthesized by neurons from amino acid precursors and stored in vesicles for release by exocytosis. The active amines do not cross the blood-brain barrier efficiently, but their precursors are actively transported into the brain.

Acetylcholine

Acetylcholine is present in certain autonomic nerves and in nerve endings in the brain, where its vesicular localization has been demonstrated. Acetylcholine is synthesized by the cytoplasmic enzyme choline acetyltransferase (CAT).

$$\text{Choline} + \text{Acetyl coenzyme A} \xrightarrow{\text{CAT}} \text{Acetylcholine} + \text{Coenzyme A}$$

The compound *hemicholinium* blocks synthesis of the mediator by interfering with transport of choline across the neuronal membrane. Acetylcholine also inhibits choline uptake; thus its release enhances choline transport.[25] The compound *vesamicol* interferes with uptake of acetylcholine into synaptic vesicles. *Botulinum toxin* blocks release of acetylcholine, whereas *black widow spider toxin* enhances release.

During nerve stimulation, recently synthesized acetylcholine appears to be preferentially released. Acetylcholine released by one nerve impulse must be destroyed rapidly so that transmitter released by the next impulse can act within a few milliseconds on a repolarized postsynaptic membrane. Hydrolysis of acetylcholine reduces the potency of the compound a hundred-thousandfold.

Destruction of acetylcholine is accomplished by two types of *cholinesterase*. *Acetylcholinesterase*, or specific cholinesterase, hydrolyzes acetyl esters of choline more rapidly than butyryl esters. *Pseudocholinesterase*, or nonspecific cholinesterase, is also called *butyrylcholinesterase* because it hydrolyzes butyrylcholine more rapidly than the acetyl ester. Acetylcholinesterase is localized primarily at pre- and post-junctional sites of cholinergic transmission and, surprisingly, in membranes of red blood cells where its function is unknown; nonspecific cholinesterase is more widely distributed. Plasma cholinesterase is of the nonspecific type. Its titer in plasma is not related to neural activity but can be a useful measure of exposure to anticholinesterase pesticides. Because plasma cholinesterase is manufactured in the liver, its titer is also depressed in advanced hepatic disease.

Catecholamines

The collective term for norepinephrine, epinephrine, and dopamine is *catecholamine*, since these neurotransmitters are catechols (*ortho*-dihydroxybenzenes) and contain an amine group in their aliphatic side chain.

LOCALIZATION

The distribution of catecholamines in the body is well understood, thanks to suitable methods for their determination, such as fluorometric assay. Histochemical fluorescence microscopy techniques developed by Swedish investigators have allowed visualization of catecholamine-containing structures (see Fig. 18-1), their precise localization, and their susceptibility to drug actions.

Norepinephrine is present in postganglionic sympathetic fibers and in certain pathways within the central nervous system. *Epinephrine* constitutes most of the catecholamine in the human adrenal medulla, though adrenal medullary tumors (pheochromocytomas) may contain primarily norepinephrine. Cells that secrete these amines, which stain brown if exposed to chromium salts, are referred to as *chromaffin* cells. Other organs and the central nervous system may contain small amounts of epinephrine. *Dopamine* is found in relatively high concentrations in the brain, particularly in the caudate nucleus and the putamen (Table 13-2).

TABLE 13-2 Distribution of norepinephrine and dopamine in the human brain (micrograms/gram)

	Norepinephrine	Dopamine
Frontal lobe	0.00-0.02	0.00
Caudate nucleus	0.04	3.12
Putamen	0.02	5.27
Hypothalamus (anterior part)	0.96	0.18
Substantia nigra	0.04	0.40
Pons	0.04	0.00
Medulla oblongata (dorsal part)	0.13	0.00
Cerebellar cortex	0.02	0.02

Based on data from Bertler Å: *Acta Physiol Scand* 51:97, 1961.

The distribution of norepinephrine corresponds well with the adrenergic innervation of various organs. Although there is considerable species variation, the heart, arteries, and veins of most mammals contain norepinephrine on the order of 1 μg/g of tissue. The liver, lungs, and skeletal muscle contain considerably less, whereas the vas deferens has about 5 to 10 times as much.

BIOSYNTHESIS

Synthesis of catecholamines is a small but very important component of tyrosine metabolism. Other metabolic pathways of this amino acid lead to formation of thyroxin, melanin, proteins, and peptides.

Tyrosine is actively taken up by neurons. The subsequent steps in synthesis of catecholamines are shown in Fig. 13-6.

Tyrosine hydroxylase, a cytoplasmic enzyme, catalyzes the rate-limiting step in catecholamine synthesis. Its inhibition by the amino acid analog metyrosine (α-methyl-*p*-tyrosine) depletes catecholamines from brain and sympathetic nerves.

Aromatic L*-amino acid decarboxylase* is a cytoplasmic enzyme that decarboxylates several substrates besides dopa (3,4-dihydroxyphenylalanine).

Dopamine-β-hydroxylase, a copper-containing enzyme bound to membranes of axoplasmic granules, catalyzes conversion of dopamine to norepinephrine. This enzyme is inhibited by copper reagents such as disulfiram and diethyldithiocarbamate. The enzyme is associated primarily with larger catecholamine vesicles. Sufficient sympathetic stimulation leads to its release into the circulation.

*Phenylethanolamine-*N*-methyltransferase* is a cytoplasmic enzyme present primarily in the adrenal medulla where it catalyzes transfer of a methyl group from S-adenosylmethionine to norepinephrine for the formation of epinephrine.

Negative feedback of catecholamine biosynthesis and release. Sympathetic nerve stimulation does not deplete axonal catecholamine; production keeps up with loss. Because norepinephrine inhibits tyrosine hydroxylase,[20] increased sympathetic activity, by decreasing intraneuronal norepinephrine, accelerates catecholamine formation. In contrast, monoamine oxidase (MAO) inhibitors, which elevate catecholamine levels in adrenergic neurons, reduce catecholamine synthesis. Thus regulation of norepinephrine formation is achieved by end-product inhibition. In addition, stimulation of

---

FIG. 13-6 *Pathway of synthesis of catecholamines. Enzymes catalyzing various reactions are as follows:* 1, *tyrosine hydroxylase;* 2, *aromatic* L*-amino acid decarboxylase;* 3, *dopamine-β-hydroxylase;* 4, *phenylethanolamine-*N*-methyltransferase.* Dopa, *3,4-Dihydroxyphenylalanine.*

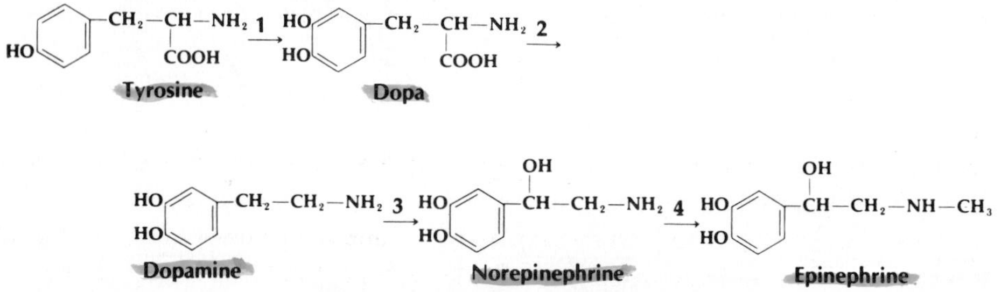

presynaptic α_2-autoreceptors on axon terminals by endogenous or exogenous norepinephrine or related agents inhibits release of the amine. Stimulation of presynaptic receptors for neurotransmitters other than the one released by a particular neuron may also affect transmitter release.

STORAGE AND RELEASE

Catecholamines are stored in both large and small vesicles in association with adenosine triphosphate.[29] The large vesicles, formed in the cell body before transport to the terminals by axoplasmic flow, also contain dopamine-β-hydroxylase, soluble proteins called *chromogranins*, and opioid peptides. These vesicles appear primarily responsible for conversion of dopamine to norepinephrine, some of which escapes into the axoplasm where it is taken up by the smaller vesicles or metabolized.

Reserpine indirectly depletes amines from neurons by blocking uptake into vesicles. Amine that escapes is no longer replaced but is deaminated by MAO (see below) within axonal mitochondria.

Release of catecholamines occurs by exocytosis.[29] In addition to the catecholamine, chromogranin and dopamine-β-hydroxylase are released by sympathetic nerve stimulation. Although this finding indicates that the larger vesicles empty their contents, other evidence indicates that recently synthesized catecholamine is released preferentially, probably from the small vesicles.

DISPOSITION OF THE RELEASED CATECHOLAMINE

Reuptake. The relative constancy of catecholamine stores in adrenergic or dopaminergic neurons is a consequence not only of feedback regulation of synthesis but also of a remarkable ability to transport the amine back into these neurons. This "reuptake," which conserves a major portion of the released catecholamine, is achieved by a carrier (called uptake$_1$), located in the axonal membrane, that requires Na^+ and Cl^- and is thought to work as follows.[4,11]

In its free form the carrier moves about within the membrane. Attachment of Na^+ prevents movement. In a quiescent state most of the carrier molecules will be fixed at the extracellular surface where the Na^+ concentration is high. Binding of amine to the carrier-Na^+ complex restores mobility. There is then net movement of the carrier-Na^+-amine complex (with Cl^- as well) to regions of lesser concentration. Physiologically this mechanism is most important in moving norepinephrine back into the neuron, although it also contributes to leakage of transmitter from the neuron. Drugs interact with this mechanism in two ways. Cocaine, tricyclic antidepressants, ouabain, and even certain antihistamines attach to the carrier extracellularly but are not themselves transported. The carrier is then unable to transport norepinephrine and uptake is inhibited. Such agents enhance the potency of catecholamines. When so-called *indirectly acting* amines, such as tyramine and amphetamine, bind to the carrier, the complex traverses the axonal membrane. These agents not only inhibit uptake of norepinephrine, they also release norepinephrine by making more carrier available at the inner surface of the membrane. Consequently, more axoplasmic norepinephrine is transported into the neuroeffector junction, where it can stimulate receptors.

Several observations indicate the importance of uptake by nerves in termination of catecholamine action. Physiologic doses of tritiated norepinephrine are rapidly cleared from blood by organs that are innervated by adrenergic fibers. This uptake is into adrenergic fibers as demonstrated by in vitro histochemistry. Furthermore, subsequent sympathetic nerve stimulation or reserpine treatment releases tritiated catecholamine in vivo. Denervated organs take up only very small quantities of tritiated norepinephrine.

Some amines, such as metaraminol, that are taken up by the relatively nonspecific carrier are retained by the axon terminal and released on nerve stimulation, thereby acting as *false transmitters*. If the false transmitter is a relatively weak agonist, transmission may be impaired.

Despite the low specificity of the transport mechanism, the adrenergic neuron is protected from accumulation of numerous amines by the much greater specificity of the granular storage mechanism. Thus, when tyramine is taken up, it is not only deaminated by MAO but is also rejected by the granules, since only β-hydroxylated amines are stored. After MAO inhibition, however, tyramine is protected from deamination and is transformed by dopamine-β-hydroxylase into the β-hydroxy derivative *octopamine*. This amine, which is stored in the granules, acts as a false transmitter. Adrenergic nerve terminals can also take up injurious compounds such as 6-*hydroxydopamine* (see below).

Extraneuronal metabolism. The portion of released catecholamine that diffuses away and escapes reuptake by the neuronal amine carrier is metabolized, after transport into other cells by another carrier (uptake$_2$), by two enzymes: *catechol-O-methyltransferase* (COMT) and MAO.[16,24] The latter is widely distributed, not only in adrenergic axonal mitochondria, where it metabolizes cytoplasmic norepinephrine, but also in nonneural structures, particularly the liver and kidneys. MAO-A, the form primarily involved in metabolism of norepinephrine, is found in adrenergic neurons and adrenergic nuclei in the brain. MAO-B is localized to serotonergic neurons and astrocytes. COMT is also widely distributed but is concentrated in the liver and kidneys. Although the precise relationship of these enzymes to sympathetic function is not understood, it is clearly not so crucial as the acetylcholine-cholinesterase interdependence; inhibition of COMT does not significantly increase sympathetic activity or potentiate injected catecholamines. Similarly, drugs that inhibit MAO fail to potentiate endogenous catecholamines and do not enhance sympathetic functions in the periphery. These relationships are depicted in Fig. 13-7.

The detailed metabolic pathways of norepinephrine and epinephrine are shown in Fig. 13-8. MOPEG, metanephrine, and normetanephrine are excreted primarily as conjugates. The role of many of these pathways is inferred from data on urinary elimination of the metabolites; the proportions of norepinephrine metabolites have been estimated as follows[16]:

Normetanephrine	3%-5%
4-Hydroxy-3-methoxyphenyl(ethylene) glycol (MOPEG)	30%-40%
4-Hydroxy-3-methoxymandelic acid (VMA)	55%-65%

Fate of norepinephrine released from adrenergic nerve. 1, *Release and interaction with receptor on effector cell;* 2, *reuptake into the nerve of a portion of released norepinephrine;* 3, *metabolism by COMT and MAO;* 4, *metabolic degradation within the nerve by MAO of norepinephrine released within the axoplasm (as after ingestion of reserpine).* *FIG. 13-7*

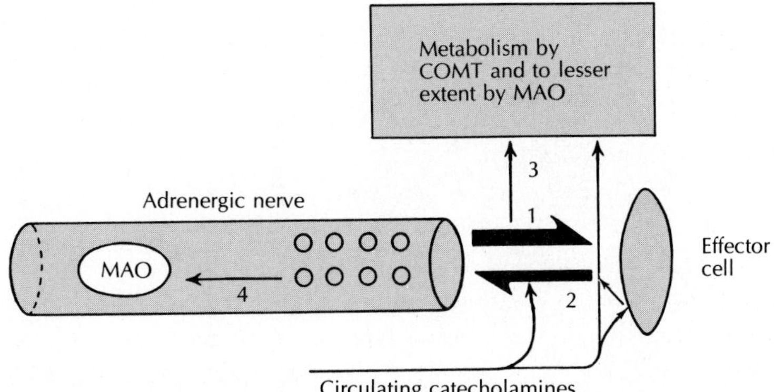

The 24-hour excretion of VMA in normal persons is about 3 mg. Much larger amounts may be eliminated by patients with adrenal medullary tumors (p. 148). Small amounts of unmetabolized catecholamines are also excreted. The particular pattern of metabolites in the urine depends on the source of amines, that is, neuronal, adrenal medullary, or exogenous.

CHEMICAL SYMPATHECTOMY: 6-HYDROXYDOPAMINE

The administration of 6-hydroxydopamine, an interesting experimental tool, causes an extremely long-lasting depletion of catecholamines from sympathetically innervated organs. Electron microscopic studies indicate that the drug selectively destroys adrenergic nerve terminals. In newborn animals the entire neuron is destroyed irreversibly, whereas in adults only terminals are affected and regeneration of the fibers is possible. Pretreatment with desipramine, an inhibitor of amine uptake, prevents damage.

Serotonin

In humans serotonin (5-hydroxytryptamine) is found in high concentrations in the enterochromaffin cells of the intestinal tract, in various brain regions, and in platelets. Several receptor subtypes have been described.[9] Daily excretion of 5-HIAA, a serotonin metabolite, may increase greatly in patients with malignancy of enterochromaffin cells. Serotonergic neurons contain MAO-B even though the amine is a better substrate for MAO-A. The amine is likely to have major central roles in sleep, modulation of nociceptive input, and in various psychologic states.

MISCELLANEOUS POTENTIAL NEUROTRANSMITTERS

In addition to the transmitters discussed above, many other compounds play a role in neuronal function,[21] although evidence for characterizing them as mediators of neurotransmission is often less than complete. The activity of an organ may be influenced by several neurotransmitters in addition to the classic agents.[23]

FIG. 13-8 *Pathways of metabolism of norepinephrine. Enzymes catalyzing various reactions are as follows:* 1, *mono-amine oxidase (MAO) and aldehyde dehydrogenase;* 2, *MAO and aldehyde reductase;* 3, *catechol-O-methyltransferase;* DOPEG, *3,4-dihydroxyphenyl(ethylene) glycol;* DOMA, *3,4-dihydroxymandelic acid;* MOPEG, MHPG, *4-hydroxy-3-methoxyphenyl(ethylene) glycol;* VMA, *vanillylmandelic acid, 4-hydroxy-3-methoxymandelic acid.*

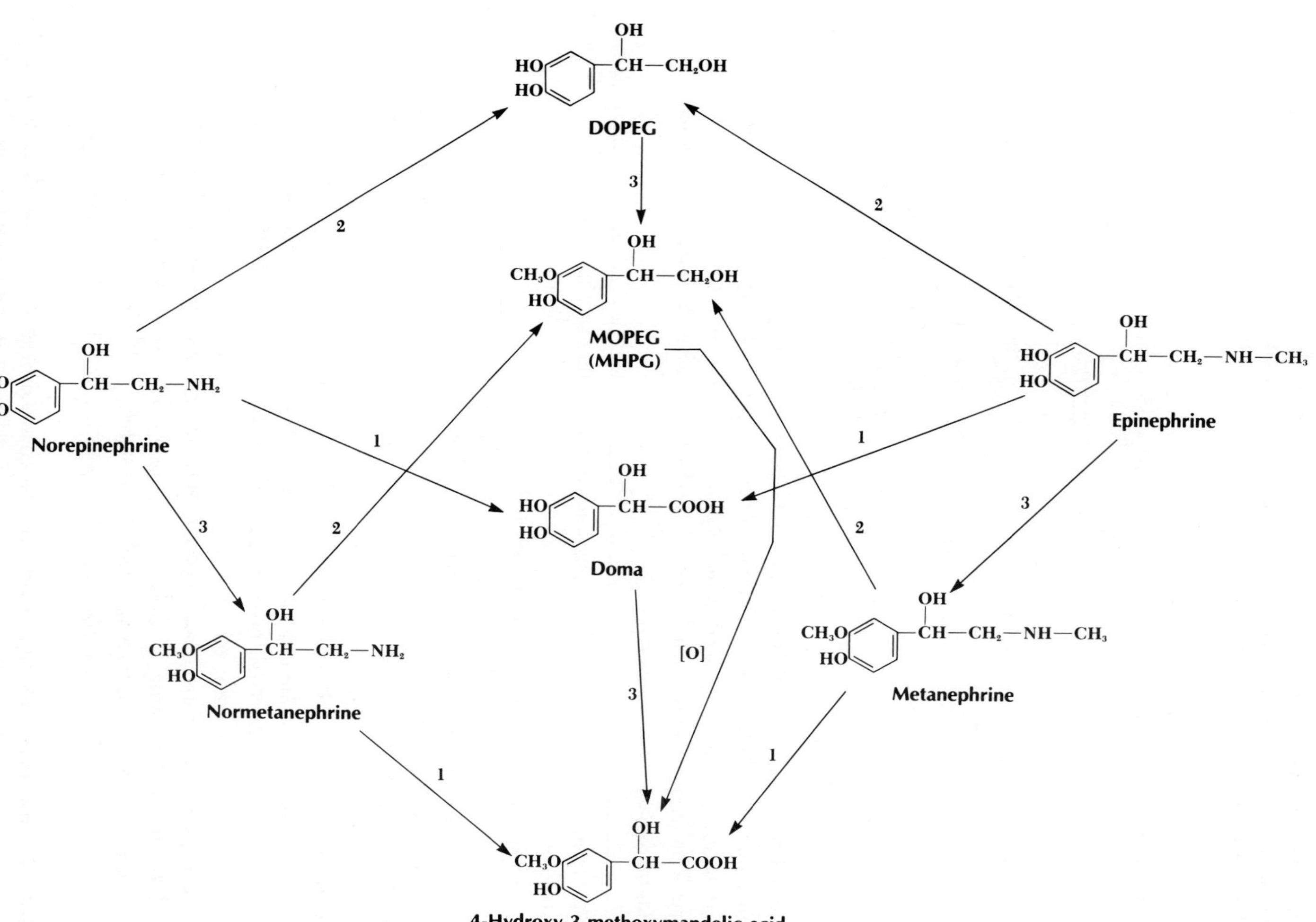

The hypothalamus contains relatively high concentrations of **histamine** along with serotonin and catecholamines. The brain can form histamine by decarboxylation of histidine and is rich in the methylating enzyme that inactivates the amine. The second messenger for H_1-receptors is the phosphoinositide system; that for H_2-receptors is adenylyl cyclase.

Glutamic and **aspartic acids** are remarkably potent in depolarizing nerve cells when applied by iontophoresis. Analogs of these acidic amino acids, *N*-methyl-*D*-aspartic acid (NMDA), quisqualic acid, and kainic acid, are relatively selective agonists at three distinct receptors associated with neuronal cation channels. Currently, there is interest in the potential benefit of NMDA-receptor antagonists in minimizing brain damage that may occur during ischemia, secondary to accumulation of excitatory amino acids.[1]

Glycine is a major inhibitory transmitter in the spinal cord; its receptor is a Cl^- channel. This simple amino acid hyperpolarizes motoneurons. Since strychnine antagonizes the naturally occurring inhibitory transmitter released from Renshaw cells onto motoneurons, the possible relationship between the alkaloid and glycine was of great interest. Antagonism of the hyperpolarizing effect of glycine by strychnine, applied by microelectrophoresis, has been clearly demonstrated.

γ-Aminobutyric acid (GABA) is now believed to be the primary inhibitory neurotransmitter in the brain. It is formed by decarboxylation of glutamic acid and is destroyed by transamination. The $GABA_A$ receptor is a Cl^- channel, whereas the $GABA_B$ receptor governs K^+ and Ca^{++} channels via G proteins.

$$HOOC{-}\underset{\displaystyle |}{\overset{NH_2}{CH}}{-}CH_2{-}CH_2{-}COOH \qquad H_2N{-}CH_2{-}CH_2{-}CH_2{-}COOH$$

Glutamic acid | **γ-Aminobutyric acid**

Adenosine is formed extracellularly, from ATP and related nucleotides, or released from cells when the cytoplasmic concentration increases during stress. Activation of presynaptic A_1-adenosine receptors decreases release of several neurotransmitters. Both A_1- and A_2-receptors, which are usually postsynaptic, are coupled to G proteins.[28] Caffeine and other methylxanthines (see Chapter 31) appear to cause many of their effects by competitively blocking the action of adenosine.

Several **peptides** are implicated as important transmitters or neuromodulators in the central nervous system.[17] Much of the impetus in this area was provided by discoveries with the opioid peptides (see Chapters 24 and 33). Immunocytochemical studies have shown that spinal ganglia and the spinal cord contain substance P, somatostatin, cholecystokinin, and other peptides. Substance P appears to be a sensory neurotransmitter with an important role in nociception. Capsaicin, obtained from red pepper, depletes substance P from the spinal cord and elevates the threshold to painful stimuli.

Autonomic and related drugs

Classification by site of action and mode of action

- I. Drugs acting on autonomic receptors in end organs
  - A. Agonists mimicking postganglionic transmitters
    - 1. Cholinergic drugs (parasympathomimetics)
      - a. Direct action on effector cell (effective after denervation)—acetylcholine, pilocarpine
      - b. Indirect action (potentiate endogenous ACh; ineffective after denervation)
        - (1) Competitive cholinesterase inhibitors—physostigmine
        - (2) Noncompetitive cholinesterase inhibitors—isoflurophate (DFP) (enzyme reactivated by pralidoxime)
    - 2. Adrenergic drugs (sympathomimetics)
      - a. Direct action on effector cell (effective after denervation)—norepinephrine, epinephrine, isoproterenol
      - b. Indirect action (release norepinephrine from adrenergic nerve endings; ineffective peripherally after denervation)—tyramine, amphetamine
      - c. Mixed action (direct and indirect)—ephedrine, metaraminol
  - B. Antagonists acting on end-organ receptors
    - 1. Cholinergic receptor antagonists (cholinergic blocking drugs)
      - a. Competitive antagonists at muscarinic receptors—atropine
    - 2. Adrenergic receptor antagonists (adrenergic blocking drugs)
      - a. Antagonize at α-adrenergic receptors
        - (1) Competitive—phentolamine
        - (2) Noncompetitive—phenoxybenzamine
      - b. Antagonize at β-adrenergic receptors
        - (1) Competitive—propranolol
- II. Drugs acting on autonomic nerve endings
  - A. Agonists that cause the release of transmitters
    - 1. Cholinergic neurons—carbachol
    - 2. Adrenergic neurons—indirect and mixed acting sympathomimetics
  - B. Drugs that inhibit the release of transmitters
    - 1. Cholinergic neurons—botulinum toxin
    - 2. Adrenergic neurons—bretylium, guanethidine
  - C. Drugs that inhibit the synthesis of transmitters
    - 1. Cholinergic neurons (inhibits synthesis of ACh)—hemicholinium
    - 2. Adrenergic neurons (deplete norepinephrine)—metyrosine
  - D. Drugs that inhibit the storage of transmitters in neurons
    - 1. Cholinergic neurons—vesamicol
    - 2. Adrenergic neurons (deplete norepinephrine)—reserpine, guanethidine
  - E. Drugs that cause the formation of false transmitters in neurons
    - 1. Cholinergic neurons—none
    - 2. Adrenergic neurons—methyldopa, metaraminol
  - F. Drugs that inhibit the uptake of transmitters into neurons
    - 1. Cholinergic neurons—none
    - 2. Adrenergic neurons—cocaine, tricyclic antidepressants
- III. Drugs acting on autonomic ganglia
  - A. Agonists that stimulate postganglionic neurons ("nicotinic" stimulants)
    - 1. Both cholinergic and adrenergic neurons—nicotine
  - B. Antagonists that inhibit nicotinic receptors on postganglionic neurons
    - 1. Both cholinergic and adrenergic neurons (competitive antagonists)—hexamethonium, mecamylamine

Nonautonomic drugs

- I. Drugs acting on the skeletal muscle neuromuscular junction
  - A. Agonists mimicking the motor nerve transmitter acetylcholine
    - 1. Direct action on muscle cell—neostigmine
    - 2. Indirect action (cholinesterase inhibitors)
      - a. Competitive—neostigmine, physostigmine
      - b. Noncompetitive—isoflurophate
  - B. Antagonists that block skeletal muscle receptors
    - 1. Depolarizing—succinylcholine
    - 2. Nondepolarizing (competitive)—tubocurarine
- II. Drugs acting on sensory nerve endings
  - A. "Sensitize" stretch receptors monitoring blood pressure—Veratrum alkaloids
- III. Drugs acting on all nerves to block conduction of action potentials
  - A. Local anesthetics
- IV. Drugs acting on vascular smooth muscle
  - A. Vasoconstrictors—angiotensin, vasopressin
  - B. Vasodilators—nitrites, papaverine
  - C. Antihypertensive drugs—hydralazine, diazoxide
- V. Other endogenous biologically active compounds
  - A. Serotonin, histamine, bradykinin, prostaglandins, adenosine, peptides, etc.

CLASSIFICATION OF NEUROPHARMACOLOGIC AGENTS

A rational classification of neuropharmacologic agents should be based on their site and mode of action, reflecting drug-receptor interactions. This can be done satisfactorily for drugs acting on autonomic end organs, nerve endings, and ganglia and at skeletal neuromuscular junctions. There are agonists and antagonists or drugs that promote or inhibit the release of neurotransmitters at each site.

REFERENCES

1. Albers GW: Potential therapeutic uses of *N*-methyl-D-aspartate antagonists in cerebral ischemia, *Clin Neuropharmacol* 13:177, 1990.
2. Angus JA, Cocks TM: Endothelium-derived relaxing factor, *Pharmacol Ther* 41:303, 1989.
3. Axelrod J: The metabolism of catecholamines *in vivo* and *in vitro*, *Pharmacol Rev* 11:402, 1959.
4. Bönisch H, Trendelenburg U: The mechanism of action of indirectly acting sympathomimetic amines, *Handb Exp Pharmacol* 90/I:247, 1988.
5. Brodie BB, Spector S, Shore PA: Interaction of drugs with norepinephrine in the brain, *Pharmacol Rev* 11:548, 1959.
6. Cannon WB, Uridil JE: Studies on the conditions of activity in endocrine glands. VIII. Some effects on the denervated heart of stimulating the nerves of the liver, *Am J Physiol* 58:353, 1921.
7. Dale HH: The action of certain esters and ethers of choline, and their relation to muscarine, *J Pharmacol Exp Ther* 6:147, 1914.
8. Fatt P, Katz B: Spontaneous subthreshold activity at motor nerve endings, *J Physiol (Lond)* 117:109, 1952.
9. Frazer A, Maayani S, Wolfe BB: Subtypes of receptors for serotonin, *Annu Rev Pharmacol Toxicol* 30:307, 1990.
10. Goyal RK: Muscarinic receptor subtypes: physiology and clinical implications, *N Engl J Med* 321:1022, 1989.
11. Graefe K-H, Bönisch H: The transport of amines across the axonal membranes of noradrenergic and dopaminergic neurones, *Handb Exp Pharmacol* 90/I:193, 1988.
12. Hausdorff WP, Caron MG, Lefkowitz RJ:

Turning off the signal: desensitization of β-adrenergic receptor function, *FASEB J* 4:2881, 1990.

13. Hökfelt T, Millhorn D, Seroogy K, et al: Coexistence of peptides with classical neurotransmitters. In Polak JM, editor: *Regulatory peptides*, Basel, 1989, Birkhäuser Verlag, p 154.
14. Johnson SM, Fleming WW: Mechanisms of cellular adaptive sensitivity changes: applications to opioid tolerance and dependence, *Pharmacol Rev* 41:435, 1989.
15. Katz B, Miledi R: Propagation of electric activity in motor nerve terminals, *Proc R Soc Lond [Biol]* 161:453, 1965.
16. Kopin IJ: Catecholamine metabolism: basic aspects and clinical significance, *Pharmacol Rev* 37:333, 1985.
17. Kow L-M, Pfaff DW: Neuromodulatory actions of peptides, *Annu Rev Pharmacol Toxicol* 28:163, 1988.
18. Loewi O: Über humorale Ubertragbarkeit der Herznervenwirkung, *Pflugers Arch Ges Physiol* 189:239, 1921.
19. Maelicke A: Structure and function of the nicotinic acetylcholine receptor, *Handb Exp Pharmacol* 86:267, 1988.
20. Masserano JM, Vulliet PR, Tank AW, Weiner N: The role of tyrosine hydroxylase in the regulation of catecholamine synthesis, *Handb Exp Pharmacol* 90/II:427, 1989.
21. Nicoll RA, Malenka RC, Kauer JA: Functional comparison of neurotransmitter receptor subtypes in mammalian central nervous system, *Physiol Rev* 70:513, 1990.
22. Silinsky EM: The biophysical pharmacology of calcium-dependent acetylcholine secretion, *Pharmacol Rev* 37:81, 1985.
23. Taylor GS, Bywater RAR: Novel autonomic neurotransmitters and intestinal function, *Pharmacol Ther* 40:401, 1989.
24. Trendelenberg U: The extraneuronal uptake and metabolism of catecholamines, *Handb Exp Pharmacol* 90/I:279, 1988.
25. Tuček S: Choline acetyltransferase and the synthesis of acetylcholine, *Handb Exp Pharmacol* 86:125, 1988.
26. Van der Kloot W: Acetylcholine quanta are released from vesicles by exocytosis (and why some think not), *Neuroscience* 24:1, 1988.
27. von Euler US: *Noradrenaline: chemistry, physiology, pharmacology and clinical aspects*, Springfield, Ill, 1956, Charles C Thomas, Publisher.
28. White TD: Role of adenine compounds in autonomic neurotransmission, *Pharmacol Ther* 38:129, 1988.
29. Winkler H: Occurrence and mechanism of exocytosis in adrenal medulla and sympathetic nerve, *Handb Exp Pharmacol* 90/I:43, 1988.

Chapter 14

Cholinergic drugs

Cholinergic agents can be divided into two major groups: directly acting cholinergic agonists and indirectly acting agents that inhibit cholinesterase (anticholinesterases).

DIRECTLY ACTING CHOLINERGIC AGONISTS

Choline esters

Although acetylcholine is essential for normal neural control of function of many organs in the body, two characteristics render it unsuitable as a drug. First, its action is very brief, even when it is injected intravenously, because of rapid destruction by ubiquitous cholinesterases. Second, it causes such diverse effects that no selective therapeutic endpoint is possible. Derivatives of acetylcholine, however, are more resistant to the action of cholinesterases and may exhibit greater selectivity in their sites of action.

From the acetylcholine-cholinesterase interaction depicted in Fig. 14-1, it is apparent that changes in the structure of the ester should alter its union with the enzyme. Relatively slight modifications can reduce or prevent hydrolysis of the molecule but still allow the ester to stimulate cholinergic receptors. Agents in this category are as follows:

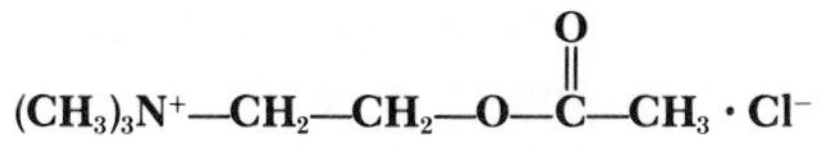

$$(CH_3)_3N^+{-}CH_2{-}CH_2{-}O{-}\overset{\overset{\displaystyle O}{\|}}{C}{-}CH_3 \cdot Cl^-$$

Acetylcholine chloride

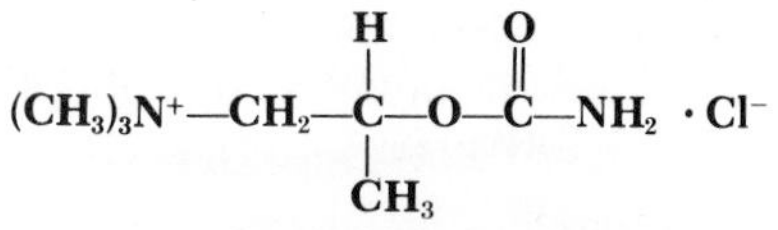

$$(CH_3)_3N^+{-}CH_2{-}\underset{\underset{\displaystyle CH_3}{|}}{\overset{\overset{\displaystyle H}{|}}{C}}{-}O{-}\overset{\overset{\displaystyle O}{\|}}{C}{-}NH_2 \cdot Cl^-$$

Bethanechol chloride

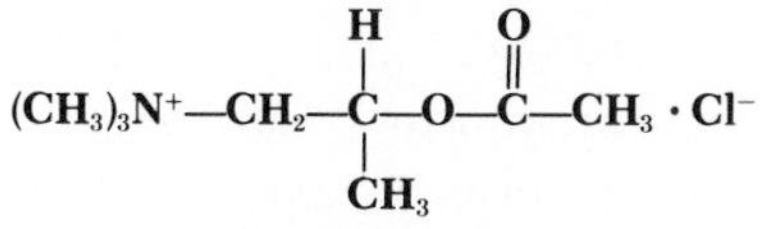

$$(CH_3)_3N^+{-}CH_2{-}\underset{\underset{\displaystyle CH_3}{|}}{\overset{\overset{\displaystyle H}{|}}{C}}{-}O{-}\overset{\overset{\displaystyle O}{\|}}{C}{-}CH_3 \cdot Cl^-$$

Methacholine chloride

$$(CH_3)_3N^+{-}CH_2{-}CH_2{-}O{-}\overset{\overset{\displaystyle O}{\|}}{C}{-}NH_2 \cdot Cl^-$$

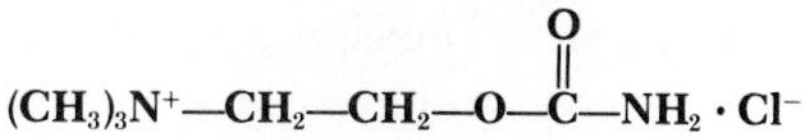

Carbachol chloride

All drugs in this group are quaternary amines. Substitution on the β carbon, as in acetyl-β-methylcholine (methacholine), protects preferentially against the action of nonspecific cholinesterase. Because methacholine is an acetyl ester, it is still hydrolyzed by acetylcholinesterase, although more slowly than acetylcholine. Replacement of the acetyl group by carbamate protects the drug (bethanechol or carbachol) from both types of cholinesterase.

Bethanechol and methacholine act like acetylcholine on smooth muscles and exocrine glands without significantly affecting ganglionic and skeletal neuromuscular transmission. Methacholine chloride (Provocholine, 100 mg in 5 ml vial) is available, as

FIG. 14-1 *Interaction of acetylcholine and acetylcholinesterase. The quaternary nitrogen of acetylcholine forms an ionic bond with the negatively charged anionic site, and the other portion of the molecule covalently acetylates a serine residue, G, at the* esteratic site. *After initial hydrolysis of choline from the molecule, the acetate in turn is rapidly hydrolyzed from the enzyme.*

From Wilson IB: Neurology 8(suppl 1):41, 1958.

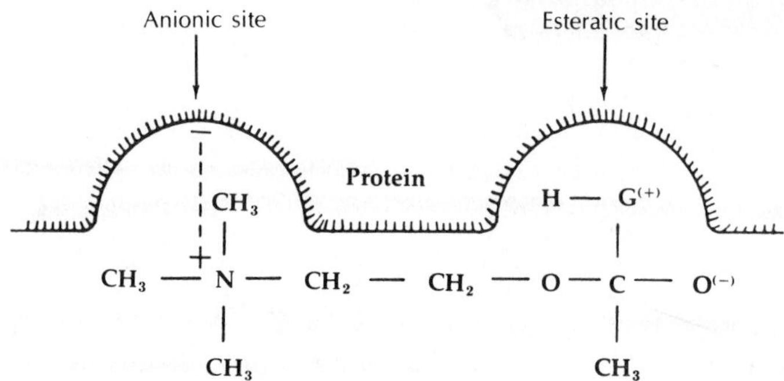

a powder for reconstitution and administration with a nebulizer, as a provocative test for asthma when the disorder is not otherwise apparent. Its use requires caution and is best reserved for specialists.

Bethanechol chloride (Urecholine, others) relatively selectively affects the gastrointestinal and urinary tracts and is the cholinergic drug of choice for treatment of postoperative, postpartum, or neurogenic urinary retention. It has also been used to relieve reflux esophagitis and postoperative abdominal distention. The cholinergic side effects include sweating, cutaneous vasodilatation with flushing, salivation, nausea, vomiting, and diarrhea. There are variable changes in heart rate and blood pressure. There may be a precipitous fall in blood pressure of some persons, whereas in others, alterations in pressure and heart rate are slight because of more effective compensatory reflexes. It must be remembered that asthmatic patients are particularly susceptible to the bronchoconstrictor action of these compounds.

Contraindications to the use of bethanechol include asthma, peptic ulcer, parkinsonism, pregnancy, severe cardiac disease, hyperthyroidism (wherein atrial fibrillation may occur), and mechanical obstruction or impairment of the structural integrity of the gastrointestinal or urinary tracts. These contraindications generally apply to all the cholinergic agents discussed in this chapter. Preparations include tablets of 5 to 50 mg and a solution for subcutaneous injection, 5 mg/ml. The recommended dosage for adults is 10 to 50 mg by mouth or 2.5 to 5 mg by subcutaneous injection three or four times daily, but rarely more frequent or larger doses may be necessary.

Carbachol (Isopto Carbachol) is a very potent choline ester with both muscarinic and nicotinic activity. Its only uses at present are in open-angle glaucoma and after cataract surgery to reduce intraocular pressure and cause miosis. Solutions of 0.75% to 3%, 1 or 2 drops, are applied to the conjunctiva at 6- to 8-hour intervals. A very dilute solution (Miostat, 0.01%) may also be instilled into the anterior chamber of the eye to induce miosis after cataract removal. Acetylcholine chloride (Miochol, 20 mg for reconstitution in a volume of 2 ml) is also used for this purpose.

FIG. 14-2

Effect of acetylcholine on blood pressure before and after atropine. The following drugs were administered intravenously to a dog that was anesthetized with pentobarbital: A, *acetylcholine, 10 μg/kg; between* A *and* B, *atropine, 1 mg/kg;* B, *acetylcholine, 10 μg/kg;* C, *acetylcholine, 100 μg/kg; between* C *and* D, *phentolamine, 5 mg/kg;* D, *acetylcholine, 100 μg/kg. Notice that atropine prevented the decrease in blood pressure in response to the low dose of acetylcholine. The larger dose of acetylcholine then increased blood pressure because of its nicotinic action in ganglia. This hypertensive response was blocked by phentolamine, an α-adrenergic blocking agent.*

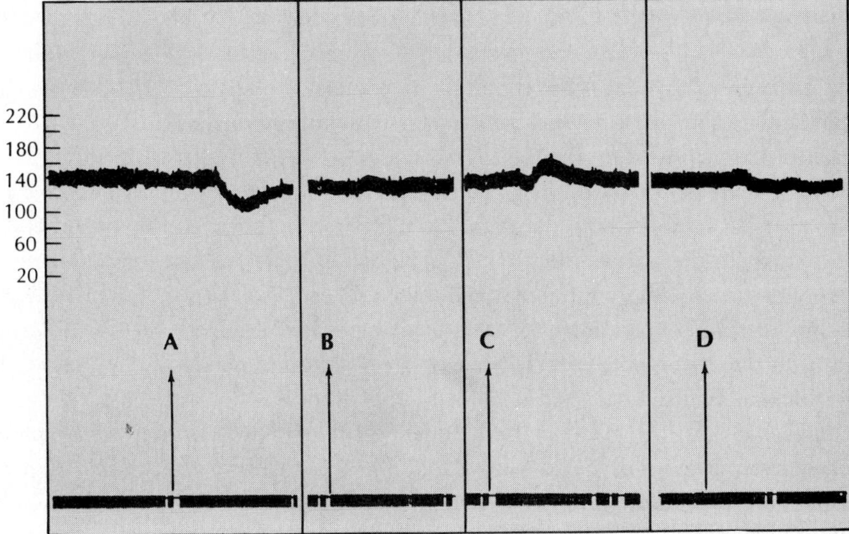

The muscarinic and nicotinic actions of choline esters can be illustrated by a simple experiment. Fig. 14-2 shows the effect of acetylcholine injection on the blood pressure of a dog before and after atropine administration.

Pilocarpine and muscarine

The alkaloids pilocarpine and muscarine have the curious property of acting like acetylcholine on receptors of smooth muscles, exocrine glands, and heart. A small amount of muscarine is present in the mushroom *Amanita muscaria*, hence its name, but much higher concentrations are found in other toxic mushrooms, such as *Inocybe* and *Clitocybe* species.[2] Pilocarpine is found in the leaves of the plant *Pilocarpus jaborandi*.

HO, H_3C, O, $CH_2—N^+(CH_3)_3$

Muscarine

H_5C_2, CH_2, CH_3, N, N, O, O

Pilocarpine

Both alkaloids elicit the so-called muscarinic effects of acetylcholine without having significant nicotinic action. Atropine blocks these muscarinic effects. It is not surprising that muscarine, a quaternary ammonium compound, shows some similarity to acetylcholine, but it is puzzling why pilocarpine, a tertiary amine, should also be similar. It is well established, however, that this is not the result of cholinesterase inhibition.

Of these two agents, muscarine has only historic and toxicologic interest. However, **pilocarpine hydrochloride** (Isopto Carpine, others; 0.25% to 10%) or nitrate (Pilagan, 1% to 4%) is employed in ophthalmology to reverse the effects of mydriatic and cycloplegic agents and is the cholinergic agent most often used to lower intraocular pressure in glaucoma.[11] Contraction of the ciliary muscle by cholinergic drugs is believed to enhance outflow of aqueous humor from the anterior chamber of the eye (Table 14-1) by improving flow through the trabecular network.[5,11] Ciliary muscle contraction can also cause myopia in younger patients and is thought responsible for headaches that may be a problem early in therapy.

In open-angle glaucoma pilocarpine is commonly taken every 6 to 8 hours as drops, initially in a 1% solution; both duration and effect can be enhanced by eyelid closure and occlusion of the nasolacrimal duct during administration. Concentrations above 4% are not usually more effective but increase the likelihood of toxicity.[5] Two controlled-release preparations are also available. One (Ocusert Pilo-20 or -40) is placed into the conjunctival sac for release of pilocarpine over a 7-day period. The other (Pilopine HS) is a gel used once daily at bedtime.

Acute angle-closure glaucoma is a much more serious disorder in which the trabecular network is obstructed by the iris. The miotic effect of a weak cholinergic drug can be useful as an emergency measure to relieve the obstruction until iridectomy can be performed. However, too much drug may increase intraocular pressure if ciliary muscle contraction allows excessive bulging of the lens into the anterior chamber.[13] Application of a drop of 2% pilocarpine four times at 5-minute intervals and then once every 3 hours should be maximally effective, with minimal toxicity,[5] if intraocular pressure is not more than 50 to 60 mm Hg. At higher pressures the iris becomes ischemic and pilocarpine is ineffective. The miotic response should return if the pressure is first reduced by other agents, often used in combination; these include osmotic diuretics and acetazolamide, a carbonic anhydrase inhibitor, and topical β-adrenergic receptor antagonists.[13]

Pilocarpine has also been used to promote salivation in patients with dryness of the mouth after radiation therapy for head or neck cancer.

TABLE 14-1 Pharmacologic approaches to chronic management of open-angle glaucoma

Drug or class	Likely mechanism
Muscarinic agonists, anticholinesterases	Improved drainage of aqueous humor
Epinephrine	Improved drainage of aqueous humor
β-Adrenergic antagonists	Decreased formation of aqueous humor
Carbonic anhydrase inhibitors	Decreased formation of aqueous humor

PROBLEM 14-1. The fixed dilated pupil may be an ominous sign caused by involvement of the third nerve in an intracranial disease. How can this be distinguished from accidental application to the eye of an anticholinergic drug? Topical application of pilocarpine can be used to establish the diagnosis.[15] The pupil responds well to pilocarpine in the case of nerve damage, whereas it is unresponsive if dilatation is caused by application of a muscarinic antagonist. Could an anticholinesterase such as physostigmine be substituted for pilocarpine in this diagnostic test?

ANTICHOLINESTERASES

Some drugs enhance cholinergic transmission indirectly by inhibiting destruction of acetylcholine, thereby increasing and prolonging its effects. Cholinesterase inhibitors are useful in management of glaucoma and, especially, myasthenia gravis (Table 14-2). This group of compounds also includes some of our most potent insecticides and several chemical warfare agents.

Whereas moderate decreases of acetylcholinesterase may have little physiologic consequence, a severe reduction in the brain can be lethal. In contrast, plasma cholinesterase can be reduced to very low levels without important consequences, and the physiologic role of this esterase is unknown. Nevertheless, it is important in metabolism of exogenous acetylcholine, the neuromuscular blocker succinylcholine (see p. 134), and local anesthetics of the ester type (see Chapter 37). Plasma cholinesterase activity may be reduced by liver disease or by previous administration of anticholinesterases. Measurements of this activity are used in industrial medicine to evaluate the extent of exposure to anticholinesterases, thus minimizing risk of poisoning.

Reversible anticholinesterases

Physostigmine and neostigmine, like acetylcholine, are esters that bind to cholinesterases. However, they are more slowly hydrolyzed from the enzyme, which is

TABLE 14-2 Anticholinestrase preparations

Drug	Preparations*	Usual route of administration
For glaucoma		
Demecarium bromide (Humorsol)	S:0.125, 0.25%	Topical
Echothiophate (Phospholine) iodide	P:1.5-12.5 mg	Topical
Isoflurophate (Floropryl)	O:0.025%	Topical
Physostigmine salicylate (Isopto Eserine)	S:0.25, 0.5%	Topical
Physostigmine (Eserine) sulfate	O:0.25%	Topical
For myasthenia gravis		
Ambenonium chloride (Mytelase)	T:10 mg	Oral
Edrophonium chloride (Tensilon, others)	I:10 mg/ml	Intravenous, intramuscular
Neostigmine bromide (Prostigmin)	T:15 mg	Oral
Neostigmine methylsulfate (Prostigmin)	I:0.25-1.0 mg/ml	Intravenous, intramuscular, subcutaneous
Pyridostigmine bromide (Mestinon)	T:60, 180 mg	Oral
	Sy:60 mg/5 ml	Oral
(Mestinon, Regonol)	I:5 mg/ml	Intravenous, intramuscular

**I*, Injectable; *O*, ointment; *P*, powder for reconstitution to 0.03% to 0.25%; *S*, ophthalmic solution; *Sy*, syrup; *T*, tablet.

unavailable to inactivate acetylcholine so long as the inhibitor remains attached. Physostigmine is a tertiary amine used to lower intraocular pressure and as an antidote to poisoning with atropine-like drugs. Neostigmine is a quaternary ammonium compound used to treat myasthenia gravis, to reverse skeletal muscle paralysis caused by curare-like drugs, and as a urinary tract stimulant.

Physostigmine, an alkaloid obtained from seeds of the calabar or ordeal bean *Physostigma venenosum*, has been familiar to pharmacologists since the latter part of the nineteenth century. In 1934 the British physician, Mary Walker, successfully used physostigmine to treat myasthenia gravis because of the clinical similarity of this disease to a curarized state. Synthesis of compounds related to physostigmine led to development of neostigmine in 1931.

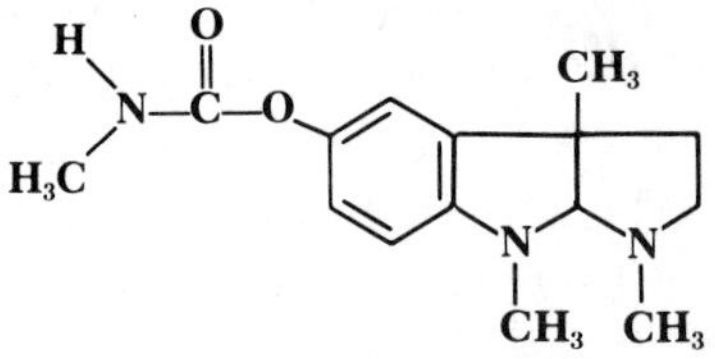

Physostigmine

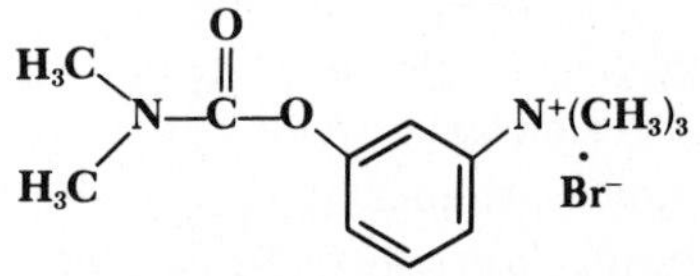

Neostigmine bromide

PHYSOSTIGMINE

The effects of physostigmine are attributable solely to cholinesterase inhibition, on the basis of the following considerations. The drug inhibits cholinesterase in vitro. Its affinity for the enzyme is about 10,000 times greater than that of acetylcholine. It has a potent action on structures with normal innervation because it protects released acetylcholine, but it does not act on denervated pupils or on denervated skeletal muscle, even when given by local intra-arterial injection. After combination with the enzyme, physostigmine is first hydrolyzed to leave a carbamyl group covalently attached to the enzyme. As this group is gradually hydrolyzed from the enzyme, activity is restored. Consequently, the drug is a reversible inhibitor of the cholinesterases.

Physostigmine salicylate (Antilirium, 1 mg/ml) injection or infusion, the specific antidote for anticholinergic intoxication, can be added to supportive management of poisoning by atropine and perhaps other agents that have appreciable anticholinergic activity. However, this antidote should be reserved for severe intoxications and must be given carefully to avoid seizures, excessive cardiac slowing, or other manifestations of cholinergic over-stimulation.[7] Physostigmine can also be used to treat primary open-angle glaucoma, although pilocarpine is preferred.

NEOSTIGMINE AND RELATED COMPOUNDS

Some effects of neostigmine are caused solely by cholinesterase inhibition, whereas others result from a combination of enzyme inhibition plus a direct acetylcholine-like action. Neostigmine, like physostigmine, produces no pupillary constriction in the denervated eye. On the other hand, intra-arterially injected neostigmine will stimulate the neuromuscular junction even after the nerves have degenerated and all cholinesterase has been destroyed. This evidence indicates that muscarinic effects of neostigmine are due to cholinesterase inhibition, whereas the nicotinic effect at the neuromuscular site is in part caused by direct stimulation.

Intramuscular or subcutaneous injection of 0.5 to 1 mg of **neostigmine methylsulfate** into a normal human will elicit common cholinergic effects. Intestinal contractions and contraction of smooth muscle of the urinary bladder can alleviate postoperative abdominal distention or urinary retention. Other responses may include elevation of skin temperature, sweating, salivation, slowing of the heart rate with possible hypotension, and skeletal muscle fasciculations. Atropine will inhibit the muscarinic, but not the nicotinic, effects of neostigmine. *As a general rule, atropine pretreatment or simultaneous parenteral administration is recommended whenever cholinergic drugs are injected for their* nicotinic *effects* (for example, to reverse paralysis induced by a nondepolarizing neuromuscular blocking agent), to avoid unnecessary and potentially dangerous muscarinic effects. *When cholinergic agents are injected for their* muscarinic *effects* (for instance, to relieve urinary retention), *a syringe containing a muscarinic antagonist should be available* as a precaution against overdose.

For chronic therapy, **neostigmine bromide** is given several times daily. An oral dose of 15 to 30 mg, sometimes as often as every 3 hours, is necessary because much of the drug is inactivated in the gastrointestinal tract. Absorption may be quite variable, and untoward reactions will occur if too much is suddenly absorbed.

Neostigmine substitutes. **Pyridostigmine bromide** is used in chronic management of myasthenia gravis and may be preferred by patients. Its duration of action is 3 to 6 hours. Sustained-release tablets containing 180 mg are available for administration at bedtime. Preparations for injection can be used to treat acute myasthenia gravis or to reverse paralysis caused by nondepolarizing neuromuscular antagonists. Rarely, bromide intoxication has been reported.[14]

Ambenonium is also used to treat myasthenia gravis. Its duration of action is 3 to 8 hours.

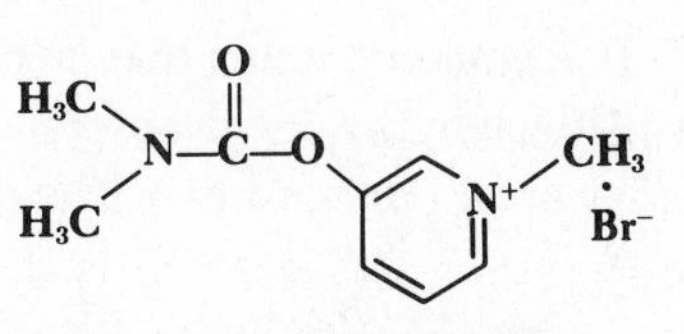

H_3C, H_3C, N—C(=O)—O, N^+, CH_3, Br^-

Pyridostigmine bromide

NH—CH_2CH_2—N^+(C_2H_5)(C_2H_5)—CH_2—(Cl-phenyl); C=O; C=O; NH—CH_2CH_2—N^+(C_2H_5)(C_2H_5)—CH_2—(Cl-phenyl) · 2 Cl^-

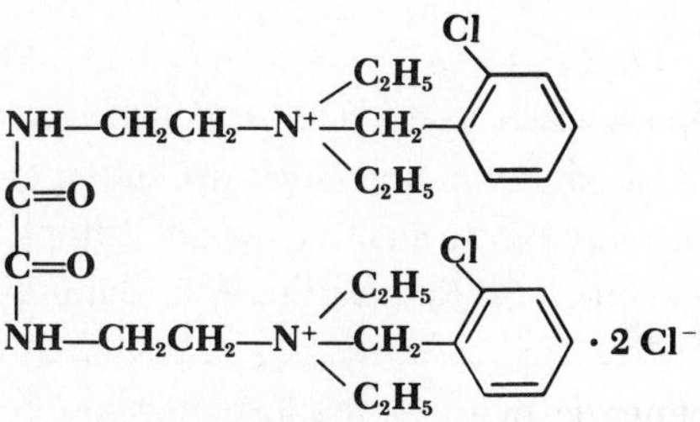

Ambenonium chloride

Demecarium is applied twice daily or less often for management of open-angle glaucoma. Minimally effective dosage is necessary to limit local and systemic reactions.

EDROPHONIUM

Edrophonium differs structurally from neostigmine primarily in not being an ester. It does not bind covalently to the enzyme, and the action of a typical intravenous dose lasts only 5 to 10 minutes in a normal subject. Although edrophonium was introduced as an antagonist of neuromuscular blockade by agents such as tubocurarine, it is especially useful as a diagnostic and investigative tool in myasthenia. In an untreated myasthenic patient, intravenous injection of 2 mg of edrophonium may cause a rapid but transient increase in muscular strength. If there is no immediate improvement, after a brief pause an 8 mg dose is given. This test may be used for diagnostic purposes and also to assess the status of therapy. Because myasthenia is a disorder of nicotinic receptors, either too little or too much neurotransmitter can cause weakness. Extreme cases have been termed *myasthenic crisis* and *cholinergic crisis* respectively. In the latter there are likely to be muscarinic indications of intoxication as well. The physician may be uncertain whether to increase or to decrease the dosage of neostigmine for a myasthenic patient. If edrophonium improves strength, it is likely that previous therapy was inadequate. On the other hand, if the reaction to this "edrophonium test" is unfavorable, indicative of overtreatment, a reduction in neostigmine dosage should be beneficial. The action of edrophonium in this test usually lasts only a few minutes. If the patient is in crisis with respiratory difficulty, measures to normalize respiration, such as assisted ventilation, must be instituted first, and the dose of edrophonium is reduced to 1 mg, given twice if necessary with a 1-minute interval. An alternative diagnostic approach is simply to stop anticholinesterase medication while beginning mechanical ventilation. If respiration improves spontaneously, the patient was receiving too much drug; if respiration does not improve, therapy can be reinstituted at a higher dosage.

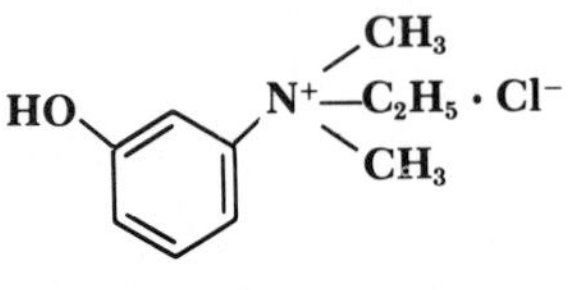

HO–C₆H₄–$N^+(CH_3)_2(C_2H_5) \cdot Cl^-$

Edrophonium chloride

Edrophonium is an effective antidote to curare. It acts more rapidly than neostigmine, but multiple injections are often needed. Although the mechanism is not understood, an intravenous bolus of edrophonium has been proposed as a diagnostic test to elicit chest pain arising from the esophagus.[12]

Irreversible organophosphorus anticholinesterases

Isoflurophate (diisopropyl fluorophosphate, DFP) and a variety of other organophosphates are highly toxic compounds that irreversibly inactivate cholinesterases. They were developed as chemical warfare agents and have had some therapeutic application, but their principal interest is toxicologic because of widespread use as insecticides. Except for echothiophate, most of these compounds are highly lipid soluble, can be absorbed through the skin as well as after inhalation or ingestion, and readily enter the central nervous system.

The structural formulas of some of the organophosphorus compounds are as follows:

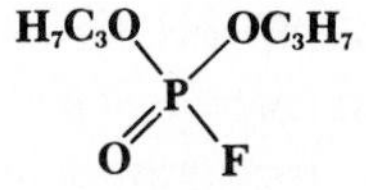

Isoflurophate

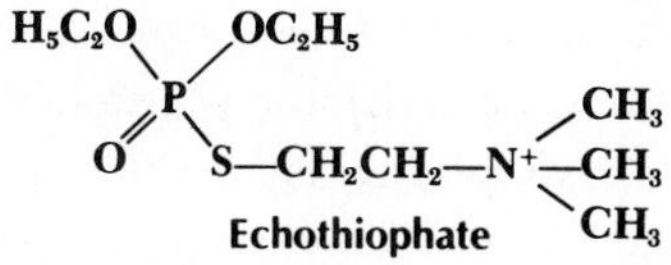

Echothiophate

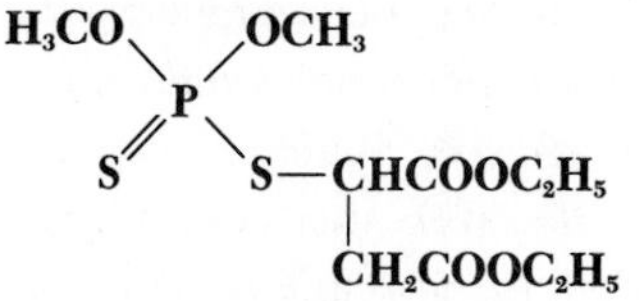

Malathion

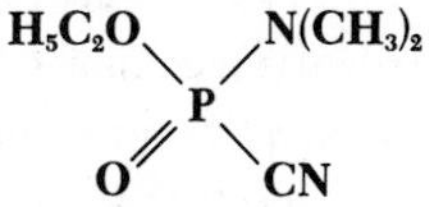

Tabun

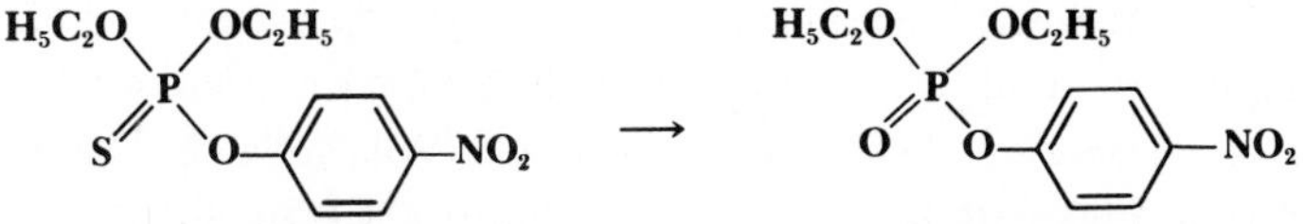

Parathion → Paraoxon

Whereas reversible anticholinesterases depress enzymatic activity up to a few hours after a single administration, the effect of organophosphates may persist for weeks or months. When the organophosphorus compounds combine with cholinesterase, the enzyme becomes permanently phosphorylated and is inactive against acetylcholine. As a consequence, enzymatic activity is reduced until new enzyme can be synthesized, unless a reactivator of cholinesterase is employed as an antidote. Although the acetylcholinesterase in red blood cells has no obvious physiologic role, its measurement can be used to assess the severity of anticholinesterase intoxication.[1] Regeneration of activity in red blood cells after administration of an irreversible anticholinesterase is directly proportional to production of new cells.

Medical uses of organophosphates

Isoflurophate and **echothiophate** are used to treat open-angle glaucoma mainly because their prolonged action improves compliance. Echothiophate, the preferred agent, is usually applied twice a day. Their action should remain localized if administered so as to minimize drainage through the lacrimal ducts into the nasal passages, where systemic absorption can occur. Discomfort associated with ciliary spasm is more of a problem with these drugs than with pilocarpine and occurs more frequently in younger than in older patients. The risk of cataract development is increased with these agents, but they can be very useful after a lens has been removed. Although most often used as an insecticide, **malathion** can be applied to the scalp as a lotion (Ovide, 0.5%) to eliminate head lice.[9]

General pharmacologic effects and toxicity

Organophosphates are used most widely as insecticides (**malathion**, **parathion**, and **diazinon**) so that acute and chronic poisoning by these agents is not uncommon. Many extremely potent chemical warfare agents (**soman** and **tabun**) are organophosphates. When an organophosphate anticholinesterase is injected or inhaled, the nonspecific cholinesterase of plasma is affected preferentially. With a sufficient dose, however, there is also inactivation of acetylcholinesterase in red blood cells and in neural tissue. Whereas plasma cholinesterase may be regenerated by the liver in 2 weeks, it may take 1 to 3 months to completely restore acetylcholinesterase activity at synapses and neuromuscular junctions.[1] The clinical picture in intoxication is a combination of peripheral cholinergic effects and involvement of the central nervous system (Table 14-3). Death is usually secondary to respiratory complications. In a group of 16 intoxicated field workers, nausea, dizziness, vomiting, abdominal pain, weakness, blurred vision, and headache were the most common symptoms initially; altered vision and headache tended to persist for more than a month.[10] A delayed, perhaps permanent, neurotoxicity may follow exposure to organophosphates.[1]

ANTIDOTAL ACTION OF PRALIDOXIME

Pralidoxime (*N*-methylpyridinium-2-aldoxime, 2-PAM) is a tailor-made molecule developed on the basis of a mechanism postulated by Wilson[16] to explain the action of organophosphate anticholinesterases. Experimental studies had shown that hydroxylamine and oximes could regenerate the enzyme after it was phosphorylated. With this in mind, a more efficient regenerator molecule was designed.

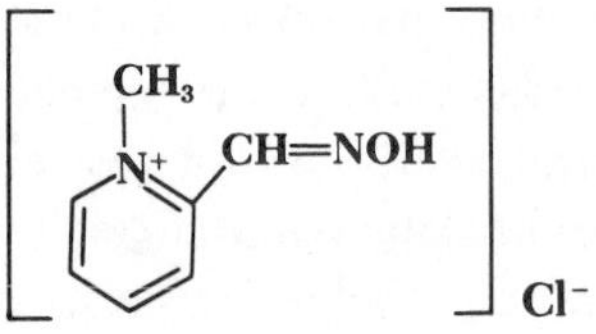

CH_3 N+ CH=NOH Cl^-

Pralidoxime chloride

Pralidoxime (Protopam) chloride must be administered parenterally in severe intoxications. It is supplied in 20 ml vials containing 1 g, and 1 to 2 g is usually dissolved in sterile water for intravenous infusion. Administration may be repeated if

TABLE 14-3 Signs and symptoms of organophosphate poisoning

Muscarinic manifestations	Nicotinic manifestations	CNS manifestations
Bronchoconstriction	Muscular fasciculation	Restlessness
Increased bronchial secretions	Tachycardia	Insomnia
Sweating	Hypertension	Tremors
Salivation		Confusion
Lacrimation		Ataxia
Bradycardia		Convulsions
Miosis		Respiratory depression
Blurring of vision		Circulatory collapse
Urinary incontinence		Hypotension

Modified from Namba T, Nolte CT, Jackrel J, Grob D: *Am J Med* 50:475, 1971.

necessary after an hour and again later if symptoms persist. Pralidoxime has some anticholinesterase activity of its own and is not used in intoxication by reversible anticholinesterases.

TREATMENT OF ORGANOPHOSPHORUS INTOXICATION

If the patient is cyanotic, mechanical ventilation should be started even before an antimuscarinic agent is given. In an adult an intravenous test dose of 2 mg of atropine can be repeated or increased at 15- to 60-minute intervals as needed, with careful observation to avoid excessive administration.[4] Atropine protects against the peripheral muscarinic actions and involvement of the central nervous system; there is some evidence that scopolamine may be more effective against the latter.[6] Antimuscarinic drugs do not protect against muscle fasciculations and skeletal muscle weakness. Pralidoxime is administered primarily to reverse the neuromuscular involvement. Pralidoxime, a quaternary amine, is of no benefit against the central nervous symptoms. The skin, stomach, and eyes should be decontaminated. Other measures are symptomatic and supportive.

PHARMACOLOGIC ASPECTS OF MYASTHENIA GRAVIS

Myasthenia gravis is an autoimmune neuromuscular disease[8] characterized by muscle fatigability. The density of acetylcholine receptors at the neuromuscular junction is reduced, and the junction undergoes extensive morphologic modifications.[3]

Repetitive stimulation of a motor nerve in a myasthenic patient leads to a rapid decrease in the force of contraction of muscles innervated by that particular nerve. Intra-arterial injection of acetylcholine, neostigmine, or edrophonium increases the strength of such fatigued muscles. In normal persons, however, such injections produce fasciculation and weakness, probably as a result of persistent depolarization of the neuromuscular end-plates. Myasthenic patients are susceptible to the relaxant activity of doses of tubocurarine or quinine that scarcely affect normal persons.

Reversible anticholinesterases are useful for diagnosis and management of myasthenia. For diagnostic purposes, edrophonium may be used as discussed above. Alternatively, neostigmine may be injected by the intramuscular route or intravenously.

For chronic management of weakness, oral administration of neostigmine and related drugs is most useful (see Table 14-2). Atropine may be necessary initially to minimize unwanted muscarinic effects.

Drug interactions

The following drugs require special caution and are probably best avoided in myasthenic patients, since they may aggravate the symptoms of the disease:

1. Aminoglycoside antibiotics and perhaps bacitracin and tetracyclines
2. Quinidine, quinine, and procainamide
3. Local anesthetics, such as procaine and lidocaine
4. Inhalational anesthetics, particularly ether
5. Skeletal muscle relaxants, such as curare and succinylcholine
6. Respiratory depressants, such as opioid analgesics and hypnotics

REFERENCES

1. Abou-Donia MB, Lapadula DM: Mechanisms of organophosphorus ester-induced delayed neurotoxicity: Type I and Type II, *Annu Rev Pharmacol Toxicol* 30:405, 1990.
2. Chilton WS: Chemistry and mode of action of mushroom toxins. In Rumack BH, Salzman E, editors: *Mushroom poisoning: diagnosis and treatment,* West Palm Beach, Florida, 1978, CRC Press, p 87.
3. Drachman DB: Myasthenia gravis: immunobiology of a receptor disorder, *Trends Neurosci* 6:446, 1983.
4. Haddad LM: Organophosphates and other insecticides. In Haddad LM, Winchester JF, editors: *Clinical management of poisoning and drug overdose,* ed 2, Philadelphia, 1990, WB Saunders, p 1076.
5. Havener, WH: *Ocular pharmacology,* ed 5, St Louis, 1983, Mosby–Year Book.
6. Janowsky D, Ziegler M, Risch SC, Gillin JC: Antagonistic effects of scopolamine and atropine on the physostigmine response in man, *Milit Med* 152:579, 1987.
7. Kirk M, Kulig K, Rumack BH: Anticholinergics. In Haddad LM, Winchester JF, editors: *Clinical management of poisoning and drug overdose,* ed 2, Philadelphia, 1990, WB Saunders, p 861.
8. Lindstrom J, Shelton D, Fujii Y: Myasthenia gravis, *Adv Immunol* 42:233, 1988.
9. Malathion for head lice, *Med Lett Drugs Ther* 31:110, 1989.
10. Midtling JE, Barnett PG, Coye MJ, et al: Clinical management of field worker organophosphate poisoning, *West J Med* 142:514, 1985.
11. Nardin GF, Zimmerman TJ, Zalta AH, Felts K: Ocular cholinergic agents. In Ritch R, Shields MB, Krupin T, editors: *The glaucomas,* St Louis, 1989, Mosby–Year Book, p 515.
12. Richter JE, Hackshaw BT, Wu WC, Castell DO: Edrophonium: a useful provocative test for esophageal chest pain, *Ann Intern Med* 103:14, 1985.
13. Ritch R, Lowe RF, Reyes A: Therapeutic overview of angle-closure glaucoma. In Ritch R, Shields MB, Krupin T, editors: *The glaucomas,* St Louis, 1989, Mosby–Year Book, p 855.
14. Rothenberg DM, Berns AS, Barkin R, Glantz RH: Bromide intoxication secondary to pyridostigmine bromide therapy, *JAMA* 263:1121, 1990.
15. Thompson HS, Newsome DA, Loewenfeld IE: The fixed dilated pupil. Sudden iridoplegia or mydriatic drops? A simple diagnostic test, *Arch Ophthalmol* 86:21, 1971.
16. Wilson IB: A specific antidote for nerve gas and insecticide (alkylphosphate) intoxication, *Neurology* 8(suppl 1):41, 1958.

Chapter 15

Cholinergic (muscarinic) blocking agents

GENERAL CONCEPTS

Atropine and scopolamine are competitive antagonists of acetylcholine in organs innervated by postganglionic cholinergic neurons. They have been extremely useful as pharmacologic tools. These alkaloids and related drugs are used in ophthalmology and anesthesia and in cardiac and gastrointestinal diseases. In addition to their peripheral anticholinergic activity, many of these agents act on the central nervous system. They are used to treat Parkinsons disease and to prevent motion sickness and were once found in many over-the-counter sleep aids. As antidotes for anticholinesterase intoxication, both peripheral and central actions of atropine are of great benefit.

ATROPINE AND SCOPOLAMINE

Origin and Chemistry

Atropine and scopolamine are among the oldest drugs in medicine. Many solanaceous plants have been used for centuries because of their active principles *l*-hyoscyamine and *l*-hyoscine (scopolamine). Atropine is *dl*-hyoscyamine; racemization occurs during the extraction process. The name *hyoscyamine* is derived from *Hyoscyamus niger* (henbane; literally 'black hog-bean'). It is of toxicologic interest that the common jimson weed, *Datura stramonium*, contains these alkaloids. They are also found in the deadly nightshade, *Atropa belladonna*. Hence these compounds are often referred to collectively as *belladonna alkaloids*. Compounds of the belladonna group are esters of complex organic bases with tropic acid. Atropine and scopolamine differ only slightly in the structure of the organic base part of the molecule.

```
H2C—CH——CH2          CH2OH            HC—CH——CH2          CH2OH
 |   |    |             |             /|   |    |            |
 |  NCH3  CH—O—CO—CH                 O< |  NCH3 CH—O—CO—CH
 |   |    |             |             \|   |    |            |
H2C—CH——CH2            C6H5            HC—CH——CH2           C6H5
```

Atropine **Scopolamine**

Pharmacologic effects

Atropine and scopolamine compete with acetylcholine for binding to muscarinic receptors in smooth and cardiac muscles and in exocrine glands (Fig. 15-1). They tend to inhibit responses to injected cholinergic drugs more easily than vagally mediated responses. There is a definite gradation in the sensitivity to inhibition by these alkaloids of the various peripheral functions mediated by acetylcholine. An oral dose of 0.6 mg of atropine may dry the mouth and inhibit sweating, whereas blockade of parasympathetic input to the eye and heart requires somewhat larger doses. Gastrointestinal and urinary tract smooth muscles are even more resistant. Because of

FIG. 15-1 *Effect of acetylcholine on tension development of guinea pig ileum. Atropine, a competitive antagonist, causes a parallel shift of the log dose-response curve.*

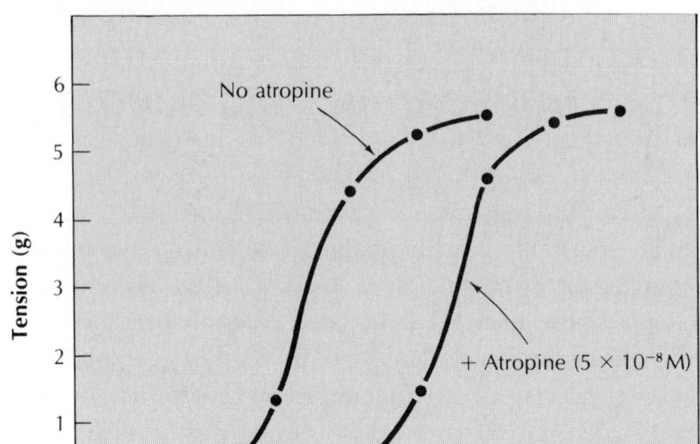

such differences in sensitivity, use of atropine to inhibit gastric secretion, the most resistant, is generally impractical; the dose required will cause side effects from more sensitive organs. Atropine and scopolamine differ in that the eye is more sensitive to scopolamine, and scopolamine can produce considerable sleepiness and even amnesia. In large enough doses both stimulate the central nervous system; very high doses may cause delirium or coma.

Cardiovascular system. The effect of atropine on heart rate in humans is complex. With high therapeutic or slightly larger doses, tachycardia develops, as expected, from blockade of the vagal influence to slow firing of the sinoatrial node. With smaller doses, paradoxically, heart rate may decrease slightly. Ablation experiments have shown that atropine stimulates vagal nuclei in the medulla. This stimulation results in bradycardia unless enough drug is given to block the peripheral action of acetylcholine at cardiac muscarinic receptors. Similarly, bradycardia has been observed in subjects given a small intravenous bolus of scopolamine or during recovery from larger doses after the tachycardia has dissipated.[4]

The effects of atropine and scopolamine on blood pressure are not impressive because most vascular beds do not receive parasympathetic innervation. However, by unclear mechanisms large doses of atropine may cause very noticeable flushing of the skin.[8]

Gastrointestinal and urinary tracts. In large enough doses, belladonna alkaloids reduce motility and tone of the gastrointestinal tract. Gastric motility is more easily reduced than secretion is, particularly if a peptic ulcer is present. Atropine has little effect on the ureters. It relaxes the fundus of the bladder but promotes contraction of the sphincter, thus favoring urinary retention.

Eye. Atropine and scopolamine produce prolonged (up to 2 weeks) mydriasis and

Autonomic innervation of iris. *FIG. 15-2*

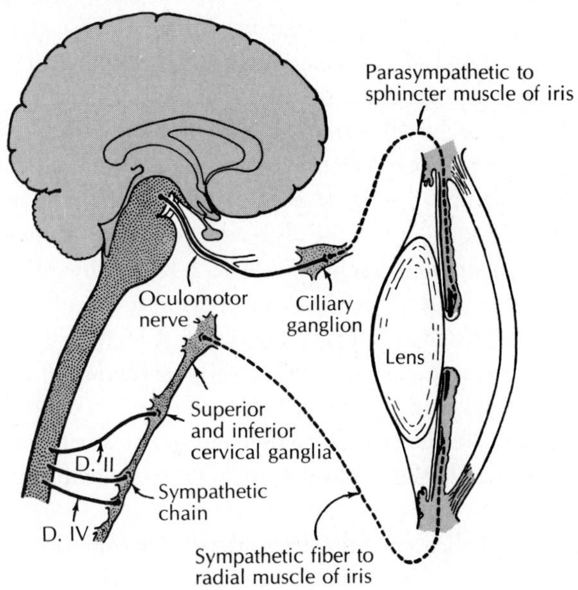

paralysis of accommodation (cycloplegia). The sphincter muscle of the iris receives cholinergic innervation from the third cranial nerve (Fig. 15-2). Atropine blocks the action of acetylcholine on this muscle, and the resulting dominance of the radial muscle causes mydriasis. The atropinized pupil does not react to light. Cycloplegia is caused by paralysis of the ciliary muscle, which is also innervated by cholinergic fibers. It should be noted that adrenergic agonists can also produce mydriasis. They act, however, by contracting the radial muscle of the iris and do not impair accommodation.

Muscarinic blocking drugs are generally contraindicated for topical use in patients subject to glaucoma. The subject most at risk is one with an undiagnosed narrow angle in whom an anticholinergic drug may precipitate an acute attack with a catastrophic increase in intraocular pressure. However, systemic anticholinergic medication for other purposes will seldom harm patients already receiving therapy for glaucoma.[6]

Central nervous system. In anticholinergic poisoning, central nervous system effects are very striking; patients most often become excited and may hallucinate or be delirious. Anticholinergic drugs were once primary therapy in management of Parkinsons disease. Scopolamine in particular is valuable in prevention of motion sickness; as preanesthetic medication, it may cause amnesia[7] in addition to sedation.

Absorption, excretion, and metabolism

Atropine and scopolamine are well absorbed from the gastrointestinal tract and after injection. Scopolamine is even absorbed after dermal application. Systemic toxicity may occur after ophthalmologic use, particularly in children, if the drug reaches the nasal mucosa through the nasolacrimal duct.

Atropine is rapidly excreted and about half of an injected dose appears in the urine within 4 hours as metabolites and unchanged drug. The remainder is eliminated within 24 hours. The duration of action reflects the rapidity of excretion except for dilatation of the pupils and paralysis of accommodation, which may persist for a long time, particularly when the alkaloids are applied to the conjunctiva.

Preparations and clinical uses

Belladonna alkaloids are used either in pure form or in galenic preparations. (Galenic preparations contain one or more active botanical ingredients as contrasted with pure chemical substances.) Belladonna tincture is given orally in a dose of 0.6 to 1.0 ml, equivalent to 0.18 to 0.3 mg of the alkaloids. Tablets of atropine sulfate contain 0.4 or 0.6 mg for administration to adults at 4- to 6-hour intervals. Atropine can be inhaled from a nebulizer (Dey-Dose). It is instilled into the conjunctival sac as an ointment or in solution (Atropisal, others). The usual strength is 0.5% or 1%, though higher concentrations are available in solution. L-Hyoscyamine sulfate is available in several forms. Scopolamine hydrobromide is available as an ophthalmic solution of 0.25% (Isopto Hyoscine). For more rapid action and preanesthetic medication, injectable solutions of atropine sulfate (0.05 to 1 mg/ml) and scopolamine hydrobromide (0.3 to 1 mg/ml) are used.

Ophthalmologic use. Anticholinergic drugs are applied topically to produce mydriasis and cycloplegia. Atropine has such a long action that its use in ophthalmology is often impractical. However, it is used to produce maximal cycloplegia for refraction in young children with accommodative esotropia and to break adhesions (synechiae) between the iris and the lens in iridocyclitis.

Perioperative uses. When ether was a commonly used anesthetic, it was necessary to premedicate surgical patients with atropine or scopolamine to protect them from salivary and bronchial secretions and from reflex vagal bradycardia. Ether has been replaced by anesthetics that do not cause excessive secretions, and the need for preanesthetic anticholinergics has greatly lessened,[1] at least in adults. However, they are still given intravenously during surgery to prevent bradycardia. Scopolamine is used in obstetrics for its sedative and amnesic effects. When an anticholinesterase is administered near the end of anesthesia to reverse muscle paralysis induced by a neuromuscular blocking agent, atropine or a related drug is also given to prevent muscarinic effects.

Cardiac uses. Atropine is used after myocardial infarction if heart rate falls below 60 and the bradycardia is associated with hypotension or arrhythmias.[5] The drug can cause dangerous tachycardia and ventricular arrhythmias in cardiac patients and should be used cautiously. It may also be useful in digitalis-induced heart block.

Uses in gastrointestinal disease. Anticholinergic drugs were once frequently used to treat peptic ulcer. They can diminish vagally mediated secretion, relieve spasm, and, by slowing gastric emptying, prolong the time during which antacids remain in the stomach. However, effective doses usually cause unpleasant side effects, and more effective agents are now available (see Chapter 45).

Motion sickness. Scopolamine was the first drug to be administered by means of a patch placed behind one ear. The disk (Transderm Scōp) is designed to release a priming dose and then about 5 μg/hour for 72 hours. It should be applied a minimum of 6 to preferably 8 hours before exposure to an emetic stimulus,[9] and the hands should be thoroughly washed to avoid transfer of the drug to the eyes. Clinical trials indicate that this preparation is as effective as 50 mg of oral dimenhydrinate and less sedative. Dry mouth is a common side effect, and heart rate tends to decrease, rather than increase.[9] Far-sighted individuals may experience blurred near vision, especially with repeated application. Motion seems to counteract the tendency to drowsiness.

Other uses. The antidotal benefit of antimuscarinic agents in anticholinesterase intoxication is discussed in Chapter 14. Treatment of Parkinsons disease is discussed in Chapter 30. Atropine-like drugs also counteract parkinsonian side effects of neuroleptic agents (see p. 245). Atropine is included in antidiarrheal preparations to prevent abuse of the opioid diphenoxylate. Asthmatics may benefit from judicious use of antimuscarinic drugs, though several other modalities of treatment are preferred (see Chapter 44).

Toxicity and antidotes

The belladonna alkaloids and other atropine-like drugs are generally safe medications. Large therapeutic doses in a healthy person may cause unpleasant effects, such as blurred vision, tachycardia, dry mouth, constipation, and urinary retention, but are not life threatening. Normal persons have survived oral doses as high as 1 g. Muscarinic blockade, by agents in several therapeutic classes, may be especially troublesome to elderly patients.[10] Subtle drug-induced impairment of mental functions is often attributed to aging. Those with glaucoma and prostatic hypertrophy can have disastrous reactions.

Severe anticholinergic poisoning[11] is characterized by hot dry skin and hyperthermia,[3] hyperactivity, confusion, delirium, and hallucinations and eventually by coma, respiratory depression, and cardiovascular collapse. Infants have died after application of eye drops. Intoxication with certain antihistamines and tricyclic antidepressants, which also have antimuscarinic activity, may mimic atropine poisoning.

Patients with atropine intoxication should be managed with supportive care, including gastric lavage or induction of emesis if the agent was ingested. Sedatives such as chlordiazepoxide or diazepam may help control violent excitement. The use of physostigmine as an antidote to atropine poisoning is discussed on p. 108.

PROBLEM 15-1. Why is physostigmine preferable to neostigmine in reversing the CNS effects of atropine? The answer undoubtedly has some connection with the relative rates of penetration of the two drugs across the blood-brain barrier. Physostigmine is not a quaternary compound, but neostigmine is.

ATROPINE SUBSTITUTES

Atropine substitutes fall into three groups based on primary indications for their use: the mydriatics; the antispasmodics, which are of minimal usefulness today; and antiparkinson drugs (see Chapter 30).

Atropine-like mydriatics

For examination of the fundus and measurement of refractive errors, relatively short-acting agents are preferred. Alternatively, topical application of α-adrenergic agonists, such as phenylephrine, produces mydriasis without cycloplegia. Combinations of phenylephrine with scopolamine or cyclopentolate are also available.

Homatropine hydrobromide (Isopto Homatropine, others), the oldest of the atropine-like mydriatic drugs, differs from atropine only in that it is an ester of mandelic rather than of tropic acid. It is applied to the eye in 2% or 5% solutions. Mydriasis develops fairly rapidly and may persist up to 4 days.

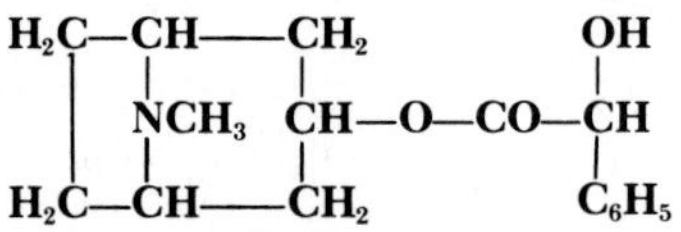

```
H2C—CH——CH2              OH
 |   |    |               |
 |  NCH3  CH—O—CO—CH
 |   |    |               |
H2C—CH——CH2              C6H5
```

Homatropine

Cyclopentolate hydrochloride (Cyclogyl, others) produces mydriasis and cycloplegia in 15 to 45 minutes, with return of normal vision in less than 24 hours. It is used in 0.5% to 2% solutions. The 2% solution may be necessary for deeply pigmented eyes. Adverse reactions are not uncommon with this higher concentration, which has evoked seizures in children.

Tropicamide (Mydriacyl, others), a more short-acting mydriatic and cycloplegic, is effective in less than 30 minutes and lasts less than 4 to 6 hours. It is used in 0.5% and 1% solutions.

Anticholinergic smooth muscle relaxants

Many atropine substitutes have been synthesized in attempts to obtain some selective action on the gastrointestinal tract. The rationale for development of such compounds includes the prevalence of peptic ulcer, the idea that reduction of smooth muscle tone and hypersecretion are beneficial in ulcer management, and the need to minimize side effects. These drugs have been replaced by more effective and better tolerated agents, including histamine H_2-receptor antagonists (see Chapter 22), sucralfate, and omeprazole (see Chapter 45).

Conversion of tertiary atropine-like drugs to quaternary amines converts them to less lipid-soluble agents that do not readily cross the blood-brain barrier. Thus atropine methylbromide does not enter the central nervous system as efficiently as atropine sulfate. The difference between the two in regard to passage across biologic membranes is illustrated in Fig. 15-3. The quaternary agents also cause some ganglionic blockade that may reinforce their action on muscarinic receptors in the gastrointestinal tract but also contributes to unwanted side effects. Methscopolamine bromide, propantheline bromide, and the tertiary compound dicyclomine hydrochloride are examples of these drugs. Urinary incontinence is another indication for such agents, in particular propantheline. The quaternary glycopyrrolate (Robinul, 0.2 mg/ml) is a popular anticholinergic for perioperative use.

Pirenzepine

Unlike other muscarinic antagonists, pirenzepine, first marketed in Germany in 1971, can reduce the volume of gastric acid and pepsin secretion at doses that cause minimal antimuscarinic side effects, dry mouth being the most common.[2] Pirenzepine is a more potent antagonist of vagally mediated secretion than of bethanechol-induced secretion. This has been attributed to its blockade of *ganglionic* muscarinic receptors (subtype M_1) in the stomach rather than to a direct action on the muscarinic receptors

Effect of atropine sulfate and atropine methylbromide on maternal and fetal heart rates. The lesser effect of the quaternary anticholinergic drug on fetal heart rate illustrates a basic difference between the two types of drugs as regards their passage across biologic membranes. *FIG. 15-3*

From dePadua CB, Gravenstein JS: JAMA 208:1022, 1969.

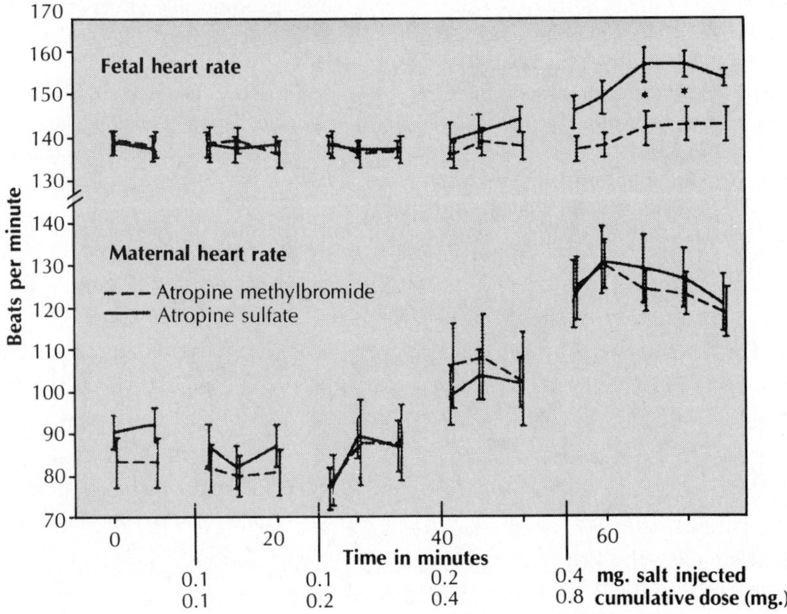

(probably subtype M_3) on parietal cells. Although histamine H_2-antagonists and antacids now constitute the primary therapy for peptic ulcer, pirenzepine may prove useful in some patients. Not yet approved for use in the United States, pirenzepine is taken in doses of 100 to 150 mg per day, divided at bedtime and before breakfast.

Pirenzepine

REFERENCES

1. Alpert CC, Baker JD, Cooke JE: A rational approach to anaesthetic premedication, *Drugs* 37:219, 1989.
2. Carmine AA, Brogden RN: Pirenzepine: a review of its pharmacodynamic and pharmacokinetic properties and therapeutic efficacy in peptic ulcer disease and other allied diseases, *Drugs* 30:85, 1985.

3. Clark WG, Lipton JM: Drug-related heatstroke, *Pharmacol Ther* 26:345, 1984.
4. Gravenstein JS, Thornby JI: Scopolamine on heart rates in man, *Clin Pharmacol Ther* 10:395, 1969.
5. Greenblatt DJ, Shader RI: Anticholinergics, *N Engl J Med* 288:1215, 1973.
6. Havener WH: *Ocular pharmacology*, ed 5, St Louis, 1983, Mosby–Year Book.
7. Izquierdo I: Mechanism of action of scopolamine as an amnestic, *Trends Pharmacol Sci* 10:175, 1989.
8. Kolka MA, Stephenson LA: Cutaneous blood flow and local sweating after systemic atropine administration, *Pflugers Arch* 410:524, 1987.
9. Parrott AC: Transdermal scopolamine: a review of its effects upon motion sickness, psychological performance, and physiological functioning, *Aviat Space Environ Med* 60:1, 1989.
10. Peters NL: Snipping the thread of life: antimuscarinic side effects of medications in the elderly, *Arch Intern Med* 149:2414, 1989.
11. Shader RI, Greenblatt DJ: Uses and toxicity of belladonna alkaloids and synthetic anticholinergics, *Semin Psychiatry* 3:449, 1971.

Chapter 16

Ganglionic blocking agents

GENERAL CONCEPT

Neurotransmission at nicotinic receptors can be inhibited either by agents that produce initial stimulation and depolarization followed by persistent receptor desensitization (nicotine) or by compounds that prevent depolarization by acetylcholine. The latter agents act in one of two ways. Hexamethonium, a classic ganglionic blocker, becomes trapped within ionic channels, thereby preventing Na^+ influx.[5] In contrast, mecamylamine and trimethaphan, the only ganglionic blocking drugs still used clinically, competitively inhibit the action of acetylcholine at nicotinic receptors on postganglionic neurons.

Sympathetic ganglia are relatively accessible and simple structures that are useful for research on neurotransmission. Nicotinic receptors are mainly responsible for transmission through intact ganglia. Muscarinic, adrenergic, and peptide receptors can also be demonstrated under certain experimental circumstances[8,10] (Fig. 16-1). Although pharmacologic blockade of muscarinic and catecholamine receptors alters ganglionic action potentials, the fast excitation of autonomic neuroeffectors mediated by nicotinic receptors is unimpeded.

GANGLIONIC STIMULANTS

Certain ganglionic stimulants, such as tetra*methyl*ammonium, and small doses of nicotine cause vasoconstriction and raise blood pressure by their action on sympathetic ganglia. This effect has not found therapeutic application. However, some drugs that were used in the past to diagnose pheochromocytoma (for example, methacholine) cause catecholamine release from the adrenal. This is analogous to ganglionic stimulation.

Nicotine

The alkaloid nicotine is a highly toxic liquid, absorbed readily through the skin. It is found in some pesticides. Symptoms of intoxication, which include nausea, vomiting, sweating, diarrhea, skeletal muscular fasciculations and weakness, fluctuations in blood pressure and heart rate, seizures, and eventually respiratory depression, result from sequential stimulation and then inhibition of transmission at nicotinic receptors in ganglia, at the neuromuscular junction, and in the central nervous system.

Chewing gum (Nicorette) containing 2 mg of nicotine per piece is available by prescription for use by persons who are addicted to cigarette smoking. The gum must be used chronically to maintain steady-state concentrations of nicotine. If patients wait until symptoms of withdrawal occur before using the gum, slow absorption of the alkaloid results in a long period of inadequate symptomatic relief. In addition, absorption of nicotine requires an alkaline pH at the oral mucosa. Soft drinks are sufficiently

FIG. 16-1 *Impulse transmission in partially curarized sympathetic autonomic ganglia. Acetylcholine* (ACh) *interacts with nicotinic receptors* (N) *on postganglionic neurons* (Principal cells) *to cause rapid depolarization, the fast excitatory postsynaptic potential* (f-EPSP). *ACh also binds to muscarinic receptors* (M) *on these cells to cause a late (l-)EPSP and on small intensely fluorescent* (SIF) *interneurons,*[3] *which release dopamine* (DA). *Dopamine interaction with* α_2*-adrenergic catecholamine receptors* (C) *initiates an inhibitory postsynaptic potential* (IPSP). *Sites of action of the antagonists are also shown.* GF, *Ganglionic fiber.*

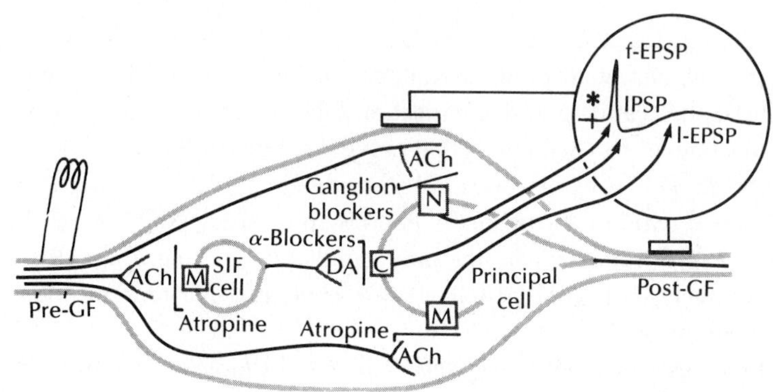

acidic that drinking one prevents nicotine absorption for about an hour. Long-term benefit is likely to be minimal without concurrent psychologic intervention,[6] and patients using nicotine gum should be counseled as to its proper use. Adverse effects include a burning sensation in the throat, belching, nausea, dizziness, and hiccups. Contraindications include recent myocardial infarction, life-threatening arrhythmias, severe angina, and pregnancy. In nonsmokers the dose is sufficient to increase heart rate and blood pressure.

GANGLIONIC BLOCKING AGENTS

Development

The ability of nicotine to block ganglionic transmission after initial stimulation has been known for many years. During the latter part of the nineteenth century, Langley and Dickinson[7] charted the distribution of fibers emanating from sympathetic ganglia by selectively blocking the ganglia with local applications of nicotine.

The fact that tetra*ethyl*ammonium prevented the effect of ganglionic stimulants received little attention until 1946, when its mode of action on mammalian circulation was thoroughly investigated.[1] This study indicated that ganglionic transmission can be blocked in a fairly selective manner. Several ganglionic blocking agents were then developed and used to treat hypertension or to produce controlled hypotension. Among these were pentolinium, chlorisondamine, and pempidine.

Chemistry

The chemical formulas of some of these agents are as follows:

$$(C_2H_5)_3N^+\text{—}CH_2\text{—}CH_3 \cdot Cl^-$$

Tetraethylammonium chloride

$$(CH_3)_3\,N^+\text{—}CH_2\text{—}(CH_2)_4\text{—}CH_2\text{—}N^+(CH_3)_3 \cdot 2Cl^-$$

Hexamethonium chloride

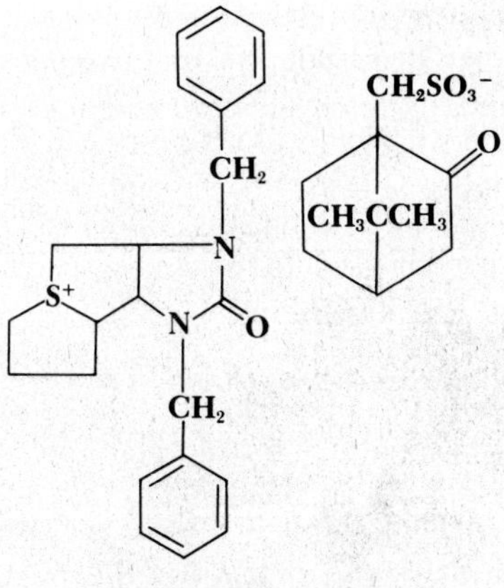

Trimethaphan camsylate

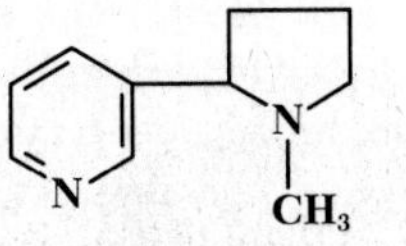

Nicotine

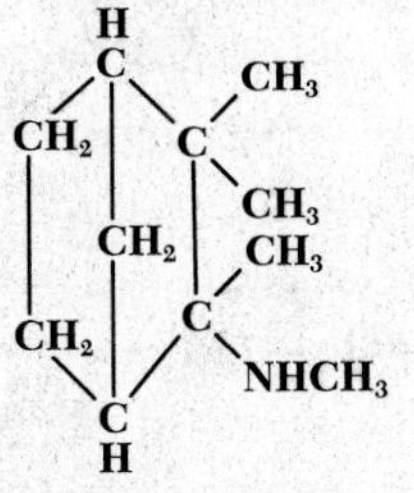

Mecamylamine

Like acetylcholine, most ganglionic blocking drugs are quaternary ammonium compounds. However, of the two agents in current though infrequent use, trimethaphan contains a tertiary sulfur, and so it too is a strong electrolyte, and mecamylamine is a secondary amine.

Clinical pharmacology

Ganglionic blocking agents have been used principally to decrease sympathetic control of vascular smooth muscle tone. They were first-line drugs for management of hypertension until more specific compounds with fewer adverse effects became available. Although ganglionic blockers are selective in that they have little if any action elsewhere, they are nonspecific by comparison with other antihypertensive drugs because they block transmission in both sympathetic and parasympathetic ganglia. For this reason their effects depend on the autonomic tone prevailing in each organ at the time of administration.

PROBLEM 16-1. Before reading the rest of this chapter, predict the effects of a typical ganglionic blocking agent in a resting subject. Keep in mind that in the resting state the parasympathetic influence is usually dominant in organs innervated by both parasympathetic and sympathetic branches of the autonomic nervous system. How did your predictions compare with Paton's description below?

A picturesque description of a person without a functioning autonomic nervous system was given by Paton in his account of the "hexamethonium man."

> He is a pink-complexioned person, except when he has stood in a queue for some time, when he may get pale and faint. His handshake is warm and dry. He is a placid and relaxed companion; he may laugh, but he can't cry because the tears cannot come. Your rudest story will not make him blush and the most unpleasant circumstances will fail to make him turn pale. His . . . collars and socks stay very clean and sweet. He wears corsets and may, if you meet him out, be rather fidgety (the corsets compress his splanchnic vascular pool, the fidgets keep the venous return going from his legs). He dislikes speaking much unless helped with something to moisten his dry mouth and throat. He is rather long-sighted and easily blinded by bright light. The redness of his eye-balls may suggest irregular habits and in fact his head is rather weak. But he always behaves like a gentleman and never belches nor hiccups. He tends to get cold

> and keeps well wrapped up. But his health is good; he does not have chilblains and those diseases of modern civilization, hypertension and peptic ulcer pass him by. He is thin because his appetite is modest; he never feels hunger pains and his stomach never rumbles. He gets rather constipated so that his intake of liquid paraffin is high. As old age comes on frequency, precipitancy and strangury will not worry him, but he will suffer from retention of urine and impotence. One is uncertain how he will end, but perhaps, if he is not careful, by eating less and less and getting colder and colder, he will sink into a symptomless, hypoglycemic coma and (like the universe) die a sort on entropy death.*

Circulatory effects. Ganglionic blocking drugs lower blood pressure primarily by decreasing sympathetic tone to various vascular regions. The intensity of this hypotensive action depends on several factors, in particular the position of the patient. Pressure may decrease only slightly when the patient is recumbent. Upon standing, however, the patient may experience a precipitous fall in blood pressure and faint. This orthostatic (postural) hypotension results from pooling of blood in the extremities in the absence of compensatory venoconstriction.

Other side effects and complications. Reduction of smooth muscle tone of the gastrointestinal and urinary tracts by ganglionic blocking agents can cause constipation or difficulty in voiding. The pupils may dilate, and accommodation for near vision is impaired. Salivary secretion is inhibited, and dry mouth may be sufficiently uncomfortable to require administration of pilocarpine. Sweating is also inhibited (not an atropine-like effect) because of decreased sympathetic activity. Impotence is another problem. The high incidence of such effects contributed to poor compliance by patients. Although many of the adverse effects can be alleviated by concurrent management with cholinergic drugs, such as pilocarpine, by laxatives, and by physical measures such as supportive stockings, newer antihypertensive drugs (see Chapter 21) have virtually eliminated the use of these unpleasant agents.

Mecamylamine and trimethaphan

Because **mecamylamine hydrochloride** (Inversine) is a secondary amine, it may cause central nervous system effects, including insomnia, confusion, depression, and even seizures. It has a duration of action of 4 to 12 hours. The initial oral dosage is 2.5 mg twice daily; this is gradually increased until a satisfactory response is obtained, usually at about 25 mg/day. The drug is available in 2.5 mg tablets.

Trimethaphan camsylate (Arfonad) is a short-acting ganglionic blocking agent that is actively secreted by the kidney. It is used to reduce blood pressure rapidly in hypertensive emergencies and in cases of acute dissecting aneurysm of the aorta and to minimize bleeding during certain types of surgery.[2,9] Although histamine release by an intravenous bolus of trimethaphan can cause feelings of warmth, dizziness, headache, and flushing of the face, this release does not contribute to the hypotensive response.[4] Intravenous infusion at rates from 0.3 to 5 mg/min can effectively lower blood pressure, but elevation of the head of the patient's bed is usually required so that pooling of blood in the extremities can occur. When the infusion is stopped, blood pressure

---

*From Paton WDM: The principles of ganglionic block. In *Lectures on the scientific basis of medicine*, vol 2, London 1954, Athlone Press.

returns to its normal level in about 10 minutes. This drug is available as a 50 mg/ml solution, which must be diluted fiftyfold before intravenous infusion.

Nowadays mecamylamine is rarely if ever used. Trimethaphan is used primarily for the indications mentioned above and then only by some physicians. For the most part, ganglionic blocking agents remain only of historic interest.

REFERENCES

1. Acheson GH, Moe GK: The action of tetraethylammonium ion on the mammalian circulation, *J Pharmacol Exp Ther* 87:220, 1946.
2. Calhoun DA, Oparil S: Treatment of hypertensive crisis, *N Engl J Med* 323:1177, 1990.
3. Eränkö O: Small intensely fluorescent (SIF) cells and nervous transmission in sympathetic ganglia, *Annu Rev Pharmacol Toxicol* 18:417, 1978.
4. Fahmy NR, Soter NA: Effects of trimethaphan on arterial blood histamine and systemic hemodynamics in humans, *Anesthesiology* 62:562, 1985.
5. Gurney AM, Rang HP: The channel-blocking action of methonium compounds on rat submandibular ganglion cells, *Br J Pharmacol* 82:623, 1984.
6. Hughes JR, Gust SW, Keenan RM, et al: Nicotine vs placebo gum in general medical practice, *JAMA* 261:1300, 1989.
7. Langley JN, Dickinson WL: On the local paralysis of peripheral ganglia, and on the connexion of different classes of nerve fibres with them, *Proc R Soc Lond* [series A] 46:423, 1889.
8. Libet B: Nonclassical synaptic functions of transmitters, *Fed Proc* 45:2678, 1986.
9. Miller ED, Jr: Deliberate hypotension. In Miller RD, editor: *Anesthesia*, vol 3, ed 2, New York, 1986, Churchill Livingstone, p 1949.
10. Skok VI: Ganglionic transmission: morphology and physiology, *Handb Exp Pharmacol* 53:9, 1980.

Chapter 17

Neuromuscular blocking agents and muscle relaxants

GENERAL CONCEPT

Neuromuscular blocking drugs act on nicotinic receptors located in the specialized end-plate region of skeletal muscle. Most clinically useful neuromuscular blockers (the *nondepolarizing* drugs) compete with acetylcholine for these receptors, whereas succinylcholine depolarizes the end-plate region and initially stimulates the muscle.

Skeletal muscle relaxation may be achieved by other mechanisms as well. Agents such as mephenesin and the antianxiety drug diazepam cause relaxation primarily by actions within the central nervous system. Dantrolene, in contrast, acts within the muscle fiber to interfere with excitation-contraction coupling. Botulinum toxins impair neurotransmitter release from cholinergic neurons.

Many other drugs impair neuromuscular transmission as an unwanted side effect. For example, local anesthetics and certain antibiotics may cause postoperative respiratory depression or may aggravate myasthenia gravis.

NEUROMUSCULAR BLOCKING AGENTS

Development

Experimentation with the South American arrow poison *curare* was one of the earliest examples of scientific pharmacology. In the nineteenth century Magendie and his pupil, Claude Bernard, studied its effects on nerve-muscle preparations. Bernard demonstrated that the drug prevented the response of skeletal muscle to nerve stimulation. Its inability to keep the muscle from responding to electrical stimulation and its failure to block conduction in the nerve indicated an action at the junction of nerve and muscle.

The active principle of *Chondodendron tomentosum* roots is (+)-tubocurarine, a bulky molecule in which two nitrogen atoms, one of which is quaternary, are separated by a distance of about 1.1 nm; at physiologic pH the tertiary nitrogen also becomes charged, as depicted on page 131. Most nondepolarizing blockers in current use exhibit a similar separation between paired quaternary structures. To open the ion channel of muscular nicotinic receptors (see Fig. 13-1), two molecules of agonist are required, one acting on each of the α subunits. Binding of a nondepolarizing antagonist to either of these subunits prevents influx of Na^+. Other actions of these antagonists at the neuromuscular junction, such as physical occlusion of ion channels (tubocurarine)[5] or prejunctional impairment of transmitter release (tubocurarine, pancuronium),[3] appear to contribute little to clinical neuromuscular blockade.

Unlike curare, succinylcholine mimics the neurotransmitter in stimulating the receptor and paralyzes much like an excess of acetylcholine, as in a myasthenic patient during anticholinesterase overtreatment.

Clinical pharmacology

The first consideration in choosing a neuromuscular blocker is the duration of paralysis needed. For brief paralysis to allow tracheal intubation, succinylcholine is most often used. For longer paralysis a nondepolarizing agent is generally preferred. The drugs are usually given intravenously, though tubocurarine and succinylcholine can be injected intramuscularly. Respiration must be assisted or controlled by the anesthetist. The most important antidotal measure is to maintain mechanical respiration until recovery. None of these agents appreciably affect the central nervous system because of the blood-brain barrier to quaternary ammonium compounds, and they are neither anesthetic nor analgesic. Since the paralyzed patient cannot speak or otherwise indicate perception of pain, the anesthetist must pay careful attention to other indications of the depth of anesthesia. The beneficial effect on pain in conditions such as strychnine intoxication or tetanus is ascribed to relaxation of contracted muscles. Nondepolarizing blockers are also used to facilitate mechanical ventilation, as in patients with tetanus, and to prevent motor manifestations of electroconvulsive therapy.

Intravenous injection of 5 to 10 mg of tubocurarine produces flaccid paralysis. Doubling the dose may produce apnea. There is a characteristic progression of effects, with the extrinsic muscles of the eye affected first, then those of the face, the extremities, and finally the diaphragm. This progression parallels the sequence of muscle involvement in myasthenia gravis.

NONDEPOLARIZING NEUROMUSCULAR BLOCKING AGENTS

Mode of action. Packets, or quanta, of acetylcholine are released from synaptic vesicles of motoneurons spontaneously or with the arrival of a nerve impulse.[2] The transmitter stimulates receptors in the end-plate region of muscle fibers to produce an electrical change known as the *end-plate potential*. If depolarization is sufficient to reach threshold, a propagated *action potential* leads to muscle contraction. In a partially curarized preparation the small end-plate potential is clearly visible, since it is not followed by the larger action potential. The effect of curare on the end-plate potential and the anticurare action of physostigmine are illustrated in Fig. 17-1.

General characteristics. Certain characteristics of individual neuromuscular blocking agents are listed in Table 17-1. Maximum paralysis develops within 2 to 5 minutes after intravenous administration. The first four drugs are relatively long acting; however, the duration of paralysis (1 to 2 hours) can vary considerably among patients. A dose beyond that necessary for paralysis prolongs relaxation but also increases the likelihood of side effects. To extend paralysis with these agents, it is better to give supplemental drug as needed. Such supplements are limited to a fraction, ranging from one eighth to one half, of the initial dose because they are given before the previous dose is completely inactivated. Accumulation after supplemental doses is unlikely to be a problem with atracurium or vecuronium, which have a shorter action; single doses provide paralysis for 30 to 50 minutes. A major advantage of the nonde-

FIG. 17-1 *Effect of tubocurarine on the end-plate potential of the frog sartorius muscle and the antagonistic action of physostigmine.* 1, *After 6 μM of curarine;* 2, *after 9 μM of curarine;* 3, *after 9 μM of curarine plus physostigmine 10^{-5}.*

From Eccles JC, et al: J Neurophysiol 5:211, 1942.

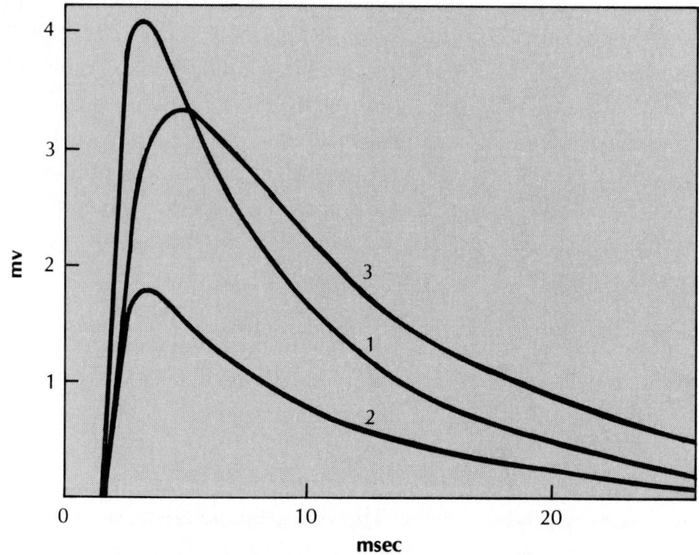

TABLE 17-1 Characteristics of neuromuscular blocking agents

Type	Intubation dose[1] (mg/kg)	Commercial preparation (mg/ml)	Typical duration[1] (min)	Histamine release	Cardiac vagal block	Prolonged by renal impairment
Nondepolarizing (competitive)						
Tubocurarine	0.5-0.6	3	80-100	++		+
Metocurine	0.3-0.4	2	80-100	+		+
Pancuronium	0.08-0.1	1,2	80-100		+	+
Gallamine	3-4	20	80-100		++	++
Atracurium	0.4-0.5	10	30-40	±		
Vecuronium	0.1-0.12	1,2*	40-50			
Depolarizing						
Succinylcholine	1.0	20-100	8-10	+		

*Powder for reconstitution.

polarizing drugs over succinylcholine is that, in addition to mechanical respiration, reversible anticholinesterases are effective antagonists, especially if given after the twitch response to nerve stimulation (see p. 134) has recovered spontaneously to 10% to 25% of normal. However, the patient must be monitored to ensure that apnea does not recur if anticholinesterase activity wears off before the blocker is inactivated.

Atropine or a related drug is given before or with the anticholinesterase to minimize muscarinic effects.

Interactions with other agents that enhance paralysis are of great importance.[1] General anesthetics such as halothane, enflurane, and isoflurane have some relaxant activity of their own, so that less neuromuscular blocker is necessary. The dose of antagonist may be reduced approximately 50% with halothane and somewhat more with the other two anesthetics. Aminoglycosides and some other antibiotics, such as polymyxin B, colistin, and lincomycin, also potentiate neuromuscular blockade, as do quinidine and magnesium salts. Finally, patients with myasthenia gravis or acidosis are exquisitely sensitive to usual doses of neuromuscular blockers. The longer-acting nondepolarizing blockers are primarily excreted intact in the urine and should be used cautiously in patients in shock or with impaired renal function. However, pancuronium and tubocurarine are partially metabolized and excreted in bile so that caution is necessary with patients who have liver disease.

Adverse reactions to nondepolarizing neuromuscular blocking drugs include prolonged apnea, bronchospasm, hypotension, and tachycardia. Those agents that release histamine (Table 17-1) are generally contraindicated in patients with asthma or who have previously experienced an anaphylactoid reaction. Fentanyl, an opioid analgesic used in balanced anesthesia, does not release histamine. This agent is probably safer for combination with tubocurarine than morphine, which can release histamine. Patients with severe cardiovascular disease may also suffer adverse responses to some of these agents. Histamine release and ganglionic blockade are both believed to contribute to hypotension. Muscarinic blockade can elicit tachycardia.

Specific agents. **Tubocurarine** [(+)-tubocurarine] **chloride** may be given initially as a divided dose, with the first two thirds over a minute or so and the remainder 3 to 5 minutes later; this reduces histamine release and ganglionic blockade. About half of the drug is excreted unchanged in the urine, whereas the rest is metabolized. Although curare is still an important neuromuscular blocking agent, newer drugs have reduced its use considerably. Rarely, tubocurarine is used very cautiously to aid diagnosis of myasthenia gravis. **Metocurine** (Metubine) **iodide**, a derivative of tubocurarine with a lower potential for cardiovascular effects, is also available.

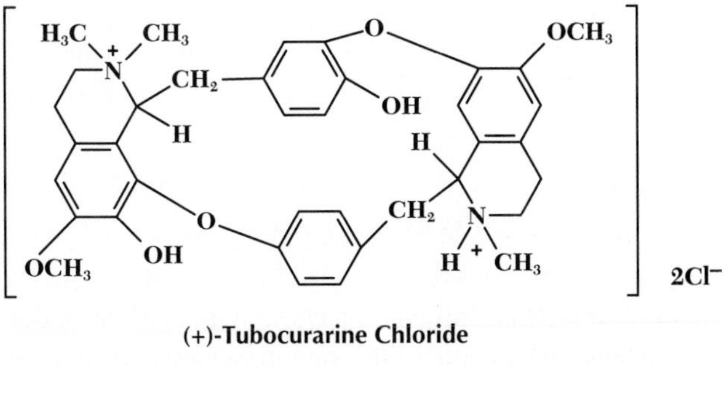

(+)-Tubocurarine Chloride

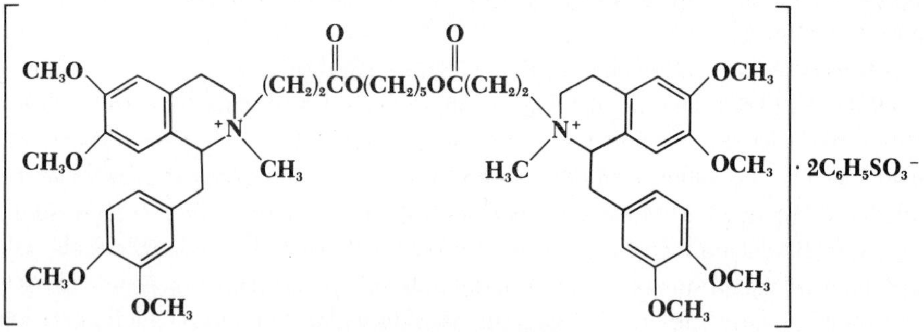

Atracurium besylate

Pancuronium bromide (Pavulon) differs from tubocurarine in its greater potency and lack of histamine-releasing or ganglionic blocking actions. It may increase heart rate if vagal tone is high. Attached to its steroid nucleus are two quaternary amines and two acetyl ester groups. About 20% of the drug is metabolized in the liver by hydrolytic cleavage of the ester linkages. Both hepatic and renal changes in elderly patients can considerably reduce clearance of pancuronium.

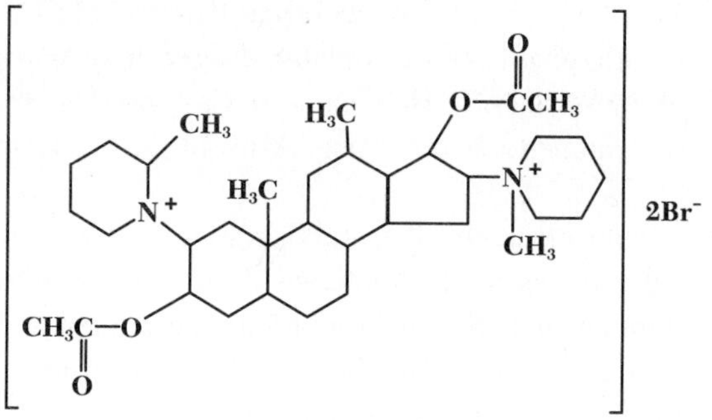

Pancuronium bromide

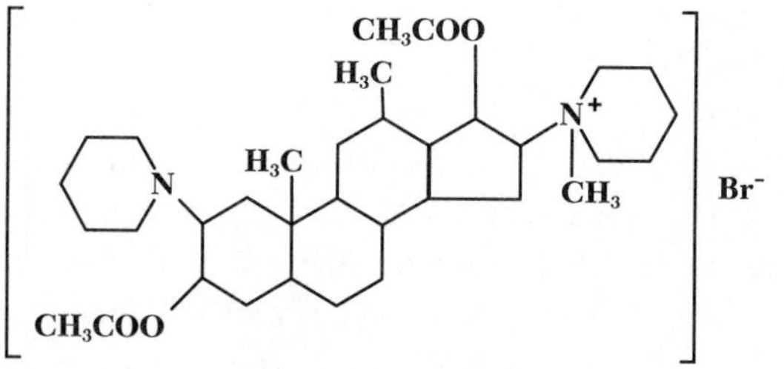

Vecuronium bromide

Gallamine triethiodide (Flaxedil) may have a slightly shorter duration of action than tubocurarine. It has an atropine-like action selectively at cardiac muscarinic receptors and may induce considerable tachycardia, a disadvantage in some patients; however, this action tends to minimize bradycardia induced by agents such as fentanyl or β-adrenergic antagonists.

Atracurium besylate (Tracrium) has an intermediate duration of action and minimal vagolytic activity or tendency to release histamine. It is rapidly inactivated by hydrolysis and by a nonenzymatic process called *Hofmann elimination*[10]; this drug can be used safely in patients with impairment of either liver or renal function. Inactivation is slowed in patients undergoing controlled hypothermia.

Vecuronium bromide (Norcuron) differs structurally from pancuronium in having only one quaternary nitrogen; the tertiary nitrogen, as in tubocurarine, can become protonated in the body. The drug has an intermediate duration of action and lacks significant ganglionic blocking, vagolytic, or histamine-releasing activity. Its pharmacokinetics are not appreciably affected by renal impairment. It is partially deacetylated in the liver and excreted in the bile; its action may be prolonged in patients with cirrhosis. Vecuronium is available as powder for reconstitution.

SUCCINYLCHOLINE

The only available short-acting neuromuscular blocking agent is the depolarizing drug succinylcholine, which consists of two acetylcholine molecules joined together. When this drug is injected intravenously, there may be considerable muscular fasciculation for several seconds before paralysis. Muscles remain paralyzed for approximately 5 minutes with full recovery after 10 to 15 minutes. Many patients will later experience muscle soreness that does not clearly correlate with the occurrence of fasciculation.

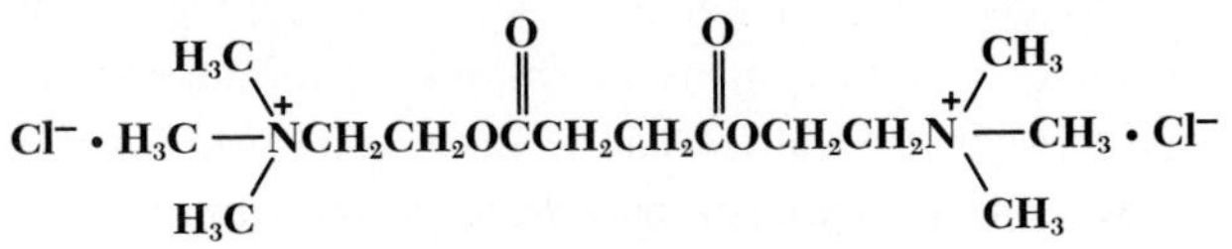

$$Cl^- \cdot (H_3C)_3\overset{+}{N}CH_2CH_2OC(=O)CH_2CH_2C(=O)OCH_2CH_2\overset{+}{N}(CH_3)_3 \cdot Cl^-$$

Succinylcholine chloride

Succinylcholine is rapidly hydrolyzed by plasma cholinesterase to choline and succinylmonocholine. The latter is then hydrolyzed to succinic acid and choline. In patients with a genetic abnormality that results in quantitative or qualitative differences in plasma cholinesterase (p. 55), succinylcholine can cause apnea for hours.

The action of succinylcholine is inhibited by prior administration of a nondepolarizing blocker. After succinylcholine is used to facilitate tracheal intubation, a sufficient interval is usually allowed for it to wear off before a nondepolarizing blocker is given.

Neostigmine is not an antidote to succinylcholine during depolarization but rather enhances early paralysis. However, with prolonged exposure to succinylcholine, as during an infusion, the characteristics of the block change, a phenomenon termed *dual block*. After initial stimulation and paralysis during depolarization (phase I block), paralysis is sustained even though repolarization has occurred (phase II block). Anticholinesterase drugs can be effective antidotes in phase II, which is not well understood but has been attributed to gradual *desensitization*, that is, a change of receptors to a conformation that cannot be activated by agonist.[5]

Succinylcholine can contribute to problems other than postoperative soreness. In the absence of muscarinic blockade, stimulation of ganglionic receptors can elicit bradycardia, whereas tachycardia occurs with large doses or after adequate treatment with atropine. Tissue loss of K^+ during depolarization may cause life-threatening hyperkalemia after extensive trauma (burns, spinal cord transection, crush injury). The potential for development of *malignant hyperthermia*, a fulminant and often fatal disorder characterized by myoglobinuria and a rapid increase in temperature, is enhanced when succinylcholine is used with potent inhalational anesthetics.

Succinylcholine chloride (Anectine, others) may be given in single intravenous doses or by infusion. Preparations for injection include powder, 0.1 to 1 g for reconstitution, and solutions of 20 to 100 mg/ml. Facilities for mechanical respiration are essential, since this is the only certain antidotal measure to apnea.

Monitoring with peripheral nerve stimulation

Many anesthesiologists, especially in the United States, use peripheral nerve stimulation as one means to assess the level of paralysis.[11] A direct postjunctional endpoint is the percent reduction in twitch height after a single stimulus. Twitch height begins to diminish when about 75% of the end-plate receptors have been blocked by a nondepolarizing drug. Patients can vary widely in sensitivity; a given dose of antagonist may not affect twitch height in some, yet completely abolish twitch in others.

Less direct approaches take advantage of actions on neuronal, rather than end-plate, receptors. Blockade of prejunctional nicotinic receptors is thought to inhibit neurotransmitter release.[3] Since responses to repetitive stimuli are more dependent on sustained availability of acetylcholine than is the response to a single stimulus, contractions evoked by a brief tetanus or by a *train of four* stimuli given at 0.5 second intervals diminish (fade) within the stimulus period. Because fade can still be demonstrated after twitch height has returned to normal, its disappearance indicates further recovery from neuromuscular blockade. Tetanus is well sustained during phase I of succinylcholine-induced paralysis; the appearance of fade is an indication that phase II block has developed.

SKELETAL MUSCLE RELAXANTS THAT ACT ON THE SPINAL CORD

Some drugs may relax muscle by acting on internuncial spinal neurons to depress polysynaptic pathways (Fig. 17-2). Such relaxants also act on higher centers, and some, such as the benzodiazepines (see Chapter 29), are commonly used to relieve anxiety or to induce sleep. Although experimentally these drugs depress the spinal cord at doses that do not cause sleep or anesthesia, it is unclear to what extent the clinical benefit is attributable to their antianxiety or sedative effects. Only those agents promoted primarily as relaxants are mentioned below. Indications for these drugs include treatment of muscle spasm resulting from sprains, arthritis, myositis, and fibrositis. They may also cause drowsiness, lethargy, ataxia, and allergic manifestations.

Innervation of skeletal muscle. *FIG. 17-2*

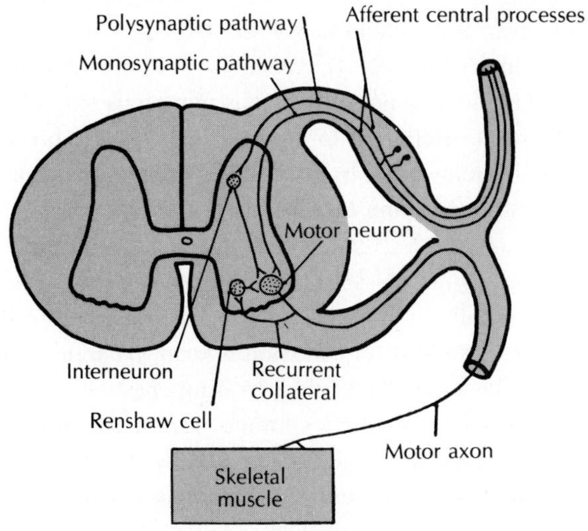

Mephenesin and mephenesin carbamate were the first drugs introduced as centrally acting muscle relaxants. Their selective action on spinal neurons was shown by abolition of strychnine-induced convulsions in animals by doses that did not cause sleep. **Methocarbamol** (Robaxin, others), closely related to mephenesin carbamate, is available in tablets of 500 and 750 mg and in a solution of 100 mg/ml for injection. **Chlorphenesin carbamate** (Maolate), also related to mephenesin, is available in tablets, 400 mg.

H_2—C—O—CONH$_2$
H—C—OH
H_2—C—O—(phenyl, H_3CO)

Methocarbamol

H_2—C—O—CONH$_2$
H_7C_3—C—CH$_3$
H_2—C—O—CON(H)—CH(CH$_3$)$_2$

Carisoprodol

Cl, N, OH, O

Chlorzoxazone

CHCH$_2$CH$_2$N(CH$_3$)$_2$

Cyclobenzaprine

Carisoprodol (Soma, others) is provided as 350 mg tablets.

Chlorzoxazone (Paraflex, Parafon Forte DSC) was developed on the basis of the observation that benzimidazole depressed polysynaptic spinal pathways. Rarely, jaundice has developed in patients taking this drug. It is available in tablets, 250 and 500 mg, and 500 mg caplets.

Metaxalone (Skelaxin) is available in 400 mg tablets.

Cyclobenzaprine hydrochloride (Flexeril) is used for short-term treatment of acute, painful musculoskeletal conditions. It has numerous side effects, as one might expect from its chemical similarity to tricyclic antidepressants (see Chapter 28). Cyclobenzaprine should be avoided by patients receiving monoamine oxidase inhibitors. The drug is available in 10 mg tablets.

APPROACHES TO MANAGEMENT OF SPASTICITY OR SPASM

Baclofen

Baclofen is a relatively new skeletal muscle relaxant that mimics GABA (γ-aminobutyric acid) at so-called $GABA_B$ (bicuculline-insensitive) receptors. Unlike the agents above, it appears to inhibit transmission in monosynaptic as well as in polysynaptic spinal pathways. Baclofen is useful in treating spasticity associated with spinal cord lesions, as in multiple sclerosis.[8] Chronic intrathecal infusion of the drug is sometimes beneficial, with a lower incidence of adverse effects, in patients who do not respond favorably to oral administration.[7] Baclofen also may be preferred for initial treatment of trigeminal or glossopharyngeal neuralgia.[6] Side effects include drowsiness, dizziness, confusion, weakness, and a variety of gastrointestinal effects. Abrupt withdrawal after long-term use has caused seizures and hallucinations. Baclofen (Lioresal, Vitarine) is supplied in 10 and 20 mg tablets.

$H_2NCH_2CH_2CH_2COOH$

γ-Aminobutyric acid

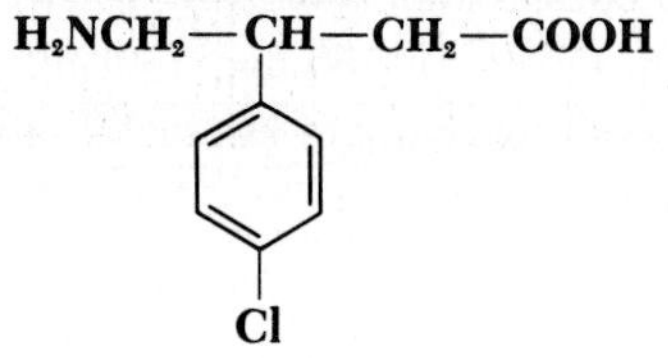
H₂NCH₂—CH—CH₂—COOH
Cl

Baclofen

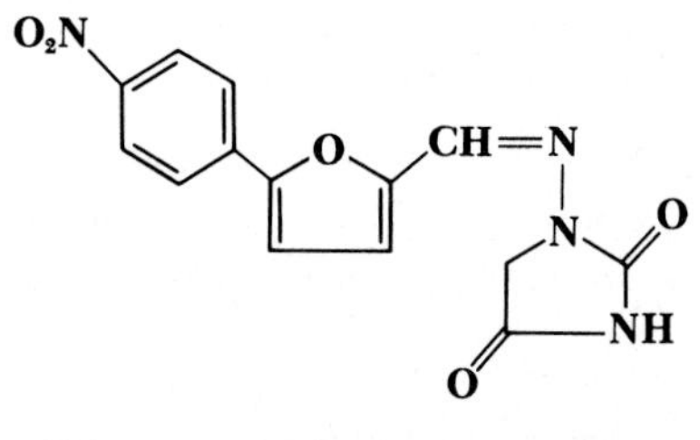
O₂N
O
CH=N
N
O
NH
O

Dantrolene

Dantrolene

Dantrolene is a hydantoin derivative that acts on skeletal muscle beyond the neuromuscular junction.[12] It reduces the cytoplasmic availability of Ca^{++} for muscle contraction. Dantrolene has produced improvement in patients with spinal cord injury, cerebral palsy, and, less consistently, multiple sclerosis. The drug has become the agent of choice for reducing heat production by muscle in anesthetic-induced malignant hyperthermia and has also been beneficial in the *neuroleptic malignant syndrome*.

Dantrolene can cause numerous serious reactions and side effects. Seizures, pleural effusion, pericarditis, and skin reactions have been noted with chronic use. Periodic liver function tests are recommended to monitor for liver damage. Drowsiness, dizziness, weakness, and gastrointestinal effects are relatively common.

For oral administration of dantrolene sodium (Dantrium), capsules of 25 to 100 mg are available. The starting dose in adults of 25 mg a day can be increased gradually to 100 mg two to four times daily. Relief of spasticity may require treatment for a week. For reconstitution and intravenous injection the drug is available in vials containing 20 mg. Dantrolene is also given before surgery to patients susceptible to malignant hyperthermia (4 to 8 mg/kg/day orally for 1 to 2 days or 2.5 mg/kg intravenously).

BOTULINUM TOXIN

There are several serologic types of botulinum toxin. They apparently enter cholinergic nerve endings after binding to the outer surface, with subsequent inhibition of exocytosis of acetylcholine-containing vesicles by mechanisms that are yet unclear and may vary with the toxin subtype.[9] In 1990, botulinum toxin type A (Oculinum) was produced for treatment of strabismus and blepharospasm associated with dystonia, by injection into muscles around the eyes. Transient side effects include excessive tearing and unilateral ptosis.[4] Benefit is prolonged and may last as long as 3 months in blepharospasm. The toxin is provided as a powder (100 units) for reconstitution and dilution.

REFERENCES

1. Ali HH: Neuromuscular block and its antagonism: clinical aspects. In Nunn JF, Utting JE, Brown BR, Jr, editors: *General anaesthesia*, ed 5, London, 1989, Butterworths, p 164.
2. Bowman WC: Neuromuscular block and its antagonism: basic concepts. In Nunn JF, Utting JE, Brown BR, Jr, editors: *General anaesthesia*, ed 5, London, 1989, Butterworths, p 151.
3. Bowman WC, Gibb AJ, Harvey AL, Marshall IG: Prejunctional actions of cholinoceptor agonists and antagonists, and of anticholinesterase drugs. In Kharkevich DA, editor: *New neuromuscular blocking agents*, Berlin, 1986, Springer-Verlag, p 141.
4. Cohen DA, Savino PJ, Stern MB, Hurtig HI: Botulinum injection therapy for blepharospasm: a review and report of 75 patients, *Clin Neuropharmacol* 9:415, 1986.
5. Colquhoun D: On the principles of postsynaptic action of neuromuscular blocking agents. In Kharkevich DA, editor: *New neuromuscular blocking agents*, Berlin, 1986, Springer-Verlag, p 59.
6. Fromm GH: Clinical pharmacology of drugs used to treat head and face pain, *Neurol Clin* 8:143, 1990.
7. Penn RD, Savoy SM, Corcos D, et al: Intrathecal baclofen for severe spinal spasticity, *N Engl J Med* 320:1517, 1989.
8. Rudick RA, Schiffer RB, Herndon RM: Drug treatment of multiple sclerosis, *Sem Neurol* 7:150, 1987.
9. Simpson LL: Peripheral actions of the botulinum toxins. In Simpson LL, editor: *Botulinum neurotoxin and tetanus toxin*, San Diego, 1989, Academic Press, Inc, p 153.
10. Stenlake JB: Biodegradation and elimination of neuromuscular blocking agents. In Kharkevich DA, editor: *New neuromuscular blocking agents*, Berlin, 1986, Springer-Verlag, p 263.

11. Viby-Mogensen J: Clinical assessment of neuromuscular transmission, *Br J Anaesth* 54:209, 1982.
12. Ward A, Chaffman MO, Sorkin EM: Dantrolene: a review of its pharmacodynamic and pharmacokinetic properties and therapeutic use in malignant hyperthermia, the neuroleptic malignant syndrome and an update of its use in muscle spasticity, *Drugs* 32:130, 1986.

Chapter 18

Adrenergic (sympathomimetic) drugs

Adrenergic or sympathomimetic drugs comprise a large group of compounds that act *directly* on adrenergic receptors or that act presynaptically, and thus *indirectly*, to release norepinephrine from nerve endings. Some of these drugs have a *mixed effect*, acting directly on receptors and also releasing catecholamine. The adrenergic group includes the endogenous catecholamines, ephedrine, and many synthetic amines. These agents are used for their cardiovascular effects and as bronchodilators, central nervous system stimulants, mydriatics, and appetite suppressants (anorexiants).

The effects of these drugs can be predicted from a knowledge of (1) the type of adrenergic receptor with which they interact, (2) the direct, indirect, or mixed nature of their action, and (3) their penetration or lack of penetration into the central nervous system.

CATECHOLAMINES

The catecholamines norepinephrine, epinephrine, and dopamine occur naturally in the body, whereas isoproterenol is a synthetic analog.

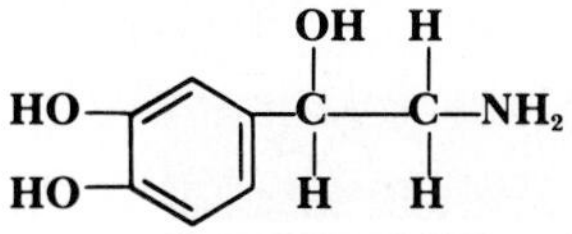

Norepinephrine 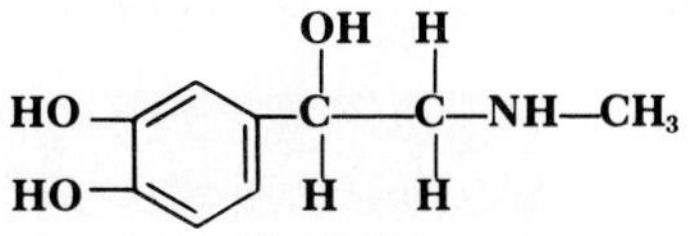 **Epinephrine**

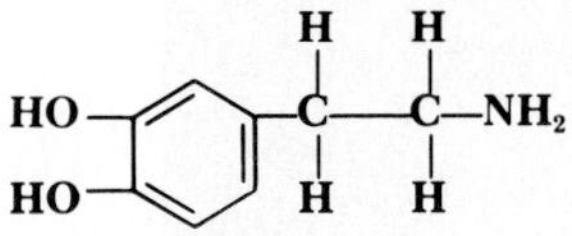

Dopamine 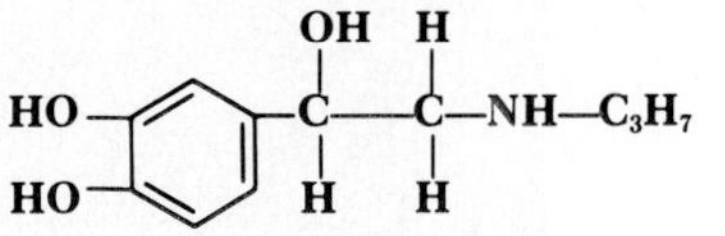 **Isoproterenol**

Epinephrine differs from norepinephrine in having a methyl group on the nitrogen, whereas isoproterenol has an isopropyl group on the nitrogen, and dopamine lacks the β-hydroxyl on the side chain. The prefix *nor-* in norepinephrine is derived from German chemical terminology. It is the abbreviation of *Nitrogen ohne Radikal* (nitrogen without radical), which means that some attached group has been removed from the nitrogen. In the body, however, epinephrine is formed from norepinephrine (rather than the other way around as the nomenclature implies) by addition of a methyl group to the nitrogen.

Occurrence and physiologic functions

The presence of norepinephrine in adrenergic nerve fibers was demonstrated by von Euler in 1946. The relationship between adrenergic nerves and blood vessels and the presence of catecholamine in the nerves is strikingly demonstrated by the fluorescence technique of the Swedish investigators Falck, Hillarp, and Carlsson, as shown in Fig. 18-1.

Epinephrine is highly concentrated in *chromaffin* granules of the adrenal medulla. It is also present in many other organs, probably in chromaffin cells. Sympathetic denervation affects the norepinephrine content of an organ without a significant decrease in epinephrine concentration. From this observation it is believed that epinephrine is limited to chromaffin cells and is not located in adrenergic neurons.

Adrenal medullary granules and adrenergic axonal vesicles contain catecholamines along with adenosine triphosphate, in the proportion of 4:1 or perhaps higher in the nerve terminals.[4] They also contain a special soluble protein, *chromogranin*, and the enzyme dopamine β-hydroxylase.

In the human adrenal medulla, norepinephrine contributes as much as 20% to the total catecholamine content. It may constitute a much higher percentage in the medulla of the newborn infant and in pheochromocytoma, a tumor of the adrenal medulla.

The main functions of norepinephrine are maintenance of normal sympathetic tone and adjustment of circulatory dynamics. Epinephrine, in contrast, is a hormone that releases substrates for metabolism and in emergencies promotes blood flow to skeletal muscles, preparing the individual for "fight or flight."

FIG. 18-1 *Fluorescent adrenergic terminals around small arteries and a vein in the rat mesentery.*

From Falck B: Acta Physiol Scand 56(suppl 197):19, 1962.

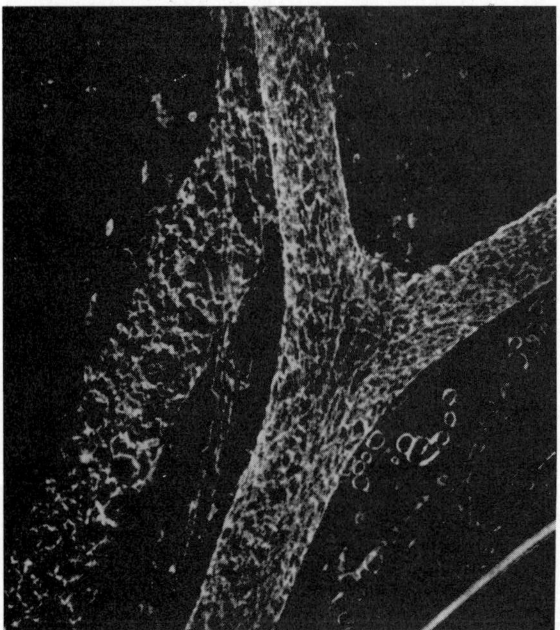

Dopamine is localized in certain regions of the central nervous system where it is an important transmitter. It is also the precursor of norepinephrine and epinephrine at other sites and may contribute to peripheral control of renal and mesenteric blood flow. The role of dopamine in the actions of psychoactive drugs and in Parkinsons disease is discussed on pp. 234 and 286.

Adrenergic receptors

The classification of adrenergic receptors as *alpha* (α) and *beta* (β), originally proposed by Ahlquist[1] in 1948, is now generally accepted. The concept was based on the order of activity of a series of sympathomimetic drugs at various effector sites and was greatly strengthened when specific blocking agents were developed for each receptor. Functions associated with α-adrenergic receptors include vasoconstriction, mydriasis, and intestinal relaxation (Table 18-1). β-Adrenergic receptors mediate bronchial and intestinal relaxation, vasodilatation, cardioacceleration, and a positive inotropic effect.

Norepinephrine acts on α- and some β-receptors. Epinephrine also acts on both receptor types, but in an organ with both types (such as vascular smooth muscle within skeletal muscle) the β-receptors are more sensitive at physiologic concentrations. Isoproterenol is a virtually pure β-receptor agonist, and its activity is blocked by

TABLE 18-1 Predominant receptors mediating selected adrenergic drug effects

Effector organ	Receptor	Response
Heart		
Sinoatrial node	β_1	Tachycardia
Atrioventricular node	β_1	Increase in conduction rate and shortening of functional refractory period
Atrial and ventricular muscle	β_1	Increased contractility
Blood vessels		
To skeletal muscle	α, β_2	Contraction, relaxation
To skin	α	Contraction
Bronchial muscle	β_2	Relaxation
Eye		
Iris radial muscle	α_1	Contraction (mydriasis)
Ciliary muscle	β_2	Relaxation
Gastrointestinal tract		
Smooth muscle	α and β	Decreased motility
Sphincters	α_1	Contraction
Urinary bladder		
Detrusor muscle	β_2	Relaxation
Trigone and sphincter	α_1	Contraction
Uterus	α_1, β_2	Contraction, relaxation
Male sex organs	α	Ejaculation, detumescence
Pancreas	α_2, β_2	Decreased, increased insulin secretion
Kidney	β_1	Renin secretion
Skeletal muscle	β_2	Tremor, glycogenolysis

propranolol, a β-adrenergic receptor antagonist. Drugs such as methoxamine and phenylephrine act selectively on α-receptors and are antagonized by the α-adrenergic blocking agents phenoxybenzamine and phentolamine. Thus there is a gradation from essentially pure α-agonists to pure β-agonists.

Subclasses of α- and β-Adrenergic Receptors

In addition to postsynaptic α-receptors that mediate vasoconstriction and mydriasis, there are *presynaptic* α-receptors on adrenergic and other neurons that mediate inhibition of neurotransmitter release[16] (Fig. 18-2). This finding, based on the relative potencies of a series of agonists,[8] led to division of α-receptors into α_1 and α_2 subtypes. The decreasing order of selectivity of agonists for α_2- versus α_1-receptors is clonidine, epinephrine, norepinephrine, and phenylephrine.[9] For antagonists this order is yohimbine, phentolamine, phenoxybenzamine, and prazosin. These facts have practical importance in antihypertensive therapy and probably explain why tachycardia is a greater problem with phentolamine than with prazosin (see p. 161). It was later found that there are also *postsynaptic* α_2-receptors that mediate other effects: vasoconstriction and inhibition of lipolysis, insulin release, and renin release.[9,11]

Drugs, such as clonidine, methyldopa, and guanabenz, that stimulate central nervous system α_2-receptors are used in management of hypertension (see Chapter 21). There is also considerable interest in use of clonidine to minimize symptoms of withdrawal from drugs of abuse (see Chapter 34), as prophylaxis for migraine headaches, in glaucoma, and in Gilles de la Tourettes syndrome.[11]

β-Adrenergic receptors are also of two subtypes. β_1-Receptors mediate cardiac

FIG. 18-2 *Autoinhibition of norepinephrine release from sympathetic nerves mediated by presynaptic α_2-receptors and facilitation of release through presynaptic β_2-receptors. Epinephrine* (A) *from the adrenal medulla is taken up by the neuron* (dotted arrows) *and acts as a false transmitter when released together with norepinephrine* (NA). *Notice that the facilitatory influence of β_2-receptor stimulation is indicated as weak relative to the effect of α_2-receptor stimulation.* +, *Facilitation of release;* −, *inhibition of release.*

From Göthert M: Arzneimittelforschung 35:1909, 1985.

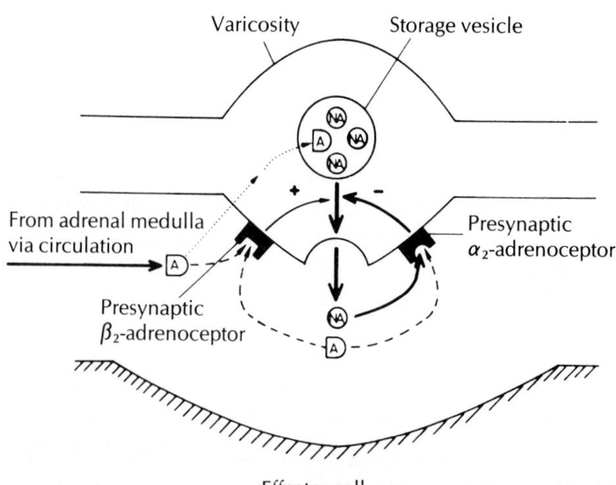

effects of catecholamines and also lipolysis. β_2-Receptors mediate bronchodilatation and vasodilatation, and on presynaptic membranes they may facilitate norepinephrine release[12] (Fig. 18-2). β_2-Agonists are especially useful in treatment of asthma (see p. 154 and Chapter 44) and have been used to prevent premature labor (see p. 598). Some β-blockers are not selective for either β_1- or β_2-receptors (propranolol); others interact preferentially with β_1-receptors (metoprolol).

The relative potencies of the three prototypic catecholamines on adrenergic receptors are as follows:

$$\alpha\text{: epinephrine} \geq \text{norepinephrine} >>> \text{isoproterenol}$$
$$\beta_1\text{: isoproterenol} > \text{epinephrine} = \text{norepinephrine}$$
$$\beta_2\text{: isoproterenol} \geq \text{epinephrine} >>> \text{norepinephrine}$$

Experimental evidence indicates that postsynaptic α_2- and β_2-receptors are located in proximity to the vascular lumen so that, rather than responding primarily to neuronal norepinephrine, they may be hormonal receptors for circulating epinephrine.[9] Events believed to occur after stimulation of α- and β-receptors are depicted in Fig. 18-3. From a biochemical standpoint, the α_2- and β-receptors mediate changes in adenylyl cyclase (Fig. 18-3 and Chapter 3), the α_2-receptor mediating inhibition and the β-receptor mediating activation.

Norepinephrine and epinephrine

Various aspects of the pharmacology of norepinephrine (levarterenol) and epinephrine (adrenaline) are discussed first, followed by those of dopamine, ephedrine, and other adrenergic drugs.

Cardiovascular effects

The cardiovascular system responds differently to norepinephrine and epinephrine, whether released physiologically or given in small doses intended to mimic physiologic activity, as a consequence of the minimal influence of norepinephrine on β_2-receptors at which epinephrine is a potent agonist.

Net effects of small doses in humans. When norepinephrine is infused intravenously so that the normal subject receives about 10 to 20 μg/min, the hemodynamic changes listed in Table 18-2 are observed. If epinephrine is infused at the same rate, the changes listed in Table 18-3 are generally observed. These changes in heart rate and blood pressure are illustrated in Fig. 18-4.

Norepinephrine has widespread vasoconstrictor (α-receptors) properties, in skeletal muscle as well as elsewhere, and increases blood pressure. This effect elicits, through a baroreceptor-mediated mechanism, a reflex bradycardia that is prevented by atropine. On the other hand, epinephrine constricts (α-receptors) some vascular beds and dilates (β_2-receptors) others. At low concentrations in blood vessels of skeletal muscle epinephrine primarily stimulates β_2-receptors. The vasodilatation and increased blood flow to the muscle is beneficial for "fight or flight" and tends to offset the effect on peripheral resistance of α-receptor—mediated constriction in other vascular beds; mean blood pressure may be only minimally affected. Blood is shunted to skeletal muscle from splanchnic and other regions of the body. If epinephrine does not elevate mean pressure, no reflex mechanism comes into play to slow the heart, and

FIG. 18-3 *Postulated α_1-, α_2-, and β-adrenergic receptor-coupled signal-transduction mechanisms leading to cellular responses. Agonist binding to the α_1-receptor activates hydrolysis of phosphatidylinositol-4,5-bisphosphate* (PIP_2) *to myo-inositol-1,4,5-trisphosphate* (IP_3) *and diacylglycerol* (DG). *IP_3 releases intracellular Ca^{++}, which activates responses such as actin-myosin coupling or together with diacylglycerol promotes protein kinase* (C-kinase) *activation. The latter may limit* (broken arrow) *further signal transduction through the α_1-receptor. Activation of α_2- or β-receptors inhibits or stimulates, respectively, the membrane-bound enzyme adenylyl cyclase (not shown); responses are mediated by independent inhibitory* (G_i) *and stimulatory* (G_s) *guanine nucleotide-binding regulatory proteins. Increased adenylyl cyclase activity promotes hydrolysis of ATP to cyclic adenosine 3',5'-monophosphate* (cAMP), *which activates cAMP-dependent protein kinase* (A-kinase).

From Homcy CJ, Graham RM: Circu Res 56:635, 1985, by permission of the American Heart Association, Inc.

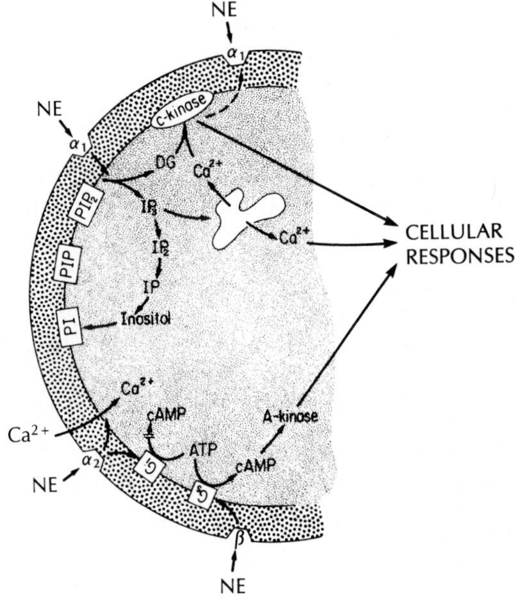

TABLE 18-2 Cardiovascular effects of small dose of norepinephrine in humans	
Systolic pressure	Increased
Diastolic pressure	Increased
Mean pressure	Increased
Heart rate	Slightly decreased
Cardiac output	Slightly decreased
Peripheral resistance	Increased

the direct stimulant action of the drug (β-receptors) increases cardiac rate. These differences between epinephrine and norepinephrine tend to disappear when large, unphysiologic doses are administered. In this case, epinephrine will also stimulate α-receptors in skeletal muscle. Both drugs will then reduce blood flow through skeletal muscles and increase total peripheral resistance and diastolic pressure.

TABLE 18-3 Cardiovascular effects of small dose of epinephrine in humans

Systolic pressure	Increased
Diastolic pressure	Decreased (increased by large dose)
Mean pressure	Unchanged
Heart rate	Increased
Cardiac output	Increased
Peripheral resistance	Decreased

FIG. 18-4 *Effect of norepinephrine and epinephrine infusion on blood pressure and heart rate in humans. Notice increased mean pressure and decreased heart rate after infusion of norepinephrine and essentially unchanged mean pressure, increase in pulse pressure, and elevated heart rate after infusion of epinephrine.*

From Barcroft H, Konzett H: Lancet 1:147, 1949.

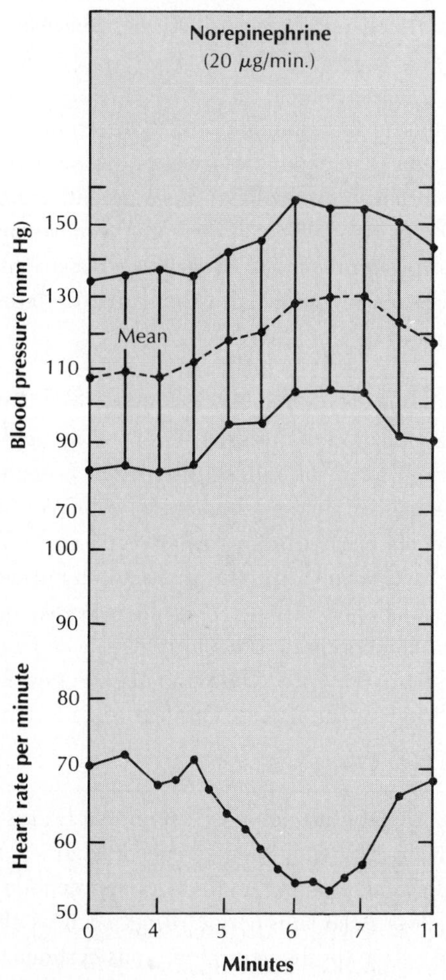

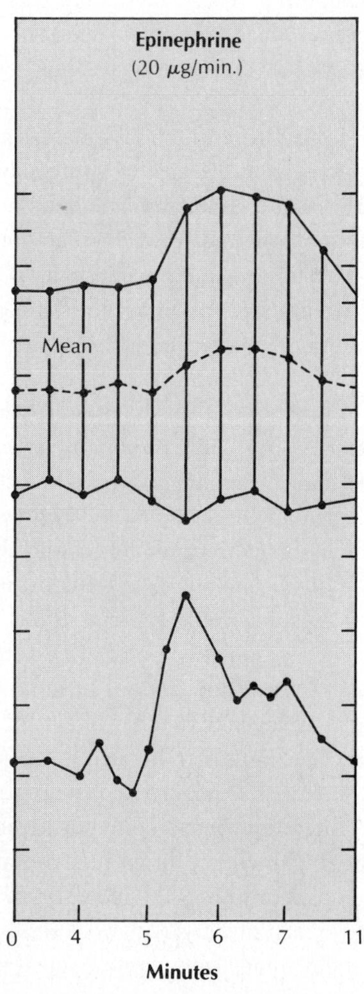

Response of heart and various vascular areas. Epinephrine increases heart rate, force of contraction, and irritability predominantly through stimulation of β_1-receptors, although a significant fraction (25% to 35%) of β-receptors in the human heart are of the β_2 subtype. Norepinephrine has a cardiac accelerator action also, but this is opposed, as noted above, by reflex slowing secondary to elevated blood pressure.

Increased coronary blood flow after administration of epinephrine is largely attributable to increased cardiac work and metabolism, though β-receptor stimulation also dilates coronary arterioles. The drug increases myocardial oxygen demand more than it increases supply, and it may precipitate anginal attacks in patients with coronary atherosclerosis.

The effects of epinephrine on renal hemodynamics have received considerable attention. It is generally accepted that the drug decreases renal plasma flow but does not influence glomerular filtration. Large doses of epinephrine, however, may decrease glomerular filtration also.

Cerebral blood flow is affected in a complex manner by norepinephrine and epinephrine. These mediators can directly constrict cerebral vessels. Nevertheless, cerebral blood flow often does not significantly change or even increases because of the primary elevation of systemic pressure.

BRONCHODILATOR EFFECT

Epinephrine dilates bronchial smooth muscle by stimulation of β_2-receptors. As expected from its lack of appreciable action on β_2-receptors elsewhere, norepinephrine is not a useful bronchodilator. Isoproterenol is a somewhat more potent dilator than epinephrine. Bronchodilatation is not important when β_2-receptor agonists are administered to a normal person. It becomes prominent when bronchi are constricted by agents such as histamine or methacholine or in bronchial asthma. In the latter condition epinephrine is a time-honored remedy.

OTHER SMOOTH MUSCLE EFFECTS

Epinephrine causes mydriasis by contracting the radial muscle of the iris. This effect is not usually prominent with direct application of the drug. Drops of epinephrine and related agents, including the prodrug dipivefrin, reduce intraocular pressure in open-angle glaucoma by improving drainage of aqueous humor.[18] Local pain or stinging may occur, and systemic absorption can cause cardiovascular reactions.

Catecholamines have a modest inhibitory action on gastrointestinal smooth muscle. The evidence indicates that β-receptor stimulation is directly relaxant, whereas α_2-receptor stimulation acts presynaptically on cholinergic neurons to inhibit acetylcholine release. These actions have no therapeutic importance. The same may be said for the complex and variable effects of epinephrine on the uterus. Ejaculation and detumescence appear to involve α-receptors.[7]

NEURAL EFFECTS

Alterations in norepinephrine content in the central nervous system can be associated with altered brain function and behavior. Although injected catecholamines do not efficiently cross the blood-brain barrier to exert prominent effects, some recipients experience anxiety and weakness. Clearly, less polar adrenergic drugs such as the amphetamines have a pronounced stimulant action on the central nervous system.

METABOLIC EFFECTS

Oxygen consumption may be increased by 25% after injection of a therapeutic dose of epinephrine. Norepinephrine has considerably weaker actions on both oxygen consumption and lactic acid production in man.

Epinephrine and isoproterenol, and to a lesser degree norepinephrine, exert complex effects on carbohydrate metabolism. They elevate blood glucose by glycogenolysis, through activation of receptors that vary with the organ. Glucose is released from the liver and lactic acid from muscle. The influence on phosphorylase was studied extensively by Sutherland and Rall.[19] Epinephrine stimulation of β-receptors promotes formation of the second messenger cyclic AMP. Characterization of the membrane components involved in control of adenylyl cyclase, which catalyzes the conversion of ATP to cyclic AMP, has progressed considerably in recent years (see Chapter 3).

Catecholamines promote release of fatty acids from adipose tissue via β_1-receptors and elevate the level of unesterified fatty acids in the blood. Thus the sympathetic nervous system, through catecholamine release, provides not only glucose but also free fatty acids as energy sources.

The distribution of K^+ between extracellular and intracellular spaces is influenced by catecholamines. β_2-Receptor agonists cause distribution into muscle, thereby decreasing plasma K^+. Transient elevation of plasma K^+ after injection of epinephrine reflects initial efflux from the liver.

THERAPEUTIC APPLICATIONS

The therapeutic uses of epinephrine and norepinephrine are based primarily on their vasoconstrictor, cardiac stimulant, and bronchodilator properties.

Vasoconstriction. Epinephrine is commonly added to local anesthetic solutions to delay absorption of the anesthetic, thereby prolonging anesthesia in the desired region and minimizing potential systemic toxicity. Epinephrine is also used to treat urticaria and angioneurotic edema, and it can be applied topically to reduce superficial bleeding.

Norepinephrine infusions have been given for management of hypotension and shock. The initial enthusiasm decreased considerably once it was realized that sympathetic activity is already greatly increased in shock and that correction of underlying abnormalities such as decreased blood volume is more important. On the other hand, epinephrine is very useful for reversing hypotension associated with anaphylactic shock, and pressor amines are also used to maintain blood pressure during spinal anesthesia.

Cardiac. Epinephrine can be injected directly into the heart in asystole in an attempt to achieve resuscitation. However, external cardiac massage and electrical defibrillation are now favored before epinephrine resuscitation is tried.

Bronchodilatation. Epinephrine was once frequently given subcutaneously or intramuscularly (0.3 to 0.5 ml of a 1:1000 solution) for relief of asthmatic attacks. More potent and specific bronchodilators are now available (see Chapter 44).

ADVERSE REACTIONS

Overdosage with norepinephrine or epinephrine may cause severe hypertension with possible cerebral hemorrhage, pulmonary edema, and arrhythmias, including ventricular fibrillation. Reactions that are less serious, such as palpitation, headache, tremor, and difficult breathing, may be very distressful to a patient who has not been forewarned. In addition, extravasation can cause ischemia at the site of intravenous infusion of norepinephrine. Such damage may be reduced by infiltration of phentolamine, an α-adrenergic blocking agent, or a local anesthetic.

Patients receiving tricyclic antidepressants or guanethidine, which block the amine uptake mechanism in adrenergic neurons, may develop exaggerated responses to norepinephrine and epinephrine.

PHEOCHROMOCYTOMA

An unusual form of hypertension is caused by tumors of adrenomedullary tissue that secrete norepinephrine with variable amounts of epinephrine. Although pheochromocytoma is a rare tumor, its detection is very important because it represents one of the few curable forms of hypertension. Most of these tumors that have been examined by chemical methods have contained a very high concentration of norepinephrine and a smaller amount of epinephrine. There may be as much as 10 to 15 mg/g of tissue, and the total catecholamine content of a large tumor may be more than 1 g.

Several methods, some based on neuropharmacologic principles and others on determination of catecholamines or their metabolites in urine or plasma, have been used to diagnose pheochromocytoma.[5] Although it is rare to use pharmacologic tests today because they are less accurate and relatively hazardous as compared with chemical tests, they illustrate interesting principles.

Pharmacologic tests. Drug tests for pheochromocytoma have been of two types: provocative and antagonistic. A provocative agent promotes secretion of catecholamines from a tumor and further increases blood pressure. Conversely, in normal persons a number of the drugs used (histamine, methacholine, tetraethylammonium) cause hypotension.

An antagonistic test employs the α-adrenergic receptor antagonist phentolamine. A dose of 2.5 mg (or if negative, 5 mg) is injected intravenously. If systolic blood pressure falls more than 35 mm Hg and diastolic pressure more than 25 mm Hg, the test is considered positive. However, false positive and negative reactions may occur.

Chemical tests. The diagnosis of pheochromocytoma is now almost always established by determination of (1) plasma amine concentrations or (2) the amount of the amines, their metabolites (normetanephrine, metanephrine, and VMA), or a combination of these in a 24-hour urine specimen. Methyldopa, tetracycline, and quinidine are among several agents that can falsely increase norepinephrine and epinephrine values, whereas MAO inhibitors will increase normetanephrine and metanephrine. Acute myocardial infarction, surgical trauma, and shock may also cause abnormally high urinary outputs of catecholamines and their metabolites.

When chemical tests alone are not definitive, they may be combined with pharmacologic approaches. If circulating catecholamines are moderately elevated due to anxiety in a normal patient, clonidine will lower free amine concentrations, through its action on central α_2 receptors (see Chapter 21). Because the tumor is not innervated, this response to clonidine does not occur in patients with pheochromocytoma. Glucagon evokes catecholamine release from pheochromocytomas; a 35/25 mm Hg elevation of blood pressure and markedly increased plasma amine concentrations 2 minutes after intravenous injection of glucagon are considered diagnostic.

PREPARATIONS

Norepinephrine (Levophed) **bitartrate** is available for injection as 1 mg of base per milliliter in 4 ml ampules. For intravenous infusion in adults the contents of one ampule are added to 0.25 to 1 liter of 5% dextrose injection.

Ethylnorepinephrine hydrochloride (Bronkephrine; 2 mg/ml) is given subcutaneously or intramuscularly to relieve bronchospasm.

Epinephrine hydrochloride is provided in solutions containing 0.01 to 1 mg/ml epinephrine for injection, 1 mg/ml for nasal administration, and 10 mg/ml for nebulization.

Epinephrine bitartrate aerosols (Medihaler-Epi, Primatene Mist Suspension, others) deliver 160 μg per metered spray.

Epinephrine hydrochloride (0.1% to 2%), bitartrate (2%), and borate (Epinal, Eppy/N; 0.5% to 2%) solutions are used in ophthalmology.

Epinephrine itself is available as aerosols and as an aqueous suspension (Sus-Phrine) containing 5 mg/ml for subcutaneous injection.

Dipivefrin hydrochloride (Propine), a prodrug that is hydrolyzed to epinephrine, is used as an 0.1% solution for management of glaucoma. Because both phenolic hydroxyls of epinephrine are esterified in this agent, it penetrates more readily into ocular tissues. Another agent used topically to reduce intraocular pressure is **apraclonidine hydrochloride** (Iopidine), an α_2-receptor agonist.

Dopamine

This catecholamine is an important neurotransmitter in certain parts of the central nervous system (Chapter 26). In the periphery, dopamine acts on β-receptors in the heart to increase contractility and, to a lesser degree, heart rate. In large doses it acts on α_1-receptors to cause vasoconstriction. On the other hand, dopamine-induced dilatation of renal and mesenteric vessels is inhibited by haloperidol and phenothiazines rather than by propranolol. These results indicate the presence of dopamine receptors that have been designated DA_1 (D_1).[10] Other peripheral dopamine receptors in ganglia or receptors that function presynaptically to inhibit norepinephrine release have been designated DA_2 (D_2).

The hemodynamic effects of dopamine depend on the dose, with some individual variation. Intravenous infusion of 1 to 5 μg/kg/min increases cardiac contractility, cardiac output, and renal blood flow. Heart rate and mean blood pressure do not change appreciably. With higher rates of infusion, arterial pressure rises and heart rate reflexly decreases.

Dopamine infusion is used in some cases of shock, in which its lack of constrictor action in the kidney and mesentery is an advantage. In this setting dopamine should be administered only if blood volume is adequate. Orally effective dopaminergic agonists are potentially of benefit in treating congestive heart failure and hypertension.

Ventricular arrhythmia is the most serious adverse effect. Nausea and vomiting may also occur. If hypertension develops, the action of the drug lasts only a few minutes.

Dopamine hydrochloride (Intropin, Dopastat) is available in ampules, vials, and syringes that contain 40 to 160 mg/ml. The drug should be diluted in 250 to 500 ml of sterile solution. Usually an intravenous infusion of 2 to 5 μg/kg/min is given initially, with subsequent adjustment of dosage as needed.

Dobutamine hydrochloride (Dobutrex) is a racemic mixture. The (+)-enantiomer preferentially stimulates β-receptors, whereas the (−)-enantiomer preferentially stimulates α_1-receptors. Infusion of the drug increases force and, to a lesser extent, rate of cardiac contraction. Typically, there is minimal change in blood pressure, presumably because β_2-receptor–mediated vasodilatation offsets α_1-receptor–mediated vasoconstriction.[15] Dobutamine is used in acute myocardial infarction with congestive failure and after coronary bypass operations. Because of its very short half-life, it is given intravenously, usually at rates of 2.5 to 10 μg/kg/min. The drug is available in 20 ml vials containing 250 mg, for eventual dilution to 250 to 1000 μg/ml.

MISCELLANEOUS ADRENERGIC DRUGS

Classification based on mechanism of action

Sympathomimetic drugs may act *directly* on α- and β-receptors, or they may act *indirectly* by releasing endogenous catecholamine. Some have a *mixed* action, both direct and indirect. Important examples are given below:

	α-RECEPTOR AGONISTS	β-RECEPTOR AGONISTS
Direct-acting drugs	Methoxamine	Isoproterenol
Mixed-acting drugs	Metaraminol	Ephedrine (indirect on α-receptors)
Indirect-acting drugs	Tyramine Amphetamine	

This classification is based mainly on two types of experiments. In one type, drugs are administered to animals in which tissue norepinephrine has been depleted by reserpine. In these animals responses to adrenergic agonists such as norepinephrine, epinephrine, and phenylephrine are normal or augmented. These drugs act directly on receptors. Other adrenergic agents, including tyramine and amphetamine, act indirectly (see p. 95) and are therefore inactivated by norepinephrine depletion (Fig. 18-5); an infusion of norepinephrine restores the capacity of the animals to react. Other adrenergic drugs are intermediate (mixed) in that some but not all of their effects are prevented by reserpine pretreatment. Ephedrine and phenylpropanolamine are examples.

The other line of support for norepinephrine release as the mode of action of indirectly acting amines is the observation that they are inactive on chronically denervated organs. Because of receptor upregulation, such organs become supersensitive to directly acting amines.

Classification based on clinical usage

Discussion of sympathomimetic amines may be simplified if they are subdivided by clinical usage into three major categories. **Vasoconstrictors**, several of which are used as eye drops or nasal decongestants, and **central nervous system stimulants**, which are commonly used as appetite suppressants, are listed in Table 18-4. Most of the **bronchodilators** are discussed in detail in Chapter 44. There is some overlap in these

FIG. 18-5 *Blood pressure response to tyramine.* **A**, *Reserpinized cat.* **B**, *Control cat. Dose of reserpine: 7 mg/kg subcutaneously. Dose of tyramine: 0.5 mg/kg intravenously. Arrows indicate times of tyramine injection.*

From Carlsson A, Rosengren E, Bertler Å, Nilsson J: In Garattini S, Ghetti V, editors: Psychotropic drugs, Amsterdam, 1957, Elsevier Publishing Co.

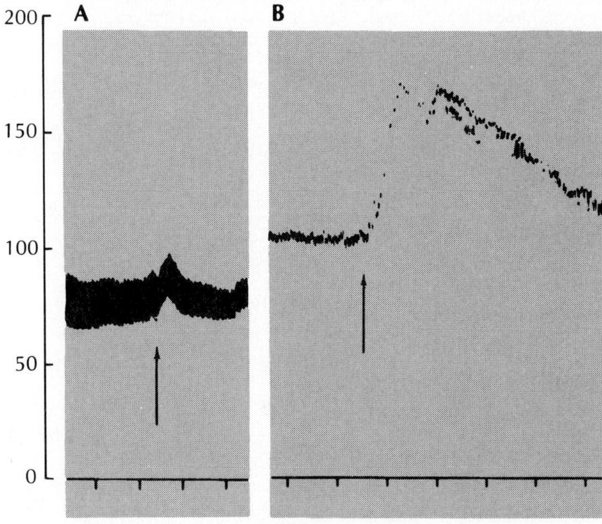

Tyramine (0.5 mg/kg)

activities, especially in the case of ephedrine, which is used for its cardiovascular, bronchodilator, and stimulant properties. It is considered separately.

Ephedrine

Used in China for centuries and introduced into the United States in 1923, ephedrine is a naturally occurring sympathomimetic drug now used primarily in over-the-counter products. Ephedrine is similar to epinephrine and norepinephrine except that it has a much longer duration of action, it is effective by the oral route, it penetrates into and stimulates the central nervous system, and it causes tachyphylaxis on frequent administration. On a weight basis, ephedrine is about one hundredth as potent as the catecholamines.

Ephedrine acts partially indirectly. Many of its peripheral actions are reduced by pretreatment with reserpine or by sympathetic denervation. Its bronchodilatory action must be direct, since norepinephrine is not a potent agonist at β_2-receptors. In addition to its vasopressor effect, ephedrine can increase heart rate and causes mydriasis when applied to the eye.

OH CH$_3$ H; CH—CH—N—CH$_3$

Ephedrine

TABLE 18-4 Indications and dosage forms for miscellaneous adrenergic drugs

Use / Drug	Tablets (mg)	Capsules (mg)	Nose drops (or spray %)	Eye drops %	Injection (mg/ml)	Miscellaneous* (mg)
	Dosage forms					
Vasoconstriction						
Ephedrine sulfate (Vatronal, others)		25, 50	0.5		25, 50	J:0.6%; S:11, 20/5 ml
Phenylephrine hydrochloride (Neo-Synephrine, others)			0.125-1	0.12-10	10	J:0.5%
Methoxamine hydrochloride (Vasoxyl)					20	
Mephentermine (Wyamine) sulfate					15, 30	
Metaraminol bitartrate (Aramine)					10	
Nasal decongestion						
Phenylpropanolamine hydrochloride	25-75	25-75				
Propylhexedrine (Benzedrex)						I:250
Oxymetazoline hydrochloride (Afrin, others)			0.025, 0.05	0.025		
Naphazoline hydrochloride (Privine, others)			0.05	0.012-0.1		
Tetrahydrozoline hydrochloride (Murine, others)			0.05, 0.1	0.05		
Xylometazoline hydrochloride (Otrivin)			0.05, 0.1			
Pseudoephedrine hydrochloride (Sudaphed, others)	30, 60	120				DO:7.5/0.8 ml; S:15,30/5ml
Pseudoephedrine sulfate (Afrinol)	120					
L-Desoxyephedrine (Vicks)						I:50
Appetite suppression						
Amphetamine sulfate	5, 10					
Dextroamphetamine sulfate (Dexedrine, others)	5,10	5-15				S:5/5 ml
Methamphetamine hydrochloride (Desoxyn)	5-15					
Diethylpropion hydrochloride (Tenuate, Tepanil)	25, 75					
Phenmetrazine hydrochloride (Preludin)	75					
Benzphetamine hydrochloride (Didrex)	25, 50					
Phentermine hydrochloride (Fastin, others)	8-37.5	15-37.5				
Phendimetrazine tartrate (Obalan, others)	35	35, 105				
Fenfluramine hydrochloride (Pondimin)	20					
Mazindol (Sanorex, Mazanor)	1, 2					

**DO*, Drops (oral); *I*, inhaler; *J*, jelly; *L*, lozenge; *S*, solution, syrup, or elixir (oral).

Adrenergic vasoconstrictors related to epinephrine or ephedrine

Phenylephrine is primarily a direct-acting α-receptor agonist. Subcutaneous or intramuscular injection of 2 to 5 mg is used to prevent hypotension during spinal anesthesia and to manage orthostatic hypotension. It can be added to local anesthetic solutions to prolong anesthesia and is applied topically as a nasal decongestant and as a mydriatic.

Methoxamine is a direct-acting α-receptor agonist that lacks cardiac stimulant properties. Both methoxamine and phenylephrine may be given intravenously to induce reflex cardiac slowing in patients with paroxysmal supraventricular tachycardia.

Two other compounds are less often used nowadays. Mephentermine is both a direct and indirect vasoactive drug acting on both α- and β-receptors. The duration of its vasoconstrictor and myocardial stimulant actions is about 60 minutes after subcutaneous injection of 10 to 30 mg. Metaraminol resembles phenylephrine in its properties but acts both directly and indirectly. It is taken up by sympathetic fibers and released as a false transmitter. The drug is usually administered subcutaneously or intramuscularly in doses of 2 to 10 mg.

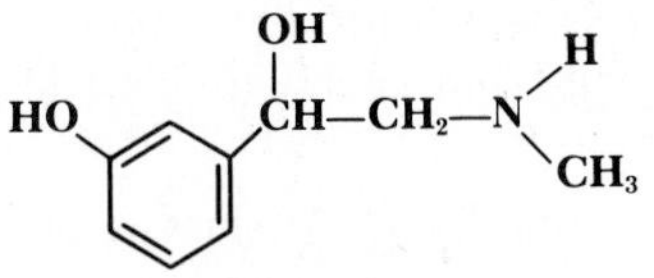

Phenylephrine

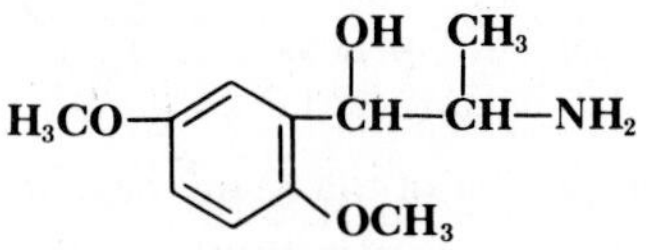

Methoxamine

NASAL DECONGESTANTS

Nasal vasoconstrictors (Table 18-4) are widely used medications that are not harmless. Their continued use to relieve symptoms of nasal congestion may actually induce chronic rhinitis and exacerbate congestion of the nasal mucosa, probably because ischemia leads to rebound swelling. In excessive doses these drugs can evoke systemic effects, such as hypertension, dizziness, palpitation, and in some cases central nervous system stimulation. Several of these agents are available over the counter. **Oxymetazoline** and **xylometazoline** are relatively longer acting and need be taken no more than two or three times daily, respectively.

The decongestants are frequently combined with antihistamines. Preparations containing pseudoephedrine, phenylpropanolamine, or phenylephrine with an antihistamine have become very popular as nasal decongestants that are taken orally.

Phenylpropanolamine is also used as an anorexiant. This over-the-counter drug is widely used and is usually safe, but moderate overdosage may cause severe hypertension.[6] **Propylhexedrine**, which is commonly administered by inhalation, has many of the properties of amphetamine, but it has less pressor activity and causes much less central nervous system stimulation. **Naphazoline**, an imidazoline derivative, may cause profound drowsiness and coma in children and also rebound swelling of the mucosa and cardiac irregularities when used excessively. **Tetrahydrozoline** is chemically similar to naphazoline and causes similar adverse effects.

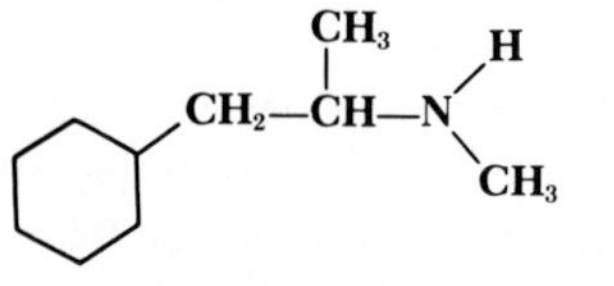

Propylhexedrine

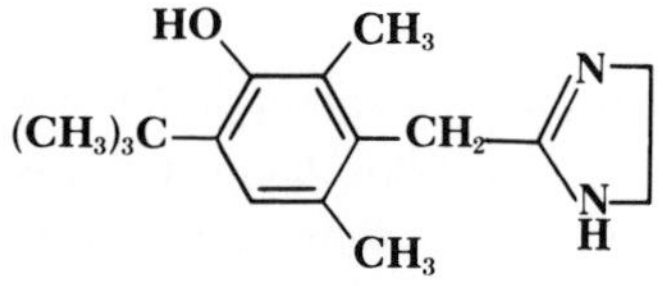

Oxymetazoline

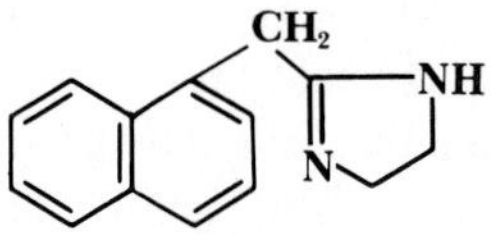

Naphazoline

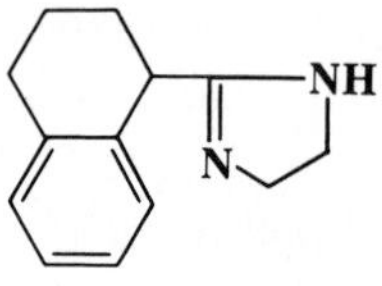

Tetrahydrozoline

Adrenergic bronchodilators

Isoproterenol

Isoproterenol (isopropylnorepinephrine) is a potent β-receptor agonist. It dilates bronchial smooth muscle and increases heart rate and contractility. It also dilates blood vessels, particularly in skeletal muscle.

Historically, isoproterenol has been used primarily for treatment of bronchial asthma, atrioventricular block, and cardiac arrest. Palpitation, tachycardia, arrhythmias, hypotension, angina, and headache may occur after its administration. Cyclopropane, halogenated anesthetics, and propellants can sensitize the myocardium to isoproterenol.

Isoproterenol hydrochloride (Isuprel) is available in solutions of 0.031% to 1% for nebulization, a solution containing 0.2 mg/ml for injection, and sublingual tablets of 10 and 15 mg. The drug can also be taken as an 0.25% aerosol or one that delivers 131 μg per metered spray. The sulfate is available as an aerosol (80 μg per spray) and a powder for oral insufflation (45 or 110 μg per inhalation).

Other bronchodilators

Theophylline derivatives and several adrenergic drugs besides isoproterenol are also used as bronchodilators. Epinephrine and ephedrine have already been discussed. More selective β_2-receptor agonists, such as albuterol and metaproterenol, are preferred for management of asthma because they cause fewer adverse cardiac effects. These agents are discussed in Chapter 44 in connection with drug effects on the respiratory tract.

Adrenergic vasodilators

Nylidrin and isoxsuprine, which dilate peripheral blood vessels experimentally, appear to act primarily as direct vasodilators with perhaps some β-agonist activity. They have been used in dementia and in peripheral vascular disease to increase blood flow. There is no evidence that they have any salutary effect, and their use for these conditions should be abandoned.

Adrenergic central nervous system stimulants and anorexiants

AMPHETAMINES

The amphetamines are powerful stimulants of the central nervous system. *Dextro*amphetamine has considerably more central, and somewhat less cardiovascular, activity than the *levo* isomer has. Medically amphetamines are used and also abused for their anorexiant effect, an indication questioned by many authorities. In addition, they find application in management of children with *attention-deficit hyperactivity disorder* (see Chapter 31) and as stimulants in treatment of narcolepsy. Amphetamine, which lacks the phenolic hydroxyl groups of the catecholamines, is well absorbed from the gastrointestinal tract and readily reaches the brain. Its main metabolite is phenylacetone, a product of microsomal deamination. A minor metabolite, *p*-hydroxyamphetamine, is taken up by adrenergic nerves and transformed to *p*-hydroxynorephedrine, which is stored in vesicles to become a false transmitter.

Numerous anorexiants have been developed and are used by the medical profession, often indiscriminately and without the realization that they are essentially relatives of dextroamphetamine that lack significant advantages over this prototype. These anorexiant drugs are believed to act at a common receptor,[13] and experimental evidence indicates that hypothalamic D_1-dopamine receptors and β-adrenergic receptors are subsequently involved in development of anorexia.[17] Except for phenylpropanolamine, which is a component of many over-the-counter "diet pills," these agents are controlled substances placed in Schedules II, III, or IV (see Table 71-1).

Disadvantages in use of anorexiants are related to development of psychic dependence, to untoward effects resulting from adrenergic actions, and to rapid development of tolerance; the anorexiant action is useful for only a week or two. Hence these agents at best are likely to serve only as a short-term adjunct to management of obesity. Large and repeated doses of amphetamines may produce a psychosis that has many of the characteristics of paranoid schizophrenia (see p. 345).

C_6H_5—CH_2—CH(CH_3)—NH_2

Amphetamine

The vascular effects of amphetamines are attributed to catecholamine release because the drugs do not elevate blood pressure in reserpinized animals. In contrast, central effects of amphetamine are not prevented by catecholamine depletion. Instead, blockade of catecholamine synthesis quickly inhibits its behavioral effects. These findings indicate that these effects may be mediated through a newly synthesized fraction of brain catecholamines.

Dextroamphetamine is available with amphetamine in a 50:50 resin complex (Biphetamine) that contains 12.5 or 20 mg of total amine. **Methamphetamine** is closely related from a structural standpoint to both ephedrine and amphetamine. It is a potent central nervous system stimulant and has considerable pressor action on blood vessels. It is used for the same purposes as amphetamine. **Diethylpropion** is basically an amphetamine-like drug, though it is claimed to cause less jitteriness and insomnia and also fewer cardiovascular effects than amphetamine. Other appetite suppressants are listed in Table 18-4.

MISCELLANEOUS ANOREXIANTS

Fenfluramine, which is related structurally to amphetamine, and **mazindol**, which is not a phenethylamine, are comparable to other anorexiants in suppressing appetite, but they appear to act by other mechanisms. They may be used as short-term adjuncts to other measures that include caloric restriction, exercise, and psychotherapy. Fenfluramine, a racemate, appears to reduce appetite, at least partially, by altering serotonergic neurotransmission.[14,17] Studies in animals indicate that, after active transport into neurons, the drug releases serotonin, reduces its turnover, and depletes it by interfering with storage; other actions of fenfluramine or norfenfluramine, its active metabolite, include inhibition of serotonin uptake and stimulation of postsynaptic serotonin receptors. The relative therapeutic importance of such actions and of the parent compound versus the metabolite is not yet clear. The *d*-enantiomer has generally been more potent; however, the *l*-enantiomer is responsible for drowsiness, an unusual characteristic among appetite suppressants. Diarrhea and dry mouth are other common side effects. Fluoxetine, an antidepressant drug that selectively inhibits serotonin uptake, may also prove to be a useful anorexiant.[3] The appetite-suppressant action of mazindol requires intact catecholamine stores and is probably independent of serotonergic neurotransmission. This drug inhibits uptake of norepinephrine and dopamine and appears to release the latter amine, but the relation of these actions to the therapeutic benefit is unknown.

The possibility that anorexiants act by a common mechanism, despite the differences in their actions enumerated above, is supported by a high correlation in the rat between the potencies of mazindol and several phenethylamines, including fenfluramine, in binding to a common receptor in hypothalamic synaptosomal membranes and in inhibiting food intake.[2]

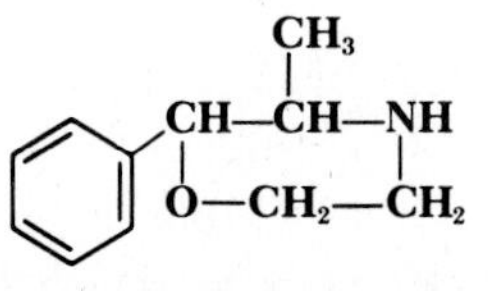

CH_3 / $CH—CH—NH$ / $O—CH_2—CH_2$

Phenmetrazine

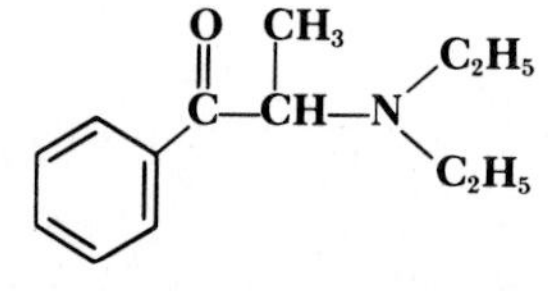

O CH_3 / $C—CH—N(C_2H_5)_2$

Diethylpropion

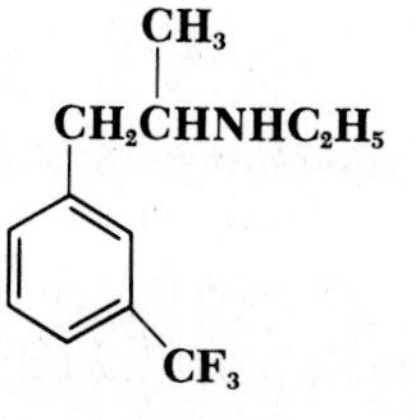

CH_3 / $CH_2CHNHC_2H_5$ / CF_3

Fenfluramine

N / N / HO / Cl

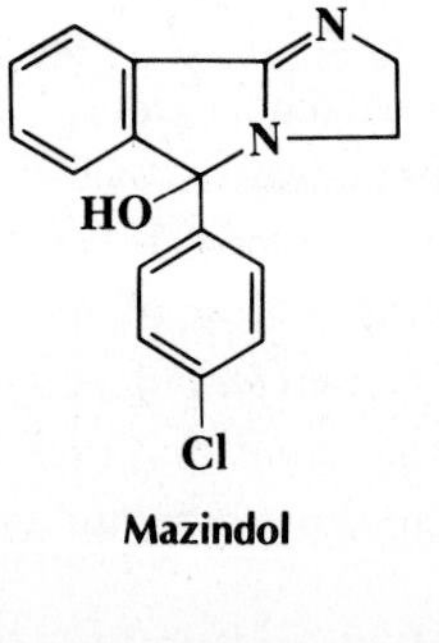

Mazindol

DRUG INTERACTIONS

All of these central stimulants and anorexiants may cause hypertensive crises in patients taking MAO inhibitors. All, except fenfluramine, antagonize the antihypertensive action of guanethidine. Fenfluramine may instead potentiate the antihypertensive action of guanethidine and methyldopa. Fenfluramine, being sedative, may enhance depression by alcohol and other central nervous system depressants. Mazindol potentiates the vasopressor effect of norepinephrine in dogs, and vasopressor medications must be used with caution in patients taking mazindol.

Structure-activity relationships in adrenergic series

A great deal is known about the relationships between structure and activity of adrenergic drugs. Such knowledge in general is important to the pharmaceutic chemist as a guide to synthesis of new drugs. Structure-activity relationships are also of fundamental importance in that they should reflect basic characteristics of receptor-drug interactions. In the case of adrenergic drugs the problem is complicated by the fact that many sympathomimetic drugs act through release of endogenous catecholamines. The differences in action of these drugs may be related to the predominant site of catecholamine release. A few generalities may serve to illustrate the concept of structure-activity relationships.

The basic adrenergic structure is β-phenethylamine.

$$\overset{\beta}{CH_2}-\overset{\alpha}{CH_2}-NH_2$$

β-Phenethylamine

Hydroxyl groups on the benzene ring or on the side chain influence the metabolism and absorption of the drugs, as well as their actions on receptors. Sympathomimetics that are not catechols are generally less polar and therefore absorbed better and are, of course, not O-methylated by COMT.

Substitutions on the nitrogen have a great influence on the type of receptor with which the drug will interact. Thus norepinephrine, lacking substitutions, acts on α- and β_1-receptors, epinephrine with one methyl group acts on α-receptors and both types of β-receptor, and isoproterenol acts virtually exclusively on β-receptors.

Substitutions on the α carbon tend to prolong the action of the drug by protecting against destruction by MAO. The hydroxyl group on the β carbon is necessary for granular storage in adrenergic neurons.

REFERENCES

1. Ahlquist RP: A study of the adrenotropic receptors, *Am J Physiol* 153:586, 1948.
2. Angel I, Paul SM: Demonstration of specific binding sites for [^{3}H]mazindol in rat hypothalamus: correlation with the anorectic properties of phenylethylamines, *Eur J Pharmacol* 113:133, 1985.
3. Bray GA, Cairella M, editors: Drugs regulating food intake and energy balance, *Int J Obes* 11(suppl 3), 1987.
4. Fried G, Lagercrantz H, Klein R, Thureson-Klein Å: Large and small noradrenergic vesicles: origin, contents, and functional significance. In Usdin E, Carlsson A, Dahlström A, Engel J, editors: *Catecholamines.* Part A: Basic and

peripheral mechanisms, New York, 1984, Alan R Liss, p 45.

5. Keiser HR, Doppman JL, Robertson CN, et al: Diagnosis, localization, and management of pheochromocytoma. In Lack EE, editor: *Pathology of the adrenal glands*, New York, 1990, Churchill Livingstone, p 237.
6. Kelley MT: Sympathomimetics. In Haddad LM, Winchester JF, editors: *Clinical management of poisoning and drug overdose*, ed 2, Philadelphia, 1990, WB Saunders, p 1392.
7. Krane RJ, Goldstein I, Saenz de Tejada I: Impotence, *N Engl J Med* 321:1648, 1989.
8. Langer SZ: Presynaptic regulation of catecholamine release, *Biochem Pharmacol* 23:1793, 1974.
9. Langer SZ, Duval N, Massingham R: Pharmacologic and therapeutic significance of α-adrenoceptor subtypes, *J Cardiovasc Pharmacol* 7(suppl 8):S1, 1985.
10. Lokhandwala MF, Hegde SS: Cardiovascular dopamine receptors: role of renal dopamine and dopamine receptors in sodium excretion, *Pharmacol Toxicol* 66:237, 1990.
11. MacDonald E, Ruskoaho H, Scheinin M, Virtanen R: Therapeutic applications of drugs acting on alpha-adrenoceptors, *Ann Clin Res* 20:298, 1988.
12. Misu Y, Kubo T: Presynaptic β-adrenoceptors, *Med Res Rev* 6:197, 1986.
13. Paul SM, Hulihan-Giblin B, Skolnick P: (+)−Amphetamine binding to rat hypothalamus: relation to anorexic potency of phenylethylamines, *Science* 218:487, 1982.
14. Rowland NE, Carlton J: Neurobiology of an anorectic drug: fenfluramine, *Prog Neurobiol* 27:13, 1986.
15. Ruffolo RR, Jr: Review: the pharmacology of dobutamine, *Am J Med Sci* 30:244, 1987.
16. Starke K, Göthert M, Kilbinger H: Modulation of neurotransmitter release by presynaptic autoreceptors, *Physiol Rev* 69:864, 1989.
17. Sugrue MF: Neuropharmacology of drugs affecting food intake, *Pharmacol Ther* 32:145, 1987.
18. Sugrue MF: The pharmacology of antiglaucoma drugs, *Pharmacol Ther* 43:91, 1989.
19. Sutherland EW, Rall TW: The relation of adenosine-3',5'-phosphate and phosphorylase to the actions of catecholamines and other hormones, *Pharmacol Rev* 12:265, 1960.

Chapter 19

Adrenergic blocking agents

GENERAL CONCEPT

Adrenergic blocking agents, with one exception, compete with catecholamines and related agonists for binding to adrenergic receptors. They are relatively specific *alpha* (α)- or *beta* (β)-receptor antagonists. In vivo the α-adrenergic blocking drugs cause vasodilatation by reducing sympathetic tone; some also relax smooth muscle directly. In contrast, β-receptor blockers usually have little effect on vascular tone in resting subjects because β_2-receptors are not being stimulated by epinephrine. However, β-blockers do prevent the vasodilator action of epinephrine or isoproterenol. In organs, such as the heart, that are controlled primarily by β-receptor activation, the β-receptor blockers oppose the excitatory action of norepinephrine.

Drugs that deplete catecholamines or prevent their release from adrenergic nerves are considered in the next chapter and should not be confused with the antagonists, which act on α- and β-receptors.

α-ADRENERGIC BLOCKING AGENTS

General features

A characteristic feature of α-adrenergic blocking agents is their ability to convert the pressor effect of pharmacologic doses of epinephrine into a depressor response. This *epinephrine reversal* by phentolamine is shown in Fig. 19-1. Vascular smooth muscle, particularly in skeletal muscle, has both α- and β_2-receptors. Since epinephrine acts on both receptors, it causes vasodilatation if the α-receptors are blocked. Because norepinephrine does not stimulate β_2-receptors, its pressor effect is decreased by an α-blocker but is not converted to a depressor response.

The drugs in this group differ from each other in potency, duration of action, and relative ability to block α_1- and α_2-receptors. Some also possess pharmacologic properties entirely unrelated to adrenergic blockade.

Phenoxybenzamine

Phenoxybenzamine hydrochloride (Dibenzyline), administered in doses of 10 to 40 mg two or three times daily, lowers blood pressure and inhibits the reflex vasoconstriction that normally occurs in the capacitance vessels upon standing; orthostatic hypotension may occur. The effects of the drug last more than 24 hours. It is available in 10 mg capsules.

The long duration of phenoxybenzamine action is a consequence of a stable combination between the drug and the α-receptor. Although there is competition between the drug and catecholamines for the receptor during the early stage of blockade, competition becomes less effective as blockade develops. The term *non-*

FIG. 19-1 *Epinephrine reversal by phentolamine. Effect of epinephrine on blood pressure before and after injection of phentolamine. A dog was anesthetized with pentobarbital. At* A, *Epinephrine was injected intravenously, 1 μg/kg. At* B, *Phentolamine was injected, 5 mg/kg. At* C, *Epinephrine injection was repeated. Notice the lowering of pressure by epinephrine after the adrenergic blocking agent. The increased pulse pressure under these circumstances is an indication that the adrenergic blocking agent does not prevent the cardiac stimulant effect of epinephrine.*

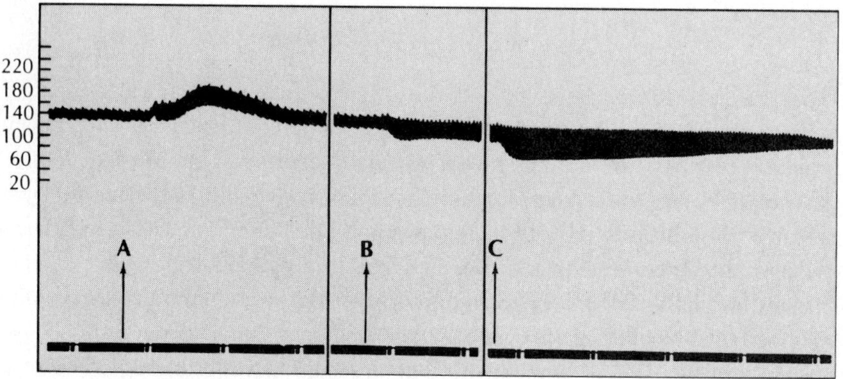

equilibrium blockade has been applied to such an interaction between agonist and antagonist. Phenoxybenzamine is converted to a highly reactive aziridinium-ion intermediate that spontaneously forms a covalent bond with the α-receptor.[4]

C_6H_5—O—CH_2—CH(CH_3)—N(CH_2—C_6H_5)—CH_2—CH_2Cl

Phenoxybenzamine

Phenoxybenzamine is used in management of pheochromocytoma both before and during surgical removal.[12] Patients with this tumor are often treated for several days or weeks to allow stabilization before surgery. Phenoxybenzamine is particularly useful in this setting because of its availability in oral form and its long duration of action.

Among the many adverse effects that may be caused by phenoxybenzamine, orthostatic hypotension, nasal congestion, and miosis are common and predictable. Tachycardia, a reflex response to hypotension, may be further enhanced by presynaptic α_2-receptor blockade, which increases release of norepinephrine. Phenoxybenzamine can also block histamine, serotonin, and cholinergic receptors.

Tolazoline

Tolazoline (Priscoline) hydrochloride, a weak reversible α-blocker related structurally to histamine, causes peripheral vasodilatation largely by a direct relaxant action on vascular smooth muscle. The drug often elicits tachycardia, both reflexly and by stimulating the heart directly. Although used infrequently, tolazoline relieves vasospasm in peripheral vascular diseases and is indicated for relief of persistent pulmonary hypertension in neonates. Tolazoline is available as a solution for injection, 25 mg/ml.

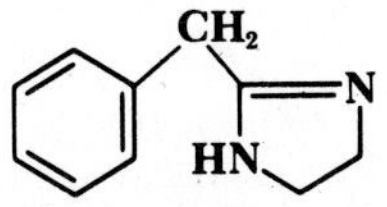

Tolazoline 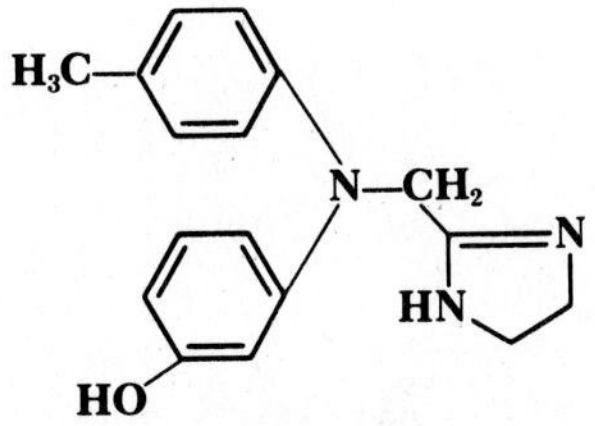 **Phentolamine**

Phentolamine

Phentolamine is a direct vasodilator and reversible α-receptor blocker used primarily to prevent hypertension during surgical removal of pheochromocytoma[12] and rarely for diagnosis of the tumor (see p. 148). Phentolamine mesylate (Regitine) is available for reconstitution and injection, 5 mg. Adverse effects include orthostatic hypotension, tachycardia, nasal stuffiness, and gastrointestinal disturbances such as nausea, vomiting, and diarrhea. The drug cannot be used for chronic management of pheochromocytoma because it is poorly absorbed after oral administration.

Reversible α_1-selective antagonists

Prazosin was initially believed to relax vascular smooth muscle directly. It was later found, however, to be a selective α_1-receptor blocking agent. Prazosin is an important antihypertensive that seldom causes the pronounced tachycardia seen with less selective α-antagonists. Because its weak action on presynaptic receptors does not greatly increase norepinephrine release, there is little cardiac stimulation. Prazosin is also used by urologists to reduce symptoms and improve voiding in patients with prostatism.

Prazosin hydrochloride (Minipress) is available in 1 to 5 mg capsules for administration two or three times daily. Adverse effects include headache, dizziness, drowsiness, and, primarily after the first dose or a dosage increment, orthostatic hypotension. The orthostatic response does not generally persist and can be minimized by giving the first dose at bedtime or by slowly titrating the dosage upward. Mental and sexual functions and exercise capacity are usually spared by this drug.[24] In contrast to some classes of antihypertensive drugs, prazosin lacks adverse actions on plasma lipids and may actually be of benefit.[1,23] **Terazosin hydrochloride** (Hytrin) is very similar to prazosin;[13] it has the advantages of more predictable absorption and once daily administration, as 1 to 5 mg tablets.

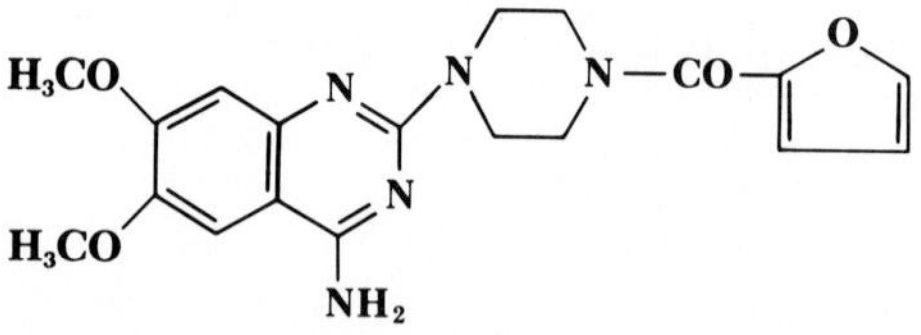

Prazosin

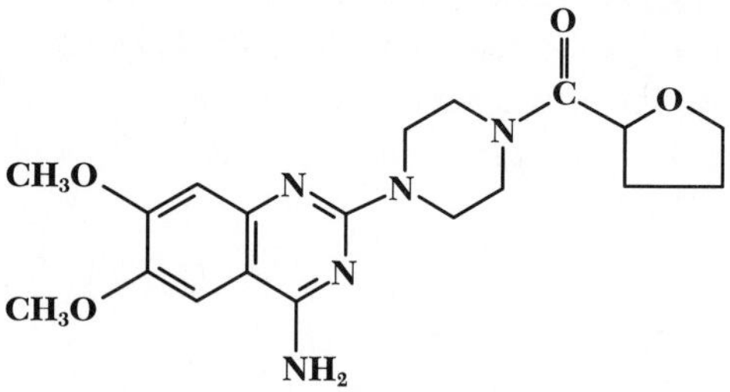

Terazosin

Yohimbine

Yohimbine, widely used as an experimental tool for its selective α_2-receptor antagonistic activity, was reported recently to improve erectile capability in impotent males.[18] Yohimbine hydrochloride (Yohimex, others) is available in 5.4 mg tablets.

Ergot alkaloids

Certain alkaloids of ergot, such as ergotamine, have α-adrenergic blocking activity. However, they are used for their direct vasoconstrictor and oxytocic actions rather than as adrenergic blocking agents. Their pharmacology is discussed in Chapters 23 and 52.

β-ADRENERGIC BLOCKING AGENTS

These drugs are competitive inhibitors of catecholamines at β-adrenoceptors.[7] Their general effects are listed in Table 19-1. They have a spectrum of potencies at β_1-receptors in the heart, and they differ from each other in their duration of action. A summary of their individual properties is given in Table 19-2.

Although β-receptor blockers were first approved to treat angina pectoris, they have numerous other clinical indications. These include hypertension, arrhythmias, thyrotoxicosis, hypertrophic cardiomyopathy, migraine, and glaucoma. The first β-blocker, dichloroisoproterenol, was made by substitution of chlorine for both phenolic hydroxyls on the ring of the agonist isoproterenol. Propranolol, however, was the first agent sufficiently selective for β-receptor blockade to be useful clinically.

TABLE 19-1 Effects of β-adrenergic receptor blockade

Heart rate	Decreased
Myocardial contractility	Decreased
Cardiac output	Decreased
Arterial blood pressure	Unaffected or decreased
Effect of exercise on heart rate and cardiac output	Decreased
β-Adrenergic drug effects (myocardial, arterial, bronchial, metabolic)	Blocked

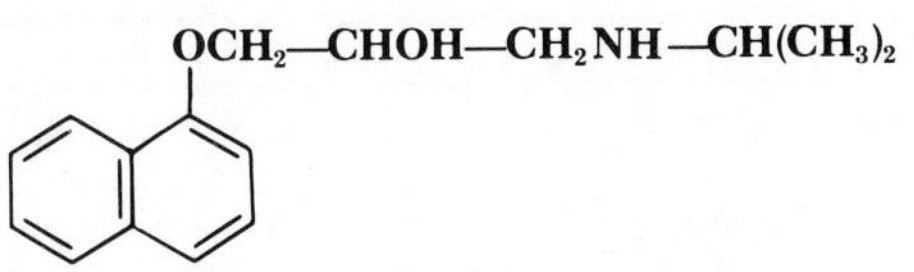

Propranolol

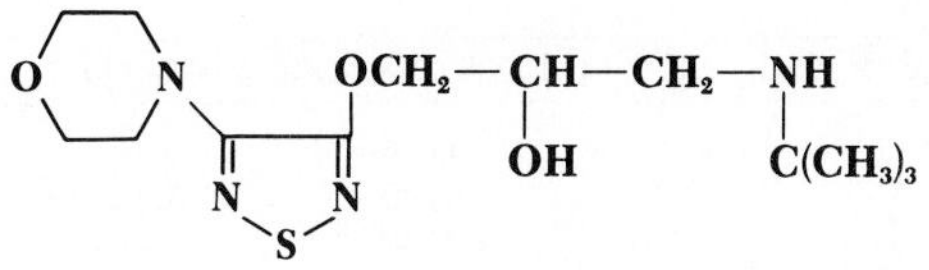

Timolol

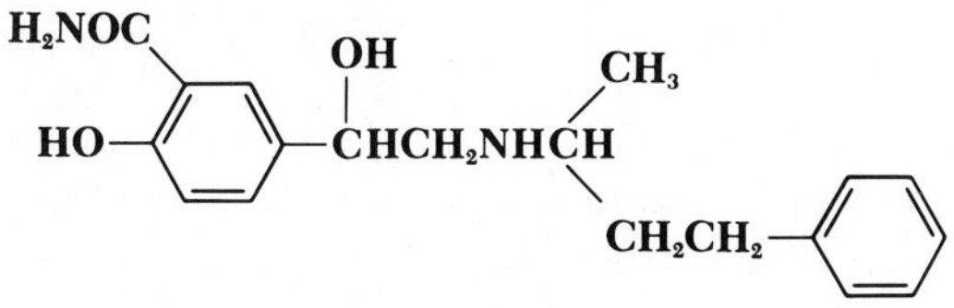

Labetalol

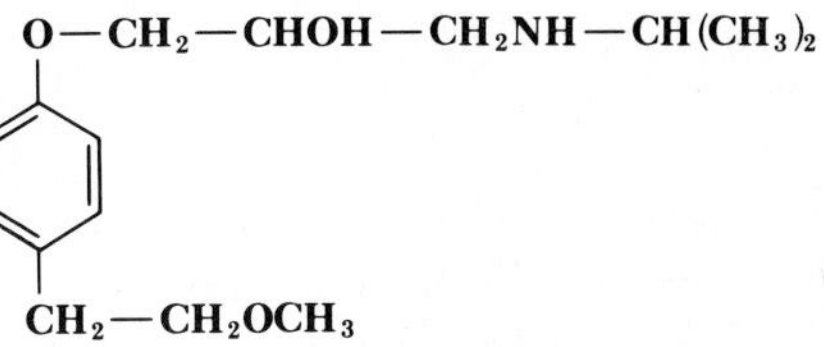

Metoprolol

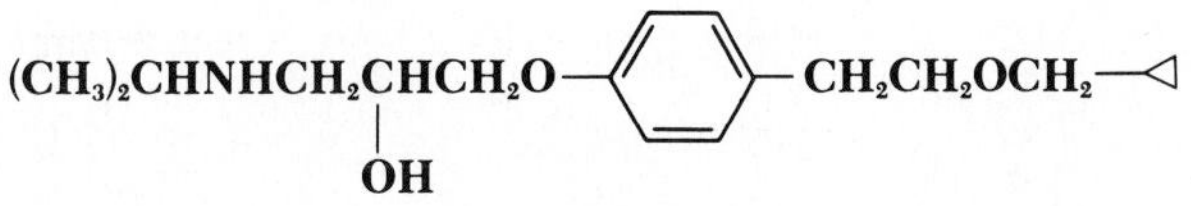

Betaxolol

Propranolol

PHARMACOLOGIC EFFECTS

Propranolol competitively antagonizes the action of catecholamines on all β-receptors. As a consequence the drug exerts negative chronotropic and inotropic actions on the heart, slows atrioventricular conduction, promotes bronchoconstriction, lowers plasma renin activity, and may cause hypoglycemia. It also exerts a quinidine-like (membrane-stabilizing) action on the heart at high doses. Propranolol is a racemic mixture. The *levo* (S) form is the β-blocker, but the *dextro* (R) form has a greater membrane effect.

The effects of propranolol may be overcome by sufficiently large doses of β-agonists, such as isoproterenol, or by glucagon, which acts on a different receptor but also activates adenylyl cyclase.

PHARMACOKINETICS

Propranolol is well absorbed from the gastrointestinal tract, but about two thirds is inactivated in the first pass through the liver.[20] Acebutolol, labetalol, and metoprolol also undergo significant first-pass metabolism, whereas nadolol and atenolol are poorly absorbed. Propranolol, metoprolol, and labetalol are somewhat unusual in that ingestion with food improves their bioavailability.[16]

Despite its short half-life, propranolol may be administered at 6- to 12-hour intervals, depending partially on the indication. 4-Hydroxypropranolol, its major active metabolite, has an even shorter half-life. Altered renal function has little effect on the dosage regimen. On the other hand, cirrhosis and drugs like cimetidine that diminish

TABLE 19-2 β-Receptor blockers: properties, uses, and dosage forms

	Relative cardio-selectivity (β_1)	β-Receptor agonist activity	Half-life (hr)	Therapeutic uses*	Dosage forms† (mg)
Propranolol hydrochloride‡ (Inderal, Ipran)			3-5	HT, AN, MI, AR	T: 10-90; C: 60-160; S: 4, 8, 80/ml; I: 1/ml
Nadolol (Corgard)			20-24	HT, AN	T: 20-160
Pindolol (Visken)		+	3-4	HT	T: 5, 10
Penbutolol sulfate (Levatrol)		+	5	HT	T: 20
Carteolol (Cartrol)		+	6	HT	T: 2.5, 5
Timolol maleate (Blocadren, Timoptic)			4	HT, MI, GL	T: 5-20; D: 0.25%, 0.5%
Labetalol hydrochloride (Normodyne, Trandate)		+	6-8	HT	T: 100-300; I: 5/ml
Metoprolol tartrate (Lopressor)	+		3-7	HT, AN, MI	T: 50, 100; I: 1/ml
Atenolol (Tenormin)	+		6-9	HT, AN, MI	T: 50, 100; I: 5/10 ml
Acebutolol hydrochloride (Sectral)	+	+	3-4	HT, AR	C: 200, 400
Esmolol hydrochloride (Brevibloc)	+		0.15	AR	I: 10,250/ml
Betaxolol hydrochloride (Kerlone, Betoptic)	+		14-22	HT, GL	T: 10, 20; D: 0.25%, 0.5%
Levobunolol hydrochloride (Betagan)				GL	D: 0.5%
Metipranolol hydrochloride (OptiPranolol)				GL	D: 0.3%

**AN,* Angina pectoris; *AR,* cardiac arrhythmias; *GL,* glaucoma; *HT,* hypertension; *MI,* myocardial infarction.
†*C,* Capsules; *D,* eye drops; *I,* injection; *S,* solution (oral); *T,* tablets.
‡Also marketed for use in patients with hypertrophic subaortic stenosis, migraine, and pheochromocytoma.

hepatic metabolism not only decrease clearance but also increase the bioavailability of propranolol (by decreasing the first-pass effect).

CLINICAL USES

The *antiarrhythmic effect* of propranolol results largely from β-receptor blockade, although a component of membrane stabilization may also contribute.[11] The drug is used against supraventricular tachyarrhythmias, as in thyrotoxicosis. Ventricular tachycardias caused by catecholamines or digitalis are also important indications, but propranolol is not the first choice for other types of ventricular tachycardias.

Angina pectoris is relieved by propranolol in selected patients who do not respond to conventional measures such as sublingual nitroglycerin. The benefit derives from the decrease in heart rate and reductions in left ventricular contractility and wall tension, all of which diminish myocardial oxygen demand.

The *antihypertensive effect* of propranolol has not been explained in a completely satisfactory manner. Reduction of cardiac output is most likely primary, but inhibition of renin release and some central nervous system actions have been suggested as other possible mechanisms of its antihypertensive action. Blockade of presynaptic β-receptors with a subsequent decrease in norepinephrine release over long-term therapy has also been proposed.[14] When propranolol is used with a peripheral vasodilator such as hydralazine, its beneficial effect is more easily understandable. Peripheral vasodilatation leads to reflex cardiac stimulation, which is blocked by propranolol.

Hypertrophic subaortic stenosis is accompanied by symptoms, such as angina, that are worsened by increased cardiac contractility. The usefulness of propranolol then becomes obvious.

Propranolol may be needed, as an adjunct to α-receptor blockade, to minimize cardiac stimulation during surgical removal or chronic management of *pheochromocytoma*.[12] β-Receptor blockade alone, by preventing catecholamine-induced vasodilatation (mediated by β_2-receptors), may cause a dangerous rise in arterial pressure in these patients. Therapy with an α-receptor antagonist must be initiated beforehand.

Treatment with β-receptor blockers for a year or more after a *myocardial infarction*[25] decreases the likelihood of death or a recurrence of infarction. Immediate intravenous administration of β-blockers upon admission followed by oral treatment for 7 days can also be beneficial, with a reduction in mortality primarily occurring within the first 2 days after infarction.

Prophylactic management of migraine is another important use of propranolol.[2] It can also reduce action tremors and autonomic symptoms of stage fright[22] and alcohol withdrawal.[7]

ADVERSE EFFECTS

The major adverse effects of propranolol result from bronchial constriction, heart block, and depression of cardiac contractility. β-Adrenergic antagonists are generally contraindicated in patients with asthma. Cardiac, metabolic, and central nervous system changes may contribute to fatigue, which is reported by about 20% of patients.[7]

Propranolol may cause hypoglycemia or interfere with recovery from hypoglycemia after insulin administration, and it can prevent the tachycardia that signals diabetics of their developing hypoglycemia. Recent reports of changes in plasma lipid profile (increased triglyceride concentration and decreased high density lipoprotein) by propranolol are reason for concern.[1,10]

Central effects of β-blockers include drowsiness, sleep disturbances, such as vivid dreams or nightmares, and possibly depression.[7] Although there is some controversy about their effects on the sensorium, the drugs probably do not cause significant cognitive impairment.[8]

PROPRANOLOL WITHDRAWAL

Abrupt withdrawal of propranolol and other short-acting β-receptor blockers can lead to increased cardiac excitability, exacerbation of angina, or even myocardial infarction.[19] These changes begin within 2 days, and the patient's condition returns to normal in 10 to 14 days. This syndrome has been attributed to upregulation of β-receptors as a consequence of prolonged suppression by the drugs. It is important to withdraw β-blockers gradually and to warn patients not to interrupt therapy. β-Blockers can also mask thyrotoxicosis, which may emerge in an exaggerated form (thyroid storm) when the drug is withdrawn.

Newer β-adrenergic blocking drugs

More recently developed β-blockers may differ from propranolol in several respects (see Table 19-2).[5,7] Those that are labeled *cardioselective*, that is, they exhibit preferential blockade of β_1- as opposed to β_2-receptors, potentially have advantages in asthmatic and diabetic patients; their most consistent effect on plasma lipid concentrations is an increase in triglycerides.[1,10] Agents with intrinsic β-receptor agonist activity[6] have minimal effects on resting cardiac output and heart rate or on plasma lipids. Those with lower lipid solubility (atenolol and nadolol more so than pindolol and the active metabolite of acebutolol) are excreted totally or partially unmetabolized[20]; it is not clear that they cause fewer central nervous system side effects,[8] although sleep may be less impaired.[15] In addition to propranolol, several of these drugs exhibit membrane-stabilizing activity. Despite differences in half-lives, once or twice daily administration of any of these agents is usually effective for antihypertensive therapy.

Nadolol, **pindolol**, **penbutolol**, and **carteolol**, like propranolol, readily block both β_1- and β_2-receptors. **Labetalol** is an unusual antihypertensive agent in that it blocks α_1-receptors in addition to β-receptors; however, these activities are distributed unequally among four stereoisomers.[3]

Timolol also is not cardioselective. In addition to their usefulness for cardiovascular indications, β-receptor blockers can reduce the formation of aqueous humor.[17,21] Although not proved, this effect is attributed to β_2-receptor blockade in ciliary epithelial cells. Propranolol is not used on the eye because of its local anesthetic action, but many ophthalmologists consider timolol the drug of choice for initial treatment of open-angle glaucoma.

Metoprolol, **atenolol**, **acebutolol,** and **esmolol** differ from the above agents in their relative cardioselectivity. Such agents are safer in asthmatics than those without β_1-receptor selectivity but still carry considerable risk because they may block β_2-receptors in therapeutic doses. Even when they are used cautiously in patients with bronchospastic disease, concomitant administration of a β_2-receptor agonist may be necessary. Because cardioselective antagonists have little activity on the β_2-receptors that mediate vasodilatation, the use of these agents may be associated with minimal increase in blood pressure when epinephrine is released during exercise or hypoglycemia. Esmolol, which is rapidly hydrolyzed by red cell esterases, is given intravenously for readily reversible control of ventricular rate in patients with supraventricular tachycardia. It comes in two strengths; the higher requires dilution before use.

Betaxolol, another cardioselective antagonist, is used for management of hypertension and glaucoma. As used topically for glaucoma, it is reported to have minimal effect on respiration in asthmatics and less cardiac activity than timolol; transient irritation is relatively common. **Levobunolol**[9] and **metipranolol** are nonselective β-blockers provided for treatment of open-angle glaucoma. It remains to be seen if any of these compounds will replace timolol in ophthalmology.

REFERENCES

1. Amery A, Lijnen P: Alterations in lipid metabolism induced by antihypertensive therapy, *Drugs* 36(suppl 2):1, 1988.
2. Andersson K-E, Vinge E: β-Adrenoceptor

blockers and calcium antagonists in the prophylaxis and treatment of migraine, *Drugs* 39:355, 1990.

3. Brittain RT, Drew GM, Levy GP: The α- and β-adrenoceptor blocking potencies of labetalol and its individual stereoisomers in anaesthetized dogs and in isolated tissues, *Br J Pharmacol* 77:105, 1982.
4. Cho AK, Takimoto GS: Irreversible inhibitors of adrenergic nerve terminal function, *Trends Pharmacol Sci* 6:443, 1985.
5. Choice of a beta-blocker, *Med Lett Drugs Ther* 28:20, 1986.
6. Cruickshank JM: Measurement and cardiovascular relevance of partial agonist activity (PAA) involving β_1- and β_2-adrenoceptors, *Pharmacol Ther* 46:199, 1990.
7. Cruickshank JM, Prichard BNC: *Beta-blockers in clinical practice,* Edinburgh, 1988, Churchill Livingstone.
8. Dimsdale JE, Newton RP, Joist T: Neuropsychological side effects of β-blockers, *Arch Intern Med* 149:514, 1989.
9. Gonzalez JP, Clissold SP: Ocular levobunolol: a review of its pharmacodynamic and pharmacokinetic properties, and therapeutic efficacy, *Drugs* 34:648, 1987.
10. Holtzman E, Rosenthal T, Goldbourt U, Segal P: Do β-blockers alter lipids and what are the consequences? *J Cardiovasc Pharmacol* 10(suppl 2):S86, 1987.
11. IJzerman AP, Soudijn W: The antiarrhythmic properties of β-adrenoceptor antagonists, *Trends Pharmacol Sci* 10:31, 1989.
12. Keiser HR, Doppman JL, Robertson CN, et al: Diagnosis, localization, and management of pheochromocytoma. In Lack EE, editor: *Pathology of the adrenal glands,* New York, 1990, Churchill Livingstone, p 237.
13. Luther RR: Terazosin: a new antihypertensive agent with favorable effects on lipids, *Int J Clin Pharmacol Ther Toxicol* 27:313, 1989.
14. Man in't Veld AJ, van den Meiracker A, Schalekamp MADH: The effect of β blockers on total peripheral resistance, *J Cardiovasc Pharmacol* 8(suppl 4):S49, 1986.
15. McAinsh J, Cruickshank JM: Beta-blockers and central nervous system side effects, *Pharmacol Ther* 46:163, 1990.
16. Melander A, Lalka D, McLean A: Influence of food on the presystemic metabolism of drugs, *Pharmacol Ther* 38:253, 1988.
17. Mittag TW: Adrenergic and dopaminergic drugs in glaucoma. In Ritch R, Shields MB, Krupin T, editors: *The glaucomas,* St Louis, 1989, Mosby–Year Book, p 523.
18. Morales A, Condra MS, Owen JE, et al: Oral and transcutaneous pharmacologic agents in the treatment of impotence, *Urol Clin North Am* 15:87, 1988.
19. Psaty BM, Koepsell TD, Wagner EH, et al: The relative risk of incident coronary heart disease associated with recently stopping the use of β-blockers, *JAMA* 263:1653, 1990.
20. Riddell JG, Harron DWG, Shanks RG: Clinical pharmacokinetics of β-adrenoceptor antagonists: an update, *Clin Pharmacokinet* 12:305, 1987.
21. Sugrue MF: The pharmacology of antiglaucoma drugs, *Pharmacol Ther* 43:91, 1989.
22. Tyrer P: Current status of β-blocking drugs in the treatment of anxiety disorders, *Drugs* 36:773, 1988.
23. Weber MA, Graettinger WF, Drayer JIM: The adrenergic inhibitors, *Med Clin North Am* 71:959, 1987.
24. Weinberger MH: Lowering blood pressure in patients without affecting quality of life, *Am J Med* 86(suppl 1B):94, 1989.
25. Yusuf S, Wittes J, Friedman L: Overview of results of randomized clinical trials in heart disease. I. Treatments following myocardial infarction, *JAMA* 260:2088, 1988.

Chapter 20

Drugs acting on the adrenergic neuron

GENERAL CONCEPT

Certain drugs that affect synthesis, storage, release, and inactivation of catecholamines[1] provide additional pharmacologic approaches to modification of the nervous system. Such agents find application as *antihypertensive agents* and in *psychopharmacology*.

The seminal discovery was that reserpine, a *Rauwolfia* alkaloid, depletes serotonin (5-hydroxytryptamine) from storage sites in various tissues, including the brain. It was then discovered that reserpine also depletes norepinephrine and dopamine. Reduction of sympathetic function by reserpine, which causes hypotension and bradycardia, is attributed to norepinephrine depletion from nerve endings. Changes in brain amine content are thought responsible for the antipsychotic and depressive effects of the drug.

Drugs are available that affect virtually all functional aspects of adrenergic neurons. Guanethidine depletes peripheral amine stores but does not reach the brain. Bretylium, on the other hand, blocks transmission without depleting neuronal norepinephrine. Methyldopa is metabolized within adrenergic neurons. Monoamine oxidase (MAO) inhibitors, which increase the amine content of neural tissues, lower blood pressure but are used clinically as antidepressants. Metyrosine inhibits the rate-limiting step in synthesis of norepinephrine. Tricyclic drugs used as antidepressants (see Chapter 28) block amine reuptake into neurons.

PHARMACOLOGIC ALTERATION OF NEURONAL AMINE CONTENT

Two basic mechanisms by which neuronal norepinephrine content is altered and some drugs that illustrate them are as follows:

- Interference with granular uptake mechanism
  - Reserpine
  - Guanethidine
- Displacement of the catecholamine
  - Tyramine
  - Amphetamine
  - Metaraminol
  - Methyldopa (through its metabolite α-methylnorepinephrine)

Interference with granular storage mechanism. As depicted in Fig. 20-1, when the contents of a norepinephrine-containing granule are released into the neuroeffector junction, the amine acts on postsynaptic receptors. There is also a certain amount of passive leakage of norepinephrine from storage granules into the axoplasm. This is normally offset by active transport of norepinephrine and its precursor, dopamine, into the granules. However, when this transport is prevented by reserpine or guanethidine, the amine that escapes into the axoplasm is subject to attack by MAO; none can be salvaged by transport back into granules. The amine appears outside the neuron mostly in the form of inactivated metabolites. This explains why ingestion of reserpine, though causing massive depletion of catecholamines, does not elevate blood pressure.

When the catecholamine content of a nerve decreases to below 50% of normal, release by nerve stimulation is reduced. The rate of depletion varies in different organs. Cardiac catecholamines decline rapidly; adrenal stores are more resistant. The rate of depletion is a function not only of the dose of reserpine but also of the rate of turnover of the amine at the various sites. The half-life of catecholamines in the heart is much shorter than in the adrenal medulla. Depletion is relatively rapid in arterioles and venules.

Displacement of catecholamine. Indirectly acting sympathomimetic agents, such as tyramine and amphetamine, release norepinephrine from adrenergic neurons (see p. 95). Other amines not only displace the catecholamine but also are incorporated as false transmitters into the granule (see p. 96).

Catecholamine release can be modified by at least four additional pharmacologic influences.

MAO inhibitors protect intraneuronally released catecholamines from inactivation. Unlike reserpine alone, injection of reserpine in the presence of MAO inhibition will increase blood pressure.

Bretylium, and other agents such as debrisoquin, guanethidine, and guanadrel, can prevent catecholamine release by nerve stimulation in the absence of depletion. The drugs appear to anesthetize adrenergic neurons. Indeed, they do have local anesthetic activity and concentrate in adrenergic fibers.

Drugs that inhibit the membrane amine pump (Fig. 20-1), such as cocaine and the tricyclic antidepressant imipramine, block the actions of indirectly acting amines,

Schematic representation of nerve ending and effector cell. (For details see text.)

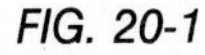
FIG. 20-1

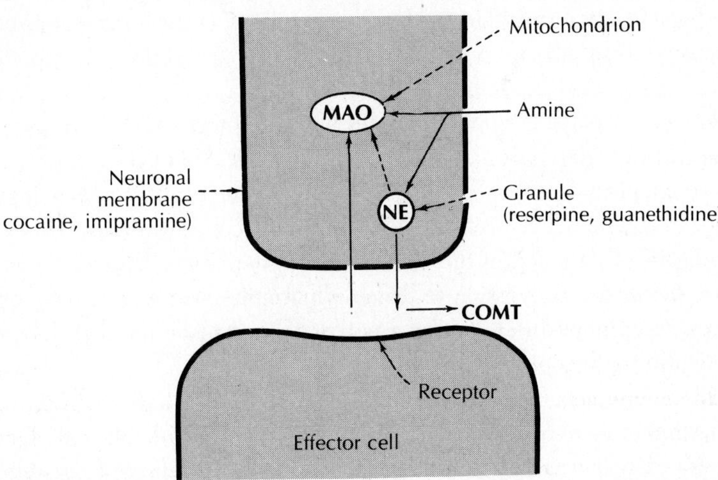

guanethidine, and bretylium by preventing their uptake into neurons. In addition, they potentiate the neurotransmitter by allowing its accumulation in the neuroeffector junction in the vicinity of postsynaptic receptors. They do not affect the action of reserpine.

Finally, *drugs may act on presynaptic α- or β-receptors*, which modulate catecholamine release (see p. 142).

RESERPINE

Alkaloids of *Rauwolfia serpentina* have antihypertensive and antipsychotic properties. Reserpine depletes norepinephrine, dopamine, and serotonin from the brain and peripheral nerves[3] by inhibiting their uptake into storage vesicles.[2] The place of reserpine in treatment of hypertension is discussed in the next chapter.

GUANETHIDINE

Guanethidine, as well as debrisoquin and guanadrel, decreases sympathetic activity by dual mechanisms. Both reserpine and guanethidine deplete catecholamine by blocking granular storage, but guanethidine has an additional *bretylium-like* action that causes early sympathetic blockade before norepinephrine depletion. Guanethidine fails to cross the blood-brain barrier and has no effect on brain amines.

Unlike reserpine, to reach its intraneuronal site of action guanethidine must be transported by the membrane amine pump. As with indirectly acting amines, transport of quanethidine is associated with release of norepinephrine, the *tyramine-like* effect, and can be blocked by cocaine and tricyclic antidepressants. Intravenous injection of guanethidine can release enough norepinephrine to transiently increase blood pressure. For this reason, guanethidine is not used parenterally for management of hypertensive emergencies.

Guanadrel, a pharmacologically similar agent with a short duration of action, is also available for control of hypertension (see Chapter 21).

BRETYLIUM

Bretylium is similar to guanethidine except that it does not deplete neurons of their catecholamine content. It apparently acts as a local anesthetic after concentration in adrenergic fibers. It also releases norepinephrine and sometimes causes transient, mild hypertension after injection. Although bretylium is no longer approved as an antihypertensive drug, it is used to control ventricular arrhythmias (see p. 434).

METHYLDOPA

Methyldopa, an analog of dopa, competes with the precursor of norepinephrine for the enzyme that decarboxylates aromatic L-amino acids. Although it inhibits synthesis of both norepinephrine and serotonin, norepinephrine concentrations in the brain remain low for a much longer time than serotonin concentrations. This and other evidence indicates that much of the catecholamine depletion induced by methyldopa is caused by the drug's conversion to α-methylnorepinephrine. α-Methylnorepinephrine replaces norepinephrine to act as a potent false transmitter that, like clonidine, stimulates central α_2-receptors (Chapter 21).

MAO INHIBITORS

MAO inhibitors were introduced as antidepressants (see Chapter 28). One of their surprising side effects was orthostatic hypotension, which indicated possible interference with sympathetic function. Experimentally, MAO inhibitors elevate concentrations of norepinephrine and serotonin in the brain, in ganglia, and in other peripheral tissues. Hypotension that occurs after use of these agents may be related to accumulation of a weak false transmitter, such as octopamine (see p. 96) in adrenergic fibers. MAO inhibitors prevent intraneuronal metabolism and the associated depletion of the amine released from storage granules after reserpine treatment. One of the serious disadvantages of MAO inhibitors is the likelihood of adverse reactions to ingested foods and to drugs that release monoamines in the body (see p. 255).

METYROSINE

Metyrosine is used only for its ability to prevent hypertensive responses, preoperatively or chronically, in patients with pheochromocytoma. This drug inhibits tyrosine hydroxylase, which catalyzes the rate-limiting step in formation of norepinephrine (see Chapter 13). Metyrosine (Demser) is available as 250 mg capsules.

REFERENCES

1. Maxwell RA, Wastila WB: Adrenergic neuron blocking drugs, *Handb Exp Pharmacol* 39:161, 1977.
2. Philippu A, Matthaei H: Transport and storage of catecholamines in vesicles, *Handb Exp Pharmacol* 90(part 1):1, 1988.
3. Rand MJ, Jurevics H: The pharmacology of Rauwolfia alkaloids, *Handb Exp Pharmacol* 39:77, 1977.

Chapter 21

Antihypertensive drugs

GENERAL CONCEPTS

Effective treatment of hypertension is a major development in medicine. Since 1949 when ganglionic blocking agents were introduced, a series of important discoveries led to development of numerous drugs that extend life expectancy and ameliorate, if not prevent, complications of hypertension.[1,16,27,39]

Among the most significant developments were the introduction of hydralazine in 1952, reserpine in 1953, the thiazide diuretics in 1959, guanethidine in 1960, methyldopa and clonidine in 1967, β-adrenergic blocking drugs in 1968, and, more recently, α-adrenergic blocking drugs, angiotensin-converting-enzyme inhibitors, and Ca^{++}-channel blockers.

Antihypertensive drugs act by many different mechanisms, as summarized in Table 21-1. Delineation of their sites of action is important for optimal use of these compounds, for understanding the pathophysiology of hypertension itself and for development of new drugs.

For clinical treatment of hypertension, however, a more simple schema can be used, one that shows hypertension in terms of its cardiovascular hemodynamics. As such, blood pressure (BP) equals cardiac output (CO) times peripheral vascular resistance (PVR):

$$BP = CO \times PVR$$

In turn, CO and PVR can be subdivided into their determinants:

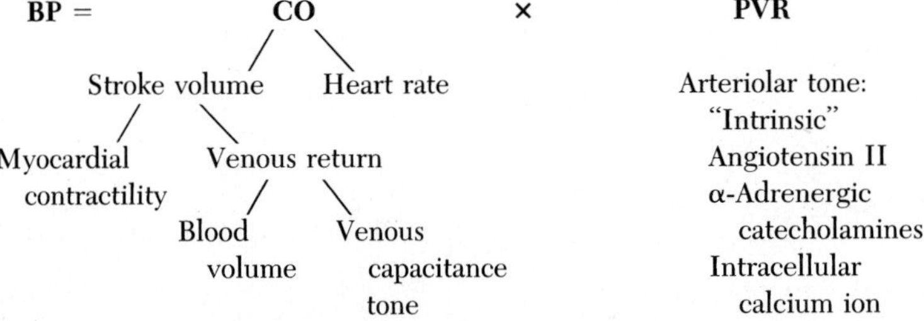

A fundamentally important concept inherent in the above schema is that an antihypertensive agent that acts on one component of the system induces reflex changes in other components, the net effect of which can be maintenance of blood pressure at an elevated level despite therapy. For example, a drug that decreases peripheral vascular resistance may initially lower blood pressure; however, this effect can dissipate if reflex tachycardia and retention of Na^+ (with an expanded blood

TABLE 21-1 Site of action of antihypertensive drugs

Site of action	Mode of action	Drug	Trade name
Arteriolar smooth muscle	Direct vasodilatation	Hydralazine	Alazine, Apresoline
		Minoxidil	Loniten, Minodyl
		Diazoxide	Hyperstat
		Nitroprusside	Nipride, Nitropress
		Thiazide diuretics	
Converting enzyme	Decreased angiotensin II formation	Captopril	Capoten
		Enalapril	Vasotec
		Lisinopril	Prinivil, Zestril
Sympathetic neurons	Blockade of norepinephrine release (also depletion)	Reserpine	
		Guanethidine	Ismelin
		Guanadrel	Hylorel
α-Adrenergic receptors	Receptor blockade (vasodilatation)	Phentolamine	Regitine
		Phenoxybenzamine	Dibenzyline
		Prazosin	Minipress
		Terazosin	Hytrin
		Doxazosin	Cardura
Central α_2-receptors	Receptor stimulation (decreased peripheral sympathetic tone)	Methyldopa	Aldomet, Amodopa
		Clonidine	Catapres
		Guanabenz	Wytensin
		Guanfacine	Tenex
Ca^{++} channel	Channel block (vasodilatation)	Verapamil	Calan, Isoptin, Verelan
		Diltiazem	Cardizem
		Nifedipine	Adalat, Procardia
		Nicardipine	Cardene
β-adrenergic receptors	Decreased cardiac output		
	Nonselective β-receptor blockade	Propranolol	Inderal, Ipran
		Nadolol	Corgard
		Timolol	Blocadren
	Cardioselective (β_1-receptor) blockade	Metoprolol	Lopressor
		Atenolol	Tenormin
	Decreased peripheral vascular resistance		
	Nonselective β-receptor blockade + ISA*	Pindolol	Visken
	Cardioselective β_1-receptor blockade + ISA	Acebutolol	Sectral
β- and α-adrenergic receptors	Blockade (decreased cardiac output and peripheral vascular resistance)	Labetalol	Normodyne, Trandate
Kidney	Sodium excretion, volume depletion	Many diuretics	
Autonomic ganglia	Ganglionic blockade	Trimethaphan	Arfonad

*Intrinsic sympathomimetic activity.

volume) increase cardiac output sufficiently to nullify the benefit from vasodilatation. This scenario frequently occurred with use of hydralazine (a direct vasodilator) as a single agent. Its efficacy was not optimized until β-adrenergic antagonists and diuretics were used concomitantly to block the reflex tachycardia and to prevent volume expansion respectively.[43] The foregoing emphasizes that in patients with moderate and severe hypertension, who often require therapy with multiple agents, the drugs used should affect different components of the hemodynamic system schematized earlier. For example, if a patient requires three antihypertensives, it is far more logical to use a vasodilator, a β-blocker, and a diuretic than to use three different vasodilators.

A second important consideration when one uses the hemodynamic schema is that peripheral vascular resistance increases in most patients with hypertension. Hence the initial agents to be used (and the single agent for those patients who need only one drug) should lower peripheral resistance.

A final consideration is that drugs that affect venous capacitance tone also cause orthostatic hypotension. In fact, effects on venous tone primarily diminish upright pressures and do not contribute to lowering of supine blood pressure. If such drugs also have an effect on supine blood pressure, it is by a concomitant decrease in arteriolar tone. Effects on capacitance tone are unwanted and constitute an adverse effect that limits the utility of the drug. The guanidinium antihypertensives (guanethidine and guanadrel) and the ganglionic blockers are the drugs of particular concern in this regard. The current availability of a variety of effective antihypertensives that do not affect capacitance tone has relegated those that do to historic interest.

RELATION OF ANGIOTENSIN AND ALDOSTERONE TO HYPERTENSION

The demonstration that renal ischemia leads to hypertension resulted in the discovery of a kidney enzyme, *renin*, in granules of the juxtaglomerular apparatus. When this enzyme is released, it acts on a substrate in blood and eventually yields angiotensin II, a potent vasopressor polypeptide. This sequence of events is shown in Table 21-2.

The amino acid composition of angiotensin I is as follows:

Asp-Arg-Val-Tyr-Ile-His-Pro-Phe-His-Leu

Converting enzyme, which is on the luminal surface of blood vessels, removes the terminal histidyl-leucine to form angiotensin II. Angiotensin I has little biologic activity, though, like angiotensin III, it may have some effect on aldosterone release.

Saralasin (1-sarcosyl-8-alanyl-angiotensin II) is an angiotensin antagonist with essentially no other pharmacologic action. Given intravenously it serves as an investigational tool for assessment of the contribution of angiotensin to blood pressure elevation. It is not available for clinical use.

Renin release

Lowering of blood pressure and renal perfusion pressure or a decrease in access of Cl^- to the macula densa of the juxtaglomerular apparatus promotes release of renin. Part of the effect of lowered pressure on renin release may be sympathetically mediated through β-receptors, since propranolol blocks catecholamine-induced renin release. Prostaglandins (presumably PGI_2) also induce renin release; the stimulus in

TABLE 21-2 Metabolism of angiotensin

Sequence	Inhibitors
Renin in kidney	
↓	β-Receptor blockers
Renin released	
+	
Angiotensinogen	
↓	
Angiotensin I (decapeptide)	
+	
Converting enzyme	Inhibitors (captopril, enalapril, lisinopril)
↓	
Angiotensin II (octapeptide)	Antagonists (saralasin)
+	
Angiotensinases A, B, C	
↓ ↓	
Angiotensin III (heptapeptide) Split product	

this case is unclear. Some argue that prostaglandins are the final common pathway for all stimuli of renin release; others disagree, particularly with regard to participation of the macula densa.

Pharmacologic effects

Effects of angiotensin II are as follows: (1) contraction of vascular smooth muscle, (2) release of aldosterone, which promotes Na^+ retention, and (3) release of catecholamines from the adrenal medulla and adrenergic nerves. Not only does angiotensin release catecholamines, it also prevents their reuptake by adrenergic nerves and thereby potentiates their activity. In addition, angiotensin is a potent central dipsogenic agent in animals, and it can alter vasopressin secretion. All of these effects contribute to an elevation of blood pressure.

The vasopressor actions of angiotensin are exerted primarily on peripheral resistance vessels in the skin, splanchnic area, and kidney. It has little cardiac stimulant action. Capacitance vessels are not greatly affected; they differ in this respect from their sensitivity to catecholamines. As one would predict, inhibition of formation of angiotensin II is an effective means of lowering blood pressure. This fact accounts for the current availability of three drugs that inhibit converting enzyme; still others are under development.

CLASSIFICATION OF ANTIHYPERTENSIVE DRUGS

The various antihypertensive compounds may be grouped according to their actions on cardiovascular hemodynamics. They will be discussed under the headings of direct vasodilators, converting-enzyme inhibitors, agents that interfere with α-adrenergic mechanisms, Ca^{++}-channel blockers, β-adrenergic receptor blocking drugs, and diuretics, with a brief mention of ganglionic blocking agents.

DIRECT VASODILATORS

Direct vasodilators act on vascular smooth muscle. Diazoxide and sodium nitroprusside are reserved for acute treatment of hypertensive emergencies. Hydralazine and minoxidil are used chronically. Thiazide diuretics may also be considered in this group. When these diuretics are administered acutely to patients with hypertension, the initial decrease in pressure is attributable to diuresis, which shrinks blood volume.[11] With chronic therapy, however, the vascular volume is restored, and the persistent antihypertensive effect is the result of a decrease in peripheral vascular resistance, the mechanism of which is unknown.[23] The vasodilating action of thiazides is the rationale for their traditional use as a first step or single agent in patients with hypertension. The diuretic and natriuretic effects of these drugs are discussed in detail in Chapter 42; their use as antihypertensives is discussed below.

Hydralazine

Hydralazine, a direct relaxant of vascular smooth muscle (the mechanism is unclear), is used commonly in management of hypertension.[25] Although it is available in combination products advocated for use in mild hypertension, hydralazine is best reserved for patients with more severe hypertension (those with diastolic blood pressures above 105 mm Hg) who will probably require multiple medications to attain blood pressure control. Usually hydralazine is sufficiently powerful to elicit reflex tachycardia and fluid retention, and other drugs must be added to blunt these homeostatic responses.

ADVERSE EFFECTS

Headache, palpitations, and gastrointestinal disturbances are the most frequent adverse effects. With daily doses larger than 200 mg many patients develop a syndrome resembling systemic lupus erythematosus. This syndrome is reversible in most cases. Since the incidence of this effect is low if the dose is kept below 200 mg per day, this amount should only rarely be exceeded.

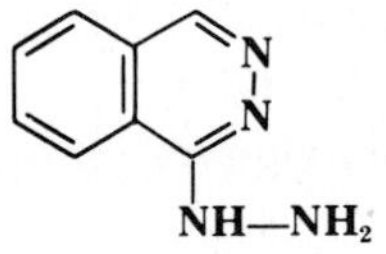

N
N
NH—NH$_2$

Hydralazine

PREPARATIONS

Hydralazine hydrochloride is available in tablets of 10 to 100 mg. Twice-daily dosing is often adequate for maintenance. The drug is also available as a solution for injection, 20 mg/ml, in hypertensive emergencies. Currently, other drugs have more predictable pressure-lowering effects in this setting, and hydralazine is not a primary choice. Hydralazine in small amounts is also available in many combination preparations, the benefit of which compared with newer agents has not been established.

Minoxidil

Minoxidil is indicated only for patients with severe hypertension who do not respond to other drugs.[6] It is such a powerful vasodilator that it causes considerable

Na^+ retention and tachycardia, which necessitate concomitant use of large doses of potent diuretics and β-adrenergic receptor antagonists. Minoxidil also causes hirsutism, a side effect that has prompted its development as a treatment (Rogaine) for baldness.

Minoxidil is available in tablets, 2.5 and 10 mg. The initial dose should be 5 mg; the dosage can be increased gradually to 40 mg a day in single or divided doses. Despite a half-life of 3 hours, the antihypertensive effect of the drug lasts at least 12 hours.

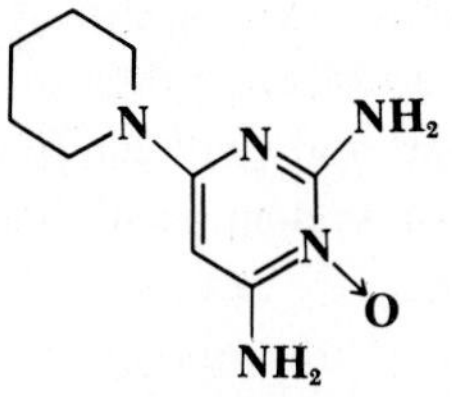

N NH₂ N N O NH₂

Minoxidil

Diazoxide

Diazoxide is a nondiuretic congener of the thiazide drugs.[19] Paradoxically, though derived from these diuretics, it causes Na^+ retention. Administered intravenously in hypertensive emergencies, it rapidly lowers blood pressure. The drug is supplied in ampules containing 15 mg/ml. Initial guidelines for its use advocated rapid bolus doses of 300 mg. It was mistakenly believed that rapid dosing would cause a greater response by overcoming a high degree of binding to plasma proteins. This myth combined with overzealous dosing resulted in an alarming incidence of hypotension. Subsequent studies showed that blood pressure can be lowered in a more controlled and predictable fashion by use of individual doses of 1 mg/kg every 10 minutes until the desired pressure is reached. Once this occurs the antihypertensive effect can last as long as 12 hours. Diazoxide can cause sufficient hyperglycemia, as a consequence of inhibition of insulin release, to require treatment with insulin. Whenever diazoxide is used, serum glucose concentration should be monitored.

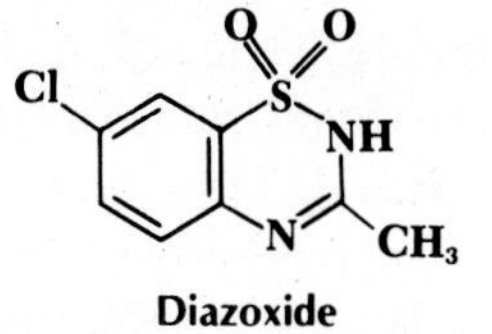

O O Cl S NH N CH₃

Diazoxide

Sodium nitroprusside

Sodium nitroprusside is the "gold standard" for use in hypertensive crises because it provides smooth and predictable blood pressure control.[32] The mechanism of its vasodilating effect is similar to that of the nitrates (Chapter 40); that is, in the vascular endothelium it forms an active nitrosothiol that increases cyclic GMP, thereby causing vasodilatation.

Adverse effects of nitroprusside include nausea, disorientation, and muscle spasms. A metabolic product of nitroprusside is cyanide, which is quickly metabolized to thiocyanate, which in turn is excreted by the kidney. When infused for prolonged periods in high doses or when given to patients with hepatic or renal disease, toxic concentrations of thiocyanate and cyanide may occur. Such patients should be monitored closely.

Sodium nitroprusside is available in amber-colored vials containing 50 mg for reconstitution with dextrose in water. A dose of 1 μg/kg/min is first administered by intravenous infusion. The infusion rate must then be adjusted by monitoring of blood pressure, preferably by an intra-arterial cannula. The drug is very sensitive to degradation by light, and so the infusion system should be shielded.

CONVERTING-ENZYME INHIBITORS

As discussed previously, the multitude of mechanisms by which the renin-angiotensin system could influence blood pressure has stimulated development of drugs that inhibit formation of angiotensin II.[41] Currently, captopril, enalapril, and lisinopril are marketed, but many similar compounds are being developed. These drugs are not only used widely to treat hypertension, they also constitute the only class of drugs shown to decrease mortality in congestive heart failure.[7] Thus they have become a primary modality of therapy in that condition as well. Drugs in this class have a unique side effect—a low incidence of dry, nonproductive cough that is sometimes sufficiently bothersome to necessitate their withdrawal. The mechanism of this effect is unknown but may relate to enhanced bradykinin activity because converting enzyme also degrades bradykinin in the lung.

Captopril

Captopril was the first converting-enzyme inhibitor available for clinical use.[4,8] Initially, dosing recommendations were too high, and therapy was associated with some alarming side effects, including neutropenia, proteinuria, and skin rash. It is now clear that total daily dosages above 200 mg are superfluous and that lower dosages are only infrequently associated with adverse effects. Consequently, use of the drug has expanded. The initial indication for captopril was as therapy in patients who had not responded to other drugs. Because its therapeutic margin has widened with the use of lower doses, captopril is now frequently and effectively used as a single agent in patients with mild hypertension.

Captopril is absorbed quickly and reaches peak activity in about 1 hour; in contrast enalapril and lisinopril require 4 or more hours to cause maximal effects. This difference can be used to advantage if a quick action is needed from a converting-enzyme inhibitor.

Captopril is supplied in tablets of 12.5 to 100 mg. Dosing should begin with 12.5 or 25 mg twice daily. The drug is eliminated by the kidney; therefore in patients with decreased renal function one should start with low doses and slowly titrate upward.

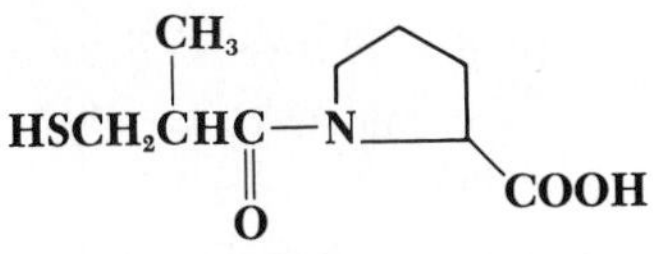

Captopril

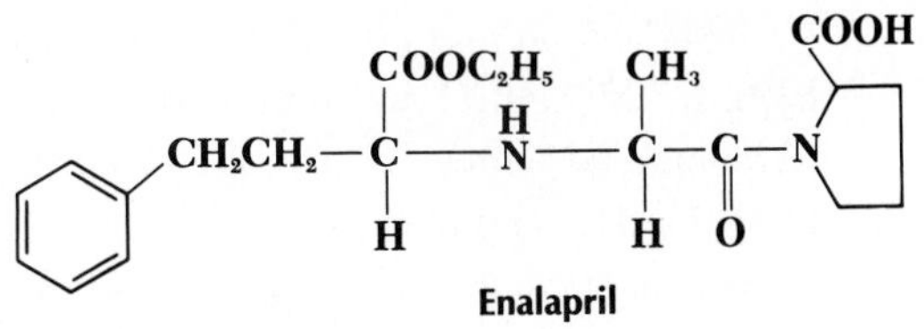

Enalapril

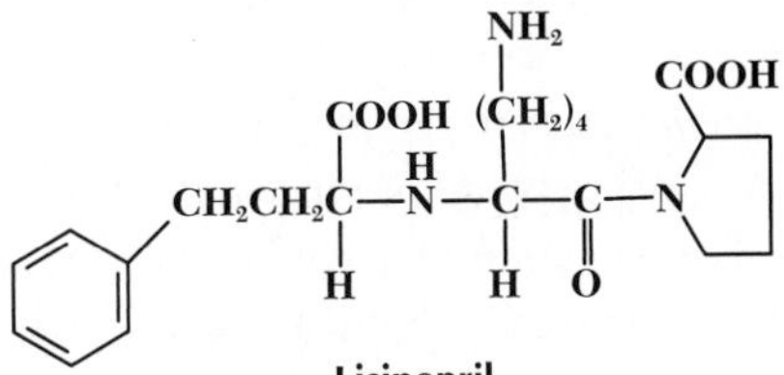

Lisinopril

Enalapril

Enalapril, a prodrug, is hydrolyzed in the liver to the active compound enalaprilat.[38] The active component has a half-life of about 11 hours and can be given once a day to most patients. Enalaprilat is excreted by the kidney, and dosage should be reduced in patients with renal insufficiency. Enalapril, like smaller doses of captopril, has a low incidence of nonspecific adverse effects; it is therefore frequently used as a single agent in patients with mild hypertension, as well as in multidrug regimens in patients with more severe disease.

Enalapril maleate is available in tablets, 2.5 to 20 mg. The initial dose is usually 10 mg. Patients with decreased renal function and the elderly should begin with 5 mg. The maximal dose is usually 40 mg but may be as high as 80 mg in some patients.

Lisinopril

Lisinopril is simply the lysine analog of enalaprilat.[21] Because its bioavailability is about half that of enalapril, it is administered in doses twice as large. Otherwise, its kinetic properties and effects are virtually identical to those of enalapril, and they can be used interchangeably. Lisinopril is available as tablets, 5 to 20 mg.

AGENTS THAT INTERFERE WITH α-ADRENERGIC MECHANISMS

α-Adrenergic functions are inhibited by a variety of agents that can be grouped into those with predominant actions in the periphery and those for which the site of action is the central nervous system. The latter stimulate α_2-adrenergic receptors in the brain and as a result diminish concentrations of circulating catecholamines. The net effect is diminished adrenergic activity.

Peripheral impairment of sympathetic neuronal function

RESERPINE

Reserpine is the prototype of several alkaloids present in *Rauwolfia serpentina*, an Indian snakeroot. Used in India for centuries, it was introduced into Western medicine in the 1950s. At first reserpine seemed as important for its tranquilizing properties as for its usefulness in the treatment of hypertension. It was gradually replaced as an antipsychotic drug by the phenothiazines. Newer antihypertensives have now relegated reserpine to historic interest because they are easier to use and have wider therapeutic margins.

Basic action and effects. Reserpine causes depletion of catecholamines and serotonin in the central and peripheral nervous systems. Depletion is a consequence of intraneuronal amine release, followed by prevention of reaccumulation. In addition, reserpine is speculated to interfere with catecholamine synthesis.

Parasympathetic effects of reserpine are in part a result of decreased sympathetic activity. Bradycardia, aggravation of peptic ulcer, increased gastrointestinal motility, and miosis may be attributable to parasympathetic predominance when sympathetic effects are prevented.

The *central nervous system effects* of the drug are among its greatest disadvantages in treatment of hypertension. An unpleasant type of drowsiness and lethargy is particularly disliked by those who must be intellectually alert and creative. Depression and suicides have occurred during chronic administration of reserpine at higher dosages than those now used. Central nervous system depression is a particular problem in patients also taking drugs such as barbiturates and alcohol. Reserpine also predisposes patients to severe hypotension during surgery and anesthesia.

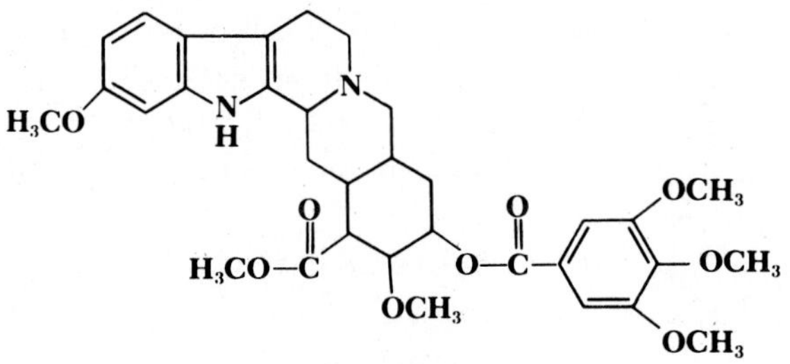

Reserpine

Preparations. The dried root of *Rauwolfia serpentina* Benth (Raudixin, others) is available in tablets containing 50 and 100 mg. *Reserpine* can be taken as tablets of 0.1 to 1 mg. The use of combination preparations should be discontinued. The reserpine derivatives deserpidine (Harmonyl) and rescinnamine (Moderil) are also available.

GUANETHIDINE AND GUANADREL

Several drugs, such as guanethidine, other guanidine compounds, and bretylium (Bretylol), block release of norepinephrine from adrenergic nerve fibers.

Guanethidine is an adrenergic neuronal blocking agent that is a highly effective antihypertensive drug. In addition to blocking adrenergic neurons, guanethidine causes catecholamine release and depletion. In this respect it resembles reserpine. Guanadrel is a newer guanidine compound that has a shorter action than guanethidine.[9] Although these drugs produce adrenergic effects similar to those of reserpine, they share an important difference; they do not cross the blood-brain barrier, and so the adverse central effects associated with reserpine do not occur. Bretylium, another intraneuronal blocking agent, was first used as an antihypertensive drug but was abandoned because of adverse side effects. Subsequently, it was noted to be effective treatment for refractory ventricular tachyarrhythmias, and it is now used for this purpose (see Chapter 39).

Mode of action. Guanethidine and guanadrel block adrenergic neurons selectively because they are concentrated within these neurons by the membrane transport system responsible for norepinephrine reuptake. Tricyclic antidepressants oppose the antihypertensive actions of these drugs by blocking their entry into adrenergic neurons.

In addition to their adrenergic neuron-blocking or *bretylium-like* action and their *reserpine-like* action, guanethidine and guanadrel may exhibit a *tyramine-like* action to cause release of catecholamine and a *cocaine-like* action, which refers to competition for the membrane amine pump.

Clinical pharmacology. The onset of action of guanethidine is slow; that for guanadrel is more rapid. Maximum effects may not occur for 2 or 3 days after initiation of treatment with guanethidine, whereas effects of guanadrel maximize within 1 or 2 days. With guanethidine, then, patients are started on small dosages, such as 10 mg once daily, which are maintained for 5 to 7 days before being increased. With guanadrel the dose can be titrated upward on a daily basis. The actions of guanethidine may persist for 7 days after its discontinuation, whereas those of guanadrel dissipate quickly. The delay of effect and long duration of action of guanethidine make it difficult to use.

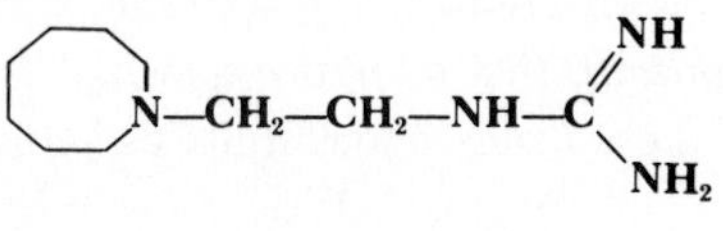

N—CH_2—CH_2—NH—C(=NH)NH_2

Guanethidine

$CH_2NHC(=NH)NH_2$

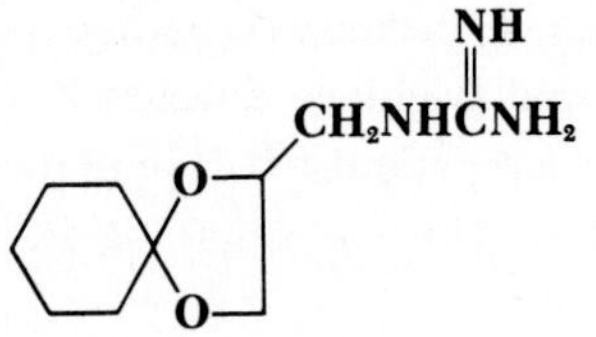

Guanadrel

Although guanethidine and guanadrel do not cause sedation and depression, both drugs cause substantial orthostatic hypotension, and they can cause retrograde ejaculation (passage of ejaculate into the bladder) without affecting erection. These adverse effects are sufficiently limiting that these drugs are rarely used today.

Preparations. Guanethidine monosulfate and guanadrel sulfate are available in tablets, 10 and 25 mg.

GANGLIONIC BLOCKING AGENTS

Ganglionic blocking drugs (Chapter 16) such as hexamethonium, pentolinium, and mecamylamine received extensive trial in hypertensive diseases. They block both sympathetic and parasympathetic activity. Reduction of blood pressure, particularly in the standing position, can be achieved, but the inevitable side effects of orthostatic hypotension and parasympathetic blockade complicate this approach to management of hypertension. Trimethaphan continues to be used by some clinicians for hypertensive emergencies, particularly if associated with dissecting aortic aneurysm.

α-ADRENERGIC RECEPTOR ANTAGONISTS

The α-adrenergic receptor blocking drugs phenoxybenzamine and phentolamine (Chapter 19) are not useful in management of hypertension because of their tendency to produce orthostatic hypotension and pronounced reflex tachycardia. Newer α_1-receptor blockers that cause less tachycardia have proved to be more useful antihypertensive agents.[13,40]

α_1-selective antagonists. Prazosin, terazosin, and doxazosin produce their antihypertensive effect by blocking postsynaptic α_1-adrenergic receptors in blood vessels. Superiority over other α-receptor antagonists is attributed to their greater affinity for postsynaptic receptors than for presynaptic α_2-adrenergic receptors. Blockade of presynaptic receptors by phenoxybenzamine or phentolamine increases release of norepinephrine. Because the α_1-selective drugs have little action on presynaptic receptors, they do not increase norepinephrine concentrations, and reflex sympathetic activity (tachycardia) is less likely to occur.

Prazosin, which is eliminated with a half-life of about 4 hours, must be administered at least twice daily. Terazosin and doxazosin have longer half-lives (about 15 and 20 hours respectively) and can be given once a day.[37,42] After oral administration, plasma concentrations of these compounds peak between 1 and 3 hours; all of them are eliminated mainly through biliary excretion.

Drugs of this class are particularly useful when treatment with a single agent is desirable in patients with mild hypertension. They have a low incidence of adverse effects and thereby a wide therapeutic margin. Prazosin was initially used to treat heart failure because it reduced both preload and afterload. Subsequent studies showed that tolerance developed to the action on preload, and the drug is no longer used in such patients. It is important to emphasize that tolerance does not develop to the antihypertensive action (on afterload) of these drugs; their utility as antihypertensives persists.

Untoward effects. A commonly encountered response to prazosin is called the *first-dose phenomenon*.[13,40] It is characterized by weakness and occasional syncope, which occur within 1 hour after the first dose is taken. This response, believed secondary to orthostatic hypotension, is aggravated by exercise and Na^+ depletion. The effect is due to venodilatation (preload reduction) to which tolerance quickly develops. One can avoid this first-dose response by having the patient take this dose before going to bed. This phenomenon seems to be less prevalent with terazosin and doxazosin, though the latter can cause persistent orthostatic hypotension in some patients.

Preparations. Prazosin and terazosin are available in 1 to 5 mg tablets. Initial dosage of prazosin should be 1 mg two times a day. The maximal daily dose is usually 20 mg, but some patients may require 40 mg. The initial dosage of terazosin is 1 mg at bedtime. Most patients respond to 1 to 5 mg daily, but dosages as high as 20 mg may be needed. Doxazosin, though approved for marketing, is not yet available.

Central α_2-adrenergic receptor agonists

METHYLDOPA

Methyldopa was introduced as an antihypertensive drug on the theory that since it is an inhibitor of aromatic L-amino acid decarboxylase it should lower catecholamine concentrations in the body. It was found, however, that the drug is taken up and metabolized to α-methylnorepinephrine. It was then postulated that this metabolite acts as an inactive or weak neurotransmitter, thereby diminishing overall sympathetic function. However, it is now apparent that α-methylnorepinephrine is an effective neurotransmitter that stimulates central α_2-adrenergic receptors.[29] This action in turn diminishes peripheral α-adrenergic activity.

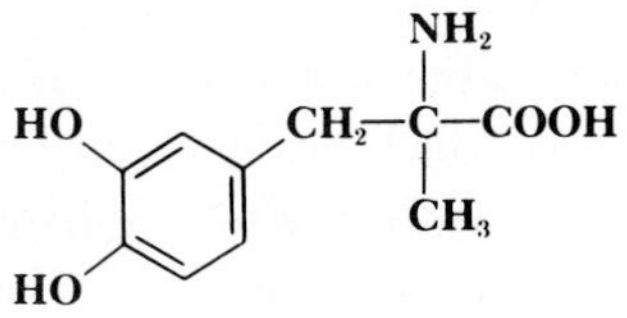

$$\text{HO},\text{HO}-C_6H_3-CH_2-C(NH_2)(CH_3)-COOH$$

Methyldopa

Methyldopa can be used for mild or more severe forms of hypertension. It causes little orthostatic hypotension.

Adverse reactions. Adverse reactions to methyldopa include pronounced drowsiness and dry mouth in many patients, depression, and nightmares. These side effects are clearly dose related. Early guidelines for use of methyldopa (and other central adrenergic stimulants) advocated doses that caused a high incidence of central nervous system side effects. Current recommendations are to use lower doses of methyldopa (for example, 250 mg twice daily) in which case central side effects are infrequent. If they do occur, they usually dissipate with continued therapy. In some patients administration of methyldopa for about a week causes an influenza-like reaction. In some of these persons subsequent administration of small doses of methyldopa will elicit the same reaction, suggestive of sensitization. Methyldopa has also been associated with other immunologic phenomena. Twenty percent of patients develop a positive Coombs test, but it is rare for the drug to cause hemolytic anemia. Rarely, cholestatic hepatitis occurs; this also may be immunologic in nature.

Pharmacokinetics. Methyldopa is absorbed well from the gastrointestinal tract. Although its elimination half-life is 2 hours, it is effective with twice daily dosing. Cumulation may occur when renal function is inadequate. The drug and its metabolites may give false-positive tests in the diagnosis of pheochromocytoma.

Preparations. Methyldopa is available in 125 to 500 mg tablets. The ethyl ester of methyldopa, methyldopate hydrochloride, is available in solution for intravenous injection, 250 mg/5 ml, in patients with hypertensive emergencies. Other drugs are currently preferred in this setting however.

CLONIDINE

Intravenous administration of clonidine is followed by a transient pressor response attributable to stimulation of peripheral α-receptors; there is then a more sustained depressor effect accompanied by bradycardia. The antihypertensive effect results from stimulation of α_2-receptors within the central nervous system, which diminishes circulating norepinephrine.[24]

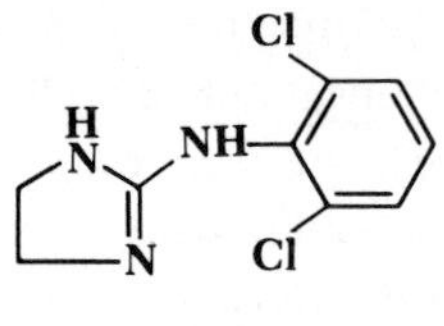

Clonidine

Adverse reactions and drug interactions. Drowsiness and dryness of the mouth are common dose-related side effects, which can be avoided in most patients by use of low doses. Constipation occurs occasionally. Orthostatic hypotension is rare. Withdrawal symptoms on discontinuation of clonidine therapy include restlessness, tachycardia, and a rebound increase in blood pressure. These usually occur after abrupt withdrawal of large doses, particularly if β-receptor blockade is present. They can be reversed quickly by reinstitution of clonidine or another α_2-adrenergic stimulant and can be blocked by peripheral adrenergic antagonists. Such withdrawal reactions are not unique to clonidine or, indeed, to this class of antihypertensives.

Pharmacokinetics. Clonidine is well absorbed after oral administration. Plasma concentration peaks within 3 to 5 hours, and the elimination half-life is 12 to 16 hours. Most of the drug is eliminated by hepatic metabolism, though sufficient renal excretion occurs to mandate dosage reduction in patients with renal dysfunction.

Preparations and dosages. Clonidine hydrochloride is available as tablets, 0.1 to 0.3 mg, and as a transdermal delivery system. The initial dose for adults is 0.1 mg two times daily. Dosage must be adjusted to the patient's requirement. Excessive doses increase the incidence of central nervous system side effects. If low doses of oral medication are effective, the transdermal system allows maintenance of stable plasma concentrations for a week. It may be most helpful in noncompliant patients.

GUANABENZ AND GUANFACINE

Guanabenz and guanfacine also stimulate central α_2-adrenergic receptors.[15,28,36] Their use in hypertension is identical to that of clonidine and methyldopa. Guanabenz acetate is supplied as tablets, 4 and 8 mg. Guanfacine hydrochloride is available as tablets, 1 mg. As with clonidine and methyldopa, low doses are advocated.

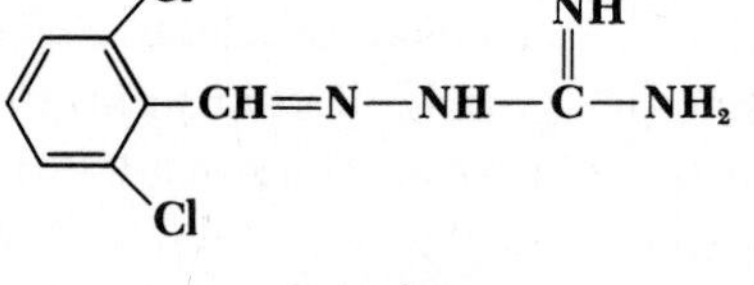

Guanabenz 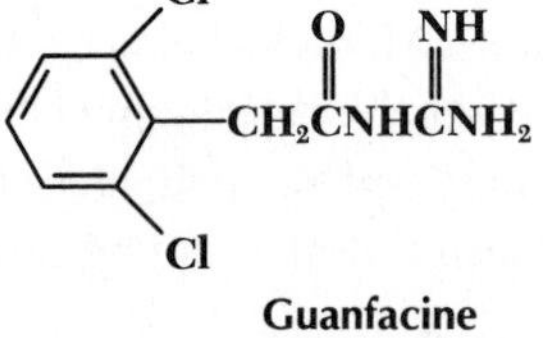 **Guanfacine**

Ca++-CHANNEL BLOCKERS

Ca^{++}-channel blockers are discussed in more detail as antianginal agents (Chapter 40). These drugs are also effective vasodilators and are therefore used frequently as antihypertensives.[2,17] Although all block the Ca^{++} channel, they differ in their pharmacologic profiles. *Nifedipine* and *nicardipine* are primarily vasodilators.[18,34,35] At the other end of the spectrum, *verapamil* has less effect on peripheral vascular resistance and has a major action to slow cardiac conduction.[26] *Diltiazem* exhibits intermediate activity.[5]

An early drawback to use of Ca^{++} antagonists was their brief action, which required dosing three or four times a day. To circumvent this problem, sustained-release preparations of all but nicardipine have been released, and other Ca^{++}-channel blockers with longer durations of action are under investigation. With availability of these newer preparations and agents, Ca^{++} antagonists are increasingly used both as single agents in mild hypertension and in combination regimens in patients with more severe disease.

In addition, nifedipine has proved effective in hypertensive emergencies.[18,35] Administration of 10 mg, either swallowed or sublingual, can promptly reduce blood pressure in this setting; the response occurs within 30 minutes and can be extreme. In some patients this pattern is helpful, but in others it can be problematic. For example, patients with cerebrovascular insufficiency may suffer ischemic insult. Thus use of this therapy should be individualized.

Nimodipine (Nimotop) is similar pharmacologically to nifedipine but is used to treat subarachnoid hemorrhage because of its relatively selective action on cerebral vasculature.[22] It is available as capsules (liquid, 30 mg); 60 mg is given every 4 hours for 21 days after such an event.

β-ADRENERGIC RECEPTOR BLOCKING DRUGS

The β-receptor antagonists have been used extensively to treat hypertension.[30] The antihypertensive effect of propranolol, the first widely used β-blocker, was discovered accidentally in England when patients with both hypertension and angina were treated with the drug. With recognition of the existence of β_1-, or cardiac, receptors efforts were made to develop specific β_1-receptor antagonists that would not affect the β_2-receptors mediating vasodilatation and catecholamine effects on the bronchial tree. Further development produced β-blockers that possess *intrinsic sympathomimetic activity* (ISA). These compounds act as partial agonists at β-receptors at low endogenous levels of sympathetic activity and function as antagonists when β-adrenergic activity increases. Such drugs do not appreciably affect resting heart rate or cardiac output but block exercise- or stress-induced increases in heart rate and output.

Mechanism of action

Despite extensive investigations, the mechanism of the antihypertensive action of the β-adrenergic receptor blocking drugs is not precisely known,[30] and there is no obvious mechanism of action to encompass *all* β-blockers in *all* hypertensive patients. Main theories for this drug class center on (1) *central nervous system effects* (for example, propranolol), (2) *decreased renin release*, (3) *reduced cardiac output*, and (4) *diminished peripheral vascular resistance* (for example, β-blockers with ISA). One or more of these effects is probably relevant in each individual patient.

The following issues illustrate the difficulty that exists when one tries to fit a single theory to the effects in all patients. (1) *Central nervous system effects*: Some β-blockers are believed not to penetrate the blood-brain barrier yet are fully effective. On the other hand, entry into the brain might occur with chronic use or, alternatively, small amounts of such drugs may reach a localized site. (2) *Decreased renin release*: Reductions in blood pressure can be dissociated from plasma renin activity; thus this action alone cannot be an *absolute* necessity for a hypotensive effect. Nevertheless, there are patients who respond to β-receptor blockade with a clear fall in plasma renin activity. (3) *Reduced cardiac output*: Nonselective β-blockers reduce cardiac output in *essentially all subjects*, but not all respond with a chronic hypotensive effect. (4) *Diminished peripheral vascular resistance*: β-Blockers with ISA tend to decrease peripheral vascular resistance, but on average this effect is small, and some patients who respond with decreased blood pressure exhibit a negligible effect on vascular resistance.

Nonselective β-adrenergic receptor blockers

Propranolol

Propranolol has historically been the most widely used β-blocker in hypertension. Although the drug blocks renin release and reduces cardiac output, these effects cannot fully account for its usefulness as an antihypertensive agent.[30]

Pharmacokinetics. Propranolol is well absorbed from the intestine, but 50% to 70% of an oral dose is extracted and metabolized by the liver during the first pass. The major metabolite, 4-hydroxypropranolol, is active, but its contribution to the overall pharmacologic effect is likely minor. Propranolol has a half-life of 4 to 6 hours. Despite its short half-life, twice-daily dosage suffices for most patients. Patients with cirrhosis exhibit both increased bioavailability (diminished first-pass effect) and reduced clearance of propranolol. Therefore they need much smaller doses of propranolol (on average one fourth normal) or, preferably, are prescribed a β-blocker eliminated by the kidney.

Effectiveness. Blood pressure is well controlled in only about one half of patients when propranolol is taken alone.[30] In combination with a diuretic the percentage increases to about 80%, and the addition of a vasodilator to the propranolol-diuretic combination achieves good results in over 90% of patients. These figures are applicable to other β-blockers as well. β-Blockers therefore have a major role in combination therapy, particularly because they can counteract the reflex tachycardia of vasodilating agents.[43] As a single treatment in patients with mild hypertension, agents that lower peripheral vascular resistance are preferable to propranolol.

Adverse effects. β-Blockers do not cause orthostatic hypotension. They may precipitate congestive heart failure and asthmatic attacks in susceptible persons, with nonselective agents theoretically more prone to do so. Bradycardia occurs but per se is not a contraindication to continued therapy unless clinically relevant. Gastrointestinal side effects, Raynauds phenomenon, and worsening of claudication occur rarely. A disadvantage of β-blockers in insulin-dependent diabetic patients is that they may mask symptoms of hypoglycemia. Propranolol, in particular, has been associated with central effects, such as sleep disturbances, vivid dreams, fatigue, and depression. These were once thought related to propranolol's high lipid solubility, which allows greater access to the brain. However, other β-blockers that enter the brain in comparable amounts cause fewer central nervous system problems.

Dosage. The initial dosage of propranolol is 40 mg twice daily. The usual effective maintenance range is 160 to 480 mg daily. See Table 19-2 for information regarding dosage forms of β-blockers.

NADOLOL

Nadolol is characterized by slow elimination, having a plasma half-life of about 12 hours[14]; it may be used once a day. The drug is excreted primarily by the kidney and thereby requires downward dose adjustment in patients with renal dysfunction.

TIMOLOL

Timolol is very similar to propranolol in its pharmacologic and kinetic profile, differing predominantly in its potency so that lower doses are used. Topical use of timolol for glaucoma (see p. 166) occasionally causes systemic β-blockade.

Cardioselective β-blockers

METOPROLOL

Metoprolol preferentially blocks β-receptors in the heart.[3,20,31] It is therefore preferable to nonselective β-blockers in patients with asthma and in those having intermittent claudication, though β-blockers in general are still best avoided in these conditions. The elimination half-life of metoprolol is 3 to 6 hours, but the antihypertensive effect is longer; the drug may be given twice daily in a total daily dosage of 50 to 200 mg. At dosages greater than this, selectivity disappears. Metoprolol is metabolized by the liver, and patients with cirrhosis have both increased bioavailability and decreased clearance. Like propranolol and timolol, dosage should be decreased drastically in such patients, or alternative agents should be used.

ATENOLOL

Atenolol is a cardioselective β-blocker with a half-life of 6 to 9 hours.[10] It can be administered once a day. It is eliminated by the kidney and requires dosage reduction in patients with renal compromise.

β-Blockers with intrinsic sympathomimetic activity

PINDOLOL

Pindolol is not cardioselective but has ISA. By stimulating vascular β_2-receptors, the drug diminishes peripheral vascular resistance; it does not suppress resting heart rate or cardiac output. Although its half-life is 3 to 4 hours, it is effective when given twice daily.

ACEBUTOLOL

Acebutolol differs from pindolol in having cardioselective β-blocking features.[33] It is metabolized to diacetolol, which is also active and cardioselective. The latter is eliminated by the kidney and accounts for the need to decrease dosage of acebutolol in patients with renal insufficiency. Acebutolol has an elimination half-life of 3 to 4 hours, whereas that of the active metabolite is 8 to 12 hours. The latter allows once daily dosing in most patients.

Combined β- and α-receptor blockade

Labetalol combines nonselective β- and α_1-adrenergic receptor blockade (in an approximate 7:1 ratio) with ISA.[12] The drug's hemodynamic actions decrease both cardiac output and peripheral vascular resistance. Labetalol has two asymmetric carbon atoms, and thus the racemate consists of four separate stereoisomers—one possesses the β-receptor blocking property with ISA, one is the α-blocker, and the other two forms are relatively less active. The β-blocking enantiomer (called dilevalol) was withdrawn from clinical trials after the appearance of hepatitis. Clinicians should be alert for changes in liver function tests in patients taking labetalol and should discontinue the drug if enzyme concentrations increase.

Labetalol is eliminated by the liver with a half-life of 3 to 4 hours. Patients with cirrhosis exhibit both an increase in bioavailability and a decrease in clearance.

The usual starting dose of labetalol is 200 mg twice daily with upward titration to 2400 mg per day. The drug is also supplied as a solution for use in hypertensive emergencies. As such, it can be given as a continuous intravenous infusion at a rate of 2 mg/min or as successive intravenous bolus doses every 10 to 20 minutes. Twenty milligrams is administered first, followed by 40 mg and then repeated doses of 80 mg until the desired blood pressure or a maximum total dose of 300 mg is reached.

DIURETICS

Drugs that promote salt excretion, such as the thiazides, are a mainstay in the treatment of hypertension. This implies that Na^+ is involved in the pathogenesis of the disease.[11] Other lines of evidence support the role of Na^+ in hypertension: (1) rats of some strains develop hypertension on a high salt intake, (2) the hypertensive effect of deoxycorticosterone and aldosterone seems attributable to salt retention, and (3) the antihypertensive action of a low salt diet is generally acknowledged. Despite these data, however, the mechanism whereby an excess of salt contributes to hypertension is not known. Expansion of extracellular fluid volume and alterations in the salt concentration in arteriolar walls, thereby increasing peripheral vascular resistance, have been suggested as important factors.

Thiazides and related drugs

Most investigators believe that thiazide diuretics initially exert their antihypertensive action through salt depletion. With chronic therapy they also lower peripheral vascular resistance.

The most useful oral diuretics, discussed in detail in Chapter 42, are the thiazides and the related drugs chlorthalidone (Hygroton, others), quinethazone (Hydromox), and metolazone (Zaroxolyn, others).[23] They are widely used to treat mild hypertension because of their safety and effectiveness and their ability to enhance the antihypertensive effect of other drugs. They differ only in their durations of action and potency.

Adverse effects of thiazide diuretics include hypokalemia, hyperuricemia, and aggravation of diabetes. A more recent concern that limits their use as single agents, particularly in young patients with hypertension, is their effect on plasma cholesterol. It appears that these drugs, by unknown mechanisms, increase low-density lipoprotein cholesterol about 10%. There is concern that over many years of treatment this will enhance cardiovascular risk. As a result, many patients who heretofore would have been prescribed thiazide diuretics as a single agent are now being treated with other drugs that lower peripheral vascular resistance.

Potassium ion-sparing diuretics

Spironolactone (Aldactone, Alatone), triamterene (Dyrenium), and amiloride (Midamor) have only weak antihypertensive activity as single agents and should not be used as primary drugs in this disorder.[23] They have been promoted for use in combination with thiazides to prevent development of hypokalemia. However, hypokalemia is an infrequent adverse effect of thiazides used alone for hypertension; it occurs in only about 5% of patients. There is no good evidence that the combination formulations diminish this incidence, but it is clear that they entail a risk of hyperkalemia. Hence these products are indicated only in patients in whom K^+ depletion develops while they are receiving other diuretics.

Loop diuretics

Loop diuretics are less effective than thiazides in patients with uncomplicated essential hypertension. They should be reserved for hypertensive patients with diminished renal function in whom thiazides are less effective.[23]

REFERENCES

1. Amery A, Birkenhäger W, Brixko P, et al: Mortality and morbidity results from the European Working Party on High Blood Pressure in the Elderly trial, *Lancet* 1:1349, 1985.
2. Antman EM, Stone PH, Muller JE, Braunwald E: Calcium channel blocking agents in the treatment of cardiovascular disorders, *Ann Intern Med* 93:875 and 886, 1980.
3. Benfield P, Clissold SP, Brogden RN: Metoprolol: an updated review of its pharmacodynamic and pharmacokinetic properties, and therapeutic efficacy, in hypertension, ischaemic heart disease and related cardiovascular disorders, *Drugs* 31:376, 1986.
4. Brogden RN, Todd PA, Sorkin EM: Captopril: an update of its pharmacodynamic and pharmacokinetic properties, and therapeutic use in hypertension and congestive heart failure, *Drugs* 36:540, 1988.
5. Buckley MM-T, Grant SM, Goa KL, et al: Diltiazem: a reappraisal of its pharmacological properties and therapeutic use, *Drugs* 39:757, 1990.
6. Campese VM: Minoxidil: a review of its pharmacological properties and therapeutic use, *Drugs* 22:257, 1981.
7. Deedwania PC: Angiotensin-converting enzyme inhibitors in congestive heart failure, *Arch Intern Med* 150:1798, 1990.
8. Duchin KL, McKinstry DN, Cohen AI, Migdalof BH: Pharmacokinetics of captopril in healthy subjects and in patients with cardiovascular diseases, *Clin Pharmacokinet* 14:241, 1988.
9. Finnerty FA, Jr, Brogden RN: Guanadrel: a review of its pharmacodynamic and pharmacokinetic properties and therapeutic use in hypertension, *Drugs* 30:22, 1985.
10. Fitzgerald JD, Ruffin R, Smedstad KG, et al: Studies on the pharmacokinetics and pharmacodynamics of atenolol in man, *Eur J Clin Pharmacol* 13:81, 1978.
11. Freis ED: Salt in hypertension and the effects of diuretics, *Annu Rev Pharmacol Toxicol* 19:13, 1979.
12. Goa KL, Benfield P, Sorkin EM: Labetalol: a reappraisal of its pharmacology, pharmacokinetics and therapeutic use in hypertension and ischaemic heart disease, *Drugs* 37:583, 1989.
13. Graham RM, Pettinger WA: Prazosin, *N Engl J Med* 300:232, 1979.
14. Heel RC, Brogden RN, Pakes GE, et al: Nadolol: a review of its pharmacological properties and therapeutic efficacy in hypertension and angina pectoris, *Drugs* 20:1, 1980.
15. Holmes B, Brogden RN, Heel RC, et al: Guanabenz: a review of its pharmacodynamic properties and therapeutic efficacy in hypertension, *Drugs* 26:212, 1983.
16. Hypertension Detection and Follow-up Program Cooperative Group: Five-year findings of the hypertension detection and follow-up program. I. Reduction in mortality of persons with high blood pressure, including mild hypertension, *JAMA* 242:2562, 1979.

17. Kates RE: Calcium antagonists: pharmacokinetic properties, *Drugs* 25:113, 1983.
18. Kleinbloesem CH, van Brummelen P, Breimer DD: Nifedipine: relationship between pharmacokinetics and pharmacodynamics, *Clin Pharmacokinet* 12:12, 1987.
19. Koch-Weser J: Diazoxide, *N Engl J Med* 294:1271, 1976.
20. Koch-Weser J: Metoprolol *N Engl J Med* 301:698, 1979.
21. Lancaster SG, Todd PA: Lisinopril: a preliminary review of its pharmacodynamic and pharmacokinetic properties, and therapeutic use in hypertension and congestive heart failure, *Drugs* 35:646, 1988.
22. Langley MS, Sorkin EM: Nimodipine: a review of its pharmacodynamic and pharmacokinetic properties, and therapeutic potential in cerebrovascular disease, *Drugs* 37:669, 1989.
23. Lant A: Diuretics: clinical pharmacology and therapeutic use, *Drugs* 29:57 and 162, 1985.
24. Lowenthal DT, Matzek KM, MacGregor TR: Clinical pharmacokinetics of clonidine, *Clin Pharmacokinet* 14:287, 1988.
25. Ludden TM, McNay JL, Jr, Shepherd, AMM, Lin MS: Clinical pharmacokinetics of hydralazine, *Clin Pharmacokinet* 7:185, 1982.
26. McTavish D, Sorkin EM: Verapamil: an updated review of its pharmacodynamic and pharmacokinetic properties, and therapeutic use in hypertension, *Drugs* 38:19, 1989.
27. Medical Research Council Working Party: MRC trial of treatment of mild hypertension: principle results, *Br Med J* 291:97, 1985.
28. Mosqueda-Garcia R: Guanfacine: a second generation α_2-adrenergic blocker, *Am J Med Sci* 299:73, 1990.
29. Myhre E, Rugstad HE, Hansen T: Clinical pharmacokinetics of methyldopa, *Clin Pharmacokinet* 7:221, 1982.
30. Nadelmann J, Frishman WH: Clinical use of β-adrenoceptor blockade in systemic hypertension, *Drugs* 39:862, 1990.
31. Regårdh C-G, Johnsson G: Clinical pharmacokinetics of metoprolol, *Clin Pharmacokinet* 5:557, 1980.
32. Schulz V: Clinical pharmacokinetics of nitroprusside, cyanide, thiosulphate and thiocyanate, *Clin Pharmacokinet* 9:239, 1984.
33. Singh BN, Thoden WR, Ward A: Acebutolol: a review of its pharmacological properties and therapeutic efficacy in hypertension, angina pectoris and arrhythmia, *Drugs* 29:531, 1985.
34. Sorkin EM, Clissold SP: Nicardipine: a review of its pharmacodynamic and pharmacokinetic properties, and therapeutic efficacy, in the treatment of angina pectoris, hypertension and related cardiovascular disorders, *Drugs* 33:296, 1987.
35. Sorkin EM, Clissold SP, Brogden RN: Nifedipine: a review of its pharmacodynamic and pharmacokinetic properties, and therapeutic efficacy, in ischaemic heart disease, hypertension and related cardiovascular disorders, *Drugs* 30:182, 1985.
36. Sorkin EM, Heel RC: Guanfacine: a review of its pharmacodynamic and pharmacokinetic properties, and therapeutic efficacy in the treatment of hypertension, *Drugs* 31:301, 1986.
37. Titmarsh S, Monk JP: Terazosin: a review of its pharmacodynamic and pharmacokinetic properties, and therapeutic efficacy in essential hypertension, *Drugs* 33:461, 1987.
38. Todd PA, Goa KL: Enalapril: an update of its pharmacological properties and therapeutic use in congestive heart failure, *Drugs* 37:141, 1989.
39. Veterans Administration Cooperative Study Group on Antihypertensive Agents: Effects of treatment on morbidity in hypertension. II. Results in patients with diastolic blood pressure averaging 90 through 114 mm Hg, *JAMA* 213:1143, 1970.
40. Vincent J, Meredith PA, Reid JL, et al: Clinical pharmacokinetics of prazosin—1985, *Clin Pharmacokinet* 10:144, 1985.
41. Williams GH: Converting-enzyme inhibitors in the treatment of hypertension, *N Engl J Med* 319:1517, 1988.

42. Young RA, Brogden RN: Doxazosin: a review of its pharmacodynamic and pharmacokinetic properties, and therapeutic efficacy in mild or moderate hypertension, *Drugs* 35:525, 1988.

43. Zacest R, Gilmore E, Koch-Weser J: Treatment of essential hypertension with combined vasodilation and beta-adrenergic blockade, *N Engl J Med* 286:617, 1972.

Chapter 22

Histamine and antihistaminic drugs

Histamine is important in pharmacology and medicine not because of its usefulness as a drug but because of its potent pharmacologic activities. Histamine is widely distributed in tissues and induces both physiologic and pathologic effects. As examples, it plays a role in central neurotransmission, is important in gastric secretion, and contributes to inflammation and to anaphylaxis, allergies, and adverse reactions to drugs.

Antihistaminic drugs competitively antagonize histamine at specific receptor sites. Two distinct histamine receptors, H_1 and H_2, serve different functions and are blocked by different groups of antihistamines.

HISTAMINE

Distribution

Histamine was synthesized in the laboratory before its biologic actions were known. It was later identified in ergot, a rye fungus, as a product of bacterial contamination. Observations of several physiologists suggested possible roles for this curious amine. Sir Henry Dale noted striking similarities between anaphylaxis and the effects of histamine injection in several animal species, including man. Sir Thomas Lewis suggested that injury releases a histamine-like substance that mediates evanescent cutaneous inflammation. Research in the 1950s revealed a correlation between the distribution of tissue mast cells and histamine, and many investigations focused on mechanisms of histamine release from these cells. Fig. 22-1, A, shows normal mast cells. Mast cells can also function as antigen-presenting cells in immune reactions.[2]

There are physiologically important non–mast cell pools of histamine as well. Basophils, which closely resemble mast cells, contain a high concentration of histamine and, like mast cells, may participate in allergic and inflammatory reactions.[11] Platelets normally contain very little histamine unless stimulated by thrombin or platelet-activating factor (PAF) or by contact with collagen. The response to stimulation is blocked by inhibitors of histidine decarboxylase and precedes platelet aggregation; this suggests that the newly formed histamine is a second messenger in the platelet-aggregation reaction.[13]

Other non–mast cell pools of histamine include the central nervous system, where histamine is associated with neural elements, and the gastric mucosa. Histamine turnover is rapid in these pools, and they are resistant to agents that release histamine from mast cells.

Formation and degradation

The chemical structure of histamine, or 2-(4-imidazolyl)ethylamine, is shown on the next page.

$$\text{Imidazole ring (N, N)}-CH_2-CH_2-NH_2$$

Histamine

In man, synthesis of histamine is catalyzed by L-histidine decarboxylase. The enzyme aromatic L-amino acid decarboxylase, which acts on several different amino acid substrates, can also catalyze formation of histamine from histidine. Although this enzyme is more prevalent than L-histidine decarboxylase, it is less specific. The observation that histidine decarboxylase can be induced in some tissues suggested possible roles for histamine, for example, in regulation of blood flow within the microcirculation or in stimulation of growth and repair of tissues.

Histamine is degraded through two main enzymatic pathways. In man, histamine is metabolized primarily to 1-methylhistamine by imidazole-*N*-methyltransferase. The methylated product is then converted to 1-methylimidazole-4-acetic acid by monoamine oxidase. Histamine is also oxidized by diamine oxidase to imidazole-4-acetic acid, much of which is conjugated with ribose and excreted as the riboside. In addition, some histamine is excreted as *N*-acetylhistamine after acetylation by bacteria in the intestine.

In a normal person 2 to 3 mg of histamine is released daily from tissues and excreted in urine. Allergic or chemically induced release of histamine from mast cells or basophils markedly increases urinary excretion.

Binding and release of mast cell histamine

Release of histamine from mast cells is a prominent feature of immediate hypersensitivity reactions and also contributes to adverse effects of certain compounds. Mast cell histamine is confined within subcellular granules in a complex with protein and heparin. Histamine is released when mast cells are perturbed by physical or chemical stimuli or by antigen-antibody reactions. Membrane stimulation evokes influx of Ca^{++}, activation of membrane phospholipase, contraction of the cytostructure, and fusion of perigranular membranes in the process of exocytosis. Next, sodium ions from the extracellular environment displace cationic amines from anionic groups within the granular matrix and also displace cationic peptides such as the eosinophil chemotactic factor. The release reaction is accompanied by formation of leukotrienes, prostaglandin D_2, and release or activation of mast cell proteases. Histamine release requires energy and is modulated by cyclic nucleotides. In addition, arachidonic acid metabolites may also regulate the release process.

Certain types of vascular headache may be caused by released histamine. Histamine injection can reproduce symptoms of migraine, and repeated administration produces a certain amount of "desensitization" and symptomatic improvement.

RELEASE BY DRUGS AND OTHER CHEMICALS

Large polymers, such as polysaccharides or lectins, as well as basically charged peptides activate mast cell degranulation. Use of some drugs is limited by histamine release; intracutaneous injection of morphine in man can cause localized erythema and edema, and curare alkaloids cause a similar response. Episodes of bronchial constriction after intravenous injection of curare or polypeptide antibiotics, such as polymyxin, have also been attributed to histamine release. However, an experimental histamine-releasing agent, compound 48/80, is a valuable tool for study of the mast cell release response. Fig. 22-1, *B*, shows degranulation of mast cells by this agent.

Compound 48/80

Release in anaphylaxis and allergy

Histamine release is clearly involved in the symptomatology of anaphylactic shock in several species, including the human. The primary pathway involves interaction of antigen with IgE bound to the mast cell surface. This reaction does not require complement, but it may be accentuated by concomitant release of complement-derived peptides (anaphylatoxins), kinins, or other inflammatory mediators.

Histamine release from mast cells in the skin and mucosa can cause cutaneous and laryngeal edema, and bronchoconstriction and hypotension can occur if there is sufficient release into the systemic circulation.

In human leukocytes histamine release by ragweed extract is inhibited by cyclic AMP and drugs that activate adenylyl cyclase. Similar studies on mast cells from human lungs support the concept of control by cyclic nucleotides. Catecholamines and

FIG. 22-1 *Mast cells in tongue.* ***A****, Normal cells;* ***B****, cell degranulated after treatment with compound 48/80.*

From Enerbäck L, Lundin PM: Cell Tissue Res 150:95, 1974.

A

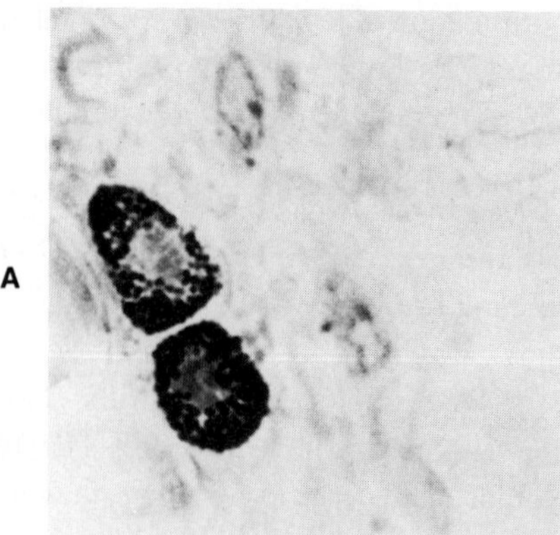

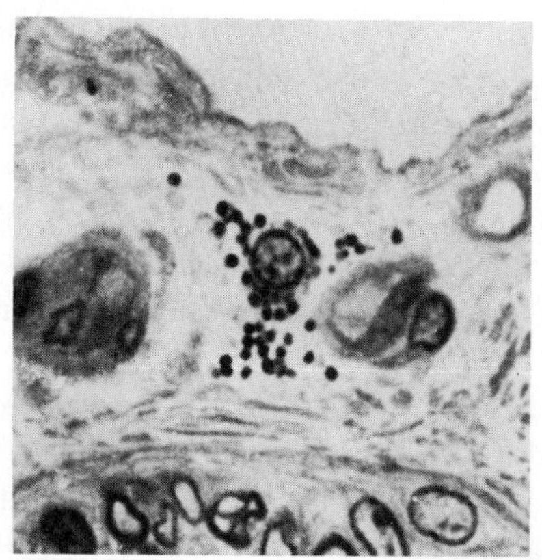

B

theophylline, drugs widely used in allergic diseases, are believed to inhibit histamine release in addition to antagonizing many of its actions. Disodium cromoglycate (see Chapter 44) inhibits both release of histamine and formation of leukotrienes (Chapter 25) by a mechanism independent of cyclic nucleotides. Some antihistamines also inhibit antigen-induced release of histamine from mast cells or basophils, but it is not clear how much this contributes to their therapeutic effect.[16]

Pharmacologic effects of histamine

Once liberated, histamine has potent actions on smooth muscles, blood vessels, and secretory glands. Histamine taken by mouth has no effect because it is rapidly metabolized by bacteria in the gastrointestinal tract, by the gastrointestinal mucosa, and by the liver.

If injected intravenously, however, as little as 0.1 mg of histamine causes vasodilatation with a rapid fall in blood pressure, reflex acceleration of heart rate, elevation of cerebrospinal fluid pressure, flushing of the face, and headache. Gastric acid secretion is stimulated severalfold. These responses last only a few minutes, but in allergic reactions histamine release may continue for several hours.

CIRCULATORY EFFECTS

The heart has both H_1- and H_2-receptors, but their function remains obscure. Histamine-induced activation of adenylyl cyclase in the human heart is not blocked by propranolol. Histamine increases the rate and force of cardiac contraction in several species, but most circulatory effects of histamine are probably due to changes in vasomotor tone.

Blood vessels also have both H_1- and H_2-receptors; H_1-receptors are generally more important, except for specific vascular beds. For example, vasodilatation of the temporal artery in humans appears mediated by H_2-receptors. The combination of arteriolar dilatation and increased capillary permeability induced by histamine promotes loss of plasma from the circulation and development of tissue edema.

OTHER SMOOTH MUSCLE EFFECTS

Histamine also affects smooth muscle in many nonvascular structures. Its action on bronchiolar smooth muscle is the most important clinically. Individuals with asthma are particularly sensitive and may exhibit severe bronchoconstriction to a dose of histamine that would only slightly reduce vital capacity in a normal person. Asthmatic individuals are also highly sensitive to methacholine, leukotrienes, and many airway irritants.

The limited benefit of antihistaminic therapy for asthmatic patients suggested that other mediators are involved. Slow-reacting substance of anaphylaxis (SRS-A) is released with histamine from IgE-sensitized fragments of human lung. This potent bronchoconstrictor is actually a family of acidic lipids formed from arachidonic acid by lipoxygenase (see Chapter 25). Leukotrienes C_4 and D_4, constituents of SRS-A, are believed to be the primary mediators of the bronchoconstrictive response in asthmatics. Prostaglandin D_2, formed in mast cells during the histamine-release reaction, is also a potent bronchoconstrictor.[8]

EFFECT ON GASTRIC SECRETIONS

Histamine is a potent stimulant of gastric acid and pepsin secretion. Subcutaneous injection of as little as 25 μg will increase gastric secretion in humans. This response is used as a test for achlorhydria, the lack of gastric hydrochloric acid production. Histamine-resistant achlorhydria has diagnostic importance in conditions such as pernicious anemia.

The concentration of histamine is particularly high in the acid-secreting part of the stomach; both mast cells in the submucosa and granule-containing cells in the lamina propria contain histamine. The amine released from cells in the lamina propria by carbachol, gastrin, or food then acts on H_2-receptors to stimulate secretion from parietal cells. The secretory response requires activation of adenylyl cyclase. The precise relationship of histamine to the stimulus for gastric secretion is still unknown. The polypeptide gastrin, another stimulant, is about 500 times more potent than histamine. Its effect is inhibited by H_2-antagonists, which suggests a functional relationship between gastrin and histamine. A similar finding for cholinergic stimulation of gastric secretion further suggests that histamine is the final common mediator of secretion.

Role in health and disease

Several physiologic roles for histamine seem likely in addition to stimulation of gastric secretion. It is probably a neurotransmitter[9]; the brain has histamine receptors, as well as enzymes for its synthesis and inactivation. Histamine can stimulate autonomic ganglia, and it releases catecholamines from the adrenal medulla.

Histamine holds a firmly established place among mediators of inflammation, but this amine also modifies immune and inflammatory responses. For example, histamine limits its own release from basophils and mast cells, inhibits chemotaxis of basophils and neutrophils, and reduces secretion of enzymes and oxidants from neutrophils. In addition, it inhibits cytokine production and proliferation in T lymphocytes. These phenomena are believed to be linked to elevation of cyclic AMP through interaction with H_2-receptors.[3]

Histamine also stimulates release of arachidonic acid in various cells, an effect mediated through H_1-receptors.[1] Thus histamine released in an area of inflammation may also modify the local response by generating prostaglandins or leukotrienes (see Chapter 25).

ANTIHISTAMINIC DRUGS

Diphenhydramine and tripelennamine, the first H_1-antihistamines, were introduced many years ago in response to the discovery that histamine causes some effects of allergy and inflammation. Although these antagonists protected experimental animals against anaphylactic shock or histamine injection, they did not block all actions of histamine. Now it is known that histamine acts on at least two distinct receptors. Contraction of smooth muscle of the bronchi and intestine is mediated by H_1-receptors and is antagonized by conventional "antihistamines" or H_1-receptor blocking agents. H_2-receptors mediate the action of histamine on gastric secretion and cardiac acceleration.[5] Stimulation of these receptors is antagonized by drugs such as cimetidine, ranitidine, famotidine, and nizatidine.

Histamine H_1-receptor antagonists

CHEMISTRY

The basic structure of H_1-antagonists is a substituted ethylamine:

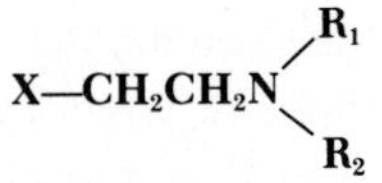

$$X{-}CH_2CH_2N\begin{matrix}R_1\\R_2\end{matrix}$$

Since histamine is 2-(4-imidazolyl)ethylamine, it is likely that the ethylamine portion of histamine and H_1-receptor antagonists is important for interaction with this receptor. The R groups in the ethylamine structure are usually CH_3. Structural formulas of several H_1-receptor antagonists are shown below.

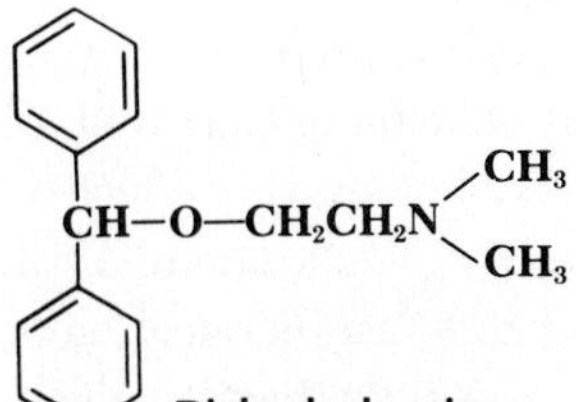

Diphenhydramine

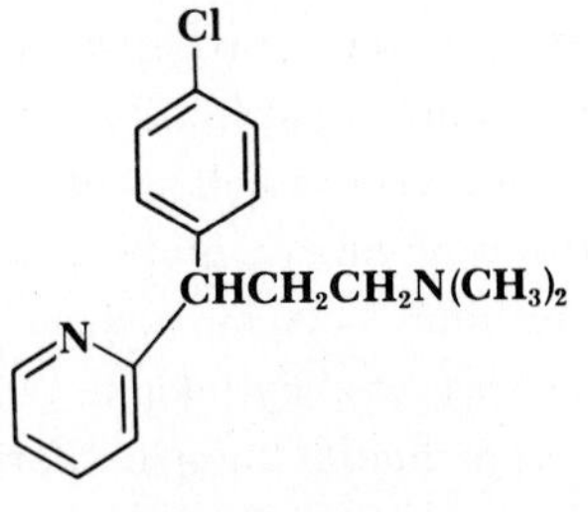

Chlorpheniramine

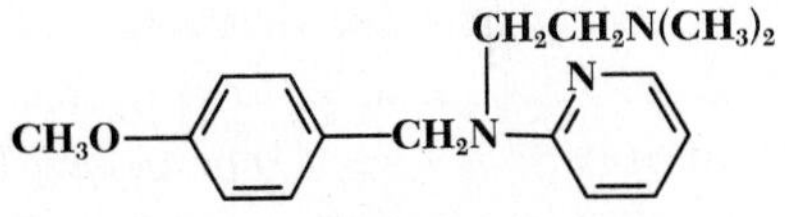

Pyrilamine

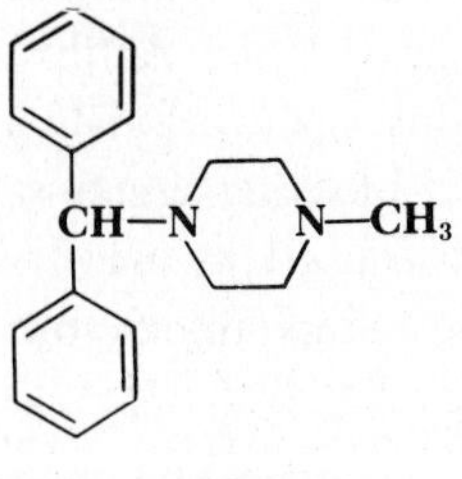

Cyclizine

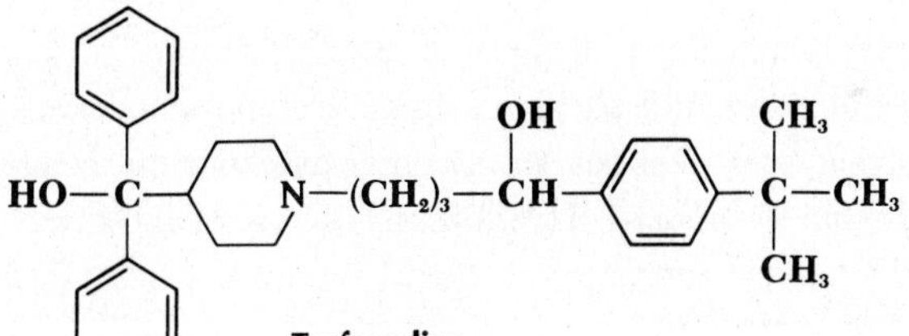

Terfenadine

All H_1-antihistamines cause a parallel shift to the right of the log dose-response curve for a given histamine effect with no change in the maximal response. In therapeutic doses, none of them affect histamine metabolism, but some are reported to inhibit its release.[16]

CLINICAL PHARMACOLOGY

Many H_1-antihistamines are marketed today, partially with the goal of improved selectivity. Nevertheless, to varying degrees they have potential for sedative, antimuscarinic, antiserotonin, and local anesthetic activities.

Their sedative action is at least additive with that of other central depressants such as barbiturates or alcohol. Some newer agents that do not readily cross the blood-brain barrier are less sedating (see Table 22-1). Terfenadine, used for prevention of allergic rhinitis, causes little impairment of the sensorium.[15] Astemizole, recently marketed in the United States, has no sedative action or synergistic interaction with alcohol.

Phenindamine is unusual because it stimulates the central nervous system in some persons, even at therapeutic doses.

Antihistamines with prominent anticholinergic actions, such as diphenhydramine, can dry salivary and bronchial secretions, which may adversely affect patients with asthma. However, some clinicians reported that chlorpheniramine and certain other H_1-blocking drugs improved lung function in asthmatic patients.[10]

The anticholinergic action of some antihistamines probably accounts for their usefulness in treatment of Parkinsons disease (see Chapter 30) and prevention of motion sickness. Dimenhydrinate, a widely used combination of diphenhydramine with 8-chlorotheophylline, owes its anti–motion sickness property to the former component. Neither terfenadine nor astemizole has anticholinergic activity. Some antihistamines, such as cyproheptadine, also block serotonin receptors, but this activity offers no advantage over compounds that block only histamine receptors.

The prominence of the various actions depends, in part, on structure. For example, ethanolamines, such as diphenhydramine, have significant anticholinergic, as well as sedative, actions. Piperazines, such as cyclizine, are less sedative but are very effective in preventing motion sickness. Pyrilamine, an ethylenediamine, has a strong local anesthetic action. Terfenadine, a complex derivative of cyclizine, has minimal anticholinergic or antiserotonin activity and little or no sedative effect. In contrast, alkylamines, such as chlorpheniramine, are sedative, even at therapeutic doses.

THERAPEUTIC USES

There are many conditions in which H_1-antihistamines are helpful. Antihistaminic therapy may relieve or prevent allergic rhinitis, urticaria, insect envenomation, some types of asthma (of allergic origin), and motion sickness. H_1-blocking agents suppress sneezing and changes in mucosal vascular permeability caused by nasal antigen challenge in humans. In addition, several of the drugs also reduce release of allergic mediators and formation of kinins within the nasal passages.[16]

Antihistamines alone are of little or no benefit in acute anaphylactic emergencies; in most types of asthma; in inflammatory disorders of the skin, eyes, and nose; or in the common cold. They are administered with epinephrine, however, to treat anaphylactic reactions, and they may be combined with other therapeutic modalities for reactions of the skin or airways in which there is clearly an allergic component.[12]

Selection of an antihistamine is usually based on its other effects, especially the degree of sedation. Three antihistamines, diphenhydramine, pyrilamine, and doxylamine, are sold over-the-counter as sleep aids. The duration of action of most antihistamines in therapeutic doses is about 4 hours. The usual adult dose and sedative activity of several antihistamines are listed in Table 22-1.

ABSORPTION AND METABOLISM

H_1-receptor antagonists are absorbed rapidly and completely from the gastrointestinal tract. Onset of action is usually within 30 minutes, and absorption is complete in 4 hours. When diphenhydramine is administered orally, peak blood concentration is achieved in 1 hour; the concentration is negligible by 6 hours. H_1-antagonists are metabolized in the liver by hydroxylation. Some studies indicate that metabolism is much slower and duration of action is prolonged in elderly patients.

TABLE 22-1 Doses and sedative property of various H_1-antihistamines

Drug	Trade name	Usual adult dose (mg)	Degree of sedation
Phenindamine tartrate	Nolahist	25	−*
Astemizole	Hismanal	10	±
Terfenadine	Seldane	60	±
Brompheniramine maleate	Dimetane, others	4	+
Chlorpheniramine maleate	Chlor-Trimeton, others	4	+
Cyproheptadine hydrochloride	Periactin	4	+
Dexchlorpheniramine maleate	Polaramine, others	2	+
Diphenylpyraline hydrochloride	Hispril	5	+
Methdilazine hydrochloride	Tacaryl	8	+
Pyrilamine maleate	Nisaval	25-50	+
Triprolidine hydrochloride	Actidil, Myidyl	2.5	+
Azatadine maleate	Optimine	1-2	++
Carbinoxamine maleate	Clistin	4-8	++
Clemastine fumarate	Tavist	1	++
Trimeprazine	Temaril	2.5	++
Tripelennamine hydrochloride	PBZ, Pelamine	25-50	++
Diphenhydramine hydrochloride	Benadryl, others	25-50	+++
Doxylamine succinate	Unisom	25	+++
Promethazine hydrochloride	Phenergan, others	12.5-25	+++

*Stimulation possible.

TOXICITY

H_1-antihistamines have a wide margin of safety; several times the recommended dose can be absorbed without danger of respiratory depression. They may contribute to automobile and other accidents, however, if combined with depressant drugs such as barbiturates, benzodiazepines, or alcohol.

Acute poisoning has occurred after ingestion of very large doses of antihistamines. The symptoms resemble those of atropine intoxication, including central nervous system excitation and convulsions. The management of acute poisoning is supportive.

Topical application of antihistamines was used in the past for symptomatic relief from acute cutaneous allergic reactions, probably because of the local anesthetic action of some compounds. Unfortunately, contact dermatitis often developed when patients became sensitized to the topically applied antihistamine.

Some antihistamines that were originally used to prevent motion sickness were later shown to be teratogenic in laboratory animals. However, the teratogenic effect has not been reported in humans. If use of such an agent is considered essential, meclizine (Antivert, others) may be safer than cyclizine (Marezine).

Histamine H_2-receptor antagonists

In 1972, Black and co-workers described the first agent, burimamide, that competitively antagonized the action of histamine on gastric parietal cells, guinea pig atria, and rat uteri,[5] thereby identifying H_2-receptors. The realization that histamine stimulation of gastric acid and pepsin secretion might be involved in peptic ulcer disease led to an extensive search for other compounds to block H_2-receptors. Cimetidine, in which the thiourea in the side chain was changed to cyanoguanidine, was the first such drug to be marketed successfully.

Differences between H_1- and H_2-Antihistamines

In addition to acting on different receptors, these two groups of drugs differ substantially in their chemistry, pharmacokinetics, and clinical uses. The H_1-antihistamines differ from histamine primarily in that the imidazole ring structure is modified or replaced by other substituents, whereas in the H_2-antagonists the side chain is extensively modified.

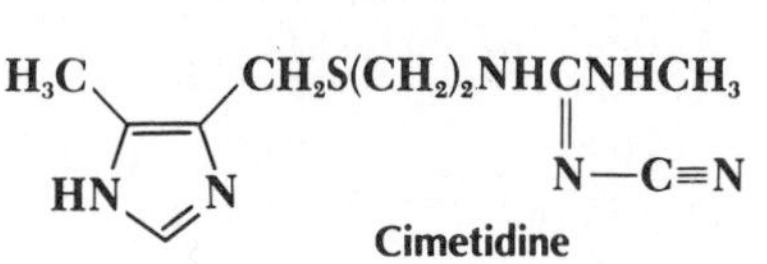

Cimetidine

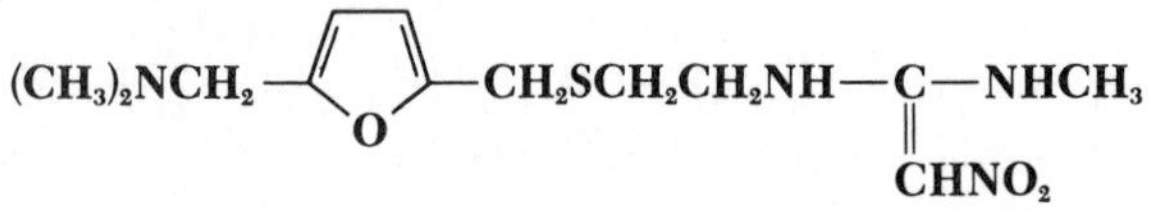

Ranitidine

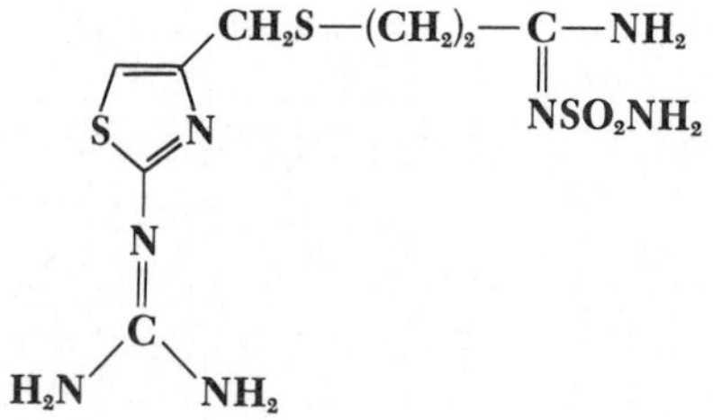

Famotidine

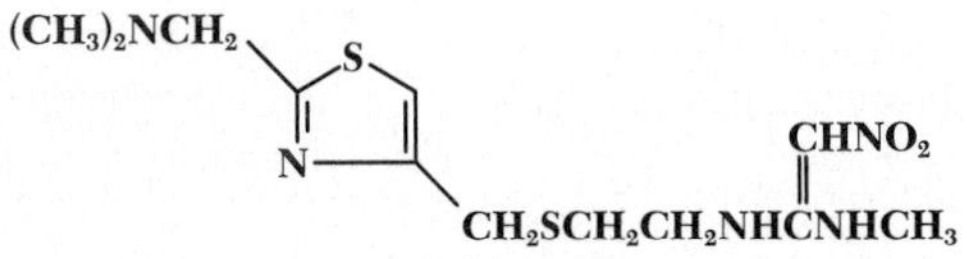

Nizatidine

In contrast to H_1-receptor antagonists, H_2-antihistamines are generally less lipid soluble. At therapeutic doses, they do not have prominent sedative, anticholinergic, or local anesthetic activities. They were originally assumed to have minimal central actions. However, there are H_2-receptors within the brain, and central effects, including mental confusion, agitation, and depression, have been reported. The incidence of such effects appears to be less common with famotidine than with either cimetidine or ranitidine.[4]

Mechanism of Inhibition of Gastric Secretion

The H_2-receptor antagonists inhibit gastric secretion caused by histamine, gastrin, and acetylcholine, as well as by food.[14] There are several possible explanations for this apparent lack of specificity. Histamine may be the final mediator for the other stimuli. Alternatively, there could be separate receptors on the parietal cell for histamine, gastrin, and acetylcholine, linked so that blockade of the histamine receptor interferes with the activity of the others. Thus histamine may have a "permissive" effect on the actions of the other stimuli.

Clinical Pharmacology

The H_2-receptor antagonists have had a tremendous impact on management of peptic ulcer disease. Cimetidine reduces diurnal gastric acid secretion; after 6 weeks of treatment, most ulcer patients are cured as compared with subjects treated with a placebo. When the drug is administered in a dose of 200 or 300 mg four times a day (with meals and at bedtime), basal and food- or gastrin-stimulated gastric secretion is inhibited. A 300 mg dose of cimetidine at bedtime significantly reduces gastric acidity for at least 8 hours. Administration of 600 mg twice a day is also adequate, and in many patients a single 800 mg dose at bedtime may be sufficient.

Ranitidine, famotidine, and nizatidine are very similar in action and indications to cimetidine, and they have comparable efficacy.[7] These drugs differ mainly in their effects on metabolism of other compounds (see the next page) and in the formulations that are available.

Ranitidine is more potent than cimetidine and also has a longer duration of action, which permits less frequent dosing. Famotidine is reported to be up to 100 times more potent than cimetidine and three times more potent than ranitidine, and it has a longer duration of action than either of these other antagonists.[6]

Cimetidine (Tagamet) can be administered as tablets, 200 to 800 mg, or as the hydrochloride as a liquid, 300 mg in 5 ml, or by injection, 300 mg in 2 or 50 ml. **Ranitidine** (Zantac) **hydrochloride** is available in tablets, 150 and 300 mg, a syrup containing 15 mg/ml, and in solution for injection, 0.5 or 25 mg/ml. **Famotidine** (Pepcid) is usually taken orally, in 20 or 40 mg tablets or as a suspension reconstituted from powder; a solution of 10 mg/ml can be injected. **Nizatidine** (Axid) is available in capsules, 150 and 300 mg.

THERAPEUTIC USES

Approved indications for H_2-receptor antagonists include (1) hypersecretory states such as Zollinger-Ellison syndrome and mastocytosis, (2) short-term treatment (up to 8 weeks) of active duodenal ulcer or benign gastric ulcer, which tends to be somewhat less responsive, and (3) prolonged therapy to prevent recurrence of duodenal ulcer. These agents are used widely in intensive care units to prevent "stress"-induced ulceration. Other applications include reflux esophagitis, pancreatic insufficiency, and prevention of NSAID-induced gastric damage.

ABSORPTION AND METABOLISM

Cimetidine is well absorbed when taken orally, has a plasma half-life of 2 hours, and about half is excreted unchanged in the urine. Either renal or hepatic insufficiency requires dosage modification.

The newer drugs have similar characteristics. A single oral or parenteral dose of famotidine has a rapid onset of action (within 1 hour) and persists for 10 to 12 hours. Like cimetidine, it is primarily excreted in the urine, and 70% of an intravenous dose or 25% to 30% of an oral dose appears in the urine unchanged.[7]

TOXICITY

Cimetidine and ranitidine have now been used by millions of patients for more than 13 years. Serious adverse effects are unusual. As wide use of cimetidine continues, adverse effects, such as dizziness, confusion (usually in elderly patients), leukopenia, rashes, or myalgias, have been reported. In addition, a mild antiandrogenic action causes breast enlargement (gynecomastia) and tenderness in some persons. Impotence reported by a few patients on cimetidine probably results from the antiandrogenic actions. The newer H_2-blocking drugs do not have this action.

Drug interactions are the primary limitation of cimetidine therapy. Cimetidine inhibits cytochrome P-450 and can decrease the metabolism of many other compounds (see Table 70-3). Dosage of propranolol, labetalol, and metoprolol should be reduced when cimetidine is added to treatment, because the H_2-blocker reduces both presystemic metabolism and systemic clearance of these agents. Drugs that may require a reduction in dosage when cimetidine is added include theophylline, phenytoin, and lidocaine.

Clinical experience thus far indicates that ranitidine, famotidine, and nizatidine generally do not inhibit hepatic drug-metabolizing microsomal enzymes, although such an effect may occur in occasional patients. As a consequence, there is less potential for toxicity due to accumulation of other drugs.

REFERENCES

1. Alhenc-Gelas F, Tsai SJ, Callahan KS, et al: Stimulation of prostaglandin formation by vasoactive mediators in cultured human endothelial cells, *Prostaglandins* 24:723, 1982.
2. Banovac K, Neylan D, Leone J, et al: Are the mast cells antigen presenting cells? *Immunol Invest* 18:901, 1989.
3. Beer DJ, Matloff SM, Rocklin RE: The influence of histamine on immune and inflammatory responses, *Adv Immunol* 35:209, 1984.
4. Berlin RG: Effects of H_2-receptor antagonists on the central nervous system, *Drug Dev Res* 17:97, 1989.
5. Black JW, Duncan WAM, Durant CJ, et al: Definition and antagonism of histamine H_2-receptors, *Nature* 236:385, 1972.
6. Dammann H-G, Müller P, Simon B: 24 Hour intragastric acidity and single night-time dose of three H_2-blockers, *Lancet* 2:1078, 1983.
7. Famotidine (Pepcid), *Med Lett Drugs Ther* 29:17, 1987.
8. Hardy CC, Robinson C, Tattersfield AE, Holgate ST: The bronchoconstrictor effect of inhaled prostaglandin D_2 in normal and asthmatic men, *N Engl J Med* 311:209, 1984.
9. Hough LB: Cellular localization and possible functions for brain histamine: recent progress, *Prog Neurobiol* 30:469, 1988.
10. Meltzer EO: To use or not to use antihistamines in patients with asthma, *Ann Allergy* 64:183, 1990.
11. Osler AG, Lichtenstein LM, Levy DA: In vitro studies of human reaginic allergy, *Adv Immunol* 8:183, 1968.
12. Popa V: The classic antihistamines (H_1 blockers) in respiratory medicine, *Clin Chest Med* 7:367, 1986.
13. Saxena SP, McNicol A, Brandes LJ, et al: A role for intracellular histamine in collagen-induced platelet aggregation, *Blood* 75:407, 1990.
14. Schlippert W: Cimetidine. H_2-Receptor blockade in gastrointestinal disease, *Arch Intern Med* 138:1257, 1978.
15. Sorkin EM, Heel RC: Terfenadine. A review of its pharmacodynamic properties and therapeutic efficacy, *Drugs* 29:34, 1985.
16. Togias AG, Proud D, Kagey-Sobotka A, et al: In vivo and in vitro effects of antihistamines on mast cell mediator release: a potentially important property in the treatment of allergic disease, *Ann Allergy* 63:465, 1989.

Chapter 23

Serotonin and serotonin antagonists

Serotonin (5-hydroxytryptamine) occupies a prominent position in the medical literature, despite limited knowledge of its functions in normal and abnormal conditions. This endogenously produced amine is believed to be a central neurotransmitter, and it has local actions in various tissues. Serotonin has been implicated in disease states ranging from mental disease and migraine to the carcinoid syndrome.

Studies of serotonin in the central nervous system have contributed to understanding the biochemical basis of psychopharmacologic phenomena. Receptor relationships between serotonin and hallucinogens, such as lysergide (lysergic acid diethylamide, LSD), suggested that abnormalities in brain serotonin may cause abnormal brain function and aberrant behavior. The discovery that serotonin stores are depleted by reserpine focused additional attention on the role of this amine in the central nervous system. More recently, attention has focused on the role of serotonin in depression, and there is evidence for specific involvement of serotonin in the emetic response to drugs that affect the chemoreceptor trigger zone.

OCCURRENCE AND DISTRIBUTION OF SEROTONIN

Serotonin is widely distributed in the body and also in various insect venoms from which it contributes to pain and the inflammatory reaction to stings. Some fruits, such as bananas and pineapples, contain a high concentration of serotonin, but little is absorbed from the gastrointestinal tract, and excretion of serotonin metabolites is normally low. When serotonin is produced in large amounts within the body, however, metabolites (in particular 5-hydroxyindoleacetic acid, 5-HIAA) can be detected in the urine. Increased urinary metabolites provide diagnostic evidence for a carcinoid tumor, composed of *enterochromaffin* cells, that releases large amounts of serotonin and other mediators.[10]

Approximately 90% of the total serotonin in mammalian tissues is in enterochromaffin cells in the intestine, about 8% is in platelets, and the rest is in the central nervous system, primarily in the pineal gland, brainstem, midbrain, and hypothalamus. In some animal species serotonin is also in granules of mast cells. Human mast cells probably do not contain serotonin, since increased urinary excretion of 5-HIAA is not associated with mastocytosis, in which there is proliferation of mast cells.

BIOSYNTHESIS AND METABOLISM

Serotonin is synthesized in neurons and enterochromaffin cells by hydroxylation and decarboxylation of the amino acid tryptophan. Normally only a small fraction of dietary tryptophan is converted to serotonin. However, this fraction increases greatly in patients with carcinoid tumors. Platelets do not synthesize serotonin, but they actively concentrate it from the circulation into granules released during platelet aggregation. The mechanisms of storage and release are similar to those for catecholamines, and drugs that affect catecholamine storage also affect the disposition of serotonin. There is rapid turnover of serotonin within neurons of the central nervous system and in enterochromaffin cells of the intestine. In contrast, the amine stored in platelets has a very slow turnover. Most of the serotonin released into blood is metabolized by monoamine oxidase (MAO) in the liver; the lung is also an active site for metabolism. Serotonin that escapes metabolism in these organs is taken up by platelets.[1] In addition, serotonin is converted in the pineal gland to *N*-acetylserotonin and its O-methylated derivative *melatonin*. Steps in biosynthesis and degradation of serotonin are shown below:

Tryptophan → 5-Hydroxytryptophan → 5-Hydroxytryptamine → 5-Hydroxyindoleacetic acid

Tryptophan hydroxylase

Aromatic L-amino acid decarboxylase

Monoamine oxidase

Tryptophan

5-Hydroxytryptophan

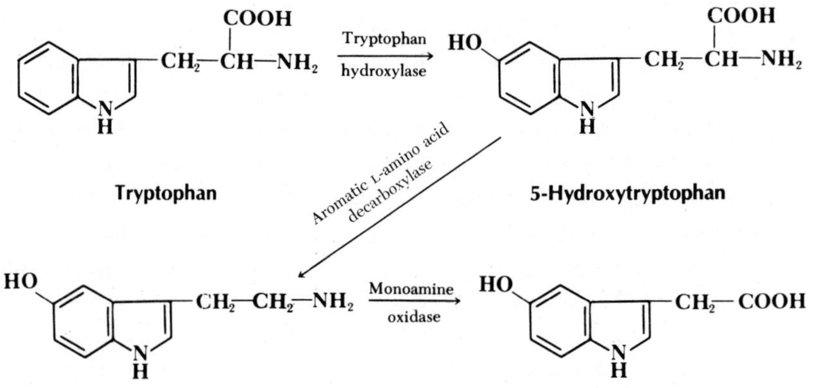

5-Hydroxytryptamine (serotonin)

5-Hydroxyindoleacetic acid (5-HIAA)

Several centrally acting drugs affect concentrations of brain serotonin. Its biosynthesis is blocked by *p*-chlorophenylalanine, which inhibits tryptophan hydroxylase, the rate-limiting synthetic enzyme. Degradation of serotonin is blocked by MAO inhibitors, which can double the serotonin content of brain in less than 1 hour. Certain tricyclic antidepressants (see Chapter 28) inhibit membrane uptake and increase the amount of free synaptic serotonin within the central nervous system. *Fluoxetine* (Prozac) inhibits neuronal reuptake of serotonin without affecting norepinephrine or dopamine.[3] This agent is used to treat depression and various forms of compulsive behaviors (see Chapter 28).

Daily excretion of 5-HIAA in urine (from 3 to 10 mg in a normal adult) increases when serotonin is produced by a carcinoid tumor or after administration of drugs that inhibit uptake into storage granules. Excretion is decreased by MAO inhibitors.

PHARMACOLOGIC EFFECTS

Serotonin acts on smooth muscle and nerve elements, including afferent nerve endings. Receptor binding studies and pharmacologic antagonists have identified multiple serotonin receptors, including 5-HT_1- and 5-HT_2-receptors in the central nervous system, the 5-HT_2-receptor in smooth muscle, and a distinct 5-HT_3-receptor in both peripheral and central nervous systems. Actions on smooth muscle account for most effects on the cardiovascular system and gastrointestinal tract. Despite the presence of serotonin receptors in the heart and throughout the circulatory system, only cerebral and mesenteric vessels receive innervation from serotonergic neurons.[4]

The responses of the cardiovascular system are complex. Serotonin, like acetylcholine (see p. 86), promotes vasodilatation through release of EDRF.[5] Other effects include receptor-mediated venoconstriction, amplification of vasoconstriction by other mediators, postjunctional inhibition of peripheral α-adrenergic neurotransmission, indirect sympathomimetic effects, and release of vasoactive mediators from platelets.

Effects of serotonin depend on the particular vascular bed, and effects of endogenously released serotonin may differ from those following its injection. Intravenous injection of a few micrograms of serotonin typically causes a *triphasic* change in blood pressure: (1) a transient decrease, (2) a period of hypertension that lasts several minutes, and (3) a prolonged period of lowered pressure. The early depressor phase is probably due to reflex stimulation of chemoreceptors within the coronary arteries (Bezold-Jarisch reflex). The hypertensive phase reflects receptor-mediated constriction of blood vessels in many regions, including splanchnic and renal vascular beds. The final depressor phase is attributed to a vasodilator action on vessels in specific vascular beds, as in skeletal muscle. Continuous infusion of serotonin causes a prolonged reduction of peripheral resistance and blood pressure.

Serotonin is a particularly potent constrictor of collateral vessels that develop after experimental arterial occlusion. This effect is blocked by ketanserin, a 5-HT_2-antagonist that has been used to relieve symptoms of intermittent claudication[5] (see p. 302).

Serotonin stimulates gastrointestinal and bronchial smooth muscles through 5-HT_2-receptors. The gastrointestinal actions include indirect stimulation through excitation of ganglion cells within the intestinal wall. Serotonin-receptor antagonists block the actions on intestinal motility. The bronchial stimulant action of serotonin is probably of little physiologic importance in humans, but asthmatic persons are particularly sensitive to this amine.

Serotonin can stimulate afferent nerve endings, ganglion cells, and adrenal medullary cells. Although it is a central neurotransmitter, serotonin does not cross the blood-brain barrier. Peripheral administration of serotonin agonists suppresses sleep in rats,[2] whereas oral administration to humans of a 5-HT_2-receptor antagonist, ritanserin, increases slow wave sleep.[6] Thus in contrast to an earlier belief that serotonin induces sleep,[7] present evidence indicates that serotonin is a sleep suppressant.

ROLE IN HEALTH AND DISEASE

Participation of serotonin in determination of mood and behavior would be anticipated from its role as a central neurotransmitter. Changes in serotonin concentrations within the brain are believed to occur in various mental disorders, such as depression, but the mechanisms are still not established. In both the brain and the gastrointestinal tract, serotonin is found in cells that secrete polypeptides. Serotonin is believed to regulate release of peptide hormones within the anterior pituitary by an action on hypothalamic neuroendocrine pathways. Although not yet certain, it may influence intestinal motility, as well, through release of peptide hormones. Serotonin in enterochromaffin cells of the intestine is released by distention or by hypertonicity.

Serotonin release probably causes some of the symptoms of the carcinoid syndrome, such as increased intestinal motility. However, catecholamines or kinins are the likely cause of the vascular phenomenon (flushing) that occurs with this condition.

Because serotonin is a potent constrictor of cerebral vessels, it has been implicated in migraine headaches. Although some serotonin antagonists may prevent migraine, there is no direct evidence that serotonin is a causal agent.

Serotonin released from platelets has potentially important roles in several disease states, particularly because of synergism among released mediators, such as thromboxane, for aggregation and vasoconstriction. This mechanism may contribute to coronary or cerebral vasospasm. Animal models indicate that atherosclerotic vessels exhibit enhanced sensitivity to serotonin, possibly due to an increased number of serotonin receptors.[5] Furthermore, serotonin released from platelets along with platelet-derived growth factor (PDGF) stimulates proliferation of vascular smooth muscle cells, possibly an additional mechanism for forming the lesions of atherosclerosis.[11]

Serotonin alters responsiveness of blood vessels to vasoactive mediators in models of chronic hypertension,[12] and it might have a role in that disease as well. Some investigators believe that interaction with G protein–coupled receptors could be the unifying mechanism for potentiating actions of serotonin on blood vessels and neurotransmission.[5]

SEROTONIN ANTAGONISTS

Drugs that compete with serotonin for tissue receptors have helped define the actions of the amine in normal and pathologic conditions. Only a few are used in therapy. The earliest recognized antagonists include ergot alkaloids and derivatives of lysergic acid. Ergotamine and methysergide are used to treat migraine, but their primary action is on α-adrenergic receptors rather than on serotonin receptors. Some antihistamines also block serotonin receptors on smooth muscles. Although many serotonin antagonists are relatively nonselective, they have aided in definition of two subclasses of serotonin receptors (5-HT_1 and 5-HT_2) in the central nervous system. Peripheral 5-HT_2-receptors appear to be associated with effects such as smooth muscle contraction. A new class of receptors (5-HT_3) has been defined that mediates excitatory responses to serotonin. Drugs that affect these receptors are still experimental but will perhaps have many uses.

Individual agents

The **ergot alkaloids**, products of fungi that grow on grains, provided the first serotonin receptor antagonists, including several compounds with partial agonist actions on adrenergic, dopaminergic, and serotonin receptors. The ergot derivative LSD proved valuable for exploring effects of serotonin within the central nervous system.

Ergot derivatives cause three major effects: (1) smooth muscle contraction, which is particularly evident on blood vessels and the uterus, (2) α-adrenergic blockade, and (3) various adverse central nervous system responses, including nausea, headache, dizziness, confusion, and even dementia. Although some ergot compounds affect serotonin receptors, their therapeutic effects are not obviously linked to serotonergic mechanisms.

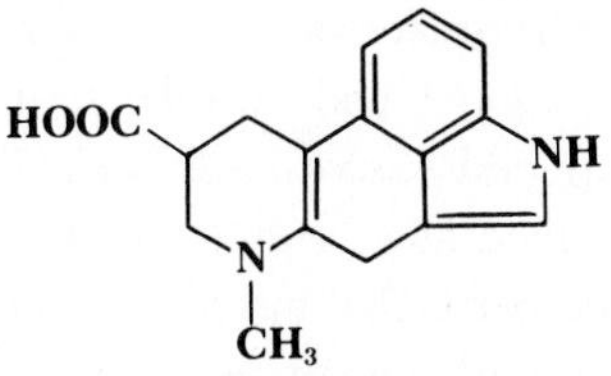

HOOC — NH — N — CH_3

Lysergic acid

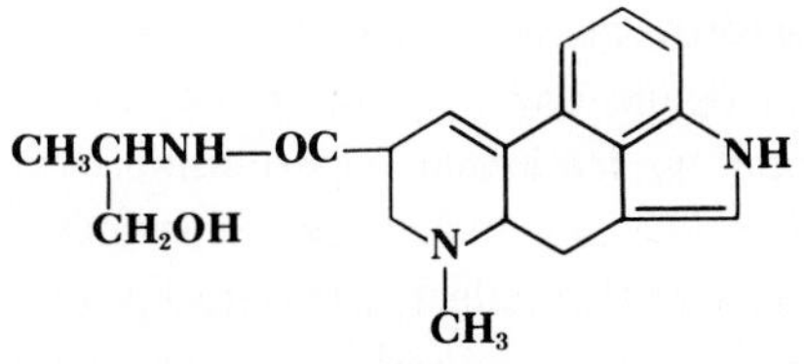

$CH_3CHNH—OC$ — CH_2OH — NH — N — CH_3

Ergonovine

Ergot alkaloids have limited application in the treatment of vascular headaches. Ergotamine is used in diagnosis and initial treatment of migraine headache. A common explanation is that its vasoconstrictor action reduces pain caused by dilatation and pulsation of cerebral arteries. Ergotamine is not indicated for long-term treatment or prevention of migraine because severe constriction of peripheral vessels and even gangrene can result from continued use.

Methysergide, a congener of methylergonovine and LSD, is a potent antagonist of serotonin in various experimental preparations. It has been used to prevent migraine headache with some degree of success, but it is not effective in treatment of established migraine.

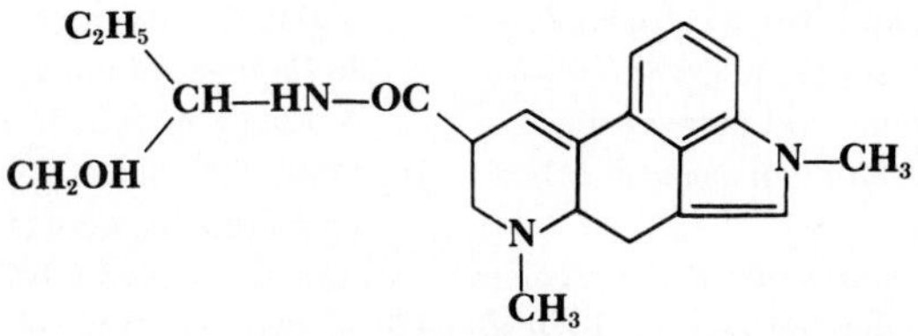

C_2H_5 — CH—HN—OC — CH_2OH — N—CH_3 — N — CH_3

Methysergide

Methysergide may cause various adverse reactions, including nausea, dizziness, insomnia, and behavioral changes. A serious but infrequent complication after long-term use is development of an inflammatory fibrosis that may affect the lungs or other organs.

Methysergide maleate (Sansert) is available in tablets containing 2 mg.

Cyproheptadine is an antihistamine that also blocks serotonin receptors. In addition to use to relieve itching in a variety of skin disorders, cyproheptadine has been given for prophylaxis of migraine. Cyproheptadine is effective against the intestinal hypermotility associated with carcinoid syndrome; when administered to a patient with malignant carcinoid syndrome, it also decreased urinary excretion of serotonin metabolites and reduced the size of liver metastases.[8]

Adverse effects are similar to those of other antihistamines; drowsiness is the most prominent. In addition, cyproheptadine has been reported to cause weight gain and increased growth in children, possibly by an effect on growth hormone secretion.

Preparations of cyproheptadine hydrochloride (Periactin) include tablets, 4 mg, and syrup, 2 mg/5 ml.

Ketanserin, an investigational antagonist that is selective for 5-HT_2-receptors, helped to define many of the actions of serotonin on blood vessels. It may have therapeutic application in hypertension and peripheral vascular diseases, including Raynauds syndrome, a cold-induced reduction of blood flow in the extremities.[5]

Antagonists that affect 5-HT_3-receptors are of particular interest for control of nausea and vomiting caused by cancer chemotherapeutic agents because serotonin is postulated to be a neurotransmitter in the emetic reaction. **Metoclopramide** (also a dopamine antagonist, see p. 248) was the first of these agents, but **ondansetron**, a newer drug, was reported superior to metoclopramide in controlling the emetic reaction to cisplatin.[9] The 5-HT_3-antagonists cause headache in some patients.

REFERENCES

1. De Clerck FF, Herman AG: 5-Hydroxytryptamine and platelet aggregation, *Fed Proc* 42:228, 1983.
2. Fornal C, Radulovacki M: Sleep suppressant action of fenfluramine in rats. I. Relation to postsynaptic serotonergic stimulation, *J Pharmacol Exp Ther* 225:667, 1983.
3. Fuller RW, Wong DT: Serotonin reuptake blockers in vitro and in vivo, *J Clin Psychopharmacol* 7(6 suppl):36S, 1987.
4. Göthert M: Serotonin receptors in the circulatory system, *Prog Pharmacol* 6:155, 1986.
5. Hollenberg NK: Serotonin and vascular responses, *Annu Rev Pharmacol Toxicol* 28:41, 1988.
6. Idzikowski C, Mills FJ, Glennard R: 5-Hydroxytryptamine-2 antagonist increases human slow wave sleep, *Brain Res* 378:164, 1986.
7. Jouvet M: Biogenic amines and the states of sleep, *Science* 163:32, 1969.
8. Leitner SP, Greenberg P, Danieu LA, Michaelson RA: Partial remission of carcinoid tumor in response to cyproheptadine, *Ann Intern Med* 111:760, 1989.
9. Marty M, Pouillart P, Scholl S, et al: Comparison of the 5-hydroxytryptamine$_3$ (serotonin) antagonist ondansetron (GR 38032F) with high-dose metoclopramide in the control of cisplatin-induced emesis, *N Engl J Med* 322:816, 1990.
10. Oates JA, Butler TC: Pharmacologic and endocrine aspects of carcinoid syndrome, *Adv Pharmacol* 5:109, 1967.
11. Seuwen K, Pouysségur J: Serotonin as a growth factor, *Biochem Pharmacol* 39:985, 1990.
12. Vanhoutte PM: 5-Hydroxytryptamine and vascular disease, *Fed Proc* 42:233, 1983.

Chapter 24

Kinins and other peptides

KININS

The polypeptides *bradykinin* and *kallidin* (lysylbradykinin) are potent vasodilators that can increase vascular permeability, stimulate bronchial and gastrointestinal smooth muscle, and affect various organ systems by interactions with neural pathways and with other mediators. Recognition that kinins affect prostaglandin synthesis and metabolism emphasizes their potential for a wide range of activities. The effects of kinins on blood vessels and other smooth muscles are similar to those of histamine. Kinins are thought to contribute to inflammation, but they do not interact with receptors for histamine or serotonin. Research on enzymes that form kinins, the kallikreins, and their substrates, the kininogens, suggests that kinins are involved in normal functioning of many different organ systems. Abnormalities of the kallikrein-kinin system in experimental models of hypertension and diabetes indicate that kinins play a role in these diseases as well.

Formation and metabolism

KININOGEN

Kinins are formed by cleavage from a protein substrate. Bradykinin is cleaved from the α_2-globulin *kininogen* by the enzymatic action of *kallikrein*. In addition to serving as a substrate for kallikrein, kininogen can inhibit certain proteases and serve as a cofactor in contact activation processes. Because of these diverse activities and because kinins were generated from proteins of different sizes, it was assumed that there were two different kininogens. Sequencing of the human kininogen gene indicated, however, that differences in RNA processing could account for the functional diversity of kininogen.

Gene sequencing technology identified structural similarities between kininogen and other proteins and suggested previously unknown functions. Sequence identity between a portion of the kininogen molecule, a major acute phase protein, and a proteinase inhibitor suggests that kininogen may inhibit acid proteases in an area of inflammation,[12] thereby prolonging actions of the kinins.

KALLIKREINS

Kallikreins from blood and tissues differ with respect to structure and preferred substrates. It appears that the kallikrein gene is part of a large gene family. In humans there is more than one gene for kallikrein-like activities, but in animals "true" kallikrein is encoded by a single gene. Recent research indicates that kallikrein-gene expression is controlled by various hormones and neurotransmitters. Analysis of restriction fragment length polymorphisms (RFLPs) in the kallikrein gene may improve understanding of the role of kallikrein in human disease.[12]

Glandular tissues, such as salivary glands or pancreas, are the richest source of tissue kallikrein. Kallikrein is also found in urine and in plasma, primarily in the form of a zymogen, prekallikrein. Enzymatically active plasma kallikrein is generated from prekallikrein in an activation sequence similar to that described for blood coagulation (see Chapter 54). As depicted below, contact activation of coagulation factor XII (Hageman factor) initiates kallikrein generation from prekallikrein. Plasma kallikrein is inhibited by several protease inhibitors in blood and tissues, including C1-inactivator, α_2-macroglobulin, and antithrombin III.

Activation of kallikrein and generation of kinins

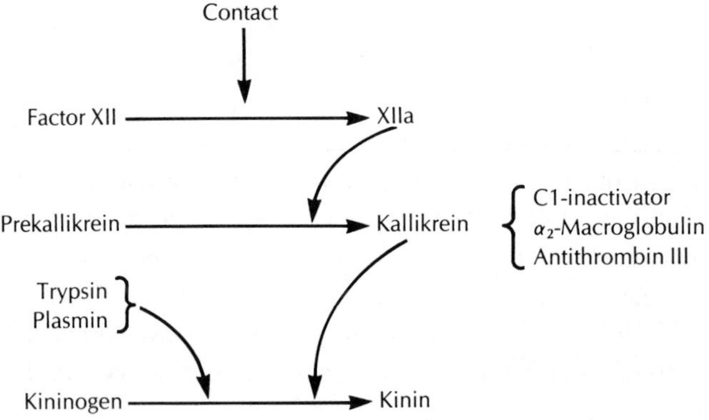

GENERATION OF KININS

Kallikrein, as well as trypsin, plasmin, and similar enzymes, can release kinins from kininogen. Human plasma kallikrein acts on high molecular weight (HMW) kininogen to produce the nonapeptide bradykinin. Human tissue kallikrein acts on either high or low molecular weight (LMW) kininogen to produce the decapeptide kallidin, which is identical to bradykinin except for an additional N-terminal lysine residue.[14]

KININASES

Kinins are inactivated by peptidases in blood and in tissues where the enzymes are concentrated on cell surfaces. Kininase I (carboxypeptidase N), the major inactivating enzyme in blood, cleaves a single arginine from the carboxyl terminal. A membrane-bound kininase I type enzyme (carboxypeptidase M) is found in many tissues and cells. Kininase II (angiotensin I converting enzyme) is found both in blood and in tissues. It is concentrated on the luminal surface of endothelial cells and also on many epithelial surfaces, including the microvilli of the intestine, placenta, and renal tubules. Kininase II cleaves the two carboxyl-terminal amino acids, just as it does to activate angiotensin I to angiotensin II.[3] Neutral endopeptidase 24.11 (enkephalinase) found in brain, lung, kidney, and other tissues inactivates kinins by cleavage at the same site as kininase II. Other brain peptidases cleave kinins elsewhere within the polypeptide chain.

INACTIVATION BY KININASES I AND II

Bradykinin: $ARG_1—PRO_2—PRO_3—GLY_4—PHE_5—SER_6—PRO_7 \underset{II}{\uparrow} PHE_8 \underset{I}{\uparrow} ARG_9$

Kallidin: $LYS_1—ARG_2—PRO_3—PRO_4—GLY_5—PHE_6—SER_7—PRO_8 \underset{II}{\uparrow} PHE_9 \underset{I}{\uparrow} ARG_{10}$

Kinin-induced effects

Kinins have many potent biologic activities, including dilatation of blood vessels, contraction of smooth muscles, and enhancement of capillary permeability. They influence eicosanoid synthesis, ion transport, and cell growth. Bradykinin injected into skin causes pain, and it may be a neurotransmitter in pathways for nociceptive stimuli. Kinins may be important in such functions as vasodilatation after exercise, metabolic processing of glucose, ion and water transport, and sperm motility, but difficulty in identifying and classifying kinin receptors and the lack of specific antagonists has delayed definition of specific mechanisms. Peptides that block bradykinin binding to so-called B_1- and B_2-receptors may help unravel the role of kinins in these processes.

Kinins cause many effects similar to those of histamine. They are about 10 times more potent than histamine on blood vessels. Release or injection of bradykinin in humans causes arteriolar dilatation and a loss of fluid from capillaries and venules, as shown in Fig. 24-1. Like histamine, bradykinin reduces blood pressure by shunting blood from large resistance vessels into mucosal and cutaneous capillary beds.

Although kinins constrict airway smooth muscle, they do not appear to be major mediators in asthma even though afflicted persons are particularly sensitive to them. Indirect kinin effects on lung (release of arachidonic acid and formation of leukotrienes and prostaglandins) may contribute.

Kinins constrict isolated preparations of uterine smooth muscle and most gastrointestinal smooth muscles. The gastrointestinal tract is rich in enzymes that form or inactivate kinins; such findings suggest a regulatory role for kinins, perhaps through release of catecholamines or generation of prostaglandins.

Experimental evidence from human studies indicates that kinins may regulate uptake of glucose in skeletal muscle under conditions of hypoxia or during muscle work. Other studies support a role for kinins in functional hyperemia, but, as noted above, it is difficult to exclude indirect effects caused by kinin-induced release of other mediators such as "endothelium-derived relaxing factor" (EDRF, see p. 86).[13,20]

Many investigators have sought a role for the kallikrein-kinin system in reproduction. The enzymes and substrates for kinin generation and degradation are present in male and female genital tracts, and there is some evidence that kinins affect sperm maturation and motility. Vascular effects of kinins are evident during transformation of the fetal circulation to neonatal conditions, when kinins constrict the umbilical artery and promote closure of the ductus arteriosus. Effects of kinins on the uterus and on

FIG. 24-1 *Micrograph of hamster cheek pouch microvasculature in fluorescent light. Upper: prior to application of bradykinin. Lower: same area 5 minutes after application of bradykinin. Notice leakage at many sites.*

From Svensjö, E: Prostaglandins Med 1:397, 1978. With permission from Churchill Livingstone.

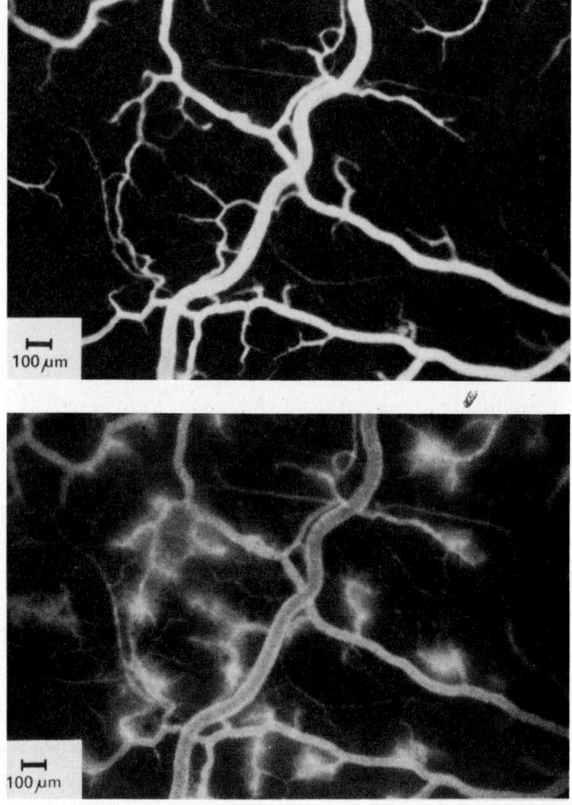

blood flow in the fetal-maternal circulation are likely attributable to production of prostaglandins.

Kinin receptors

The actions of kinins on various organs implies the presence of specific kinin receptors. A variety of synthetic peptide agonists and antagonists have identified a receptor linked to classic kinin effects, such as hypotension, smooth muscle contraction, and pain perception in intact animals. This receptor is designated as B_2; other kinin receptors have been described but are probably not involved in the general response to kinins. The less common B_1-receptor can bind bradykinin after its carboxyl terminal arginine has been removed by a carboxypeptidase.

Kinins interact with cell membrane receptors to activate phospholipases A_2 and C and trigger formation of second messengers. Studies of isolated tissues and cultured cells indicate that the B_2-receptor is coupled directly or indirectly to cell messenger systems that involve Ca^{++} movement, G proteins, and phosphoinositide metabolism.

Many, but not all, of the effects of kinins involve eicosanoid production.[12] Kinin receptor blocking drugs have obvious therapeutic potential, but none of the various peptide derivatives known to block kinin action are available for clinical use.

Clinical significance of kinins

In view of the ease with which plasma and tissue prekallikreins are activated, it is not surprising that numerous physiologic mechanisms have been attributed to kinin products. It is sometimes difficult to discriminate the singular effect of these peptides, however, as there is interregulation of the kinin-forming system with other mediators. Both coagulation and complement systems have control factors in common with the kinin system. For example, plasma prekallikrein can be activated by activated Hageman factor, antigen-antibody reactions, proteases, and endotoxins. In turn, kallikrein can activate Hageman factor.[14] Anaphylatoxins, the products of complement activation, are inactivated by kininase I.

Kinin formation is implicated in endotoxin shock, carcinoid syndrome, hereditary angioneurotic edema, anaphylaxis, arthritis, and acute pancreatitis. A role in early stages of inflammation is likely because kinins both vasodilate and increase vascular permeability. They may be responsible for the vascular flushing that occurs in the carcinoid syndrome. A deficiency of a kallikrein inhibitor, as in hereditary angioneurotic edema, permits kinin formation that would ordinarily be suppressed.

Experiments in genetically hypertensive rats indicate a link between abnormalities in the components of the kallikrein-kinin system and hypertension. Although kinin receptor antagonists are still not available for therapy, they are used to explore the role of kinins in experimental models of hypertension.

PEPTIDES OF THE BRAIN AND GASTROINTESTINAL TRACT

Several peptides, including substance P, the enkephalins, neurotensin, vasoactive intestinal polypeptide (VIP), gastrin, and cholecystokinin, are found in both the gastrointestinal tract and in neural tissue. This observation implies a common origin of hormone-secreting gastrointestinal and neuroendocrine cells. In addition, secretory cells in the lung have structural and cytochemical features similar to neuroendocrine cells. It seems likely that the array of biologically active peptides that modulate function in the brain, gut, lung, and other organs arises from a common type of progenitor cell during embryonic development.

Abnormalities in concentration of neuropeptides might disturb neuronal function, and indeed various studies have linked changes in concentration of certain peptides to specific disease states. However, nerve cells contain much lower concentrations of peptides than of amino acid or monoamine transmitters. Peptides are synthesized not within synaptic nerve terminals but as part of a larger precursor molecule within the neuronal cell body and are then transported to and processed within secretory granules. Thus many different processes can potentially influence the final concentration of a peptide mediator or neuromodulator.[9]

Substance P

Substance P is an undecapeptide (11 amino acids) member of a family of peptides called *tachykinins*, defined by their common pharmacologic properties and similar carboxyl-terminal sequences. Substance P was originally discovered in extracts of brain and intestine when von Euler and Gaddum attempted to isolate acetylcholine.[8] It was named "substance P" because it was extracted and stored in powdered form.

ARG—PRO—LYS—PRO—GLN—GLN—PHE—PHE—GLY—LEU—MET—NH_2

Substance P

Substance P is found in neurons throughout the body, including the autonomic nervous system. The highest concentrations are in the dorsal horn of the spinal cord, the trigeminal nucleus, and the substantia nigra. It is also found in nerves of tooth pulp, the myenteric plexus of the gut, and in enterochromaffin cells. In these structures substance P often coexists with other neurotransmitters or neuromodulators. For example, enterochromaffin cells and certain neurons contain substance P and serotonin.[7] Several sites in the hypothalamus and the anterior pituitary contain both substance P and neurotensin, and experiments in animals indicate that these peptides influence functions of the anterior pituitary through paracrine action on neuroendocrine cells.[1] In the myenteric plexus, neurons contain either substance P or VIP, suggestive that these two peptides have opposing actions.[11]

Actions on Organ Systems

Substance P has several activities in common with kinins. Like bradykinin, it vasodilates and lowers blood pressure. Patients with carcinoid tumors may experience hypotension when substance P is released along with kinins and serotonin. Substance P directly stimulates lymphocytes and other leukocytes that participate in the inflammatory response,[16] and its ability to cause bronchoconstriction suggests that it is a mediator of asthmatic reactions.[6] Substance P can stimulate nerves, and it is very potent in evoking salivary secretion, an effect not blocked by atropine.

Receptors

Peptide agonists and antagonists have helped define receptors for tachykinins, including substance P. Three tachykinin receptors have been identified, and one has been cloned and sequenced. A substance P receptor that appears to be linked to G proteins and to involve inositol phosphatides as second messengers has been isolated from human lymphoblasts and membranes from animal brain tissue.[16]

Role in Health and Disease

Substance P is probably a neurotransmitter in the central and peripheral nervous systems. Localization of the peptide in various hormone-secreting cells of the anterior pituitary suggests that it also plays a role in regulating neuroendocrine mechanisms.[1]

Substance P is believed to transmit nociceptive signals from small primary afferents entering the dorsal horn. Regulation of the action of substance P by enkephalins may contribute to control of various neural circuits (Fig. 24-2).[7]

The high concentration of substance P in the substantia nigra, a region concerned with movement, suggested that abnormalities of this peptide are linked to movement disorders. The concentration of substance P and the number of substance P–containing neurons are reduced in specific regions of the brain in Huntingtons chorea, perhaps evidence that these neurochemical defects contribute to the abnormal movement that characterizes the disease. However, Met^5-enkephalin, cholecystokinin, and

Hypothetical gating mechanism at first synaptic relay in spinal cord. Enkephalin released from interneuron inhibits release of substance P. ***FIG. 24-2***

From Iversen LL: The chemistry of the brain, Sci Am 241:134, copyright 1979 by Scientific American, Inc; all rights reserved.

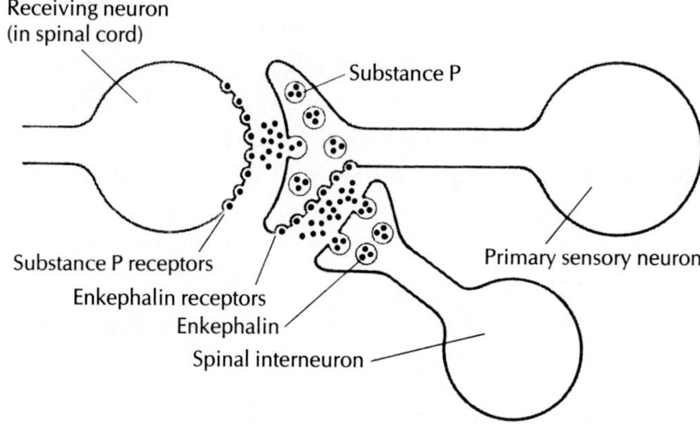

prodynorphin-derived peptides are also reduced in the globus pallidus and substantia nigra in Huntingtons disease, and several other peptides are increased in related brain structures. Detailed neurochemical and immunohistologic studies of peptide distribution indicate that the critical defect is most likely a disruption of neuronal circuits between cortical, basal ganglia, and thalamic structures rather than to altered levels of peptide neurotransmitters.[9]

Senile plaques in the cerebral cortex of patients with Alzheimers disease contain substance P along with other peptides. The recent observation that a portion of the amyloid β protein found in brains of Alzheimer patients had homology with tachykinins strengthens the assumption that these peptides contribute to the disease.[21]

Several effects of substance P could contribute to inflammation. Along with release of histamine from mast cells, it enhances formation of leukotrienes and stimulates chemotaxis and mediator release from monocytes. Substance P also binds to both helper and suppressor-cytotoxic classes of T lymphocytes, and it stimulates proliferation of human T lymphocytes. It has been linked to various inflammatory diseases, including arthritis, bullous pemphigoid, asthma, inflammatory bowel disease, and carcinoid tumor.[16] Demonstration of substance P in nasal secretions after antigen challenge suggests that the peptide may also contribute to allergic reactions. Substance P is inactivated by neutral endopeptidase, and experiments in animals with an inhibitor of this enzyme indicate that substance P is a potent bronchoconstrictor with a possible role in asthma.[19]

Enkephalins and endorphins

It is well known that opiates affect specific receptors in the brain and that electrical stimulation of certain brain regions can produce analgesia. Naloxone, a specific opiate antagonist, can prevent this analgesia, indicative of release of naturally occurring opiate-like compounds in the brain. The enkephalins, two very similar pentapeptides from the brain, were shown to mimic opiate activity. β-Endorphin, a larger, 31-residue peptide containing the sequence of methionine enkephalin, also has opioid activity.

The endorphins are a family of peptides whose sequences contain an enkephalin pentapeptide sequence. These peptides have common actions at opioid receptors as indicated by naloxone antagonism, and they are derived from the precursor pro-opiomelanocortin.[2] The common N-terminal sequence of Tyr-Gly-Gly-Phe conveys opioid activity, and the C-terminal extension affects potency and receptor specificity.[5]

The enkephalins are members of another family of peptides derived from a proenkephalin.[4,10] The active sequence is released by proteolysis; the extent and sites at which proteolysis occurs produces peptides with affinity for different opioid receptors.[4]

TYR—GLY—GLY—PHE—MET

Met^5—Enkephalin

TYR—GLY—GLY—PHE—LEU

Leu^5—Enkephalin

TYR—GLY—GLY—PHE—MET—THR—SER—GLU—LYS—SER—GLN—THR—PRO—LEU—VAL—
THR—LEU—PHE—LYS—ASN—ALA—ILE—ILE—LYS—ASN—ALA—TYR—LYS—LYS—GLY—GLU

β-Endorphin

Enkephalins and endorphins are found in separate and distinct regions of the central nervous system. β-Endorphin–containing cell bodies are localized primarily within the arcuate nucleus, whereas enkephalin-containing neurons are found throughout the brain. The distribution of enkephalin-containing neurons indicates that enkephalins may be neurotransmitters in many regions.[2]

Enkephalins are also found in the gastrointestinal tract, pancreas, sympathetic ganglia, and adrenal medulla. It is now accepted that they are endogenous opioid mediators that are released and cause analgesia upon electrical stimulation of certain regions of the brain; they may also be responsible for the analgesia from acupuncture. The precise mechanisms through which they relieve pain are still unclear, although interactions between enkephalins and substance P may be involved. Enkephalins are very rapidly degraded by peptidases, which explains some of the difficulty in defining their physiologic roles. An aminopeptidase attacks the N-terminal end of the peptide, and neutral endopeptidase 24.11 (enkephalinase) cleaves it to a di- and tri-peptide.

Endorphins are less readily inactivated, and there is considerable speculation about their involvement in blood pressure regulation, temperature regulation, and intake of food and water. It is still not clear, however, if endorphins mediate these functions or if they act through peripheral or central mechanisms.[2]

VIP

VIP (vasoactive intestinal polypeptide) is widely distributed in the central and peripheral nervous systems, but it is concentrated in certain regions of the brain (cerebral cortex, hypothalamus), in the intestine, exocrine glands, and in some endocrine glands. It is also found in certain neuroendocrine tumors. This 28-residue peptide was first discovered in lung as a smooth muscle–relaxing, vasodilator peptide. It was later isolated from the intestine and found to be structurally related to glucagon and secretin. All three of these peptides stimulate adenylyl cyclase in specific target cells, an action that may account for most if not all of the activities of VIP.

ACTION ON ORGAN SYSTEMS

VIP acts synergistically with norepinephrine to increase cyclic AMP in neurons of the cerebral cortex. It also releases hormones from the hypothalamus and pituitary and may thus modulate neural function through endocrine mechanisms. VIP contributes to sexual arousal through its actions on nerves and blood vessels, and it has been linked to various immune responses, including production of antibodies by B lymphocytes and release of cytokines by T lymphocytes.[18]

VIP is a potent vasodilator and relaxes nonvascular smooth muscle of gastrointestinal, respiratory, and genitourinary tracts. VIP-containing nerve fibers are found in the nasal mucosa and in the tracheobronchial wall (Fig. 24-3). Stimulation of the vidian nerve dilates small vessels in the nasal mucosa and increases the amount of VIP in the venous effluent. Hence VIP may control vascular tone within the airways. A recent finding that nerves in the lungs of asthmatics lack VIP underscores a potentially important role for this peptide in the pathogenesis of asthma.[15] VIP appears to act in concert with acetylcholine to regulate blood flow and secretion in sweat and salivary glands.

Nearly half of the neurons in the myenteric plexus of the gut contain VIP. The peptide stimulates secretion of water and electrolytes from the intestine but inhibits gastric acid secretion. The relaxation component of peristaltic movement in the intestine is thought to be mediated primarily by VIP. Enkephalins and somatostatin likely modulate peristalsis by inhibiting release of VIP from the myenteric nerve endings.[11]

FIG. 24-3 *Nerve fibers immunoreactive to VIP in the bronchial smooth muscle of a subject without asthma (×660). Varicosities along the fibers are indicated by the arrows.*

From Ollerenshaw S, Jarvis D, Woolcock A, et al. Reprinted by permission of The New England Journal of Medicine 320:1244, 1989.

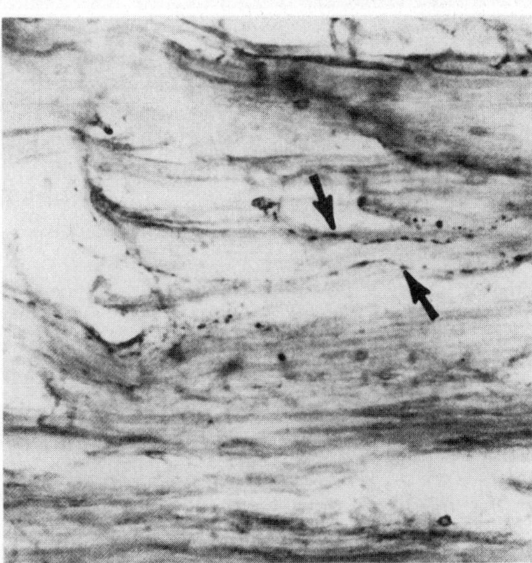

HIS—SER—ASP—ALA—VAL—PHE—THR—ASP—ASN—TYR—THR—ARG—LEU—ARG—LYS—

GLN—MET—ALA—VAL—LYS—LYS—TYR—LEU—ASN—SER—ILE—LEU—ASN

VIP

VIP has an additional role in smooth muscle relaxation of sphincters of the digestive and urogenital tracts. Release of the peptide from intramural neurons around the esophageal sphincter promotes relaxation. VIP also acts in the gall bladder to relax the sphincter of Oddi.[11]

Clinical Significance

The potent actions of VIP on blood vessels, smooth muscle, secretory cells, and nerves suggest that it is involved in regulation in many organ systems. The widespread distribution of VIP-containing nerves and its codistribution with other peptides and neurotransmitters implicates multiple and complex regulatory mechanisms.

VIP is postulated to be a causative agent in several diseases of the gastrointestinal tract. VIP is produced by nerves and endocrine cells in the pancreas and by pancreatic islet cell and neurogenic tumors. Patients with these tumors may have a high concentration of VIP in the circulation and present with a profuse watery diarrhea, supportive of the conclusion that VIP causes the "pancreatic cholera" syndrome. Achalasia, which is characterized by defective movement of the esophagus and its failure to relax with swallowing, is associated with reduced or absent VIP-containing nerves in the sphincter and in the esophageal body. A similar defect in VIP innervation in the large intestine has been linked to Hirschsprungs disease, or congenital megacolon, and lack of VIP innervation has been postulated as an organic mechanism for impotence.[18] Most recently a deficiency of VIP was suggested to be a cause of bronchial hyperreactivity.[15] These observations suggest that VIP or related peptides might be used to promote bronchial relaxation. There is also considerable interest in the relationship of the VIP sequence to peptides that appear to block the infectivity of the AIDS virus.[17]

References

1. Aronin N, Coslovsky R, Leeman SE: Substance P and neurotensin: their roles in the regulation of anterior pituitary function, *Annu Rev Physiol* 48:537, 1986.
2. Bloom FE: The endorphins: a growing family of pharmacologically pertinent peptides, *Annu Rev Pharmacol Toxicol* 23:151, 1983.
3. Erdös EG: Angiotensin I converting enzyme and the changes in our concepts through the years, *Hypertension* 16:363, 1990.
4. Höllt V: Opioid peptide processing and receptor selectivity, *Annu Rev Pharmacol Toxicol* 26:59, 1986.
5. Howlett TA, Rees LH: Endogenous opioid peptides and hypothalamo-pituitary function, *Annu Rev Physiol* 48:527, 1986.
6. Gerard NP: Characterization of substance P contractile activity on isolated guinea pig lung tissues, *J Pharmacol Exp Ther* 243:901, 1987.
7. Iversen LL: The chemistry of the brain, *Sci Am* 241(3):134, 1979.
8. Leeman SE, Mroz EA: Substance P, *Life Sci* 15:2033, 1974.
9. Lewis DA, Bloom FE: Clinical perspectives on neuropeptides, *Annu Rev Med* 38:143, 1987.
10. Lewis RV, Stern AS: Biosynthesis of the enkephalins and enkephalin-containing polypeptides, *Annu Rev Pharmacol Toxicol* 23:353, 1983.
11. Makhlouf GM: Neural and hormonal regulation of function in the gut, *Hosp Pract* 25(2):79, 1990.

12. Margolius HS: Tissue kallikreins and kinins: regulation and roles in hypertensive and diabetic diseases, *Annu Rev Pharmacol Toxicol* 29:343, 1989.

13. Moncada S, Radomski MW, Palmer RMJ: Endothelium-derived relaxing factor: identification as nitric oxide and role in the control of vascular tone and platelet function, *Biochem Pharmacol* 37:2495, 1988.

14. Movat HZ: The plasma kallikrein-kinin system and its interrelationship with other components of blood, *Handb Exp Pharmacol* 25(suppl):1, 1979.

15. Ollerenshaw S, Jarvis D, Woolcock A, et al: Absence of immunoreactive vasoactive intestinal polypeptide in tissue from the lungs of patients with asthma, *N Engl J Med* 320: 1244, 1989.

16. Payan DG: Neuropeptides and inflammation: the role of substance P, *Annu Rev Med* 40:341, 1989.

17. Ruff MR, Martin BM, Ginns EI, et al: CD4 receptor binding peptides that block HIV infectivity cause human monocyte chemotaxis. Relationship to vasoactive intestinal polypeptide, *FEBS Lett* 211:17, 1987.

18. Said SI, Mutt V, editors: Vasoactive intestinal peptide and related peptides, *Ann NY Acad Sci* 527:1, 1988.

19. Stimler-Gerard NP: Neutral endopeptidase-like enzyme controls the contractile activity of substance P in guinea pig lung, *J Clin Invest* 79:1819, 1987.

20. Vane JR, Änggård EE, Botting RM: Regulatory functions of the vascular endothelium, *N Engl J Med* 323:27, 1990.

21. Yankner BA, Duffy LK, Kirschner DA: Neurotrophic and neurotoxic effects of amyloid β protein: reversal by tachykinin neuropeptides, *Science* 250:279, 1990.

Chapter 25

Prostaglandins and leukotrienes

The name "prostaglandin" was first applied to the substance in human seminal fluid that was responsible for its potent hypotensive and spasmogenic activities. Subsequent studies showed that these activities are caused by acidic lipids. Prostaglandins, thromboxanes, leukotrienes, and hydroperoxyeicosatetraenoic acids are derived from fatty acids released from cell membrane phospholipids. Collectively, these compounds are termed eicosanoids because they are derived from 20-carbon fatty acids. Although eicosanoids affect many biologic processes, their importance as mediators and regulators of complex cellular functions has only recently been appreciated. The naturally occurring eicosanoids have only limited application in therapeutics, but stable derivatives and synthesis inhibitors are valuable therapeutic agents.

PROSTAGLANDINS AND THROMBOXANE

History

The history of prostaglandins underscores many of their important properties. In the 1930s von Euler in Sweden and Goldblatt in England independently described the hypotensive and smooth muscle–stimulating properties of lipid extracts of seminal fluid. Von Euler soon recognized that these activities could not be attributed to any known substance. Because he believed that it originated in the prostate gland, he named the active substance *prostaglandin*. After a lapse of more than 10 years, Bergström isolated a hydroxy fatty acid fraction from lipid extracts of seminal vesicles. Almost 10 more years passed before he was able to purify from this fraction two components that had the biologic activities attributed to the original extracts; they were designated "prostaglandins E and F." Bergström and Samuelsson subsequently isolated additional compounds from sheep vesicular gland extracts and identified the pathways for their formation.[20] The active compounds were derived from oxygenation of arachidonic acid, a precursor released from membrane phospholipids.

A signal achievement was the demonstration by Vane and by Smith and Willis that aspirin and related drugs block the synthesis of prostaglandins.[22,24] It was proposed that this action might account for the anti-inflammatory and analgesic effects of aspirin. Furthermore, these studies provided a pharmacologic method to determine the role of prostaglandins in normal physiology and disease.

Through studies of the metabolism of arachidonic acid, Samuelsson and co-workers identified two cyclic endoperoxide intermediates (PGG_2 and PGH_2) that are transformed enzymatically into prostaglandins and into a labile, platelet-aggregating, vasoconstrictor compound designated thromboxane A_2. Vane and co-workers found that in vascular tissue the cyclic endoperoxides are also metabolized to a potent but transiently acting vasodilator. They recognized that this activity differed from that of known prostaglandins, and they attributed it to "PGX."[13] PGX was produced primarily by vascular endothelium. It also inhibited platelet aggregation, both in vivo and in vitro. When the structure of PGX was determined, it was renamed *prostacyclin*, or PGI_2. For their discoveries in this field, Samuelsson, Bergström, and Vane were awarded the Nobel Prize in Physiology and Medicine.

Structures

The prostaglandins are 20-carbon carboxylic acids containing a five-membered ring (Fig. 25-1). Naturally occurring prostaglandins are classified according to their ring substituents as E and D (β-hydroxyketones), F (1,3-diols), or A, B, and C (α or β unsaturated ketones). They also have one, two, or three double bonds in their side chains. Biologic activity requires a carboxyl group at carbon position 1, a double bond at C-13, and a β-hydroxyl at C-15. When there are additional double bonds, they are at positions 5 and 17. The number of double bonds is indicated by the subscript, for example, PGE_1, PGE_2.

Synthesis and metabolism

The main precursor of the naturally occurring prostaglandins and thromboxane is the 20-carbon, unsaturated, essential fatty acid 5,8,11,14-eicosatetraenoic acid (arachidonic acid) (Fig. 25-2, **B**). The structurally related 8,11,14-eicosatrienoic acid is converted to prostaglandins with one double bond, for example, PGE_1. The polyunsaturated fatty acid 5,8,11,14,17-eicosapentaenoic acid (EPA) is converted to triene prostanoids, such as PGE_3.

The precursor fatty acids are derived from the diet. They are not free within cells but are esterified in the form of phospholipids, triglycerides, or cholesterol esters. The first step in prostaglandin synthesis is release of arachidonic acid from phospholipid stores by phospholipases within the cell membrane (Fig. 25-3).[5] Various stimuli, including mechanical distortion of the membrane, changes in ion fluxes, ischemia, hormones, and drugs, can activate tissue phospholipases by a process that depends on Ca^{++} from extracellular and intracellular stores. The availability of arachidonic acid is limited by two opposing reactions: (1) its liberation from and (2) its reacylation back into membrane phospholipids.

Once arachidonic acid is released, a portion that escapes reacylation is oxidized by either cyclooxygenase or lipoxygenases. Oxidation by cyclooxygenase forms labile prostaglandin endoperoxides (PGG_2 and PGH_2), which are further metabolized to prostaglandins and thromboxane. Importantly, cyclooxygenase is inhibited by aspirin and other *nonsteroidal anti-inflammatory drugs* (see Chapter 35). By inhibiting this enzyme, synthesis of all of the prostaglandins and thromboxane is reduced. The particular arachidonic acid product formed in a given tissue depends on which endoperoxide-metabolizing enzymes are present. For example, PGH_2 is converted to PGE_2 by endoperoxide isomerase or to $PGF_{2\alpha}$ by endoperoxide reductase. Both PGH_2 and PGG_2 are converted to prostacyclin by prostacyclin synthase or to thromboxane A_2 by thromboxane synthase. Platelets produce thromboxane A_2 rather than prostacyclin because they have thromboxane synthase but lack prostacyclin synthase. Thromboxane is also produced in the lung, probably by cells in the interstitium. Endothelial cells produce primarily prostacyclin, and also PGE_2 and $PGF_{2\alpha}$, but no thromboxane.[14]

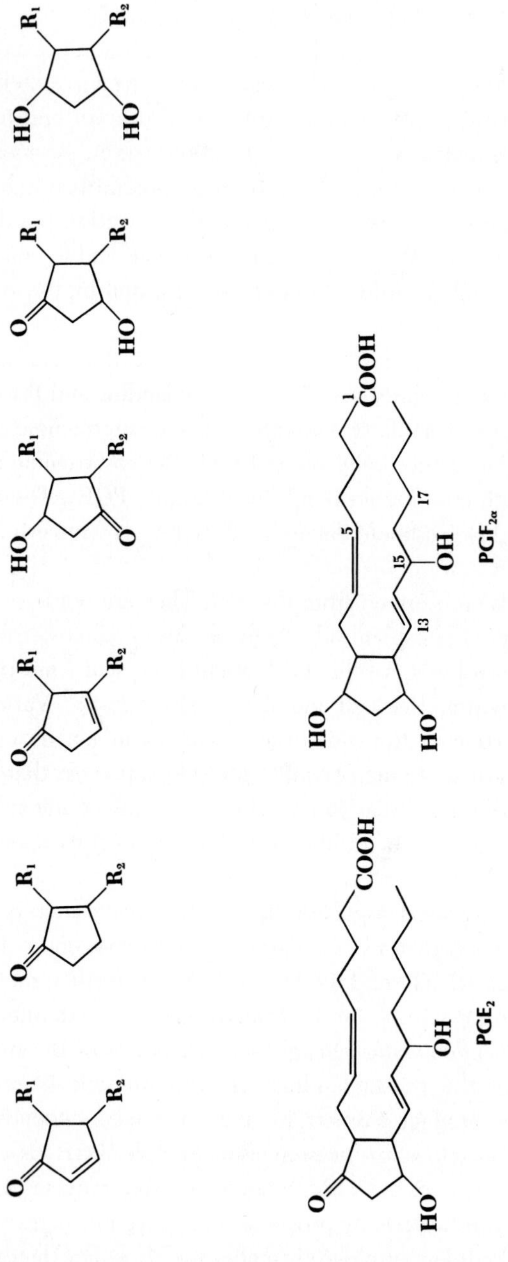

FIG. 25-1 Basic structures of prostaglandins.

FIG. 25-2

Precursors of prostaglandins.

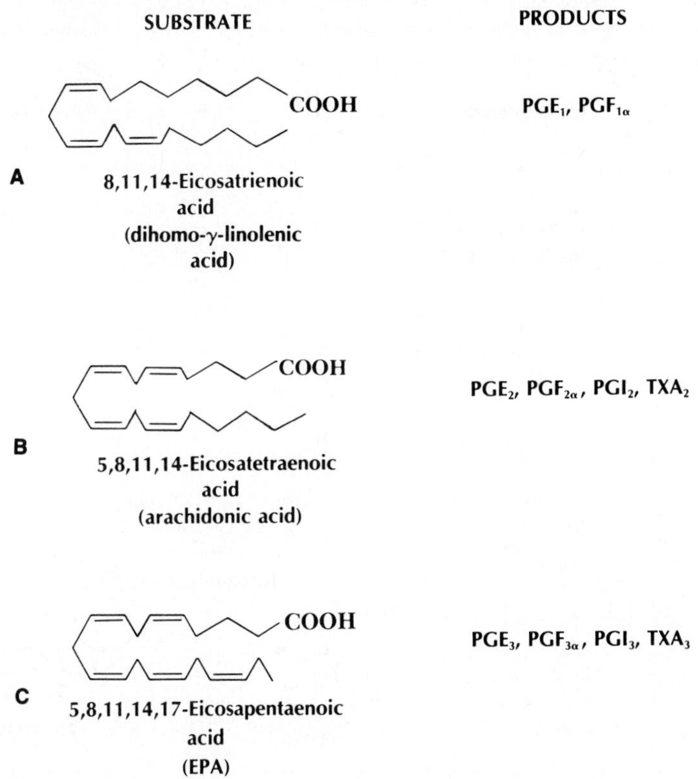

Lipoxygenation of arachidonic acid results in formation of hydroperoxyeicosatetraenoic acids and leukotrienes[21] (see below).

Prostaglandins are not stored. They are synthesized in response to membrane stimuli and then act locally as mediators or regulators of biologic events. Newly formed prostaglandins affect target tissues through distinct receptors (see below).

Prostaglandins are rapidly metabolized to inactive compounds by 15-hydroxyprostaglandin dehydrogenase (PGDH) and Δ^{13} reductase; this accounts in part for their brief duration of action. These enzymes are found in most tissues, but their activity is greatest in lung, kidney cortex, and liver. The strategic location of these enzymes in the lung prevents passage of prostaglandins from the venous to the arterial circulation. PGE_2 and $PGF_{2\alpha}$ are almost entirely removed during one passage through the pulmonary circulation.[1] In contrast, circulating PGI_2 and TXA_2 are rapidly converted nonenzymatically to the inactive products 6-keto $PGF_{1\alpha}$ and TXB_2 respectively, which are further oxidized by PGDH.[14] After metabolism by PGDH, the prostaglandin and thromboxane metabolites may be further metabolized by β-oxidation in the liver.

FIG. 25-3 *Conversion of arachidonic acid to prostaglandins and intermediates. The enzymes at each synthetic step are designated as: 1, phospholipase A_2; 2, cyclooxygenase; 3, prostacyclin synthase; 4, thromboxane synthase; 5, endoperoxide isomerase; 6, endoperoxide reductase.*

Modified from Dunn MJ, Hood VL: Am J Physiol 233:F169, 1977.

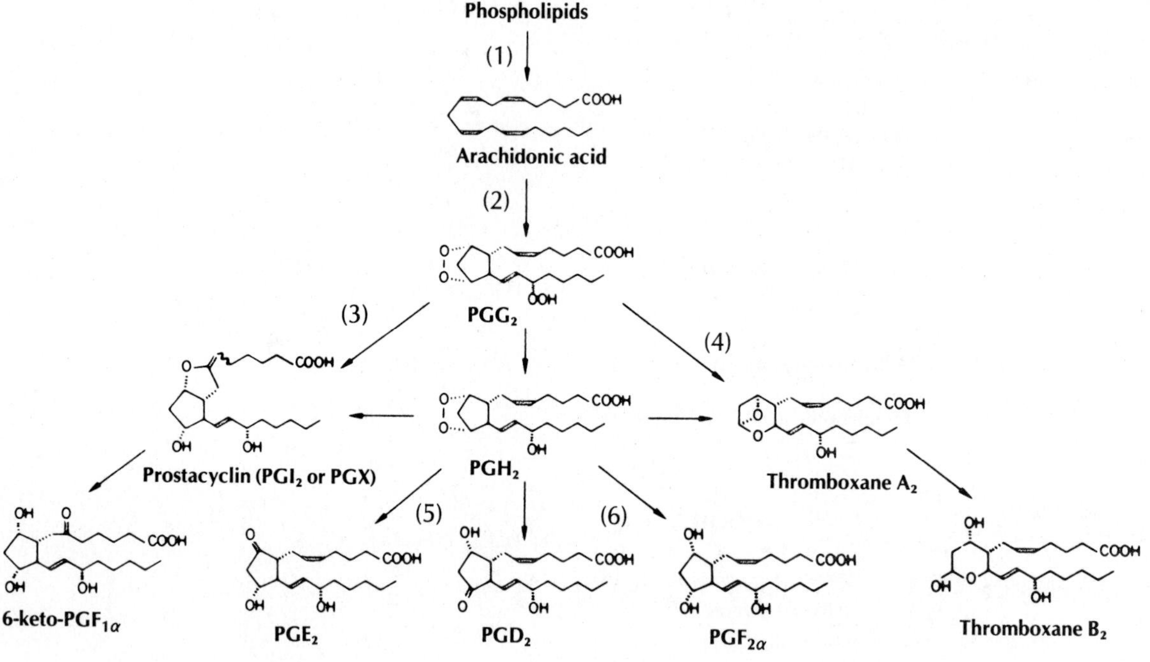

Actions of prostaglandins and thromboxane

The cellular mechanisms of action of the prostaglandins are not completely known. Prostaglandins interact with cell-surface receptors. Such receptors have been identified for PGD_2 (DP-receptor), $PGF_{2\alpha}$ (FP-receptor), PGI_2 (IP-receptor), PGE_2 (EP_1-, EP_2-, and EP_3-receptors), and thromboxane (TP_α- and TP_τ-receptors).[4,8] Prostaglandins, particularly in pharmacologic concentrations, may interact with several eicosanoid receptors. For example, $PGF_{2\alpha}$ may contract smooth muscle by interacting with the FP-, EP_1-, or TP_τ-receptors. Prostaglandins are believed to influence concentrations of cyclic nucleotides and Ca^{++} within cells.[7,8]

Much information about the effects of eicosanoids on intracellular processes comes from studies on platelets. An increase in free Ca^{++} within platelets promotes aggregation; conversely, decreased free Ca^{++} inhibits aggregation. Prostacyclin activates adenylyl cyclase, which increases cyclic AMP. This in turn decreases the free intracellular Ca^{++} concentration and inhibits aggregation. Thromboxane A_2 activates phospholipase C, which catalyzes the formation of the second messenger inositol trisphosphate (IP_3).[17] Intracellular Ca^{++} is mobilized by IP_3 and promotes aggregation. The cellular cyclic AMP concentration is not changed by thromboxane A_2. Postreceptor events in other cells and with other eicosanoids are not as well defined, but there is evidence for modulation of cyclic nucleotides and intracellular Ca^{++} concentration by prostaglandins in several cell types.

TABLE 25-1 Major effects of prostanoids and leukotrienes

	Eicosanoid	Effect
Cardiovascular	PGD_2, PGE_2, PGI_2	Vasodilatation
	$PGF_{2\alpha}$, TXA_2	Vasoconstriction
	LTC_4, LTD_4	Increased capillary permeability
Gastrointestinal	PGE_2, PGI_2	Inhibition of acid secretion, stimulation of mucus secretion
	PGE_2, $PGF_{2\alpha}$, TXA_2	Increased motility, smooth muscle contraction
Renal	PGD_2, PGE_2, PGI_2	Vasodilatation, natriuresis, diuresis, renin release
Pulmonary	TXA_2	Vasoconstriction
	PGE_2, PGI_2	Bronchodilatation, vasodilatation
	PGD_2, $PGF_{2\alpha}$, TXA_2, LTC_4, LTD_4	Bronchoconstriction
Platelet	TXA_2	Aggregation
	PGD_2, PGI_2	Inhibition of aggregation
Reproductive organs	PGE_2	Contraction of pregnant uterus
	$PGF_{2\alpha}$	Contraction of pregnant or nonpregnant uterus; lysis of corpus luteum
Leukocytes	LTB_4	Chemotaxis

Table 25-1 lists some of the prominent effects of the naturally occurring prostaglandins and thromboxane A_2.

Role in physiology and disease

In general, the potent activity of prostaglandins on blood vessels, smooth muscles, and secretory glands indicates that any disorder of normal prostaglandin generation would alter physiologic function. There are several diseases in which prostaglandins and thromboxane play a role. PGI_2, PGD_2, and PGE_2 reduce blood pressure and dilate coronary, renal, and mesenteric vascular beds. Vasodilatation induced by PGE_2 and PGI_2 helps maintain renal perfusion in clinical states of decreased cardiac output. The vasodilator and natriuretic effects of prostaglandins have led some investigators to speculate that some forms of hypertension result from reduced prostaglandin production in the kidney.[3]

The effects of thromboxane and prostaglandins on coronary vessels are of particular interest. Studies in patients with unstable angina pectoris have revealed that local release of thromboxane A_2 into the coronary circulation may contribute to anginal episodes by causing platelet aggregation and possibly vasospasm.[10] These findings have stimulated interest in thromboxane synthase inhibitors and thromboxane receptor antagonists for use as therapeutic adjuncts in patients with coronary ischemia.[17] Normally PGI_2 is the major arachidonic acid metabolite in coronary vessels and in cells cultured from coronary arteries.[18] It inhibits platelet aggregation and causes vasodilatation, which may help prevent myocardial ischemia.[14] When given intravenously in man, PGI_2 lowers blood pressure and causes a reflex tachycardia, effects that preclude its use in angina. PGE_2 also has a direct vasodilatory action. In addition, it modulates vessel sensitivity to constrictors and inhibits release of norepinephrine from nerve endings.[12]

Another important function of prostaglandins is in the prenatal circulation. The maintenance of a patent ductus arteriosus by continued production of PGI_2 or PGE_2 is necessary for circulation of oxygenated maternal blood through the fetal heart. PGE_1 has a similar effect, and alprostadil (PGE_1, Prostin VR Pediatric; 500 μg/ml) is available for administration, usually by intravenous infusion, to neonates in whom temporary maintenance of a patent ductus arteriosus is desirable. On the other hand, cyclooxygenase inhibitors are sometimes used to promote closure when the ductus remains patent after birth.

Prostaglandins E_2 and I_2 are 75 to 100 times more potent than isoproterenol in reversing bronchoconstriction caused by inhalation of a cholinergic agonist.[23] These prostaglandins are not particularly useful clinically because their action is so brief; stable derivatives may be more useful. Such bronchodilators may be of particular value in patients who become resistant to the action of β-adrenergic agonists. In contrast, other eicosanoids may contribute to acute airway constriction in asthma.[23] TXA_2, PGD_2, the primary prostanoid formed in mast cells, and $PGF_{2\alpha}$ are potent bronchoconstrictors (as are some leukotrienes discussed below). Studies with TXA_2-receptor antagonists and thromboxane synthase inhibitors indicate that TXA_2 may be an important regulator of bronchial tone. PGD_2 is synergistic with other mediators in contracting airway smooth muscle and promoting inflammatory changes. Thus it too is of considerable interest as a potential mediator of asthma.[9]

Prostaglandins are believed to have an important regulatory function in gastric secretion. PGE_2 and PGI_2 inhibit gastric acid and pepsin secretion that is stimulated by foods, secretogogues, or irritants, and they also promote mucus secretion. Thus these endogenous prostaglandins are cytoprotective for the gastric mucosa.[19] Irritants, such as alcohol, stimulate prostaglandin formation. Aspirin, other cyclooxygenase inhibitors, and glucocorticoids may promote or worsen peptic ulcer disease because inhibition of prostaglandin synthesis blocks normal cytoprotective mechanisms. In contrast, **misoprostol**, a stable PGE_1 analog, promotes healing of duodenal and gastric ulcers[15] and is comparable to cimetidine in effectiveness. It is indicated for use in patients who are treated chronically with aspirin-like drugs and are at risk for developing gastric ulcers. Diarrhea is a common side effect with this drug. It is contraindicated in pregnancy. Misoprostol (Cytotec) is taken as tablets, 200 μg.

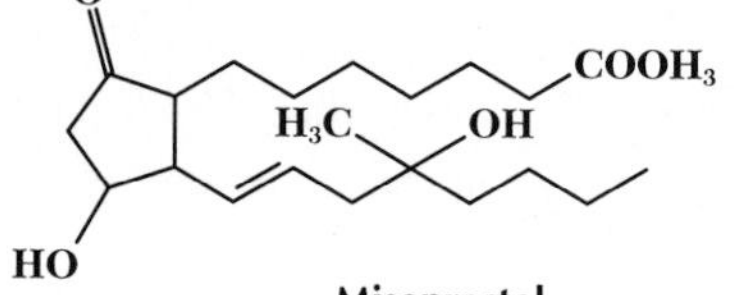

O COOH$_3$ H$_3$C OH HO

Misoprostol

Prostaglandins have several activities that can interfere with pregnancy. $PGF_{2\alpha}$ causes lysis of the corpus luteum and enhances uterine motility. These actions have led to use of prostaglandins to terminate pregnancy. Luteolysis decreases the progesterone production that is necessary to maintain early pregnancy, and so treatment is effective in the first trimester. PGE_2 has been used to stimulate uterine motility at parturition. Available preparations include carboprost tromethamine (Prostin/15 M; 250 μg/ml) for injection and dinoprostone (PGE_2, Prostin E2; 20 mg) vaginal suppositories.

When injected into the corpus cavernosum in impotent patients, PGE_1 will cause partial or complete erection. It causes erection without priapism. Because of its shorter duration of action, PGE_1 appears superior to papaverine for this indication.

Unfortunately, receptors for prostaglandins are ubiquitous, and systemic administration of any of these agents can cause several undesirable effects. For example, in studies in which $PGF_{2\alpha}$ was used to terminate an early pregnancy or to stimulate labor, it caused diarrhea, nausea, and changes in blood pressure as well as increased uterine motility. Similarly, misoprostol, used in healing gastric ulcers, is contraindicated in women of child-bearing age as it may induce miscarriage.

Inhibitors

Enzymatic steps at which synthesis of prostaglandins or thromboxane can be inhibited include (1) the release of arachidonic acid, (2) the oxygenation of arachidonic acid to endoperoxides, and (3) the conversion of endoperoxides to active prostanoids. Drugs that inhibit these steps are listed in Table 25-2. In addition, antagonism at the thromboxane receptor, for example by sulotroban, blocks the action of this mediator.

LEUKOTRIENES AND HYDROPEROXY-EICOSATETRAENOIC ACIDS

Formation and chemistry

Arachidonic acid is transformed by lipoxygenases to another family of compounds that includes the active leukotrienes.[21] The lipoxygenase reaction involves addition of a hydroperoxy group at a double bond of arachidonic acid to form the hydroperoxyeicosatetraenoic acids (HPETEs) (Fig. 25-4). 5-, 12-, and 15-HPETE are commonly found as metabolic products and are pharmacologically active.

The position of the hydroperoxy group may vary with the particular tissue and will influence activity. Effects attributed to HPETEs include vasoconstriction, platelet aggregation, chemotaxis of neutrophils, inhibition of immune lymphocyte responses, and regulation of arachidonic acid metabolism. The physiologic importance of these effects is not yet established, and receptors for these eicosanoids have not been identified. The available evidence suggests that 12-HPETE or a metabolite of it may

TABLE 25-2 Inhibitors of prostanoid synthesis

Enzyme inhibited	Inhibitor
Phospholipase A_2	Glucocorticoids, mepacrine*
Cyclooxygenase	Nonsteroidal anti-inflammatory agents, including aspirin
Prostacyclin synthase	Tranylcypromine*
Thromboxane synthase	Dazoxiben,* pirmagrel,* imidazole*

*Agents used experimentally.

FIG. 25-4 *Oxygenation of arachidonic acid by 12-lipoxygenase to form 12-HPETE. A peroxidase converts 12-HPETE to 12-HETE.*

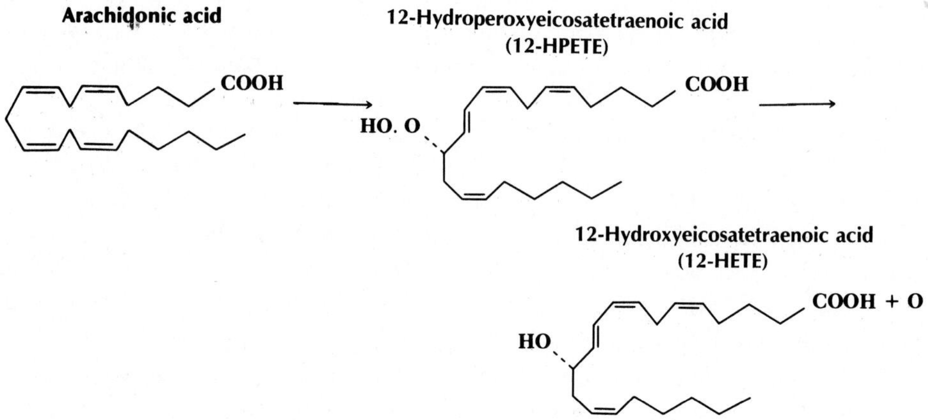

Arachidonic acid COOH → **12-Hydroperoxyeicosatetraenoic acid (12-HPETE)** HO. O COOH → **12-Hydroxyeicosatetraenoic acid (12-HETE)** HO COOH + O

act intracellularly to regulate K^+ channels in neural tissue. The HPETEs are inactivated by conversion to the corresponding hydroxyeicosatetraenoic acids (HETEs) by a peroxidase.

Leukotriene synthesis is initiated by the metabolism of arachidonic acid, by 5-lipoxygenase, to 5-HPETE.[21] It is then converted to the unstable epoxide leukotriene A_4 (LTA_4) by a dehydrase, leukotriene synthase (Fig. 25-5). LTA_4 may be metabolized in two ways: (1) hydration and rearrangement to form leukotriene B_4 (LTB_4) or (2) conjugation of LTA_4 to glutathione to form the peptidolipid leukotriene C_4 (LTC_4). Active leukotrienes D_4 and E_4 (LTD_4 and LTE_4) are formed stepwise by hydrolysis of the glutathione peptide bonds of LTC_4.

Biologic activities

LTB_4 is a prominent mediator of inflammation because of its chemotactic and phagocyte-activating actions.[21] It is produced by neutrophils and macrophages and, to a lesser extent, by eosinophils. LTB_4 can be released in anaphylactic reactions, and it has been linked to bronchospasm in man and experimental animals, possibly through release of thromboxane A_2.[16] LTB_4 also promotes attachment of neutrophils to vascular endothelium and may thus contribute to inflammation.[6]

Leukotrienes C_4 and D_4 are the active components of the *slow-reacting substance of anaphylaxis* (SRS-A).[11] These mediators are formed primarily by mast cells, monocytes, and eosinophils. They are recognized for their prominent bronchoconstrictor action, which may be involved in asthma. Furthermore, minute amounts of LTD_4 enhance bronchiolar sensitivity to histamine. In addition, LTC_4 and LTD_4 contract gastrointestinal and vascular smooth muscle and constrict coronary arteries and vessels of the skin. They are approximately 100 times more potent than histamine in increasing permeability within the microcirculation and may contribute to development of edema in inflammation. LTE_4 has actions similar to LTC_4 and LTD_4, but it is less potent in some tissues. Distinct receptors for LTB_4 and LTC_4 have been identified.

Biosynthesis of leukotrienes from arachidonic acid. *FIG. 25-5*

Modified from Lewis RA, Austin KF: J Clin Invest 73:889, 1984.

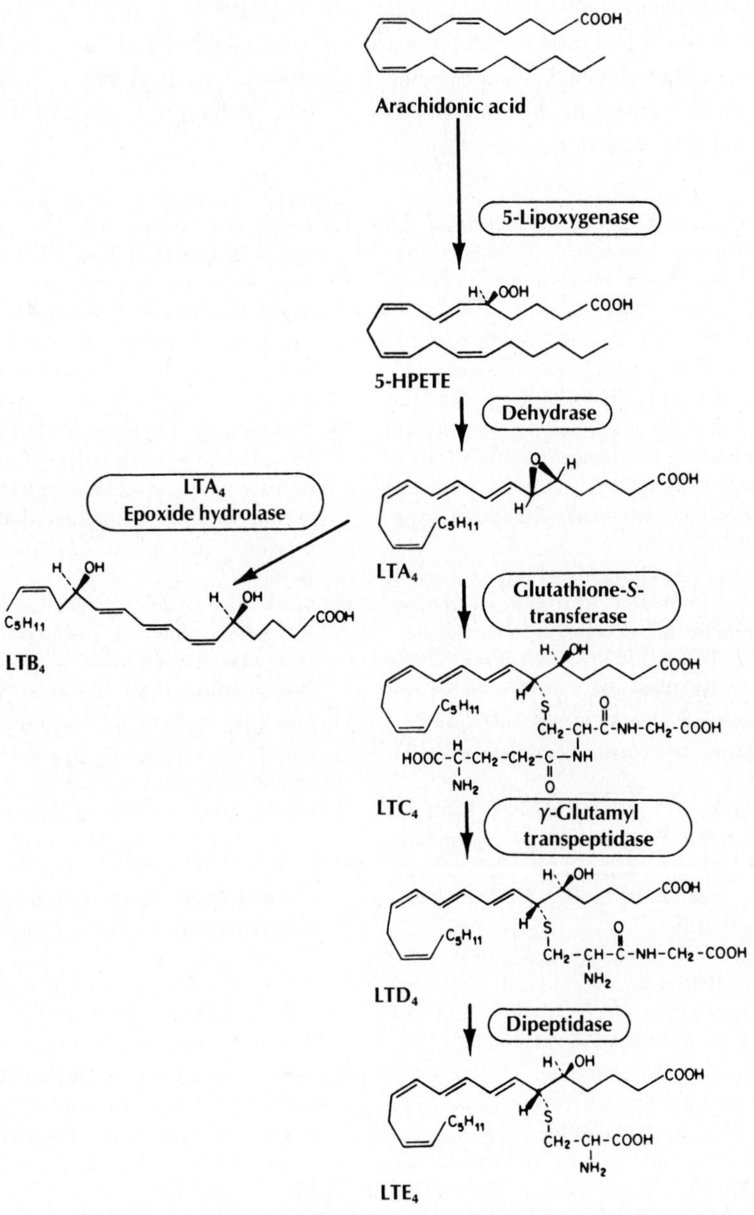

Arachidonic acid

5-Lipoxygenase

5-HPETE

Dehydrase

LTA_4

LTA_4 Epoxide hydrolase

LTB_4

Glutathione-*S*-transferase

LTC_4

γ-Glutamyl transpeptidase

LTD_4

Dipeptidase

LTE_4

Inhibitors

Although formation of lipoxygenase products can be decreased by inhibition of arachidonic acid release, with glucocorticoids or by a competing substrate such as eicosatetraynoic acid (ETYA), there are still no drugs specific for inhibition of lipoxygenase as there are for cyclooxygenase. Many different compounds are being studied with the goal of specifically inhibiting 5-lipoxygenase. There is some indication that analogs of prostacyclin might block conversion of LTA_4 to LTC_4.[2] Such analogs might be used to prevent the bronchoconstrictor action of SRS-A.

Antagonists at leukotriene receptors are not yet available for clinical use, but there is evidence that the actions of specific leukotrienes can be blocked with certain experimental compounds. Such agents will likely be applied to therapy of asthma and inflammatory disease in the near future.

REFERENCES

1. Anderson MW, Eling TE: Prostaglandin removal and metabolism by isolated perfused rat lung, *Prostaglandins* 11:645, 1976.
2. Bach MK, Brashler JR, Smith HW, et al: 6,9-Deepoxy-6,9-(phenylimino)-$\Delta^{6,8}$-prostaglandin I_1, (U-60,257), a new inhibitor of leukotriene C and D synthesis: in vitro studies, *Prostaglandins* 23:759, 1982.
3. Baer PG, McGiff JC: Hormone systems and renal hemodynamics, *Annu Rev Physiol* 42:589, 1980.
4. Coleman RA, Humphrey PPA, Kennedy I, Lumley P: Prostanoid receptors—the development of a working classification, *Trends Pharmacol Sci* 5:303, 1984.
5. Flower RJ, Blackwell GJ: The importance of phospholipase-A_2 in prostaglandin biosynthesis, *Biochem Pharmacol* 25:285, 1976.
6. Gimbrone MA, Jr, Brock AF, Schafer AI: Leukotriene B_4 stimulates polymorphonuclear leukocyte adhesion to cultured vascular endothelial cells, *J Clin Invest* 74:1552, 1984.
7. Gorman RR: Modulation of human platelet function by prostacyclin and thromboxane A_2, *Fed Proc* 38:83, 1979.
8. Halushka PV, Mais DE, Mayeux PR, Morinelli TA: Thromboxane, prostaglandin and leukotriene receptors, *Annu Rev Pharmacol Toxicol* 29:213, 1989.
9. Hardy CC, Robinson C, Tattersfield AE, Holgate ST: The bronchoconstrictor effect of inhaled prostaglandin D_2 in normal and asthmatic men, *N Engl J Med* 311:209, 1984.
10. Hirsh PD, Hillis LD, Campbell WB, et al: Release of prostaglandins and thromboxane into the coronary circulation in patients with ischemic heart disease, *N Engl J Med* 304: 685, 1981.
11. Lewis RA, Austen KF: The biologically active leukotrienes: biosynthesis, metabolism, receptors, functions, and pharmacology, *J Clin Invest* 73:889, 1984.
12. Messina EJ, Weiner R, Kaley G: Prostaglandins and local circulatory control, *Fed Proc* 35:2367, 1976.
13. Moncada S, Gryglewski R, Bunting S, Vane JR: An enzyme isolated from arteries transforms prostaglandin endoperoxides to an unstable substance that inhibits platelet aggregation, *Nature* 263:663, 1976.
14. Moncada S, Vane JR: Pharmacology and endogenous roles of prostaglandin endoperoxides, thromboxane A_2, and prostacyclin, *Pharmacol Rev* 30:293, 1979.
15. Monk JP, Clissold SP: Misoprostol: a preliminary review of its pharmacodynamic and pharmacokinetic properties, and therapeutic efficacy in the treatment of peptic ulcer disease, *Drugs* 33:1, 1987.
16. O'Byrne PM, Leikauf GD, Aizawa H, et al: Leukotriene B_4 induces airway hyperresponsiveness in dogs, *J Appl Physiol* 59:1941, 1985.
17. Ogletree ML: Overview of physiological and pathophysiological effects of thromboxane A_2, *Fed Proc* 46:133, 1987.
18. Revtyak GE, Johnson AR, Campbell WB: Cultured coronary artery endothelial cells synthesize monohydroxyeicosatetraenoic acids and prostacyclin, *Am J Physiol* 254:C8, 1988.
19. Robert A, Nezamis JE, Lancaster C, et al: Mild irritants prevent gastric necrosis through "adaptive cytoprotection" mediated by prostaglandins, *Am J Physiol* 245:G113, 1983.
20. Samuelsson B: Biosynthesis of prostaglandins, *Fed Proc* 31:1442, 1972.
21. Samuelsson B: Leukotrienes: mediators of

immediate hypersensitivity reactions and inflammation, *Science* 220:568, 1983.

22. Smith JB, Willis AL: Aspirin selectively inhibits prostaglandin production in human platelets, *Nature New Biol* 231:235, 1971.

23. Spannhake EW, Hyman AL, Kadowitz PJ: Bronchoactive metabolites of arachidonic acid and their role in airway function, *Prostaglandins* 22:1013, 1981.

24. Vane JR: Inhibition of prostaglandin synthesis as a mechanism of action for aspirin-like drugs, *Nature New Biol* 231:232, 1971.

section three

Psychopharmacology

Chapter 26

General concepts of psychopharmacology

Before the 1950s there were no effective drugs for treatment of the major mental illnesses.[11] Large doses of barbiturates were used to calm agitated psychotic patients, and amphetamine was used to combat acute depression. In the early 1950s, reserpine and chlorpromazine were introduced for management of psychotic patients. These drugs have since been major investigational tools for assessment of roles of central neurotransmitters and neuronal circuits in the antipsychotic effects of drugs and in the pathophysiology of the disease process itself. Many agents (see Chapters 27 to 29) are now available for management of schizophrenia, affective disorders (depression and mania), and anxiety states.

MONOAMINE BASIS OF PSYCHOPHARMACOLOGY

Antipsychotic agents

Reserpine, the major active substance of *Rauwolfia serpentina* and related plants, provided the earliest insights into possible roles of specific brain amines in mental disease. It was initially found that this drug depletes stores of serotonin in the brain and peripheral organs and that only the psychoactive alkaloids of *Rauwolfia* share this activity. Later, it was discovered that reserpine likewise depletes stores of norepinephrine and epinephrine. After identification of dopamine stores in the brain, it was established that reserpine depletes these as well. These findings, coupled with observations that monoamine oxidase (MAO) inhibitors interfere with metabolism of these amines and also alter behavioral effects of reserpine in animals, implicated one or more of the amines in the central actions of reserpine.

The inability of chlorpromazine, a phenothiazine antipsychotic, to affect brain amine concentrations was at first an obstacle to further advances. However, it was soon demonstrated that chlorpromazine and related drugs are antagonists at dopamine receptors in various brain regions. It now appears that the major antipsychotic action of phenothiazines and related drugs is blockade of dopamine receptors (specifically the D_2 subtype) in mesolimbic and mesocortical pathways, whereas blockade of D_2 receptors in the corpus striatum is responsible for major motor side effects of these drugs.

Some of the evidence for involvement of dopamine in the therapeutic action of antischizophrenic drugs may be summarized as follows:

1. Ligand-binding studies show a close association between clinical potency and the affinity of antipsychotic drugs for dopamine receptors on brain membrane fractions (Fig. 26-1).

2. The potencies of antipsychotic drugs for initially enhancing brain concentrations of the dopamine metabolites homovanillic acid and dihydroxyphenylacetic acid (Fig. 26-2) in dopamine neuronal brain regions, in general, correlate well with their clinical

Concentrations of various antipsychotic drugs that produce 50% inhibition of binding of haloperidol to a preparation of caudate nucleus are plotted against the average clinical dose in humans to control schizophrenic symptoms. ***FIG. 26-1***

From Seeman P, Lee T, Chau-Wong M, Wong K: Reprinted by permission from Nature 261:717, copyright 1976, Macmillan Journals Ltd.

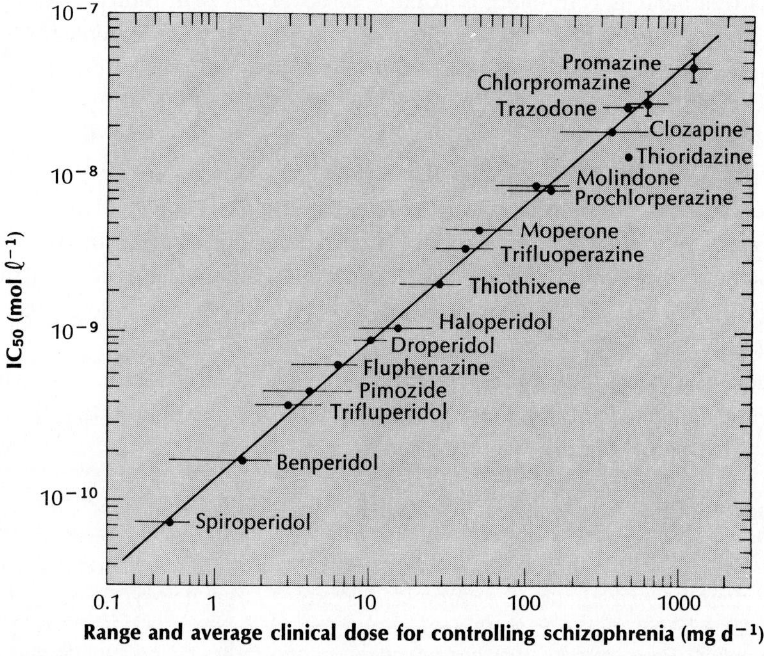

Metabolism of dopamine in the brain. MAO, *Monoamine oxidase;* COMT, *catechol-O-methyltransferase.* ***FIG. 26-2***

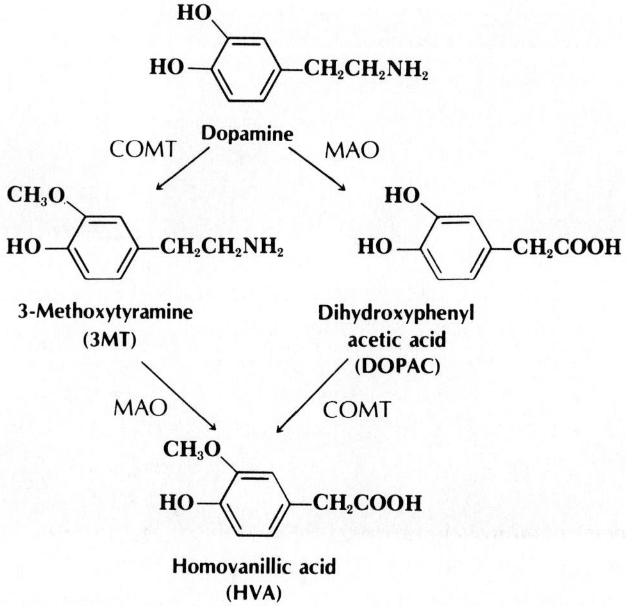

HO
HO—⟨ring⟩—$CH_2CH_2NH_2$

Dopamine

COMT ↙ ↘ MAO

CH_3O
HO—⟨ring⟩—$CH_2CH_2NH_2$

3-Methoxytyramine (3MT)

HO
HO—⟨ring⟩—CH_2COOH

Dihydroxyphenyl acetic acid (DOPAC)

MAO ↘ ↙ COMT

CH_3O
HO—⟨ring⟩—CH_2COOH

Homovanillic acid (HVA)

potencies. Thus blockade of dopamine receptors appears to cause a compensatory increase in dopamine synthesis. This change has been attributed (1) to a reduction of normal inhibitory feedback to presynaptic dopaminergic neurons through collaterals from the postsynaptic neurons or (2) to blockade of presynaptic dopamine autoreceptors.[2] As treatment is continued, dopamine turnover tends to return toward normal.

3. Similarly, electrophysiologic studies on dopamine neurons demonstrate a correlation between clinical antipsychotic potency and the ability of the drugs to increase neuronal firing rate. Some examples are given in Fig. 26-3.

4. Of less specific evidence, inhibition of tyrosine hydroxylase, the rate-limiting enzyme in the biosynthesis of catecholamines, allows a major reduction in the dose of antipsychotic drug required to control symptoms in schizophrenic patients (Fig. 26-4).

5. Drugs such as the amphetamines, which release dopamine in the brain, can exacerbate schizophrenic symptoms or even initiate symptoms of paranoid schizophrenia (see Chapter 34). These responses are blocked by dopamine antagonists such as chlorpromazine.

Although there is an impressive array of evidence for a role of dopamine in therapeutic actions of antipsychotic drugs, it should be remembered that these agents

FIG. 26-3 ***A***, *Antagonism by chlorpromazine* (CPZ) *of* d-*amphetamine* (AMP)*-induced slowing of dopaminergic cell activity in a nonanesthetized animal. AMP significantly decreased firing rate. After CPZ, cell firing resumed and increased.* ***B***, *Effect of haloperidol on a dopaminergic cell in a nonanesthetized animal. Haloperidol increased basal activity.* ***C***, Lack of effect of promethazine (PRO) *on cell firing rate subsequent to AMP-induced depression in an anesthetized animal. Promethazine, which is not antipsychotic, failed to increase the rate, whereas perphenazine* (PER) *rapidly increased rate to above baseline values.*

From Bunney BS, et al: J Pharmacol Exp Ther 185:560, copyright 1973, Williams & Wilkins.

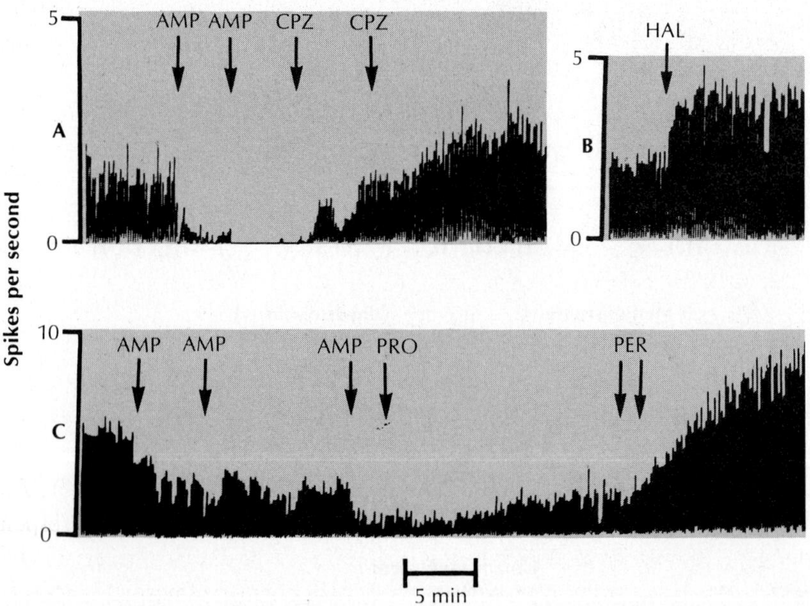

Social behavior (solid lines) *and mental symptoms* (dashed lines) *in a patient with chronic schizophrenia. Patient had been receiving 1000 mg of chlorpromazine daily. The patient's condition worsened when this dosage was reduced but improved when α-methyltyrosine (metyrosine) was given with a small dose of chlorpromazine.* *FIG. 26-4*

From Carlsson A, Persson T, Roos B-E, Walinder J: J Neural Transm 33:83, 1972.

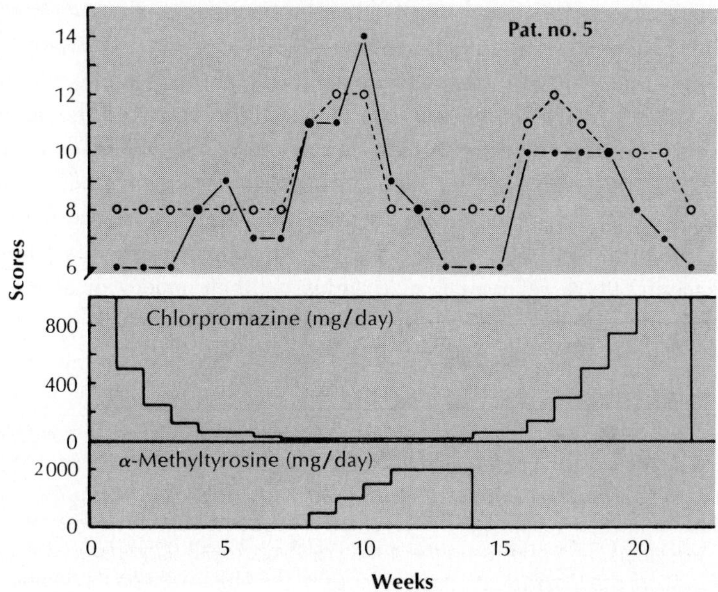

do not immediately alleviate psychotic illness; some adaptation to persisting dopamine receptor blockade, perhaps at presynaptic receptors, apparently contributes to their action. Furthermore, these findings do not, in themselves, constitute evidence that schizophrenia per se is caused by abnormalities in dopamine neurotransmission.[6]

Antidepressant drugs

Basic and clinical investigations have led to development of drugs for treatment of depression and have improved understanding of their basic actions. The MAO inhibitors were tried because they altered central depressant effects evoked in animals by reserpine and because of their unusual effect on mood in patients with tuberculosis. Their beneficial effect in depression has been attributed to downregulation of adrenergic or serotonergic receptors, secondary to chronic inhibition of MAO subtype A in mitochondria of the terminals of monoamine neurons.[12]

MAO inhibitors have largely been replaced in clinical practice by tricyclic and second-generation antidepressants, such as imipramine and fluoxetine respectively. The latter drugs inhibit amine reuptake into neurons. This property reinforced an early hypothesis that depression is caused by a functional deficiency of amines, which is corrected by slowing removal of amine from the synaptic cleft. However, the effect of these drugs on amine uptake is immediate, whereas the therapeutic response is considerably delayed (weeks). Accordingly, there is more recent interest in the idea that depression arises from hyperactivity, or perhaps failure of normal homeostasis,[16] of amine pathways, rather than a deficiency, and that a therapeutic response depends on secondary adaptation to a chronic excess of neurotransmitter in the synapse after inhibition of uptake. Effects of chronic treatment with antidepressants have been studied primarily in peripheral tissues and in rat brain. Changes with chronic treatment have included: desensitization (downregulation) of postsynaptic β- and presynaptic α_2-adrenergic receptors and sensitization (upregulation) of α_1-adrenergic receptors.[17] Links to the serotonergic system also appear important.[4,14] Some antidepressants inhibit uptake of both norepinephrine and serotonin, whereas others preferentially affect one or the other of the pumps.[9] Bupropion, on the other hand, is nearly devoid of uptake-blocking activity, except for weak blockade of dopamine uptake. Amineptine is an investigational drug that selectively inhibits dopamine reuptake; chronic administration of this agent also downregulates β-adrenergic receptors. Thus antidepressants may act at a variety of points in complex pathways that modulate mood. Future refinement of theories on their modes of action will, one hopes, further integrate their seemingly selective actions at various synapses. Fig. 26-5

FIG. 26-5 *Synaptic effects of different types of antidepressant or stimulant drugs as conceptualized in the biogenic amine hypothesis of mental illness. Four aminergic axon varicosities are in synaptic contact with a target cell. Depicted is an association between intraneuronal and extraneuronal transmitter* (stippling) *as governed by incorporation into vesicles* (shading), *release by exocytosis, and uptake via the amine pump* (arrows). *Compared with the normal, drug-free condition, the terminal altered by a tricyclic antidepressant has a greater proportion of transmitter in the synaptic cleft because of inhibition of uptake mechanisms. The terminal subjected to an MAO inhibitor has a greater accumulation of transmitter outside and inside the terminal as a result of decreased breakdown of the amine. Psychomotor stimulants of the amphetamine type increase the concentration of transmitter in the cleft by enhancing release and blocking reuptake. Although the neurotransmitter is probably released from the cytoplasm, amine synthesis and incorporation into vesicles may not keep pace with release; therfore some vesicles are shown empty.*

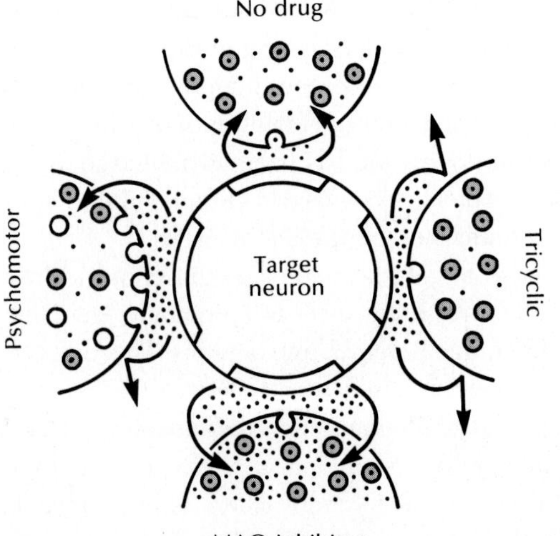

illustrates the modes of action of different types of antidepressants as these relate to acute changes in amine distribution at the synaptic level.

Many of the side effects of these agents depend on their antagonistic actions at muscarinic (dry mouth), histaminic (sedation), and α-adrenergic (orthostatic hypotension) receptors.

LITHIUM ION

Recent interest in the mechanism of action of Li^+ in mania and depression has focused on its effects on second-messenger systems. The ion reduces brain concentrations of inositol in animals by inhibiting inositol monophosphatase, thus preventing the final steps in regeneration of free inositol from inositol 1,4,5-trisphosphate (see Fig. 3-3). It has been proposed that the beneficial effects of this ion relate to insufficient synthesis of phosphatidylinositol from inositol,[3] especially in a highly active state, with subsequent impairment of the phosphoinositide system. Alternatively, there is evidence that Li^+ can affect both the phosphoinositide and cyclic AMP systems by interfering with interactions between receptors and G proteins.[1] Li^+ also competes with sodium, potassium, calcium, and magnesium ions at a variety of sites, and actions on a number of neurotransmitter systems have been studied.[15]

ANTIANXIETY AGENTS

Receptors for benzodiazepines, the primary agents used today to reduce anxiety and alleviate insomnia, are found within a complex (Fig. 26-6) that contains a Cl^- channel, $GABA_A$ receptors for the inhibitory amino acid γ-aminobutyric acid (GABA), and receptors that bind barbiturates and the convulsant picrotoxin. A characteristic of the $GABA_A$ receptor is that the convulsant agent (+)-bicuculline is a competitive antagonist. GABA increases the affinity of benzodiazepine receptors for benzodiazepines, and electrophysiologic effects of GABA are enhanced in the presence of benzodiazepines.

FIG. 26-6 *Schematic representation of postulated sites of action of several neuronal depressants and stimulants within the $GABA_A$ receptor/chloride ionophore. Drugs that tend to close the Cl^- channel are stimulants and convulsants. Drugs that open or facilitate opening of the channel are depressants.* BDZ, *Benzodiazepine;* PICRO, *picrotoxinin.*

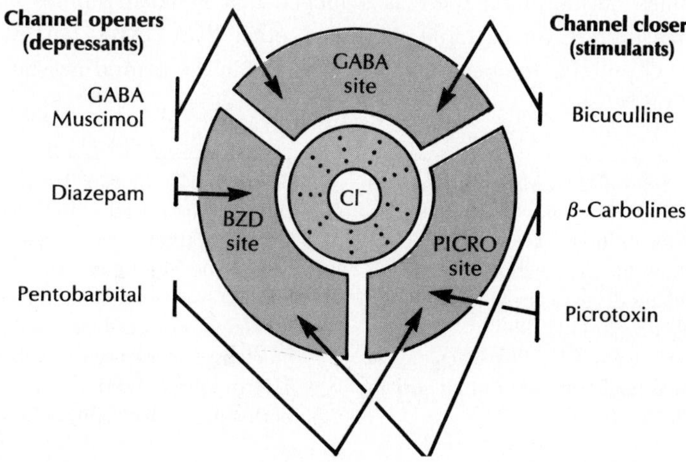

Among the structures proposed for the complex is a tetramer composed of two α and two β subunits, with GABA receptors on the β subunits and benzodiazepine receptors on the α subunits. More recent evidence indicates that there are also γ and δ subunits and even subtypes of the various subunits,[8,13] which include at least two types of benzodiazepine receptor. Whether four or five subunits comprise the channel complex is not yet certain.

Most commonly, GABA-induced channel opening promotes influx of Cl^- from the extraneuronal to the intraneuronal compartment and, thus, hyperpolarization and stabilization of the membrane. GABA appears to evoke closely spaced openings, or bursts, of individual Cl^- channels. In the absence of GABA, benzodiazepines will not open the channel. In the presence of GABA, however, benzodiazepines increase the *frequency* of bursts.[18] In contrast, the more generally depressant barbiturates act on the so-called *picrotoxinin* site to *prolong* burst duration. In high enough concentrations they may open the channel independently of GABA.

The ability of various benzodiazepines to displace labeled, bound diazepam parallels their clinical potency. An unusual feature of benzodiazepine receptors is that a spectrum of agonists has been discovered, from those that favor an open Cl^- channel to those that favor a closed channel. The benzodiazepines relieve anxiety and are anticonvulsant, whereas certain β-carboline derivatives that also bind to benzodiazepine receptors can cause seizures and appear to elicit "anxiety" in animals. The latter compounds have been called *inverse* agonists, or *contragonists*. Flumazenil is a competitive antagonist that produces little or no effect alone but prevents the actions of both benzodiazepines and β-carbolines. One explanation is that there are multiple states of the benzodiazepine receptor;[10] benzodiazepine binding promotes a conformation that allosterically enhances GABA-receptor function, β-carboline binding promotes a conformation with the opposite effect, and flumazenil maintains the receptor in an inactive configuration. Efforts are ongoing to identify possible endogenous ligands for benzodiazepine-binding sites.[7]

It should be noted that there are also $GABA_B$ receptors that are stimulated by (-)-baclofen (see Chapter 17) but are unaffected by bicuculline or the presence of benzodiazepines; furthermore, there is evidence that benzodiazepines can interact with neurotransmitters, for example adenosine, other than GABA. $GABA_B$ receptors are linked by G proteins to opening of K^+ channels in the central nervous system or to closure of Ca^{++} channels in the periphery.[5]

REFERENCES

1. Avissar S, Schreiber G: Muscarinic receptor subclassification and G-proteins: significance for lithium action in affective disorders and for the treatment of the extrapyramidal side effects of neuroleptics, *Biol Psychiatry* 26:113, 1989.
2. Bannon MJ, Roth RH: Pharmacology of mesocortical dopamine neurons, *Pharmacol Rev* 35:53, 1983.
3. Berridge MJ: Inositol trisphosphate, calcium, lithium, and cell signaling, *JAMA* 262:1834, 1989.
4. Blier P, de Montigny C, Chaput Y: A role for the serotonin system in the mechanism of action of antidepressant treatments: preclinical evidence, *J Clin Psychiatry* 51(4 suppl):14, 1990.
5. Bormann J: Electrophysiology of $GABA_A$

and $GABA_B$ receptor subtypes, *Trends Neurosci* 11:112, 1988.

6. Carlsson A: The current status of the dopamine hypothesis of schizophrenia, *Neuropsychopharmacology* 1:179, 1988.
7. De Robertis E, Peña C, Paladini AC, Medina JH: New developments on the search for the endogenous ligand(s) of central benzodiazepine receptors, *Neurochem Int* 13:1, 1988.
8. Dingledine R, Myers SJ, Nicholas RA: Molecular biology of mammalian amino acid receptors, *FASEB J* 4:2636, 1990.
9. Goodman WK, Charney DS: Therapeutic applications and mechanisms of action of monoamine oxidase inhibitor and heterocyclic antidepressant drugs, *J Clin Psychiatry* 46[10, sec 2]:6, 1985.
10. Haefely W: The GABA-benzodiazepine interaction fifteen years later, *Neurochem Res* 15:169, 1990.
11. Jacobsen E: The early history of psychotherapeutic drugs, *Psychopharmacology* 89:138, 1986.
12. McDaniel KD: Clinical pharmacology of monoamine oxidase inhibitors, *Clin Neuropharmacol* 9:207, 1986.
13. Olsen RW, Tobin AJ: Molecular biology of $GABA_A$ receptors, *FASEB J* 4:1469, 1990.
14. Price LH, Charney DS, Delgado PL, et al: Clinical data on the role of serotonin in the mechanism(s) of action of antidepressant drugs, *J Clin Psychiatry* 51(4, suppl):44, 1990.
15. Price LH, Charney DS, Delgado PL, Heninger GR: Lithium and serotonin function: implications for the serotonin hypothesis of depression, *Psychopharmacology* 100:3, 1990.
16. Siever LJ, Davis KL: Overview: toward a dysregulation hypothesis of depression, *Am J Psychiatry* 142:1017, 1985.
17. Smith CB, Hollingsworth PJ: Adrenergic receptors and the mechanism of action of antidepressant treatments. In Tipton KF, Youdim MBH, editors: *Biochemical and pharmacological aspects of depression*, London, 1989, Taylor & Francis, 69.
18. Twyman RE, Rogers CJ, Macdonald RL: Differential regulation of γ-aminobutyric acid receptor channels by diazepam and phenobarbital, *Ann Neurol* 25:213, 1989.

Chapter 27

Antipsychotic drugs

Antipsychotic drugs improve the mood and behavior of psychotic patients without excessive sedation and without causing drug dependence. They relieve signs and symptoms of schizophrenia in a large percentage of affected persons.[14] So-called *positive* or *productive* symptoms (thought disorder, agitation, hostility, delusions, hallucinations) tend to respond better than *negative* or *defect* symptoms (blunted affect, diminished capacity for pleasure, lack of drive, poverty of speech).[19] The relapse rate for schizophrenics maintained on antipsychotic agents during remission is much lower than the rate for patients given placebo. Antipsychotic drugs were previously termed "major tranquilizers" to distinguish them from the antianxiety drugs discussed in Chapter 29.

DEVELOPMENT

Greatly improved pharmacologic management of psychotic patients, which enables most of them to function as outpatients, began with the almost simultaneous introduction of two powerful drugs, chlorpromazine and reserpine. Preparations of *Rauwolfia serpentina*, a wild shrub, were used in India for centuries to treat various illnesses. **Reserpine** (see Chapters 20 and 26), one of its alkaloids, was isolated in 1952.

Chlorpromazine, the prototype *phenothiazine* antipsychotic drug, originated in France from a search for new antihistamines. Chlorpromazine and related drugs bind to adrenergic, muscarinic, serotonergic, and histaminic (H_1) receptors to varying degrees. Their relative antagonistic activities at these receptors may influence the choice of medication for a particular patient.[3] However, their antipsychotic potencies correlate best with antagonism of dopamine. Blockade of dopamine appears to be particularly important in D_2-receptor pathways that lead into the limbic system or cortex. On the other hand, interference with regulation of endocrine and motor pathways normally mediated by dopamine is responsible for some of their undesirable effects.

Calming of wild animals and disturbed patients by reserpine and chlorpromazine can be quite striking. Once the unusually beneficial effect of chlorpromazine in psychotic patients was recognized, many related compounds were introduced. Several of these compounds are also used as antiemetics, and some are antipruritic.

From a chemical standpoint the available antipsychotic drugs include *phenothiazines*, *thioxanthenes*, *butyrophenones*, and individual agents from other classes. Their properties are quite similar; this discussion emphasizes the phenothiazines. Reserpine has essentially been abandoned in psychiatric practice. Its limited use as an antihypertensive is discussed in Chapter 21.

The term *neuroleptic* is often used synonymously with *antipsychotic* because all antischizophrenic drugs used at the present time cause psychomotor slowing, emotional quieting, and in higher doses psychic indifference to the environment. If the term is taken to mean, alternatively, that the drugs cause acute and long-term extrapyramidal motor problems, then clozapine (see p. 251) is the first clinically available nonneuroleptic antipsychotic drug. There is considerable interest in agents that selectively block dopamine autoreceptors, D_1-dopamine receptors, and 5-HT_3-receptors, in hopes of obtaining drugs that control symptoms of schizophrenia without motor abnormalities.

PHENOTHIAZINE DERIVATIVES

The phenothiazines in current use differ from chlorpromazine primarily in potency, special clinical indications, and incidence of side effects.

Antipsychotic phenothiazines are classified on the basis of their structures and pharmacology into three groups (Table 27-1). The *three*-carbon link between the nitrogen on the ring and the nitrogen on the side chain is necessary for antipsychotic activity.

The piperazines are more potent than other phenothiazines, more likely to cause significant extrapyramidal effects, and not very sedative. The piperidines are less potent, least likely to induce extrapyramidal effects, and cause sedation and weight gain. The aliphatic compounds are somewhat intermediate but tend to resemble the piperidines. Relative potencies are often indicated as *chlorpromazine equivalents*, in Table 27-1 as doses approximately equieffective to 500 mg of chlorpromazine.

Chlorpromazine

Chlorpromazine, an aliphatic phenothiazine, is a sedative antipsychotic drug. It is also used for prevention of nausea and vomiting and relief of intractable hiccups. The structures of chlorpromazine and the antihistaminic drug promethazine are quite similar. However, promethazine and other phenothiazines that have only a *two*-carbon link between the nitrogens lack antipsychotic activity.

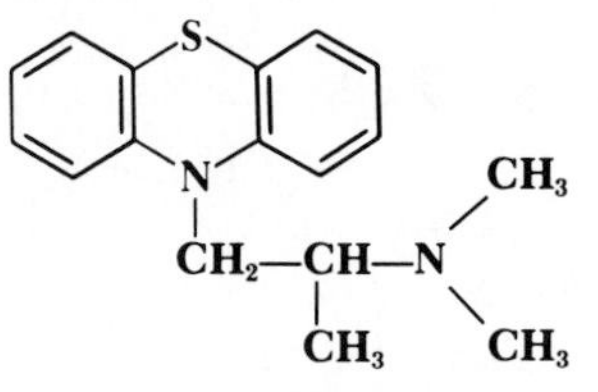

S, N, CH_2—CH—N, CH_3, CH_3, CH_3

Promethazine

S, N, Cl, CH_2—CH_2—CH_2—N, CH_3, CH_3

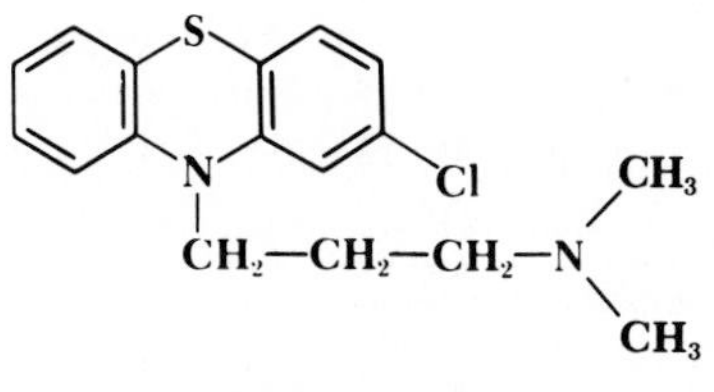

Chlorpromazine

PHARMACOLOGIC EFFECTS

The original French proprietary name for chlorpromazine, Largactil, reflects the fact that it has a great many actions.

Antipsychotic effects. In addition to the quieting and slowing effects mentioned above, phenothiazines tend to decrease paranoid ideation, fear, hostility, and agitation. They lessen the intensity of delusions and hallucinations of schizophrenia. Even though brain dopamine D_2-receptors are blocked within a few hours, improvement

TABLE 27-1 Classification of phenothiazines and other drugs used as antipsychotic agents

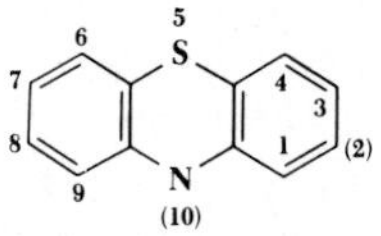

Phenothiazine nucleus

	Substitution in (2)	Substitution in (10)	Equivalent daily dose (mg)*	Daily dose range[10] (mg)	Summary of effects by groups
A. Phenothiazines					
Piperazines					
Acetophenazine (Tindal)	$C(=O)-CH_3$	$CH_2-CH_2-CH_2-N(piperazine)N-CH_2-CH_2-OH$	115	60-120	Most potent antipsychotic and antiemetic; highest incidence of extrapyramidal effects and catalepsy; least sedative
Fluphenazine (Prolixin; Permitil)	CF_3	$CH_2-CH_2-CH_2-N(piperazine)N-CH_2-CH_2-OH$	6	0.5-40	
Perphenazine (Trilafon)	Cl	$CH_2-CH_2-CH_2-N(piperazine)N-CH_2-CH_2-OH$	44	12-64	
Trifluoperazine (Stelazine)	Cl	$CH_2-CH_2-CH_2-N(piperazine)N-CH_3$	14	2-40	
Aliphatics					
Chlorpromazine (Thorazine)		$CH_2-CH_2-CH_2-N-(CH_3)_2$	500	30-800	Less antipsychotic and antiemetic potency; notable parkinsonian side effects; hypotension, sedation, and antihistaminic activity
Promazine (Sparine)		$CH_2-CH_2-CH_2-N-(CH_3)_2$		40-1200	

*Equivalent to 500 mg of chlorpromazine; calculated from analysis of double-blind trails.[9]

Continued.

may not be apparent for 3 or more weeks after initiation of therapy, especially in chronic schizophrenia. However, acute mania can be brought under control more quickly by neuroleptics than by lithium ion. In normal subjects phenothiazines induce dysphoria and impair intellectual function.

Changes in extrapyramidal motor function. Phenothiazines can precipitate an unusual variety of motor disorders,[5] presumably as a result of acute and chronic blockade of dopamine receptors in the basal ganglia. When it occurs, *acute dystonia* (painful, sustained twisting or contraction of muscles) typically appears within 5 days

TABLE 27-1 Classification of phenothiazines and other drugs used as antipsychotic agents—cont'd

	Substitution in (2)	Substitution in (10)	Equivalent daily dose (mg)*	Daily dose range[10] (mg)	Summary of effects by groups
Piperidines					
Mesoridazine (Serentil)	SCH_3 ↓ O	$CH_2—CH_2$— (N-methylpiperidin-2-yl), N—CH_3	280	30-400	Less antipsychotic and antiemetic potency but lowest incidence of extrapyramidal effects; most anticholinergic; most electrocardiographic changes
Thioridazine (Mellaril)	SCH_3	$CH_2—CH_2$— (N-methylpiperidin-2-yl), N—CH_3	485	150-800	
B. Nonphenothiazines					
Chlorprothixene (Taractan)			220	75-600	See p. 249.
Thiothixene (Navane)			44	8-30	See p. 249.
Haloperidol (Haldol)			8	1-15	See p. 250.
Loxapine (Loxitane)			87	20-250	See p. 250.
Molindone (Moban)			30	15-225	See p. 250.
Clozapine (Clozaril)			250	300-900	See p. 251.

of initiating neuroleptic therapy. Young male patients are particularly susceptible. Intravenous administration of benztropine or diphenhydramine can rapidly alleviate the spasm. *Parkinsonian signs* (tremor, rigidity, and bradykinesia) may be encountered after continuous administration of phenothiazines for several weeks or more. They can limit dose escalation but respond well to drugs used to manage true Parkinsons disease (see Chapter 30). A possible variant with rhythmic tremors about the mouth, which may develop anytime, has been termed the *rabbit syndrome*. *Akathisia*, which includes motor restlessness and subjective feelings of tension or unease, can be very stressful. It tends to occur in the first month of therapy, but occasionally within hours. Because it responds relatively poorly to anticholinergic therapy, akathisia may arise from some brain site other than the basal ganglia. If reduction of neuroleptic dosage does not help, treatment with propranolol may be beneficial.[12] These "early" motor abnormalities are common, reversible, and dose dependent (that is, severity decreases if daily neuroleptic intake is reduced).

Tardive dyskinesia is a serious problem in long-term use of antipsychotic drugs.[5] Unlike the motor disorders discussed above, no particular type of antipsychotic, with the exception of clozapine, seems less likely to evoke this disorder. A prevalence of about 15% in excess of spontaneous dyskinesias has been estimated, with increased risk with increasing age, female sex, and the presence of mental disease such as an affective disorder.[1,5] The dyskinesia most often appears as grossly abnormal orofacial movements (oro-buccal-lingual dyskinesia), but tardive dystonia and tardive akathisia also occur, often in combinations. Tardive dyskinesia may first appear or worsen when the dose of neuroleptic is reduced. If the drug is discontinued, the dyskinesia may subside over a period of years.

Unlike the other neuroleptic-induced motor problems, anticholinergic drugs do not reverse, and may exacerbate, tardive dyskinesia. Increasing neuroleptic dosage may suppress the clinical signs but is likely to worsen the problem eventually. It is preferable to minimize the hazard from the beginning by using the lowest effective dose, perhaps in short courses. Use of the lowest necessary dosage of any concurrent anticholinergic medication and treatment with noradrenergic antagonists and GABAergic agonists may be of benefit.[13] Dyskinetic responses have generally been attributed to dopamine receptor supersensitivity, but other mechanisms may be important.[17] Fig. 27-1 summarizes current perceptions of the complex relationships between transmitter activities and motor abnormalities in response to antipsychotic drugs and in true Parkinsons disease.

Anticholinergic and antiadrenergic effects. The atropine-like activity of chlorpromazine can cause dry mouth, constipation, urinary retention, and paralysis of accommodation. Thioridazine, a more potent muscarinic antagonist, is likely to dilate the

FIG. 27-1 *Consequences of perturbations in the functional balance between dopaminergic and cholinergic activity in the basal ganglia (neostriatum). Imbalances are depicted as though dopaminergic transmission* (DA) *is altered while cholinergic transmission* (ACh) *is unchanged. This depiction is greatly simplified; not only may cholinergic transmission also be altered, but additional neurotransmitters may be involved. Obviously, such disparate disorders as Parkinsons disease, dystonia, and akathisia cannot all be caused by precisely the same mechanism.*

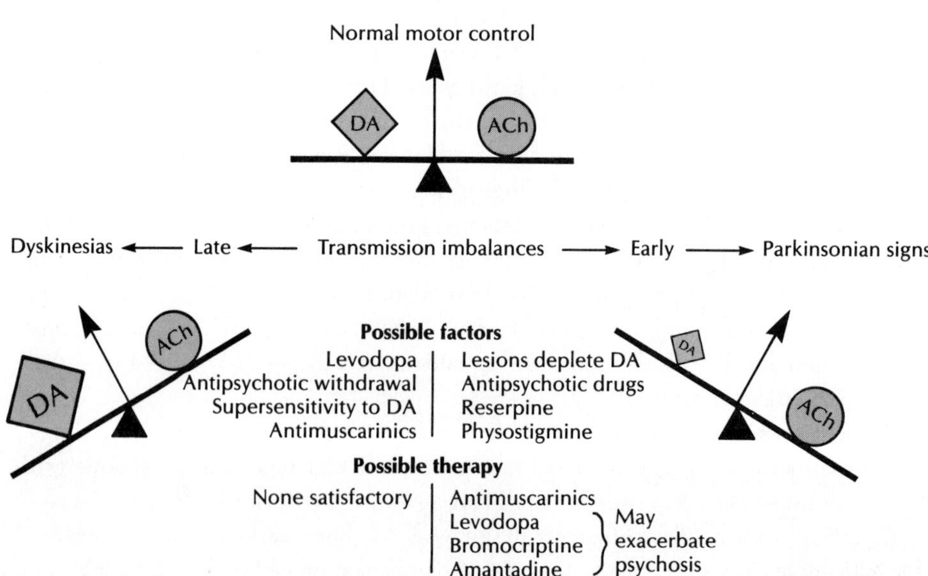

pupils, whereas α-adrenergic blockade by chlorpromazine contributes to miosis. Pronounced orthostatic hypotension and reflex tachycardia may occur after parenteral administration of phenothiazines. Use of thioridazine in particular has been associated with a variety of sexual dysfunctions, including impotence and priapism.[18]

Temperature regulation. Chlorpromazine depresses thermoregulation. It has been used to prevent shivering and thereby facilitate development of a deeply hypothermic state for surgery. Neuroleptics are also the leading cause of drug-related heatstroke.[6] Dangerous elevations in temperature can occur in hot environments due to impairment of heat-loss mechanisms. In ordinary thermal environments, life-threatening hyperthermia may develop in the context of the *neuroleptic malignant syndrome*, in which excessive motor tone or activity is apparently responsible for the temperature increase. Treatment with dantrolene or bromocriptine may be beneficial in such cases.

Antiemetic effect. Chlorpromazine blocks the emetic action of the dopamine agonist apomorphine and certain other agents at the chemoreceptor trigger zone (CTZ) in the area postrema on the floor of the fourth cerebral ventricle (Fig. 27-2). The

FIG. 27-2 *Survey of mechanisms for emesis and the sites of action for several drugs or chemicals that initiate or control vomiting.*

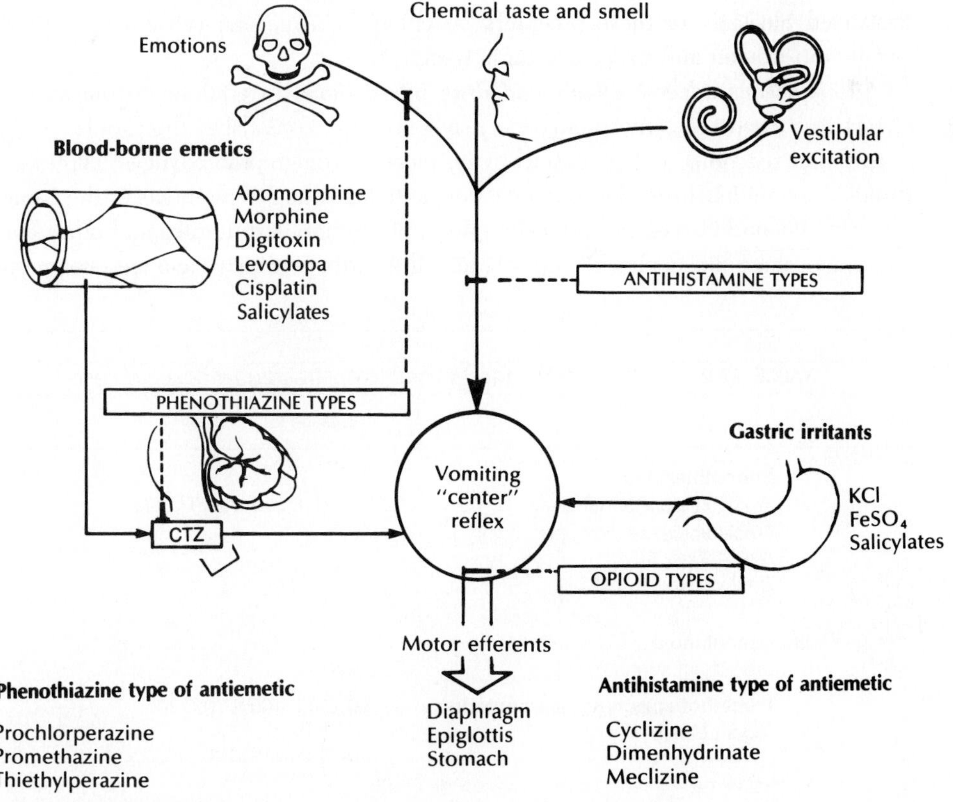

blood-brain barrier is weak in this region, and stimulation of chemoreceptors by circulating toxins and emetic drugs initiates the complex vomiting reflex. Table 27-2 lists some agents used primarily as antiemetics. Trimethobenzamide, though not a phenothiazine, may have similar antiemetic activity. Nonphenothiazine dopamine antagonists and cannabinoids appear more useful for alleviating emetic responses to cancer chemotherapeutic drugs. Combination therapy may be required for maximal benefit.[16] The antiemetic properties of **metoclopramide** (see p. 513) are believed to result from blockade of dopamine receptors in the CTZ and in the enteric nervous system. The drug is effective against nausea and vomiting induced by cisplatin, a chemotherapeutic agent and powerful emetic against which phenothiazines are not very effective.[8] Trials with domperidone, an investigational drug that acts similarly but does not appreciably enter the brain, indicate that it too is an effective antiemetic. Dronabinol (Δ^9-tetrahydrocannabinol), the major active component of marijuana, is also available for use with cancer chemotherapy; its mechanism of action is not understood. None of the above agents is useful in preventing motion sickness, for which muscarinic antagonists and antihistamines with strong atropine-like activity are more beneficial (see p. 118).

Endocrine effects. Chlorpromazine may cause galactorrhea, delayed menstruation, amenorrhea, and weight gain. It is generally believed that these effects are due to disruption of hypothalamic control over the pituitary gland. Dopamine release at synapses in the tuberoinfundibular pathway normally inhibits prolactin secretion. Prolonged blockade of these receptors by chlorpromazine can cause inappropriate lactation in women and gynecomastia in men.

Miscellaneous adverse effects and drug interactions. In addition to the adverse effects just discussed, chlorpromazine may lower the convulsive threshold.[7] It also causes skin reactions and photosensitivity, electrocardiographic changes, cholestatic jaundice, agranulocytosis, skin pigmentation, and deposition of pigments in the cornea and lens. Phenothiazines can intensify effects of alcohol, barbiturates and other hypnotics, morphine-like analgesics, anesthetics, and antihypertensive and anticholinergic

TABLE 27-2 Miscellaneous agents used to control drug-induced emesis

Drug	Dosage forms* (mg)
Phenothiazines	
Prochlorperazine maleate	C: 10-30;I: 5;S: 2.5-25;T: 5-25
Prochlorperazine edisylate (Compazine)	I: 5;Sy: 5
Triethylperazine maleate (Torecan)	I: 5;S: 10;T: 10
Cannabinoid	
Dronabinol (Marinol)	C: 2.5-10
Trimethobenzamide hydrochloride (Tigan, others)	C: 100,250;I: 100;S: 100,200

*C, Capsule; I, injection (per ml); S, suppository; Sy, syrup (per 5 ml); T, tablet.

drugs. The patient and close relatives should be advised of potential problems, especially the extrapyramidal disorders, that may arise with continued therapy.

PHARMACOKINETICS

Chlorpromazine is absorbed erratically when given by mouth. The drug is highly bound to plasma proteins; peak plasma concentration occurs in 2 to 4 hours. The elimination half-life is extremely variable but averages about 30 hours. Measuring concentrations has not yet proved to be useful as a guide to therapy. In a particular patient the optimum dosage is the smallest that relieves psychotic symptoms without causing intolerable side effects. In general, a single daily dose of neuroleptic can be given at bedtime.

The distribution of chlorpromazine in various tissues is quite uneven, and its volume of distribution is large. The brain contains about four times more drug than does the plasma. Chlorpromazine has numerous dealkylated, hydroxylated, and conjugated metabolites. The drug is also excreted in milk.

Antihistaminic activity

Some phenothiazines with powerful antihistaminic activity are used to relieve the pruritus of various skin diseases. Examples are **promethazine** hydrochloride (Phenergan, others), **trimeprazine** tartrate (Temaril), and **methdilazine** hydrochloride (Tacaryl). In general, these compounds can cause drowsiness and the toxic effects described above so that precautions applicable to the other phenothiazines should be observed.

Preparations

The phenothiazines, as well as other neuroleptics, are available in several dosage forms including tablets, capsules, syrups, elixirs, injectables, and rectal suppositories. Fluphenazine, as the decanoate and enanthate esters, has an extended duration of action after intramuscular injection. These dosage forms are useful for managing combative or noncompliant patients, because the effects of a single injection persist for 1 to 4 weeks.

THIOXANTHENE DERIVATIVES

The thioxanthene derivatives **chlorprothixene** and **thiothixene** are structurally and pharmacologically similar to the phenothiazines. The side chain on the central ring influences activity in the same way. Thus thiothixene, which has a piperazine side chain, is more potent than the aliphatic chlorprothixene.

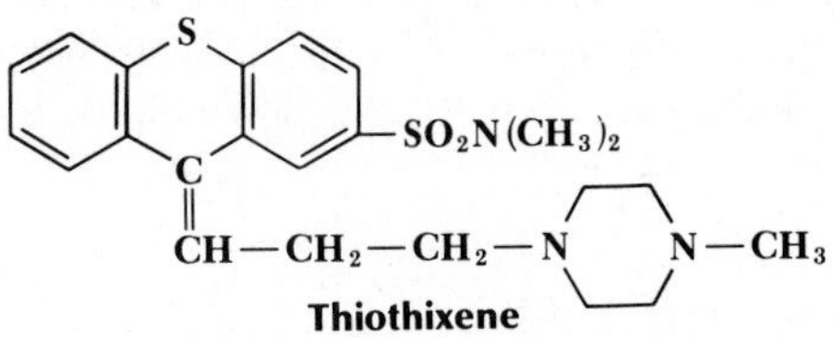

S; $SO_2N(CH_3)_2$; C; $CH-CH_2-CH_2-N$ (piperazine) $N-CH_3$

Thiothixene

S; Cl; C; $CH-CH_2-CH_2-N(CH_3)_2$

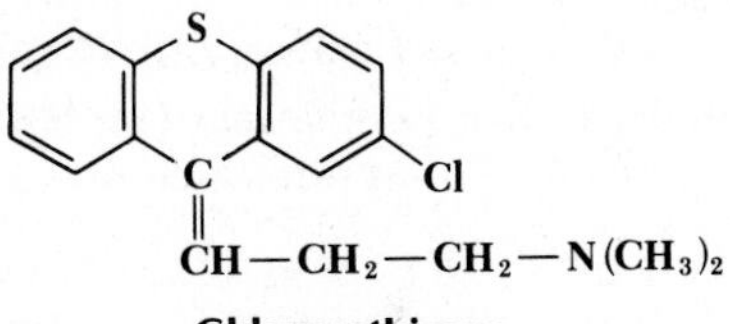

Chlorprothixene

Chlorprothixene is available in tablets of 10 to 100 mg, in an oral concentrate containing 20 mg/ml, and for injection as the hydrochloride in a solution of 12.5 mg/ml. Thiothixene is available in capsules of 1 to 20 mg, as the hydrochloride in a concentrate containing 5 mg/ml, and in vials for injection.

BUTYROPHENONES

Substituted butyrophenones have been used increasingly as antipsychotic agents and in anesthesiology. **Haloperidol**, the prototype of this series, is a potent antipsychotic and antiemetic, available in tablets, 0.5 to 20 mg; as the lactate in an oral concentrate of 2 mg/ml; and for intramuscular injection as the lactate, 5 mg/ml; or the long-acting decanoate, 50 and 100 mg/ml. Although there is no obvious chemical similarity, haloperidol pharmacologically resembles piperazine phenothiazines; it can cause extrapyramidal reactions and has been associated with several cases of neuroleptic malignant syndrome.[6] Haloperidol is less sedating than many other antipsychotics and is useful for temporary management of acute mania. It is also the first-line drug for control of the tics of Gilles de la Tourettes syndrome. **Pimozide** (Orap), a structurally unrelated neuroleptic, can be used in patients for whom haloperidol is intolerable or ineffective. Although pimozide causes side effects common to neuroleptics, it has also caused sudden death in some patients taking doses well in excess of the recommended maximum of 10 mg daily. Baseline and periodic ECG monitoring is recommended, with dosage reduction if the QT interval exceeds 0.47 seconds in children or 0.52 seconds in adults. The drug is taken as tablets containing 2 mg.

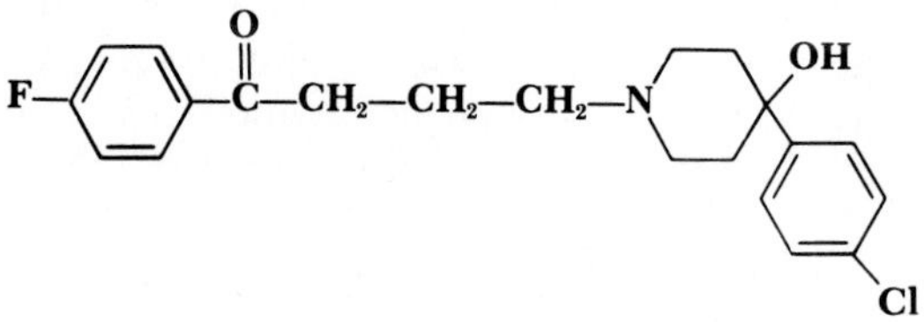

F—C(=O)—CH_2—CH_2—CH_2—N, OH, Cl

Haloperidol

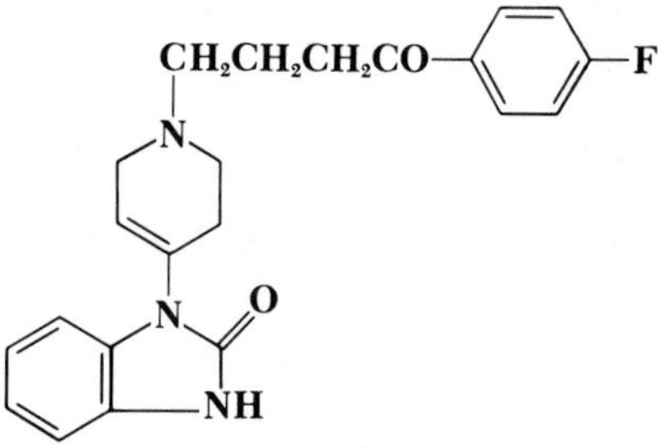

$CH_2CH_2CH_2CO$—F, N, N, O, NH

Droperidol

The butyrophenone **droperidol** (Inapsine) in combination with fentanyl, a meperidine-like analgesic, is often employed in *neuroleptanalgesia* and, with the addition of nitrous oxide, in *neuroleptanesthesia*. Although a fixed-ratio combination is available (Innovar), for repeated administration droperidol and fentanyl are usually administered separately because droperidol has a much longer duration of action.

OTHER ANTIPSYCHOTIC DRUGS

Although **molindone** and **loxapine** are structurally different, their pharmacology is similar to that of other antipsychotic drugs. Molindone, in particular, has a side effect profile like that of other potent neuroleptics.

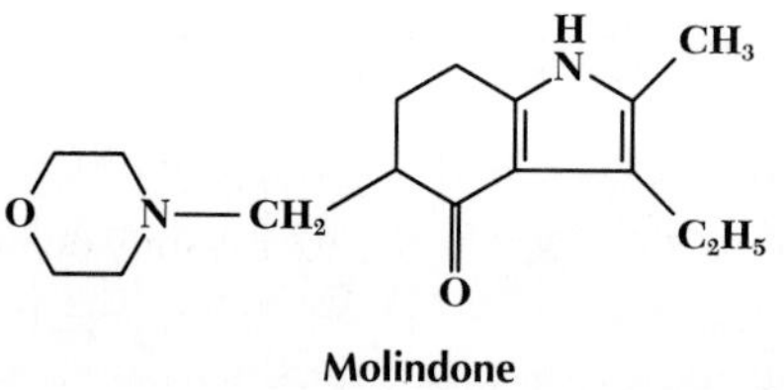

H, N, CH_3, O, N—CH_2, C_2H_5, O

Molindone

Clozapine, which is closely related structurally to loxapine, is an unusual (also called *atypical*) antipsychotic agent[11] that was approved for use in the United States in 1989, although it had been available in some countries for several years. It appears to differ from other antipsychotics in (1) having minimal propensity to cause acute extrapyramidal motor problems or tardive dyskinesia,[4] (2) being more effective therapy for both positive and negative symptoms of schizophrenia,[15] and (3) causing agranulocytosis with an estimated cumulative incidence of 1.3% to 1.6% after 1 year. The mechanism for the relative lack of extrapyramidal effects is unclear. To minimize the likelihood of life-threatening agranulocytosis, it is recommended that the drug be reserved for severely disturbed schizophrenics who do not respond to adequate trials with at least two other antipsychotics or for whom side effects have been intolerable.

The drug can be obtained only through the *Clozaril Patient Management System*, which provides for a 1 week supply and weekly white cell counts. Therapy should be interrupted if white blood cell and granulocyte counts fall below 3000 and 1500 per mm^3 respectively, in which case recovery is the rule. Agranulocytosis has occurred most commonly between 6 weeks and 6 months after initiation of therapy[14]; it should be possible to determine before this period of time whether or not a patient will respond favorably. Other adverse effects include drowsiness, dizziness, salivation, antimuscarinic effects, hypotension, mild temperature elevations, and dose-related seizures.[11] Clozapine is available as tablets, 25 and 100 mg; daily dosage should be increased gradually.

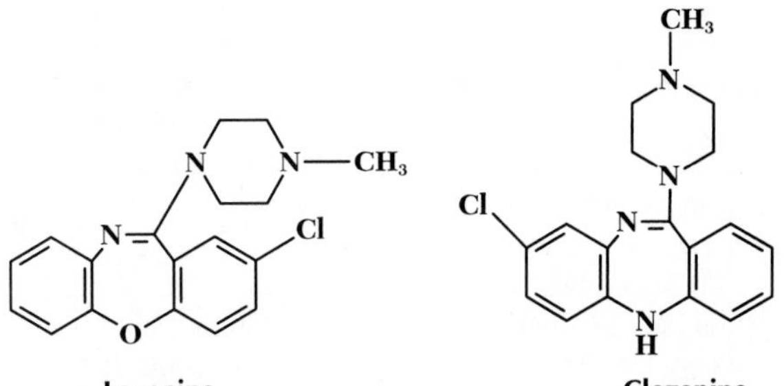

Loxapine

Clozapine

CHOOSING ANTIPSYCHOTIC DRUGS

Although the many antipsychotic drugs differ considerably in potency, relative propensity for particular side effects, and duration of action, aside from clozapine perhaps, there is little or no difference in therapeutic benefit when they are used in optimal dosage regimens. Thus it is generally accepted best for a clinician to become familiar with a few drugs representative of the various structural classes, rather than to use a great number of them. In order, thioridazine, haloperidol, and chlorpromazine are currently the most widely prescribed antipsychotics. Haloperidol has been favored for use in older patients and in hospitals and nursing homes.[20] There has been an unfortunate tendency toward greater use of the more potent agents in relatively high doses, even though moderate doses should be sufficient for most patients.[2]

REFERENCES

1. Awouters F, Niemegeers CJE, Janssen PAJ: 'Tardive' dyskinesia: etiological and therapeutic aspects, *Pharmacopsychiatry* 23:33, 1990.
2. Baldessarini RJ, Cohen BM, Teicher MH: Significance of neuroleptic dose and plasma level in the pharmacological treatment of psychoses, *Arch Gen Psychiatry* 45:79, 1988.
3. Black JL, Richelson E, Richardson JW: Antipsychotic agents: a clinical update, *Mayo Clin Proc* 60:777, 1985.
4. Casey DE: Clozapine: neuroleptic-induced EPS and tardive dyskinesia, *Psychopharmacology* 99:S47, 1989.
5. Casey DE, Keepers GA: Neuroleptic side effects: acute extrapyramidal syndromes and tardive dyskinesia. In Casey DE, Christensen AV, editors: *Psychopharmacology: current trends*, Berlin, 1988, Springer Verlag, p 74.
6. Clark WG, Lipton JM: Drug-related heatstroke. In Schönbaum E, Lomax P, editors: *Thermoregulation: pathology, pharmacology and therapy*, London, 1991, Pergamon Press, p 125.
7. Cold JA, Wells BG, Froemming JH: Seizure activity associated with antipsychotic therapy, *DICP Ann Pharmacother* 24:601, 1990.
8. Craig JB, Powell BL: Review: the management of nausea and vomiting in clinical oncology, *Am J Med Sci* 293:34, 1987.
9. Davis JM, Barter JT, Kane JM: Antipsychotic drugs. In Kaplan HI, Sadock BJ, editors: *Comprehensive textbook of psychiatry*, vol 2, ed 5, Baltimore, 1989, Williams & Wilkins, p 1591.
10. Drug Facts and Comparisons: St Louis, 1990, JB Lippincott Co.
11. Ereshefsky L, Watanabe MD, Tran-Johnson TK: Clozapine: an atypical antipsychotic agent, *Clin Pharm* 8:691, 1989.
12. Fleischhacker WW, Roth SD, Kane JM: The pharmacologic treatment of neuroleptic-induced akathisia, *J Clin Psychopharmacol* 10:12, 1990.
13. Jeste DV, Lohr JB, Clark K, Wyatt RJ: Pharmacological treatments of tardive dyskinesia in the 1980s, *J Clin Psychopharmacol* 8 (4, suppl):38S, 1988.
14. Kane JM: The current status of neuroleptic therapy, *J Clin Psychiatry* 50:322, 1989.
15. Kane J, Honigfeld G, Singer J, et al: Clozapine for the treatment-resistant schizophrenic: a double-blind comparison with chlorpromazine, *Arch Gen Psychiatry* 45:789, 1988.
16. Kris MG, Gralla RJ: Management of vomiting caused by anticancer drugs, *Adv Pain Res Ther* 16:337, 1990.
17. Lieberman J, Pollack S, Lesser M, Kane J: Pharmacologic characterization of tardive dyskinesia, *J Clin Psychopharmacol* 8:254, 1988.
18. Sitsen JMA: Prescription drugs and sexual function. In Sitsen JMA, editor: *Handbook of sexology*, vol 6: The pharmacology and endocrinology of sexual function, Amsterdam, 1988, Elsevier Science Publishers BV, p 425.
19. Wyatt RJ, Alexander RC, Egan MF, Kirch DG: Schizophrenia, just the facts: what do we know, how well do we know it? *Schizophrenia Res* 1:3, 1988.
20. Wysowski DK, Baum C: Antipsychotic drug use in the United States, 1976-1985, *Arch Gen Psychiatry* 46:929, 1989.

Chapter 28

Antidepressant and antimanic drugs

GENERAL CONCEPT

Affective disorders are the most frequent of the serious psychiatric illnesses. Most depressed persons are treated as outpatients by physicians who are not psychiatrists, partly because there are not enough psychiatrists to care for all such patients. For example, as many as 20% of elderly patients are estimated to be clinically depressed. The greatest danger to depressed patients is suicide, although the disease may also be characterized by severe physical and psychiatric debilitation.

A simple definition of severe depression is that it is sadness of duration and intensity that makes it incapacitating. Emotional complaints, which may not surface without probing, include apathy, hopelessness, guilt, disinterest in work or family, and preoccupation with tragedy or death. Physical complaints voiced frequently include abnormal eating and sleeping patterns, fatigue, headache, decreased libido, and vague gastrointestinal disturbances. There may be either psychomotor agitation or retardation.

According to the revised third edition of *Diagnostic and Statistical Manual of Mental Disorders*,[6] affective disorders fall into two major divisions. *Depressive disorders* include *major depression*, often referred to as unipolar, and *dysthymia*, a less severe but more continual problem with only brief periods of remission. *Bipolar disorders* include *bipolar disorder*, in which episodes of both mania and depression occur, and *cyclothymia*, again a milder but more continual disorder. Mania or less severe *hypomania* may appear when patients with bipolar disorder are treated with antidepressant drugs. There have been many other classifications, including *reactive* depression for lingering reactions to an identifiable personal disaster or setback and *endogenous* depression, which occurs without an established cause. Although an episode of major depression may include psychotic symptoms, depression associated with schizophrenia is just one of the numerous signs of psychosis. In the latter case, neuroleptics are the drugs of choice. Benzodiazepines may initially relieve some of the symptoms of depression but, except for alprazolam, are not likely to be of benefit for long-term relief.

Some depressed persons, especially those who have a reactive type, may respond to simple reassurance from family, friends, or physician. At the other extreme, profoundly depressed, delusional, catatonic, or suicidal persons may benefit from a course of electroconvulsive therapy. Antidepressant drugs are indicated for many of the rest.

Cyclic shifts between depression and normal affect tend to occur, even without medical intervention. Some patients need therapy only during episodes of depression. Others may benefit from maintenance treatment to decrease the incidence of relapse.

It is essential that patients be closely monitored initially and that they understand that drug-induced relief of depression is not immediate.

Monoamine oxidase (MAO) inhibitors were introduced as the first antidepressants. *Iproniazid*, the first MAO inhibitor used clinically, has been replaced by less toxic drugs. MAO inhibitors are generally reserved for depressed patients who respond poorly to other antidepressants.

The *tricyclic antidepressant* imipramine was discovered during clinical testing for antipsychotic drugs. Many related compounds then appeared, including two (desipramine and nortriptyline) that are active metabolites of other tricyclics. Later, a number of *second-generation* antidepressants were introduced. One of these, fluoxetine, quickly became the most often prescribed antidepressant drug. Current ideas about the mechanisms of action of antidepressants are discussed in Chapter 26.

A *central stimulant*, such as amphetamine or methylphenidate (see Chapter 31), may occasionally be used to provide more rapid relief from depression.[24]

MAO INHIBITORS

Types and actions

All of the MAO inhibitors currently approved as antidepressants are irreversible and nonspecific inhibitors of both MAO-A and MAO-B. Their initial attachment to the enzyme converts them to reactive compounds that bind covalently with the enzyme; such enzyme-activated agents are also termed mechanism-based or suicide inhibitors. Structurally, these compounds are hydrazines or nonhydrazines. Hydrazine drugs in current use are **phenelzine** and **isocarboxazid**. Phenelzine also appears effective in management of panic disorders,[15] which are classified as a form of anxiety. Adverse effects of these drugs include orthostatic hypotension, insomnia or sedation, hypertensive crises, and rare, but serious, hepatic necrosis,[30] associated with the hydrazine structure. Phenelzine may promote weight gain.

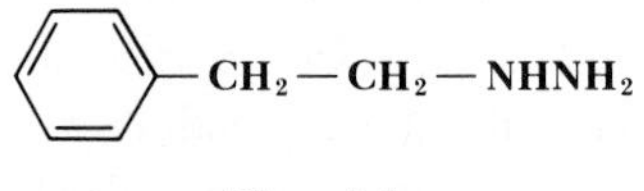

$C_6H_5-CH_2-CH_2-NHNH_2$

Phenelzine

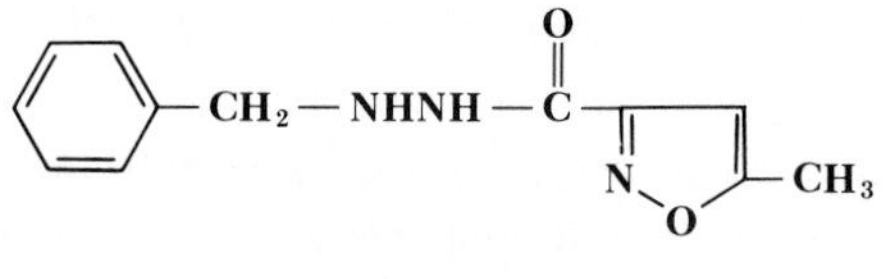

$C_6H_5-CH_2-NHNH-C(=O)-$ (isoxazole ring, N, O) $-CH_3$

Isocarboxazid

Tranylcypromine is a potent *nonhydrazine* MAO inhibitor related structurally to amphetamine; an amphetamine-like stimulant action may account for somewhat more rapid behavioral improvement. Like other MAO inhibitors tranylcypromine can cause orthostatic hypotension or, after ingestion of certain foods, hypertensive crisis. Its use should be closely supervised.

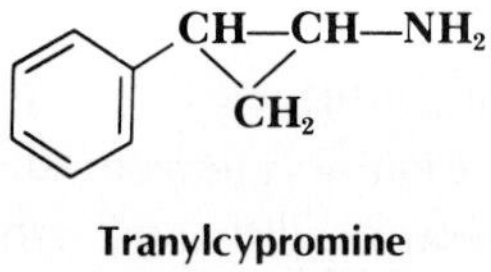

$C_6H_5-CH-CH-NH_2$ (cyclopropane ring with CH_2)

Tranylcypromine

The irreversible MAO-B inhibitor selegiline (L-deprenyl) is used to treat parkinsonism (see Chapter 30).

Potential for hypertensive crises during treatment with MAO inhibitors greatly limits their use. This response is usually associated with ingestion of foods or drinks that have fermented and so contain a high concentration of tyramine, or possibly another amine. Foods such as aged cheeses and some sausages, wines, and beer must be avoided.[4] Dietary monoamines are normally inactivated by MAO in the intestine (mostly MAO-A) and liver (predominately MAO-B). When both enzymes are inhibited irreversibly, sufficient tyramine may be absorbed to release norepinephrine from neurons that contain additional neurotransmitter because of MAO-A inhibition. Theoretically, a selective inhibitor of MAO-A would alleviate depression with less risk of hypertensive crisis; unaffected MAO-B in the liver should be sufficient to inactivate dietary tyramine. Unfortunately, clorgyline, an irreversible MAO-A inhibitor, has not exhibited greatly improved safety. However, recent studies of *reversible* MAO inhibitors, such as moclobemide, are more promising.[4] Ingestion of this short-acting compound after meals, so that its concentration in the gut is minimal while food is being absorbed, is unlikely to cause significant hypertension, even if a meal is rich in tyramine. Such reversible agents may benefit patients who cannot tolerate other antidepressant drugs or who exhibit a poor therapeutic response.

Interactions with other drugs

Combination with sympathomimetic drugs or levodopa, just as with tyramine in food, can cause hypertension,[13] whereas concurrent administration with agents that depress the brain can greatly lower blood pressure. Use of an MAO inhibitor with a tricyclic antidepressant or with the opioid meperidine may cause hyperthermia, delirium, convulsions, and coma. A withdrawal period of about 2 weeks is currently recommended for either MAO inhibitors or tricyclics before elective surgery or before initiating therapy with the other class of drugs. The same is true when shifting from one MAO inhibitor to another or before administration of meperidine. Nevertheless, there is evidence that tranylcypromine and amitriptyline can be safely taken together if the drugs are introduced concurrently. A tricyclic antidepressant may protect against a hypertensive response if tyramine is ingested.

TRICYCLIC ANTIDEPRESSANTS

The tricyclic antidepressants, which have in common two benzene rings separated by a seven-membered ring, are the agents most widely used in treating depression. Fig. 28-1 summarizes the chemical structures of the tricyclic drugs available in the United States. Major effects of these antidepressants derive from their ability to impair amine reuptake into neurons; to block transmission at muscarinic, α-adrenergic, and histamine receptors; and to mimic quinidine in the heart. Their adverse effect profiles overlap those of the phenothiazine neuroleptics, to which they are closely related structurally.

Pharmacokinetics

Tricyclic antidepressants are quite lipid-soluble. They are completely absorbed after ingestion but undergo considerable first-pass metabolism.[23] Inactivation is almost

FIG. 28-1 *Structural formulas of tricyclic antidepressants. Clomipramine differs from imipramine only in having a chlorine atom on one of the aromatic rings.*

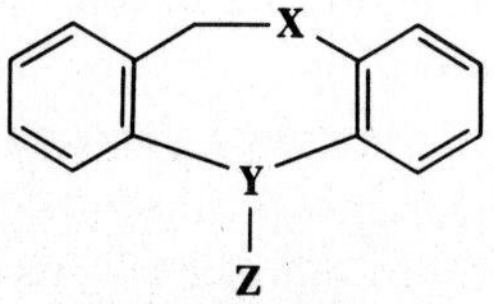

	X	Y	Z
Amitriptyline	C	C	$=CH(CH_2)_2N(CH_3)_2$
Desipramine	C	N	$(CH_2)_3NHCH_3$
Doxepin	O	C	$=CH(CH_2)_2N(CH_3)_2$
Imipramine	C	N	$(CH_2)_3N(CH_3)_2$
Nortriptyline	C	C	$=CH(CH_2)_2NHCH_3$
Protriptyline	$=C$	C	$(CH_2)_3NHCH_3$
Trimipramine	C	N	$CH_2\underset{CH_3}{\underset{\vert}{C}}HCH_2N(CH_3)_2$

Amoxapine

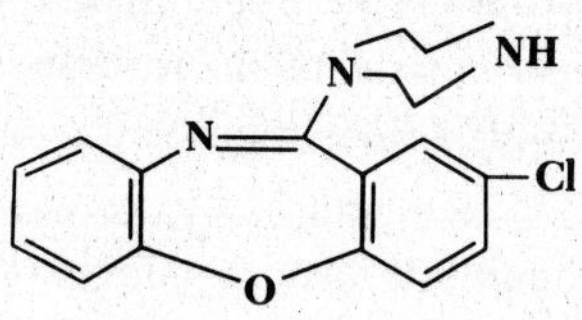

entirely hepatic. Tertiary amines may be demethylated to active secondary amines, for example, imipramine to desipramine (desmethylimipramine). Their rates of metabolism can vary greatly among individuals,[23] and determination of optimal dosage may be facilitated by monitoring plasma concentration.[19] Variability is due in part to the fact that these compounds are also hydroxylated by the same cytochrome P-450 isoenzyme that metabolizes debrisoquin and sparteine. Thus 8% to 10% of Caucasian patients hydroxylate the tricyclics poorly. The influence of this phenotype likely differs among the drugs. For example, due to reduced hydroxylation of imipramine, its demethylation to desipramine is likely to be enhanced in such patients, who would have higher plasma concentrations of the active metabolite, which itself is poorly metabolized. The net effect on efficacy becomes difficult to predict, and a higher plasma concentration would increase risk of toxicity. The frequency of the poor metabolizer phenotype provides a rationale for prospective phenotyping in Caucasian patients. In a patient known to be a poor metabolizer, doxepin, which does not appear to be metabolized by this isoenzyme, might be a good choice. In monitoring, if the prescribed drug has an active metabolite, concentrations of both are measured. Because the tricyclics bind extensively in tissues, as well as to plasma proteins, they have large volumes of distribution; hemodialysis is not an efficient treatment of intoxication.

Antidepressant effect

After a delay of 1 to 2 weeks, the tricyclic compounds elevate mood, increase alertness, and improve appetite in about 80% of depressed patients. Maximal benefit usually develops over 3 to 5 weeks of treatment. Unsatisfactory responses may be attributable to inadequate dosage, administration for too short a period, or lack of compliance; the last is often related to unacceptable side effects or lack of perceived improvement.

Dosage forms and side effect profiles of antidepressant drugs are summarized in Table 28-1. Imipramine pamoate (Tofranil-PM), in 75 to 150 mg capsules, is intended for once daily ingestion. The daily oral dosages are for otherwise healthy, adult outpatients. Gradually escalating from the lower dosages should minimize side effects. In general, lower dosages are indicated for adolescents, the elderly, or other patients with disorders that would be exacerbated by the anticholinergic, quinidine-like, or sedative actions of tricyclic antidepressants. On the other hand, larger dosages may be necessary for many patients.[19] Use in preadolescents[12] has not been approved except for the use of imipramine in management of enuresis. Sudden death of three children taking desipramine has been reported.[27]

Other uses and effects

In children 6 years of age or older, enuresis responds quickly to imipramine administration,[22] in contrast to the delay in antidepressant effect. The drug also alleviates agoraphobia, decreases the frequency of attacks in panic disorder,[15] and controls the cataplectic component of narcolepsy.[10] In the United States, obsessive-compulsive disorder is the only approved indication for clomipramine (chlorimipramine)[16]; it has responded best to this compound and perhaps other antidepressants that preferentially block serotonin uptake. Tricyclics may also prove beneficial in certain types of chronic pain, attention-deficit hyperactivity disorder in children, laughing or weeping spells in patients with multiple sclerosis, bulimia, and some types of drug abuse.

The anticholinergic action of the tricyclics causes dry mouth, blurred vision, constipation, and urinary retention. Disorientation and confusion are apparently related to a central anticholinergic action, since they can be counteracted with physostigmine. Cholinergic effects such as salivation and sweating may appear when tricyclic use is discontinued unless withdrawal is gradual.

Sedation may be considerable, and tricyclic drugs are often prescribed as a single maintenance dose at bedtime, once a satisfactory response has developed. Most persons eventually become tolerant to the sedative action. Excessive weight gain can occur. The frequency of extrapyramidal side effects is much lower than that with phenothiazines.

Orthostatic hypotension is the most common cardiovascular side effect in healthy patients receiving therapeutic doses of tricyclic antidepressants. Nortriptyline and, perhaps, trimipramine seem to be the safest in this regard.[2,20] A modest increase in heart rate is common and partially attributable to muscarinic blockade. Slowing of atrioventricular (His-ventricular) conduction can culminate in heart block if the patient already has a conduction disorder.[20] Actions on the heart may be beneficial in some patients with ventricular arrhythmias, but intoxication is characterized by arrhythmias typical of quinidine. Extra caution and initiation of therapy with lower doses is important in the elderly and in patients with preexisting cardiovascular disease.

TABLE 28-1 Antidepressants: synopsis of clinical response and dose

Compound	Adverse effects*			Usual daily oral dose (mg)	Dosage forms‡ (mg)
	Cardiovascular†	Anticholinergic	Sedative		
MAO inhibitors					
Isocarboxazid (Marplan)	H	L§	±	10-30	T: 10
Phenelzine sulfate (Nardil)	H	L§	±	15-60	T: 15
Tranylcypromine sulfate (Parnate)	H	L§	±	30-60	T: 10
Tricyclics					
Amitriptyline hydrochloride (Elavil, Endep)	H	H	H	50-150	T: 10-50 ;V: 100/10 ml
Amoxapine (Asendin)	L	M	M	100-300	T: 25-150
Clomipramine hydrochloride‖ (Anafranil)	M	H	H	25-250	C: 25-75
Desipramine hydrochloride (Norpramin, Pertofrane)	M	L	L	100-200	C: 25, 50 ;T: 10-150
Doxepin hydrochloride (Adapin, Sinequan)	H	M	H	75-150	C: 10-150; S: 1200/120 ml
Imipramine hydrochloride (Tofranil, others)	H	M	M	50-150	T: 10-50 ;A: 25/2 ml
Nortriptyline hydrochloride (Aventyl, Pamelor)	M	M	L	75-100	C: 10-75 ;S: 10/5 ml
Protriptyline hydrochloride (Vivactil)	H	H	L	15-40	T: 5,10
Trimipramine maleate (Surmontil)	M	M	H	75-150	C: 25-100
Miscellaneous					
Trazodone hydrochloride (Desyrel)	M	±	M	150-400	T: 50-300
Fluoxetine hydrochloride (Prozac)	±	±	±	20-80	C: 20; S:20/5 ml
Maprotiline hydrochloride (Ludiomil)	L	M	M	75-150	T: 25-75
Bupropion hydrochloride (Wellbutrin)	L	M	M	200-300	T: 75,100

*Incidence: *H*, High; *M*, moderate; *L*, low; ±; minimal or none.
†Labile blood pressure or abnormal electrocardiographic tracing.
‡*A*, Ampule; *C*, capsule; *S*, solution (oral); *T*, tablet; *V*, vial.
§Not due to direct muscarinic receptor block.
‖For obsessive-compulsive disorder.

Intoxication Based on reports from poison control centers, acute tricyclic poisoning carries a relatively high risk of death.[14] As one would expect, acute intoxication may be characterized by anticholinergic effects and in severe cases by quinidine-like disturbances in cardiac rhythm, such as a prolonged Q-T interval and widened QRS complex.[18,20] QRS prolongation to more than 0.1 second may portend arrhythmias or seizures. Patients with such an ECG change should be admitted and monitored closely, even if other symptoms have not developed. Respiratory depression and other problems such as pneumonia and pulmonary edema, acidosis, hyperthermia, and coma can also occur. Treatment includes gastric lavage, alkalinization with bicarbonate, and support of respiration and blood pressure.[8,18] Administration of activated charcoal and a cathartic may also reduce absorption of the drug. Diazepam can be given to control seizures. Lidocaine or phenytoin may control ventricular arrhythmias, but Class III and quinidine- or flecainide-like Class I antiarrhythmics (see Chapter 39) should be avoided. Although physostigmine can reverse central nervous system and peripheral manifestations of anticholinergic activity, the drug should probably not be used to treat tricyclic intoxication because of its potential for severe bradycardia, hypotension, and seizures.[11]

Interactions with other drugs

Tricyclic antidepressants prevent the antihypertensive actions of guanethidine and the hypertensive action of amphetamine by blocking the amine pump that transports these compounds into the adrenergic neuron. Anticholinergic drugs and central nervous system depressants should be used cautiously in patients taking a tricyclic antidepressant because of additive actions. The interaction with MAO inhibitors is discussed on p. 255.

SECOND GENERATION ANTIDEPRESSANTS

The tricyclic antidepressants are effective and relatively inexpensive, but they are less than optimal on the issues of safety, patient acceptance, and speed of onset. Several new drugs with diverse structures, known collectively as *second-generation* antidepressants, are now available or are in clinical trials.[21] In particular, fluoxetine has a more favorable side effect profile and is widely used.

The tricyclic **amoxapine** is a demethylated congener of the neuroleptic loxapine. It blocks dopamine receptors, and extrapyramidal responses have been reported. Seizures during intoxication are relatively common with this agent.

Alprazolam (Zanax), a benzodiazepine, differs from other members of its class (see Chapter 29) in being useful against depression.[21] In treatment of panic disorder[1] it causes fewer side effects and perhaps a more rapid response than classic antidepressants do. Problems with dependence and withdrawal are a concern with all benzodiazepines.

Fluoxetine

The chief action of fluoxetine is selective inhibition of serotonin, rather than norepinephrine or dopamine, uptake. Unlike tricyclic antidepressants, this drug lacks antagonistic activity at muscarinic, adrenergic, and histaminic receptors. Its effects on the autonomic and cardiovascular systems are correspondingly benign. Adverse effects include insomnia, more often than drowsiness; anorexia with weight loss, rather than weight gain; as well as anxiety, nausea, and diarrhea.[3,7] Akathisia, adverse interactions with MAO inhibitors, and a preoccupation with suicide have been reported recently.[7] Fluoxetine may prove to be of benefit in obsessive-compulsive disorder and as an appetite suppressant. It has a long half-life (1 to 3 days) and an even longer acting active metabolite, norfluoxetine; half-life is prolonged with chronic use.

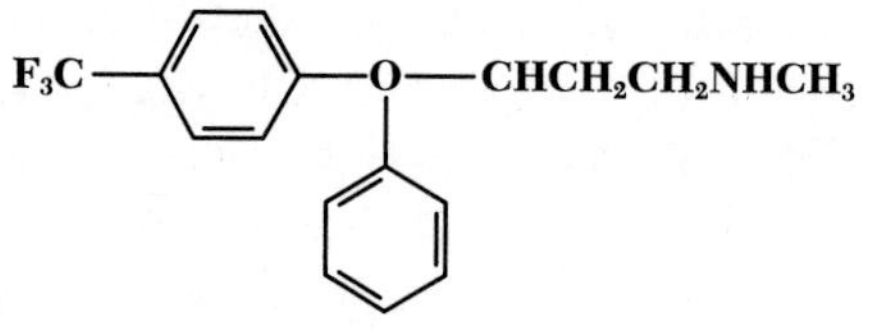

Fluoxetine

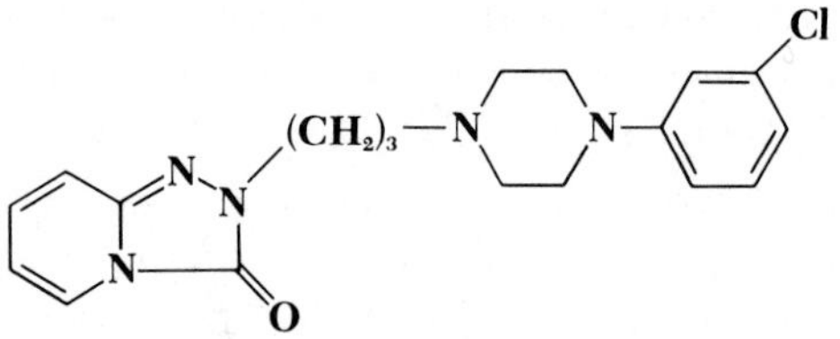

Trazodone

Trazodone

Trazodone also inhibits serotonin uptake and, perhaps partially as the longer acting metabolite *m*-chlorophenylpiperazine (*m*-CPP), stimulates serotonin receptors. Advantages are its lack of appreciable antimuscarinic activity and relative safety in acute intoxication. The primary serious effects of intoxication are hypotension and central nervous system depression. No deaths have been reported from trazodone intoxication alone. Males should discontinue trazodone if they develop abnormal erectile activity, estimated to occur in one of 6000 patients. More than 100 cases of priapism, which has often required surgery, have been reported.[21] This response is generally attributed to α-adrenergic receptor blockade, unopposed by muscarinic blockade.

Maprotiline

Maprotiline has a long half-life and a spectrum of activities intermediate to those of the tricyclics. It is recommended that outpatient treatment be initiated at a low dosage for 2 weeks, then slowly escalated to no more than 225 mg per day; this cautious approach should minimize precipitation of seizures, which occurred disproportionately in early studies. As with amoxapine, seizures occur relatively often in intoxication.

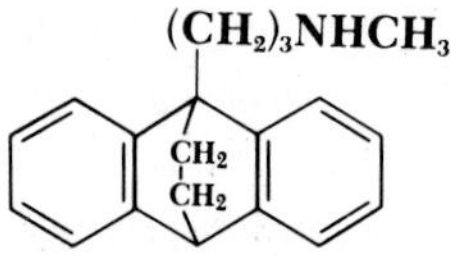

Maprotiline

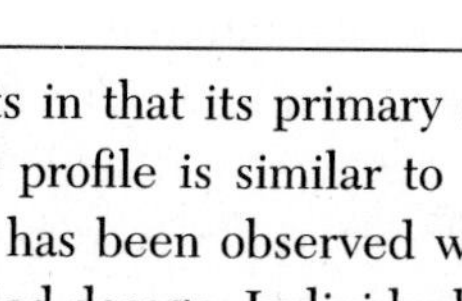

Bupropion

Bupropion

Bupropion is unique among antidepressants in that its primary action is interference with uptake of dopamine. Its side effect profile is similar to that of fluoxetine except that a seizure incidence of about 0.4% has been observed when daily dosage was 450 mg or less,[5] the maximum recommended dosage. Individual doses should not exceed 150 mg (100 mg initially).

LITHIUM CARBONATE IN TREATMENT OF MANIA

Lithium ion lessens the intensity of the manic phase of manic-depressive (bipolar) psychosis. In 1949 Cade[9] of Australia studied its effect on psychotic behavior after the observation that lithium carbonate caused lethargy in guinea pigs. Li^+ may also be of benefit as prophylaxis for both unipolar and bipolar disorders[17] and in depressed (unipolar) patients who have responded poorly to an antidepressant alone.[25]

Li^+ is distributed in total body water, and its renal elimination is proportional to its concentration in plasma. The ion is reabsorbed only in the proximal tubule, in proportion to Na^+ and water reabsorption.[28] Li^+ retention and the potential for toxicity are increased by factors that enhance fractional reabsorption in the proximal tubule. These are primarily dehydration and Na^+ depletion and, secondarily, certain diuretics, such as the thiazides.

Patients in an acute manic phase require about 600 mg of lithium carbonate three times a day to produce a target serum Li^+ concentration, determined 8 to 12 hours after the previous dose, of 0.9 to no more than 1.4 mEq/L. Continuous therapy for a week or more may be needed before manic signs abate, and more rapid control may be achieved by temporary coadministration of a neuroleptic or possibly carbamazepine (see Chapter 32). Dosage is reduced for maintenance; a concentration of 0.6 to 0.8 mEq/L is sufficient for most patients.[17,29]

Chronic Li^+ therapy causes nephrogenic diabetes insipidus in a substantial number of patients. Impaired renal concentrating ability manifests as increased thirst, urine volume, and frequency of urination. Glomerular function is unimpaired.[26] Hypothyroidism may develop after prolonged treatment.

Nausea, weight gain, diarrhea, memory impairment, tremor, and ataxia are mild adverse effects of Li^+. Moderately severe symptoms include hyperactive reflexes and spasticity. Very severe reactions such as peripheral circulatory collapse, convulsions, coma, and death are associated with serum Li^+ concentrations of 2.5 mEq/L or more. One can hasten Li^+ elimination by increasing Na^+ excretion, but hemodialysis is the most effective method for removing Li^+ in an emergency.

Lithium carbonate is available in capsules (Eskalith, Lithonate) containing 150 to 600 mg, regular tablets (Eskalith, others) containing 300 mg, and in controlled-release tablets containing 300 mg (Lithobid) or 450 mg (Eskalith-CR). A syrup (Cibalith-S) of lithium citrate is also available; it provides the equivalent of 300 mg of lithium carbonate in 5 ml.

REFERENCES

1. Ballenger JC, Burrows GD, DuPont RL, Jr, et al: Alprazolam in panic disorder and agoraphobia: results from a multicenter trial. I. Efficacy in short-term treatment, *Arch Gen Psychiatry* 45:413, 1988.
2. Cole JO, Bodkin JA: Antidepressant drug side effects, *J Clin Psychiatry* 51(1, suppl):21, 1990.
3. Cooper GL: The safety of fluoxetine—an update, *Br J Psychiatry* 153(suppl 3):77, 1988.
4. Da Prada M, Zürcher G, Wüthrich I, Haefely WE: On tyramine, food, beverages and the reversible MAO inhibitor moclobemide, *J Neural Transm* 26(suppl): 31, 1988.
5. Davidson J: Seizures and bupropion: a review, *J Clin Psychiatry* 50:256, 1989.
6. *Diagnostic and statistical manual of mental disorders*, ed 3, revised, Washington, 1987, The American Psychiatric Association.
7. Fluoxetine (Prozac) revisited, *Med Lett Drugs Ther* 32:83, 1990.
8. Frommer DA, Kulig KW, Marx JA, Rumack B: Tricyclic antidepressant overdose: a review, *JAMA* 257:521, 1987.
9. Johnson FN: *The history of lithium therapy*, London, 1984, The Macmillan Press Ltd.
10. Kales A, Vela-Bueno A, Kales JD: Sleep disorders: sleep apnea and narcolepsy, *Ann Intern Med* 106:434, 1987.
11. Kirk M, Kulig K, Rumack BH: Anticholin-

ergics. In Haddad LM, Winchester JF, editors: *Clinical management of poisoning and drug overdose*, ed 2, Philadelphia, 1990, WB Saunders Co, p 861.

12. Lapierre YD, Raval KJ: Pharmacotherapy of affective disorders in children and adolescents, *Psychiatr Clin North Am* 12:951, 1989.
13. Lippman SB, Nash K: Monoamine oxidase inhibitor update: potential adverse food and drug interactions, *Drug Safety* 5:195, 1990.
14. Litovitz TL, Schmitz BF, Bailey KM: 1989 annual report of the American Association of Poison Control Centers National Data Collection System, *Am J Emerg Med* 8:394, 1990.
15. Lydiard RB, Ballenger JC: Antidepressants in panic disorder and agoraphobia, *J Affective Disord* 13:153, 1987.
16. McTavish D, Benfield P: Clomipramine: an overview of its pharmacological properties and a review of its therapeutic use in obsessive compulsive disorder and panic disorder, *Drugs* 39:136, 1990.
17. NIMH/NIH Consensus Development Panel: Mood disorders: pharmacologic prevention of recurrences, *Am J Psychiatry* 142:469, 1985.
18. Pentel PR, Keyler DE, Haddad LM: Tricyclic and newer antidepressants. In Haddad LM, Winchester JF, editors: *Clinical management of poisoning and drug overdose*, ed 2, Philadelphia, 1990, WB Saunders Co, p 636.
19. Preskorn SH: Tricyclic antidepressants: the whys and hows of therapeutic drug monitoring, *J Clin Psychiatry* 50(7, suppl):34, 1989.
20. Roose SP, Glassman AH: Cardiovascular effects of tricyclic antidepressants in depressed patients with and without heart disease, *J Clin Psychiatry Monogr* 7(2):1, 1989.
21. Rudorfer MV, Potter WZ: Antidepressants: a comparative review of the clinical pharmacology and therapeutic use of the 'newer' *versus* the 'older' drugs, *Drugs* 37:713, 1989.
22. Rushton HG: Nocturnal enuresis: epidemiology, evaluation, and currently available treatment options, *J Pediatr* 114:691, 1989.
23. Sallee FR, Pollock BG: Clinical pharmacokinetics of imipramine and desipramine, *Clin Pharmacokinet* 18:346, 1990.
24. Satel SL, Nelson JC: Stimulants in the treatment of depression: a critical overview, *J Clin Psychiatry* 50:241, 1989.
25. Schöpf J: Treatment of depressions resistant to tricyclic antidepressants, related drugs or MAO-inhibitors by lithium addition: review of the literature, *Pharmacopsychiatry* 22:174, 1989.
26. Schou M, Vestergaard P: Prospective studies on a lithium cohort. 2. Renal function: water and electrolyte metabolism, *Acta Psychiatr Scand* 78:427, 1988.
27. Sudden death in children treated with a tricyclic antidepressant, *Med Lett Drugs Ther* 32:53, 1990.
28. Thomsen K: Excretion. In Johnson FN, editor: *Depression and mania. Modern lithium therapy*, Oxford, 1987, IRL Press, p 75.
29. Vestergaard P, Schou M: Prospective studies on a lithium cohort. 1. General features, *Acta Psychiatr Scand* 78:421, 1988.
30. Zimmerman HJ, Ishak KG: The hepatic injury of monoamine oxidase inhibitors, *J Clin Psychopharmacol* 7:211, 1987.

Chapter 29

Antianxiety and hypnotic drugs and alcohol

GENERAL CONSIDERATIONS

Many compounds from two chemical classes allay anxiety and promote sleep. The newer *benzodiazepines* have largely replaced the *barbiturates* for these indications, primarily because they are much safer in acute intoxication[29] and because their potential for chronic abuse, and the severity of withdrawal associated with such abuse, is less. Specific barbiturates still have important uses in control of epilepsy (see Chapter 32) and for induction of anesthesia. The therapeutic agents from both classes are general central nervous system depressants. They produce some, if not all, of their effects via interactions with the $GABA_A$ receptor complex (see Chapter 26).

Anxiety

Anxiety is a familiar disorder that is ordinarily productive. It merits medical attention only when it becomes so counterproductive that it is psychologically paralyzing. Administration of antianxiety drugs is the most common means for reducing anxiety to a level with which patients can cope. However, certain disorders classified as anxiety, such as agoraphobia (with or without panic attacks) or panic disorder, respond better to drugs considered to be primarily antidepressants.[1] Anxieties that are prominent components of painful or paroxysmal organic diseases, such as angina pectoris or thyrotoxicosis, often vanish with treatment directed at the underlying condition.

Although benzodiazepines used to relieve anxiety were once called "*minor* tranquilizers," the term is misleading. It implies that they are simply less efficacious versions of phenothiazines. In fact, antipsychotic and antianxiety drugs differ greatly in their mechanisms of action (see Chapter 26), in the beneficial and untoward effects they induce, and in indications for their use.

Benzodiazepine derivatives are currently the dominant drugs for management of *generalized anxiety disorder*. The structures of the benzodiazepines currently available in the United States are summarized on the next page. The last three compounds contain an additional ring in their structure. Alprazolam and triazolam are termed *triazolo*benzodiazepines because this ring contains three nitrogens.

Insomnia

Insomnia is by far the most prevalent sleep disorder; over 40% of the population report a current or past problem. This complaint is more frequent with increasing age, in women, and in persons with high levels of psychologic distress.

Transient sleep disturbances are extremely prevalent and may relate to situational problems at home or at work or involving finances. Jet travel or changes in work shift may disrupt circadian rhythms and disturb sleep. Medical conditions with significant

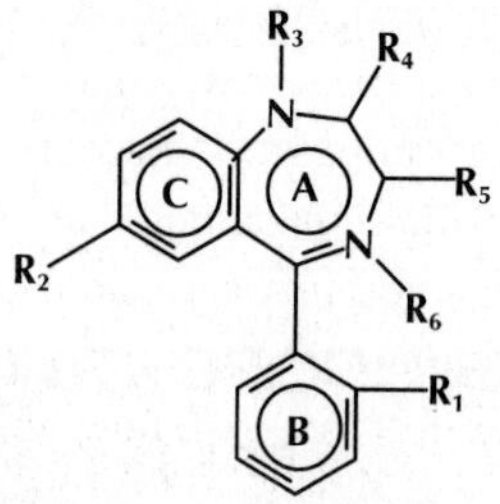

	R_1	R_2	R_3	R_4	R_5	R_6
Chlordiazepoxide		Cl		$NHCH_3$		$\rightarrow O$
Clonazepam	Cl	NO_2		$=O$		
Clorazepate		Cl		$(OH)_2$	COOH	
Diazepam		Cl	CH_3	$=O$		
Flurazepam	F	Cl	$CH_2CH_2N(C_2H_5)_2$	$=O$		
Halazepam		Cl	CH_2CF_3	$=O$		
Lorazepam	Cl	Cl		$=O$	OH	
Oxazepam		Cl		$=O$	OH	
Prazepam		Cl	CH_2—◁	$=O$		
Quazepam	F	Cl	CH_2CF_3	$=S$		
Temazepam		Cl	CH_3	$=O$	OH	

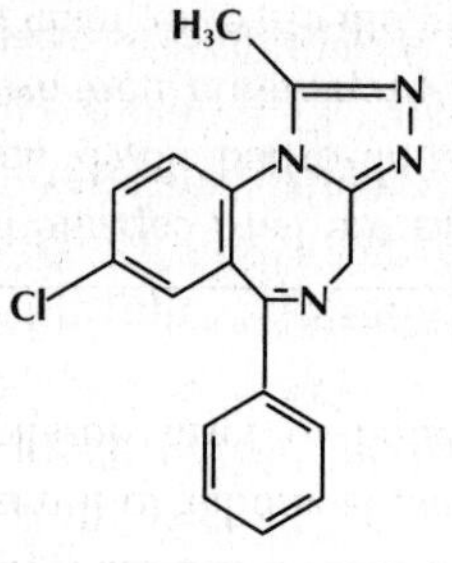

Alprazolam 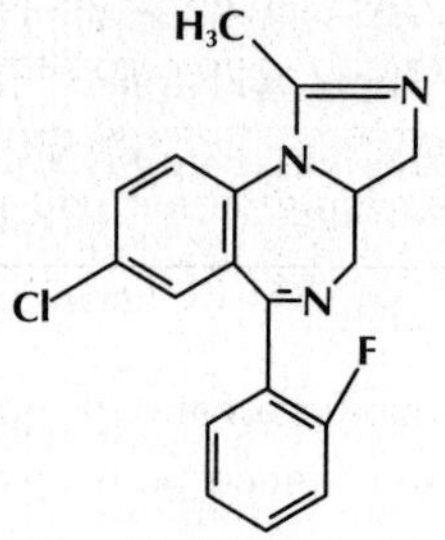 **Midazolam** 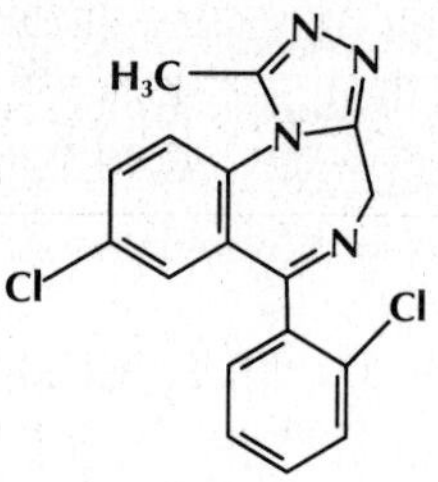 **Triazolam**

pain, physical discomfort, anxiety, or depression are likely to produce complaints of insomnia. Furthermore, elderly people sleep less and have very little of the deeper sleep at stages 3 and 4. A change in sleep pattern that is a physiologic component of aging may be misinterpreted by an elderly patient as being abnormal and requiring treatment. Reassurance and an appropriate explanation often suffices in this setting.

Pharmacologic agents, such as stimulants, steroids, antidepressants, or β-adrenergic antagonists, can disrupt sleep, particularly when taken near bedtime. Coffee or cola drinks as well as cigarette smoking may delay sleep. Abrupt withdrawal of high doses of drugs used to promote sleep can cause an abstinence syndrome that may include both insomnia and nightmares. Alcohol consumption or use of benzodiazepines with a rapid elimination rate may produce early morning insomnia.

Although medical conditions and aging may often contribute to chronic insomnia, psychopathology is the predominant etiologic factor. Personality patterns of most patients with chronic insomnia are characterized by an internalization of emotions. Retrospective studies indicate that chronic insomnia may develop in persons who have inadequate coping mechanisms for life-stress factors.

A thorough evaluation of patients with chronic insomnia includes taking sleep, drug, and psychiatric histories. The sleep history should include determination of the specific sleep problem and assessment of its clinical course, exclusion of other sleep disorders, evaluation of sleep/wakefulness patterns, questioning of close family members, and evaluation of the impact of the sleep problem on the patient's life.

The drug history should include information on current use of prescribed and nonprescribed medication and the timing of its administration, particularly in relation to bedtime, as well as on dosage and length of administration of any sedative-hypnotics recently discontinued. Also included should be a review of current or past use of alcohol, caffeine, and nicotine.

TREATMENT

By definition, hypnotic drugs are used to promote sleep. Such agents are only an adjunctive component of the overall therapy of insomnia[9,15] and, if used at all, are best taken only for brief periods. Since transient insomnia usually develops in reaction to some immediate stress, it can be expected to subside when patients adapt through their own coping mechanisms. If the stress-generating situation cannot be eliminated, the physician is best able to help over the long term by identifying adaptive coping mechanisms and by aiding the patient to strengthen them.

Treatment of chronic insomnia is more complex because it is multifaceted. In general, the most effective treatment for chronic insomnia combines the following elements: (1) nonpharmacologic treatment, including improvement of sleep hygiene (regularizing schedules including time for bed, gradually increasing levels of physical exercise during the day, restricting use of caffeinated beverages, and avoiding use of alcohol as a sedative), supportive counseling, behavioral therapy, and psychotherapy and (2) pharmacologic treatment consisting in adjunctive use of hypnotic medication or possibly antidepressant medication. A hypnotic with an intermediate elimination half-life of 8 to 10 hours may be the best choice.

Hypnotic compounds are also sedative at lower doses. For about 100 years the bromides and, after the turn of the century, the barbiturates and chloral hydrate were the only medications available to calm agitated patients, from the anxious neurotic to the most disturbed psychotic.

Tolerance to the hypnotic action of barbiturates develops fairly rapidly and may lead to use of higher doses. This increases the potential for dependence and an abstinence syndrome after abrupt withdrawal. Another concern with these substances is their rather narrow margin of safety.

Currently the most commonly used hypnotics are benzodiazepines. Flurazepam was the first of these marketed specifically to relieve insomnia. Triazolam and temazepam are now more often prescribed for this indication. Barbiturates and a few other nonbenzodiazepine drugs are still used as hypnotics, albeit to a much lesser extent.

BENZODIAZEPINES

The clinical effects of biologically active benzodiazepines are qualitatively similar, even though certain benzodiazepines are approved and marketed specifically for purposes other than relief of anxiety. Flurazepam and quazepam (long half-life metabolites), temazepam (intermediate half-life), and triazolam (short half-life) are promoted as hypnotics, midazolam is used for diagnostic or perioperative situations, and clonazepam is offered as an anticonvulsant (see p. 314).

In animal models of epilepsy, convulsant compounds are antagonized by benzodiazepines. In this respect benzodiazepines are similar to phenobarbital but different from phenothiazines or reserpine, which lower seizure threshold. Intravenous diazepam has been the primary treatment for status epilepticus and seizures induced by drugs or toxins, but many neurologists now prefer lorazepam for this indication. Diazepam, which is believed to relax skeletal muscle by depressing reflex pathways, is also prescribed to relieve spontaneous muscle spasms and those associated with procedures such as endoscopy. Alprazolam, perhaps the most prescribed benzodiazepine, has clinically useful antidepressant activity.[28] It is also beneficial in alleviating agoraphobia and panic disorder.[33]

Kinetics

Circulating concentrations of benzodiazepines taken orally generally peak between 1 and 3 hours. Chlordiazepoxide is poorly absorbed after intramuscular injection. Diazepam is well absorbed from the deltoid but less well absorbed from gluteal sites; such injections may cause considerable pain if propylene glycol is the solvent. Lorazepam is well absorbed by the intramuscular route, but may also be painful. Highly lipid soluble agents such as diazepam and midazolam readily distribute into tissues; an intravenous bolus will have a rapid but relatively short action in the brain because the drug quickly distributes to other organs (similar to thiopental, p. 272). Benzodiazepines readily cross the placenta and, with chronic administration, tend to accumulate in the fetus.

Several benzodiazepines, including chlordiazepoxide, diazepam, halazepam, chlorazepate, and prazepam, are converted in the stomach or by the hepatic microsomal system to one or more active metabolites; of these desmethyldiazepam has an elimination half-life of 36 to 200 hours.[10] This metabolite is responsible for much or all of the activity of the last two compounds. Flurazepam is converted to two rapidly eliminated metabolites (hydroxyethylflurazepam and flurazepam aldehyde) and one that is slowly eliminated (desalkylflurazepam with a half-life of 40 to 250 hours). Factors such as age, liver disease, or concurrent therapy with cimetidine can decrease the clearance of such benzodiazepines. Lorazepam, oxazepam, and temazepam are excreted as glucuronide conjugates, and their metabolism is relatively unaffected by these factors. Active metabolites of triazolam and alprazolam probably contribute little to their therapeutic effect.[7] The half-lives of active benzodiazepines range from 2 hours or less for triazolam and midazolam to as long as 250 hours for desalkylflurazepam (Table 29-1).

Mechanism of action

In animals, benzodiazepines cause calming and taming effects similar to those of barbiturates. However, in contrast to the barbiturates, these effects occur at doses

TABLE 29-1 Characteristics of benzodiazepine anxiolytics and hypnotics

Drug	Elimination half-life*[10] (hr)	Anxiolytic dose (mg/day)	Hypnotic dose (mg)	Dosage forms† (mg)	Contribution from active metabolite(s)‡
Long acting					
Diazepam (Valium, others)	20-200	4-40	2-10	C: 15; T: 2-10; S: 5/ml; I: 5/ml	+
Chlordiazepoxide (Librium, others)	5-200	15-100		C: 5-25; T: 5-25; P: 100	+
Chlorazepate dipotassium (Tranxene, Gen-Xene)	36-200	15-60		C: 3.75-15; T: 3.75-22.5	+ +
Halazepam (Paxipam)	14-200	60-160		T: 20, 40	+
Prazepam (Centrax)	36-200	20-60		C: 5-20; T: 10	+ +
Flurazepam hydrochloride (Dalmane)	40-250		15-30	C: 15, 30	+ +
Quazepam (Doral)	40-250		7.5-15	T: 7.5, 15	+
Clonazepam (Klonopin)	30-60	1.5-20§		T: 0.5-2	–
Intermediate acting					
Alprazolam (Xanax)	8-15	0.75-4		T: 0.25-1	–
Lorazepam (Ativan)	10-20	2-6		T: 0.5-2; I: 2,4/ml	–
Oxazepam (Serax, Zaxopam)	4-15	30-120		C: 10-30; T: 15	–
Temazepam (Restoril)	8-22		15-30	C: 15,30	–
Short acting					
Midazolam hydrochloride (Versed)	<5		7.5-15‖	I: 1,5/ml	–
Triazolam (Halcion)	<5		0.125-0.5	T: 0.125, 0.25	–

*$T_{1/2}$ of β phase of elimination from plasma; pertains to parent compound and any active metabolites.
†*C*, Capsule; *I*, injection; *P*, powder for reconsitution and injection; *S*, solution (oral); *T*, tablet.
‡+ +, Metabolite(s) primarily account for activity; +, metabolites contribute to activity; –, contribution from metabolites negligible.
§For anticonvulsant activity.
‖Not available for oral administration.

considerably lower than those that decrease activity or induce sleepiness. Benzodiazepines consistently attenuate the effects of punishment or lack of reward on animal behavior; again, sedation is not a necessary component. Benzodiazepines usually reduce both evoked and spontaneous hostility and aggressive behavior, but their disinhibitory effects may also increase aggression.

High-affinity binding of benzodiazepines has been demonstrated in several brain sites, such as the cortex, hippocampus, amygdala, and reticular formation. Understanding of the physiologic importance of these receptors awaits definitive demonstration of an endogenous ligand(s). The interaction between benzodiazepines and GABA regulation of Cl^- channels is discussed in Chapter 26.

Adverse effects

Benzodiazepines cause drowsiness, ataxia, paradoxical excitement, and altered libido. With continued therapy, tolerance develops to drowsiness, the most common unwanted effect, whereas anxiolytic effectiveness is apparently retained. Even with massive overdose the victim can often be aroused, but caution should be exercised in using benzodiazepines with other central nervous system depressants. In elderly patients, diminished alertness from these drugs may be mistaken for signs of senility or contribute to falling and risk of fractures. It is recommended that benzodiazepines be avoided in the first trimester of pregnancy to minimize risk of congenital malformations.

When used for brief periods (weeks) to promote sleep, *rebound insomnia* and *rebound anxiety* (noticeable increases in wakefulness and in daytime anxiety, respectively) may appear. The potential for rebound is related to rate of benzodiazepine elimination and to rate of change in occupancy of benzodiazepine receptors. Thus after abrupt discontinuation of a short-acting benzodiazepine these symptoms usually occur and may be severe.[14] When a long-acting benzodiazepine is withdrawn, such effects occur infrequently and are relatively mild, possibly because the brain has sufficient time to adapt as the drug is slowly eliminated.

Dependence is a proper concern when benzodiazepines are taken for months to years,[31] although psychologic dependence is uncharacteristic of patients without a history of drug abuse.[36] Regular long-term use of therapeutic doses is usually a response to chronic physical (cardiovascular, arthritic) and emotional problems rather than abuse of the drug for pleasurable mental effects. Physical dependence develops when usage is prolonged, or dosage is excessive, or both. Abrupt discontinuation then evokes an abstinence syndrome (gastrointestinal and sleep disturbances, anxiety, tremor, sweating, headache, hypersensitivity to various sensory stimuli, and so forth) that is occasionally severe.[24] If mild, it may be very difficult to distinguish from rebound phenomena or recurrence of the original anxious state. Seizures have occurred in dependent persons who took larger than therapeutic doses for many months. The addictive liability of benzodiazepines is lower than that of meprobamate or barbiturates. Nevertheless, a prudent prescriber takes certain precautions: (1) benzodiazepines should be used cautiously, if at all, for persons with a history of drug abuse; (2) dosage should be titrated so that daily intake is not needlessly large; (3) an expected duration of treatment should be identified at the outset so that drug taking is not prolonged through lack of planning.

Anterograde amnesia from a benzodiazepine is not uncommon,[11,25] especially after parenteral administration. This response, though usually undesirable, is one of the reasons for including a benzodiazepine in the presurgical regimen of balanced anesthesia and for their use in outpatient invasive procedures such as endoscopy.

Life-threatening reactions like agranulocytosis are very rare, and deaths from benzodiazepines alone seldom occur. Considering the extent to which benzodiazepines are used worldwide, the incidence of toxicity must be very low indeed.

Benzodiazepines used primarily for hypnosis

FLURAZEPAM

Flurazepam has been studied more extensively than any other hypnotic agent. With short-term administration of 30 mg, there is appreciable improvement in sleep, both in terms of induction and maintenance.[14] When used on consecutive nights, peak effectiveness occurs on the second and third nights. The metabolites of the drug with a short elimination half-life largely account for activity on the first night, but the long half-life metabolite desalkylflurazepam is the most active agent thereafter.[21]

An important consideration is that the effectiveness of flurazepam, in contrast to that of most nonbenzodiazepine hypnotics and shorter acting benzodiazepines, is maintained with consecutive nightly administration over a 2-week period.[14] This apparent lack of tolerance may reflect accumulation of desalkylflurazepam, which should require 10 to 20 days to reach steady state.

During the first 2 to 3 nights after withdrawal of flurazepam, there is clear-cut evidence of carry-over effectiveness; that is, levels of total awake time remain somewhat below the baseline values.[14] Serious rebound insomnia has not been demonstrated after withdrawal of the drug; sleep disturbances have been mild and delayed.[23]

The incidence of adverse effects with flurazepam is generally low. However, daytime sedation and performance decrements are greater with flurazepam than with more rapidly eliminated benzodiazepines.[23] These problems are most common after the first several nights of administration and then decrease. Since daytime sedation and performance decrement are mild with a 15 mg dose,[11] therapy should perhaps be initiated with this dose in the majority of patients, particularly in the elderly.

QUAZEPAM

Quazepam, the most recently introduced benzodiazepine, is similar to flurazepam because its initial metabolite, 2-oxoquazepam, is dealkylated to form desalkylflurazepam.

TEMAZEPAM

Temazepam has an intermediate elimination half-life. In the hard capsule formulation initially marketed in the United States, the drug was absorbed slowly and was relatively ineffective for inducing sleep. The reformulated preparation now available should minimize this problem.[11] Temazepam is moderately effective for maintaining sleep. Rebound insomnia often occurs after withdrawal, is moderate in intensity, and may be somewhat delayed.

TRIAZOLAM

Triazolam, the agent currently most prescribed for hypnosis, is absorbed rapidly, including after sublingual administration. It is also quickly inactivated[7] and so is unlikely to cause daytime drowsiness and performance decrements. With short-term use, the drug is effective both for inducing and maintaining sleep and may be useful for overcoming "jet-lag." An initial dose of 0.25 mg, or in the elderly even 0.125 mg, may suffice and cause only minimal adverse effects. However, sustained effectiveness with long-term nightly administration has not been clearly demonstrated. In one study[23] the drug appeared to maintain effectiveness for 5 weeks of therapy, but the sleep duration of the control group steadily increased over the same period. Data from some studies in which efficacy is claimed actually show that total sleep time increased by only 5 to 15 minutes.

Triazolam has certain disadvantages.[30] Memory impairment and anterograde amnesia have been reported after administration of as little as 0.125 mg of the drug.[11,14] Relatively rapid development of tolerance can increase wakefulness during the final hours of drug nights (early morning insomnia) and may enhance daytime anxiety. Because the compound is quickly eliminated, discontinuance may be accompanied by an immediate and intense rebound insomnia. Total awake time may increase two to three times over the predrug level. Early morning insomnia, daytime anxiety, and

FIG. 29-1 *Efficacy and withdrawal of triazolam. Changes in total wake time with administration and after withdrawal of triazolam, 0.5 mg. The ± standard error of the minutes of total wake time is represented by the vertical bars. Values are plotted for the following conditions: baseline (nights 2-4), initial (nights 5-7), and continued (nights 16-18) drug administration, and drug withdrawal (nights 19-21). The baseline mean is indicated by the broken line. The mean degree of worsening of sleep after withdrawal is considerably greater than even the maximum degree of improvement of sleep with drug administration.*

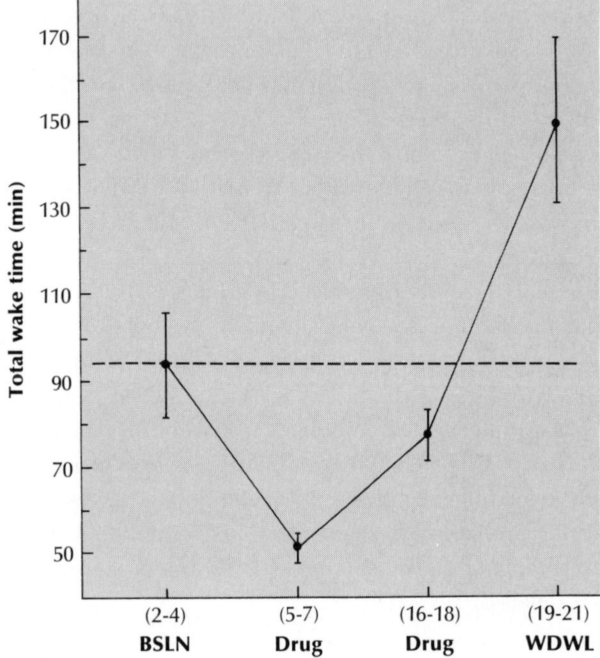

rebound insomnia are all factors that may reinforce drug-taking behavior and contribute to development of dependence (Fig. 29-1). Serious side effects (confusional states, depersonalization, severe anxiety, delirium, or hallucinations) associated with use of excessive doses are probably withdrawal phenomena.

MIDAZOLAM Midazolam is a short-acting compound that is less irritating than other injected benzodiazepines. It is used intravenously or intramuscularly to facilitate short diagnostic procedures and in anesthesia for preoperative sedation, for induction, and with other agents for balanced anesthesia. Though not approved for such use, the drug is also being given as a continuous infusion to maintain sedation in adults and especially children receiving assisted ventilation. A small percentage of patients metabolize midazolam relatively slowly, probably on a genetic basis, and its elimination may also be delayed with cirrhosis and in the elderly.[7] Midazolam is available in solution in 2 ml disposable syringes and in 1 to 10 ml vials so that reconstitution is unnecessary.

Flumazenil Flumazenil (Anexate) is a competitive antagonist of both benzodiazepines and inverse agonists.[16] It has been used to reverse depressant effects of benzodiazepines postoperatively and in intoxicated subjects and may aid differential diagnosis of the cause of an intoxication. Because flumazenil is rapidly metabolized by the liver, bioavailability is low and its antagonistic action after oral or intravenous administration lasts only 2 to 3 hours; patient monitoring is necessary to avoid recurrence of depression. The drug is best given intravenously, in small bolus doses at brief intervals as necessary, until reversal is obtained, usually within a minute or two. Excessive doses may evoke indications of agonist activity, principally anxiety. There is experimental and anecdotal evidence that flumazenil lessens hepatic encephalopathy, presumably by preventing the action of an endogenous benzodiazepine receptor agonist.[13] The drug is not yet approved for use in the United States.

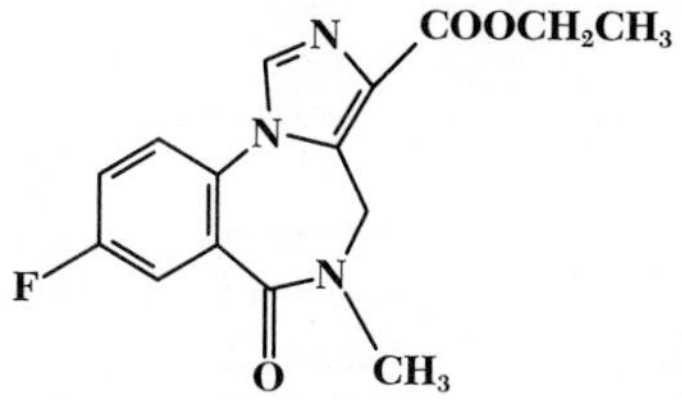

$COOCH_2CH_3$, N, N, F, N, O, CH_3

Flumazenil

BARBITURATES

Chemistry and pharmacokinetics

Barbituric acid, the parent compound of the barbiturate series, is synthesized through the combination of urea and malonic acid.

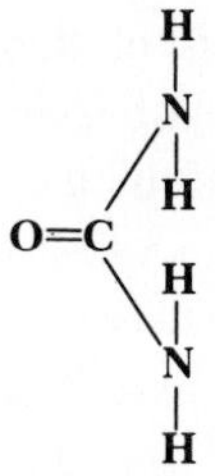

Urea 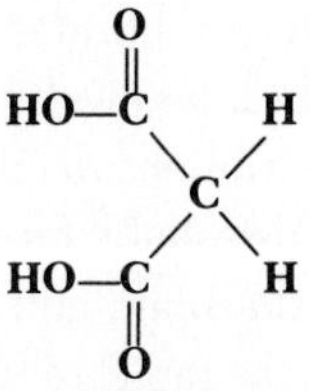 **Malonic acid** 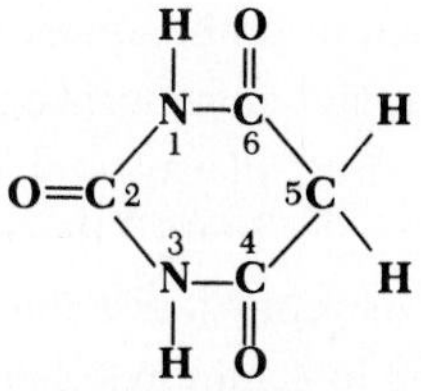 **Barbituric acid**

Barbituric acid has no hypnotic activity. Clinically useful barbiturates are synthesized by replacing the hydrogens at carbon position 5 with alkyl or aryl groups. The resulting weak acids are at least 50% unionized in the body, except possibly in an alkaline urine. The onset of central depression is determined by the rapidity of their entry into the brain, which in turn is influenced primarily by lipid solubility. Substitution of sulfur for the oxygen at position 2 of pentobarbital and secobarbital yields thiopental and thiamylal respectively, which are much more lipid soluble than the former two agents. The latter *ultrashort-acting* barbiturates reach the brain very rapidly and are used as anesthetics. In contrast, barbital, a poorly lipid-soluble barbiturate, reaches the brain much more slowly but is very long-acting; it is now obsolete. In Table 29-2 the barbiturates are classified as ultrashort-, intermediate-, and long-acting drugs.

TABLE 29-2 Barbiturates: elimination half-life and clinical data

Generic name	Trade name	Elimination half-life (hr)	Clinical use	Dosage (mg)	Route of administration
Long acting					
Butabarbital	Butisol	34-42	Hypnotic	50-100	Oral
Phenobarbital	Luminal	24-140	Hypnotic	100-200	Oral
Intermediate acting					
Amobarbital	Amytal	8-42	Hypnotic	100-200	Oral
Aprobarbital	Alurate	14-34	Hypnotic	40-160	Oral
Pentobarbital	Nembutal	20-25	Hypnotic	100	Oral
Secobarbital	Seconal	19-34	Hypnotic	100	Oral
Ultrashort acting					
Thiopental	Pentothal	3-8	Anesthetic	2.5%*; 0.3%†	Intravenous
Thiamylal	Surital		Anesthetic	2.5%*; 0.3%†	Intravenous
Methohexital	Brevital	4-8	Anesthetic	1.0%*; 0.2%†	Intravenous

*Concentration of intravenous solution for induction of anesthesia.
†Concentration of a continuous intravenous drip when used as sole anesthetic.

The duration of action of a dose of the ultrashort-acting drugs is not determined by metabolism or excretion. Because of their extreme lipid solubility, there is virtually no barrier to penetration into tissues. Therefore the major factor affecting uptake is blood flow to each organ. After an intravenous bolus of thiopental, its concentration in brain almost immediately equilibrates with the plasma concentration of free drug, and anesthesia occurs. As other, less well vascularized tissues continue to take up the drug, plasma and brain concentrations decrease. Within a few minutes the concentration in brain falls below the threshold for anesthesia and consciousness returns. Thus rapid *redistribution* out of the brain and into other tissues (distribution half-life of 2 to 4 minutes) is responsible for rapid recovery.

Barbiturates are metabolized by liver microsomal enzymes to less lipid-soluble compounds that are excreted in urine. This process accounts for eventual removal of ultrashort-acting agents as well. Long-acting phenobarbital is metabolized slowly, and a significant amount is excreted unchanged in urine. Its excretion is enhanced in an alkaline urine, a fact that is important in management of acute intoxication. Diseases of the liver or kidneys may prolong the action of barbiturates.

Sites and mechanism of action

Barbiturates depress the activity of all brain cells; they do not selectively concentrate in specific regions. However, the reticular activating system in the brainstem is especially sensitive. Low doses of the drugs appear to enhance the effects of the inhibitory neurotransmitter GABA or to have GABA-like activity, presumably by acting at the *picrotoxinin* receptor (see Chapter 26).

Clinical uses and miscellaneous effects

Ultrashort-acting barbiturates are used to induce anesthesia and to supplement inhalation agents. Intermediate-acting barbiturates were once extensively used as hypnotics. However, much of their effectiveness is lost with continued administration over a 2-week period, and the potential for escalation of dosage and development of dependence is greater than for the benzodiazepines.

The available barbiturates, in general, inhibit development of seizures. They can abolish convulsions secondary to tetanus and eclampsia and are effective antidotes for convulsant drugs. Phenobarbital is more selectively antiepileptic, however, in that it is often useful for chronic management of generalized tonic-clonic and simple partial forms of epilepsy without excessive drowsiness (see Chapter 32).

Paradoxically, in certain persons, or if pain is present, barbiturates may produce restlessness, excitement, and delirium. Elderly people are generally more prone to manifest carry-over effects and to become confused or agitated.

Intoxication

The most serious drawback of barbiturates as hypnotics relates to their narrow margin of safety; only 10 times the therapeutic dose may be lethal. Barbiturates were implicated in over 21% of all drug-related (not including carbon monoxide) deaths in Maryland from 1975 through 1980.[3] Since insomnia may be a symptom of depression with suicidal potential, safety is an important issue in prescribing barbiturates as hypnotics.

Large doses of barbiturates depress the respiratory center and especially decrease its responsiveness to carbon dioxide. Low blood pressure in barbiturate poisoning may be secondary to hypoxia or, in very severe cases, may result from direct depression of central and peripheral elements of the autonomic nervous system. These effects are commonly the cause of early death. As with opiate intoxication, miosis and coma also occur, but barbiturate poisoning is not dramatically reversed by naloxone. A flat electroencephalographic tracing in this setting does not denote brain death. Treatment of intoxication is symptomatic and supportive,[35] with particular attention to maintenance of patent airways, along with oxygen administration and assisted ventilation as necessary. Additional measures include removal (emesis, lavage) and inactivation (activated charcoal) of residual drug in the stomach, restoration of blood pressure if improved ventilation does not reverse hypotension, and maintenance of urine flow and body temperature. There is no specific chemical antidote, and the use of analeptic drugs (see Chapter 31) is not recommended and may be harmful. A clinically beneficial increase in excretion can be achieved *for long-acting barbiturates only* by alkalinization of the urine and forced diuresis. Hemodialysis and particularly hemoperfusion increase clearance of any barbiturate, though again it is easier to remove longer-acting agents.

Drug interactions

When drugs such as alcohol, reserpine, and neuroleptics, as well as sedative-hypnotics from other drug classes, are administered with barbiturates, additive effects of the combination may enhance risk. Such interactions may seriously impair daytime performance or respiratory function with relatively low doses of barbiturates.

Other significant interactions with barbiturates arise from their ability to induce hepatic microsomal enzymes. Chronic administration of phenobarbital can increase metabolism of drugs such as phenytoin and coumarin anticoagulants. Moreover, if the dosage of a drug is then increased to compensate for enhanced metabolism, discontinuation of the barbiturate may cause an exaggerated response to this other drug as its rate of metabolism reverts toward normal.

Barbiturates may also induce a mitochondrial enzyme, δ-aminolevulinic acid synthetase, and for this reason are contraindicated in patients with *acute intermittent* or *variegate porphyrias* in whom they can precipitate neuronal demyelination.

Chronic abuse

Barbiturates can produce both psychologic and physiologic dependence. A mild abstinence syndrome after abrupt withdrawal from a barbiturate-dependent person is similar to that after benzodiazepine withdrawal. However, dependence is likely to be much more pronounced in a barbiturate abuser, in which case withdrawal can be very severe, with seizures, and even more dangerous than withdrawal from an opiate. (See Chapter 34 for further discussion of abuse of this type of drug.)

NONBENZODIAZEPINE, NONBARBITURATE AGENTS

Before development of the benzodiazepines, several compounds besides barbiturates were used as hypnotics. In general, their use is no longer recommended. Ethchlorvynol (Placidyl) is short-acting and less effective than most of the commonly used hypnotics. Glutethimide (Doriden) is an intermediate-acting drug. Poisoning with glutethimide presents a particular hazard because the drug depresses the cardiovascular system and is not effectively removed by hemodialysis or hemoperfusion. Methaqualone is frequently abused and is now a Schedule I drug no longer manufactured legally in the United States. Other hypnotic drugs that remain available are meprobamate, chlormezanone (Trancopal) and hydroxyzine (Atarax, others). Chloral hydrate, and paraldehyde occasionally, may still be useful. Recently introduced buspirone may become an important antianxiety medication.

Chloral hydrate

Chloral hydrate was first used in 1869. It is rapidly reduced in vivo to active trichloroethanol, CCl_3CH_2OH. Chloral hydrate is short acting and can be useful in pediatric and geriatric patients in whom it is less likely than barbiturates to cause excitation. The recommended dose is 0.5 to 1 g, but 2 g may be required. Preparations for oral (Noctec) and rectal (Aquachloral) administration are available. Tolerance to its hypnotic effect occurs after about 2 weeks of use. In its concentrated form, chloral hydrate can cause gastric irritation.

$$\mathrm{Cl_3C{-}CH(OH)OH}$$

Chloral hydrate

The lethal dose of chloral hydrate may range between 3 and 30 g. Overdosage can adversely affect cardiac muscle, and the drug should be avoided in patients with heart disease. Chloral hydrate can displace other protein-bound drugs; trichloroethanol is partially metabolized to trichloroacetic acid, which is tightly bound to plasma albumin and displaces other drugs from their binding sites.

Paraldehyde

Paraldehyde (Paral) is a cyclic trimer of acetaldehyde, to which it decomposes on exposure to light and oxygen. In the liver both paraldehyde and ethanol are transformed initially to acetaldehyde, and paraldehyde should not be given to patients taking disulfiram (see p. 280).

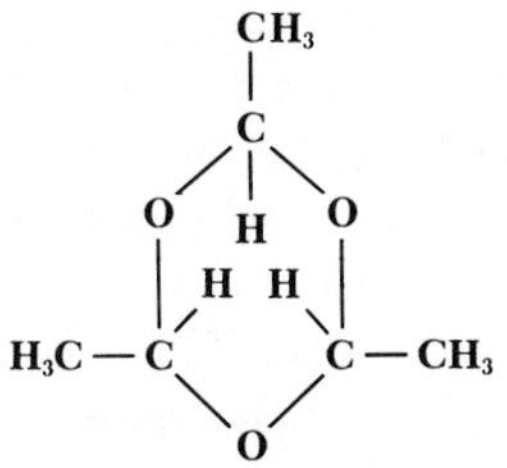

Paraldehyde

The drug is a liquid with a strong odor. It is usually administered in a cold beverage to disguise its disagreeable taste. An effective oral hypnotic dose is 4 to 8 ml. Currently, paraldehyde is almost exclusively used in management of hospitalized patients undergoing alcohol withdrawal, though benzodiazepines have been shown in at least one double-blind, controlled trial to be superior. Paraldehyde has also been used in patients with convulsive states such as eclampsia or tetanus and in patients with renal shutdown. Up to a third of the drug is eliminated through the lungs, and the remainder is metabolized ultimately to carbon dioxide and water.

Because of its irritant effect, paraldehyde should not be administered orally to patients suffering from inflammatory conditions or ulcers in the esophagus, stomach, or duodenum. Similarly, rectal administration should be avoided in patients with inflammatory conditions in this region.

Buspirone

Buspirone, the first of a series of *azapirones* to be released, was introduced as an anxiolytic in 1986. Its place in therapy is not yet established. Reported advantages include minimal drowsiness and lack of physical dependence or potentiation of ethanol. However, full benefit appears to be relatively delayed, for 2 or more weeks, perhaps because the drug lacks hypnotic and muscle relaxant properties that contribute to perceived early relief of anxiety.[32] Buspirone lacks an action on the GABA/benzodiazepine complex, but it is a relatively potent agonist or partial agonist at serotonergic ($5\text{-}HT_{1A}$) receptors.[32,38] Buspirone hydrochloride (BuSpar) is available in tablets, 5 and 10 mg, for daily administration of 15 to 30 mg.

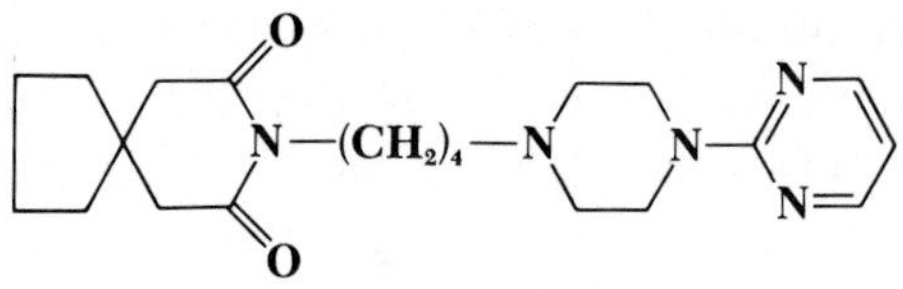

Buspirone

Meprobamate

Meprobamate, introduced shortly before the benzodiazepines, is best regarded as a nonspecific sedative similar to the barbiturates. It is believed that meprobamate also has a blocking action on spinal interneurons, because it has no effect on knee jerk but diminishes flexor and crossed extensor reflexes. Its central muscle relaxant effect is also illustrated by reduction of experimental tremors induced by strychnine.

Drowsiness and ataxia occur when fairly large doses of meprobamate are used. It may cause rash, purpura, and gastrointestinal disturbances. Coma, hypotension, hypothermia, and pulmonary edema have been observed after large doses. Addiction resembling that caused by barbiturates can develop; serious muscle twitching and convulsions may occur when meprobamate is discontinued abruptly. It should be withdrawn slowly, if used at all.

Meprobamate is available in 200 to 600 mg tablets (Equanil, others) and in capsules (Meprospan) containing 200 or 400 mg. Oral administration of 400 mg causes only mild sedation. Larger doses tend to cause drowsiness and to reduce muscle spasm without interference with normal proprioception.

Over-the-counter hypnotics

In the past, nonprescription sleep medications often contained scopolamine or bromide. Nowadays they contain an antihistamine, usually diphenhydramine or pyrilamine. The manufacturers' intent is that the sedative side effect will facilitate sleep. Such over-the-counter medications are less consistent than prescription preparations in relieving insomnia and may also cause undesirable antimuscarinic effects.

Insomniacs who fear addiction to prescription hypnotics may turn to nonprescription medications in the belief that they are safer. However, even recommended doses of antihistamine preparations may precipitate glaucoma in elderly patients prone to narrow-angle glaucoma. Two to three times the recommended dosage can induce transient disorientation or hallucinations, especially in emotionally unstable persons. A considerable overdose (15 to 30 tablets) may cause a stuporous state, confusion, extreme psychiatric disturbance, coma, and even death.

ETHYL ALCOHOL

As a medicinal agent, ethyl alcohol (**alcohol, ethanol**) is only of moderate importance. It is of great toxicologic interest, however, and chronic alcoholism is one of the great social problems of humankind. Alcoholic beverages contain a variety of *congeners*, determined by the ingredients and procedures for preparation and storage, that confer different qualities of taste, aroma, and color.[20] Congeners like tyramine and histamine may cause adverse reactions in susceptible individuals.

Pharmacologic effects

The main action of alcohol is exerted on the central nervous system. It may be regarded as an unusual hypnotic and as an anesthetic with a very low margin of safety. There is general agreement that the apparent stimulant action of the drug is a consequence of primary depression of higher centers, resulting in uninhibited behavior. A variety of mechanisms, including interactions with $GABA_A$ and excitatory amino acid receptor systems, have been proposed to account for its effects[4] and for central tolerance. In addition to actions on behavior and consciousness, alcohol influences cardiovascular, gastrointestinal, and renal functions.

Cutaneous vasodilatation and a feeling of warmth are generally observed after ingestion of an alcoholic beverage. Vasodilatation is attributable, at least partially, to central nervous system actions affecting thermoregulation, though a direct action on blood vessels may contribute as well. There is a popular impression that alcohol dilates coronary vessels, but it does not prevent electrocardiographic evidence of coronary insufficiency after exercise. Adverse myocardial responses, in particular congestive cardiomyopathy, are commonly associated with chronic alcoholism.

Low concentrations of alcohol promote secretion of acid gastric juice. Small doses may improve appetite, whereas excessive concentrations, either acutely or chronically, can disrupt the mucosal barrier to acid diffusion and cause gastritis. Adverse effects on the esophagus and on lower esophageal sphincter pressure contribute to reflux and esophagitis.

The diuresis observed in persons who drink alcoholic beverages is partly caused by ingestion of water, but alcohol also inhibits release of antidiuretic hormone (ADH) from the posterior pituitary. On the other hand, liver disease associated with chronic abuse may cause an elevated ADH level and water retention.

The influence of alcohol on carbohydrate and lipid metabolism has received much attention. Alcoholism is a common cause of hypoglycemia, which can be induced in humans by ingestion of 35 to 50 ml of ethanol after a 2-day fast. Such persons have low liver glycogen. Animal studies indicate that alcohol inhibits gluconeogenesis.

It is quite likely that acute hyperlipemia after alcohol ingestion and the hyperlipemia of the chronic alcoholic develop through different mechanisms. The acute hyperlipemia is probably mediated by sympathetic activation, with subsequent lipolysis from fat depots, because it can be prevented by β-adrenergic blocking agents. In contrast, hyperlipemia in the chronic alcoholic may depend largely on deficient removal of lipid from the blood. There is also evidence for decreased lipoprotein lipase activity in alcoholic patients.

A great many structural and functional changes in the liver have been reported to occur with chronic exposure to alcohol.[18] Alcoholic patients commonly have enlarged livers with increased protein and deposits of fat. Functional changes include (1) reduced availability of NAD (see equation below) for oxidation of fatty acids, (2) enhanced glycerolipid and triglyceride synthesis, (3) induction of microsomal enzymes, (4) glutathione depletion, (5) decreased protein secretion, (6) an increase in fatty acid-binding protein, (7) swelling and other changes in mitochondria, and (8) formation of antibodies against acetaldehyde-protein adducts.

Excessive exposure of a fetus to alcohol, especially in the first trimester but throughout pregnancy, can cause the *fetal alcohol syndrome*.[12] This syndrome is characterized by retarded growth, facial deformities, and central nervous system problems such as mental retardation; defects in sight, hearing, and cardiac function occur as well. Alcohol readily crosses the placenta and equilibrates between fetal and maternal circulations. Proposed mechanisms for damage include fetal hypoxia and altered hormone and prostaglandin metabolism.

Local injection of alcohol can destroy neural pathways and is used to provide permanent, or at least prolonged, nerve block in such conditions as trigeminal neuralgia and terminal cancer. Sponging of alcohol on the skin to enhance heat loss in fever has led to acute intoxication in children and is no longer recommended. Alcohol is also used as a disinfectant and as a solvent for many drugs.

Kinetics

On an empty stomach an alcoholic beverage produces a peak blood concentration in less than an hour. Absorption is delayed if the stomach is filled with food. In men about 20% of a moderate dose is metabolized in the stomach; such presystemic clearance is less in women and after prolonged exposure.[5]

Once absorbed, alcohol is distributed in total body water. If its concentration in blood is assigned the value of 1.0, the value for plasma (serum) and saliva is approximately 1.15 and for cerebrospinal fluid 1.1.[2] A value of about 0.0005 has often been used as standard for alveolar air, but individual ratios range from 0.0003 to 0.0011. Urine values are likely to vary considerably.

The concentration of alcohol in blood has great medicolegal importance; it is generally accepted that a concentration of 0.10% or 100 mg/100 ml (range in United States: 0.08% to 0.15%) indicates intoxication.[26] Coma and even death may occur at concentrations as low as 0.4%. The concentration will depend on (1) the quantity and rate of ingestion, (2) speed of absorption, (3) body weight and percentage of total body water, and (4) rate of alcohol metabolism.

The quantity of alcohol excreted in the urine, exhaled through the lungs, and lost in perspiration ordinarily represents less than 10% of the total. The remainder is metabolized.

In the liver of a nonalcoholic subject (Fig. 29-2, *A*), a low concentration of ethanol is first converted to acetaldehyde by the cytosolic enzyme *alcohol dehydrogenase*.[18]

$$CH_3CH_2OH + NAD^+ \longrightarrow CH_3CHO + NADH^+ + H^+$$

The acetaldehyde is further metabolized to acetate by *acetaldehyde dehydrogenase* within mitochondria. At high concentrations alcohol is converted to acetaldehyde partially by the microsomal ethanol-oxidizing system or MEOS (Fig. 29-2, *B*). If exposure to alcohol is prolonged, several microsomal enzyme systems, including the MEOS, are induced. This enhances metabolism of alcohol (metabolic tolerance) and of other drugs normally metabolized by these enzymes (Fig. 29-2, *C*). In general, acute ingestion of alcohol tends to decrease metabolism of other drugs, whereas chronic alcoholism tends to increase their metabolism (Fig. 29-2, *C* and *D*), until hepatic impairment supervenes.[17]

FIG. 29-2

Hepatic ethanol-drug metabolism interactions. **A**, *Low concentration of alcohol is metabolized by alcohol dehydrogenase, drugs by microsomes.* **B**, *Microsomal drug metabolism is inhibited in the presence of high concentration of ethanol, as in acute inebriation, in part through competition for a common microsomal process.* **C**, *Microsomal induction after long-term alcohol consumption enhances drug metabolism and contributes to accelerated ethanol metabolism at high blood ethanol concentration.* **D**, *Increased drug metabolism persists after cessation of long-term alcohol consumption. Hatching indicates high blood alcohol concentration.*

From Lieber CS: Reprinted by permission of the New England Journal of Medicine 319:1639, 1988.

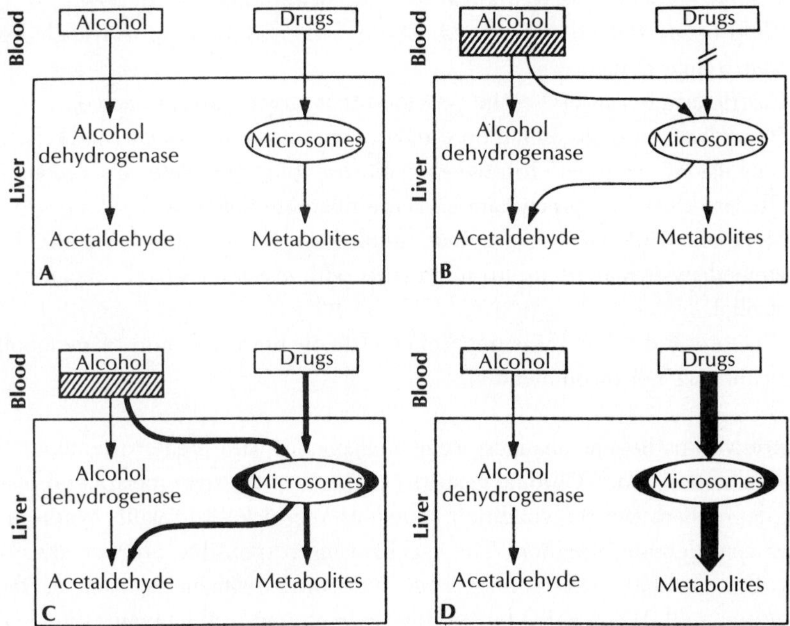

The average person metabolizes 6 to 8 g (7.5 to 10 ml) of alcohol per hour. This figure is fairly constant for a given individual and is independent of the quantity present in the body, a *zero-order reaction* (provided the concentration is not high enough to involve the MEOS appreciably). Metabolism of 1 g of alcohol yields 7 calories. Since the maximal amount that can be metabolized in 24 hours is approximately 170 g, alcohol can contribute up to 1200 calories per day to a person's metabolic requirement.

Tolerance and acute intoxication

It is well known that the experienced drinker shows fewer and less noticeable responses to moderate amounts of alcohol than does an abstainer. This "tolerance" cannot be explained on the basis of pharmacokinetic differences. It is thought that the experienced drinker has learned to perform habitual tasks at alcohol concentrations that would seriously disturb an unaccustomed person. This apparent tolerance does not appear to extend to the lethal actions of alcohol, and even a chronic alcoholic may die when blood concentration exceeds 0.55%. If a person has taken another central nervous system depressant, such as a barbiturate, death may occur at even lower alcohol concentrations. Acute intoxication with alcohol alone was implicated in 14% of drug- and chemical-related deaths (not including carbon monoxide) in Maryland from 1975 through 1980, and alcohol was present in over a third of the intoxications overall.[3]

The severely intoxicated patient represents a medical emergency and should be managed according to the following recommendations[27]:

1. Respiratory support should be given if necessary.
2. Aspiration of vomitus should be prevented by placement of the patient in the semilateral decubitus position with head forward and mouth down.
3. Fluid needs should be assessed. The patient may be fluid overloaded or may have a fluid deficit.
4. Gastric lavage can be helpful provided that airways are protected.
5. Hypoglycemia is suspected on the basis of unusual neurologic findings, such as convulsions or coma. Intravenous glucose plus thiamine are recommended (glucose alone can precipitate an acute thiamine deficiency).
6. Metabolic acidosis, if severe, may require use of sodium bicarbonate.
7. Hemodialysis may be useful in patients with excessive blood concentrations of alcohol.
8. Fructose and other measures believed to increase the rate of metabolism of alcohol are not recommended.

Chronic alcoholism

A variety of pathologic changes occur in alcoholics with greater frequency than in the general population.[22] Chronic gastritis, cirrhosis of the liver, peripheral polyneuropathy, depression, and the condition known as Wernicke-Korsakoffs syndrome have received considerable attention. The mechanisms responsible are not always clear because the alcoholic often suffers from nutritional deficiencies, such as thiamine deficiency, as well. When aided by psychiatric treatment or the organization known as Alcoholics Anonymous, about 50% of alcoholics may be able to abstain from drinking.

Another treatment modality, which complements other approaches to abstinence in the well-motivated patient, is the administration of a drug that makes the response to subsequent alcohol ingestion extremely unpleasant. The best known of these is disulfiram.[37] Because the reaction can be dangerous, such agents should not be used in pregnancy and should be used very cautiously, if at all, in patients with severe myocardial, pulmonary, liver, or renal disease. A relatively recent trial in outpatients showed that, although it reduced the mean number of drinking days, disulfiram did not affect the incidence of total abstinence over a 1-year period relative to control groups.[6] Those subjects, regardless of their treatment group, who were compliant were more likely to have abstained as well. Other agents that may elicit a similar reaction include **calcium carbamide, nitrefazole, hypoglycemic sulfonylureas, chloramphenicol, furazolidone, metronidazole, pargyline, quinacrine**, and **cephalosporins** with a methyltetrazolethio group, such as cefoperazone.

DISULFIRAM

The development of the disulfiram approach followed a chance discovery. While certain new drugs were being tested as potential anthelmintics, it was observed that after ingestion of disulfiram even a few bottles of beer caused very unpleasant side effects. Disulfiram (Antabuse) irreversibly inactivates aldehyde dehydrogenase and thus the second step in metabolism of alcohol. (It also inhibits dopamine-β-hydroxylase and some other enzymes.) If alcohol is ingested several hours after a high dose of disulfiram, within 5 to 15 minutes the person develops an *Antabuse reaction* characterized by nausea, vomiting, flushing, palpitation, and headache; the severity varies with the dosage of both disulfiram and alcohol. There may be ECG changes, a fall in blood pressure, metabolic acidosis, and possibly shock. If the symptoms are potentially unpleasant enough, hopefully the patient will avoid alcohol while maintained on disulfiram. Intolerance to alcohol may remain for a week or more after disulfiram is withdrawn. Disulfiram by itself can cause drowsiness, a metallic taste, diminished libido, and perhaps a toxic psychosis with excessive dosage.

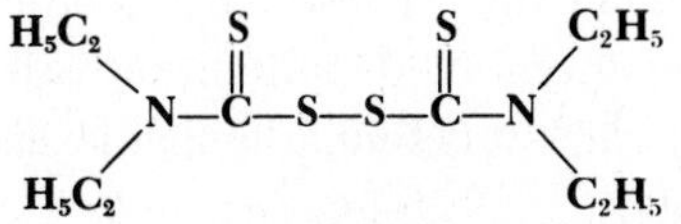

$$(H_5C_2)_2N-C(=S)-S-S-C(=S)-N(C_2H_5)_2$$

Disulfiram

When a patient ingests alcohol while taking disulfiram, acetaldehyde accumulates. The blood concentration in this condition may be of the order of 0.001%. Intravenous infusion of acetaldehyde to produce a comparable concentration reproduces the manifestations of the Antabuse reaction. Acetaldehyde has both vasoconstrictor and vasodilator actions, but hypotension characterizes the Antabuse reaction. Acetaldehyde also releases catecholamines to increase heart rate and cardiac output and may affect the pharmacokinetics of other amines that contribute to symptoms of the reaction.

Initially, after a patient is alcohol free, disulfiram is usually administered as a single morning dose of 250 or 500 mg. After a week or two, the dose is maintained at 250 or even 125 mg.

OTHER ALCOHOLS

Aliphatic alcohols other than ethanol are of interest in medicine largely because they are sometimes involved in cases of poisoning.

Methanol

Generally the toxicity of the alcohols increases with chain length, an exception being methanol,[19] which causes pronounced acidosis and blindness. Methanol may be found in "denatured" alcohol, that is, ethanol to which methanol (wood alcohol, methyl alcohol) has been added expressly to prevent its use as a beverage. Other sources include windshield de-icer and washing solutions, paint remover, and model airplane fuel, as well as "bootleg" whiskey. Methanol is slowly converted by alcohol dehydrogenase to formaldehyde, which is rapidly oxidized to formic acid. The presence of ethanol slows the metabolism of methanol so that poisoning may be obscured until the ethanol is largely inactivated. Death has been reported after as little as 6 ml of methanol, but 30 ml is an accepted lethal dose. In addition to acidosis, methanol intoxication involves the central nervous system, with development of headache, dizziness, delirium, seizures, and coma. Blindness appears to be a consequence of formic acid toxicity on the retina.

Treatment of the life-threatening acidosis is based primarily on its correction with sodium bicarbonate. Therapeutic administration of ethanol, based on the competition between the alcohols for metabolism, can be lifesaving and is likely to provide protection from blindness. It may be necessary to maintain ethanol concentrations of 0.1% or higher for several days. If blood methanol concentration exceeds 0.05%, hemodialysis can efficiently remove the methanol while ethanol is used to block methanol metabolism. In so doing, ethanol administration must be increased because it too is removed by the dialysis.

Miscellaneous alcohols or glycols

Ethylene glycol, found in antifreeze, brake fluid, and windshield de-icer,[19] is another alcohol metabolized by alcohol dehydrogenase. Intoxication results in formation of glycolate, lactate, and oxalate.[34] These cause central nervous system depression, systemic acidosis, and calcium oxalate deposition in tissues such as the kidney, with subsequent renal failure. Treatment is similar to that for methanol intoxication, including administration of ethanol.

Isopropyl alcohol (isopropanol), a major component of rubbing alcohol and windshield de-icers, is of toxicologic interest also. It is metabolized to acetone. Gastrointestinal (abdominal pain, irritation, vomiting) and central nervous (ataxia, confusion, coma) effects predominate.[19] Severe renal damage has occurred in patients who recovered from ingestion of a few ounces of isopropyl alcohol. Supportive treatment and gastric lavage usually suffice but hemodialysis is indicated in serious intoxications. The lethal dose is estimated as 150 to 240 ml.

A variety of adverse central nervous system effects and death in 10 premature infants was attributed to benzyl alcohol, a preservative added to intravenous solutions.[8]

REFERENCES

1. Breier A, Charney DS, Heninger GR: The diagnostic validity of anxiety disorders and their relationship to depressive illness, *Am J Psychiatry* 142:787, 1985.
2. Caplan YH: Blood, urine, and other fluid and tissue specimens for alcohol analyses. In Garriott JC, editor: *Medicolegal aspects of alcohol determination in biological specimens*, Littleton, Mass, 1988, PSG Publishing Co, p 74.
3. Caplan YH, Ottinger WE, Park J, Smith TD: Drug and chemical related deaths: incidence in the state of Maryland—1975 to 1980, *J Forens Sci* 30:1012, 1985.
4. Deitrich RA, Dunwiddie TV, Harris RA, Erwin VG: Mechanism of action of ethanol: initial central nervous system actions, *Pharmacol Rev* 41:489, 1989.
5. Frezza M, di Padova C, Pozzato G, et al: High blood alcohol levels in women: the role of decreased gastric alcohol dehydrogenase activity and first-pass metabolism, *N Engl J Med* 322:95, 1990.
6. Fuller RK, Branchey L, Brightwell DR, et al: Disulfiram treatment of alcoholism: a Veterans Administration cooperative study, *JAMA* 256:1449, 1986.
7. Garzone PD, Kroboth PD: Pharmacokinetics of the newer benzodiazepines, *Clin Pharmacokinet* 16:337, 1989.
8. Gershanik J, Boecler B, Ensley H, et al: The gasping syndrome and benzyl alcohol poisoning, *N Engl J Med* 307:1384, 1982.
9. Gillin JC, Byerley WF: The diagnosis and management of insomnia, *N Engl J Med* 322:239, 1990.

10. Greenblatt DJ: Pharmacokinetics and pharmacodynamics, *Hosp Pract* 25(suppl 2):9, 1990.
11. Greenblatt DJ, Harmatz JS, Engelhardt N, Shader RI: Pharmacokinetic determinants of dynamic differences among three benzodiazepine hypnotics: flurazepam, temazepam, and triazolam, *Arch Gen Psychiatry* 46:326, 1989.
12. Hoyseth KS, Jones PJH: Ethanol induced teratogenesis: characterization, mechanisms and diagnostic approaches, *Life Sci* 44:643, 1989.
13. Jones EA, Basile AS, Mullen KD, Gammal SH: Flumazenil: potential implications for hepatic encephalopathy, *Pharmacol Ther* 45:331, 1990.
14. Kales A, Kales JD: Sleep laboratory studies of hypnotic drugs: efficacy and withdrawal effects, *J Clin Psychopharmacol* 3:140, 1983.
15. Kales A, Soldatos CR, Kales JD: Sleep disorders: insomnia, sleepwalking, night terrors, nightmares, and enuresis, *Ann Intern Med* 106:582, 1987.
16. Klotz U, Kanto J: Pharmacokinetics and clinical use of flumazenil (Ro 15-1788), *Clin Pharmacokinet* 14:1, 1988.
17. Lane EA, Guthrie S, Linnoila M: Effects of ethanol on drug and metabolite pharmacokinetics, *Clin Pharmacokinet* 10:228, 1985.
18. Lieber CS: Biochemical and molecular basis of alcohol-induced injury to liver and other tissues, *N Engl J Med* 319:1639, 1988.
19. Litovitz T: The alcohols: ethanol, methanol, isopropanol, ethylene glycol, *Pediatr Clin North Am* 33:311, 1986.
20. McAnalley BH: Chemistry of alcoholic beverages. In Garriott JC, editor: *Medicolegal aspects of alcohol determination in biological specimens*, Littleton, Mass, 1988, PSG Publishing Co, p 1.
21. Miller LG, Greenblatt DJ, Abernethy DR, et al: Kinetics, brain uptake, and receptor binding characteristics of flurazepam and its metabolites, *Psychopharmacology* 94:386, 1988.
22. Miller NS, Gold MS, Cocores JA, Pottash AC: Alcohol dependence and its medical consequences, *NY State J Med* 88:476, 1988.
23. Mitler MM, Seidel WF, van den Hoed J, et al: Comparative hypnotic effects of flurazepam, triazolam, and placebo: a long-term simultaneous nighttime and daytime study, *J Clin Psychopharmacol* 4:2, 1984.
24. Noyes R, Jr, Garvey MJ, Cook BL, Perry PJ: Benzodiazepine withdrawal: a review of the evidence, *J Clin Psychiatry* 49:382, 1988.
25. O'Boyle CA: Benzodiazepine-induced amnesia and anaesthetic practice: a review. In Hindmarch I, Ott H, editors: *Benzodiazepine receptor ligands, memory and information processing*, Berlin, 1988, Springer-Verlag, p 146.
26. Pilchen NB: State and federal regulations concerning driving while intoxicated with alcohol. In Garriott JC, editor: *Medicolegal aspects of alcohol determination in biological specimens*, Littleton, Mass, 1988, PSG Publishing Co, p 180.
27. Redetzki HM: Treatment of ethanol intoxication, *Hosp Formulary*, p 934, Oct 1979.
28. Rickels K, Chung HR, Csanalosi IB, et al: Alprazolam, diazepam, imipramine, and placebo in outpatients with major depression, *Arch Gen Psychiatry* 44:862, 1987.
29. Roberts JR, Tafuri JA: Benzodiazepines. In Haddad LM, Winchester JF, editors: *Clinical management of poisoning and drug overdose*, ed 2, Philadelphia, 1990, WB Saunders, p 800.
30. Schneider PJ, Perry PJ: Triazolam—an "abused drug" by the lay press? *DCIP Ann Pharmacother* 24:389, 1990.
31. Task Force on Benzodiazepine Dependency: *Benzodiazepine dependence, toxicity, and abuse*, Washington, 1990, American Psychiatric Association.
32. Taylor DP: Buspirone, a new approach to the treatment of anxiety, *FASEB J* 2:2445, 1988.
33. Tesar GE: High-potency benzodiazepines for short-term management of panic disorder: the U.S. experience, *J Clin Psychiatry* 51(5, suppl):4, 1990.
34. Winchester JF: Methanol, isopropyl alcohol, higher alcohols, ethylene glycol, glycol, cellosolves, acetone, and oxalate. In

Haddad LM, Winchester JF, editors: *Clinical management of poisoning and drug overdose*, ed 2, Philadelphia, 1990, WB Saunders, p 687.

35. Winchester JF: Barbiturates, methaqualone, and primidone. In Haddad LM, Winchester JF, editors: *Clinical management of poisoning and drug overdose*, ed 2, Philadelphia, 1990, WB Saunders, p 718.

36. Woods JH, Katz JL, Winger G: Use and abuse of benzodiazepines: issues relevant to prescribing, *JAMA* 260:3476, 1988.

37. Wright C, Moore RD: Disulfiram treatment of alcoholism, *Am J Med* 88:647, 1990.

38. Yocca FD: Neurochemistry and neurophysiology of buspirone and gepirone: interactions at presynaptic and postsynaptic 5-HT_{1A} receptors, *J Clin Psychopharmacol* 10(3, suppl):6S, 1990.

section four

Other drugs with prominent central actions

Chapter 30

Drugs for treatment of movement disorders

GENERAL CONCEPTS

Disturbances in function of nuclei in the basal ganglia cause major movement disorders such as Parkinsons disease, Huntingtons disease, Wilsons disease, dystonia, and ballismus. Relevant structures are the striatum (caudate nucleus and putamen), globus pallidus, subthalamic nucleus, and substantia nigra.[17] Disorders in neurotransmission or lesions within these nuclei or connecting pathways can cause either diminished mobility (a bradykinesia, as in Parkinsons disease) or excessive movement (a dyskinesia, as in chorea). Unfortunately, understanding of the pathology of movement disorders is often limited by incomplete knowledge of the normal functions of these nuclei and their integration with other brain regions.

The basal ganglia contain several neurotransmitters.[7,25] Thus movement disorders likely arise from changes in multiple neurotransmitter systems. Nevertheless, dopamine, acetylcholine, and γ-aminobutyric acid (GABA) are emphasized in this chapter, for two reasons: (1) there is abundant evidence that they are critically important in movement disorders,[7] and (2) current therapy of these disorders relies primarily on drugs that alter dopaminergic or cholinergic neurotransmission.

PARKINSONS DISEASE

Parkinsons disease is a progressive neurologic disorder characterized by four major symptoms; slowness or lack of movement (bradykinesia), resting tremor, muscle rigidity, and abnormal posture. Symptoms tend to appear in later life (often in the 50s), and they progress until patients can no longer care for themselves. The lack of mobility eventually leads to complications that may result in death.

The etiology of idiopathic Parkinsons disease remains to be elucidated. The disease does not appear to be genetically determined, and parkinsonian symptoms can occur secondary to encephalitis or exposure to a variety of drugs.[5] Some investigators hypothesize that external factors cause the disease. This is supported by observations that 1-methyl-4-phenyl-1,2,3,6-tetrahydropyridine (MPTP), a contaminate of certain "designer drugs" (meperidine analogs), produces irreversible parkinsonian symptoms in persons who inject it intravenously.[11] MPTP is a useful tool to study Parkinsons disease because its administration mimics the destruction of nigrostriatal dopamine neurons seen in idiopathic Parkinsons disease.[26]

The nigrostriatal dopaminergic system plays a crucial role in the pathogenesis of Parkinsons disease. Dopamine is present in relatively high amounts in striatal neurons that originate in the pars compacta of the substantia nigra.[1,17] In brains from patients with Parkinsons disease, however, its concentration is reduced at least 90%.[9] Furthermore, compounds such as reserpine, neuroleptics, and MPTP, which impair dopamin-

Schematic representation of a simple neurochemical model of Parkinsons disease (see text for details). ACh, *acetylcholine;* DA, *dopamine;* GABA, *γ-aminobutyric acid.* *FIG. 30-1.*

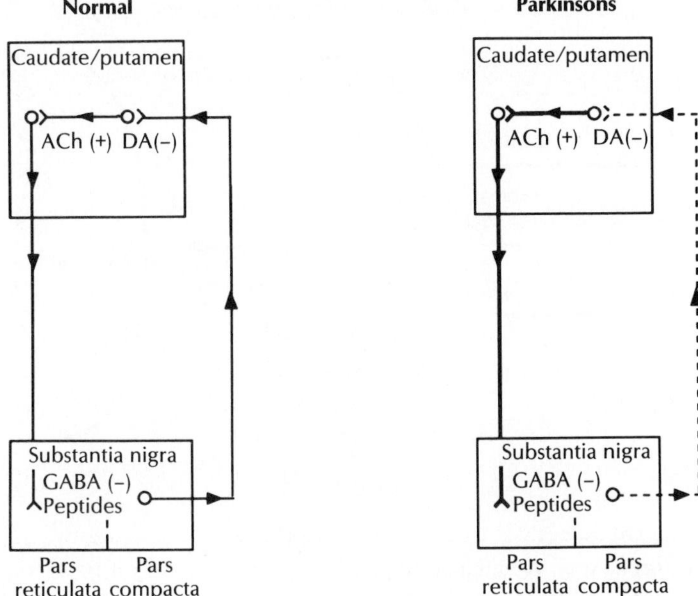

ergic transmission, can cause or exacerbate parkinsonian symptoms. Altogether, these observations indicate that loss of nigrostriatal dopamine is a major component of Parkinsons disease.

Numerous other mediators are also altered in patients with Parkinsons disease.[7,17] However, other than dopamine, only acetylcholine is clearly implicated in the disease process; muscarinic antagonists partially alleviate symptoms of Parkinsons disease, whereas muscarinic agonists exacerbate the symptoms. A simplistic neurochemical model of Parkinsons disease is illustrated in Fig. 30-1. Excitatory cholinergic interneurons in the caudate/putamen are modulated by inhibitory dopaminergic input. This "balance" maintains a normal integration between nuclei of the basal ganglia and other brain regions (Fig. 30-1, *left*). Presumably, parkinsonian symptoms develop when the inhibitory dopamine input deteriorates; uncontrolled cholinergic activity alters movement (Fig. 30-1, *right*).

Two primary strategies are currently used to treat Parkinsons disease: enhancement of dopaminergic function or attenuation of cholinergic function; they may also be used together.

Enhancement of dopaminergic activity

Fig. 30-2 illustrates therapeutic strategies to improve dopamine function in patients with Parkinsons disease. Dopamine content can be elevated by providing more precursor or by reducing its metabolism. Alternatively, release of the remaining dopamine can be increased, or dopamine-receptor agonists can be administered to stimulate postsynaptic sites.

FIG. 30-2. *Model of therapeutic strategies to treat Parkinsons disease by enhancing dopamine (DA) function. These include administration of: (1) levodopa to increase synthesis of DA, (2) drugs that enhance DA release, (3) drugs that prevent DA breakdown by monoamine oxidase (MAO), and (4) drugs that are agonists at postsynaptic dopamine receptors.*

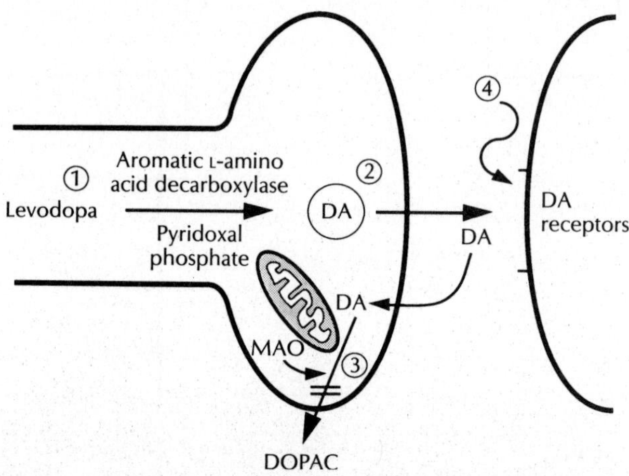

LEVODOPA The most direct way to enhance dopaminergic activity would be to supply dopamine to the basal ganglia. However, dopamine does not readily cross the blood-brain barrier. Fortunately, its precursor, the amino acid levodopa, is actively transported into the central nervous system. In a majority of parkinsonian patients, ingestion of levodopa markedly lessens symptoms of the disease; the disease process itself is unaffected. Rigidity, involuntary movements, and symptoms associated with bradykinesia, such as a speech impediment or poor handwriting, are significantly improved. In contrast, tremor and postural problems may not respond as well. After initiation of levodopa therapy, patients often exhibit elevated mood and an improved outlook, secondary to the improvement in movement. Unfortunately, levodopa is not beneficial for the dementia that develops in some patients. Although levodopa may alleviate the parkinsonian symptoms induced by antipsychotic therapy, it is rarely used in this setting because it may worsen the psychosis.

The therapeutic activity of levodopa depends on its conversion to dopamine, which in turn stimulates receptors in the striatum.[24] The favored hypothesis, although somewhat controversial, is that the D_2-receptor is more relevant than the D_1-receptor for the antiparkinson action. This conclusion is based, in part, on observations that agonists beneficial in Parkinsons disease (see p. 292) have a higher affinity for D_2-receptors. In addition, those neuroleptic drugs that more frequently cause parkinsonian side effects are potent D_2-receptor antagonists.

Adverse effects. Levodopa, via its metabolite dopamine, causes a number of side effects that may limit therapy. A majority of patients initially experience nausea, vomiting, and anorexia. Because tolerance develops to the emetic action, these effects can be minimized by slowly increasing dosage. Alternatively, the daily dosage can be subdivided, or levodopa can be given with a decarboxylase inhibitor that blocks its peripheral conversion to dopamine (see p. 291). Administration with meals or antacids may reduce nausea and vomiting but can also delay absorption and reduce peak plasma concentration.[19] Although selected phenothiazines are useful antiemetics, they are contraindicated here because they can worsen parkinsonian symptoms.

Other peripheral effects of levodopa include hypotension and cardiac arrhythmias. Orthostatic hypotension occurs in approximately 30% of patients, but tolerance gradually develops. Cardiac arrhythmias are less common and generally appear as tachycardia, ventricular ectopic beats, or, rarely, atrial fibrillation. Mydriasis, changes in hepatic enzyme concentrations, attacks of gout, and, rarely, blood dyscrasias may also develop. Levodopa is contraindicated in patients with angle-closure glaucoma.

Perhaps the most limiting problem in levodopa therapy is development of excessive involuntary movements or dyskinesias.[18] These abnormal movements can be minimal, or they can be debilitating. The emergence of dyskinesias is often associated temporally with maximal clinical benefit. They occur in a large percentage of patients on long-term levodopa therapy. Patients can fluctuate between periods of normal mobility and periods of excessive movement. They may exhibit tics, tremors, dystonia, ballismic movements of the limbs or trunk, or chorea of the face or limbs. Although the cause of the dyskinesias is unclear, it appears to involve some chronic adaptation in the brain. An increase in density of D_2-receptors in the striatum does not seem to be a factor.[8]

Unfortunately, there is no specific therapy to prevent the dyskinesias. Neuroleptic drugs, which diminish them, exacerbate the parkinsonian symptoms. The dyskinesias can be minimized by lowering the dose of levodopa, but this too can worsen the parkinsonism. Consequently, the alternatives are to titrate the dosage of levodopa carefully to maximize the therapeutic effect while minimizing the dyskinesias, to reduce levodopa dosage while supplementing therapy with drugs that are less likely to contribute to abnormal movement, or to terminate levodopa therapy.

Behavioral changes in patients receiving levodopa are less frequent than dyskinesias. Patients may experience confusion, delirium, hallucinations, nightmares, and alterations in mood or personality. Furthermore, levodopa can worsen underlying psychosis and should be avoided in psychotic patients. As with dyskinesias, the only treatment for such changes is to reduce or withdraw therapy.

Because dyskinesias and behavioral alterations increase in incidence and severity with the duration of chronic levodopa therapy, they are thought to occur secondarily to adaptive processes in the brains of parkinsonian patients. If so, withdrawal of drug treatment for a period of time could reverse the effect. This is the rationale behind the use of a "drug holiday" (a period without levodopa therapy) in patients who exhibit central nervous system toxicity. A majority of patients show an improved therapeutic response to levodopa when the drug is reinstated; the dosage of drug can often be reduced, and the potential for side effects diminishes, at least for a time. Unfortunately, there is no method for determining prospectively whether a patient will benefit from a drug holiday. In addition, the loss of mobility that occurs when levodopa is withdrawn can be demoralizing and physically harmful to the patient. Because the risks of drug withdrawal usually outweigh the potential benefits, drug holidays are no longer routinely recommended.[16] Whenever levodopa therapy is stopped, dosage should be reduced gradually under medical supervision to prevent abrupt and dramatic akinesia or symptoms reminiscent of the neuroleptic malignant syndrome.

Loss of therapeutic effect of levodopa. After years of treatment with levodopa, its efficacy diminishes. For this reason, there is some controversy about the use of levodopa early in Parkinsons disease. Some physicians believe that levodopa should be reserved until other agents prove ineffective. However, the loss of benefit from levodopa is probably related to progression of the disease rather than to the length of time on the drug.[2] Continued degeneration of the dopaminergic neurons may further impair their ability to store and release the neurotransmitter. There is also evidence that early treatment with levodopa improves prognosis.[4] In any case, levodopa treatment should be started with the lowest effective dosage whenever the patient requires the drug.[3]

Another problem with levodopa therapy is development of fluctuations in its effectiveness. These swings, often called the "on-off phenomenon," occur in over half of patients who receive the drug for a number of years.[14] They are characterized by periods of symptomatic relief followed by a "wearing off" of the beneficial effect before the next dose of levodopa. Eventually, such fluctuations may occur rather abruptly, hence the term "on-off." In many instances, the fluctuations correlate with changes in the plasma concentration of levodopa. When the concentration is low, there is a greater incidence of bradykinesia. Ingestion of dietary neutral amino acids may contribute to the variability. These compounds compete with levodopa for transport from the gut to the circulation and from the circulation to the brain.[20] Vitamin B_6 availability may also contribute to the problem because it enhances peripheral metabolism of levodopa. Control of such variables by alterations in diet and more frequent administration of levodopa may minimize the on-off phenomenon. For example, maintenance of a steady plasma concentration of levodopa by intravenous infusion significantly attenuates fluctuations in symptoms.[20] Another approach to diminish on-off periods is the addition of an agent that enhances dopamine function by another mechanism (see below).

Pharmacokinetics. Levodopa is readily absorbed by active transport from the gastrointestinal tract. Peak plasma concentration occurs within 1 to 2 hours after administration.[19] A considerable amount of levodopa is converted to dopamine in the gut; oral bioavailability is 15% to 30%. If levodopa is administered with a large dose of an anticholinergic agent (which is often the case in treatment of Parkinsons disease), its absorption can be delayed. As discussed earlier, administration of levodopa with a meal slows absorption and reduces peak plasma concentration because of the presence of other neutral amino acids.

Once absorbed, very little levodopa reaches the brain because most is decarboxylated in the periphery. This conversion to dopamine by aromatic L-amino acid decarboxylase requires the co-factor pyridoxal (vitamin B_6). Thus adding vitamin B_6 can worsen parkinsonian symptoms in a patient already controlled with levodopa.

The initial daily dosage of levodopa is 500 mg to 1 g. To minimize side effects, dosage is gradually increased, generally to no more than 8 g, until noticeable improvement occurs or adverse reactions make further increases impractical. Levodopa (Dopar, Larodopa) is available in capsules or tablets containing 100 to 500 mg.

Coadministration of levodopa with decarboxylase inhibitors. Since approximately 95% of levodopa is metabolized before it can enter the central nervous system, large doses of the amino acid must be administered. To minimize peripheral decarboxylation, levodopa is usually administered with **carbidopa** (Lodosyn), a levodopa analog. Carbidopa inhibits aromatic L-amino acid decarboxylase in the gut and other peripheral tissues but not in the brain, because it does not readily cross the blood-brain barrier. Although the dose of levodopa is considerably less in this combination, other advantages are more important. Gastrointestinal and cardiac side effects are much less bothersome because little dopamine is formed in the periphery. The levodopa/carbidopa combination diminishes the on-off phenomenon that occurs in many patients with Parkinsons disease. Finally, the combination alleviates the interaction of levodopa with vitamin B_6. Because the combination is more potent and dosage does not need to be escalated gradually to allow tolerance to peripheral actions, dyskinesias or behavioral changes may initially be somewhat worse than with levodopa alone until optimal dosage is established.

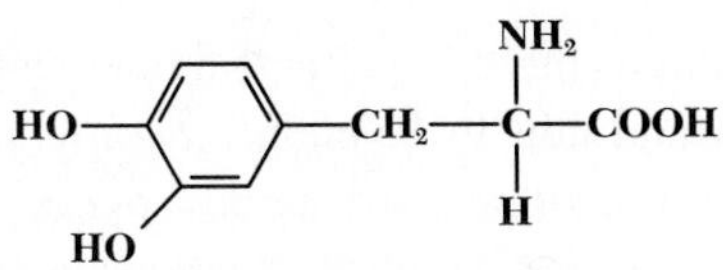

Levodopa

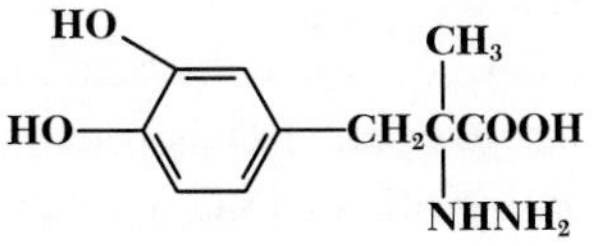

Carbidopa

Levodopa is almost always administered in a combination (Sinemet) with carbidopa. The preparation is available in tablets of three strengths: 10/100, 25/100, or 25/250 (the first number indicates the dose of carbidopa and the second of levodopa, in milligrams). Dosage for each patient must be determined by careful titration. Benserazide, another peripheral decarboxylase inhibitor, is marketed outside the United States in capsules containing 25 mg of benserazide and 200 mg of levodopa (Madopar).

AMANTADINE

Amantadine, an antiviral drug, lessens rigidity, bradykinesia, and tremor in some patients. It is about as effective as anticholinergic drugs (see p. 294) but less so than levodopa. Although its precise mechanism of action is not clear, amantadine can enhance dopamine release from neurons, prevent dopamine reuptake, and increase the number of dopamine receptors.[6] Tolerance develops to the drug after a few months of therapy and limits its usefulness.

In general, amantadine causes fewer and milder side effects than levodopa. Adverse effects of amantadine include mottling of the skin (livedo reticularis) and ankle edema. Other effects are anxiety, irritability, insomnia, and gastrointestinal disturbances. A few cases of congestive heart failure have been associated with amantadine, and convulsions have occurred after excessive doses. Amantadine hydrochloride (Symmetrel) is available in capsules of 100 mg and in a syrup containing 50 mg/5 ml. The initial dose is 100 mg twice daily.

SELEGILINE (L-DEPRENYL)

Another method to enhance dopamine activity in patients with Parkinsons disease is by preventing its breakdown by monoamine oxidase (MAO). The major problem with nonselective MAO inhibitors is their potentially lethal interaction with tyramine-containing foods and with levodopa (see p. 255). Because selegiline is a relatively selective inhibitor of MAO-B, at usual dosages it is less likely to interact with tyramine or levodopa to produce hypertension. Selegiline does, however, inhibit oxidation of dopamine in the central nervous system.

$$\begin{array}{c} \qquad\quad CH_3 \\ \qquad\quad | \\ C_6H_5CH_2CHNCH_2C{\equiv}CH \\ \quad | \\ \quad CH_3 \end{array}$$

Selegiline

Selegiline can diminish fluctuations in movement in patients treated with levodopa for more than 5 years. Furthermore, its addition to levodopa therapy substantially reduces "wearing off" in a majority of patients; often levodopa dosage can be reduced. Selegiline is not as beneficial in alleviating abrupt on-off fluctuations, and its use for this purpose has been questioned. Unfortunately, the beneficial effects of selegiline are limited, and it becomes ineffective after administration for 6 months to 2 years. Recent clinical studies suggest that selegiline is effective alone in relieving early parkinsonian symptoms[21] and may delay the need to initiate levodopa therapy. Some evidence also suggests that selegiline delays the progression of Parkinsons disease.[28] Overall, adverse effects of therapeutic doses of selegiline are minimal. The drug can potentiate the central nervous system toxicity (hallucinations, dyskinesias) that occurs with levodopa, but this problem develops early in the course of therapy and dosage can be adjusted. Patients starting selegiline sometimes experience nausea and dizziness. The drug may exacerbate peptic ulcer disease. Selegiline hydrochloride (Eldepryl) is available in 5 mg tablets. Recommended daily dosage is 10 mg, usually divided into two doses.

ERGOLINES

A fourth way to enhance striatal dopamine function is to use a dopamine agonist that can reach the brain. Ergot derivatives with these properties include bromocriptine, pergolide, and lisuride, the last of which is not yet marketed in the United States. At relatively low concentrations, bromocriptine stimulates D_2-receptors and is an antagonist at D_1-receptors. Its clinical efficacy is based on its agonist activity. The drug can be used alone as initial treatment of Parkinsons disease[22] and is useful in patients who cannot tolerate levodopa. It is not effective, however, in patients who show no response to levodopa. Bromocriptine is added for patients who do not respond adequately to levodopa alone, and it is also given with levodopa to minimize the wearing-off and on-off phenomena. When they are coadministered, the dosage of levodopa must be reduced. As with levodopa, the therapeutic activity of bromocriptine diminishes after long-term therapy.

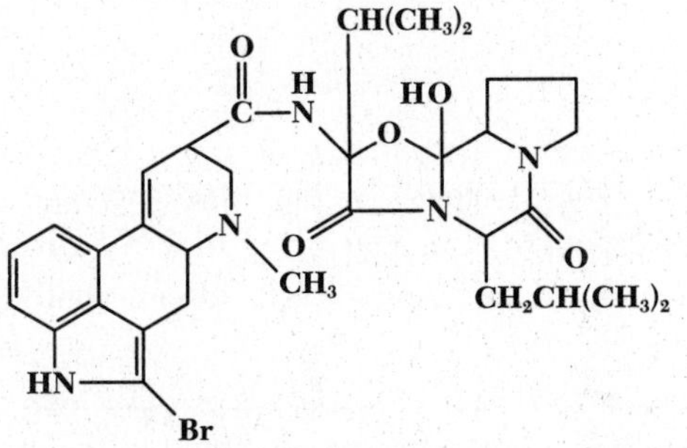

Bromocriptine

The major side effects of bromocriptine are similar to those of levodopa, except for a lower incidence of dyskinesias and a higher incidence of psychic side effects, including auditory and visual hallucinations. Peripheral effects include nausea, vomiting, postural hypotension, and, in some instances, cardiac arrhythmias. Rarely, patients exhibit a catastrophic hypotensive reaction to the first dose of bromocriptine; caution is appropriate when starting therapy.

Because bromocriptine inhibits prolactin secretion (see p. 523), it is contraindicated during pregnancy and is not given to breast-feeding mothers. Other side effects include livedo reticularis, erythromelalgia, and rebound hyperprolactinemia with galactorrhoea.

Bromocriptine mesylate (Parlodel) is administered orally with peak therapeutic effects observed in 2 to 4 hours. The drug has an extensive first-pass effect and is excreted in the bile. The usual starting dose is 2.5 mg/day given in two doses. Dosage is gradually increased to up to 100 mg/day. The drug is available in 2.5 mg tablets and 5 mg capsules.

Pergolide, a highly potent D_1- and D_2-receptor agonist, is another ergoline used as an adjunct to levodopa to improve mobility.[12] It decreases the "off" time in patients with the on-off phenomenon. When coadministered with pergolide, the dosage of levodopa can be reduced 30% to 80%. Pergolide is being studied as initial therapy in Parkinsons disease. The incidence of nausea, vomiting, and cardiovascular problems may be less than with bromocriptine. Dyskinesias, hallucinations, and other psychic disturbances are the most common adverse effects. Pergolide has actions on the endocrine system similar to those of bromocriptine and can produce first-dose cardiovascular collapse.

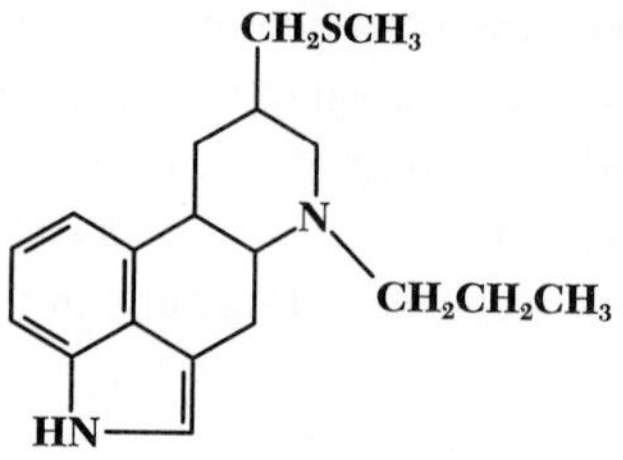

Pergolide

Initial dosage of pergolide should be low (0.05 mg/day). Dosage is then slowly increased to approximately 2 to 4 mg/day, given in 3 to 4 divided doses. Peak plasma concentration is achieved in 1 to 2 hours. **Pergolide mesylate** (Permax) is available in tablets of 0.05 to 1 mg.

Attenuation of cholinergic function

As discussed on p. 287, a deficiency of dopamine in the striatum allows excessive activity of cholinergic neurons. Indeed, the effectiveness of antimuscarinic drugs in alleviating parkinsonian symptoms supports the premise that increased activity of cholinergic neurons contributes to the disability. For many years, the naturally occurring alkaloids atropine and scopolamine were used to treat Parkinsons disease. They were replaced, however, by synthetic drugs that produce less troublesome peripheral effects without compromising efficacy. The anticholinergic drugs currently used to treat parkinsonism include trihexyphenidyl, benztropine, biperiden, procyclidine, and ethopropazine and the antihistamines, diphenhydramine and orphenadrine, as well. The latter two agents have weak antimuscarinic activity that accounts for their effectiveness.

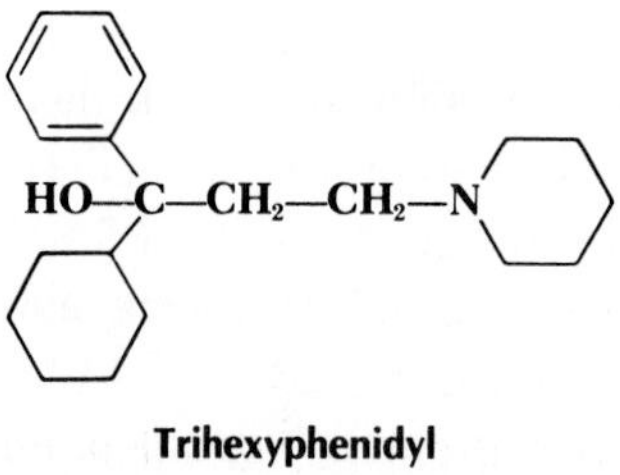

Trihexyphenidyl

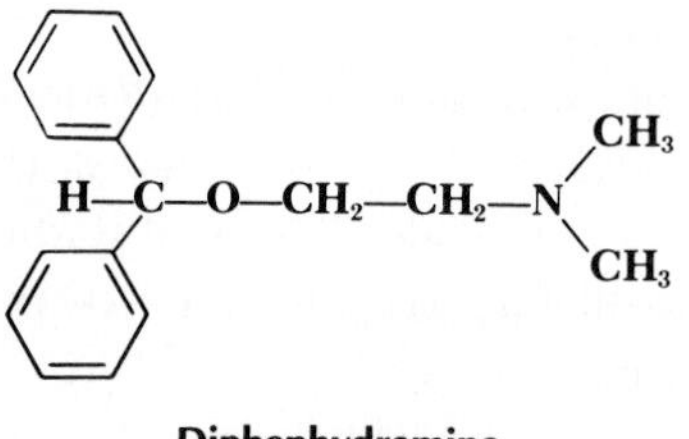

Diphenhydramine

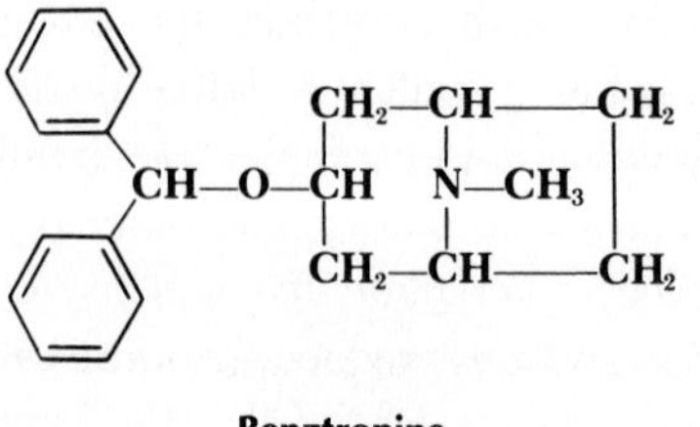

Benztropine

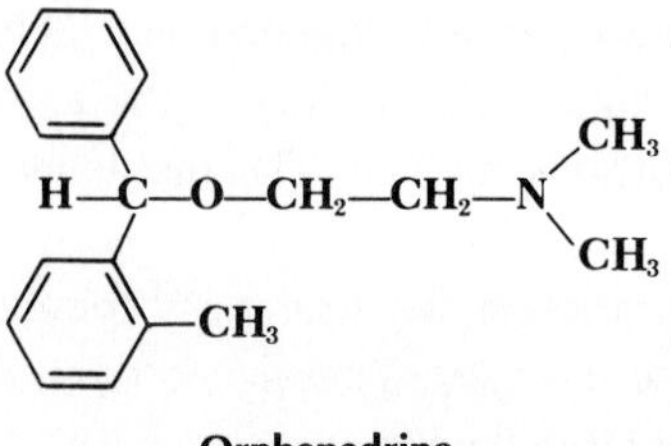

Orphenadrine

For the most part, these drugs have similar therapeutic and side effect profiles (see Chapter 15). They diminish tremor and rigidity, but are generally less effective than levodopa; overall functional improvement is about 30% in most patients. However, trihexyphenidyl is more effective than levodopa against parkinsonian tremor. Anticholinergic drugs are often used to treat mild parkinsonism prior to initiating levodopa therapy or in patients who are hypersensitive or unresponsive to levodopa. They are the preferred agents for treating parkinsonian symptoms caused by neuroleptic therapy. Antimuscarinic drugs are also coadministered with levodopa, but they may worsen levodopa-induced dyskinesias and can delay absorption of levodopa.

Aside from their peripheral antimuscarinic effects, the most serious obstacle to use of these antagonists is mental deterioration and memory loss. Loss of mental function is worse in patients over 65, and thus these drugs should be used sparingly in the elderly. They are contraindicated in patients with prostatic hypertrophy, glaucoma, or pyloric stenosis. The antihistamines, diphenhydramine and orphenadrine, produce fewer anticholinergic problems but cause drowsiness.

Dosage of the muscarinic antagonists should be increased gradually to minimize adverse effects. Concomitant use of multiple anticholinergic agents is of no benefit. Peak plasma concentration is achieved in 2 to 4 hours after oral administration; the therapeutic effect lasts 1 to 6 hours. Withdrawal of anticholinergic therapy should be gradual to avoid rebound worsening of symptoms.

Trihexyphenidyl hydrochloride (Artane, Trihexy) is available in tablets of 2 and 5 mg, timed-release capsules of 5 mg, and an elixir at 2 mg/5 ml. Daily dosage ranges from 1 mg initially to a maximum of 15 mg. **Biperiden hydrochloride** (Akineton) is provided as 2 mg tablets; biperiden lactate is available in solution, 5 mg/ml, for injection. Dosage ranges from 6 to 16 mg/day. **Procyclidine hydrochloride** (Kemadrin) is available in 5 mg tablets. **Benztropine mesylate** (Cogentin) is available in tablets of 0.5 to 2 mg and in solution for intramuscular or, occasionally, for intravenous injection, 1 mg/ml. The daily dosage range is 0.5 to 6 mg. **Ethopropazine hydrochloride** (Parsidol), a phenothiazine, may be a useful adjunct. Drowsiness is common, and the drug can cause muscle cramps, paresthesias, hypotension, or rarely, agranulocytosis. It is supplied as tablets of 10 and 50 mg.

HUNTINGTONS DISEASE

Huntingtons disease, a progressive neurologic disorder,[15,27] is inherited in an autosomal dominant manner. All persons who carry the Huntington gene ultimately develop the disease. Symptoms of Huntingtons disease usually do not occur until midlife (30 to 50 years of age). The disease is characterized by three major symptoms: (1) choreoathetosis (that is, excessive, irregular spontaneous movements), (2) dementia, and (3) psychologic or personality changes. Approximately 95% of patients develop choreiform movements that progress until the patients cannot ambulate. Dementia is eventually observed in 90% of patients with Huntingtons disease. Behavioral changes include depression, irritability, and apathy.

The major pathology in Huntingtons disease is atrophy of the striatum and cerebral cortex. As in Parkinsons disease, multiple neurotransmitter systems are affected,[15] but changes in dopamine, acetylcholine, and GABA content in the basal ganglia have attracted the most interest. On postmortem examination, the basal ganglia of patients with Huntingtons disease exhibit a substantial loss of GABA and the GABA-synthesizing enzyme, glutamic acid decarboxylase. There is also a significant reduction in acetylcholine and choline acetyltransferase. Nigrostriatal dopamine-containing neurons are not affected. Such findings have led to simple models of Huntingtons disease such as that depicted in Fig. 30-3. Presumably, the imbalance in this disease favors dopamine because cholinergic and GABAergic activities are reduced. Loss of GABA-mediated inhibition from neurons projecting from the striatum to the substantia nigra allows excessive activity of dopamine. This model is supported by observations that dopamine receptor antagonists (neuroleptics) reduce choreiform movement, whereas levodopa worsens symptoms. Unfortunately, attempts to replace GABA and acetylcholine (in a manner similar to dopamine replacement in Parkinsons disease) have not been successful. Neither GABA-receptor agonists nor drugs that prevent GABA breakdown are of benefit. Likewise, attempts to enhance cholinergic activity are ineffective. Clearly, the simple model in Fig. 30-3 does not sufficiently explain the symptoms of Huntingtons disease.

To date, there are no specific therapies for Huntingtons disease. The only effective strategy to minimize the choreoathetotic movements is to limit the activity of dopamine. Haloperidol or another potent neuroleptic (see Chapter 27) is most commonly employed. The usual daily dosage of haloperidol is 2 to 15 mg. Increasing the dose further is not beneficial. In later stages of the disease, unfortunately, neuroleptics

FIG. 30-3. Schematic representation of a simple neurochemical model for Huntingtons disease (see text for details). ACh, *acetylcholine;* DA, *dopamine;* GABA, *γ-aminobutyric acid.*

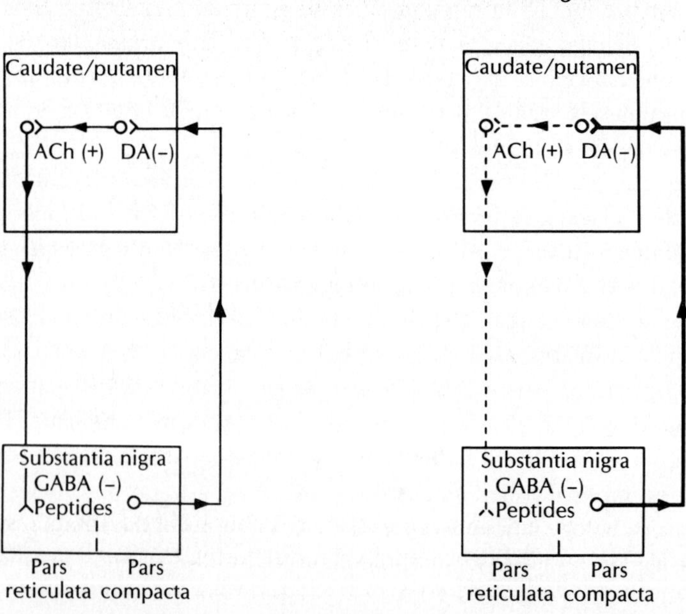

become ineffective. Treatment of the chorea with numerous other classes of drugs has been tried without success.

Tricyclic antidepressants have been used to treat the depression experienced by many patients with Huntingtons disease. Caution is essential with these agents, however, because they have anticholinergic properties that may exacerbate the chorea. Propranolol has been used with some success to treat aggression associated with the disease. Overall, however, pharmacologic intervention provides extremely limited benefit and does not retard the progress of this fatal disease. Compassion, supportive therapy, and genetic counseling are perhaps the most effective ways of dealing with this disorder.

WILSONS DISEASE

Wilsons disease (hepatolenticular degeneration)[13] is an autosomal recessive disorder that involves loss of liver function and neurologic symptoms. It is caused by a hepatic defect that impairs copper metabolism. Patients are deficient in ceruloplasmin, a copper-binding protein. Although plasma copper concentration is low, excessive amounts of copper are found in the brain (especially in the basal ganglia), the liver, and the kidneys.

Some patients with Wilsons disease present with hepatic toxicity similar to hepatitis or liver failure. Others initially exhibit psychic disturbances such as antisocial behavior, anxiety, paranoia, or depression. Three types of movement disorders may also be observed: akinesia resembling Parkinsons disease, dystonia, or tremors with ataxia.

The drug of choice to treat Wilsons disease is *D*-penicillamine (see p. 739). This agent binds copper and promotes its excretion. The goal of therapy is to remove excess copper and maintain normal concentrations in the body. Clinical improvement after initiation of penicillamine therapy usually occurs within the first 3 months, but more prolonged treatment may be necessary. Neurologic symptoms may initially be exacerbated by therapy as copper is mobilized from the liver. Starting dosages of penicillamine should, therefore, be low in patients with such symptoms. Once initiated, penicillamine therapy is continued for life. The usual daily dosage is 1 g initially, divided over four doses; it is gradually increased to 2 to 3 g. If early side effects such as fever, rash, and lymphadenopathy occur, the drug should be discontinued until they subside. Patients may develop bone-marrow depression with granulocytopenia and thrombocytopenia. Long-term toxicity includes a lupus-like syndrome, proteinuria, and possibly the nephrotic syndrome and dermatopathy.

Trientine, another chelating agent, is used to treat Wilsons disease in patients who cannot tolerate penicillamine. It may be less toxic than penicillamine, but more experience with this drug is warranted to assess potential side effects.

D-Penicillamine is available in 125 and 250 mg capsules (Cuprimine) and 250 mg tablets (Depen). **Trientine hydrochloride** (Cuprid) is available in 250 mg capsules.

ESSENTIAL TREMOR

Essential tremor is defined as rhythmic oscillations of body parts (especially the hands) that occur while maintaining posture or during action.[10] At rest, tremor is absent. The tremor may slowly worsen over time. Because essential tremor is not associated with degeneration of the central nervous system and is not fatal, it has been termed "benign." Essential tremor, however, can cause considerable discomfort and may interfere with tasks such as writing, eating, and drinking. Its etiology is unknown, but it may be inherited. Almost half of patients who develop essential tremor have a family history of the disease.

Although numerous drugs have been tested, only β-adrenergic receptor blockers and primidone are accepted as appropriate therapies. **Propranolol** (see p. 163) remains the drug of choice for treating essential tremor. It is believed to act by blocking β_2-receptors in the periphery, especially on muscle spindles and muscle afferent nerve fibers. The usual daily dosage of 240 to 320 mg is effective in 50% to 70% of patients.

The anticonvulsant **primidone** also reduces essential tremor. Although it may completely suppress the tremor, most studies suggest efficacy similar to that of propranolol. The major limitation of primidone, especially in the elderly, is a high incidence of side effects such as nausea, vomiting, headache, and ataxia. In addition, sedation can be a problem. A low dosage of primidone should be administered initially (50 mg/day), with a gradual increase to the therapeutic level. Although ethyl alcohol can reduce tremor, its use is clearly not recommended.

GILLES DE LA TOURETTES SYNDROME

Tourettes syndrome is a movement disorder characterized by daily, intermittent, motor and vocal tics.[23] Motor tics include touching, hitting, jumping, smelling objects, and other activities, whereas vocal tics include grunting, coughing, snorting, screaming, high and low pitched noises, and coprolalia (involuntary uttering of obscenities). Onset of the disorder is prior to 21 years of age, and patients often exhibit attention-deficit hyperactivity disorder, learning disabilities, antisocial behavior, obsessional disorders, and hyperkinesis. The etiology of the disease remains unknown.

Haloperidol and other potent neuroleptics are the standard treatment for symptomatic relief of the tics; approximately 85% of patients show improvement. Haloperidol is usually started at a daily dosage of 0.25 to 0.5 mg, to be increased to 3 to 8 mg if necessary. For patients who do not respond, **pimozide** (see p. 250) may provide effective relief. Unfortunately, the usefulness of such drugs is limited by their side effects. Recent indications that clonidine may help a subpopulation of patients with Tourettes syndrome warrant further studies.

MISCELLANEOUS MOVEMENT DISORDERS

There are several other movement disorders including dystonia, ballismus, and other forms of chorea. The etiology of these movement disorders remains to be determined. Dystonic patients may benefit from anticholinergic therapy; ballismic and choreic movements may benefit from neuroleptic therapy.

It is not uncommon for drug treatment to cause movement disorders.[5] Such neurologic side effects are usually treatable and remit when the offending compound is withdrawn. This is not, however, the case for tardive dyskinesias that occur secondary to neuroleptic therapy (see p. 245). Usually such dyskinesias involve involuntary movements of the mouth and tongue and widespread choreoathetosis. Currently, prevention is the only means of dealing with this disorder.

REFERENCES

1. Andén N-E, Carlsson A, Dahlström A, et al: Demonstration and mapping out of nigro-neostriatal dopamine neurons, *Life Sci* 3:523, 1964.
2. Blin J, Bonnet A-M, Agid Y: Does levodopa aggravate Parkinson's disease? *Neurology* 38:1410, 1988.
3. Calne DB, Rinne UK: Controversies in the management of Parkinson's disease, *Movement Dis* 1:159, 1986.
4. Diamond SG, Markham CH, Hoehn MM, et al: Multi-center study of Parkinson mortality with early versus later dopa treatment, *Ann Neurol* 22:8, 1987.
5. Dickey W, Morrow JI: Drug-induced neurological disorders, *Prog Neurobiol* 34:331, 1990.
6. Gianutsos G, Chute S, Dunn JP: Pharmacological changes in dopaminergic systems induced by long-term administration of amantadine, *Eur J Pharmacol* 110:357, 1985.
7. Graybiel AM: Neurotransmitters and neuromodulators in the basal ganglia, *Trends Neurosci* 13:244, 1990.
8. Guttman M, Seeman P, Reynolds GP, et al: Dopamine D_2 receptor density remains constant in treated Parkinson's disease, *Ann Neurol* 19:487, 1986.
9. Hornykiewicz O: Brain neurotransmitter changes in Parkinson's disease. In Marsden CD, Fahn S, editors: *Movement disorders, Neurology 2,* London, 1981, Butterworth Scientific, p 41.
10. Hubble JP, Busenbark KL, Koller WC: Essential tremor, *Clin Neuropharmacol* 12:453, 1989.
11. Langston JW, Ballard D, Tetrud JW, Irwin I: Chronic parkinsonism in humans due to a product of meperidine-analog synthesis, *Science* 219:979, 1983.
12. Langtry HD, Clissold SP: Pergolide: a review of its pharmacological properties and therapeutic potential in Parkinson's disease, *Drugs* 39:491, 1990.
13. Marsden CD: Wilson's disease, *Q J Med* 65:959, 1987.
14. Marsden CD, Parkes JD: "On-off" effects in patients with Parkinson's disease on chronic levodopa therapy, *Lancet* 1:292, 1976.
15. Martin JB, Gusella JF: Huntington's disease: pathogenesis and management, *N Engl J Med* 315:1267, 1986.
16. Mayeux R, Stern Y, Mulvey K, Cote L: Reappraisal of temporary levodopa withdrawal ("drug holiday") in Parkinson's disease, *N Engl J Med* 313:724, 1985.
17. McGeer PL, McGeer EG, Itagaki S, Mizukawa K: Anatomy and pathology of the basal ganglia, *Can J Neurol Sci* 14:363, 1987.
18. Nutt JG: Levodopa-induced dyskinesia: review, observations, and speculations, *Neurology* 40:340, 1990.
19. Nutt JG, Fellman JH: Pharmacokinetics of levodopa, *Clin Neuropharmacol* 7:35, 1984.
20. Nutt JG, Woodward WR, Hammerstad JP, et al: The "on-off" phenomenon in Parkinson's disease: relation to levodopa absorption and transport, *N Engl J Med* 310:483, 1984.
21. Parkinson Study Group: Effect of deprenyl on the progression of disability in early Parkinson's disease, *N Engl J Med* 321:1364, 1989.
22. Riopelle RJ: Bromocriptine and the clinical spectrum of Parkinson's disease, *Can J Neurol Sci* 14:455, 1987.
23. Robertson MM: The Gilles de la Tourette syndrome: the current status, *Br J Psychiatry* 154:147, 1989.
24. Seeman P, Grigoriadis D: Dopamine receptors in brain and periphery, *Neurochem Int* 10:1, 1987.
25. Semba K, Fibiger HC, Vincent SR: Neurotransmitters in the mammalian striatum: neuronal circuits and heterogeneity, *Can J Neurol Sci* 14:386, 1987.
26. Snyder SH, D'Amato RJ: MPTP: a neurotoxin relevant to the pathophysiology of Parkinson's disease, *Neurology* 36:250, 1986.
27. Stewart JT: Huntington's disease, *Am Fam Physician* 37(5):105, 1988.
28. Tetrud JW, Langston JW: The effect of deprenyl (selegiline) on the natural history of Parkinson's disease, *Science* 245:519, 1989.

Chapter 31

Central nervous system stimulants

GENERAL CONCEPTS

A great many drugs can stimulate the central nervous system. Stimulation may range from a mild increase in alertness or wakefulness to life-threatening seizures. Drugs at one end of the spectrum stimulate the nervous system chiefly in the setting of intoxication; examples include tricyclic antidepressants, organophosphate anticholinesterases, and salicylates. Other agents are used therapeutically or by the lay public for mild to moderate central nervous system stimulation at dosages employed for other therapeutic purposes; caffeine and amphetamines are prime examples. Again intoxication may cause seizures. Finally, *analeptic* (restorative) drugs, which are occasionally used to improve respiration, have narrow margins of safety and are known primarily for their convulsant properties.

METHYLXANTHINES

The methylxanthines, caffeine, theophylline, and theobromine, generally cause mild central nervous system stimulation, though toxic doses can elicit seizures. Theobromine is the least potent and is not used medicinally; it is the major methylxanthine in chocolate. Theophylline, used primarily for its bronchodilating action, is discussed in Chapter 44.

Caffeine

Caffeine (1,3,7-trimethylxanthine) is the stimulant most widely consumed by the lay public, and it also has some medical uses. A cup of coffee may contain from 50 to 150 mg of the alkaloid, whereas cola drinks have from 35 to 55 mg. A clinical dose for adults is 100 to 200 mg. Although coffee is believed to account for 90% of caffeine consumption in the United States, about 2 million pounds of caffeine is added yearly to other foodstuffs, mainly soft drinks.[4]

Caffeine stimulates the cerebral cortex and medullary centers. In ordinary doses it causes wakefulness, increases mental alertness, and decreases response times for simple motor tasks. These effects of caffeine are considered pleasant by most persons. It is not surprising that wherever a caffeine-containing plant grows, the inhabitants have usually learned to utilize the drug. Habituation to the use of caffeine occurs. Withdrawal symptoms, often headache or fatigue, are generally mild.[5] "Look-alike" drugs, which counterfeit the physical appearance of controlled substances, may contain caffeine. In large doses, caffeine stimulates respiration and can precipitate convulsions. The respiratory stimulant activity is beneficial in apneic, preterm infants.

Caffeine also has actions on the gastrointestinal tract and the cardiovascular system and is a diuretic (Table 31-1). Even though it stimulates gastric secretion of acid, pepsin, and gastrin, the drug is not the only active ingredient in coffee because

TABLE 31-1 Chemical structures and relative activities of methylxanthines

Xanthine

Alkaloid	Source	Methyl	Analepsis and gastric secretion	Cardiac stimulation, bronchodilatation, and diuresis
Caffeine	Coffee, tea, cocoa, cola	1,3,7	+ + +*	+
Theophylline	Tea	1,3	+ +	+ + +
Theobromine	Cocoa	3,7	+	+ +

*+, Least potent; + + +, most potent.

decaffeinated coffee may be a more potent stimulus to secretion than regular coffee or the alkaloid alone. In naive subjects, caffeine can evoke acute cardiovascular changes, such as modest increases in blood pressure, heart rate, and stroke volume; tolerance develops within a few days of chronic intake. High daily consumption of coffee or acute intoxication has been associated with ventricular premature contractions or tachyarrhythmias.[4,14] Increased coronary blood flow is probably a consequence of increased myocardial work and is not likely to be beneficial. Cerebral vessels are constricted by caffeine.

The end products of caffeine metabolism are 1-methyluric acid primarily and other methyl derivatives of xanthine and uric acid. Caffeine does not increase the miscible pool or urinary excretion of uric acid itself and is not contraindicated in gout.

For intramuscular or intravenous injection, caffeine (125 mg/ml) is provided with sodium benzoate in 2 ml ampules. For over-the-counter purchase, citrated caffeine is sold in 65 mg tablets and plain caffeine is available as tablets (100 and 200 mg) and timed-release capsules (200 and 250 mg). In addition, caffeine is often added to analgesic remedies containing salicylates or acetaminophen and, for the treatment of migraine, to ergotamine (Cafergot, others). In the latter combination, constriction of cerebral vessels by both alkaloids is believed to contribute to pain relief. An assessment of the clinical effectiveness of over-the-counter analgesic mixtures[8] indicates that addition of 130 mg of caffeine to such mixtures (in two tablets) is equivalent to a 30% to 40% increase in the dose of analgesic. However, even this modest increment in activity is unlikely with most presently available mixtures, which provide half or less of this dose of caffeine.

Visceral smooth muscle relaxation, such as bronchodilatation, is accomplished better by theophylline or by aminophylline, a soluble complex of theophylline with ethylenediamine. For many years the methylxanthines were believed to act primarily by inhibition of phosphodiesterase, the enzyme that inactivates cyclic AMP (cyclic adenosine 3',5'-monophosphate). This would account for the benefit in asthma from combinations with β-adrenergic receptor agonists, which promote the formation of this cyclic nucleotide. However, theophylline dilates bronchi at concentrations insufficient to inhibit phosphodiesterase so that some as yet unknown mechanism must be responsible for this particular effect.[9] Methylxanthines are also potent competitive antagonists of adenosine, a putative neurotransmitter that exhibits sedative, anticonvulsant, muscle relaxant, cardiac depressant, and Na^+-retaining activities. This mechanism may account for many of their other effects, such as diuresis and central nervous system and cardiac stimulation.[9]

Pentoxifylline

Pentoxifylline (Trental) is a synthetic methylxanthine with a longer side chain in place of the methyl group in carbon position 1 of caffeine. It was approved in 1984 to prevent *intermittent claudication*, in which inadequate blood flow to skeletal muscle results in pain or fatigue in the legs. The mechanisms most likely involved include improvement in red blood cell flexibility, decreased plasma fibrinogen, decreased viscosity of blood, and reduced platelet aggregation.[17] This drug is given as a controlled-release tablet of 400 mg, usually three times daily. Benefit may not be apparent until 2 to 8 weeks after initiation of therapy. The most common complaints are gastrointestinal.

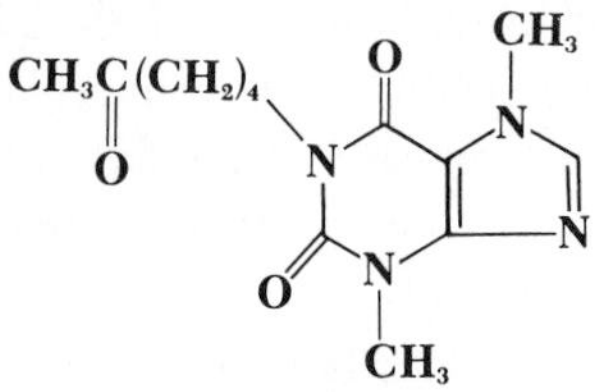

Pentoxifylline

METHYLPHENIDATE AND OTHER STIMULANTS

Some central nervous system stimulants, the amphetamines and methylphenidate, have been used for rapid elevation of mood in depressed patients, without persuasive evidence of benefit.[11] Unlike the antidepressants discussed in Chapter 28, these agents, sometimes called psychomotor stimulants, increase the general level of central nervous system excitability and lack a selective effect on psychologic depression. Hence the terms *antidepressant* and *stimulant* indicate quite different effects.

An important action of amphetamine is to promote release of monoamines from presynaptic terminals,[10] although it also inhibits amine reuptake. Its stimulant effect is blocked by metyrosine, an inhibitor of catecholamine synthesis, but not by reserpine, indications that it requires a newly synthesized (cytoplasmic) dopamine pool rather than the stored (vesicular) pool.[7,10] In contrast, methylphenidate, which also blocks amine reuptake, may facilitate amine release from storage vesicles; its stimulant effect is blocked by reserpine.

Major disadvantages of **amphetamine**, particularly the more potent *dextro* form (dextroamphetamine), include its cardiovascular effects, the letdown that follows the short period of stimulation, and its potential for abuse (see Chapter 34). Amphetamines are now used much less often than methylphenidate to treat attention-deficit hyperactivity disorder (ADHD).

Methylphenidate is primarily used in management of ADHD in children 6 years of age or older[3,15] and to alleviate the sleepiness of narcolepsy.[1,6] Daily pediatric dosage is usually 0.3 to 0.8 mg/kg in divided doses, taken on an empty stomach. Common, though often transient, side effects include insomnia, stomach aches, headaches, anorexia, and weight loss. Growth may be slowed temporarily, but final adult stature is not thought to be affected. Generally, stimulants should be avoided by patients with tics or a family history of Tourettes syndrome. Blood pressure should be monitored; methylphenidate must be used cautiously, if at all, in hypertensive persons or others in whom sympathetic stimulation may be hazardous, such as a patient taking an MAO inhibitor.

Pemoline, a longer acting stimulant, is occasionally used to treat ADHD. Potential for hepatotoxicity necessitates periodic tests of liver function.

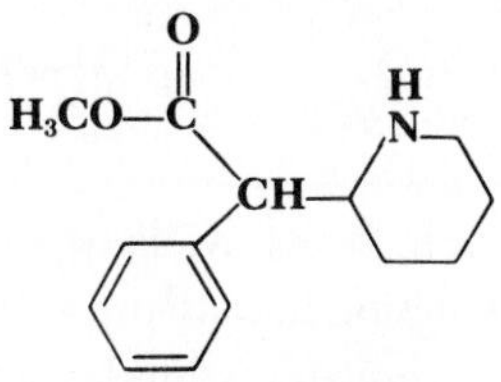

O
H
H_3CO—C
N
CH

Methylphenidate

Preparations of methylphenidate hydrochloride (Ritalin) include tablets containing 5 to 20 mg as well as a sustained-release 20 mg tablet. Pemoline (Cylert) is available in tablets of 18.75 to 75 mg and as a chewable tablet of 37.5 mg.

ANALEPTICS

Analeptic agents cause two potentially beneficial effects: they promote generalized arousal, and they increase the rate and depth of respiration. Important sites of action include the reticular activating system, vital centers in the medulla, and carotid chemoreceptors. Unfortunately, most analeptics also act on corticospinal pathways to enhance reflex excitability, which can lead to convulsions.[16] Analeptics are of toxicologic interest (strychnine), are tools for basic research on neurotransmission (bicuculline, pentylenetetrazol, picrotoxin, strychnine), or may be used as respiratory stimulants (doxapram, almitrine). They may excite neurons directly (doxapram), block presynaptic inhibition (picrotoxin), or block postsynaptic inhibition (strychnine). The older analeptics pentylenetetrazol and picrotoxin have a narrow margin of safety between their analeptic and convulsant doses and have been replaced in therapy by doxapram, a safer agent.

Doxapram

Doxapram is a powerful respiratory stimulant. Lower doses stimulate the carotid chemoreceptors; higher doses also stimulate brainstem respiratory centers. The drug increases respiratory volume more than rate. Its therapeutic index, determined in animals and expressed as "convulsant $dose_{50}$/respiratory stimulant $dose_{50}$," is considerably higher than that of the older analeptics. For improvement of postanesthetic respiration, doxapram hydrochloride (Dopram) is given as a single intravenous bolus of 0.5 to 1 mg/kg of body weight, as divided doses at 5-minute intervals, totaling up to 2 mg/kg, or as an infusion of 5 mg/minute, tapered to 1 to 3 mg/minute for maintenance. Doxapram has a duration of activity as short as 3 or 4 minutes. It causes sympathomimetic side effects such as hypertension and may be considered a very short-acting sympathomimetic stimulant.

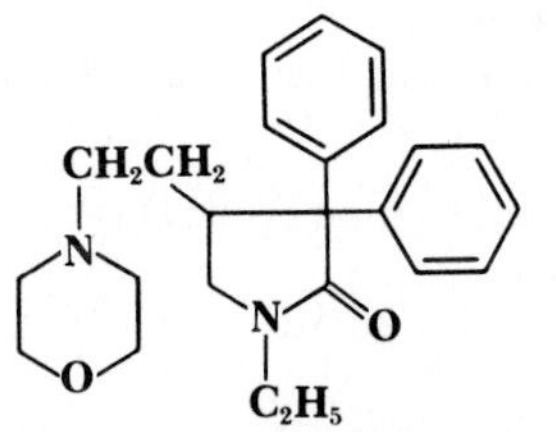

Doxapram

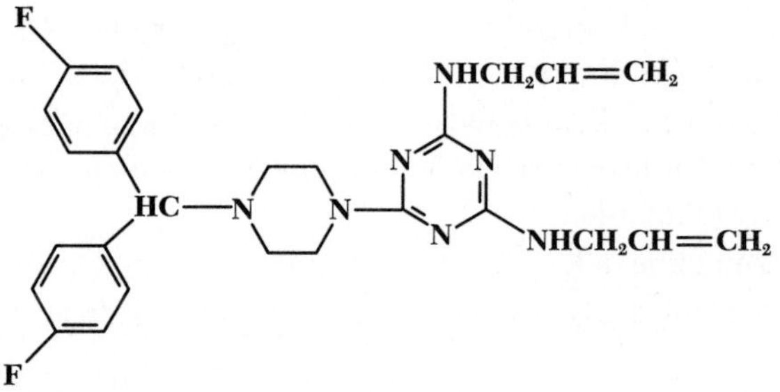

Almitrine

Almitrine

Almitrine dimesylate (Vectarion) is not available in the United States but has been used in Europe to improve oxygenation in patients with chronic obstructive pulmonary disease (COPD). Like doxapram, almitrine stimulates carotid body chemoreceptors. It also appears to redistribute pulmonary blood flow to alveoli that are relatively well ventilated.[13] Advantages over doxapram are that it is effective orally and has a prolonged action. Adverse effects include headache, diarrhea and abdominal pain, fatigue, peripheral sensory neuropathy, and, in some patients, a worsening of dyspnea. Administration with meals lessens nausea. Doses of 50 to 100 mg have generally been given twice daily.

Miscellaneous convulsants

There is much experience with the convulsant action of **pentylenetetrazol** in humans because the drug was once used in shock treatment for mental disease and, in lower doses, in diagnosis of epilepsy. When approximately 5 ml of a 10% solution of pentylenetetrazol is injected rapidly by the intravenous route, the person becomes apprehensive and in a few seconds convulses and loses consciousness. The major convulsive phase may last only a minute, to be followed by exhaustion and sleep. It was customary to premedicate patients with a muscle relaxant such as succinylcholine to prevent fractures.

Picrotoxin is a mixture of nonnitrogenous substances obtained from an East Indian shrub. The more active component is *picrotoxinin*. Picrotoxin is a convulsant of the pentylenetetrazol type. In normal animals it stimulates respiration only with doses near the convulsant dose. Barbiturate-anesthetized animals may show significant respiratory stimulation without a convulsant effect because barbiturates antagonize the convulsive tendency. Picrotoxin has been an important tool in elucidation in vitro of GABA-receptor mechanisms. See Chapter 26 for a discussion of relationships between picrotoxinin receptors and GABA-regulated Cl^- channels.

Strychnine is a complex alkaloid obtained from the seed of the plant *Strychnos nux vomica.* It affects all levels of the neuraxis but acts predominantly on the spinal cord, where glycine is the major inhibitory transmitter. Strychnine acts on a glycine/Cl^- channel complex,[2] possibly much in the way an inverse agonist acts on the $GABA_A$/Cl^- channel complex (see Chapter 26), to oppose the inhibitory influence of Renshaw cells, thereby lowering the threshold of excitability of motoneurons. Strychnine convulsions differ from pentylenetetrazol seizures in humans by the predominance of the tonic extensor phase, *opisthotonos* being characteristic of both this type of poisoning and of tetanus. The person becomes highly susceptible to various stimuli, so that a sudden noise, light, or other stimulus can precipitate a seizure.

H_2C—CH_2 N N O O

Strychnine

Toxicologic interest in strychnine[12] arises from its use as a rodenticide and its presence as a contaminant in "street drugs." Death by strychnine poisoning is secondary to asphyxia due to prolonged spasms of the respiratory musculature. Barbiturates and diazepam are effective antagonists of the convulsant and lethal actions of strychnine. Mechanical ventilation, physical cooling, correction of acidosis, and paralysis with a nondepolarizing neuromuscular blocking agent may be needed as well. Gastric lavage with activated charcoal may lessen intoxication.

REFERENCES

1. Aldrich MS: Narcolepsy, *N Engl J Med* 323:389, 1990.
2. Betz H, Becker C-M: The mammalian glycine receptor: biology and structure of a neuronal chloride channel protein, *Neurochem Int* 13:137, 1988.
3. Buttross S: Disorders of attention and vigilance, *Semin Neurol* 8:97, 1988.
4. Council on Scientific Affairs: Caffeine labeling, *JAMA* 252:803, 1984.
5. Griffiths RR, Woodson PP: Caffeine physical dependence: a review of human and laboratory animal studies, *Psychopharmacology* 94:437, 1988.
6. Kales A, Vela-Bueno A, Kales JD: Sleep disorders: sleep apnea and narcolepsy, *Ann Intern Med* 106:434, 1987.
7. Kuczenski R: Biochemical actions of amphetamine and other stimulants. In Creese I, editor: *Stimulants: neurochemical, behavioral, and clinical perspectives,* New York, 1983, Raven Press, p 31.
8. Laska EM, Sunshine A, Mueller F, et al:

Caffeine as an analgesic adjuvant, *JAMA* 251:1711, 1984.

9. Persson CGA, Andersson K-E, Kjellin G: Effects of enprofylline and theophylline may show the role of adenosine, *Life Sci* 38:1057, 1986.
10. Rebec GV: Electrophysiological pharmacology of amphetamine, *Monogr Neural Sci* 13:1, 1987.
11. Satel SL, Nelson JC: Stimulants in the treatment of depression: a critical overview, *J Clin Psychiatry*, 50:241, 1989.
12. Smith BA: Strychnine poisoning, *J Emerg Med* 8:321, 1990.
13. Smith PD, Gotz VP, Ryerson GG: Almitrine bismesylate, *Drug Intell Clin Pharm* 21:417, 1987.
14. Stavric B: Methylxanthines: toxicity to humans. 2. Caffeine, *Fd Chem Toxic* 26:645, 1988.
15. Stevenson RD, Wolraich ML: Stimulant medication therapy in the treatment of children with attention deficit hyperactivity disorder, *Pediatr Clin North Am* 36:1183, 1989.
16. Wang SC, Ward, JW: Analeptics. *Pharmacol Ther [B]* 3:123, 1977.
17. Ward A, Clissold SP: Pentoxifylline: a review of its pharmacodynamic and pharmacokinetic properties, and its therapeutic efficacy, *Drugs* 34:50, 1987.

Chapter 32

Antiepileptic drugs

GENERAL CONCEPT

Convulsions are involuntary skeletal muscular contractions. Unconsciousness may or may not occur. Convulsions can arise from pathologic processes within or outside the brain, toxins, drug overdose, or withdrawal from drug dependence. A frequent cause is the assortment of neuronal deficits grouped under the term *epilepsy*. Epileptic seizures, however, take many forms and are not necessarily convulsive; for example, in *absence* the victim may exhibit a 5- to 30-second period of staring without motor manifestations.

Epilepsies are categorized for purposes of treatment, yet epilepsy is a symptom more than a specific disease. Diagnosis is based mainly on clinical patterns of the seizure. An electroencephalogram (EEG) can be helpful. For instance, regular, symmetric, three-per-second spike-wave complexes are characteristic of absence seizures. A brief, annotated classification of epileptic seizures is given below. More detailed classifications and descriptions are offered elsewhere.[2,8]

1. *Generalized seizures* (abrupt bilateral involvement of both hemispheres)
   a. *Tonic-clonic*, or grand mal (unconsciousness, convulsions)
   b. *Absence*, or petit mal (impairment of consciousness, staring, often no motor signs; prepubertal or adolescent)
   c. *Myoclonic* (brief shocklike jerks or contractions)
   d. *Atonic* (sudden loss of muscle tone, *drop attacks*)
   e. *Infantile spasms* (short flexion spasms without loss of consciousness, *hypsarrhythmia* EEG pattern; infants, retarded development, may respond to ACTH or anti-inflammatory steroids if usual anticonvulsants fail)
2. *Partial*, or focal, *seizures* (spread contained within limits)
   a. *Simple*, includes jacksonian (consciousness not impaired; motor, somatosensory, autonomic, or psychic symptoms)
   b. *Complex*, or psychomotor (consciousness impaired; may be preceded by prodromal sensation or aura [simple partial]; automatisms may occur)
   c. *Partial becoming generalized* (focal EEG discharge before generalized seizure occurs; focal behavioral events before or after tonic-clonic seizures)

A region of abnormal neuronal discharge is an essential feature of partial epileptic seizures. This "focus" may be *functional* (arising from proximity to a tumor, hypoxic tissue, a cyst) or *cryptogenic* (abnormal synaptic connections or biochemical lesion). Neurons within this region discharge rapidly in bursts. A seizure arises when these discharges invade adjacent regions, recruiting neurons into a synchronously discharging aggregate of excited cells. Stimuli for spread of excitation may include changes in blood glucose, plasma pH, osmotic pressure, electrolytes, or circulating hormones. Fatigue, stress, or nutritional deficiencies may also trigger spread. Generalized seizures ensue if excitation extends to both cerebral hemispheres, or they may be the first manifestation of epilepsy without evidence of a specific focus. As part of the excitation process, certain neurons feed back inhibitory information to the neuronal aggregate (Fig. 32-1). Inhibitory synaptic potentials summate with time, gradually hyperpolarizing and desynchronizing the aggregate. This latter process terminates the motor or sensory manifestations (ictus) and may be partially responsible for the usual period of postictal lethargy.

MODES OF ACTION

Working hypotheses for the actions of anticonvulsants arise from the idea that drug-induced changes in permeability to specific ions may stabilize membranes, interfere with Ca^{++}-mediated release of neurotransmitters, and so forth. There is considerable information about electrophysiologic effects of antiepileptic agents and about their effects on ion fluxes.[10,14,20] Nevertheless, the relevance of the experimental observations to the therapeutic benefit remains somewhat speculative.

Phenytoin and carbamazepine are used in management of generalized tonic-clonic and partial seizures. They block Na^+ channels in voltage-, frequency-, and time-dependent fashion, probably by binding to and stabilizing the channels in their inactive, rather than their resting or open, state. In a routine screening procedure, they

FIG 32-1. *Diagram of neuronal connections believed to be important in the genesis of tonic-clonic convulsions. Excitation spreads from focal neuron* (asterisk) *through excitatory synapses* (e) *to form an aggregate of excited cells* (shaded). *Involvement of motor pathways leads to skeletal muscle contractions. Some neurons* (unshaded), *when activated, feed back inhibitory signals through synapses* (i) *on focal and other neurons in the chain to terminate the seizure episode. Intracellular recordings depicted are typical for cells in a focal region during interictal periods: bursts of action potentials on waves of depolarization. Such bursts are often coincident with spikes in electroencephalographic spike/wave combinations (three combinations are shown). A paroxysm of exaggerated amplitude, slow (3 to 5/sec) waves appears in the EEG during spread. These paroxysms can occur in the absence of clinical convulsions if spread is not extensive. The time calibration is 200 msec for the intracellular record and 1 sec for the electroencephalograms.*

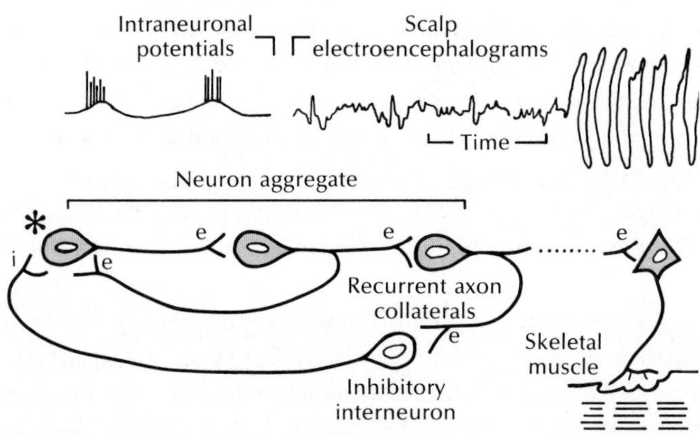

raise the threshold for electroshock-induced convulsions. At the neurophysiologic level, these agents decrease the spread of seizure discharge, probably by reducing posttetanic potentiation.

Phenobarbital and benzodiazepines promote Cl^- influx and hyperpolarization through interactions with the $GABA_A/Cl^-$ channel complex (see Fig. 26-6). Phenobarbital appears to act at the so-called picrotoxinin site. Benzodiazepines bind at a different site. Valproic acid, a broad-spectrum antiepileptic drug, in some way facilitates GABA-mediated inhibition and also blocks Na^+ channels.

Agents such as ethosuximide and trimethadione, which are primarily useful for treatment of absence seizures, block a specific type (T) of Ca^{++} channel and are relatively effective in preventing seizure production by pentylenetetrazol (see p. 304).

Many other agents that interact with the GABA complex (vigabatrin or γ-vinyl GABA, progabide), Na^+ or Ca^{++} channels, or excitatory amino acid receptors are under investigation for potential use in management of epilepsy.[13,20] Analogs of adenosine, a putative neurotransmitter with anticonvulsant activity, may provide yet another avenue for discovery of improved antiepileptic compounds.

ADVERSE EFFECTS AND DRUG INTERACTIONS

Adverse effects of antiepileptic drugs tend to be gastrointestinal, mental or behavioral, and neurologic or, less commonly, cutaneous, hematopoietic, hepatic, or teratogenic. Initial gastrointestinal disturbances usually respond to dosage reduction. Changes in personality, behavior, and cognitive performance can present special problems in children.[7,23] Drugs that control tonic-clonic seizures may exacerbate or unmask other types of seizures and vice versa. Discontinuance of benzodiazepine, barbiturate, and possibly carbamazepine medication should be gradual; abrupt withdrawal may precipitate status epilepticus. Vitamin K deficiency and bleeding in neonates can be prevented by giving the vitamin to the mother in the 2 weeks before birth. Clinically significant interactions among antiepileptics and with other drugs are numerous (Chapter 70) and frequently necessitate monitoring of serum concentration.[5] For example, all of the drugs favored for management of generalized tonic-clonic seizures can induce hepatic enzymes and enhance metabolism of themselves and other drugs.

ANTIEPILEPTIC DRUG CLASSES

From a structural standpoint the various drugs used in treating epilepsy may be categorized as follows:

BARBITURATES AND RELATED DRUGS
- Phenobarbital (Solfoton, others)
- Mephobarbital (Mebaral)
- Primidone (Mysoline, Myidone)

HYDANTOINS
- Phenytoin (Dilantin, Diphenylan)
- Mephenytoin (Mesantoin)
- Ethotoin (Peganone)

SUCCINIMIDES
- Ethosuximide (Zarontin)
- Methsuximide (Celontin)
- Phensuximide (Milontin)

OXAZOLIDINEDIONES
- Trimethadione (Tridione)
- Paramethadione (Paradione)

BENZODIAZEPINES
Clonazepam (Klonopin)
Diazepam (Valium)
Lorazepam (Activan)
Clorazepate (Tranxene)

MISCELLANEOUS ANTICONVULSANTS
Carbamazepine (Tegretol, Epitol)
Valproic acid (Depakene)
Divalproex sodium (Depakote)
Phenacemide (Phenurone)
Acetazolamide (Diamox, others)
ACTH, corticosteroids

The formulas of barbiturates, hydantoins, succinimides, and oxazolidinediones have many similarities. Whereas barbituric acid is malonylurea, hydantoins have a five-membered ring formed by condensation of acetic acid and urea. In the succinimide and oxazolidinedione series, one of the nitrogens in the hydantoin ring is replaced by carbon or oxygen respectively. Bromides were the earliest antiepileptic drugs, followed by phenobarbital in 1912 and phenytoin in 1938. Information regarding dosage, pharmacokinetics, and therapeutic spectra of the major antiepileptic agents is summarized in Table 32-1.

Carbamazepine

Carbamazepine is related structurally to the tricyclic antidepressants. It is quite useful in management of generalized tonic-clonic seizures and partial seizures[15] and in trigeminal neuralgia. The drug is also a possible alternative to neuroleptics for rapid control of acute mania in patients with bipolar disorder. Carbamazepine may produce the least cognitive impairment of any of the major antiepileptic agents.[22]

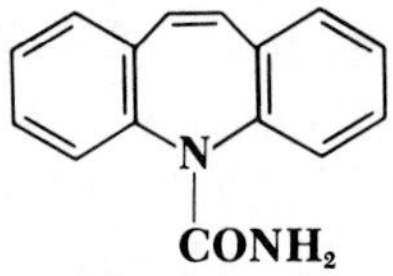

N
$CONH_2$
Carbamazepine

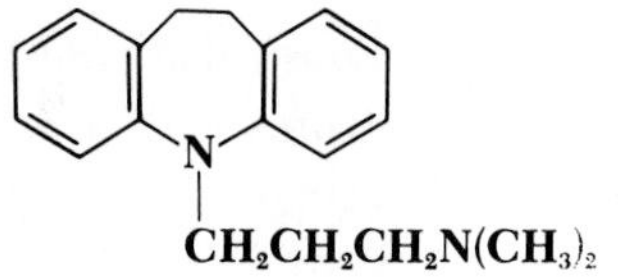

N
$CH_2CH_2CH_2N(CH_3)_2$
Imipramine

Pharmacokinetics. Carbamazepine is absorbed slowly from the gastrointestinal tract. Twice daily administration may suffice, but more frequent, smaller doses can minimize adverse effects. Unlike phenytoin and phenobarbital, only oral preparations of carbamazepine are available. The drug is oxidized primarily to carbamazepine-10,11-epoxide, an active metabolite. Carbamazepine induces drug metabolism. Its elimination half-life with chronic administration ranges from 10 to 25 hours, whereas the half-life of a single dose may be 30 to 40 hours. Such *autoinduction* is complete within 3 to 6 weeks. Autoinduction and induction from exposure to other anticonvulsants will require gradual adjustment of dosage. Valproate can slow metabolism of the epoxide and allow it to accumulate. When possible, it is preferable to avoid concurrent use of carbamazepine with other antiepileptic drugs.

Adverse effects. Carbamazepine may elicit transient drowsiness, ataxia, or dizziness and rarely hepatic damage or cardiotoxicity.[7,19] Features of overdose include dyskinetic movements, combativeness, hallucinations, seizures, and coma.[24] Symptoms may recur unexpectedly late in recovery, probably due to delayed absorption as the antimuscarinic activity of the drug wears off and gastrointestinal motility increases. Car-

TABLE 32-1 Primary antiepileptic drugs: summary of dosage, pharmacokinetics, and clinical activity

Drug	Daily maintenance dose[5] Adult (mg) / Child (mg/kg)	Therapeutic concentration[5] (μg/ml)	Days to reach steady-state	Preferred drugs for control of seizures* — Seizure type — Partial[5]: Simple, complex	Generalized: Tonic-clonic[5]	Generalized: Absence[5]	Generalized: Myoclonic, atonic§	Generalized: Infantile spasms†	Oral dosage forms‡ (mg)
Carbamazepine	600-1200 20-30	6-12	3-6	1	1				CT: 100; S: 100; T:200
Phenytoin	300-400 4-7	10-20	variable	1	1				C: 30,100; CT: 50; S: 30,125
Phenobarbital	120-250 3-5	15-35	16-21	2	2				C: 16; S: 15, 20;T: 8-100
Primidone	750-1500 10-25	6-12	1-5	2	2				S: 250; T: 50, 250
Ethosuximide	750-2000 20-40	40-100	5-12			1	3		C: 250; S: 250
Valproic acid	1000-3000 15-60	50-100	2-4		1§	1	1§	3	C: 250; S: 250
Clonazepam	1.5-20 0.01-0.2	0.013-0.072	4-5			2	2	2	T: 0.5-2
Trimethadione	900-2400 15-30	10-30	3			3			C: 300; CT: 150; S: 200

*The numbers listed for each seizure type indicate a relative order of choice for seizure management. However, the order of preference by individual clinicans varies, and definite evidence of the superiority of one drug over another is often unavailable.
†ACTH and glucocorticoids are first choice.
‡*C*, Capsules; *CT*, chewable tablets; *S*, suspension or other liquid preparation (in 5 ml); *T*, tablets.
§Approved only with concurrent absence.

bamazepine can also cause aplastic anemia or agranulocytosis.[19] Patients should be alert for such signs as sore throat, fever, ulcers in the mouth, easy bruising, and petechial or purpuric hemorrhage. A transient, or even persistent, leukopenia is fairly common but usually benign, not requiring discontinuance of the drug. Initial and periodic blood counts and liver function tests are generally recommended. An association of carbamazepine use during pregnancy with relatively frequent but minor birth defects (craniofacial malformations, hypoplastic fingernails, delayed development) has been reported.[9]

Hydantoins

Phenytoin is still one of the most valuable antiepileptic drugs.[15] It seldom causes sedation at therapeutic concentrations. It may, however, impair cognitive function.[22] Phenytoin is given intravenously in status epilepticus: 30 to 50 mg/min (adults) or 0.5 to 1.5 mg/kg/min (children) for a loading dose of 15 to 20 mg/kg.[5]

Pharmacokinetics of phenytoin.[17] The drug is slowly absorbed from the intestinal tract and is about 90% bound to albumin. Like salicylic acid (see p. 362), phenytoin exhibits *concentration-dependent* clearance; an increase in dosage within the therapeutic range may cause a disproportionate rise in plasma concentration as microsomal enzymes become saturated. Half-life increases, and small dosage increments may result in toxicity. Monitoring of serum concentration can aid adjustment of dosage. Interpretation is hampered if a drug is added that displaces phenytoin from albumin. The concentration of unbound drug is usually increased only transiently, but the monitored concentration (total phenytoin) decreases, even though the therapeutic response is maintained. Displacement by valproic acid, however, may elicit delayed toxicity, apparently because it also reduces metabolism of phenytoin. Concurrent therapy with cimetidine and several other drugs can impair metabolism of phenytoin (see Table 70-3).

Adverse effects of phenytoin. Chronic intoxication is characterized by nystagmus, ataxia, lethargy, and a paradoxical increase in seizures. These manifestations are dose related and appear at plasma concentrations of 20 to 40 μg/ml. Severe and prolonged intoxication may cause degeneration of cerebellar Purkinje cells. Acute intoxication can also induce cardiac arrhythmias and hypotension.

Osteomalacia and hypocalcemia may be attributable to enhanced vitamin D metabolism. Impaired utilization of folic acid can cause megaloblastic anemia. Hypertrophy of the gums (gingival "hyperplasia") occurs in a substantial minority of patients, is generally attributed to a disorder of fibroblastic activity, and is exacerbated by poor dental hygiene. Other "cosmetic" effects include hirsutism, acne, and a coarsening of facial features.

Although phenytoin may increase the risk of teratogenesis, other antiepileptic drugs and epilepsy itself may contribute to the teratogenesis. Current thinking is that anticonvulsant medication should be withdrawn from a pregnant woman who has had no seizures for "many years" but that otherwise seizures during pregnancy pose a greater risk to the developing fetus than antiepileptic drugs do.[1]

The hydantoins may induce blood dyscrasias and rarely a clinical picture resembling malignant lymphoma. Rash is an indication for withdrawal, to avoid rare but serious exfoliative dermatitis. The use of phenytoin as an antiarrhythmic drug is discussed in Chapter 39.

Mephenytoin is partially metabolized to ethylphenylhydantoin, which was withdrawn from the market because it produced an extraordinarily high incidence of fever and rash. Likewise a high incidence of reactions has been reported for mephenytoin. Clearly it should be used only if safer agents are ineffective. The antiepileptic effectiveness of **ethotoin**, another hydantoin, has not been well established.

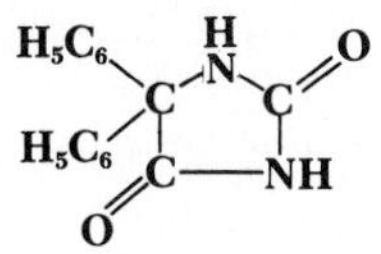

H_5C_6, H, N, O, H_5C_6, C, C, NH, O

Phenytoin

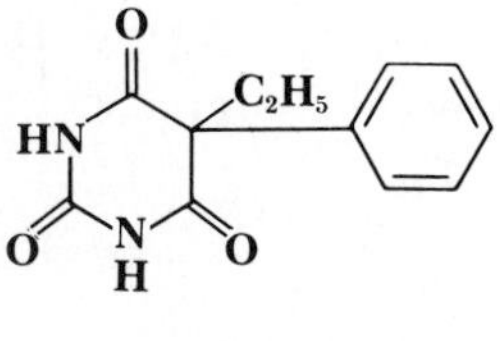

O, HN, C_2H_5, O, N, H, O

Phenobarbital

O, HN, C_2H_5, N, H, O

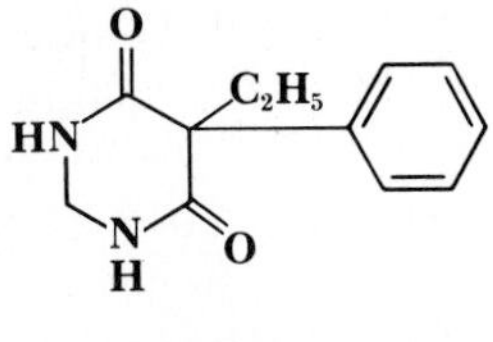

Primidone

Barbiturates and primidone

Phenobarbital is one of the oldest and least expensive antiepileptic drugs. Unlike most barbiturates, it can be antiepileptic in many patients without causing excessive drowsiness. Patients tend to become tolerant to its sedative action. The major usefulness of the drug is in preventing tonic-clonic and simple partial seizures. A single dose at bedtime is effective. In the United States, phenobarbital has been the preferred prophylactic treatment for febrile convulsions in young children at high risk, but this approach has been increasingly questioned.[6,11]

Irritability, hyperactivity, and more subtle changes in behavior and intellectual function are among its effects in children.[6,7,23] Sporadic reports of barbiturate-associated connective tissue disorders (e.g., contractures, frozen joints) were recently supported by a prospective survey of patients being treated with a single antiepileptic drug.[16] Sudden withdrawal of phenobarbital is likely to precipitate a generalized seizure or status epilepticus.

Mephobarbital, *N*-methylphenobarbital, has similar indications. The compound is partially demethylated to form phenobarbital, thus accounting for some of its antiepileptic action. The average adult dosage of mephobarbital is 400 to 600 mg/day.

Primidone, though not a true barbiturate, is similar in structure to phenobarbital. Because sedation, ataxia, and nausea can be pronounced initially, a low starting dose of 100 mg at bedtime should be used. The dose can be gradually increased, if necessary, to 250 mg or more four times daily. Although use in adults has been associated with a higher incidence of side effects than with other drugs,[15] primidone may be relatively well tolerated by children.[7] The drug is converted to two active metabolites: phenobarbital and phenylethylmalonamide. If primidone is used during pregnancy, vitamin K should be given before delivery to avoid maternal and neonatal problems with hemorrhage.

Succinimides

Ethosuximide, **methsuximide**, and **phensuximide** are useful in the order listed for management of typical and atypical absence seizures. They are less toxic than the oxazolidinediones discussed below, though transient, dose-related nausea, drowsiness, and anorexia, as well as headache, may occur. Rare cases of rash, leukopenia, and lupus-like syndromes have been reported. Monthly blood counts are recommended. Interactions with other antiepileptic agents are minimal. Ethosuximide and valproic acid are the drugs of choice for management of absence seizures; the former if hepatotoxicity is a particular concern, the latter if the patient also has tonic-clonic seizures.

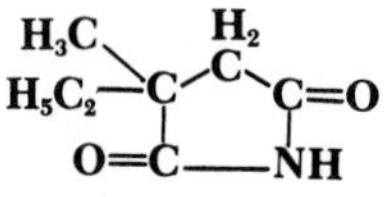

Ethosuximide

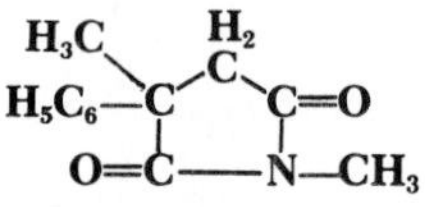

Methsuximide

Oxazolidinediones

Trimethadione and **paramethadione**, once primary agents for control of absence seizures, are now used mainly in patients who have not responded to other therapy. Toxic effects include photophobia and white halos around objects in the visual field (hemeralopia), drowsiness, ataxia, rashes, and alopecia. Bone marrow depression and kidney damage after prolonged use have been described. A fetal teratogenic trimethadione syndrome has resulted in facial abnormalities, growth retardation, cardiac and ocular problems, and microcephaly.[1] The drug should not be taken by pregnant women.

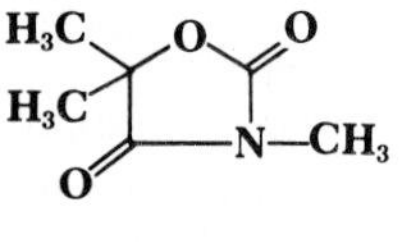

Trimethadione

Benzodiazepines

Clonazepam, **diazepam**, and **clorazepate** are the benzodiazepines approved as antiepileptic drugs. Clonazepam is useful for management of drug-resistant absence seizures and progressive myoclonic epilepsy. Tolerance may slowly diminish its effectiveness. Adverse effects include drowsiness, ataxia, and, in children, behavioral changes. Diazepam is indicated for status epilepticus. It readily enters the brain. Like thiopental, its duration of action after a single intravenous bolus is relatively short because it rapidly redistributes from the brain to peripheral tissues. Accordingly, it is more useful by infusion for control of status epilepticus. Diazepam for intravenous use is available in ampules, vials, and syringes containing 5 mg/ml. Alternatively, because it has a smaller volume of distribution, a single injection of **lorazepam** can provide more prolonged control of status.[21] Rectal administration of diazepam in solution, as needed during high fevers, has been advocated to prevent or control febrile convulsions in children.[11] Clorazepate is an approved adjunct in control of partial seizures.

Valproic acid

Valproic acid, dipropylacetic acid, is highly effective in controlling generalized seizures, both tonic-clonic and absence, is indicated also for myoclonic seizures, and has been used for prophylaxis of febrile seizures.[11] Thus it has a remarkably wide range of applications. Its use is limited somewhat by its potential for serious toxicity.

$$\begin{array}{l} CH_3-CH_2-CH_2 \\ \qquad\qquad\qquad \diagdown \\ \qquad\qquad\quad HC-COOH \\ \qquad\qquad\qquad \diagup \\ CH_3-CH_2-CH_2 \end{array}$$

Valproic acid

Pharmacokinetics. Absorption from the gastrointestinal tract is rapid, and the drug has a relatively short half-life. It is usually administered three or four times daily. **Divalproex sodium**, a combination of two valproate molecules intended to minimize gastrointestinal side effects, is available in enteric-coated tablets as equivalents of 125 to 500 mg of the active drug. At least a dozen metabolites of valproic acid are formed.[25] Some of these apparently contribute to the therapeutic effect and others, including some free radicals, to toxicity. Concomitant therapy with drugs that induce liver enzymes can enhance valproate potential for hepatotoxicity or hyperammonemia. Conversely, valproate affects the kinetics of other antiepileptic agents. It inhibits metabolism of phenobarbital and increases the plasma concentration of unbound phenytoin.

Adverse effects. Patients may experience nausea, vomiting, polyuria and thirst, tremor, transient hair loss, weight gain, and pancreatitis.[3,7] Cognitive impairment seems to be minimal.[23] Thrombocytopenia may develop with prolonged administration of high dosages, and cerebral edema seems to be a feature of severe intoxication. Transaminase concentrations are elevated in many patients, usually without clinical manifestations. However, fatal hepatotoxicity can occur, usually within 6 months of initiation of therapy. Patients should be monitored regularly during this period and reevaluated in the event of clinical indications of liver damage, such as nausea, malaise, weakness, anorexia, and loss of seizure control. In the United States the risk has been greatest with combination therapy in children under 2 years of age.[4] In addition to avoiding such usage, it is also recommended that salicylates not be given concurrently; salicylates alter valproate kinetics, and the hepatotoxicity resembles Reyes syndrome. Valproic acid is estimated to cause neural-tube defects in 1% to 2% of exposures during the first trimester of pregnancy.

Miscellaneous anticonvulsants

Metabolic acidosis induced by a ketogenic diet is occasionally used for infantile spasms and other refractory seizures. **Acetazolamide** (see Chapter 42) is used adjunctively as an anticonvulsant. It has a broad anticonvulsant spectrum, but rapid development of tolerance limits its usefulness. Its effectiveness results from inhibition of carbonic anhydrase in the brain rather than from systemic acidosis. Acetazolamide is given in doses of 250 to 500 mg two or three times a day.

Phenacemide, a quite toxic anticonvulsant, may cause severe bone marrow depression, hepatocellular damage, and toxic psychoses. It is used rarely, mostly for partial complex seizures, only after all other measures fail. Tablets of 500 mg are taken three times a day.

CLINICAL PHARMACOLOGY

The relative usefulness of the major antiepileptic drugs in management of various seizure types is indicated in Table 32-1. Their clearance is often greater in children than in adults, and so the effective dose per kilogram of body weight is usually higher in children (Table 32-1). The general incidence of side effects is less if doses are low initially and then increased slowly. Complete seizure control may not be possible because of side effects. Sufficient time to reach steady state must be allowed between increments in dosage.

Patient compliance is a major problem.[12] More often than not, "nonresponders" are not taking their medication at all or as prescribed. Periodic monitoring of serum drug concentrations is useful both for ensuring adequate but not toxic dosage and as an indication of compliance.

Management of epilepsy solely with the less sedative agents (phenytoin, carbamazepine, valproic acid, and ethosuximide) can reduce problems with daytime drowsiness, behavior, and withdrawal. It is also advantageous if seizures can be controlled by a single drug; interactions and the potential for side effects are then minimized. Although the same agents are used, complex partial seizures are generally more difficult to control than are generalized tonic-clonic seizures. After prolonged drug therapy without seizure recurrence some patients are candidates for cautious drug withdrawal to determine if antiepileptics are still needed.[18]

Status epilepticus

Status epilepticus is the occurrence of a prolonged seizure or a series of seizures, convulsive or nonconvulsive, without full recovery between episodes. Tonic-clonic status is life threatening and causes hyperthermia, metabolic acidosis, catecholamine release, and often pulmonary edema. Various treatment protocols have been proposed. One begins with intravenous lorazepam, followed by phenytoin (up to three doses) and then phenobarbital, as necessary.[21] If status continues, EEG burst suppression is induced and maintained by infusion of the barbiturate. Others prefer to initiate treatment with phenytoin, phenobarbital, or diazepam with phenytoin. In unresponsive cases, general anesthesia may be required.

REFERENCES

1. American Academy of Pediatrics Committee on Drugs: Anticonvulsants and pregnancy, *Pediatrics* 63:331, 1979.
2. Commission on Classification and Terminology of the International League against Epilepsy: Proposal for revised clinical and electroencephalographic classification of epileptic seizures, *Epilepsia* 22:489, 1981.
3. Dreifuss FE, Langer DH: Side effects of valproate, *Am J Med* 84(suppl 1A):34, 1988.
4. Dreifuss FE, Langer DH, Moline KA, Maxwell JE: Valproic acid hepatic fatalities. II. US experience since 1984, *Neurology* 39:201, 1989.
5. Drugs for epilepsy, *Med Lett Drugs Ther* 31:1, 1989.
6. Farwell JR, Lee YJ, Hirtz DG, et al: Phenobarbital for febrile seizures—effects on

intelligence and on seizure recurrence, *N Engl J Med* 322:364, 1990.

7. Herranz JL, Armijo JA, Arteaga R: Clinical side effects of phenobarbital, primidone, phenytoin, carbamazepine, and valproate during monotherapy in children, *Epilepsia* 29:794, 1988.
8. Janz D: Epilepsy: seizures and syndromes, *Handb Exp Pharmacol* 74:3, 1985.
9. Jones KL, Lacro RV, Johnson KA, Adams J: Pattern of malformations in the children of women treated with carbamazepine during pregnancy, *N Engl J Med* 320:1661, 1989.
10. Jurna I: Electrophysiological effects of antiepileptic drugs, *Handb Exp Pharmacol* 74:611, 1985.
11. Knudsen FU: Optimum management of febrile seizures in childhood, *Drugs* 36:111, 1988.
12. Leppik IE: Compliance during treatment of epilepsy, *Epilepsia* 29 (suppl 2):S79, 1988.
13. Löscher W, Schmidt D: Which animal models should be used in the search for new antiepileptic drugs? A proposal based on experimental and clinical considerations, *Epilepsy Res* 2:145, 1988.
14. Macdonald RL, Meldrum BS: General principles. Principles of antiepileptic drug action. In Levy R, Mattson R, Meldrum B, Penry JK, Dreifuss FE, editors: *Antiepileptic drugs*, ed 3, New York, 1989, Raven Press, p 59.
15. Mattson RH, Cramer JA, Collins JF, et al: Comparison of carbamazepine, phenobarbital, phenytoin, and primidone in partial and secondarily generalized tonic-clonic seizures, *N Engl J Med* 313:145, 1985.
16. Mattson RH, Cramer JA, McCutchen CB, and the Veterans Administration Epilepsy Cooperative Study Group: Barbiturate-related connective tissue disorders, *Arch Intern Med* 149:911, 1989.
17. Nation RL, Evans AM, Milne RW: Pharmacokinetic drug interactions with phenytoin, *Clin Pharmacokinet* 18:37, 1990.
18. Pedley TA: Discontinuing antiepileptic drugs, *N Engl J Med* 318:982, 1988.
19. Pellock JM: Carbamazepine side effects in children and adults, *Epilepsia* 28 (suppl 3):S64, 1987.
20. Rogawski MA, Porter RJ: Antiepileptic drugs: pharmacological mechanisms and clinical efficacy with consideration of promising developmental stage compounds, *Pharmacol Rev* 42:223, 1990.
21. Treiman DM: Pharmacokinetics and clinical use of benzodiazepines in the management of status epilepticus, *Epilepsia* 30 (suppl 2):S4, 1989.
22. Trimble MR: Anticonvulsant drugs and cognitive function: a review of the literature, *Epilepsia* 28 (suppl 3):S37, 1987.
23. Vining EPG, Mellits ED, Dorsen MM, et al: Psychologic and behavioral effects of antiepileptic drugs in children: a double-blind comparison between phenobarbital and valproic acid, *Pediatrics* 80:165, 1987.
24. Weaver DF, Camfield P, Fraser A: Massive carbamazepine overdose: clinical and pharmacologic observations in five episodes, *Neurology* 38:755, 1988.
25. Zaccara G, Messori A, Moroni F: Clinical pharmacokinetics of valproic acid—1988, *Clin Pharmacokinet* 15:367, 1988.

Chapter 33

Opioid analgesic drugs

Suffering and disability caused by unrelieved pain lower the quality of life for vast numbers of persons. Alleviation of pain is therefore a major objective in medicine. *Analgesics* are drugs with a prominent pain-relieving action. The two types, *opioid* and *nonopioid* (see Chapter 35), differ in several major respects. (1) Perhaps the most important distinctions are that only the opioids have potential for abuse and that tolerance to their actions can develop. Accordingly, opioids are usually administered for short periods, and precautions are taken to avoid their diversion to illicit use. (2) Opioids are the more powerful analgesics, but they do not reduce inflammation. In an individual patient with severe pain an opioid is likely to provide greater relief than a nonopioid. When groups of patients are treated, opioids are generally analgesic in a higher percentage. (3) Opioids undergo sufficient first-pass metabolism that a given dose is more effective by injection than after oral administration, as reflected by the differences between equianalgesic oral and parenteral doses shown in Table 33-1. Nonopioid analgesics are very seldom injected. Another difference is that opioids act mainly within the central nervous system, whereas the primary *analgesic* action of nonopioids is peripheral.

The opioid class includes alkaloids found in opium and their semisynthetic derivatives (opiates) as well as synthetic compounds that resemble the alkaloids in their pharmacology if less so in their structures. The word *narcotic* was widely used in the past to refer to these compounds. However, this term indicates a state of insensibility or stupor, which is not always induced by such agents and is preferably avoided. Accordingly, the term *opioid* is now most often used to designate this class of analgesics. The use of opioids is regulated by the Federal Controlled Substances Act of 1970. Morphine has been available for nearly 200 years, but opium has been used for thousands of years. The opioid antagonist nalorphine was introduced in 1941. Characterization of multiple types of opioid receptors and discoveries of endogenous opioid peptides have given new perspective to the topics of pain and analgesia. It must be remembered, however, that use of opioid analgesics is only one approach to pain alleviation (Fig. 33-1).

OPIOID RECEPTORS

For some time the existence of opioid receptors in the brain was suspected, based on several observations: (1) some analgesics are extremely potent, etorphine being up to 10,000 times more potent than morphine; (2) opioids are stereospecific with activity residing in the *levo* isomers; (3) there are selective competitive opioid antagonists, such as naloxone, that are not analgesic.

TABLE 33-1 Dosage information for opioids

Drug	Route*	Equieffective doses†‡ (mg) Oral	Injection	Duration[13] (hours)	Available preparations§ (mg)
Agonists					
Naturally occurring alkaloids					
Morphine sulfate	1-4	60	10	4-7	S: 10-100/5 ml, 20/ml;T: 15-100; R: 5-30;I: 0.5-15/ml;I°: 10-30; PF: 0.5,1/ml
Codeine phosphate	1,2	200	130	4-6	I: 15-60/ml;I°: 30,60
Codeine sulfate	1,2	200	130	4-6	T: 15-60;I°: 15-60
Hydrochlorides of opium alkaloids (Pantopon)	2		20	4-5	I: 20/ml
Semisynthetic opiates and other phenanthrene derivatives					
Hydrocodone bitartrate	1				Combinations only
Hydromorphone hydrochloride (Dilaudid)	1-3	7.5	1.5	4-6	T: 1-4;R: 3;I: 1-10/ml
Heroin hydrochloride	1,2	60	5	4-5	Not available in U.S.A.
Levorphanol tartrate (Levo-Dromoran)	1,2	4	2	4-7	T: 2;I: 2/ml
Nalbuphine hydrochloride‖ (Nubain)	2		10	4-6	I: 10,20/ml
Oxycodone hydrochloride (Roxicodone)	1	30		3-5	S: 5/5 ml;T: 5
Oxymorphone hydrochloride (Numorphan)	2,3		1	4-6	R: 5;I: 1,1.5/ml
Butorphanol tartrate‖ (Stadol)	2		2	4-6	I: 1,2/ml
Buprenorphine hydrochloride‖ (Buprenex)	2		0.4	4-6	I: 0.324/ml
Piperidines					
Meperidine hydrochloride (Demerol)	1,2	300	75	4-6	S: 50/5 ml; T: 50,100; I: 10-100/ml
Diphenoxylate hydrochloride (Lomotil, others)	1	5-10		3-4	T: 2.5; S: 2.5/5 ml (with atropine)
Difenoxin hydrochloride (Motofen)	1	1-2		3-4	T: 1 (with atropine)
Loperamide hydrochloride (Imodium)	1	2-4		8-12	C: 2; S: 1/5 ml
Fentanyl (citrate) (Sublimaze)	2		0.1	0.5-2	I,PF: 0.05/ml
Sufentanil (citrate) (Sufenta)	2		0.02	2-4	PF: 0.05/ml
Alfentanil (hydrochloride) (Alfenta)	2		3-10	0.5-1	PF: 0.05/ml

**1*, Oral; *2*, parenteral; *3*, rectal; *4*, extradural.
†Primary source.[13]
‡*Agonists:* acute analgesia or antidiarrheal (diphenoxylate, difenoxin, loperamide); *antagonists:* inital doses for acute opioid intoxication; or maintenance dose (naltrexone).
§*C*, Capsules; *I*, solution for injection; *I°*, soluble tablets to be dissolved for injection; *PF*, preservative-free for parenteral administration, *R*, rectal suppositories; *S*, solution, syrup for ingestion; *T*, tablets.
‖Agonist-antagonist or partial agonist.

Continued.

TABLE 33-1 Dosage information for opioids—cont'd

Drug	Route*	Equieffective doses†‡ (mg) Oral	Injection	Duration[13] (hours)	Available preparations§ (mg)
Miscellaneous					
Methadone hydrochloride (Dolophine)	1,2	20	10	3-6	S: 5,10/5ml,10/ml; T: 5-40; I: 10/ml
Propoxyphene hydrochloride (Darvon, Dolene)	1	130		4-6	C: 65
Propoxyphene napsylate (Darvon-N)	1	130		4-6	S: 10/ml; T: 100
Pentazocine hydrochloride‖ (Talwin Nx)	1	180		4-7	T: 50
Pentazocine (lactate)‖ (Talwin)	2		60	4-6	I: 30/ml
Dezocine (Dalgan)‖	2		≤10	3-6	I: 5-15/ml
Antagonists					
Naloxone hydrochloride (Narcan)	2		0.4		I: 0.02-1/ml
Naltrexone hydrochloride (Trexan)	1	50/day			T: 50

FIG. 33-1 *Correlation of neural projections and chemical mediators in pain perception with some of the different types of drugs that alleviate pain.*

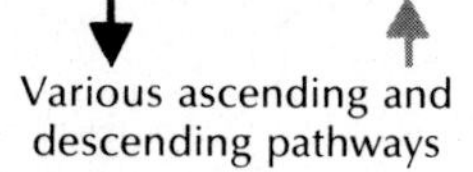

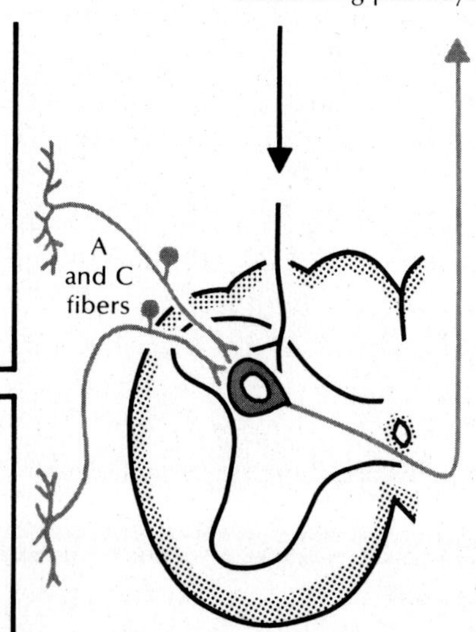

Tissue target: mixed function nociceptors

Mediators: ionic channels for membrane depolarization

Relevant drugs: local anesthetics

Tissue target: chemosensitive nociceptors

Mediators: histamine, serotonin, prostaglandins, kinins

Relevant drugs: steroidal and nonsteroidal anti-inflammatory agents

Tissue target: synapses in sensory and integrative nuclei

Mediators: opioid peptides, monoamines

Relevant drugs: narcotic analgesics, antidepressants, dissociative neuroleptics

In the early 1970s, the concept of specific opioid receptors was supported by demonstrations that opioid agonists and antagonists bind stereospecifically to membranes of pinched-off nerve terminals. Affinities of agonists for binding sites parallel closely their relative clinical potencies. In 1976 Martin and co-workers presented evidence of three types of opioid receptors, which they termed μ (for morphine), κ (for ketocyclazocine), and σ (for SKF 10,047, now named *N*-allylnormetazocine). A δ-receptor has since been widely accepted, and several other receptor types and approaches to nomenclature have been proposed.[17] Opioids depress neuronal activity and decrease neurotransmitter release.[7] Activation of μ- and δ-receptors increases K^+ conductance and causes hyperpolarization, whereas κ-receptor stimulation reduces Ca^{++} conductance and shortens action potential duration. Evidence is accumulating that G proteins are important links between the opioid receptors and the ion channels.

Receptors (stereospecific binding sites) for opioids are widely distributed within the brain, but the patterns of greatest density vary greatly among the receptor types.[16] μ-Receptors, which are thought responsible for the analgesic activity of morphine, are concentrated in the neocortex, striatum, limbic system, thalamus, and other regions involved in pain perception, such as the *substantia gelatinosa* of the spinal cord. These receptors are also found in the *nucleus tractus solitarii* and related nuclei concerned with vagal reflexes. High receptor densities in these latter regions indicate possible contributions to the cough reflex, gastric secretion, and orthostatic hypotension. Opioid receptors are also present in several peripheral organs.

ENDOGENOUS OPIOID PEPTIDES

The demonstration of opioid receptors suggested the existence of endogenous morphine-like compounds (see p. 215). Isolation of Met⁵-enkephalin and Leu⁵-enkephalin, pentapeptides with opiate-like activity, from brain tissue was reported in 1975. β-Lipotropin, a 91 amino acid peptide isolated from the pituitary some years before, contains another opioid peptide, β-endorphin, in residues 61 to 91. Although residues 61 to 65 are the same as Met⁵-enkephalin, β-endorphin is not the precursor of the enkephalin. Determination of the functions of these and other endogenous opioid peptides is a topic of major interest. Morphine, codeine, and their precursor thebaine have been identified in brain tissue from untreated animals, but their source and importance are not yet known.[14]

CURRENT CONCEPTS OF ANALGESIC ACTION

Beecher[2] had a major impact on concepts of pain and analgesia when he emphasized that two major factors contribute to pain or, perhaps more accurately, suffering. One factor is the *perception* of a noxious stimulus, which involves classic pathways that ascend in the spinal cord to the reticular substance, the thalamus, and eventually the cortex. The other factor, the *reaction component*, was invoked to account for wide variation in suffering among persons who have comparable tissue damage. Since patients given morphine may indicate that even though they feel pain it no longer bothers them, Beecher attributed the analgesic effect of morphine principally to a beneficial action on the reaction component. Patients given opioids may also be indifferent to other stimuli, such as urges to urinate or defecate. The benefit of morphine, a respiratory depressant, in patients with dyspnea secondary to acute left ventricular failure and pulmonary edema may be, at least partially, attributable to diminished reaction and anxiety. Presumably opioid receptors in the limbic system are involved in effects on reaction, whereas stimulation of brainstem and spinal receptors affect perception. Recent research on opioid-induced analgesia has focused more on perception than on reaction. Morphine given by the usual routes acts at the *supraspinal* level to activate descending pathways, in the dorsolateral funiculus,[4] that influence afferent input from Aδ and C fibers. Direct exposure of the spinal cord to opioids, given intrathecally or extradurally, can also provide analgesia by stimulating receptors in the dorsal horn. Experiments with animals in which morphine was injected into the cerebral ventricles, applied to the spinal cord, or both demonstrated marked synergism with the combination. Section of the dorsolateral funiculi or administration of an antagonist into appropriate brainstem regions inhibits the analgesic effect of morphine; whether such procedures prevent a dominant supraspinal action of the opiate or interfere with a synergistic interaction is not established. There is also some evidence that opioids can act peripherally to reduce nociceptive input associated with inflammation.[23]

Clinical comparisons of analgesics are difficult because of the complex interplay between perception and reaction. The most useful approach has been to administer analgesics to patients with pain of pathologic origin. Typically the patient is asked to rank the pain as severe, moderate, or slight, before and at intervals after treatment to arrive at a subjective estimate of pain relief. The pain-relieving efficacy of the agent in question is compared with that of a placebo or an established analgesic such as morphine or aspirin. Positive placebo responses occur in about 30% of patients tested in acute situations.

Potent opioid analgesics alleviate severe pain and are antagonized by the antagonist naloxone. Pure agonists exhibit cross-tolerance and, in contrast to mixed agonist-antagonists (see p. 331), can be substituted for each other in the addict. Their formulas contain the common moiety,γ-phenyl-*N*-methylpiperidine. The chair form of piperidine is believed to be the more realistic representation; heavy lines indicate projection from the plane of the paper. Substituent R is often quite bulky.

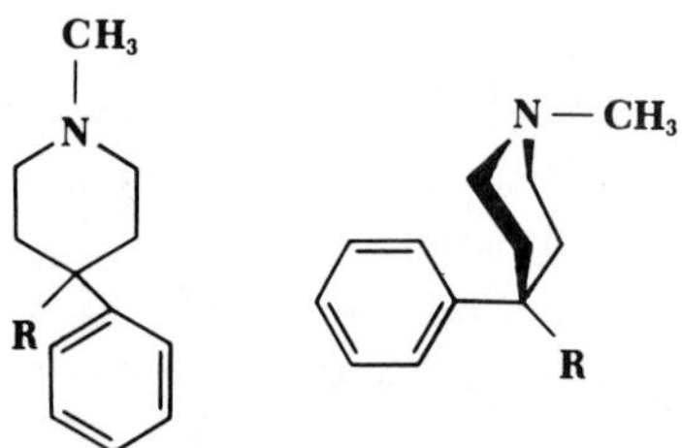

Disubstituted *N*-methylpiperidine

Opioid analgesics and antagonists can be divided into several structural categories, as in Table 33-1, which also summarizes information regarding administration of these agents. Of more practical importance, however, is their division into agonists, antagonists, and agents with both of these activities. The agonists are discussed first.

NATURAL OPIATES AND SEMISYNTHETIC DERIVATIVES

Morphine

CHEMISTRY

Morphine remains the most important opioid analgesic. It is obtained from opium, the dried juice of the poppy plant, *Papaver somniferum*. Alkaloids in opium are of two types, called *phenanthrenes* and *benzylisoquinolines*. Of the latter, noscapine has been used to relieve cough, and papaverine has been used as an antispasmodic, a vasodilator, and, by intracavernous injection, to induce penile erection. Neither agent is analgesic. Morphine and codeine in the phenanthrene group are the important analgesics. Opium contains about 10% morphine and 0.5% codeine. The phenanthrene thebaine evokes strychnine-like convulsions and has no medical uses, but it is manufactured into naloxone. In the poppy thebaine is demethylated to codeine, which in turn is demethylated to morphine.

Morphine was isolated in the first decade of the nineteenth century by Sertürner. Its total synthesis in 1952 confirmed a structure proposed by Gulland and Robinson in 1925. The two hydroxyls, one phenolic and the other alcoholic, are important because certain semisynthetic alkaloids are prepared by modifications of these groups. Codeine, for instance, is 3-methylmorphine, and heroin is 3,6-diacetylmorphine. On the other hand, the opioid antagonist nalorphine is prepared by replacement of the methyl group on the nitrogen with an allyl radical $-CH_2CH{=}CH_2$.

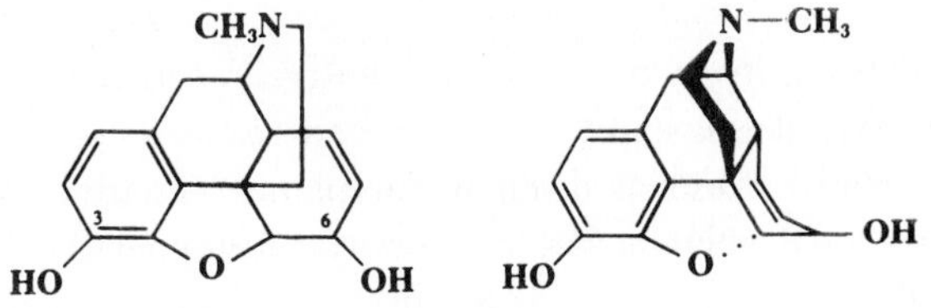

Morphine

Morphine sulfate is available in many forms (see Table 33-1 on p. 319), including tablets for prolonged-release and preservative-free solutions for spinal administration. The subcutaneous dose range is usually 8 to 15 mg.

PHARMACOLOGIC EFFECTS

When a therapeutic dose of morphine is administered to normal persons, it induces drowsiness and euphoria in some, but dysphoria and other unpleasant reactions such as nausea are not uncommon. The person may sleep, respiration may slow, and the pupils may constrict. Dysphoria is less common in patients with pain.

Analgesia. Subcutaneous or intramuscular injection of 10 mg of morphine relieves moderate to severe postoperative pain in 70% to 80% of adult patients. A placebo is effective in about 30%, whereas oral aspirin may benefit just 40%. Because of pronounced first-pass inactivation, the oral dose of morphine for comparable peak analgesia is about 60 mg. Consequently morphine is usually injected for relief of acute pain. There is increasing use of patient-controlled delivery systems for relief of postoperative pain.[11] In contrast is oral use of morphine for chronic analgesia in patients with terminal cancer.[13] The goal in any case is to provide opiate at regular intervals in a dose sufficient to *prevent* pain rather than to wait for pain to develop.

The doses required in such regimens may be surprisingly low, and the need to increase dosage does not necessarily indicate tolerance; it may reflect progression of the disease. To relieve pain by an action on the spinal cord, extradural administration of morphine appears much less likely than intrathecal administration to induce itching or dangerous respiratory depression.[3] Elderly people tend to receive more prolonged pain relief from morphine, and so their daily requirement may be less.

Gastrointestinal tract. Morphine is constipating, and opiates are time-honored remedies in management of diarrhea. Paregoric, a preparation of opium, has been used for centuries. Although morphine can act centrally to reduce gastrointestinal transit, the amount (2 to 4 mg) in a typical adult dose of paregoric is much less than that needed orally to evoke definite central effects, such as analgesia. This indicates that an action of morphine directly on the gut is primarily responsible for constipation. The dose of paregoric for children is 0.1 to 0.2 mg of morphine per kilogram of body weight.

Morphine increases the tone of intestinal smooth muscle, delays gastric emptying, and decreases propulsive peristalsis throughout the gastrointestinal tract.[15] Enhanced fluid and electrolyte absorption by the gut, decreased secretion, or both and failure to respond to sensory stimuli that would otherwise elicit defecation also may contribute to constipation.

Respiration. The sensitivity of respiratory centers to carbon dioxide is diminished by morphine; at toxic doses sensitivity to oxygen may also decrease. Cessation of respiration is the usual cause of death in morphine poisoning. Therapeutic doses moderately reduce tidal volume, but respiratory rate generally does not decrease because carbon dioxide retention tends to offset the change in sensitivity. However, larger doses will clearly lower respiratory rate. Carbon dioxide retention is responsible for cerebral vasodilatation and increased intracranial pressure after administration of morphine. As tolerance develops to its analgesic and euphoric actions, the respiratory center becomes tolerant also. For this reason an addict may tolerate otherwise lethal doses of morphine.

Emesis. The emetic action of morphine is exerted on the chemoreceptor trigger zone (CTZ) in the medulla. However, morphine also depresses the vomiting center, which is located nearby, and so subsequent doses are less likely to induce nausea and vomiting. Apomorphine, a dopamine agonist synthesized from morphine, is a potent stimulant of the CTZ. It is occasionally used clinically as an emetic.

Miscellaneous effects.

Excitation. Morphine is not a uniform depressant of neural structures. It does not oppose the action of convulsants such as strychnine or picrotoxin. Morphine may actually stimulate some persons, and it consistently stimulates cats and horses.

Pupils. The pupils are constricted by morphine, an effect inhibited by atropine and attributable to enhanced parasympathetic input from the Edinger-Westphal nucleus. Tolerance can be demonstrated, but addicts usually exhibit miosis. Their pupils maximally dilate during withdrawal. Animals, such as cats, that are excited by morphine develop mydriasis upon acute administration.

Biliary tract. Morphine can increase intrabiliary pressure by contracting smooth muscle in the biliary tract. Pain relief in biliary colic therefore must be caused by the central analgesic action of the drug. Meperidine and pentazocine, which cause less increase in pressure, are preferred opioids for analgesia in this circumstance.

Cardiovascular system. Morphine reduces arterial resistance and venous tone. These effects may lead to orthostatic hypotension, but they can be beneficial in reducing ventricular work, pulmonary congestion, and edema. Histamine release by intravenous morphine administration may contribute to the hypotensive reaction. The hemodynamic effects of morphine are unfavorable in hemorrhagic shock.

Bronchial smooth muscle. Contraction of bronchial smooth muscle by large doses of morphine may decrease airway diameter. Death in asthmatic patients has been attributed to this effect. It is possible, however, that such mortality is caused by reduction of the action of carbon dioxide on respiration; if so, carbon dioxide narcosis, rather than bronchial constriction, is the cause of death. This issue remains unsettled.

Genitourinary tract. Opiates ordinarily contract the smooth muscle of the ureter and the detrusor muscle of the bladder and increase the tone of the vesicle sphincter. The latter, along with decreased attention to the stimulus for urination, may result in urinary retention. In addition, morphine can release antidiuretic hormone (ADH), which also contributes to antidiuresis. Urinary retention is a relatively common problem when morphine is given epidurally; in this case detrusor tone is reduced. Despite its spasmogenic action, morphine is used to relieve ureteral colic, in which its effectiveness must be due to its analgesic action. Uterine contractions during labor may be slowed somewhat by a therapeutic dose of morphine.

Endocrine and immune systems. In addition to their effect on ADH release, opiates decrease release of ACTH, corticosterone, and luteinizing hormone in humans but enhance prolactin release.[27] There has been increasing interest in the ability of opioids to modulate various immune functions. As examples, they have been reported to enhance natural killer cell activity, to be chemotactic for monocytes, and to reduce resistance to infection.

PHARMACOKINETICS

Depending on route of administration, several factors may delay absorption of opioids. These include delayed gastric emptying, reduced cutaneous circulation, hypothermia, and shock. Because first-pass hepatic metabolism can be considerable, parenteral routes are preferred for relief of acute pain. The 3-glucuronide is the major metabolite of morphine. However, accumulation of morphine-6-glucuronide, a minor metabolite, may contribute to activity in patients with renal insufficiency.[21]

Morphine partitions from blood into most tissues, but very little actually reaches the brain. Its plasma half-life is about 3 hours, and the period of effective analgesia is 4 to 5 hours. In contrast, a single intrathecal dose (250 μg) of morphine may provide analgesia in obstetric procedures for 24 hours or more.

TOLERANCE

A striking feature of opioid pharmacology is the tolerance that develops to their actions. However, tolerance does not develop rapidly to all opioid actions, and addicts typically exhibit constricted pupils and constipation.

Chronic abuse (see Chapter 34) will necessitate progressively larger doses of morphine to obtain the same subjective effects. Tolerance can reach incredible proportions. Addicts have been known to take 4 g of the drug in 24 hours, and a patient with terminal cancer received over 8 g on the seventh day of continuous infusion.[8] In contrast, the lethal dose in a nontolerant person is about 100 to 200 mg. After 1 to 2 weeks of abstinence an addict is again sensitive to a small dose of morphine.

The discovery of enkephalins may clarify the mechanism or mechanisms of tolerance. The continued presence of morphine at opioid receptors could inhibit opioid peptide production or release (Fig. 33-2). Larger doses of morphine would then be required as peptide concentrations declined. When the morphine is withdrawn abruptly, the lack of immediately available endogenous peptides may cause abstinence signs. Alternatively, there is evidence of opioid receptor down-regulation and uncoupling from associated G protein upon continuous exposure to morphine.[26]

INTOXICATION

In severe *acute* morphine poisoning the person is comatose and cyanotic, respiration is very slow or absent, and the pupils are of pinpoint size, unless hypoxia is appreciable. Noncardiogenic pulmonary edema may also develop.

The discovery of specific antidotes was a major development in treatment of acute morphine poisoning. Intravenous injection of naloxone promptly improves respiration and circulation with virtually no adverse effects, if used properly. Opioid antagonists are not of benefit in overdoses with barbiturates or general anesthetics. If a course of naloxone therapy does not dramatically reverse respiratory depression, the initial

FIG. 33-2 *Possible servomechanisms in morphine tolerance and abstinence. Opioid peptides are assumed to act as neurotransmitters or neuromodulators. Peptide binding to μ receptors initiates effects on target neurons compatible with normal function. Synthesis and release of peptide commensurate with need is under feedback control. Morphine competes with the peptide either directly or indirectly. Continuously available morphine is responsible for persistent feedback signals to decrease peptide production. With time, higher concentrations of morphine are required to maintain a specified level of responsiveness in the target neuron (tolerance). If morphine is withdrawn or blocked abruptly with naloxone, the available level of "analgesia" (peptide plus morphine) is grossly inadequate to meet need. In response to the deficit, target cells enter into activities that lead to withdrawal signs. The abstinence syndrome subsides as peptide stores are replenished.*

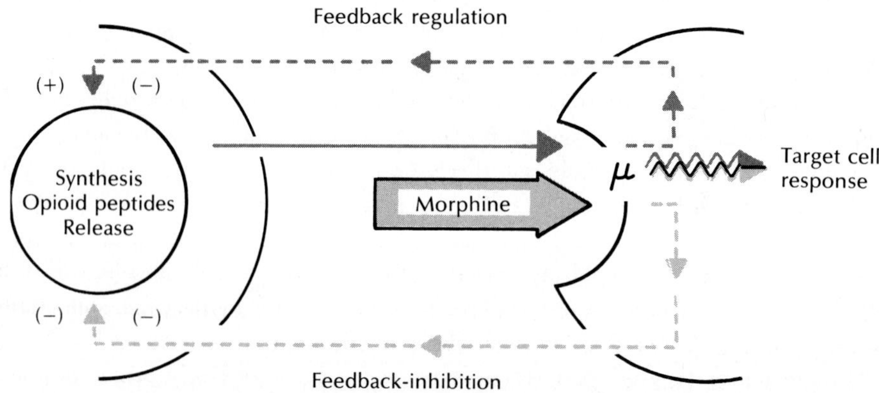

diagnosis must be questioned. In opioid-dependent persons, whether abusers or patients in chronic pain, naloxone can precipitate a severe abstinence syndrome.

Codeine

Codeine is an important oral analgesic and antitussive drug. In the usual 30 to 60 mg dose it is equally or slightly more analgesic than aspirin. Tolerance to codeine develops more slowly, and it is less likely to be abused than morphine. As used clinically, codeine is also less active on the gastrointestinal and urinary tracts and on the pupil, and it causes less nausea and constipation. In children excessive doses may cause convulsions, attributed to disinhibitory effects on spinal neurons. Codeine is the opiate most frequently prescribed, usually in combination with aspirin or acetaminophen and miscellaneous other agents. It is widely used to relieve moderate pain and can be injected if necessary. Codeine is partly demethylated to morphine, which has much greater affinity for opioid receptors, and partly to norcodeine. Metabolism of codeine involves the cytochrome P-450 isoenzyme that metabolizes debrisoquin (see p. 55)

Semisynthetic opiates and other phenanthrene derivatives

None of the semisynthetic opiate agonists (Table 33-1) are commonly used in the United States. **Hydrocodone** and **oxycodone** resemble codeine structurally. **Oxymorphone** is more potent than morphine but causes more side effects. **Hydromorphone** is also more potent than morphine in producing analgesia and respiratory depression but may be less nauseating and constipating. The **hydrochlorides of opium alkaloids** product is a concentrated preparation that contains the alkaloids of opium in the same proportion as they exist naturally.

Heroin is a highly euphoriant and analgesic drug. It is preferred by addicts, who may take it intravenously to obtain a peculiar orgiastic sensation. Heroin may not be legally manufactured in or imported into the United States, though it is used clinically elsewhere for its analgesic property. Its acetyl groups reduce its polarity, relative to morphine, so that heroin penetrates the blood-brain barrier more readily. Heroin does not bind to brain opiate receptors but is rapidly hydrolyzed to active 6-acetylmorphine and morphine. There is no evidence that heroin provides better analgesia than morphine. The greater solubility of heroin would be advantageous in reducing the volume injected in patients whose pain is not adequately relieved by oral morphine, but some other opioids, such as hydromorphone, share this attribute.

MEPERIDINE AND RELATED COMPOUNDS

Meperidine, introduced as an antispasmodic of the atropine type, is probably the opioid most frequently used for parenteral inpatient analgesia. Its action is relatively brief, and intermittent intramuscular administration may inadequately sustain analgesia. Intravenous infusion and oral administration at frequent intervals have been recommended for more consistent relief of acute pain.

Meperidine is as depressant to respiration and as addictive as morphine when compared in equianalgesic doses, though at birth neonates may exhibit somewhat less respiratory depression if the mother receives meperidine rather than morphine. It is generally believed that meperidine has relatively less activity on the gastrointestinal and biliary tracts and on bronchial smooth muscle. Meperidine lacks useful antitussive or antidiarrheal activity but may cause mydriasis in addicts and tachycardia because of muscarinic blockade.

The liver is important in metabolism of meperidine; usual doses of the drug may be toxic to persons with liver disease. Meperidine is not useful for management of chronic pain because normeperidine, a metabolite that can cause myoclonus and seizures, tends to accumulate, particularly in patients with diminished renal function. Ordinary doses of meperidine have caused severe untoward reactions and death in patients taking MAO inhibitors.

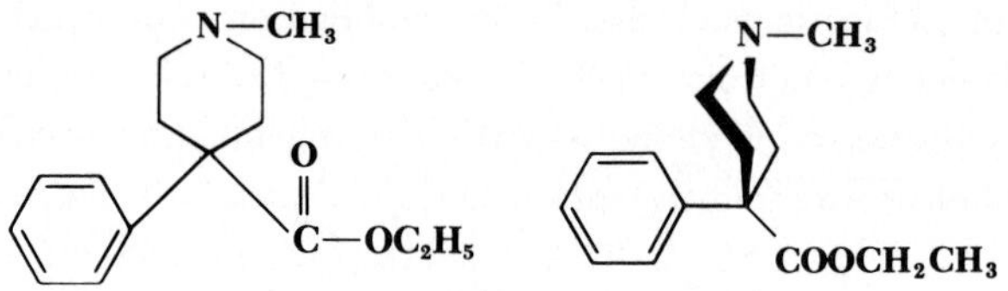

Meperidine

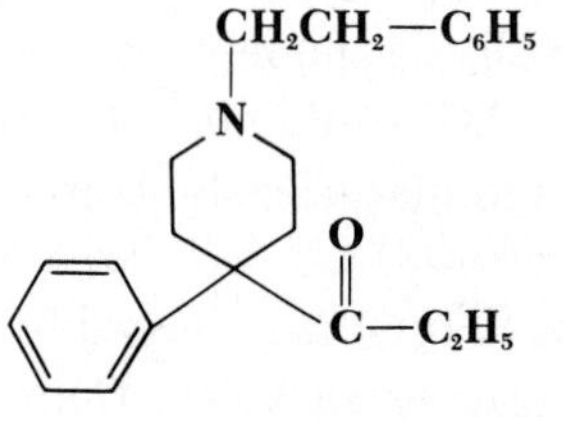

Fentanyl

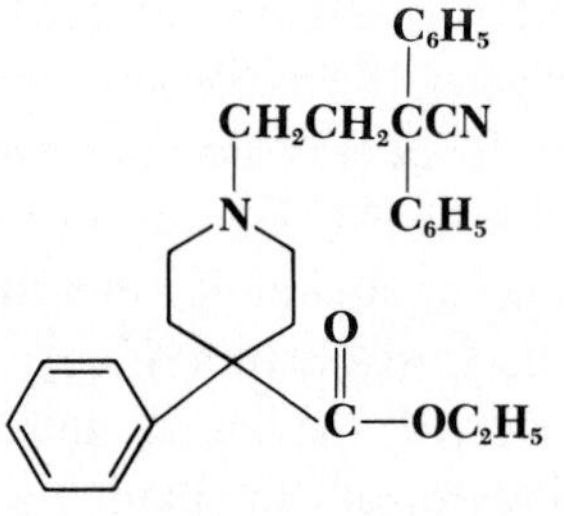

Diphenoxylate

Fentanyl is a potent, lipophilic opioid used as an intramuscular or intravenous analgesic in *balanced anesthesia* with nitrous oxide and oxygen, in *neuroleptanalgesia* with a neuroleptic, such as droperidol, or even as the primary anesthetic with oxygen alone. Such combinations maintain a relatively stable cardiovascular system and constitute a common anesthetic regimen for cardiac surgery. The dose of opioid used, up to 0.15 mg/kg in the case of fentanyl, is much larger than that necessary for analgesia. With such doses there is a high incidence of skeletal muscle rigidity, especially in the thorax and abdomen, that responds to neuromuscular blocking drugs. Residual respiratory depression may require prolonged postoperative ventilation. Anesthesia has sometimes been inadequate, as indicated by postoperative reports of patient awareness or evidence of autonomic or endocrine responses to stress.[22] Bradycardia or hypotension may also occur. A transdermal form (Duragesic) of fentanyl is available for relief of chronic pain. In another context, fentanyl has formed a starting point for manufacture of so-called *designer drugs* (see Chapter 34). **Sufentanil** is very lipid soluble and about five to ten times more potent than fentanyl. Intranasal administration has been proposed for preanesthetic medication. Unlike morphine and meperidine, fentanyl and sufentanil do not release histamine in man.[12] **Alfentanil**, another agent in this class, is less lipophilic, less potent, and shorter acting and may prove useful for short procedures. **Diphenoxylate**, its metabolite **difenoxin**, and **loperamide**, which is now available over-the-counter, are used only as antidiarrheal drugs. Atropine is combined with diphenoxylate and difenoxin ostensibly to discourage overzealous self-medication, but the amount present is quite small. The solubility of diphenoxylate is sufficiently poor as to prevent dissolution for injection. Although central nervous system effects are usually minimal, intoxication with these mixtures can be characterized by symptoms of both opioid and anticholinergic intoxication. Loperamide undergoes extensive enterohepatic circulation and has minimal, if any, abuse potential or central nervous system activity. If central nervous system depression should occur, it can be antagonized by naloxone. Such preparations are not recommended for children under 2 years of age, and they should not be used if the diarrhea is attributable to organisms, such as *Salmonella*, that penetrate the intestinal mucosa.

METHADONE AND RELATED COMPOUNDS

Methadone was developed in Germany during World War II as a substitute for morphine. The two-dimensional formula of methadone does not resemble that of morphine, but a disubstituted *pseudo*piperidine ring is evident in three-dimensional representation. Methadone undergoes less first-pass inactivation than morphine. Although a single dose of methadone has about the same duration of analgesic action as morphine, when given chronically methadone accumulates and can be given at longer intervals.

Tolerance to and dependence on methadone occur, but the abstinence syndrome is less severe, though more prolonged, than that after morphine withdrawal. Methadone has unique applications (discussed in Chapter 34) in the withdrawal or maintenance of opioid addicts. It is also employed for relief of severe chronic pain. Levomethadyl acetate (*l*-α-acetylmethadol, LAAM) is under investigation as a long-acting methadone substitute for maintenance therapy. An oral dose has a duration of action of 2 to 4 days.

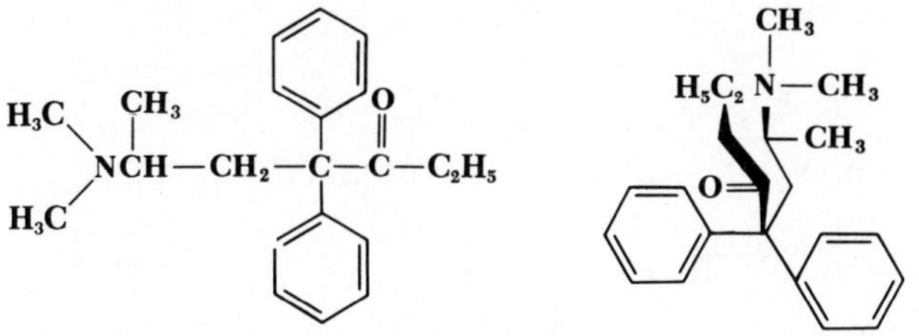

H_3C, CH_3, H_3C — $NCH-CH_2-C-C(=O)-C_2H_5$ (two phenyl groups on C)

CH_3, H_5C_2, $N-CH_3$, CH_3, $O=$

Methadone

Propoxyphene has been a widely prescribed drug despite reservations about its efficacy. It is a weak analgesic available only for oral administration, often in combinations with acetaminophen or aspirin. Occasional doses of less than 100 mg of propoxyphene alone may have placebo value only and are certainly no more analgesic than aspirin. The *dextro* isomer of propoxyphene is used for analgesia. The *levo* isomer has been used as an antitussive.

Propoxyphene overdose was once responsible for many deaths each year in the

United States. Signs of serious overdose resemble those of morphine. Convulsions are not uncommon. In addition, the metabolite norpropoxyphene is cardiotoxic and can cause sudden death. Respiratory depression responds to naloxone. The presence of aspirin or acetaminophen in the mixtures complicates management of toxicity as does concomitant ingestion of alcohol or other depressants. When its widespread use is taken into consideration, the number of persons addicted to propoxyphene is low, though tolerance and dependence are known to occur. The prudent physician will exercise caution in prescribing propoxyphene for persons with a history of substance abuse.

OPIOID ANTAGONISTS

An allyl ($-CH_2CH{=}CH_2$) substitution on the nitrogen atom of opioids yields compounds that competitively antagonize opioid actions. **Nalorphine** (*N*-allylnormorphine), once clinically important in reversing opioid intoxication, has been replaced by naloxone. Nalorphine precipitates acute withdrawal in dependent persons. In contrast, in a person who is neither intoxicated nor dependent nalorphine can be analgesic and dysphoric or depress respiration. One explanation for this pattern has been that nalorphine is a *partial agonist* at opioid receptors. However, the currently favored explanation is derived from observations that morphine and ketocyclazocine induce many of the same effects: nalorphine is an antagonist at the μ-receptor and an agonist at the κ-receptor, stimulation of which elicits weaker responses. Nalorphine mimics opiates in a person previously unexposed to an opioid (κ-receptor stimulation), but in severe intoxication replacement of morphine by nalorphine lessens depression (antagonism at μ-receptor plus weaker κ-agonist activity). Dysphoria, depersonalization, vivid dreams, hallucinations, and other adverse mental effects of nalorphine are attributed to stimulation of the σ-receptor, as defined originally.[20]

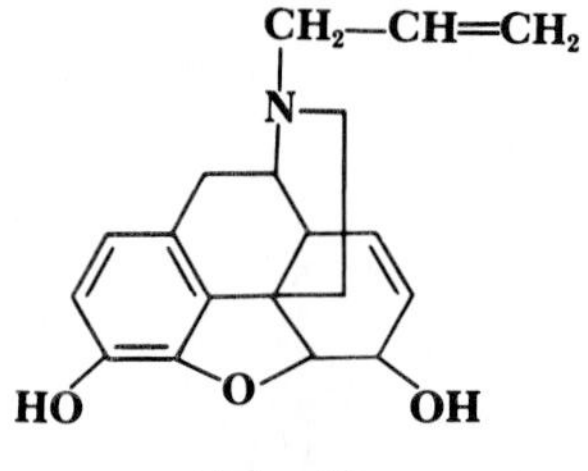

$CH_2{-}CH{=}CH_2$ N HO O OH

Nalorphine

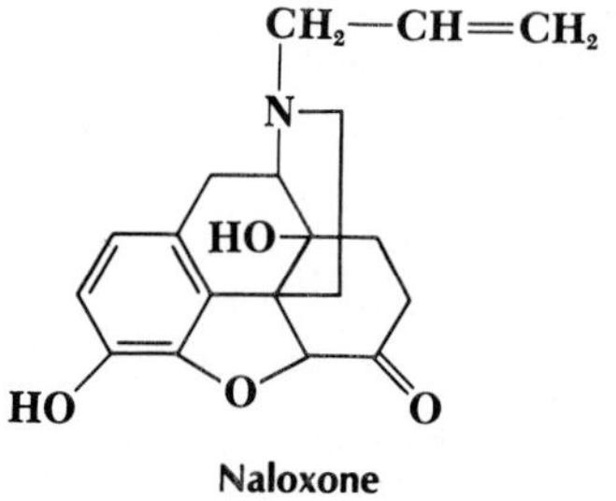

$CH_2{-}CH{=}CH_2$ N HO HO O O

Naloxone

Naloxone, the N-allyl derivative of oxymorphone, is now the most important opioid antagonist. It lacks agonist activity and hence does not depress respiration. Naloxone is a clinically useful antagonist of opioids regardless of the receptor involved, but somewhat larger doses are needed to antagonize agonist-antagonist opioids (see below) than to antagonize morphine. The drug is a major tool in studies to ascertain physiologic roles of the endogenous opioid peptides. The usual adult dosage of naloxone is 0.4 to 2 mg intravenously, at 2- to 3-minute intervals if necessary. If a cumulative dose of 10 mg of naloxone has not improved respiration, an opioid is unlikely to have contributed to the central depression. Although the approved initial dose for children is 0.01

mg/kg, 10 times that is recommended.[9] Naloxone has a nearly immediate action that lasts 45 minutes or more. Since some agonists, such as methadone, may depress respiration for a day or two, additional injections or an infusion of naloxone may be necessary. A difficult therapeutic problem is the treatment of opioid intoxication in an addict. When naloxone precipitates abstinence in such patients, the syndrome is short but may be very severe. **Naltrexone**, a longer-acting pure antagonist, has been approved to facilitate maintenance of abusers in an opioid-free state after withdrawal (detoxification). After an opioid-free period of 7 to 10 days, a naloxone challenge is given to ensure that detoxification is complete. Naltrexone doses of 50 to 150 mg, given daily to every third day respectively, can then prevent physical dependence as well as the pleasurable effects of opioid agonists. Although periodic tests of hepatic function are recommended, there is evidence that naltrexone does not adversely affect liver enzymes.[6]

MIXED AGONIST-ANTAGONISTS

A high incidence of dysphoria precluded clinical use of nalorphine as an analgesic. However, its minimal abuse potential led to the search for related compounds with less dysphoric activity. Most such agents, like nalorphine, are currently classified as *agonist-antagonist* drugs. However, because κ-receptors do not appear to mediate respiratory depression,[28] this effect of these agents probably indicates partial agonist activity at another receptor.[27] Likewise their analgesic mechanism is poorly understood, because they do not mimic more selective κ-receptor agonists in certain analgesic assays.[27] Regardless of their precise interactions with various receptors, the newer agents as a group are much less likely than nalorphine to elicit dysphoria or hallucinations. They have relatively low potential for abuse. They cause less severe maximal respiratory depression than pure agonists and are powerful enough antagonists to precipitate withdrawal in dependent abusers. Pentazocine and butorphanol tend to increase cardiac work, a disadvantage in patients with myocardial infarction, whereas nalbuphine and buprenorphine appear safe in this regard.[5]

Pentazocine was the first of these agents to be used clinically. Because of abuse of pentazocine in combination with the antihistamine tripelennamine, so-called *Ts and blues*, naloxone was added to the oral preparation of **pentazocine hydrochloride**. The dose of naloxone (0.5 mg) is too small to have an effect after oral administration, but if the tablets are dissolved for injection the naloxone can precipitate withdrawal in a dependent user. **Dezocine**, the most recently available agonist/antagonist, is a structural analog of pentazocine.

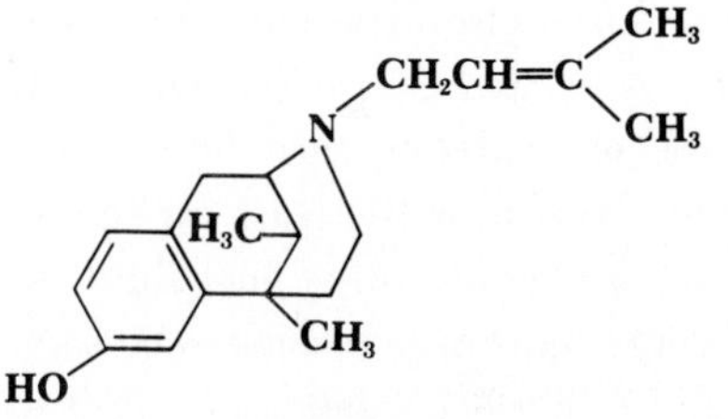

$CH_2CH{=}C(CH_3)_2$ — N — H_3C — CH_3 — HO

Pentazocine

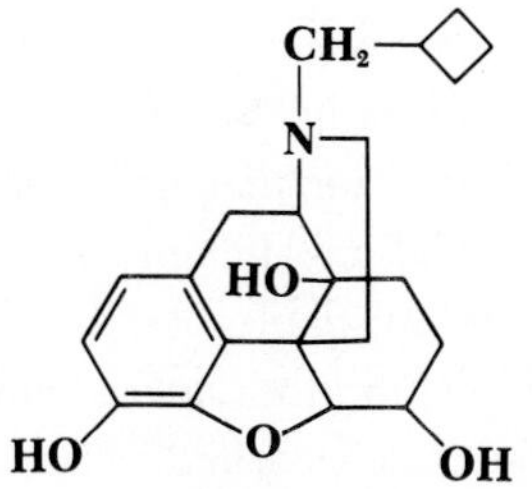

CH_2 — N — HO — HO — O — OH

Nalbuphine

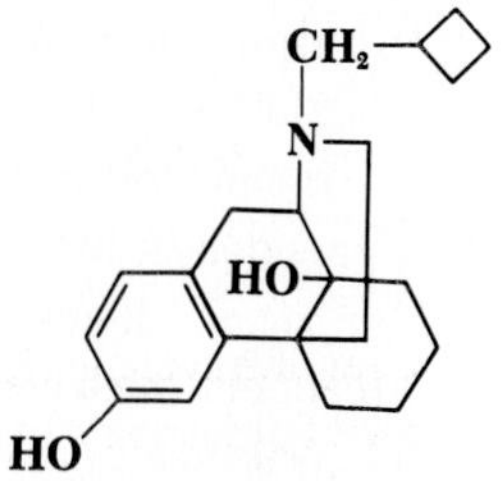

CH_2 — N — HO — HO

Butorphanol

Butorphanol has about five times the analgesic potency of morphine and one fortieth the antagonist potency of naloxone. Its clinical applications and abuse potential appear to be roughly comparable to those of pentazocine.

Nalbuphine is nearly equivalent to morphine in analgesic potency. As an antagonist, it has about one hundredth the potency of naloxone. Nalbuphine has been proposed for postoperative use to relieve opioid-induced respiratory depression while maintaining analgesia.[1] The incidence of dysphoric reactions is low.

Buprenorphine is about 30 times more potent than morphine with an analgesic action lasting perhaps 6 to 8 hours. Unlike the agonist-antagonists above, buprenorphine is a partial opioid (μ) agonist. It has a slow onset of action and, probably because it dissociates slowly from receptors, is poorly antagonized by naloxone.[5] Buprenorphine is well absorbed from the buccal mucosa[25] and is available for sublingual administration in many countries. There is interest in the potential of this drug as an alternative to methadone for detoxification and maintenance and in treatment of cocaine abuse.

CONTRAINDICATIONS TO THE USE OF MORPHINE AND RELATED AGENTS

Morphine and related drugs should be avoided entirely or used with extreme caution in the following medical conditions:

Head injuries and after craniotomy
Bronchial asthma and other hypoxic states
Acute alcohol intoxication
Convulsive disorders
Undiagnosed acute abdominal conditions

CURRENT CLINICAL APPROACHES TO PAIN RELIEF

Relief of pain may be considered in at least five clinical contexts. (1) Pharmacologic relief of *mild to moderate acute pain*, such as muscle aches or simple headache, is provided by ingestion of aspirin-like drugs discussed in detail in Chapter 35. Neither tolerance nor physical dependence is a problem with these analgesics. (2) More *severe acute pain* after surgery is typically treated initially by injections of morphine or meperidine. The goals in this case are to provide adequate pain relief and at the same time minimize exposure to the opioid. Unfortunately, excessive concern with abuse potential can lead to prescription or administration of insufficient analgesic for optimal relief of symptoms.[19] Although mild physical dependence may develop within a matter of days or a week, such patients seldom if ever become "addicted" to opioids secondary to therapeutic usage. Within a few days, as pain lessens, injections may be replaced by orally administered codeine or codeine-containing combinations and then by aspirin-like agents alone. Neonates and young children also experience pain and should be medicated accordingly.[24] (3) *Chronic pain associated with inflammation*, as in rheumatoid arthritis, can be managed for years, without tolerance or physical dependence, by nonsteroidal anti-inflammatory drugs. Aspirin is the least expensive, but many alternatives are available. As the disease progresses, other modalities of treatment, such as gold salts or other disease-modifying agents may become necessary. (4) One need not be overly concerned about dependence when opioids are used to relieve the *pain of terminal disease*. Here the objective is to extend for as long as possible the period of adequate pain relief.[18] The progression of analgesic use is therefore somewhat the reverse of that for postoperative pain, progressing from aspirin to oral codeine to oral morphine to parenteral morphine, eventually perhaps by intravenous, subcutaneous, or epidural routes. Transcutaneous nerve stimulation, local anesthetics, surgical interruption of afferent neuronal pathways, and so forth may ultimately be required. (5) Finally there are patients who experience *pain*, which may be very severe and debilitating, *for which no organic cause can be found*. Usually, one of the first goals in chronic pain clinics is to stop analgesic use. Further considerations in management of this type of pain are detailed elsewhere.[10]

CLINICAL PHARMACOLOGY OF ANTITUSSIVE DRUGS

Coughing is usually a defense mechanism for clearing the respiratory tract. However, cough accompanies cardiac dyspnea, pleurisy, hiatal hernia, and other conditions not directly related to tracheobronchial irritation. In many instances coughing should not be restrained lest its prevention lead to pneumonia or other infections. Medical intervention is indicated if coughing serves no useful purpose and interferes with sleep or other normal activities.

Antitussives may suppress the neural component of the cough reflex or may influence the quantity or viscosity of respiratory tract fluid. Drugs that act on the neural component may act in the central nervous system or on sensory endings in the mucous membrane of the respiratory tract. The effectiveness of antitussives is difficult to determine because nonspecific sedation and placebos can be of benefit. Furthermore, in many cough mixtures, the demulcent action of the vehicle may contribute to the benefit.

There is little doubt that morphine and synthetic opioid-like drugs are potent, centrally acting cough suppressants. **Codeine** is the traditional suppressant to which nonaddictive antitussives should be compared in controlled clinical trials. The usual adult antitussive dose of codeine is 15 to 20 mg every 4 to 6 hours. For cough suppression it is usually dispensed in a demulcent syrup or suspension. Mixtures of codeine with an assortment of antihistamines, antipyretics, and other drugs are common; however, these seem to have little advantage over codeine alone.

Hydrocodone bitartrate is a more potent antitussive than codeine, but its addiction liability is greater. It is available only in combinations.

Dextromethorphan hydrobromide (Pertussin, others) is a substituted *dextro* isomer of the opioid levomethorphan. Dextromethorphan is not analgesic or addictive, but toxic doses can depress the central nervous system. It equals codeine in antitussive potency but appears to act on a different receptor. The usual dose is 10 to 30 mg every 4 to 8 hours. Dextromethorphan is available in lozenges with or without benzocaine, in syrups, and in many combinations. Because of its safety dextromethorphan, another of the drugs metabolized by the cytochrome P-450 isoenzyme that metabolizes debrisoquin, has proved useful in determining the metabolic phenotype of patients.

In general, antitussive drugs may be valuable in reducing a useless cough. They are purely symptomatic medications, and their use should not obviate the necessity for treating the cause of the cough if possible.

REFERENCES

1. Bailey PL, Clark NJ, Pace NL, et al: Antagonism of postoperative opioid-induced respiratory depression: nalbuphine versus naloxone, *Anesth Analg* 66:1109, 1987.
2. Beecher HK: *Measurement of subjective responses: quantitative effects of drugs*, New York, 1959, Oxford University Press.
3. Benedetti C: Intraspinal analgesia: an historical overview, *Acta Anaesthesiol Scand* 31(suppl 85):17, 1987.
4. Bonica JJ: Biochemistry and modulation of nociception and pain. In Bonica JJ, editor: *The management of pain*, vol I, ed 2, Philadelphia, 1990, Lea & Febiger, p 95.
5. Bovill JG: Which potent opioid? Important criteria for selection, *Drugs* 33:520, 1987.
6. Brahen LS, Capone TJ, Capone DM: Naltrexone: lack of effect on hepatic enzymes, *J Clin Pharmacol* 28:64, 1988.
7. Chavkin C: Electrophysiology of opiates and opioid peptides. In Pasternak GW, editor: *The opiate receptors*, Clifton, NJ, 1988, The Humana Press Inc, p 273.
8. Citron ML, Johnston-Early A, Fossieck BE, Jr, et al: Safety and efficacy of continuous intravenous morphine for severe cancer pain, *Am J Med* 77:199, 1984.
9. Committee on Drugs: Naloxone dosage and route of administration for infants and children: addendum to emergency drug doses for infants and children, *Pediatrics* 86:484, 1990.
10. Crue BL, Jr: Multidisciplinary pain treatment programs: current status, *Clin J Pain* 1:31, 1985.
11. Ferrante FM, Ostheimer GW, Covino BG, editors: *Patient-controlled analgesia*, Boston, 1990, Blackwell Scientific Publications.
12. Flacke JW, Flacke WE, Bloor BC, et al: Histamine release by four narcotics: a double-blind study in humans, *Anesth Analg* 66:723, 1987.
13. Foley KM, Inturrisi CE: Pharmacologic approaches to cancer pain. In Foley KM, Payne RM, editors: *Current therapy of pain*, Toronto, 1989, BC Decker Inc, p 303.
14. Kodaira H, Lisek CA, Jardine I, et al: Identification of the convulsant opiate thebaine in mammalian brain, *Proc Natl Acad Sci USA* 86:716, 1989.
15. Kromer W: Endogenous and exogenous opioids in the control of gastrointestinal motility and secretion, *Pharmacol Rev* 40:121, 1988.
16. Mansour A, Khachaturian H, Lewis ME, et al: Anatomy of CNS opioid receptors, *Trends Neurosci* 11:308, 1988.
17. Martin WR: Pharmacology of opioids, *Pharmacol Rev* 35:283, 1984.
18. Melzack R: The tragedy of needless pain, *Sci Am* 262(2):27, 1990.
19. Morgan JP: American opiophobia: customary underutilization of opioid analgesics. In Hill CS, Jr, Fields WS, editors: *Advances in pain research and therapy*, vol 11, New York, 1989, Raven Press, Ltd, p 181.
20. Musacchio JM: The psychotomimetic effects of opiates and the σ receptor, *Neuropsychopharmacology* 3:191, 1990.
21. Peterson GM, Randall CTC, Paterson J: Plasma levels of morphine and morphine glucuronides in the treatment of cancer pain: relationship to renal function and route of administration, *Eur J Clin Pharmacol* 38:121, 1990.
22. Philbin DM, Rosow CE, Schneider RC, et al: Fentanyl and sufentanil anesthesia revisited: how much is enough? *Anesthesiology* 73:5, 1990.
23. Stein C, Millan MJ, Shippenberg TS, et al: Peripheral opioid receptors mediating antinociception in inflammation: evidence for involvement of *mu*, *delta* and *kappa* receptors, *J Pharmacol Exp Ther* 248:1269, 1989.
24. Tyler DC, Krane EJ, editors: *Pediatric pain*, New York, 1990, Raven Press.
25. Weinberg DS, Inturrisi CE, Reidenberg B, et al: Sublingual absorption of selected opioid analgesics, *Clin Pharmacol Ther* 44:335, 1988.
26. Werling LL, McMahon PN, Cox BM: Selective changes in μ opioid receptor properties induced by chronic morphine expo-

sure, *Proc Natl Acad Sci USA* 86:6393, 1989.

27. Wood PL, Iyengar S: Central actions of opiates and opioid peptides: in vivo evidence for opioid receptor multiplicity. In Pasternak GW, editor: *The opiate receptors*, Clifton, NJ, 1988, The Humana Press Inc, p 307.
28. Yeadon M, Kitchen I: Opioids and respiration, *Prog Neurobiol* 33:1, 1989.

Chapter 34

Drug abuse and dependence

The opioids, central nervous system depressants and stimulants, hallucinogens, cannabinoids (marijuana), and some inhalants have in common the ability to produce euphoria, and thus they provide positive reinforcement. Their reinforcing properties may lead to repeated intermittent usage or, eventually, to chronic usage. Compulsive drug taking (a form of dependence) may develop with continued use. Emphasis in this chapter is placed on the characteristics of these drugs that lead to abuse and dependence. The general pharmacology of many of the drugs is discussed elsewhere. Drugs within each class have qualitatively similar effects.

TERMINOLOGY

In contemporary society, the term drug abuse has become synonymous with the nonmedical use of drugs to alter one's mental state. Individuals self-administer both prescription and illicit drugs in attempts to alter mood, to alter perception of reality, to experience unique sensations, and/or to improve physical or mental capabilities. In general, society establishes what constitutes drug abuse by its laws and social taboos. Consequently, a particular drug-taking behavior in one society or in a particular situation may be considered drug abuse, whereas in another it may be considered appropriate.

A term that is often used in place of drug abuse is drug dependence. Dependence is defined by the World Health Organization as drug self-administration that is detrimental to the individual or society. The term encompasses the biologic interaction between drugs and an individual, independently of social norms. Use of this term may be confusing because dependence also refers to alterations in physiologic or psychologic states that occur with chronic drug use. Accordingly, in this chapter *drug abuse* will refer to detrimental drug use, and *dependence* will denote alterations in physiologic or psychologic conditions secondary to chronic drug administration.

Perhaps the term used most often when dealing with drug abuse is *addiction*. Addiction, as defined by Seevers,[26] is a state of chronic compulsive drug use characterized by an overwhelming desire to continue obtaining and taking drugs, physical dependence, a tendency to increase dose, and a detrimental effect on the individual taking the drug. Because this term is often used inappropriately and does not encompass many aspects of drug abuse, its usefulness is limited. Indeed, it is more appropriate to characterize drug use in terms of degree and type of dependence.

Chronic administration of the drugs discussed below can lead to two types of dependence: psychologic and physical. *Psychologic dependence* is an emotional and mental preoccupation with drug acquisition and use to receive some positive reinforcement. Drug usage becomes a habit necessary for the subject's well-being. All drugs discussed in this chapter can produce psychologic dependence. In contrast, not all of them produce physical dependence. *Physical dependence* is an altered physiologic condition caused by chronic exposure to a drug. It results in reproducible physiologic signs and symptoms when the drug is withdrawn abruptly. These signs and symptoms constitute the *abstinence or withdrawal syndrome* and occur after chronic use of opiates, barbiturates, antianxiety agents, ethanol, and nonbarbiturate sedatives (Table 34-1).

Chronic use of many drugs leads to development of tolerance (Table 34-1). *Tolerance* is a phenomenon in which prior exposure to a drug decreases the response to a given dose; thus more drug is necessary to produce the desired effect. Tolerance that develops as a consequence of enhanced elimination of a drug (for example, induction of hepatic enzymes) is called *dispositional or metabolic tolerance*. Tolerance that develops as a result of adaptive processes within cells is termed *functional or cellular tolerance*. In addition, persons who chronically self-administer drugs often learn to modify their behavior (usually toward normal) while under the influence of the drug. This adaptation is called *behavioral tolerance*.

When a person becomes tolerant to one drug, he often becomes tolerant to other drugs as well. This phenomenon is termed *cross-tolerance*. There are two types of cross-tolerance. *Specific cross-tolerance* occurs among drugs within a given pharmacologic class, presumably because they have similar mechanisms of action at the cellular level (that is, via the same receptors, second messengers, and so forth). *Nonspecific cross-tolerance* occurs when drugs share a common and inducible metabolic pathway. Thus enhanced metabolism produced by one drug increases metabolism of another. Note that specific cross-tolerance is related to cellular tolerance, whereas nonspecific cross-tolerance is a dispositional tolerance.

TABLE 34-1 Comparison of commonly abused drugs

Drug category	Tolerance	Psychologic dependence	Physical dependence*	Psychotogenic
Opioids	X	X	X	
Barbiturates	X†	X	X	
Antianxiety agents	X†	X	X	
Ethyl alcohol	X†	X	X	
Amphetamines	X	X		X‡
Cocaine	X	X		X‡
Nicotine	X	X		
LSD	X	X		X
Phencyclidine	X	X		X‡
Cannabinoids	X	X		X‡
Inhalants	?	X		X‡

*A defined abstinence syndrome occurs after abrupt discontinuation.
†Little tolerance with lethal effects.
‡In relatively high doses.

Finally, an individual who is physically dependent on one drug of a given class can substitute another of that class to prevent abstinence. This *cross-dependence* is used to therapeutic advantage in controlling symptoms of withdrawal while detoxifying patients who are physically dependent.

OPIOIDS

Drugs are classified as opioids (see Chapter 33) if they bind stereospecifically to opioid receptors and possess some morphine-like activity. In addition to naturally occurring opium, morphine, and codeine, this class includes semisynthetic compounds such as heroin (also known as horse, smack, junk, H), oxymorphone, and hydromorphone as well as synthetic compounds such as meperidine, methadone, pentazocine (Ts), and propoxyphene. Such opioids are used therapeutically to relieve pain, to treat diarrhea and dysentery, and to suppress cough.

Characteristics of abuse

Opioids are abused primarily for their euphoric and sedative effects. The euphoria is characterized by feelings of peace and contentment. Normal concerns and anxiety are diminished or absent. Initial use of opioids, however, may produce dysphoria rather than euphoria. Furthermore, opioids can produce some central nervous system stimulation, including activation of the chemoreceptor trigger zone and consequently nausea or vomiting.

Heroin is the most widely abused opioid. Users believe heroin is more euphoric than other opioids, but its abuse potential is equivalent to that of morphine. Indeed, after administration, heroin is rapidly hydrolyzed to morphine. It acts more rapidly than morphine, however, because it enters the brain more readily. This may largely account for the preference of users for heroin.

When heroin is administered intravenously, the user may experience a thrilling sensation, in the lower abdominal area, that has been compared to a sexual orgasm. This is accompanied by feelings of warmth and tingling. Because opioids depress the central nervous system, users may become sedated. The degree of sedation depends on the dose taken and on the user's level of tolerance to the opioid. In nontolerant individuals, opioids can induce sleep and vivid dreams. Opioids also depress respiration, and many produce marked miosis (pin-point pupils).

The patterns of opioid abuse vary widely. Some individuals use the drugs sporadically for recreation and do not become dependent. Others become both psychologically and physically dependent. Chronic use of opioids does not necessarily result in mental or physical deterioration. Many persons dependent on opioids function well in society, maintaining careers and family life provided they take the drug on a regular basis. Others tend to sacrifice "normal" lives for the sake of increased drug experiences. These individuals are consumed with drug-seeking and drug-taking behaviors and often use many different drugs. There are no known predictors of the pattern of dependence that will develop.

Tolerance and dependence

When opioids are used regularly, pronounced tolerance lessens most of their effects, including sedation, euphoria, and respiratory depression. In contrast, their miotic and constipating actions persist. The degree and rapidity of tolerance development are dependent on the opioid taken, the dose, and the frequency of administration. Because tolerance develops to the reinforcing actions of opioids, most users increase dosage over time. Upon withdrawal tolerance rapidly diminishes. Consequently, tolerant individuals often withdraw intentionally for short periods to reduce the amount of drug they need. Although a high degree of cross-tolerance develops among opioids that act at the same receptor subtype, that is μ, δ, or κ, less cross-tolerance develops between agonists that act predominantly at different receptor subtypes.

Pronounced psychologic and physical dependence develop rapidly during continuous use of opioids. As in the case of tolerance, the degree of dependence varies with the individual, the drug administered, and the dosage. It is often the psychologic dependence, rather than the physical dependence, that dictates continued use of the drug and/or recidivism after withdrawal. Upon cessation of drug usage, however, persons who are physically dependent exhibit a characteristic abstinence syndrome. For the shorter acting opioids, such as heroin or morphine, symptoms appear about 8 hours after the last dose and reach peak intensity between 36 and 72 hours. Lacrimation, rhinorrhea, yawning, and diaphoresis develop between 8 and 12 hours. At about 13 hours, restless sleep may occur. At about 20 hours, gooseflesh, dilated pupils, agitation, and tremors usually appear. During the second and third day, the abstinence syndrome is at its peak, with symptoms and signs of weakness, insomnia, chills, intestinal cramps, nausea, vomiting, diarrhea, violent yawning, muscle aches in the legs, severe low back pain, elevation of blood pressure and pulse rate, diaphoresis, and gooseflesh. Although withdrawal is generally not life-threatening (that is, convulsions do not occur), fluid depletion during the withdrawal period has resulted in cardiovascular collapse and death. At any point during the course of withdrawal, administration of an opioid agonist in adequate dosage will dramatically eliminate the symptoms and restore a state of apparent normalcy (cross-dependence). Although the duration of the syndrome is roughly 7 to 10 days, mild symptoms may persist for months, and the "craving" for opioids may continue for years.

Other opioid abstinence syndromes are qualitatively similar to that of morphine or heroin. Opioids with a longer duration of action, such as methadone, usually produce a milder and more prolonged syndrome.

Opioid abstinence syndromes also develop in babies born to opioid-dependent mothers, because these newborns are physically dependent. Withdrawal is characterized by high-pitched crying, tremors, hyperreflexia, sucking of the fist, sneezing, yawning, vomiting, and hyperthermia. With heroin dependence the abstinence syndrome usually appears in the first day of life. Withdrawal symptoms may not occur for days in babies born to methadone-dependent mothers. These babies need to be detoxified slowly by first administering sufficient opioid (usually paregoric) to control signs and symptoms; opioid dosage is then tapered.

Treatment of opioid dependence

There are two components to treatment of opioid dependence: withdrawal (detoxification) and rehabilitation. Withdrawal can be accomplished over several days by gradually reducing the dosage of the opioid on which the user is dependent. More often, however, methadone is used for detoxification. Methadone substitutes for most other opioids, is well absorbed when administered orally, and has a longer duration of action than other opioids. Thus, gradually decreasing doses need be given only once in a 24-hour period, and parenteral administration is avoided. Furthermore, the methadone abstinence syndrome is less severe than that produced by heroin or morphine.

In methadone maintenance programs, as in detoxification, methadone is substituted for the opioid that the patient has been abusing. The patient is not detoxified, however, but is given a high daily dose of methadone to maintain tolerance (and dependence). The rationales are (1) that exposure to additional opioid (superimposed on the methadone) outside the clinic environment should lack reinforcing qualities and (2) that patients who no longer need to engage in illegal and time-consuming drug-seeking behavior will pursue more useful activities. Although programs involving methadone maintenance and psychologic counseling appear somewhat successful in decreasing recidivism rates, many patients eventually return to illicit opioid use.[6,9,24]

Clonidine (see Chapter 21) reduces the severity of opioid withdrawal, probably by depressing preganglionic sympathetic nerve activity.[11] It appears to be a safe nonopioid therapy that diminishes withdrawal symptoms.[17,32] Because a major side effect of clonidine is hypotension, the drug should be used with caution.

After detoxification, rehabilitation, a far more difficult task, confronts the clinician. The craving for opioids persists for months to years after detoxification and results in exceedingly high rates of recidivism. One adjunctive approach to rehabilitation after detoxification utilizes a narcotic antagonist. Administration of a pure opioid antagonist should prevent the reinforcing effects of opioid agonists and thus diminish opioid abuse. Naltrexone, a long-acting antagonist, has been used for this purpose with some success.[15] Of course, such treatment must not be started before detoxification is complete, because the antagonist will precipitate abstinence in an opioid-dependent individual.

Medical problems of opioid abuse

Other medical problems also occur secondary to opioid use. A major problem with most illicit drugs is not knowing the amount of drug an individual is taking. Street heroin is usually 2% to 5% opioid. The remaining powder comprises adulterants that increase the volume. A user who obtains an unusually pure sample of drug may overdose unintentionally. As mentioned above, tolerance to the actions of opioids reverses quickly upon withdrawal. Consequently, overdose is likely after withdrawal if a user takes a dose that was effective previously when he was still tolerant. Overdose is characterized by respiratory and central nervous system depression and miosis (although not all overdose patients have pin-point pupils). Death occurs as a result of respiratory arrest and/or noncardiogenic pulmonary edema. The opioid antagonist naloxone (Narcan) reverses the apnea and coma caused by opioid overdose. In an opioid-dependent individual, naloxone can precipitate a full abstinence syndrome. Although the drug may be needed to treat an overdose, such patients may rapidly go from coma into withdrawal; extreme caution is essential. Naloxone neither depresses respiration nor enhances toxic effects of barbiturates or other central nervous system depressants, and it is often used in the emergency room to differentiate opioid from central depressant overdose. Because its action is short-lived, repeated administration is likely to be necessary. Patients who exhibit a salutary response to a single dose of naloxone should be observed for a prolonged period before discharge.

Additional medical problems are secondary to intravenous opioid administration with unsterile needles. These complications include AIDS, viral hepatitis, bacterial and fungal infections, chronic liver disease, thrombophlebitis, cellulitis, and local abscesses. Further danger arises from foreign substances intentionally or accidentally added by the supplier as adulterants to dilute (cut) the drug. Recently, new "designer" drugs have appeared. They are so-named because they are designed with unique chemical substitutions to circumvent the law, while producing effects similar to their illegal counterparts. One such meperidine analog was found to be contaminated with 1-methyl-4-phenyl-1,2,3,6-tetrahydropyridine (MPTP), which causes selective degeneration of nigrostriatal dopamine neurons and a syndrome similar to Parkinsons disease (see Chapter 30).[29] Finally, although opioid users are not likely to be hostile or aggressive while on the drug, their need for more drug to avoid abstinence as tolerance develops may cause many chronic users to engage in criminal activities.

CENTRAL NERVOUS SYSTEM DEPRESSANTS

Included within this class of compounds are the barbiturates, nonbarbiturate sedatives, antianxiety agents, and alcohol (see Chapter 29). Such drugs are used medically to relieve anxiety, induce sleep, and control seizures. Abuse of central depressants is more common than that of opioids and often originates with their medical use.

Barbiturates

CHARACTERISTICS OF ABUSE

In general, short-acting barbiturates are preferred by abusers. This class includes secobarbital (reds, red devils, red birds), pentobarbital (yellow jackets), and amobarbital (blues, blue heavens). They are abused for feelings of tranquility, relaxation, and disinhibition. As with opioids, patterns of abuse vary greatly from occasional to compulsive chronic use. Unlike opioids, however, long-term administration of these drugs can cause physical or mental deterioration of the user. Effects of barbiturates include sedation (without analgesia), decreased mental activity, slowed speech, and emotional lability. Individuals taking these drugs appear as if intoxicated with ethyl alcohol. Higher doses produce ataxia, diplopia, nystagmus, vertigo, stupor, sleep, and, eventually, respiratory depression, coma, and death. The risk of overdose with these agents is high because actions of central depressants are additive with one another. Furthermore, because these agents decrease mental acuity and impair memory, individuals may ingest more drug than they intend in a short period of time. Treatment of acute barbiturate overdose involves maintaining respiration and supporting the cardiovascular system. There is no specific antagonist that will reverse the apnea or coma.

TOLERANCE AND DEPENDENCE

Tolerance and cross-tolerance develop to the sedative and intoxicating actions of barbiturates. Consequently, individuals seeking the reinforcing properties of these agents must increase dosage over time. A component of the tolerance is dispositional because chronic use of barbiturates can induce hepatic microsomal enzymes. Functional tolerance also develops, but the mechanism remains unknown. Little tolerance develops to the lethal actions of these drugs. Thus, as dosage is increased, the risk of overdose becomes greater.

Chronic use of barbiturates can produce both psychologic and physical dependence, and acute withdrawal produces a dangerous abstinence syndrome. As with opioids, the onset and severity of abstinence is dependent on the drug used; withdrawal of short-acting drugs generally produces more rapid and severe symptoms. Unlike opioids, however, withdrawal from barbiturates is often life-threatening. Withdrawal symptoms progress from weakness, restlessness, tremulousness, and insomnia to abdominal cramps, nausea, vomiting, hyperthermia, orthostatic hypotension, confusion, disorientation, and, eventually, convulsions, including status epilepticus. Agitation and hyperthermia may lead to exhaustion and cardiovascular collapse. With short-acting barbiturates, convulsions are most likely to appear during the second or third day of abstinence. With long-acting barbiturates, such as phenobarbital, convulsions are less likely, but if they do occur it is usually between the third and eighth day of abstinence.

TREATMENT OF BARBITURATE DEPENDENCE

Treatment of barbiturate withdrawal requires hospitalization. First, patients are stabilized on a suitable barbiturate, usually pentobarbital. The dosage is titrated to the individual patient. Dosage is subsequently tapered over the next 7 to 14 days. The long withdrawal period is required to minimize the likelihood of an abstinence syndrome and convulsions. Babies born to mothers who are physically dependent on central nervous system depressants will also be dependent. The newborn abstinence syndrome is similar to that described for opioids, but is more dangerous. As with adults, babies are first stabilized on a central nervous system depressant, usually a benzodiazepine, then detoxified by gradually reducing the dosage.

Nonbarbiturate sedatives and antianxiety agents

There are numerous other central nervous system depressants that have the potential for abuse. These include meprobamate, methaqualone (quaalude, ludes), glutethimide, chloral hydrate, and the benzodiazepines. Like barbiturates, these drugs are abused for euphoria, feelings of tranquility, and the intoxication they produce. Effects of overdose with most of these agents are similar to those of the barbiturates. Benzodiazepines, however, are less powerful than barbiturates; severe respiratory depression and coma are unlikely, but if they occur flumazenil (see p. 270) can reverse them.[2] Methaqualone in large doses may produce convulsions, pulmonary edema, and respiratory arrest.

As with barbiturates, tolerance and cross-tolerance develop to the sedative and reinforcing properties of the nonbarbiturate sedatives including the benzodiazepines, but little tolerance is observed to the lethal effects. Strong psychologic and physical dependence can develop with chronic use of these drugs.[33] Abrupt withdrawal may produce a life-threatening abstinence syndrome. The severity of withdrawal depends on the drug used, the amount taken, and the duration of abuse. For example, withdrawal from therapeutic doses of diazepam generally produces anxiety and irritability, but rarely results in convulsions.

ETHYL ALCOHOL

Characteristics of abuse

Alcohol abuse is still the most serious drug abuse problem in Western society, if not in all countries. Alcohol is a contributing factor in 35% to 50% of cases of marital violence and 10% of occupational injuries. Some 18,000 or more traffic deaths (about 40%) in the United States are alcohol related.

Alcohol is a central nervous system depressant, and even small amounts decrease mental acuity and impair motor coordination. This compound is abused for intoxicating and euphoric feelings and for relief from anxiety. Acute ingestion of relatively small doses of alcohol produces feelings of warmth and relaxation, with only slight impairment in motor skills. Higher doses may produce paradoxic stimulation with feelings of buoyancy and exaggerated emotions. Further escalation of dosage can cause marked impairment of motor skills, slurred speech, unsteady gait, stupor, and ultimately unconsciousness.

Genetic factors appear to be important in the predisposition to alcohol dependence.[7] Familial occurrence of alcoholism is well documented, and the risk of becoming an alcoholic increases with the number of close relatives who are alcoholics. A higher rate of alcohol dependence occurs in identical twins as compared with fraternal twins. Furthermore, children from families of alcoholics, when adopted by other families show a fourfold higher risk of alcoholism than controls, whereas children of nonalcoholics reared by alcoholics are at no greater risk than controls.[25]

Tolerance and dependence

As with other central nervous system depressants, both dispositional and functional tolerance develop when alcohol is ingested chronically. Cross-tolerance between alcohol and other central nervous system depressants likewise has components of both dispositional and functional tolerance. Chronic use of alcohol can produce both psychologic and physical dependence, and the abstinence syndrome may be life threatening. Withdrawal symptoms appear within a few hours after the last dose of alcohol and are characterized by tremors, weakness, anxiety, intestinal cramps, and hyperreflexia. Between 12 and 24 hours after the last dose, patients may have visual hallucinations. By 48 hours, an acute neurologic syndrome may become apparent, with confusion, disorientation, and delusional thinking. When this syndrome is accompanied by gross tremors it is called "delirium tremens." Convulsions are less common than with barbiturate withdrawal. If the abstinence syndrome is not fatal, the patient will recover by the fifth to the seventh day after the drug is withdrawn.

Treatment of alcohol dependence

The treatment of alcohol dependence, like that of other types of drug dependence, requires detoxification and rehabilitation. Because the abstinence syndrome can be fatal, a strategy similar to that used for other central depressants should be employed. However, alcoholic patients often require fluids, nutrients, and vitamins (especially B vitamins) prior to detoxification to counter nutritional deficiencies. Patients are stabilized on another central nervous system depressant, usually a benzodiazepine, the dosage of which is gradually reduced.

For rehabilitation, Alcoholics Anonymous presents a unique and often pivotal source of help for alcoholics. In addition, the drug disulfiram (Antabuse) may help minimize recidivism by detoxified alcoholics.[12] When patients taking disulfiram ingest even a small amount of alcohol, they become physically ill due to accumulation of acetaldehyde. Presumably, this illness or the potential for it provides sufficient negative reinforcement to discourage drinking. The use of disulfiram obviously requires compliance on the part of the alcoholic.

Medical problems of alcohol abuse

Chronic use of alcohol can result in pathologic conditions and diseases not usually associated with other types of drug abuse. These include cirrhosis of the liver (with or without complications of portal hypertension), peripheral polyneuropathy, alcoholic gastritis, Korsakoffs psychosis, and Wernickes encephalopathy. Some of these are believed to be consequences of nutritional deficiencies. However, alcohol appears to contribute directly to the pathogenesis of the liver disease.

Prenatal exposure to alcohol may produce developmental defects in the brain with motor dysfunction, hypotonia, cognitive deficiencies, and microcephaly. As many as 2% of all babies born in the Western world may suffer to some extent from this *fetal alcohol syndrome*. Finally, there is evidence that alcoholism interferes with immune function and thereby predisposes individuals to infection.[23]

CENTRAL NERVOUS SYSTEM STIMULANTS

Drugs in this class include amphetamines (bennies, dex), methamphetamine (meth, speed, crystal, ice, crank), cocaine (coke, crack, rock, snow, toot), methylphenidate, and the less potent stimulants caffeine and nicotine.

Amphetamines and cocaine

CHARACTERISTICS OF ABUSE

Because the characteristics of dependence on amphetamine and cocaine are quite similar, they will be discussed together. Indeed, there is evidence that experienced users cannot distinguish between the subjective effects of these drugs.[10] The major difference between amphetamine and cocaine is in their durations of action, with cocaine being much shorter acting than amphetamine.

Amphetamines have been used medically as appetite suppressants and to treat narcolepsy and attention-deficit hyperactivity disorder. These potent stimulants are abused for their ability to cause euphoria, elevate mood, enhance a sense of well-being, and reduce fatigue. They are also taken in attempts to enhance mental or physical performance. Amphetamines are usually taken orally, sniffed, or injected intravenously. Administration by the latter route quickly produces a short-lived, extremely pleasant sensation (rush). Recently, a highly purified form ("ice") of methamphetamine that can be smoked has appeared.[5] This potent form for delivery of the drug is likely to increase the incidence of methamphetamine overdose; a large dose of drug can be absorbed quickly, without the need for intravenous injection.

In moderate doses, amphetamines produce a sense of well-being. They tend to lower anxiety and social inhibitions, to elevate mood, and to increase self-confidence. Users feel that their physical and mental abilities are heightened and that performance of simple tasks is enhanced. Amphetamines also promote insomnia and loss of appetite. At higher doses, they reduce mental acuity and impair performance of complex tasks. Users become anxious, restless, irritable, and irrational. Symptoms of amphetamine overdose include dizziness, tremor, hyperreflexia, confusion, agitation, hostility, delirium, and paranoid ideation. "Amphetamine psychosis" may develop during long- or short-term abuse of amphetamines and is characterized by visual and auditory hallucinations and paranoid delusions. It resembles paranoid schizophrenia and usually clears within a few days after the drug is discontinued.

After central stimulation by amphetamines, the user exhibits fatigue and depression. Depending on the amount of drug taken and the duration of the "spree," the user may be physically exhausted. This phase is termed "the crash" and is characterized by prolonged sleep, anxiety, agitation, and depression. The dysphoric feelings, after a period of excessive exhilaration, may lead users of amphetamine, methamphetamine, or cocaine to take large quantities over a long period termed a *run* or a *speed run*. Injection of hundreds of milligrams of drug every few hours for days, or until the supply runs out, is not uncommon.[13] After a run, the exhaustion and depression seen after acute doses may be greatly exaggerated.

Effects of amphetamines include mydriasis, hypertension, hyperreflexia, and hyperthermia. Hypertensive crisis with intracranial hemorrhage has been reported after oral and intravenous administration of methamphetamine. Cardiac arrhythmias can occur secondary to amphetamine use, as can myocardial infarction and circulatory collapse. Amphetamines also lower the seizure threshold and predispose individuals to convulsions.

Cocaine is a local anesthetic, a vasoconstrictor, and a powerful central nervous system stimulant.[18] It occurs naturally in the leaves of the coca plant, *Erythroxylon coca*, and in other species of *Erythroxylon*, which are indigenous to Peru and Bolivia. Coca leaf chewing has been a way of life for centuries among the Quechua Indians living in the Andean highlands. In recent years, abuse of cocaine has increased dramatically. By 1986, approximately 15% of the persons in the United States had tried cocaine.[13] A much smaller percentage became dependent on the drug.

Cocaine, like amphetamines, is abused for euphoria, heightened energy, self-esteem, and increased feelings of confidence.[13,18] Cocaine hydrochloride is usually sniffed (snorted) or injected intravenously. Recently, cocaine base (crack or rock) has emerged as a prominent form of the drug. It is smoked, and combustion produces a fine aerosol and volatile drug that is rapidly absorbed from the lungs. Crack is sold in small quantities that make it affordable to the young and impoverished. A high concentration of drug is rapidly reached in the brain and heart, and toxic overdoses are all too frequent. Users experience an initial rush similar to that obtained by intravenous administration of stimulants.

Acute toxicity from an excessive dose of cocaine, regardless of the route of administration, may be characterized by extreme agitation, restlessness, confusion, chest pain, anxiety, palpitations, and headache.[1] Cocaine overdose is extremely dangerous.[20] It may rapidly induce paranoid thinking, hallucinations, cerebrovascular accidents,[21] and convulsions. There are reports of acute myocardial infarction after cocaine use, even in young patients with normal coronary arteries.[16] In addition, release of epinephrine and blockade of norepinephrine reuptake may evoke cardiac arrhythmias, including ventricular fibrillation. Extreme central stimulation is followed by severe depression and possibly medullary paralysis and respiratory failure. Cocaine abuse can produce a paranoid state that is similar to amphetamine psychosis. Another complication of cocaine sniffing is ischemic necrosis and perforation of the nasal septum caused by intense and prolonged vasoconstriction as the cocaine remains in the nasal mucosa for hours after application.

Tolerance and Dependence

Marked tolerance can develop to the euphoric effects of amphetamines and some of the actions of cocaine. Consequently, users increase the amount they take to achieve the initial rush. There is, however, little tolerance to the cardiovascular effects of these agents or to the development of psychotic side effects.

Central stimulants produce a high degree of psychologic dependence. Whether physical dependence develops is still in question. A reproducible abstinence syndrome like that of opioid withdrawal is not observed. Abrupt withdrawal from chronic use or from a run, however, may cause serious depression and anxiety with possible suicidal ideation. Users will also be hypersomnolent and physically exhausted. Mood returns to normal after a number of days, but craving for drug, dysphoria, and altered sleep patterns may persist for weeks.

Treatment of Dependence

Treatment of amphetamine or cocaine overdose requires control of the various symptoms produced by the drug. For example, cardiac complications are treated with β-adrenergic receptor antagonists or, more recently, with Ca^{++}-channel blockers. β-Blockers should not be administered without α-receptor blockade to prevent unopposed α-receptor-mediated vasoconstriction. Convulsions are treated with diazepam, as is hyperactivity. Hyperthermia should be controlled. Users who have residual psychiatric complications are treated with antipsychotic or antidepressant drugs. Acidification of the urine will increase elimination of amphetamine, but this procedure is seldom used as the urine is normally acidic.

Methylphenidate

Methylphenidate (see p. 302) is used to treat attention-deficit hyperactivity disorder and narcolepsy. It is less potent than amphetamines and in normal therapeutic doses produces fewer side effects. At higher doses it produces effects similar to those from amphetamine and has similar abuse potential.

Nicotine

Nicotine is one of numerous alkaloids found in the tobacco plant *Nicotiana tabacum*. This plant is cultivated in every country where the climate permits, and smoking of tobacco is one of the most prevalent forms of drug abuse. When burned, tobacco smoke contains numerous chemicals in a mixture of gases, uncondensed vapors, liquid, and particulate matter. The products of major clinical importance are nicotine, carbon monoxide, carcinogens in the tars, and phenols.

Characteristics of Abuse

Nicotine is a mild stimulant with less powerful reinforcing properties than those of amphetamine. It produces feelings of well-being, increased alertness, and a sense of relaxation. These effects on mood appear responsible for the strong psychologic dependence that develops to the use of tobacco. Nicotine also causes stimulation of respiration, tremors, and relaxation of skeletal muscle. In extremely high doses it can produce convulsions. Acute use often produces dizziness, nausea, and vomiting. The latter is caused by nicotine-induced stimulation of the chemoreceptor trigger zone and its activation of vagal reflexes. Nicotine elevates heart rate and blood pressure, presumably by stimulation of the sympathetic nervous system and the adrenal medulla.

Chronic use of nicotine results in tolerance; many of its effects, including nausea, vomiting, dizziness, and mood alteration, are lessened. Although strong psychologic dependence develops, physical dependence does not. Subjects who discontinue taking nicotine will crave the drug, and there is a high rate of recidivism. Withdrawal from nicotine may produce impatience, irritability, anxiety, restlessness, headache, insomnia, and decreased cognitive abilities. These symptoms vary with the individual user and do not constitute a defined abstinence syndrome. Nicotine gum (Nicorette) may help nicotine-dependent individuals quit smoking (see p. 123). Clonidine also appears to be an effective aid in smoking cessation.[14]

MEDICAL PROBLEMS OF TOBACCO SMOKING

Regular heavy smoking can have a number of untoward effects on the respiratory system, including labored breathing, wheezing, shortness of breath, and frequent upper respiratory tract infections. Cessation of smoking will reverse these effects. In addition, smokers are at greater risk than non-smokers for developing chronic bronchitis, emphysema, and lung cancer. Chronic smoking also increases the risk of contracting cardiovascular diseases such as coronary artery disease and cerebrovascular disease (stroke). Over time, cessation of smoking will reverse the increased risk of respiratory and cardiovascular diseases. Chronic smoking during pregnancy is associated with lower infant birth weight and an increased likelihood of prenatal mortality.

Caffeine

Caffeine (see Chapter 31) and related methylxanthines occur naturally in the coffee bean (seeds of *Coffea arabica* and related species), the leaves of the tea plant (*Thea sinensis*), and the seeds of the chocolate tree (*Theobroma cacao*). Caffeine is the most widely used central nervous system stimulant. Ingestion of caffeine increases alertness and elevates mood. Although numerous studies have attempted to link caffeine use with other health problems, no causal relationships have been found. Psychologic dependence develops with chronic use, but little, if any, physical dependence occurs. Withdrawal after chronic use, however, may result in headache, irritability, nervousness, and lethargy.

HALLUCINOGENS

Numerous drugs can induce hallucinations when taken in sufficiently high doses. This section discusses only those that are abused primarily for their psychotogenic or hallucinogenic effects. D-Lysergic acid diethylamide (LSD, acid), mescaline (peyote), psilocybin (mushrooms), and phencyclidine (PCP, angel dust, crystal, hog) are among the most popular hallucinogens. They have diverse pharmacologic effects[3] and no current medical use.

Lysergide (LSD)

CHARACTERISTICS OF ABUSE

LSD (D-Lysergic acid diethylamide) is a highly potent hallucinogen synthesized from alkaloids of ergot (*Claviceps purpurea*) found in a fungus that attacks rye and other grains. Although it was first synthesized in 1938, its hallucinogenic activity was not discovered until 1943.

Ingestion of microgram quantities of LSD produces physiologic and psychotogenic effects that last for 8 to 12 hours. It is abused primarily for unique and altered sensory experiences, for feelings of altered reality, and for perceptions of understanding hidden truths. The psychotogenic effects of LSD (the *trip*) vary considerably and depend to some degree on the state of mind, mood, and expectations of the user. The usual trip is characterized by initial feelings of depersonalization and loss of body image. Individuals experience altered sensorium; altered perceptions of colors, shapes, and distances; and frank hallucinations. Often, sensory modalities are mixed, and the user perceives that he hears colors or sees music (synesthesias). Users may also have intense introspective experiences and believe that they have discovered new truths. Emotional states are enhanced and may range from ecstasy to profound feelings of despair. Effects of LSD include slight increases in heart rate and blood pressure, mydriasis, hyperreflexia, muscular incoordination, salivation, and lacrimation.

Unpleasant experiences with LSD are relatively frequent and may involve dissociative reactions, acute panic reactions, or acute psychotic episodes.[28] At the onset of the drug experience, the depersonalization and altered sensorium often produce anxiety and panic, leading to a negative psychotogenic experience (bad trip). In attempting to escape the bad trip the user may inadvertently harm himself or others. In some instances an acute psychotic reaction occurs, and the user becomes paranoid or suicidal. Although prolonged psychotic reactions are rare, use of LSD may worsen an underlying psychosis.

Symptoms of an LSD trip that recur days, weeks, or months after a single dose are called "flashbacks." Flashback symptoms can vary from alterations in mood to severe changes in thought processes. The reaction may be triggered by stress, fatigue, or use of other drugs. Long-term use of LSD is also associated with permanent changes in thought or behavior. Frequent users sometimes think and feel as they did under the influence of drug, even when not taking it. In addition, chronic users may develop an amotivational syndrome in which they become apathetic and lose interest in work, social life, and long-term planning.

TOLERANCE AND DEPENDENCE

Tolerance develops rapidly to the effects of LSD and reverses when users abstain for short periods of time. Cross-tolerance develops between LSD, mescaline, and psilocybin. Although psychologic dependence can develop with chronic use, no physical dependence occurs.

TREATMENT OF LSD ABUSE

In most instances, LSD intoxication resolves without incident. Acute panic attacks can be alleviated by benzodiazepines. Antipsychotic drugs are effective for treating the confusion and agitation caused by LSD, but they should be used with caution because they can potentiate side effects. A quiet and reassuring environment is often helpful in calming an individual on a bad trip.

Mescaline

The tops of the peyote cactus, *Lophophora williamsii*, contain hallucinogens and are used in religious ceremonies by Indians in northern Mexico and the southwest United States. The major psychoactive drug in peyote is mescaline (3,4,5-trimethoxyphenethylamine). Ingestion of peyote or mescaline produces both physiologic and psychotogenic effects similar to LSD, although LSD is thousands of times more potent than mescaline. The onset of effect is slow and often accompanied by nausea, profuse sweating, and tremors. Mescaline produces vivid and colorful hallucinations, and the psychic effects last for 8 to 12 hours. Tolerance and psychologic dependence develop with chronic use, but no physical dependence develops.

Psilocybin

Psilocybin and psilocin, another hallucinogen, are found in *Psilocybe* and other mushrooms indigenous to Mexico.[30] Their effects are similar to those induced by LSD. Their onset is more rapid (15 minutes), however, and their duration of action is much shorter (2 to 3 hours). Furthermore, these compounds are much less potent than LSD. Like LSD, tolerance and psychologic dependence can develop with chronic usage.

Phencyclidine

Phencyclidine (PCP, 1-[1-phenylcyclohexyl]piperidine) was first introduced as a veterinary anesthetic agent in the 1950s. It was not marketed for use in humans because of the prolonged delirium that occurred as patients emerged from anesthesia. Its illicit use became popular in the 1970s, in part because it was easily synthesized and misrepresented by suppliers as other drugs, especially LSD and tetrahydrocannabinol. Phencyclidine is an extremely dangerous compound that can produce a variety of acute and long-term toxic effects.[4,27] It has central nervous system depressant, stimulant, and hallucinogenic properties. In low doses it induces euphoria, disinhibition, intoxication, and increased emotional liability. Larger doses produce a dissociative state (lack of recognition of self), analgesia, delirium, stupor, and hallucinations. Users may appear agitated or may be withdrawn. Hostile or bizarre behavior and unprovoked aggression may be associated with a psychotic state that occurs while the user is taking the drug or possibly later.

Effects elicited by phencyclidine include tachycardia, hypertension, flushing, sweating, and miosis. Users are often hyperreflexic and exhibit nystagmus, ataxia, and rigidity. With sufficiently high doses, convulsions, status epilepticus, hypertensive crisis, cardiac or respiratory arrest, and coma may occur. Some tolerance appears to develop to the effects of phencyclidine, and psychologic dependence may occur. Physical dependence has not been demonstrated.

Treatment of phencyclidine overdose is complex and involves treating the major symptoms. For example, hypertension may require antihypertensive therapy. Antipsychotic drugs can alleviate phencyclidine-induced psychosis. If ingested orally, ingestion of charcoal or gastric emptying may limit absorption and enterohepatic reabsorption of the drug.

Other psychotogenic drugs

Numerous amphetamine derivatives produce hallucinations and other psychic effects. For example, **2,5-dimethoxy-4-methyl-amphetamine** (DOM, STP) produces mild euphoria and central nervous system stimulation in small doses and LSD-like effects in larger doses. Negative experiences (bad trips) appear to be more common with DOM than with LSD. Other agents include **3,4-methylenedioxymethamphetamine** (MDMA, ecstasy) and **3-methoxy-4,5-methylenedioxyamphetamine** (MDA).

There are three tryptamine derivatives that also produce LSD-like effects. These are **dimethyltryptamine** (DMT), **diethyltryptamine** (DET), and **dipropyltryptamine** (DPT). They differ from LSD in that their onset of action is more rapid and their duration of action is only 1 to 2 hours. Mydriasis and hypertension are more pronounced with these drugs than with LSD. DMT is present in several South American snuffs, including cohoba snuff.

CANNABINOIDS

Cannabinoids are the psychoactive substances found in marijuana. They produce sedative, euphoric, and hallucinogenic effects depending on the dose.[8] Consequently, they do not fit cleanly into any other drug category. The source of marijuana is the hemp plant *Cannabis sativa*. Marijuana (weed, pot, hash, maryjane, smoke, reefer, dope) usually refers to any part of the plant that is cultivated, because active cannabinoids are found throughout. The highest concentrations of drug are found in flowering tops of the plant, and preparations of the dried resin from this part are called "hashish" and "charas." The potency of marijuana (that is, the concentration of active cannabinoids) varies with plant strain and growth conditions. The principle psychoactive cannabinoid found in marijuana is (-)-Δ^9-*trans*-tetrahydrocannabinol (Δ^9-THC or simply THC). Δ^1-THC and Δ^9-THC represent different systems of nomenclature for the same compound. A very small amount of the active compound Δ^8-THC may also be present. Cannabinoids are used medically (see p. 248) to diminish the nausea and vomiting that occur secondary to cancer chemotherapy.

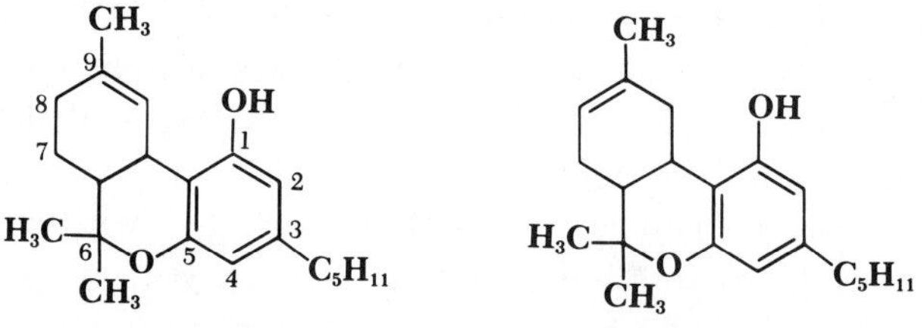

Δ^9-THC **$\Delta^{8(9)}$-THC ($\Delta^{1(6)}$-THC)**

Characteristics of abuse

Low to moderate doses of THC produce an increased sense of well-being and euphoria. Perceptions of time and space are altered and senses appear to be enhanced. This increase in sensorium often results in users being preoccupied with seemingly novel ways of seeing, hearing, touching, or tasting simple and familiar objects. In contrast to LSD, users are relaxed and sleepy rather than aroused. Short-term memory, motor skills, and performance of goal-oriented and complex tasks are diminished. At higher doses, hallucinations, delusions, and depersonalization reactions may occur. Users may also experience paranoid ideation. These effects may produce anxiety, fear, and panic reactions. Toxic psychosis secondary to marijuana use has been reported.[31]

Acute effects of marijuana include dry mouth, tachycardia, increased or decreased blood pressure depending on whether the user is supine or standing, and reddening of the conjunctiva. Hyperthermia may occur when the user is in a hot environment. THC has been shown to impair spermatogenesis, to inhibit synthesis of testosterone, and in females to suppress LH and FSH production. Whether these endocrine effects are of physiologic significance remains to be determined. THC reduces intraocular pressure, is a bronchodilator, and is an effective antiemetic.

When marijuana is smoked, the onset of psychogenic effects is rapid. The duration of these effects is usually 2 to 3 hours. Tetrahydrocannabinol accumulates in fat, and the drug can be detected for several days after a single administration.

Chronic use may cause pervasive feelings of apathy and loss of interest in goals (that is, an amotivational syndrome). Users may also exhibit some memory loss, impaired judgement, and a lack of ability to concentrate. One serious hazard of marijuana is enhancement of a paranoid thought disorder and exacerbation of psychosis in schizophrenic patients. Secondary to excessive, chronic smoking of marijuana, users may also develop asthma or bronchitis.

Tolerance and dependence

With chronic use, tolerance develops to the altered mood and sensorium produced by THC.[19] Tolerance is also observed to the cardiovascular effects, the diminished psychomotor performance, and the decrease in intraocular pressure. Strong psychologic dependence may develop to the use of marijuana, and users may not feel "normal" unless they are under the influence of the drug. Little, if any, physical dependence occurs. Withdrawal from chronic use, however, may cause irritability, restlessness, nervousness, insomnia, weight loss, chills, tremor, and increased REM sleep.

INHALANTS

Inhalants[22] can be subdivided into anesthetic agents (see Chapter 36), volatile nitrates and hydrocarbon solvents, and fluorocarbon aerosol propellants. Nitrous oxide, the most abused general anesthetic, is popular for the intoxicating effects and pleasant sensations it produces. Although its side effects are minimal, hypoxia and death because of lack of oxygen have occurred with use of nitrous oxide in confined spaces.

Volatile nitrates, principally amyl nitrite and isobutyl nitrite (poppers, snappers), are popular abused inhalants. They relax most smooth muscle. Inhalation of these agents produces transient euphoria, light-headedness, and perceptual distortions. The unsubstantiated belief that these drugs enhance sexual performance and orgasm account for much of their usage. The major side effects of the volatile nitrites are headache, dizziness, and flushing. Large doses can produce profound hypotension, nausea, vomiting, glaucoma, decreased respiration, and unconsciousness. Tolerance develops to the vasodilating properties of these agents.

Perhaps the most insidious group of inhalants are the volatile solvents and fluorocarbon propellants. These include gasoline, lacquer thinners, various glues and cements, cleaning fluids, nail-polish remover, lighter fluid, and aerosol propellants. Toluene, acetone, benzene, *n*-hexane, isobutane, and freons are among the chemicals inhaled from the above products, most of which are readily available. Because of their availability, these are the compounds most abused by children and young teenagers. In general, these agents produce dose-related central nervous system depressant effects. Users become intoxicated, ataxic, and have sensory and perceptual distortions and delusions. Higher doses cause loss of consciousness. These agents may also induce cardiac arrhythmias, nausea, vomiting, diarrhea, headache, and irritation of the eyes. Long-term toxic effects (depending on the agent used) include peripheral nerve damage, hepatotoxicity, nephrotoxicity, cerebellar atrophy, damage to the respiratory tract, lead poisoning (from the use of gasoline), and bone-marrow depression. Death is a consequence of cardiac arrhythmias, cardiac failure, and suffocation. In the latter instance, death usually occurs because the user loses consciousness while a plastic bag or other container is placed over the nose and mouth. Tolerance develops to the intoxicating effects of these agents and psychologic dependence may occur.

REFERENCES

1. Brody SL, Slovis CM, Wrenn KD: Cocaine-related medical problems: consecutive series of 233 patients, *Am J Med* 88:325, 1990.
2. Brogden RN, Goa KL: Flumazenil: a preliminary review of its benzodiazepine antagonist properties, intrinsic activity and therapeutic use, *Drugs* 35:448, 1988.
3. Brown RT, Braden NJ: Hallucinogens, *Pediatr Clin North Am* 34:341, 1987.
4. Burns RS, Lerner SE: Perspectives: acute phencyclidine intoxication, *Clin Toxicol* 9:477, 1976.
5. Cho AK: Ice: a new dosage form of an old drug, *Science* 249:631, 1990.
6. Cooper JR: Methadone treatment and acquired immunodeficiency syndrome, *JAMA* 262:1664, 1989.
7. Devor EJ, Cloninger CR: Genetics of alcoholism, *Annu Rev Genet* 23:19, 1989.
8. Dewey WL: Cannabinoid pharmacology, *Pharmacol Rev* 38:151, 1986.
9. Dole VP: Methadone treatment and the acquired immunodeficiency syndrome epidemic, *JAMA* 262:1681, 1989.
10. Fischman MW, Schuster CR: Cocaine self-administration in humans, *Fed Proc* 41:241, 1982.
11. Franz DN, Hare BD, McCloskey KL: Spinal sympathetic neurons: possible sites of opiate-withdrawal suppression by clonidine, *Science* 215:1643, 1982.
12. Fuller RK, Branchey L, Brightwell DR, et al: Disulfiram treatment of alcoholism: a Veterans Administration cooperative study, *JAMA* 256:1449, 1986.
13. Gawin FH, Ellinwood EH Jr: Cocaine and other stimulants: actions, abuse, and treatment, *N Engl J Med* 318:1173, 1988.
14. Glassman AH, Stetner F, Walsh BT, et al: Heavy smokers, smoking cessation, and clonidine: results of a double-blind, randomized trial, *JAMA* 259:2863, 1988.
15. Gonzalez JP, Brogden RN: Naltrexone: a review of its pharmacodynamic and pharmacokinetic properties and therapeutic efficacy in the management of opioid dependence, *Drugs* 35:192, 1988.
16. Howard RE, Hueter DC, Davis GJ: Acute myocardial infarction following cocaine abuse in a young woman with normal coronary arteries, *JAMA* 254:95, 1985.
17. Jasinski DR, Johnson RE, Kocher TR: Clonidine in morphine withdrawal: differential effects on signs and symptoms, *Arch Gen Psychiatry* 42:1063, 1985.
18. Johanson C-E, Fischman MW: The pharmacology of cocaine related to its abuse, *Pharmacol Rev* 41:3, 1989.
19. Jones RT, Benowitz N, Bachman J: Clinical studies of cannabis tolerance and dependence, *Ann NY Acad Sci* 282:221, 1976.
20. Lathers CM, Tyau LSY, Spino MM, Agarwal I: Cocaine-induced seizures, arrhythmias and sudden death, *J Clin Pharmacol* 28:584, 1988.
21. Levine SR, Brust JCM, Futrell N, et al: Cerebrovascular complications of the use of the "crack" form of alkaloidal cocaine, *N Engl J Med* 323:699, 1990.
22. Linden CH: Volatile substances of abuse,

Emerg Med Clin North Am 8:559, 1990.

23. MacGregor RR: Alcohol and immune defense, *JAMA* 256:1474, 1986.
24. Milby JB: Methadone maintenance to abstinence: how many make it? *J Nerv Ment Dis* 176:409, 1988.
25. Schuckit MA: Genetics and the risks for alcoholism, *JAMA* 254:2614, 1985.
26. Seevers MH: Medical perspectives on habituation and addiction, *JAMA* 181:112, 1962.
27. Showalter CV, Thornton WE: Clinical pharmacology of phencyclidine toxicity, *Am J Psychiatry* 134:1234, 1977.
28. Strassman RJ: Adverse reactions to psychedelic drugs: a review of the literature, *J Nerv Ment Dis* 172:577, 1984.
29. Snyder SH, D'Amato RJ: MPTP: a neurotoxin relevant to the pathophysiology of Parkinson's disease, *Neurology* 36:250, 1986.
30. Spoerke DG, Hall AH: Plants and mushrooms of abuse, *Emerg Med Clin North Am* 8:579, 1990.
31. Thacore VR, Shukla SRP: Cannabis psychosis and paranoid schizophrenia, *Arch Gen Psychiatry* 33:383, 1976.
32. Washton AM, Resnick RB: Clonidine for opiate detoxification: outpatient clinical trials, *Am J Psychiatry* 137:1121, 1980.
33. Woods JH, Katz JL, Winger G: Abuse liability of benzodiazepines, *Pharmacol Rev* 39:251, 1987.

section five

Nonsteroidal anti-inflammatory antipyretic analgesics

Chapter 35

Nonsteroidal anti-inflammatory antipyretic analgesics

GENERAL CONCEPT

Drugs from several diverse structural classes share analgesic, antipyretic, and anti-inflammatory activity. They have been termed *nonsteroidal anti-inflammatory drugs* (NSAIDs) to distinguish them from glucocorticoids (Chapter 47), *nonnarcotic analgesics* to distinguish them from opioids (Chapter 33), *antipyretic analgesics, aspirin-like agents,* and so forth. A widely accepted mechanism for many of their effects is their ability to inhibit *cyclooxygenase* and thereby decrease conversion of arachidonic acid to prostaglandins, thromboxane A_2, or prostacyclin (see Chapter 25). In general, adverse gastrointestinal effects may limit their use. They may also elevate plasma concentrations of hepatic enzymes, promote water and electrolyte retention, or cause acute renal insufficiency. They are highly bound to plasma albumin, from which they can displace other drugs. NSAIDs should be used with caution in pregnant women, the elderly, and patients with cardiac, hepatic, or renal disease. They should be avoided in patients with bleeding disorders, gastrointestinal ulcers, or intolerance to aspirin. Aspirin, the prototype, is considered in detail. Acetaminophen, a widely used antipyretic analgesic, differs in that it lacks useful anti-inflammatory activity.

DRUG CLASSIFICATION

The NSAIDs and other nonnarcotic analgesics are classified in the list on the next page according to their therapeutic uses and structural classes.

SALICYLATES

Salicylic acid (2-hydroxybenzoic acid) is closely related to compounds that occur naturally in willow bark and oil of wintergreen. Most compounds related to salicylic acid (salicylates) act by conversion to this acid or by similar mechanisms. The most commonly employed is aspirin (acetylsalicylic acid). Salicylamide, which is not metabolized to salicylate and lacks useful activity, is included in several combination products. Diflunisal is a long-acting salicylate analog that, likewise, is not metabolized to salicylate. Oil of wintergreen is methyl salicylate.

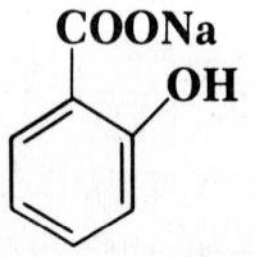

COONa, OH — **Sodium salicylate**

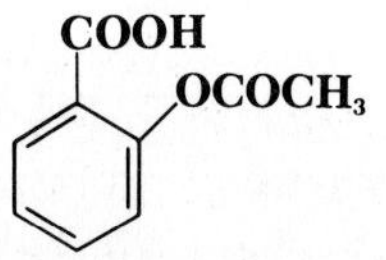

COOH, $OCOCH_3$ — **Aspirin**

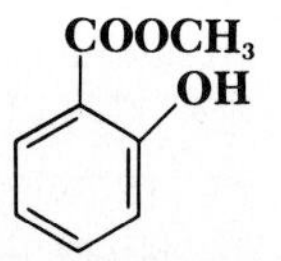

$COOCH_3$, OH — **Methyl salicylate**

Salicylates—anti-inflammatory antipyretic analgesics
- Acetylsalicylic acid (aspirin)
- Sodium salicylate (Uracel)
- Magnesium salicylate (Magan, others)
- Choline salicylate (Arthropan)
- Choline magnesium trisalicylate (Trilisate)
- Diflunisal (Dolobid)
- Salsalate (Disalcid)
- Salicylamide (Uromide)
- Sodium thiosalicylate (Rexolate, others)
- Trolamine salicylate (Aspercreme, others)

Never ingest
- Salicylic acid, used topically for wart and corn removal
- Methyl salicylate, used as a counterirritant in ointments

Salicylate-like anti-inflammatory agents
- Propionic acid derivatives
  - Ibuprofen (Motrin, others)
  - Naproxen (Naprosyn)
  - Naproxen sodium (Anaprox)
  - Fenoprofen calcium (Nalfon)
  - Flurbiprofen (Ansaid, Ocufen)
  - Ketoprofen (Orudis)
  - Suprofen (Profenal)
- Acetic acid derivatives
  - Indomethacin (Indocin, others)
  - Sulindac (Clinoril)
  - Tolmetin sodium (Tolectin)
  - Diclofenac sodium (Voltaren)
- Ketorolac tromethamine (Toradol)
- Piroxicam (Feldene)
- Phenylbutazone (Butazolidin, Azolid)
- Fenamates
  - Meclofenamate sodium (Meclomen, Meclodium)
  - Mefenamic acid (Ponstel)

Antipyretic analgesic
- Acetaminophen (Tylenol, others)

Sedative analgesic
- Methotrimeprazine (Levoprome)

Combinations with other analgesics, caffeine, sedatives, and so forth

---

Mechanisms and sites of action

When 600 mg of aspirin is ingested by healthy adults, the effects are negligible though some may complain of gastric upset. In disease states or in painful conditions, however, therapeutic effects of salicylates can be quite prominent. Most if not all mammalian cells can synthesize prostaglandins. A major action of NSAIDs is inhibition of cyclooxygenase activity (see Fig. 25-2). Since prostaglandins are not stored, their release depends on continual synthesis, and inhibition of cyclooxygenase reduces their availability. NSAIDs generally do not antagonize the actions of the end products. Unlike other NSAIDs, aspirin irreversibly acetylates and inactivates cyclooxygenase. As platelets are exposed to a relatively high concentration of aspirin in the portal circulation during absorption of a single dose,[15] their cyclooxygenase is permanently inactivated because platelets cannot synthesize new enzyme. Inhibition is not irreversible in other tissues because new enzyme can be formed and because aspirin is rapidly hydrolyzed to salicylate, a reversible and less potent inhibitor.[10] Nevertheless, chronic administration of nonacetylated salicylates, or other NSAIDs, should maintain cyclooxygenase inhibition. There is also evidence that a variety of other mechanisms, such as inhibition of neutrophil activation and reduced release of arachidonic acid, contribute to therapeutic effects of NSAIDs.

THERAPEUTIC USES

Analgesia. Prostaglandins alone induce pain only in concentrations that are unlikely to occur physiologically. However, they enhance the potency of *algesic* (pain-inducing) substances, such as bradykinin, that stimulate nerve endings of unmyelinated C fibers and small-diameter Aδ fibers to elicit noxious afferent input. Furthermore, bradykinin stimulates formation and release of prostaglandins, a positive feedback of sorts. Thus the *analgesic* action of NSAIDs appears to be primarily, if not solely, peripheral to reduce potentiation of algesic activity by prostaglandins. Aspirin is most effective in alleviating pain of mild to moderate intensity; some NSAIDs may relieve more severe pain.

Antipyresis. In contrast to analgesia, the site of antipyretic action of NSAIDs is central.[2] In fever the temperature-regulating system maintains temperature at a higher level than normal. The stimulus for the shift to a higher level is the action of an *endogenous pyrogen,* such as interleukin-1, on neurons of the thermoregulatory system in the preoptic hypothalamus (Fig. 35-1). Aspirin does not act directly on the thermoregulatory system and does not affect pyrogen release; rather it reduces the effect of the pyrogen. Inhibition of prostaglandin synthesis does not adequately account for the antipyretic action of NSAIDs. Therapeutic doses of aspirin affect neither normal body temperature nor an elevated temperature (hyperthermia), associated with exercise, drugs, or hypothalamic lesions, to which pyrogen does not contribute.

Antipyretics are best utilized when body temperature is dangerously high or when a reduction of fever provides significant relief. Temperatures to 39° C (102° F) or somewhat higher are often well tolerated, and changes in body temperature provide an indication of the progression of a disease. Salicylates, acetaminophen, and ibuprofen are the only drugs approved as antipyretics in the United States, though indomethacin and naproxen have been recommended to lower fever of neoplastic disease that is uncontrolled by other antipyretics.

Anti-inflammatory effect. Since prostaglandins induce symptoms of inflammation and enhance the effects of bradykinin and histamine, a reduction of prostaglandins at sites of inflammation should be beneficial. In rheumatic fever large daily dosages of salicylate lower temperature, relieve joint symptoms, and normalize sedimentation

Fever production. *FIG. 35-1*

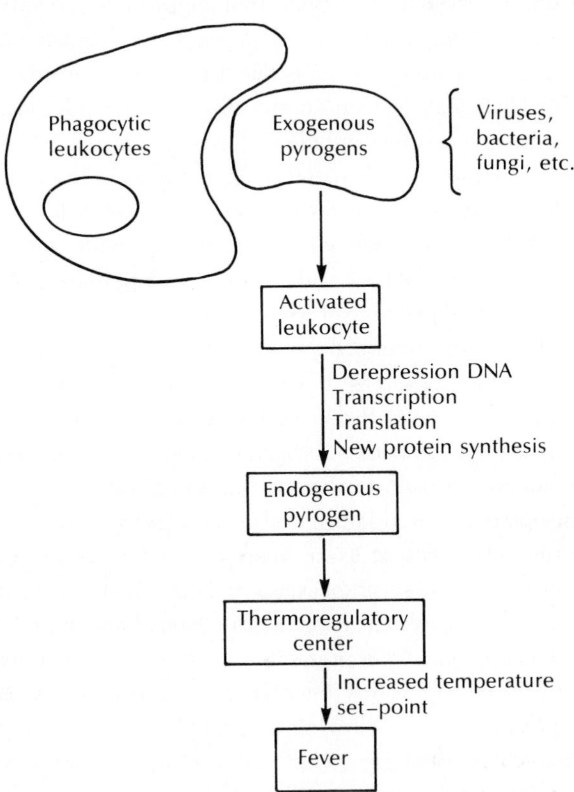

rate but have no effect on rheumatic carditis. In arthritic diseases NSAIDs reduce inflammation and swelling, to provide considerable relief. The idea that cyclooxygenase inhibition is the sole or primary mechanism for the beneficial effects of such drugs has been challenged.[1,4]

There is considerable individual variability in therapeutic response and adverse reactions to NSAIDs; treatment of arthritic patients must be individualized. Aspirin may be tried first, because it is least expensive and an excellent drug if tolerated. If aspirin is ineffective at a tolerable dosage, another NSAID is usually prescribed. Some persons will require treatment with more toxic drugs such as gold salts, penicillamine, or glucocorticoids. Only aspirin, naproxen, and tolmetin have been approved for children with rheumatoid arthritis. It is recommended that aspirin be avoided in pregnancy.

Miscellaneous clinical uses. NSAIDs have been used to treat ocular inflammation, acute and chronic glomerulonephritis, Bartters syndrome, Kawasaki disease, and traveler's diarrhea. Aspirin is recommended for prophylactic treatment of migraine. Uses based on the "antiplatelet" action of aspirin are discussed in Chapter 41. Treatment of dysmenorrhea and patent ductus arteriosus with NSAIDs, usually not aspirin, is discussed below (pp. 368 and 369 respectively). Salicylic acid has long been used topically to remove warts, and a transdermal patch containing a 15% solution (Trans-Ver-Sal) recently became available for nighttime application.

ADVERSE AND SIDE EFFECTS

Uric acid retention and excretion. The effect of aspirin on uric acid excretion is predictably variable. Salicylates given chronically in high daily dosages inhibit uric acid reabsorption from the proximal tubule of the nephron (see Fig. 53-1). Before the advent of better tolerated uricosuric agents such as probenecid (see Chapter 53), this property was used to promote uric acid excretion in patients with gout. When salicylates are given acutely, however, salicylic acid competes with uric acid for secretion into tubular fluid. This can cause uric acid retention and perhaps precipitate an attack of gouty arthritis. Patients taking other uricosuric drugs should avoid the use of aspirin, which can reduce the uricosuric effect.

Intolerance. Intolerance to aspirin develops in approximately 0.3% of the normal population. This intolerance, which does not extend to sodium salicylate, has been defined as "acute urticaria-angioedema, bronchospasm, severe rhinitis, or shock occurring within three hours of aspirin ingestion."[20] Intolerance is usually manifest as an exacerbation of the patient's preexisting problem, such as bronchoconstriction in an asthmatic, but it may also present as an anaphylactoid reaction. Aspirin should be avoided by patients with severe asthma, nasal polyps, chronic urticaria, or recurrent rhinitis. Since no specific antibodies for aspirin have been found in sera of such patients, the term "intolerance" is preferable to the term "hypersensitivity." The mechanisms of intolerance are poorly understood; for asthma, one possibility is that cyclooxygenase inhibition shifts arachidonic acid metabolism toward synthesis of bronchoconstrictor leukotrienes. Patients show cross-intolerance to varying degrees to other NSAIDs and occasionally to tartrazine, a yellow dye used in food and pharmaceutical preparations. Such agents should be avoided by patients intolerant to aspirin.

Gastrointestinal irritation and bleeding. Therapeutic doses of aspirin may irritate gastric mucosa and increase blood loss in a majority of persons, frequently without obvious symptoms. Many patients cannot tolerate the large dosages needed to manage arthritic conditions. A nonacetylated salicylate may be less irritating.[18] NSAID-associated gastropathy can extend to hemorrhage and perforation, often without warning; it has been proposed as the most frequent serious adverse drug effect in the United States.[7] Aspirin should be avoided by patients with a history of ulcers and should not be used with alcohol or other agents that promote ulcer formation. Risk is greater in elderly and debilitated patients. Esophageal injury may also occur.

The mechanisms of gastrointestinal bleeding and ulceration induced by aspirin are complex, but irritation due to direct contact with mucosal cells and cyclooxygenase inhibition after absorption are important factors. Lesions of the gastric mucosa are more common after aspirin ingestion when intragastric pH is low; thus acid is a factor. Acutely, local irritation and bleeding are reduced with enteric-coated preparations or administration of antacids; even without such measures, adaptation can lead to recovery over a week or so. Eventually, however, chronic inhibition of prostaglandin synthesis may reduce mucosal cytoprotection (see p. 507) enough that severe damage occurs. Although the prostaglandin analog misoprostol (Cytotec) was recently approved for prevention of gastric ulcers in high-risk patients taking NSAIDs (see p. 226), the rationale for its use has been questioned.[9] H_2-receptor antagonists, which are effective treatment for established gastric ulceration, have been relatively ineffective as prophylactic agents; the reason is unclear. It is likely that aspirin-induced bleeding is aggravated by its effect on platelet aggregation. After prolonged therapy, intestinal inflammation may also develop.

Reyes syndrome. Reyes syndrome is primarily a childhood illness, with a death rate of about 25%, that develops after apparent recovery from influenza or chicken pox. It is characterized by vomiting, liver abnormalities, and encephalopathy progressing from drowsiness to combative behavior and delirium to coma. Nearly all victims had received salicylates for management of the viral illness. Early "case-control" studies that indicated an association between salicylate use and Reyes syndrome were criticized on a number of grounds, but a subsequent study by the Centers for Disease Control[11] also supported a link between salicylate use and the disease. Since there is no evidence of an association between acetaminophen and Reyes syndrome, it would appear prudent, if an analgesic-antipyretic is needed, to use acetaminophen in acute viral illness in children.

Miscellaneous side effects. Prostaglandins become important for maintenance of renal function in many situations, including congestive heart failure, cirrhosis with ascites, nephrotic syndrome, and dehydration. Acute renal failure may then develop if NSAIDs are administered; recent evidence indicates that the elderly and patients with coronary artery disease exhibit increased risk, at least with ibuprofen.[14] NSAIDs can also promote fluid and electrolyte retention and may interfere with diuretic and antihypertensive therapy. By inhibiting prostaglandin-mediated renin release, they can cause a hyporenin-hypoaldosterone syndrome, manifesting as hyperkalemia. Long-term excessive use of oral analgesic mixtures can also cause renal damage (see p. 366).

Anti-inflammatory therapy with aspirin, especially if the plasma salicylate concentration exceeds 250 μg/ml, may be associated with reversible elevations in plasma aminotransferases (transaminases). Young females with rheumatoid arthritis, systemic lupus erythematosus, or other connective tissue disorders have been most commonly affected.[17]

Salicylates uncouple oxidative phosphorylation. This accounts for the hyperthermia that develops during intoxication. Disturbances in acid-base balance are discussed on p. 365. Hearing loss and tinnitus (ringing in the ears) are common in patients taking anti-inflammatory dosages of salicylates. Displacement of bilirubin from albumin by high concentrations of salicylates may contribute to kernicterus in neonates. Interference with thyroid function is more apparent than real. Salicylates interfere with binding of thyroxin to plasma proteins and alter certain tests of thyroid function.

Pharmacokinetics

Absorption

Aspirin, a weak acid with a pK_a of 3.5, is rapidly absorbed from the upper gastrointestinal tract. Dissolution of tablets, which is favored by higher pH, is the rate-limiting step. Dosage forms in which aspirin is already dissolved (for example, an effervescent preparation) speed absorption. Buffered tablets undergo more rapid dissolution, but the buffering neither prevents gastric irritation nor significantly enhances effectiveness. Several preparations (enteric coated or timed release, magnesium or choline salicylates, and salsalate[18]) have been developed in attempts to minimize irritation.

Once aspirin is dissolved, nonionized molecules diffuse into mucosal cells where the equilibrium is shifted in favor of the ionized moiety (Fig. 35-2). Although aspirin is absorbed from the stomach, more is absorbed in the duodenum and upper small intestine, despite the higher pH, because of greater surface area. Thus faster gastric emptying hastens its absorption.

Distribution

Approximately 85% to 95% of salicylate in plasma is bound to protein, primarily to albumin. The unbound fraction passively distributes throughout body fluids. Aspirin and salicylate, its metabolite, are found in saliva and in cerebrospinal, peritoneal, and synovial fluids. Salicylic acid crosses the placental barrier to reach the developing fetus and can be ingested during breast feeding.

Metabolism

Aspirin is rapidly deacetylated to pharmacologically active salicylic acid. The half-life of aspirin in plasma is only 15 to 20 minutes. Salicylic acid is then oxidized to

FIG. 35-2 *Absorption of aspirin from the stomach.* During absorption *the concentration of uncharged aspirin* (HA) *in gastric juice is greater that that in mucosal cells; the specific values given below (100 units and 1 unit, respectively) were arbitrarily assigned for illustrative purposes.*

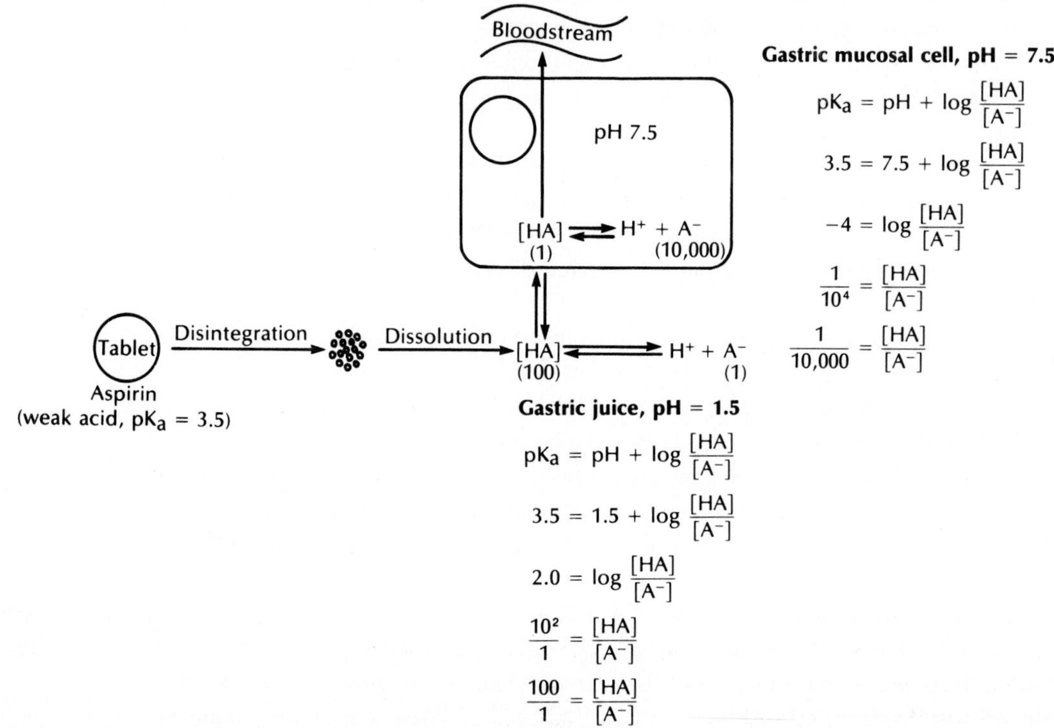

gentisic acid and conjugated with glycine to form salicyluric acid and with glucuronide to form ester and ether conjugates (Fig. 35-3). Of salicylate, 90% (after an aspirin dose of 300 mg) to 50% (after 3 g of aspirin) is excreted as salicyluric acid. The half-life of salicylate (3 to 6 hours with acute administration) increases to a range of 15 to 30 hours after chronic administration of the amounts needed to manage arthritis. The prolonged half-life results from saturation of the enzymes for conjugation of salicylate with glycine and glucuronide (ether formation). Saturation becomes important with daily dosages exceeding 2.5 to 3 g of aspirin in adults and contributes to salicylate intoxication during therapeutic administration to children.

EXCRETION

Salicylates are excreted mainly by the kidney. Clearance is increased approximately fourfold when the pH of urine is ≥8.0. At this pH, salicylate is highly ionized and cannot readily diffuse from the tubular fluid. A high rate of urine flow also decreases reabsorption; oliguria increases reabsorption. The glucuronide conjugates of salicylic and gentisic acids do not readily backdiffuse from the tubules regardless of urinary pH.

DOSAGE

The usual analgesic or antipyretic dose of aspirin is 650 mg (range 325 mg to 1 g) for adults and about 10 mg/kg for children, every 4 to 6 hours (Table 35-1). Single doses are not anti-inflammatory. When adults take 4 to 6 g daily, however, salicylate accumulates, and its plasma concentration and half-life increase, for reasons discussed above; the anti-inflammatory effect is achieved when its concentration is 150 to 250 μg/ml. With anti-inflammatory regimens, a change in dosage causes a relatively

FIG. 35-3 *Salicylate metabolism.* SAG, *Salicyl acyl glucuronide;* SPG, *salicyl phenolic glucuronide;* SU, *salicyluric acid;* GA, *gentisic acid;* GU, *gentisuric acid.*

From Needs CH, Brooks PM: Clin Pharmacokinet 10:164, 1985.

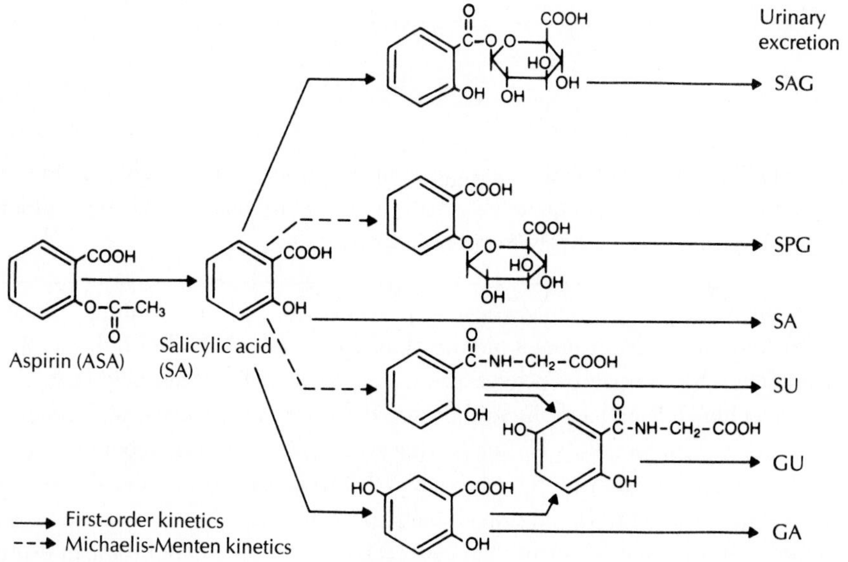

Urinary excretion

COOH
C-O O
HO
OH OH OH → SAG

COOH
COOH
O O
HO
OH OH → SPG

COOH
O-C-CH$_3$
O
Aspirin (ASA)

COOH
OH
Salicylic acid (SA) → SA

O
C-NH-CH$_2$-COOH
OH → SU

O
HO C-NH-CH$_2$-COOH
OH → GU

HO COOH
OH → GA

→ First-order kinetics
--→ Michaelis-Menten kinetics

TABLE 35-1 Dosages, dosage forms, and indications for NSAIDS and other analgesics

Drug	Usual single dose* (mg)	Usual daily dose range† (mg)	Dosage interval (hours)	Dosage forms‡ (mg)	Approved indications§ AN	AP	RA	OA	AS	PS	Dys	GA	MI
Aspirin‖	650	4000-6000	4	C: 325,500; CT: 81; T: 65-975; R: 60-1200	x	x	x	x	x	x	x		x
Diflunisal	500	500-1000	12	T: 250,500	x		x	x					
Acetaminophen‖¶	650		4-6	C: 500; CT: 80,160; T:160-650; S: 24-65; R: 120-650	x	x							
Ibuprofen	200	900-2400	6-8	C: 200; T: 200-800; S: 100	x	x	x	x			x		
Naproxen	250	500-750	12	T: 250-500; S: 25	x		x	x	x	x	x	x	
Naproxen sodium	275	550-875	12	T: 275,550	x		x	x	x	x	x	x	
Fenoprofen calcium	200	900-2400	6-8	C: 200-600; T: 600	x		x	x					
Flurbiprofen		200-300	6-12	D: 0.03%; T: 50,100			x	x					
Ketoprofen	25,50	150-300	6-8	C: 50,75	x		x	x			x		
Indomethacin		50-200	8-12	C: 10-75; S: 5; R: 50			x	x	x	x		x	
Sulindac		300-400	12	T: 150,200			x	x	x	x		x	
Tolmetin sodium		1200-1600	6-8	C: 400; T: 200,600			x	x					
Ketorolac tromethamine	15-60		6	I: 15,30/ml	x								
Diclofenac sodium		100-200	6-12	T: 25-75			x	x	x				
Piroxicam		10-20	24	C: 10,20			x	x					
Phenylbutazone		100-600	6-8	C,T: 100			x	x	x			x	
Meclofenamate sodium	50	200-400	6-8	C,T: 50,100	x		x	x					
Mefenamic acid	250		6	C: 250	x						x		
Methotrimeprazine¶	15		4-6	I: 20	x								

*For short-term simple analgesia, antipyresis (adults).
†For chronic anti-inflammatory effect (adults).
‡*C*, Capsule; *CT*, chewable tablet; *D*, drops (for intraoperative miosis); *I*, injection (per ml); *R*, rectal suppository; *S*, suspension, solution, elixir (in 5 ml); *T*, tablet.
§*AN*, Simple analgesia; *AP*, antipyresis; *RA*, rheumatoid arthritis, rheumatic fever; *OA*, osteoarthritis; *AS*, ankylosing spondylitis; *PS*, (acute) painful shoulder; *Dys*, dysmenorrhea; *GA*, (acute) gouty arthritis; *MI*, prophylaxis after myocardial infarction.
‖Children's strength (65 mg) also available.
¶Lacks anti-inflammatory activity.

greater change in steady-state plasma concentration. Accordingly, if the anti-inflammatory effect is inadequate, a small increase in dosage may be sufficient, whereas a large increase is likely to become toxic.

Intoxication

Mild salicylate intoxication (*salicylism*) is characterized by tinnitus, dizziness, headache, and mental confusion, a picture similar to *cinchonism* after quinine. Severe intoxication is characterized by hyperpnea, nausea and vomiting, acid-base disturbances, petechial hemorrhage, hyperthermia, delirium, convulsions, and coma. The lethal dose of aspirin for adults is usually over 10 g. As little as a teaspoonful of methyl salicylate may kill a child. After introduction of "child-proof" bottle caps, the incidence of pediatric intoxication declined dramatically; now the majority of cases are probably iatrogenic. Vomiting and hyperthermia caused by overdosage may be misinterpreted by a parent as manifestations of the original illness and thus evoke still more treatment with aspirin.

Disturbances in acid-base balance are quite complex. Salicylates increase the sensitivity of medullary chemoreceptors to carbon dioxide, and hyperventilation leads to respiratory alkalosis. Enhanced production of carbon dioxide also increases respiratory drive. Respiratory alkalosis is usually present in older children and adults and early in acute intoxication in infants. Secondarily, in infants, in severe acute intoxication in older children, and in chronic intoxication formation of lactic acid and ketone bodies contributes to metabolic acidosis. As intoxication increases, central nervous system depression, respiratory depression, and respiratory acidosis occur. Infants usually arrive at the emergency room in an acidotic state. Sweating, vomiting, hyperpnea, and failure to drink contribute to dehydration.

Treatment includes correction of fluid and electrolyte disturbances, replacement of K^+, and glucose administration. The severity of acute intoxication can be predicted with the Done nomogram[5] if serum salicylate concentration is known at a given time after ingestion. Correction of acidosis has two beneficial consequences: more salicylate is ionized in plasma so that it less readily enters the brain, and, if sufficient bicarbonate can be given to alkalinize the urine, elimination is enhanced. Although dialysis is efficient, a forced diuresis along with urine alkalinization can greatly shorten the period of dangerous intoxication. Other measures are directed toward removal of residual salicylate from the stomach (lavage or emesis followed by activated charcoal) and counteracting hyperthermia by physical methods (sponging with tepid water, cooling blanket).

ACETAMINOPHEN

Acetaminophen is a metabolic product of phenacetin (acetophenetidin). It lacks anti-inflammatory, antirheumatic, or uric acid excretory effects. The drug is equipotent to aspirin as an antipyretic or for simple analgesia, and it can be especially useful in patients (1) with peptic ulcer, (2) with gout who are taking a uricosuric agent, (3) taking oral anticoagulants, (4) with clotting disorders, (5) at risk of Reyes syndrome. In patients intolerant to aspirin there is a small chance of cross-intolerance to acetaminophen. Like salicylates, acetaminophen acts centrally to reduce fever. The mechanism of its analgesic action is unclear. Acetaminophen is available in a wide variety of over-the-counter and prescription combinations.

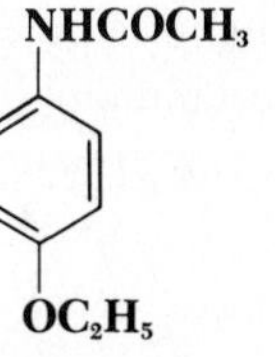

$NHCOCH_3$ — benzene ring — OC_2H_5

Phenacetin

$NHCOCH_3$ — benzene ring — OH

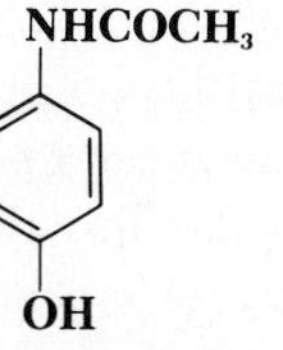

Acetaminophen

Acute intoxication and metabolism

Partially because of concern with salicylate toxicity, use of acetaminophen, especially in England, increased greatly in the mid-1960s. Liver damage from acetaminophen intoxication, virtually unknown before, then became apparent. Necrosis is localized to hepatocytes in the centrilobular region. These cells contain the highest activity of the cytochrome P-450 mixed-function oxidase system. At recommended doses acetaminophen is conjugated to glucuronide (especially in adults) and sulfate (especially in children). A small percentage is oxidized to a toxic metabolite (Fig. 35-4), most likely *N*-acetyl-*p*-benzoquinoneimine, that is normally inactivated by conjugation with glutathione. However, when the dose of acetaminophen is above about 10 g, the enzymes catalyzing conjugation become saturated, and a greater proportion of drug is converted to the reactive metabolite. Hepatic damage results when glutathione stores are depleted. A similar mechanism may also damage the kidney. Hepatic necrosis is likely if the plasma concentration of drug exceeds, respectively, 200 and 50 µg/ml at 4 and 12 hours after ingestion.[21] Evacuation of the stomach is followed by immediate treatment (within 24 hours, but optimally within 8 hours) with a substance that enhances glutathione synthesis or otherwise mimics its beneficial effect. The current choice in the United States is *N*-acetylcysteine (Mucomyst, Mucosol) by mouth, diluted in a soft drink or fruit juice, 140 mg/kg as a loading dose; therapy is continued with 70 mg/kg every 4 hours for 17 doses if the plasma acetaminophen concentration indicates potential for necrosis. Charcoal, which will adsorb acetylcysteine, is not used in this regimen, but it can be used if the acetylcysteine is administered intravenously. Acetaminophen is the most commonly reported cause of single-drug intoxication in the United States in children under 6 years of age, but, fortunately, children appear less susceptible to liver damage, even with plasma concentrations in the range toxic to older victims. In contrast, alcoholics taking therapeutic doses of acetaminophen may exhibit hepatic toxicity.

Chronic renal damage

Some people self-medicate chronically with NSAIDs for pain relief or other indications. In particular, combinations of aspirin, phenacetin, and caffeine (APC tablets) were once used excessively. Chronic toxicity begins as medullary ischemia, leading to papillary necrosis followed by chronic interstitial nephritis and ultimately to renal failure. Although phenacetin, initially believed responsible, was replaced by acetaminophen in the United States and several other countries, the use of such drugs in combinations appears to be the most dangerous. The mechanism may be similar, except for the time frame, to that responsible for acute liver damage: aspirin-induced reduction in glutathione availability (due to impaired prostaglandin formation and decreased renal blood flow) permits an acetaminophen metabolite to damage tubular cells.[24] The possibility that long-term use of acetaminophen alone is a risk factor was suggested by a recent case-control study.[19] The prognosis is perhaps best if all analgesics are discontinued, rather than any single one. Chronic analgesic abuse may also promote development of uroepithelial tumors, most commonly transitional cell carcinoma.

PROPIONIC ACID DERIVATIVES

These NSAIDs (Table 35-1), introduced into therapy since 1975, present an improvement in safety over aspirin, indomethacin, and phenylbutazone. In general gastrointestinal distress is not so likely to be a problem. Acute intoxication is less of a

Metabolism of acetaminophen. *FIG. 35-4*

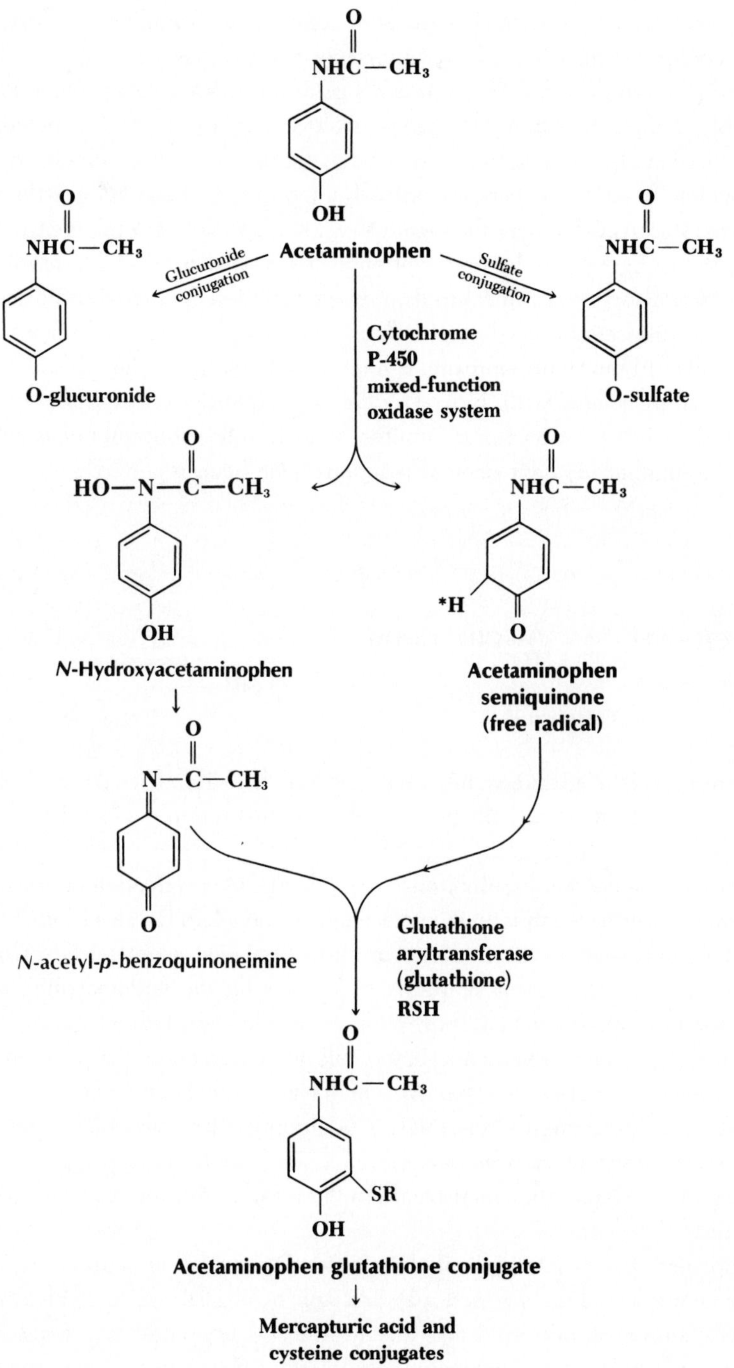

Acetaminophen

Glucuronide conjugation → **O-glucuronide**

Sulfate conjugation → **O-sulfate**

Cytochrome P-450 mixed-function oxidase system

***N*-Hydroxyacetaminophen**

Acetaminophen semiquinone (free radical)

*H

***N*-acetyl-*p*-benzoquinoneimine**

Glutathione aryltransferase (glutathione) RSH

Acetaminophen glutathione conjugate

↓

Mercapturic acid and cysteine conjugates

hazard than with aspirin and acetaminophen.[22] Unfortunately, newer agents are usually considerably more expensive than aspirin and acetaminophen, an important consideration in treatment of chronic diseases.

The propionic acid derivatives are *chiral* compounds. Naproxen is marketed in the active *S* configuration, whereas the others are available as racemates. In humans a significant proportion of the *R*-enantiomers of ibuprofen and fenoprofen is converted irreversibly to the active configuration; possible sites of this *inversion* include the gut, liver, and kidney. In contrast, inversion of flurbiprofen and ketoprofen is unimportant.

Ibuprofen is useful in patients with dysmenorrhea, rheumatoid arthritis, or osteoarthritis. It is available over the counter in 200 mg tablets or caplets (Advil, Nuprin, others) as an analgesic and by prescription as a suspension for children with fever or arthritis. After a survey of clinical trials, it was concluded that variability was such that no statistical differences in adverse effects could be demonstrated among six of the newer agents.[3] Ibuprofen, naproxen, fenoprofen, tolmetin, sulindac, and meclofenamate were all associated with, in roughly descending order of frequency: gastrointestinal disturbances > headache ≥ tinnitus = rash. Since ibuprofen was released for OTC use, a number of anaphylactoid reactions have been reported.

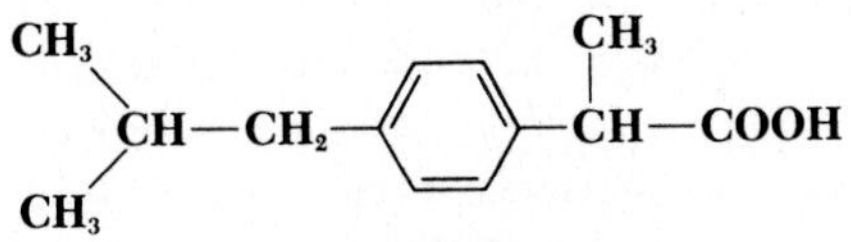

Ibuprofen

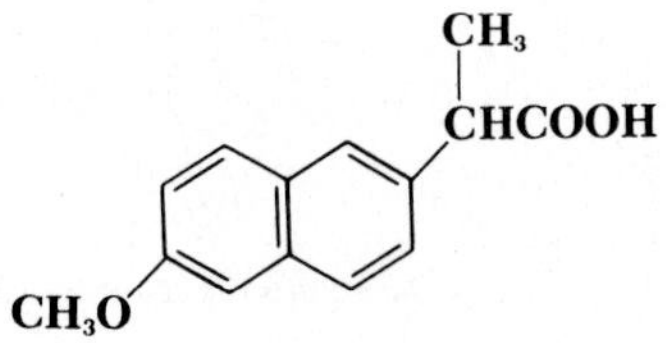

Naproxen

Naproxen has the advantage of a relatively long half-life; twice daily administration is sufficient for chronic antiarthritic therapy. Administration every 8 hours is recommended for acute relief of gouty arthritis.

Primary dysmenorrhea results from excessive uterine production of prostaglandins, which causes uterine contractions and ischemia and can also reach other organs to induce symptoms such as diarrhea and vomiting. Oral contraceptives (see Chapter 48), which decrease prostaglandin synthesis by actions on the endometrium, are highly effective therapy provided that conception is not desired. Otherwise, naproxen and ibuprofen appear as effective as and better tolerated than other NSAIDs, and they are consistently more effective than aspirin, which has usually been no better than placebo in clinical trials. Treatment with NSAIDs beginning a few days before menstruation may be most effective. However, if there is any likelihood of pregnancy the drug should be administered after menstrual flow has begun to avoid exposure of a developing fetus.

Fenoprofen has been implicated in several cases of interstitial nephritis and nephrotic syndrome. **Flurbiprofen** was first approved as drops to reduce intraoperative miosis; **suprofen,** also used topically for miosis, was withdrawn for systemic use after many reports of acute flank pain, perhaps related to uric acid deposition in renal tubules.

ACETIC ACID DERIVATIVES

Indomethacin

In many experimental studies, indomethacin has been used as the prototypic NSAID. In treatment of arthritis, adverse effects are more common than with many newer agents and include gastrointestinal symptoms, blood dyscrasias,[12] and acute renal failure. Associated with its relative lipophilicity is a greater incidence of headache and other central nervous effects. Indomethacin is now the drug most often used to relieve acute gouty attacks.

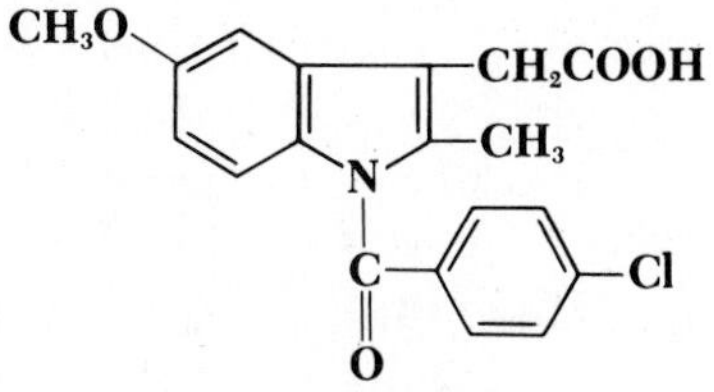

Indomethacin

PATENT DUCTUS ARTERIOSUS

The ductus arteriosus is the distal segment of the left sixth aortic arch, which connects the pulmonary artery to the descending aorta so that blood can bypass the lungs in the developing fetus. Its patency is favored by low oxygen tension and prostaglandin E_2 (see Chapter 25). This vessel normally constricts during the first day of life. However, it may remain patent after birth, especially in premature infants of low body weight. Although surgical closure is an established therapy, cyclooxygenase inhibitors can also be effective. Indomethacin, given after patent ductus arteriosus has become evident, promotes closure and alleviates the associated symptoms of cardiac failure in the neonate.[6] Sensitivity to indomethacin decreases with time after birth. Transient renal insufficiency, fluid retention, and bleeding are relatively common adverse effects.

Sulindac

Sulindac is a sulfoxide that has some structural similarity to indomethacin with similar anti-inflammatory properties but perhaps less renal toxicity. There have been reports of elevated plasma aminotransaminase concentrations and other indications of liver damage, with some deaths, in patients, usually women, taking sulindac.[17] Sulindac itself is an inactive *prodrug* that is oxidized irreversibly to an inactive sulfone and reduced reversibly to an anti-inflammatory sulfide.

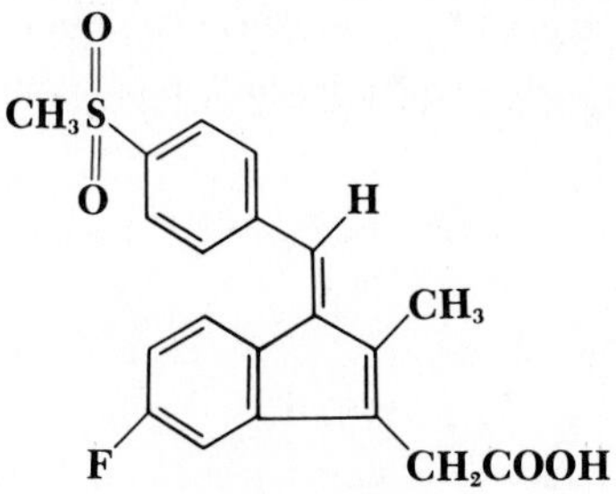

Sulindac sulfone (inactive) 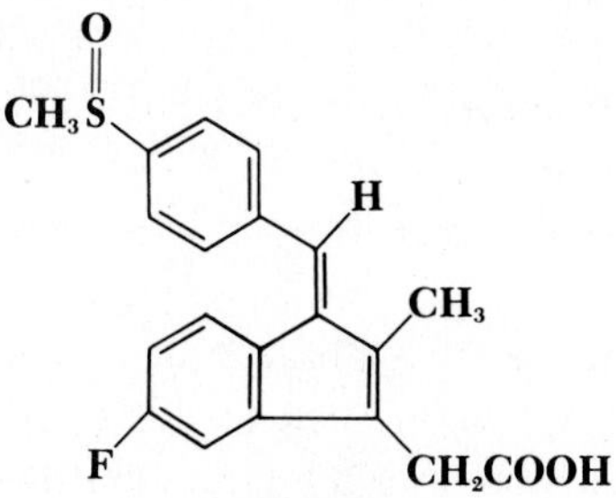 **Sulindac (inactive)** 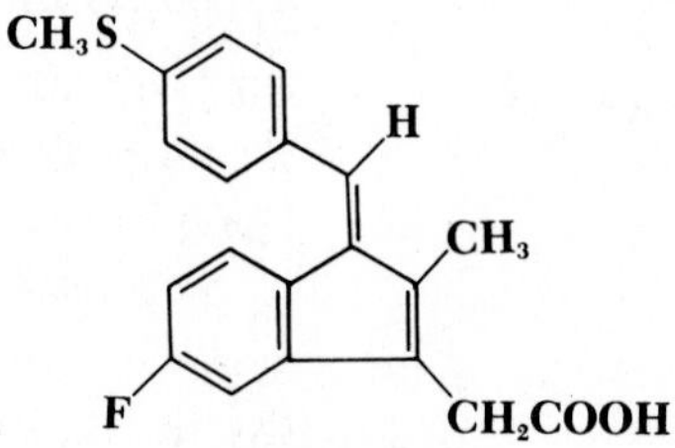 **Sulindac sulfide (active)**

Tolmetin and ketorolac

Tolmetin differs structurally from the propionic acid derivatives but is similar pharmacologically. Aside from aspirin, it and naproxen are the only drugs approved for therapy of juvenile rheumatoid arthritis. Several anaphylactoid reactions to this agent have been reported.

A structurally related agent, **ketorolac,** is the most recently introduced NSAID. At present it is given by intramuscular injection to relieve postoperative pain; unlike other NSAIDs it has been at least as effective as opioid analgesics in several clinical trials.

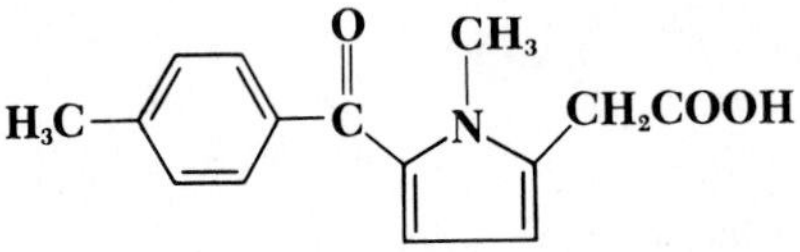

H_3C O CH_3 CH_2COOH C N

Tolmetin

O C N COOH

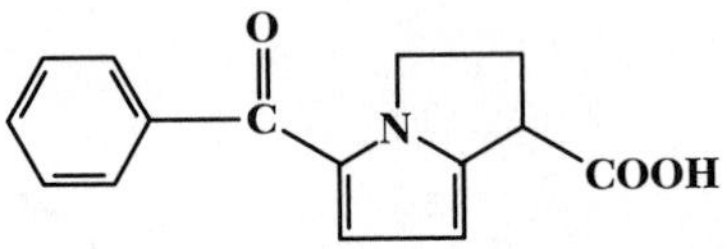

Ketorolac

Diclofenac sodium

Although not approved for use in the United States until 1988, diclofenac has been available elsewhere since 1974 and is perhaps the most widely used prescription NSAID in Europe. In addition to inhibiting cyclooxygenase, high doses may reduce formation of lipoxygenase products by altering availability of the precursor, arachidonate. The side effect profile of this drug is similar to that of NSAIDs in general. Withdrawal because of adverse reactions is relatively uncommon, even in elderly patients.[23] However, use of diclofenac may be associated with some increased risk of aplastic anemia[12] or impaired liver function[17]; periodic tests of hepatic function are recommended.

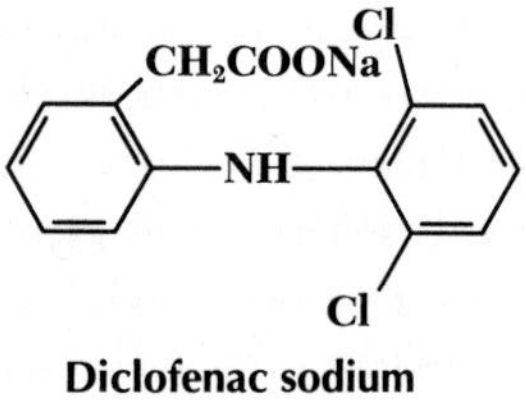

Cl CH_2COONa NH Cl

Diclofenac sodium

PIROXICAM

Piroxicam has a long half-life and can be taken once a day. It can cause cutaneous reactions including photosensitivity. The risk of gastrointestinal bleeding and ulceration with piroxicam is less than that with aspirin.

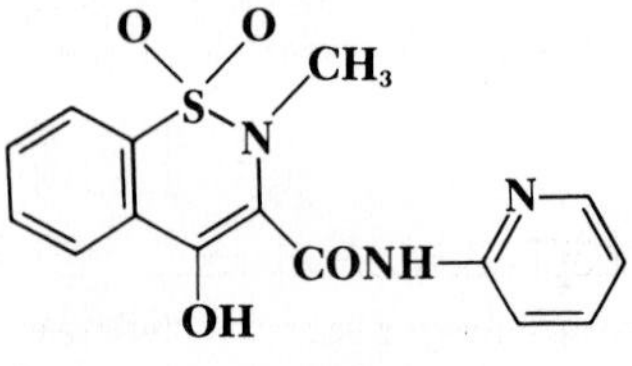

O O CH_3 S N N CONH OH

Piroxicam

MISCELLANEOUS AGENTS

Phenylbutazone

The only pyrazolone still used as an anti-inflammatory drug is phenylbutazone. It is intermediate in effectiveness for treatment of rheumatoid arthritis, ankylosing spondylitis, and osteoarthritis between salicylates and anti-inflammatory steroids. The drug has largely been replaced by less toxic agents for acute relief of gouty arthritis. Although uricosuric, it is not used for this effect.

Phenylbutazone is metabolized to two active compounds. Oxyphenbutazone has activity and toxicity similar to those of the parent compound. The other product is strongly uricosuric and is similar to sulfinpyrazone (Chapter 53).

Phenylbutazone should be used only when safer medications do not suffice. Some toxicity may appear in 25% of patients receiving the drug. These include Na^+ and water retention, visual disturbances, gastrointestinal symptoms, generalized hypersensitivity reactions that are unrelated to aspirin intolerance, bone marrow depression,[12] liver damage,[17] and acute renal failure. When this drug is used, particularly in the elderly, patients should be closely monitored for indications of toxicity.

Fenamates

Mefenamic acid is not more effective than aspirin and may produce serious adverse effects such as diarrhea, gastrointestinal bleeding, and impairment of renal function. **Meclofenamate sodium,** the most recent derivative of this class, is approved for analgesia and chronic management of arthritis. Colitis and diarrhea may develop after formation of a metabolite that is toxic to the colon.

Methotrimeprazine

This phenothiazine derivative is a novel nonaddictive and non-anti-inflammatory analgesic. It is approximately equivalent to 10 mg of morphine by the intramuscular route. Special advantages claimed for methotrimeprazine are an antiemetic action and a lack of respiratory-depressant action. On the other hand, pronounced sedation and possible orthostatic hypotension limit its use to hospitalized patients.

MISCELLANEOUS DRUGS USED IN RHEUMATIC DISEASES

In addition to the NSAIDs, several other agents are used to treat rheumatic diseases[8]; their mechanisms of action are often unknown. Gold salts are discussed briefly below. Sulfasalazine is discussed on p. 515. Adrenal corticosteroids, the antimalarial hydroxychloroquine, cyclophosphamide and methotrexate, azathioprine, and penicillamine are discussed in Chapters 47, 65, 67, 68, and 69, respectively. The benefit from such drugs, which are often grouped as *second-line, disease-modifying* or *remittive* agents, develops slowly over weeks or months and may occasionally be associated with periods of remission. However, compliance may be poor, and evidence is lacking for long-term improvement.[16] It has been argued recently (1) that a common sequence of treatment, from NSAIDs to second-line drugs to steroids, may inadequately control inflammation and (2) that in severe cases a better long-term outcome could be achieved by early therapy with steroids in combination with multiple second-line compounds, followed by gradual discontinuation of individual agents until control is maintained with a single second-line drug.[25]

Gold salts such as **aurothioglucose** (Solganal) and **gold sodium thiomalate** (Myochrysine) are given initially at weekly intervals (progressively from 10 to 50 mg) by intramuscular injection. Ultimately, monthly doses may be optimal to avoid reappearance of symptoms. In one series of over 1000 patients given the latter drug, therapy was discontinued in about 38% within the first 2 years because of toxicity, most frequently rash, pruritus, or buccal irritation.[13] An oral preparation of gold, **auranofin** (Ridaura), which is taken once or twice daily, is also available. Diarrhea is common; other side effects include abdominal cramping and anemia.

REFERENCES

1. Abramson SB, Cherksey B, Gude D, et al: Nonsteroidal antiinflammatory drugs exert differential effects on neutrophil function and plasma membrane viscosity: studies in human neutrophils and liposomes, *Inflammation* 14:11, 1990
2. Clark WG: Antipyretics. In Mackowiak PA, editor: *Fever: basic mechanisms and management*, New York, 1991, Raven Press, p 297.
3. Coles LS, Fries JF, Kraines RG, Roth SH: From experiment to experience: side effects of nonsteroidal anti-inflammatory drugs, *Am J Med* 74:820, 1983.
4. Dawson W: Theories of mechanism of action of anti-inflammatory compounds. In Williamson WRN, editor: *Anti-inflammatory compounds*, New York, 1987, Marcel Dekker, p 109.
5. Done AK: Aspirin overdosage: incidence, diagnosis, and management, *Pediatrics* 62(5, suppl):890, 1978.
6. Douidar SM, Richardson J, Snodgrass WR: Role of indomethacin in ductus closure: an update evaluation, *Dev Pharmacol Ther* 11:196, 1988.
7. Fries JF, Miller SR, Spitz PW, et al: Toward an epidemiology of gastropathy associated with nonsteroidal antiinflammatory drug use, *Gastroenterology* 96:647, 1989.
8. Furst DE: Rational use of disease-modifying antirheumatic drugs, *Drugs* 39:19, 1990.
9. Hadler NM: There's the forest: the object lesson of NSAID "gastropathy," *J Rheumatol* 17:280, 1990.
10. Higgs GA, Salmon JA, Henderson B, Vane JR: Pharmacokinetics of aspirin and salicylate in relation to inhibition of arachidonate cyclooxygenase and antiinflammatory activity, *Proc Natl Acad Sci USA* 84:1417, 1987.
11. Hurwitz ES, Barrett MJ, Bregman D, et al: Public Health Service study of Reye's syndrome and medications. Report of the main study, *JAMA* 257:1905, 1987.
12. International Agranulocytosis and Aplastic Anemia Study: Risks of agranulocytosis and aplastic anemia: a first report of their relation to drug use with special reference to analgesics, *JAMA* 256;1749, 1986.
13. Lockie LM, Smith DM: Forty-seven years experience with gold therapy in 1,019 rheumatoid arthritis patients, *Semin Arthritis Rheum* 14:238, 1985.
14. Murray MD, Brater DC, Tierney WM, et al: Ibuprofen-associated renal impairment in a large general internal medicine practice, *Am J Med Sci* 299:222, 1990.
15. Pedersen AK, FitzGerald GA: Dose-related kinetics of aspirin: presystemic acetylation of platelet cyclooxygenase, *N Engl J Med* 311:1206, 1984.
16. Pincus T: Rheumatoid arthritis: disappointing long-term outcomes despite successful short-term clinical trials, *J Clin Epidemiol* 41:1037, 1988.
17. Prescott LF: Effects of non-narcotic analgesics on the liver, *Drugs* 32 (suppl 4):129, 1986.
18. Roth S, Bennett R, Caldron P, et al: Reduced risk of NSAID gastropathy (GI mucosal toxicity) with nonacetylated salicylate (salsalate): an endoscopic study, *Semin Arthritis Rheum* 19(4, suppl 2):11, 1990.
19. Sandler DP, Smith JC, Weinberg CR, et al: Analgesic use and chronic renal disease, *N Engl J Med* 320:1238, 1989.
20. Settipane GA: Aspirin and allergic diseases: a review, *Am J Med*, 74(6A):102, 1983.
21. Smilkstein MJ, Knapp GL, Kulig KW, and Rumack BH: Efficacy of oral *N*-acetylcysteine in the treatment of acetaminophen overdose: analysis of the National Multicenter Study (1976 to 1985), *N Engl J Med* 319:1557, 1988.

22. Smolinske SC, Hall AH, Vandenberg SA, et al: Toxic effects of nonsteroidal anti-inflammatory drugs in overdose: an overview of recent evidence on clinical effects and dose-response relationships, *Drug Safety* 5:252, 1990.
23. Todd PA, Sorkin EM: Diclofenac sodium: a reappraisal of its pharmacodynamic and pharmacokinetic properties, and therapeutic efficacy, *Drugs* 35:244, 1988.
24. Walker RJ, Duggin GG: Drug nephrotoxicity, *Annu Rev Pharmacol Toxicol* 28:331, 1988.
25. Wilske KR, Healey LA: Remodeling the pyramid—a concept whose time has come, *J Rheumatol* 16:565, 1989.

section six

Anesthetics

Chapter 36

Pharmacology of general anesthesia

GENERAL CONCEPT

The scope of anesthesiology touches nearly every specialty of medicine. Drugs that allow painless, controlled surgical, obstetric, and diagnostic procedures constitute a cornerstone of modern therapy. It is estimated that 25 million anesthetics are administered annually in the United States alone.

The hallmark of anesthetic drugs is *controllability*; needed features are rapid onset and recovery and the ability to titrate effects. For this reason, most of the potent anesthetics are short-acting parenteral agents, gases, or vapors. The latter two can be administered through the lungs with rapid uptake into the systemic circulation. Elimination of these drugs is also primarily by the pulmonary route. Unlike nonvolatile drugs, elimination and termination of pharmacologic activity do not depend on hepatic biotransformation or renal excretion but rather on the rate and depth of respiration, which can be actively controlled by the anesthesiologist. The large surface area of the lungs provides a means of precise dosage administration or elimination.

Inhalation anesthetics are nonspecific in that they do not function by interacting with specific receptors. As a corollary to this generalization, there are no specific antagonists to anesthetics. Inhalation anesthetics should produce all the following effects (though there may be quantitative differences among various drugs): (1) hypnosis, (2) analgesia, (3) skeletal muscle relaxation, and (4) reduction of certain autonomic reflexes. General anesthesia is characterized by these four attributes.

Selection of a particular anesthetic or combination of anesthetics is determined by the patient's pathophysiologic state and the nature of the anticipated surgical procedure. Anesthetics differ in their abilities to depress various organ systems. They also differ in potency, in speed of induction and awakening, and in degree of skeletal muscle relaxation; thus one anesthetic may be superior to another depending on the clinical circumstances. Final selection of an anesthetic or anesthetic sequence is based on three factors, in the following order: (1) those drugs and anesthetic techniques judged safest for the patient, (2) drugs and techniques that facilitate performance of the surgical procedure, and (3) techniques most acceptable to the patient. The last factor is generally a judgment between general and regional (for example, spinal) anesthesia.

Popular potent organohalogen inhalation anesthetics include enflurane, isoflurane, and halothane. Sevoflurane and desflurane are new halogenated anesthetics soon to be introduced into clinical practice. Nitrous oxide, a weak gaseous anesthetic, is frequently used in combination with these volatile compounds or with intermittent doses of intravenous drugs such as barbiturates (for hypnosis), opioids (for analgesia), and neuromuscular blockers (for skeletal muscle relaxation). The older anesthetics cyclopropane and diethyl ether are rarely used because of their flammability; they are incompatible with the cautery and electronic monitoring equipment of modern operating suites.

Intravenous anesthetics are used for specific purposes or to supplement inhalation anesthetics, but they lack some of the controllability and other salutary features of the inhalation anesthetics. Thus they are generally ancillary drugs. Thiobarbiturates such as thiopental are still the preferred induction agents because they produce hypnosis rapidly and pleasantly. Lack of analgesic or muscle-relaxant properties and slow elimination limit both usefulness and dosage. Propofol is a new drug that produces rapid, pleasant induction and rapid awakening. Benzodiazepines, primarily midazolam (see p. 270), are also used occasionally for induction.[8] Opioids such as morphine and the more rapidly eliminated fentanyl are frequently used to supplement nitrous oxide anesthesia. The sobriquet *dissociative anesthesia* describes the effect of the drug ketamine, which is related to phencyclidine. This drug has limited scope, however, as it does not allow for other than superficial procedures and can produce worrisome side effects, including abnormal psychic reactions.

POTENCY AND EFFICACY

Because volatile and gaseous anesthetics distribute and reach equilibrium in various body compartments by virtue of their partial pressures, it is convenient to establish potency in terms of partial pressure rather than the more conventional ED_{50}. Equilibrium is defined as the state in which net transfer of anesthetic is zero, that is, the partial pressure of an anesthetic in the alveoli and blood equals that in tissues. The *minimum alveolar concentration* (MAC) is defined as *that concentration of anesthetic (in v/v percent or mm Hg) measured in end-tidal gas that prevents response to a standard painful stimulus in 50% of humans or test animals.*[11] In the clinical setting, anesthetics are usually given in multiples of MAC (1.5 to 2.5 × MAC). Several factors change MAC. These include circadian rhythm, body temperature (direct proportional decrease), age (direct proportional decrease), and other drugs (sedatives, hypnotics, anesthetics, and other central nervous system depressants decrease MAC; excitants such as cocaine increase MAC). Factors that do *not* influence MAC include sex, species, state of oxygenation, acid-base changes, and arterial blood pressure. A response to a painful stimulus is different from awareness; "MAC aware" is a measure of awareness. At this partial pressure of anesthetic, 50% of subjects are aware; 50% are not. "MAC aware" is generally about 40% of the MAC value of any anesthetic.

SOLUBILITY

The object of inhalation anesthesia is to attain a concentration (partial pressure) of drug in the brain sufficient to produce the desired degree of anesthesia. To achieve this goal, molecules of anesthetic must pass from the lungs through several biophases. Anesthetic gases and vapors are soluble in blood, tissue fluids, and tissues and are quite lipophilic. Various tissues and fluids differ in their lipid content; nevertheless, any particular gas or vapor, depending on its lipid solubility, will eventually reach partial pressure equilibrium at different concentrations in the various biophases. Table 36-1 illustrates this concept with a hypothetical inhalation anesthetic at partial pres-

TABLE 36-1 Distribution of inhalation anesthetic concentrations in various biophases after partial pressure equilibrium

	Biophase		
Anesthetic	Blood	Lean tissue	Fat
Concentration at equilibrium	3mM ⇄	6 mM ⇄	660 mM
Partial pressure at equilibrium	8 mm Hg ⇄	8 mm Hg ⇄	8 mm Hg

sure equilibrium for a given inspired concentration. Notice that although the partial pressure of the anesthetic is the same in all phases, the concentrations in those tissues differ over a hundredfold. This is attributable to differences in solubility of the drug in the various tissues. Table 36-1 also illustrates the large capacity of fat for storage of an anesthetic that is highly lipophilic.

There are three solubility coefficients germane to anesthetic distribution. All are based on Henrys law and are temperature dependent. For clinical purposes these coefficients are measured at 37° C.

1. *Blood-gas partition coefficient (λ).* This is the most important solubility parameter for understanding uptake of inhaled gases and vapors. Fig. 36-1 illustrates how this coefficient is derived. Notice in this figure that when equilibrium is reached (right side), the end-tidal concentration of the anesthetic in the alveoli is proportional to the pulmonary blood concentration. Thus end-tidal concentration or partial pressure (abbreviated F_E) can be used as a measure of degree of equilibrium at steady-state. The partial pressure of anesthetics administered via the lungs for uptake by blood is the inspired alveolar partial pressure (F_I). When

$$F_E/F_I = 1$$

blood-gas equilibrium with the inspired gas concentration has been reached.
2. *Tissue solubility.* In the lungs anesthetics enter pulmonary arterial blood and then are distributed to peripheral tissues. Obviously, those organs with the most blood flow per unit time will receive more anesthetic than organs with lower flow. Richly perfused organs include brain, heart, liver, and kidney; skeletal muscle perfusion is intermediate; the lowest perfusion is in bone, ligaments, and fat. The tissue:blood partition coefficient is between 1 and 3 for most anesthetics. Fat is an exception in which anesthetic solubility may exceed solubility in blood several hundredfold. However, as a result of the low blood flow, even though solubility is high, a long time is required before the anesthetic partial pressure in body fat achieves equilibrium with other tissues.
3. *Oil-gas partition coefficient.* This partition coefficient is an artificial one in certain respects because the oil commonly used, olive oil, is not a biologic constituent of the body. However, olive oil has solubility characteristics similar to body fat. The lipid solubility of anesthetics is proportional to potency.[10] This

Schema illustrating derivation of blood-gas partition coefficient (λ). Gas or vapor is inhaled into lungs perfused with pulmonary arterial blood. Anesthetic partial pressure in lungs is high initially and absent in blood, **A**. *Anesthetic molecules diffuse into blood and reach partial pressure equilibrium,* **B**. *Because of partition coefficient, partial pressure equilibrium results in concentration differences in anesthetic. Anesthetic of low blood-gas coefficient will have fewer molecules in blood than in gas phase; high coefficient produces fewer molecules in gas than in blood at equilibrium.* ***FIG. 36-1***

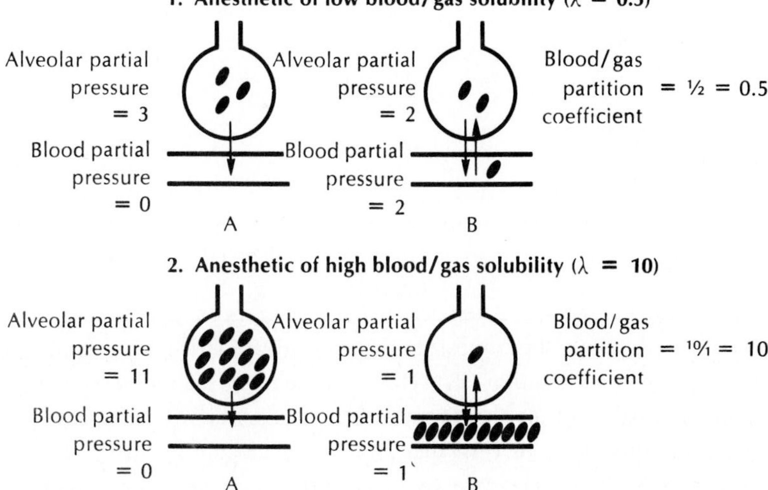

is the basis of the Meyer-Overton correlation, which demonstrates proportionality between fat solubility and anesthetic potency. Thus a high oil-gas partition coefficient indicates a potent anesthetic (that is, one with a low MAC or low partial pressure required for anesthesia). This correlation does not explain the mechanism of anesthesia, but it can be used to predict MAC. In fact, the correlation between MAC and the oil-gas partition of inhalation anesthetics is essentially linear.

Importance of blood-gas partition coefficient to speed of induction. A low λ indicates that the anesthetic's partial pressure in the alveoli will rapidly approach equilibrium with the partial pressure in blood; that is, an F_E/F_I equal to 1 will be approached quickly because such a gas or vapor is relatively insoluble in blood. Thus clinical induction of anesthesia is rapid with such an agent. On the other hand, a high λ correlates with a relatively long interval before blood-gas equilibrium is attained and thus a slower induction. Because of the higher solubility, it takes more time for the blood to take up enough anesthetic to reach the partial pressure required for anesthesia. Blood solubility differentiates inhalation anesthetics into three groups: low solubility (nitrous oxide, desflurane, sevoflurane), medium solubility (isoflurane, enflurane, halothane), and high solubility (methoxyflurane). High-solubility anesthetics are rarely used in current practice because of slow onset and recovery. Table 36-2 lists the MAC and the blood-gas and oil-gas partition coefficients for seven inhalation anesthetics.

TABLE 36-2 MAC and partition coefficients at 37°C for inhalation anesthetics[14]

Anesthetic	Blood/gas coefficient (λ)	Oil/gas coefficient	MAC (%)
Low-solubility			
Desflurane	0.42	18.7	8
Nitrous oxide	0.47	1.4	108
Sevoflurane	0.6	55	2.1
Intermediate-solubility			
Isoflurane	1.4	91	1.2
Enflurane	1.8	97	1.5
Halothane	2.3	220	0.78
High-solubility			
Methoxyflurane	11	950	0.16

MAC, Minimum alveolar concentration.

UPTAKE OF AN ANESTHETIC

Ventilation with an inhaled anesthetic causes a rapid rise in alveolar anesthetic partial pressure or concentration (F_I). However, the *rate* of increase in F_I slows as uptake into pulmonary arterial blood removes the gas or vapor from the lungs. Arterial blood containing anesthetic in turn distributes the anesthetic throughout the body. Uptake of the anesthetic by a specific tissue is a function of anesthetic solubility, blood flow to that tissue, and the arterial blood to tissue anesthetic partial pressure difference. The partial pressure difference is the driving force. When the partial pressure difference becomes zero, equilibrium has been achieved; no further net uptake occurs.[6,9]

Uptake from the lungs, as from any tissue, is directly related to three variables: (1) the blood-gas partition coefficient of the anesthetic, (2) cardiac output ($\dot{Q}$), and (3) the alveolar to venous anesthetic partial pressure difference. The time to equilibrium depends on the non-lung tissue capacity, which is related to the volume and capacity of the tissues concerned. In summary:

$$\text{Uptake} = \lambda \cdot \dot{Q} \cdot (P_A - P_V)/BP$$

where $(P_A - P_V)$ = (Alveolar − Venous partial pressure of anesthetic)
$\dot{Q}$ = Cardiac output
λ = Blood-gas partition coefficient
BP = Barometric pressure

An increase in any of these factors will increase uptake. It is worthwhile noting that if uptake of an anesthetic is plotted graphically, the resulting curve is the inverse of the equilibrium curve (Fig. 36-2). The first *knee* (bend) of the F_E/F_I curve is due to ventilatory effects. The second knee marks the end of uptake by organs with rich perfusion (heart, liver, brain). The rise then slows as skeletal muscle approaches equilibrium.

Equilibration curves for two anesthetics. Notice that the anesthetic with the lower blood-gas partition coefficient approaches equilibration much faster than the anesthetic with the higher coefficient. The anesthetic with the lower solubility in blood will induce a state of anesthesia more rapidly. The arrows indicate the approximate positions of the knees, which are not otherwise obvious from these curves. *FIG. 36-2*

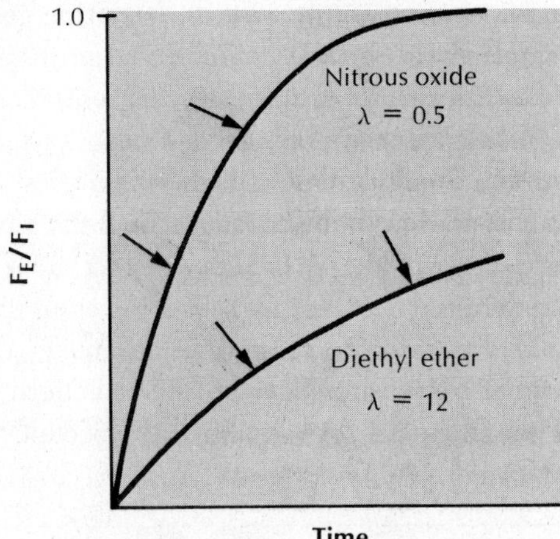

Factors that prevent attainment of equilibrium

There are several variables that prevent or slow attainment of the $F_E/F_I = 1$ state of equilibrium.

1. *Fat solubility*. Hours or even days may be required before body fat, with its poor perfusion but large storage capacity for general anesthetics, achieves equilibrium with alveolar anesthetic partial pressure.
2. *Biotransformation of anesthetics*. Inhalation anesthetics are metabolized by hepatic microsomal enzymes,[22,24,28] but the degree of metabolism is small compared with the overabundance of drug given during the course of anesthesia and has little if any effect on the conduct of anesthesia or dosage requirements of the anesthetic drug. Of more importance, biotransformation may convert certain halogenated anesthetics to metabolites that are toxic to the kidney, the liver, or both.[20,23]
3. *Diffusion through skin or into bowel or other air spaces*. Diffusion of an anesthetic through the skin into the atmosphere is another factor that delays equilibrium. Typical losses include nitrous oxide (F_I = 70%) at 2.5 ml/min/m^2 and halothane (F_I = 0.9%) at 0.006 ml/min/m^2. Anesthetics with a high F_I (nitrous oxide) replace nitrogen in the bowel and other air spaces, such as the middle ear. Since nitrous oxide is more soluble than nitrogen at the same partial pressure, when it passes from a dissolved state in blood into an air space, it expands to a larger volume than the nitrogen it replaces. Thus nitrous oxide anesthesia produces variable increases in bowel volume and can also enlarge a preexisting pneumothorax.

Concentration effect

Basically the *concentration effect*[12] denotes that the higher the inspired concentration of an anesthetic, the faster the rate of rise toward equilibrium. In theory, the equilibrium curves in Fig. 36-2 should be independent of concentration or partial pressure of the anesthetic inspired. In practice, this is not so. High concentrations give a more rapid initial rise toward the equilibrium state than low concentrations. Practically, the concentration effect is seen only with nitrous oxide given in relatively high concentrations. To understand this effect, first imagine an inspired concentration of an anesthetic to be 100% (F_I = 1.0). If this 100% concentration fills the alveoli, regardless of uptake into blood, the end-tidal alveolar concentration will remain 100% (F_E = 1.0) even though total lung volume is reduced. In this circumstance there is rapid uptake of a significant portion of the anesthetic into the blood. To maintain lung volume there is literal sucking of the anesthetic mixture from the reservoir of the anesthesia machine into the lungs. With a high concentration of nitrous oxide (F_I = 0.5 to 0.7), the nitrous oxide sucked from the machine mixes with residual alveolar nitrous oxide to increase the partial pressure of the anesthetic at end-tidal ventilation. This mixing produces a higher F_E than would be expected, and the F_E/F_I ratio approaches 1.0 more quickly.

Second gas effect

Uptake of a large volume of a *first*, or primary, gas given in high concentration (the concentration effect) accelerates the alveolar rate of rise of a *second* gas given simultaneously. The second gas, given in a low concentration, approaches equilibrium faster than if it were given in the absence of the primary, high-concentration gas. Advantage is taken of this phenomenon when nitrous oxide (the primary gas) is given with low concentrations of a potent anesthetic such as halothane or enflurane (F_I = 0.005 to 0.02). The large volume of nitrous oxide sweeps along an increased volume of the second gas and hastens anesthesia.

Effects of ventilation

An increase in minute alveolar ventilation ($\dot{V}_A$) obviously causes a more rapid rise in F_E regardless of partition coefficients because more anesthetic is presented to the alveoli per unit time. However, uptake of anesthetics of high solubility is altered relatively more by changes in ventilation than is uptake of anesthetics of low solubility.[19]

1. *High-solubility anesthetics ($\lambda > 1.0$).* Increasing $\dot{V}_A$ causes a large increase in F_E per unit time. The reason is that the blood has a large capacity for soluble anesthetics. When blood is exposed to more molecules of higher solubility anesthetics, more of these can be absorbed. This increases the partial pressure of the anesthetic in the blood, manifested as an increase in F_E partial pressure.
2. *Low-solubility drugs ($\lambda < 1.0$).* In contrast, an increase in amount of low-solubility anesthetic presented to pulmonary arterial blood per unit time does not increase uptake (or arterial blood partial pressure and F_E) to a great extent. The insoluble anesthetic rapidly reaches equilibrium with blood. Being near saturation because of its low capacity for such drugs, the blood can pick up only a few of the extra molecules presented to it by an increase in $\dot{V}_A$.

The clinical corollary of uptake changes produced by increases in $\dot{V}_A$ are obvious.

Higher solubility anesthetics are taken up more rapidly with forced artificial ventilation, and they may quickly reach dangerous concentrations in tissues. In contrast, it is generally safe to hyperventilate patients with anesthetics of low solubility, since any change in uptake is minimal.

Effects of cardiac output

An increase in cardiac output ($\dot{Q}$) lowers F_E, because there is more pulmonary arterial blood available for uptake of the anesthetic per unit time. One would expect low-solubility anesthetics to be affected to a lesser extent than those with high solubility. Clinical corollaries of these relationships are that (1) depression of cardiac output by an anesthetic can alter its own uptake because the alveolar end-tidal rate of rise (F_E) is rapid with decreased cardiac output and (2) highly soluble anesthetics more rapidly approach equilibrium when cardiac output is depressed. Use of soluble anesthetics in shock can thus excessively depress an already compromised circulation.

In summary, the blood-gas partition coefficient is the most important physical constant determining speed of induction of an inhalation anesthetic. The lower this coefficient, the faster the pulmonary blood reaches equilibrium with a given anesthetic partial pressure and hence the faster the induction of anesthesia. Awakening from anesthesia is similar. The lower the solubility, the faster the awakening as the anesthetic rapidly passes from pulmonary venous blood into alveoli and is exhaled. The concentration and second gas effects can be used to hasten induction with an inhalation anesthetic. Changes in ventilation and cardiac output have opposite effects—increasing ventilation speeds the rise to equilibrium (more prominent with soluble anesthetics), and increased cardiac output delays equilibrium. In clinical practice these factors and physiologic parameters such as ventilation/perfusion inequalities, alterations of regional blood flow, volume status, the degree of circulatory depression, and the pathophysiologic status of the patient must be taken into account during the conduct of general anesthesia.

STAGES AND SIGNS OF ANESTHESIA

With the newer agents depth of anesthesia can be categorized into two stages: (1) the stage of analgesia and delirium and (2) the stage of surgical anesthesia. The latter is divided into light, moderate, and deep. With progressive deepening of surgical anesthesia there are parallel diminutions in ventilation and circulatory integrity. Death from overdosage of potent anesthetics occurs from medullary paralysis and circulatory arrest in the absence of hypoxia. As a general rule, deepening the level of anesthesia with the newer halogenated agents produces the following effects in a dose-dependent fashion:

1. Decreased blood pressure caused by peripheral vasodilatation or a direct decrease in cardiac contractility or both.
2. Decreased alveolar minute ventilation because of reduced tidal volume. (Ventilation becomes more dependent on the diaphragm as anesthesia deepens.)
3. Constriction and centering of the pupils in medium levels of surgical anesthesia that proceeds to pupillary dilatation with onset of deep anesthesia. (Increased lacrimation is observed in light levels of surgical anesthesia, but the eyes are dry during deep anesthesia.)

METHODS OF ADMINISTRATION OF GENERAL ANESTHETICS

The anesthetic gases and vapors are customarily administered through an anesthesia machine, basic components of which include the following:

1. Steel cylinders, containing anesthetic gases and oxygen under pressure, with reduction valves to lower the extremely high pressures in the cylinders to usable pressures.
2. Accurate flowmeters.
3. Calibrated vaporizers. These are containers of a high heat capacity metal such as copper, filled with liquid anesthetic. A sintered bronze disk in the bottom of the vaporizer disperses in-flowing oxygen into small bubbles that vaporize the liquid anesthetic in a precise fashion. Volatile anesthetics such as halothane and enflurane are vaporized to permit administration of precise amounts.
4. A carbon dioxide absorber.
5. A rebreathing bag.
6. Connecting tubing.
7. Unidirectional valves.

Although open-drop and insufflation techniques were used in the past, they are now only of historic interest. Closed and semiclosed systems are used commonly for adult patients; nonrebreathing, nonvalvular systems are used for pediatric patients. A description, including the advantages and disadvantages of these systems, follows:

1. *Closed system*: Economical; prevents excess anesthetics from polluting operating room; conserves heat and respiratory moisture; more difficult to calibrate anesthetic dosage.
2. *Semiclosed system*: Easy to calibrate anesthetic dose; not economical because gases are expelled into the environment; the system loses heat and moisture.
3. *Nonrebreathing, nonvalvular system*: Low resistance highly suitable for pediatric patients; loses heat and contributes to operating room pollution with trace anesthetic concentrations. Despite the term "nonrebreathing," some rebreathing may occur depending on flow rate.

Fig. 36-3 illustrates the schemes of two of these systems. Administration of gases and vapors from the anesthesia machine is accomplished either by face mask or endotracheal tube.

THEORIES OF GENERAL ANESTHESIA

The mechanism or mechanisms by which anesthetics exert their effects is not known. Inhaled anesthetics possess no unique molecular configuration that can be associated with a particular structure-activity relationship. Interaction with cellular components is by means of van der Waals forces only. The anesthetics are nonspecific and can affect the function of all cellular constituents.

Effects of anesthetics have been attributed to blockade of ionic channels and alterations of neurotransmitter release, but these do not correlate well enough with potency to allow a unitary hypothesis of mechanism of action. Of the several proposed mechanisms of anesthesia, three are listed below.

1. *Hydrate hypothesis*: Pauling and Miller postulated that anesthetic molecules form gas hydrates or structured water, which inhibit brain function at crucial

FIG. 36-3 *Schema of,* **A,** *closed anesthesia system and,* **B,** *pediatric valveless system.* **A,** 1, *Vaporizer for volatile liquid anesthetics;* 2, *compressed gas source;* 3, *inhalation unidirectional valve;* 4, *mask;* 5, *unidirectional exhalation valve;* 6, *rebreathing bag; and* 7, *carbon dioxide absorption chamber.* **B,** 1, *vaporizer for volatile liquid anesthetics;* 2, *compressed gas source,* 3, *mask;* 4, *rebreathing bag; and* 5, *gas exhaust port.*

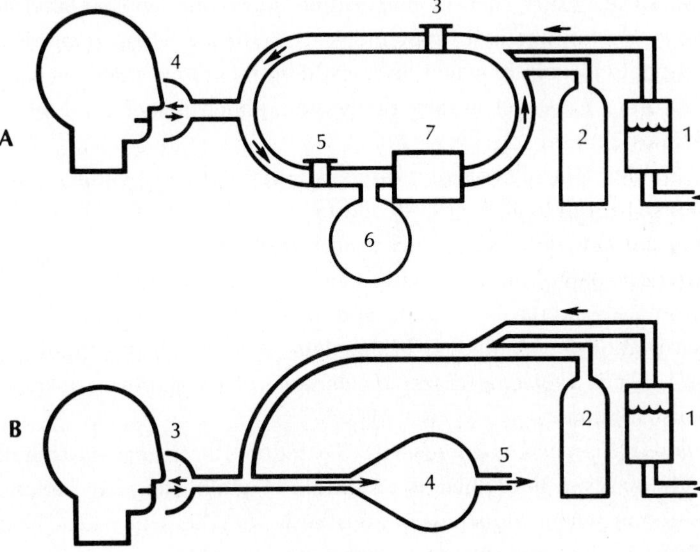

sites. However, recent studies have demonstrated little correlation between hydrate formation and potency of inhalation anesthetics.

The experimental observation that high pressures can reverse anesthesia[15] has contributed to two other ideas.

2. *Ionic pore hypothesis*: Anesthetics block ionic channels by interaction of the molecules with membranes. High pressures perhaps reverse anesthesia by changing membrane structure so that the anesthetics no longer interact at such sites.
3. *Membrane fluidity hypothesis*[27]: Anesthetics stabilize the fluidity of cell membranes. Again high pressures may reverse this action.

The Meyer-Overton correlation relating fat solubility to anesthetic potency has stood the test of time. In general, the more lipid soluble an anesthetic, the more potent it is. However, this correlation does not explain the anesthetic state. It is difficult to imagine that anesthetics act on lipids only, and many fat-soluble organic solvents lack anesthetic properties.

PREANESTHETIC MEDICATION

Several classes of drugs are frequently given before induction of anesthesia. The primary objective is to produce an anxiety-free, sedated patient. Additional reasons for such medications are to depress vagal tone and to supplement the anesthetic drugs. Individual drugs used for preanesthetic medication are described in the following categories:

1. *Anticholinergic agents*: Atropine, scopolamine, and glycopyrrolate are occasionally given intramuscularly before anesthesia to decrease vagal cardiac tone and to inhibit bronchial secretion. The use and value of such muscarinic blockers is less now than when cyclopropane and diethyl ether were used, the irritant effects of which stimulated secretion.
2. *Opioids*: Analgesics such as meperidine, morphine, and fentanyl are given to decrease anxiety and as a supplement to anesthesia. They are particularly useful for patients in pain or when an anesthetic technique involves painful stimuli. These drugs cause respiratory depression, which is increased when combined with anesthetics.
3. *Barbiturates*: The short-acting drugs secobarbital and pentobarbital were once commonly given to allay anxiety and to cause drowsiness. However, benzodiazepines are now quite frequently used instead.
4. *Benzodiazepines*: Midazolam given intravenously or diazepam given orally or intravenously produces sedation and some amnesia without significant effects on circulation or ventilation. **Midazolam** (see p. 270) is a rapidly acting compound that is replacing diazepam because of its shorter half-life and lack of venous irritation.
5. *Histamine H_2-receptor antagonists*: To reduce the threat of aspiration of acid into the lungs, a drug such as ranitidine is administered to patients who may vomit or in whom induction of anesthesia may be a problem. Nonparticulate antacids (sodium citrate) and metoclopramide, which increases gastrointestinal peristalsis, can also be beneficial in this setting.

All preanesthetic drugs possess certain disadvantages, for example, respiratory depression. Thus their proper use necessitates intimate pharmacologic and pathologic knowledge and clinical judgment. As important as the premedicant drugs are in allaying the patient's anxiety, of equal importance is psychologic rapport with the anesthesiologist.

PHARMACOLOGIC EFFECTS OF ANESTHETICS

Because of the ubiquitous nature of anesthetic distribution in the body and the nonspecific action of these drugs on all cellular functions, discussion of their specific effects on various organs is frequently incomplete. Although anesthetics in general are depressants of function, there are many quantitative differences in their activities. To add complexity, the anesthetics also differ qualitatively in their effects.

Nervous system

Central nervous system

Anesthetics depress all portions of the central nervous system. There is no single site or focus of action, but there are considerable regional differences. It is believed that the higher cortical centers and the ascending reticular activating system are the most susceptible portions of the brain. However, as anesthetic concentration in the brain increases, lower centers also become depressed.[17] This eventually leads to respiratory and circulatory arrest, the mechanism of death with overdosage.

Peripheral nervous system

Recent studies have indicated that profound effects on the spinal cord are produced by general anesthetics. The gating region for pain impulses, the substantia gelatinosa of Rolando, is depressed such that nociceptive input ascending by pathways such as the spinothalamic tract is reduced. Thus fewer pain impulses reach the brain during anesthesia. Many general anesthetics also produce skeletal muscle relaxation by effects on the internuncial pool of neurons in the spinal cord. Although there are discernible effects of general anesthetics in the region of the myoneural junction, it is believed that actions on the cord are responsible for most of the skeletal muscle relaxation seen with administration of these drugs.

AUTONOMIC NERVOUS SYSTEM

In the autonomic nervous system there are wide differences in the range of effects produced by general anesthetics, which are made more complex by the dose-response relationships involved. Nitrous oxide is the only presently employed anesthetic with sympathetic excitatory actions. In contrast, modern halogenated anesthetics inhibit the sympathetic nervous system, reduce plasma catecholamine concentration, and do not induce glycogenolysis.

Effects of inhalation general anesthetics on parasympathetic activity are quite variable. Halothane has been adjudged to be a vagal stimulant, particularly in lighter planes of anesthesia. The evidence for this is scanty, but it produces a mild degree of bradycardia that can be overcome by atropine. Further evidence for enhanced vagal activity comes from clinical reports implicating cyclopropane as a trigger for bronchial constriction in asthmatics. On the other hand, halothane and the other halogenated hydrocarbon anesthetics do not have this effect on bronchial smooth muscle and are therefore considered drugs of choice for the patient with lung disease.

Ventilation

With deep levels of anesthesia, ventilatory depression is common with all potent general anesthetics. At all planes of anesthesia there is a graded depression of medullary activity. Classically, ventilation during anesthesia is characterized by lowered tidal volume and increased frequency of breathing with a net reduction in alveolar minute ventilation. The response to arterial and alveolar carbon dioxide tensions is decreased; characteristically there is a rightward shift and eventually decreased slope of the carbon dioxide—response curve. This is a dose-dependent phenomenon. In lighter planes of surgical anesthesia, some anesthetics, such as diethyl ether, have less effect on ventilation, such that normal or near normal carbon dioxide tension is maintained. However, with most halogenated anesthetics the drop in alveolar ventilation and alveolar minute ventilation ($\dot{V}_A$) will increase Pa_{CO_2}. For this reason the administration of a general anesthetic is frequently performed with assisted or controlled ventilation. This may be done by manipulation of the rebreathing bag of the anesthesia machine or by insertion of a mechanical ventilator into the circuit.

Circulation

Anesthetics affect both the heart and the peripheral circulation. A dose-related, negative inotropic effect, which is least with nitrous oxide, is evident in the depression of twitch height in isolated animal papillary muscles[3] and in intact humans as a fall in cardiac output.[5] Peripheral vasodilatation occurs because anesthetics, particularly the halogenated ones, act on autonomic ganglia to depress sympathetic nerve activity. Vasodilatation and the negative inotropic effect combined cause dose-dependent decreases in blood pressure, by perhaps as much as 25% to 40%. Systolic blood pressure seems to be reduced more than diastolic blood pressure; during anesthesia there is a tendency for the pulse pressure to narrow. At equianesthetic concentrations, the common halogenated anesthetics differ quantitatively. Myocardial contractility is thought to be most depressed by enflurane and least by isoflurane; halothane has an intermediate effect. Peripheral resistance is decreased most by isoflurane and least by enflurane, with halothane again intermediate.[13]

Changes in cardiac rhythm and conduction are not uncommon during anesthesia[1] and often involve the pacemaker, with progression from a wandering pacemaker to nodal rhythms. These arrhythmias are usually benign. The second most common form of arrhythmia is premature ventricular contractions. Potential for arrhythmias can be enhanced by elevated plasma catecholamine concentrations. Because the straight-chain hydrocarbons, namely cyclopropane and halothane, are most likely to cause cardiac irregularities, the arrhythmias are often called "hydrocarbon anesthetic arrhythmias." The ether series of anesthetics, halogenated or not, seems to present far fewer problems in this regard.

Probably as a result of changes in automaticity, the threshold for premature ventricular contractions is lowered by many anesthetics. In light planes of anesthesia, if there is sympathetic stimulation or if exogenous sympathomimetic amines are administered, troublesome ventricular arrhythmias can develop. For example, sequential administration of cyclopropane and epinephrine is used in pharmacology for testing cardiac antifibrillatory drugs. Hypercapnia can also increase release of catecholamines and enhance the potential for ventricular arrhythmias in a myocardium "sensitized" by hydrocarbon anesthetics. These arrhythmias are frequently clues to the clinician that ventilation is not adequate. Administration of catecholamines during anesthesia with certain of these anesthetics should be done with caution, if at all. Recommendations of minimal doses of drugs such as epinephrine that can be safely injected during the course of halothane anesthesia are available, but caution should still be exercised.[16]

Uterus

The halogenated anesthetics inhibit the contractile response of the gravid uterus to administration of oxytocic drugs. Thus they may produce or allow uterine relaxation, which may be advantageous for version extractions or other intrauterine manipulations. This effect is a two-edged sword, however, because these anesthetics will also permit sufficient degrees of uterine relaxation to increase postpartum bleeding. These effects must be taken into consideration during obstetrical anesthesia. Furthermore, the gaseous and vapor anesthetics readily cross the placenta into the fetus.

Hepatic and metabolic actions

Anesthetics have several actions on the liver. They depress mitochondrial function such that total body oxygen consumption is reduced. Actually, this has a certain advantage, since reduction in hepatic blood flow with impaired oxygen delivery will have fewer adverse effects if oxygen need is diminished. The anesthetics also seem to have an "anti-insulin action" that decreases the ability of the liver to take up glucose and incorporate it into glucose-6-phosphate. If an exogenous glucose load is administered during the course of general anesthesia, a diabetic type of prolonged glucose-tolerance curve will result. This effect coupled with the enhanced glycogenolysis that occurs with some anesthetics can increase blood glucose. The activity of hepatic microsomal enzymes responsible for biotransformation of various drugs is diminished during clinical anesthesia. This effect combined with decreased hepatic blood flow, which limits access of drugs to the liver, will decrease the clearances of some drugs.[2] Recent evidence indicates that during deep anesthesia there is also impairment of certain synthetic pathways, such as the urea cycle and bilirubin conjugation. These effects quickly dissipate as the anesthetic is terminated.

Biotransformation and toxicity

Until 1965 it was believed that the general inhalation anesthetics were inert and were not extensively metabolized in the body. This concept has proved to be incorrect. The anesthetics are metabolized to various degrees, depending on their molecular structure and partition coefficient. A low partition coefficient limits the time that an anesthetic is in contact with metabolic enzymes and relatively less biotransformation would be expected. The extremes occur in the case of isoflurane and desflurane, which are less than 1% metabolized, as compared with methoxyflurane of which over 50% is metabolized. Biotransformation of certain anesthetics may be responsible for cases of toxicity reported after anesthesia. For example, methoxyflurane metabolism releases free fluoride ion. Fluoride concentrations greater than 80 μmol/L may cause nephrotoxicity, which often manifests as a so-called high-output renal failure syndrome. Metabolism of chloroform, a compound obsolete as an anesthetic, causes hepatic toxicity. Free radicals or other reactive intermediates that combine covalently with liver macromolecules are formed. The altered proteins and lipoproteins no longer function, and tissue necrosis can occur. Halothane, ordinarily a very safe anesthetic, has been implicated in unpredictable hepatic toxicity. This is a rare event that probably occurs no more often than 1:10,000 administrations. The injury is believed to be caused by biotransformation of the anesthetic to metabolites that bind covalently to hepatic macromolecules to produce a hapten. This hapten, specifically a trifluoroacetyl derivative, then induces an immunologic inflammatory response that causes hepatitis and centrolobular necrosis.[4] Repeated exposure to halothane anesthesia over short periods of time seems more likely to produce this event, particularly in obese, middle-aged women. Although this effect is rare, it is unpredictable and has a lethality approaching 50%.

Biotransformation of halogenated anesthetics varies widely. Methoxyflurane is metabolized to the greatest extent (75%), followed in descending order by halothane (20%), enflurane (3%), sevoflurane (2-3%), isoflurane (1%), and desflurane (0%). Because some cross-sensitivity to their metabolites may occur, it may be prudent to avoid any halogenated anesthetic in a patient who has had a prior unexplained hepatic reaction to one of them.

Miscellaneous effects

A reduction in renal function is commonly seen during the course of anesthesia. This is primarily caused by a decrease in renal blood flow and, consequently, a reduced glomerular filtration rate. Nausea and vomiting may occur after administration of general anesthetics. Although these effects may have a central nervous system cause, surgical stimulation and pain probably also play a role. No one inhalation anesthetic used presently seems more prone than others to cause nausea and vomiting. Because of hypothalamic depression, patients' temperatures generally decrease slightly during anesthesia. Certain anesthetics, such as halothane, may trigger a catastrophic syndrome known as *malignant hyperthermia* in genetically susceptible persons. This sudden and often lethal event can increase temperatures to 42° C or higher with severe metabolic acidosis. It can be treated or even prevented in susceptible patients with dantrolene (see p. 136). If ventilation is unassisted, many anesthetics can increase intracranial pressure.[26]

CLINICAL PHARMACOLOGY OF INDIVIDUAL ANESTHETICS

The inhalation anesthetics (Table 36-3) are divided into two major categories: gases and volatile liquids. Gaseous anesthetics are those with boiling points below room temperature and critical pressures greater than 760 mm Hg. They are usually marketed as compressed gases, in the liquid or gaseous state, under high pressure in steel cylinders. The cylinders are colored differently for each gas. The volatile anesthetics are liquids at room temperature, are usually more potent than the gases, and are ethers or halogenated hydrocarbons. Gaseous anesthetics generally possess blood-gas and oil-gas partition coefficients lower than those of the volatile anesthetics, are consequently faster for induction and recovery, and are less potent. Selection of a particular anesthetic for an individual patient is predicated on pathophysiology and the type of surgical procedure involved. Selection of the appropriate anesthetic(s) is one of the critical factors to be resolved in the presurgical rounds of the anesthesiologist.

Nitrous oxide

Nitrous oxide (N_2O) is a colorless, odorless, tasteless gas that is not metabolized. It is carried in the body in physical solution. Nitrous oxide is a weak anesthetic. It is usually supplemented in *balanced anesthesia* with hypnotics (barbiturate or benzodiazepine), analgesics (intravenous opioid), and muscle relaxants (curariform drug). Nitrous oxide is not flammable and is compatible with all other drugs, including catecholamines. Analgesia occurs with inspired concentrations greater than 20% and

TABLE 36-3 Clinical characteristics of general anesthetics

Anesthetic	Analgesia	Hypnosis	Skeletal muscle relaxation	Depression of reflexes	Flammability	Compatibility with epinephrine
Nitrous oxide	+	+	0	+	No	Yes
Cyclopropane	++	++++	+	++	Yes	No
Diethyl ether	++++	++++	++++	++++	Yes	Yes
Methoxyflurane	++++	++++	++++	++++	No	Yes
Halothane	++	++++	++	++++	No	No
Enflurane	+++	++++	+++	++++	No	Yes
Isoflurane	+++	++++	+++	++++	No	Yes

++++, Maximum effect, +, minimum effect.

hypnosis at concentrations of about 40% at sea level. However, because of its low potency, it is impossible to achieve complete surgical anesthesia with nitrous oxide without depriving the patient of oxygen.

Nitrous oxide has no significant effects on the respiratory, hepatic, renal, or autonomic nervous systems, except for slight myocardial depression and sympathomimetic effects. Because of this supposed lack of depressant effects, nitrous oxide has been called an ideal anesthetic. However, recent investigations indicate that it may not be totally benign. Nitrous oxide inhalation for only 2 hours can drastically lower levels of methionine synthetase used in vitamin B_{12} synthesis.[18] Although surgical patients given nitrous oxide do not develop pernicious anemia, persons abusing the drug chronically for long periods have developed neurologic manifestations of vitamin B_{12} deficiency.

In addition to use in the balanced technique, nitrous oxide is commonly administered with more powerful anesthetics. This hastens uptake of the more powerful agent and adds the analgesic activity of nitrous oxide without harmful systemic effects. For example, halothane depresses myocardial contractility. The MAC for halothane in oxygen alone is 0.8%. If halothane is administered in 70% nitrous oxide with 30% oxygen, the MAC of halothane is reduced to 0.35%. Hence anesthesia can be accomplished with less adverse cardiac effects.

Volatile liquid anesthetics

HALOTHANE

Halothane ($CF_3CHBrCl$, Fluothane) was the first of the truly modern, nonflammable halogenated inhalation anesthetics. It is rapid in onset, pleasant for patients, and possesses a proved record of safety. The unresolved problem of hepatotoxicity has, nevertheless, caused a decline in its use.

Halothane greatly depresses alveolar minute ventilation with the classic decrease in tidal volume but with increased inspiratory rate. Therefore assisted or controlled ventilation is commonly employed when halothane is administered. It is nonirritating to the respiratory tract and does not increase pulmonary secretion.

Halothane is an example of an anesthetic with depressant effects on the heart[3] with no increase in sympathetic nervous activity to secondarily augment contractility. Cardiac output, contractile force, and blood pressure all fall during its administration. Part of the blood pressure decline results from a decrease in sympathetic nervous activity with a consequent reduction in peripheral vascular resistance. Some degree of bradycardia is frequently seen during anesthesia with halothane. Halothane also lowers the threshold of ventricular muscle to catecholamine-induced arrhythmias. This effect is not so great as with cyclopropane, though it still warrants extreme caution when epinephrine or other sympathomimetic amines are to be administered. Uterine relaxation is good with halothane anesthesia.

Because of its low solubility, halothane is considered a rapid anesthetic. It is commonly used with nitrous oxide, though it may be given alone with oxygen. At the present time, it is regarded as the primary anesthetic for pediatric patients because of the ease of induction and rapid awakening. Although there is the specter of hepatic damage, which is occasionally reported after its use, this effect is rare in infants and children.

METHOXYFLURANE

Methoxyflurane ($CCl_2HCF_2OCH_3$, Penthrane), a potent, nonflammable anesthetic, is one of the first of a series of halogenated ethers. Its hallmark is that it produces excellent skeletal muscle relaxation. A drawback, however, is its rather high solubility, which results in slow induction and awakening. Unlike halothane, methoxyflurane does not sensitize the myocardium to catecholamines. This may be related to its ether link. Methoxyflurane is a rather pleasant-smelling liquid of low volatility and is only slightly irritating to the respiratory tract. Although it depresses ventilation, depression of cardiac contractility is probably less than that with halothane at equally effective dosages.

The great drawback to methoxyflurane, which has decreased its clinical use, is its biotransformation with release of free fluoride ions that contribute to high output renal failure. To reduce the amount of free fluoride released, it has been recommended that methoxyflurane anesthesia be limited to 2 MAC hours.

ENFLURANE

Enflurane (CF_2HOCF_2CFClH, Ethrane) is a halogenated ether that possesses many of the virtues of halothane and methoxyflurane without some of their disadvantages. Enflurane depresses myocardial contractility comparably to halothane. However, because of its ether link, it does not sensitize the myocardium to endogenous and exogenous catecholamines to the degree that halothane does. The ether link also gives enflurane its excellent skeletal muscle–relaxant properties.

Because of lower solubility parameters, no more than 2% to 3% of an absorbed dose of enflurane is metabolized. Even though free fluoride ion is a metabolic product, it does not achieve blood concentrations sufficient to produce renal disease. An exception is in patients taking the antitubercular drug isoniazid, which can specifically induce defluorination enzymes. High free fluoride concentrations may then develop. The incidence of hepatic damage with enflurane seems to be far less than with halothane so that repeated exposures are not contraindicated. Clinically the drug may be a little more difficult to use than halothane, which it largely replaced in adult anesthesia before isoflurane became widely used.

A major problem associated with enflurane is that the combination of high anesthetic concentrations and hypocapnia fosters grand mal seizures.[21] This effect does not seem to be deleterious and can be avoided by maintaining normocapnia and employing no higher concentration than that necessary for the surgery.

ISOFLURANE

Isoflurane ($CF_3CHClOCHF_2$, Forane) is an isomer of enflurane. Less than 1% of the total absorbed dose is metabolized. Therefore it may cause less renal and hepatic toxicity than any other commonly employed anesthetic. Many of its features are similar to those of enflurane. However, there is evidence that its respiratory depressant effect may be slightly greater than that of enflurane, whereas its cardiovascular depressant effect is less. Although it lacks a significant negative inotropic action, the anesthetic does produce profound peripheral vasodilatation with concomitant decreases in blood pressure. Tachycardia can result and may be bothersome in patients with coronary artery disease. Isoflurane does not cause seizures. The drug is nonflammable and is compatible, to a certain degree, with catecholamines, similarly to enflurane. Skeletal muscle and uterine relaxant properties are good. Because of a somewhat pungent odor, inductions are often not so smooth as with halothane.

SEVOFLURANE

Sevoflurane ($CFH_2OCH[CF_3]_2$), a rapidly acting, pleasant to inhale anesthetic, is in final stages of clinical experimentation. Major disadvantages lie in its degree of biotransformation (3%) to free fluoride ion and the fact that it can be absorbed by the soda lime used in anesthesia circuits to absorb carbon dioxide.

DESFLURANE

Desflurane ($CF_2HOCFHCF_3$) differs from isoflurane only in a fluorine atom substitution for a chlorine atom. The drug is very rapid acting, almost totally inert, and less potent than the other halogenated anesthetics. Its major disadvantage relates to its relatively high vapor pressure, which will necessitate use of complex vaporizers.

INTRAVENOUS ANESTHETICS

Some nonvolatile drugs are classified as anesthetics though they do not have all four attributes ascribed to general anesthetics and lack the ready controllability of the inhaled drugs.

Barbiturates

Highly lipid-soluble barbiturates are used intravenously to produce or supplement hypnosis during anesthesia. They exhibit many of the distribution characteristics of inhaled anesthetics. One must remember that barbiturates are hypnotics only and do not possess analgesic or muscle-relaxant activity except with gross overdosage. Two barbiturates, thiopental and methohexital, are commonly employed.

Thiopental sodium (Pentothal), a potent ultrashort-acting thiobarbiturate, is the sulfur analog of pentobarbital. The thio group gives the drug greater lipid solubility and hence facilitates entry into the brain.

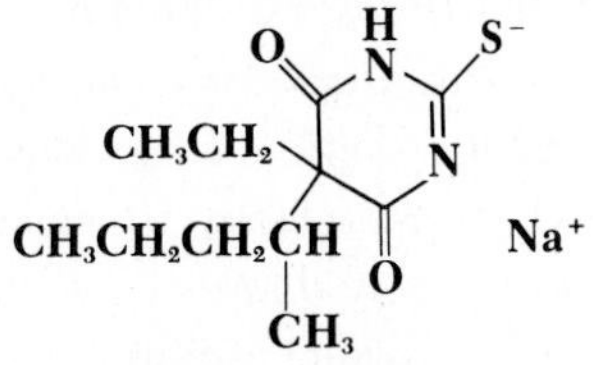

Thiopental sodium

Thiopental is used to produce a smooth, pleasant induction of anesthesia. It has no adverse effects on the viscera; overdosage is characterized by pronounced circulatory and ventilatory depression.

Termination of the action of thiopental, and other intravenously administered barbiturates, is attributed primarily to redistribution from the brain to other tissues (see p. 272). Awakening after normal therapeutic doses occurs within 15 minutes, which corresponds to the time when drug concentration in skeletal muscle becomes maximal. Metabolism of the barbiturate is extensive; less than 5% is excreted unchanged by the kidney. Although metabolism begins as soon as the drug is administered, the rate, compared with redistribution, is not sufficient to be important in terminating the activity of a single dose of thiopental. **Thiamylal sodium** (Surital) is a thiobarbiturate similar to thiopental.

Methohexital sodium (Brevital) is an ultrashort-acting oxybarbiturate. It was designed to have a slightly shorter duration of hypnosis than thiopental, but clinically this difference is not always apparent.

Contraindications to the use of intravenous barbiturates include shock and asthma. Barbiturates exacerbate acute intermittent porphyria, a metabolic disease, and should not be used in affected patients. Inadvertent intra-arterial injection of barbiturates can induce severe arterial spasm and thrombosis followed by gangrene of the extremities. Barbiturates are given intravenously in 1.0% to 2.5% solutions.

Propofol

Propofol (Diprivan) is a rapidly acting hypnotic used intravenously to produce anesthesia.[25] Its major advantage lies in its brevity of action in a dose of approximately 2 mg/kg. A disadvantage is that it can cause transient hypotension and so should be used with care, particularly in the geriatric patient.[7] Propofol is available in an emulsion that can cause minor venous irritation.

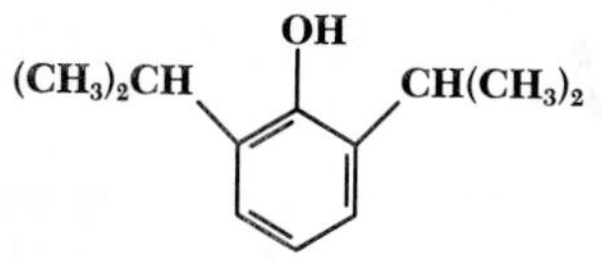

OH

$(CH_3)_2CH$ $CH(CH_3)_2$

Propofol

Opioids

The opioids **fentanyl, alfentanil,** and **sufentanil** (see p. 328) are used as analgesics during anesthesia. Conventional doses of fentanyl for routine surgery vary from 3 to 5 μg/kg. Fentanyl is now used extensively as an analgesic for open-heart procedures because it lacks some of the cardiac depressant actions of other anesthetics. For this purpose large doses of fentanyl, approximately 50 μg/kg or higher, are administered.

Fentanyl, like all narcotics, severely depresses ventilation. A peculiar increase in chest wall muscle tone, termed "wooden rigidity," is occasionally observed if the narcotic is injected rapidly. Rarely, droperidol, the neuroleptic usually used with an opioid and nitrous oxide for neuroleptanesthesia, produces a parkinsonian type of extrapyramidal reaction.

Ketamine

Ketamine is a phencyclidine derivative capable of producing a trancelike state with freedom from pain, termed "dissociative anesthesia." Ketamine produces little or no muscular relaxation. Patients under the influence of ketamine will respond to visceral pain but not to superficial pain. In adults the drug frequently produces psychic problems such as terrifying dreams and severe distortions of reality. For this reason ketamine use is usually limited to anesthesia for superficial procedures in infants and children. The drug stimulates the sympathetic nervous system and may increase blood pressure. It frequently increases salivation. Ketamine increases intracranial pressure and is relatively contraindicated in the presence of central nervous system tumors or space-occupying lesions. Ketamine hydrochloride (Ketalar) is injected intravenously or intramuscularly and is available in solutions of 10 to 100 mg/ml.

$NHCH_3$ Cl O

Ketamine

Etomidate

Etomidate (Amidate), an imidazole congener, is quite distinct from other induction agents. It is hypnotic only and possesses no analgesic properties. The dose is 0.3 to 0.4 mg/kg.

Characteristics of etomidate include rapid biotransformation by liver and kidney, a very brief duration of action, essentially no depression of cardiovascular or ventilatory function, and, in animal studies, a wider margin of safety than thiopental or methohexital. Thus etomidate may be preferable for induction in certain poor-risk patients. Adverse reactions of involuntary skeletal muscle contractions and pain on injection, with secondary thrombophlebitis, limit the use of etomidate for routine anesthetic induction. The venous irritant action is believed to be caused by the propylene glycol vehicle that is employed for solubility. Inhibition of adrenal steroid production has also seriously limited the usefulness of this drug.

REFERENCES

1. Atlee JL III: Anaesthesia and cardiac electrophysiology, *Eur J Anaesthesiol* 2:215, 1985.
2. Brown BR Jr: Drug biotransformation by the liver. In Brown BR Jr, editor: *Anesthesia in hepatic and biliary tract disease*, Philadelphia, 1988, FA Davis, p 67.
3. Brown BR, Jr, Crout JR: A comparative study of the effects of five general anesthetics on myocardial contractility: I. Isometric conditions, *Anesthesiology* 34:236, 1971.
4. Callis AH, Brooks SD, Waters SJ, et al: Evidence for a role of the immune system in the pathogenesis of halothane hepatitis. In Roth SH, Miller KW, editors: *Molecular and cellular mechanisms of anesthetics*, New York, 1986, Plenum Medical Book, p 443.
5. Calverley RK, Smith NT, Prys-Roberts C, et al: Cardiovascular effects of enflurane anesthesia during controlled ventilation in man, *Anesth Analg* 57:619, 1978.
6. Carpenter RL, Eger EI II, Johnson BH, et al: Pharmacokinetics of inhaled anesthetics in humans: measurements during and after the simultaneous administration of enflurane, halothane, isoflurane, methoxyflurane, and nitrous oxide, *Anesth Analg* 65:575, 1986.
7. Dundee JW, Robinson FP, McCollum JSC, Patterson CC: Sensitivity to propofol in the elderly, *Anaesthesia* 41:482, 1986.
8. Dundee JW, Halliday NJ, Harper KW, Brogden RN: Midazolam: a review of its pharmacological properties and therapeutic use, *Drugs* 28:519, 1984.
9. Eger EI II: *Anesthetic uptake and action*, Baltimore, 1974, Williams & Wilkins.
10. Eger EI II, Lundgren C, Miller SL, Stevens WC: Anesthetic potencies of sulfur hexafluoride, carbon tetrafluoride, chloroform and ethrane in dogs: correlation with the hydrate and lipid theories of anesthetic action, *Anesthesiology* 30:129, 1969.
11. Eger EI II, Saidman LJ, Brandstater B: Minimum alveolar anesthetic concentra-

tion: a standard of anesthetic potency, *Anesthesiology* 26:756, 1965.

12. Epstein RM: Theoretical analysis of the effect of concentration-dependent solubility upon the uptake of anesthetic agents, *Anesthesiology* 29:187, 1968.
13. Forrest JB: Comparative pharmacology of inhalational anaesthetics. In Nunn JF, Utting JE, Brown BR Jr, editors: *General anaesthesia*, ed 5, London, 1989, Butterworths, p 60.
14. Halsey MJ: Potency and physical properties of inhalational anaesthetics. In Nunn JF, Utting JE, Brown BR Jr, editors: *General anaesthesia*, ed 5, London, 1989, Butterworths, p 7.
15. Halsey MJ, Wardley-Smith B, Green CJ: Pressure reversal of general anaesthesia—a multi-site expansion hypothesis, *Br J Anaesth* 50:1091, 1978.
16. Johnston RR, Eger EI II, Wilson C: A comparative interaction of epinephrine with enflurane, isoflurane, and halothane in man, *Anesth Analg* 55:709, 1976.
17. Kendig JJ: Neuronal basis of the anaesthetic state. In Nunn JF, Utting JE, Brown BR Jr, editors: *General anesthesia*, ed 5, London, 1989, Butterworths, p 30.
18. Layzer RB: Myeloneuropathy after prolonged exposure to nitrous oxide, *Lancet* 2:1227, 1978.
19. Mapleson WW: Pharmacokinetics of inhalational anaesthetics. In Nunn JF, Utting, JE, Brown BR Jr, editors: *General anaesthesia*, ed 5, London, 1989, Butterworths, p 44.
20. McLain GE, Sipes IG, and Brown BR Jr: An animal model of halothane hepatotoxicity: roles of enzyme induction and hypoxia, *Anesthesiology* 51:321, 1979.
21. Modica PA, Tempelhoff R, White PR: Pro- and anticonvulsant effects of anesthetics (Part I), *Anesth Analg* 70:303, 1990.
22. Mukai S, Morio M, Fujii K, Hanaki C: Volatile metabolites of halothane in the rabbit, *Anesthesiology* 47:248, 1977.
23. Mazze RI, Trudell JR, Cousins MJ: Methoxyflurane metabolism and renal dysfunction: clinical correlation in man, *Anesthesiology* 35:247, 1971.
24. Rehder K, Forbes J, Alter H, et al: Halothane biotransformation in man: a quantitative study, *Anesthesiology* 28:711, 1967.
25. Sebel PS, Lowdon JD: Propofol: a new intravenous anesthetic, *Anesthesiology* 71:260, 1989.
26. Shapiro HM: Intracranial hypertension: therapeutic and anesthetic considerations, *Anesthesiology* 43:445, 1975.
27. Ueda I, Hirakawa M, Arakawa K, Kamaya H: Do anesthetics fluidize membranes? *Anesthesiology* 64:67, 1986.
28. Van Dyke RA, Chenoweth MB, Van Poznak A: Metabolism of volatile anesthetics—I: Conversion in vivo of several anesthetics to $^{14}CO_2$ and chloride, *Biochem Pharmacol* 13:1239, 1964.

ADDITIONAL READINGS

Miller RD, editor: *Anesthesia*, ed 3, New York, 1990, Churchill Livingstone.

Nunn JF, Utting JE, Brown BR Jr, editors: *General anaesthesia*, ed 5, London, 1989, Butterworths.

Stoelting RK: *Pharmacology and physiology in anesthetic practice,* Philadelphia, 1987, JB Lippincott.

Chapter 37

Pharmacology of local anesthesia

GENERAL CONCEPT

Local anesthetics are drugs employed to produce a transient and reversible loss of sensation in a circumscribed region of the body. They achieve this effect by interfering with nerve conduction.

In 1884 Köller, who had studied the drug with Sigmund Freud, introduced *cocaine* as a topical anesthetic in ophthalmology. This was the beginning of the first era in the history of local anesthesia.

The second era began in 1904 with the introduction of *procaine* by Einhorn. This was the first safe local anesthetic suitable for injection. Procaine remained the most widely used local anesthetic until the introduction of *lidocaine*, which is now considered the agent of choice for infiltration. Other local anesthetics of importance are tetracaine, mepivacaine, prilocaine, and bupivacaine. These drugs differ from each other in their toxicity, metabolism, and onset and duration of action. Lidocaine, in addition to being an important local anesthetic, has important uses as an antiarrhythmic agent (p. 430).

CLASSIFICATION

Local anesthetics may be classified according to their chemistry or on the basis of their clinical usage.

According to chemistry

Local anesthetics are generally either esters or amides (Table 37-1). They consist of an aromatic portion, an intermediate chain, and an amine portion. The aromatic portion confers lipophilic properties to the molecule, whereas the amine portion is hydrophilic. The ester or amide component of the molecule determines whether the compound will be inactivated primarily by hydrolysis in plasma or destruction in the liver.

According to clinical usage

Local anesthetics have several types of clinical application, and their suitability for these varies with their pharmacologic properties. These applications and preferred agents for each are also indicated in Table 37-1.

MODE OF ACTION

Electrophysiologic studies indicate that local anesthetics do not alter the resting membrane potential or threshold potential of nerves. They decrease the rate of rise of the depolarization phase of the action potential by impeding the initial increase in Na^+ conductance. As a consequence the cell does not depolarize sufficiently after excitation to reach threshold, and the propagated action potential is prevented.

Local anesthetics impair Na^+ influx after binding within the Na^+ channels.[1] The

TABLE 37-1 Local anesthetics and their uses

Drug	Uses in anesthesia: Infiltration and block	Surface	Spinal	Epidural and caudal	Intravenous
Esters					
Butamben (Butesin)		2			
Chloroprocaine (Nesacaine)	1			2	
Cocaine		1			
Benzocaine (ethyl aminobenzoate, Hurricaine, others)		1			
Procaine (Novocain)	1		2		
Proparacaine (Ophthaine, others)					
Propoxycaine (Ravocaine)	3				
Tetracaine (Pontocaine)	2	2	1	2	
Amides					
Bupivacaine (Marcaine, Sensorcaine)	1		2	2	
Dibucaine (Nupercainal)		2			
Etidocaine (Duranest)					
Lidocaine (Xylocaine, others)	1	2	2	1	1
Mepivacaine (Carbocaine, others)	2			1	
Prilocaine (Citanest)	3				

1, Primary agent; *2*, secondary agent; *3*, primarily dental use.

clinically used compounds are tertiary amines. Studies with these amines and with related quaternary amines (always charged) and neutral amines (never charged) indicate that these anesthetics do not enter the Na^+ channel from the exterior surface of the cell. Instead they reach the channel from within the cytoplasm (a hydrophilic pathway) or from within the cell membrane (a hydrophobic pathway). In either case, a compound must penetrate in an uncharged state into or through the membrane if it is to exhibit local anesthetic activity. Consequently an acidic external environment, which favors the charged form of tertiary amines, impairs the local anesthetic activity of these compounds.

Active form

PROBLEM 37-1. When the hydrochloride of a local anesthetic is injected, which is the active form, the uncharged base or the charged cation? When one is dealing with an intact isolated nerve, the local anesthetics such as lidocaine are more potent in an alkaline solution, an indication that the uncharged base is the active form. On the other hand, when a desheathed nerve is used, the less alkaline preparations are more efficacious. It is believed at present that the uncharged base penetrates better across the nerve sheath but that the charged cation exerts the pharmacologic action. The problem is complicated by the fact that the results are not applicable to all members of the series of local anesthetics.

TABLE 37-2 Onset and duration of action of various local anesthetics, as determined by a standardized ulnar block technique

Drug	Concentration	Relative potency	Onset in minutes	Duration of action in minutes
Procaine	1	0.5	7	19
Lidocaine	1	1	5	40
Mepivacaine	1	1	4	99
Prilocaine	1	1	3	98
Tetracaine*	0.25	4	7	135
Bupivacaine*	0.25	4	8	415

Modified from Covino BG: N Engl J Med 286:975, 1035, 1972; based on data from Albért J and Löfstöm B: Acta Anaesth Scand 5:99, 1961.
*Solutions contain epinephrine 1:200,000.

Action on various nerve fibers

According to diameter, myelination, and conduction velocities, nerve fibers can be classified into three types—A, B, and C fibers. The A fibers have a diameter of 1 to 20 μm, are myelinated, and have conduction velocities up to 100 m/sec. Somatic motor and some sensory fibers fall into this classification. Blockade of these fibers results in skeletal muscle relaxation, loss of thermal and tactile sensation, proprioceptive loss, and loss of the sensation of sharp pain. B fibers vary in diameter from 1 to 3 μm, are also myelinated, and conduct at intermediate velocities. Preganglionic fibers fall into this group, and their blockade results in autonomic paralysis. C fibers are usually under 1 μm in diameter, are not myelinated, and conduct at approximately 1 m/sec. Postganglionic fibers, as well as some somatic sensory fibers, fall into this classification. Blockade results in autonomic paralysis; loss of the sensations of itch, tickle, and dull pain; and loss of much of the thermal sensation.

Clinically the general order of loss of function (upon exposure to a local anesthetic) is as follows: (1) pain, (2) temperature, (3) touch, (4) proprioception, and (5) skeletal muscle tone. If pressure is exerted on a mixed nerve, the fibers are depressed in somewhat the reverse order.

In summary, local anesthetic drugs depress the small, unmyelinated fibers first and the larger, myelinated fibers last. The time for the onset of action is shorter for the smaller fibers, and the concentration of drug required is less.[2]

ABSORPTION, FATE, AND EXCRETION

Absorption of the various local anesthetics depends on the site of injection, the degree of vasodilatation caused by the agent itself, the dose, and the presence or absence of a vasoconstrictor. Epinephrine is frequently added to the solution to greatly increase the duration of action of procaine as an infiltration agent. The vasoconstriction caused by the sympathomimetic diminishes blood flow at the site of injection and allows the local anesthetic to persist at that site for a longer period of time.

The onset and duration of action of various local anesthetics are listed in Table 37-2.

Local anesthetics of the ester type (procaine) are hydrolyzed by plasma pseudo-

TABLE 37-3 Relative rates of local anesthetic hydrolysis by plasma esterase

Local anesthetic	Rate of hydrolysis
Piperocaine	6.5
Chloroprocaine	5.0
Procaine	1.0
Tetracaine	0.2
Dibucaine	0

cholinesterase (Table 37-3). Those having the amide linkage (lidocaine) are largely metabolized in the liver.

In humans, procaine is cleaved to *p*-aminobenzoic acid, 80% of which is excreted in the urine, and diethylaminoethanol, 30% of which is excreted in the urine. Only 2% of the drug is excreted unchanged. Procaine is hydrolyzed in spinal fluid, in which there is very little esterase, 150 times more slowly than in plasma. Hydrolysis results from the alkalinity of the spinal fluid and is approximately the same in a buffered solution of the same pH.

About 10% to 20% of lidocaine is excreted intact. The rest is metabolized in the liver by removal of one or both ethyl groups. The resulting metabolites still have pharmacologic activity and may contribute to central nervous system toxicity.

METHODS OF ADMINISTRATION

Local anesthetics may be administered by topical application, by infiltration of tissues to bathe fine nerve elements, by injection adjacent to nerves and their branches, and by injection into the epidural or subarachnoid spaces. In certain situations intravenous injections are utilized to control pain. The details of subarachnoid and epidural anesthesia are outside the scope of this discussion.

SYSTEMIC ACTIONS

Local anesthetics largely exert their action on a circumscribed region. Nevertheless, they are absorbed from the site of injection and may cause systemic effects, particularly in the cardiovascular and central nervous systems and especially when an excessive dose is utilized.

Cardiovascular effects

Since lidocaine is widely used as an antiarrhythmic drug (see Chapter 39), much has been learned about its effects on the heart. The same effects are generally also produced by other local anesthetics. At nontoxic concentrations lidocaine alters or abolishes slow diastolic depolarization in Purkinje fibers and may shorten the effective refractory period as well as the duration of the action potential. In toxic doses lidocaine decreases the maximal depolarization of Purkinje fibers and reduces conduction velocity. Toxic doses may also have a direct negative inotropic effect. Before such doses are reached, however, patients usually manifest central nervous system toxicity.

Local anesthetics tend to relax vascular smooth muscle, but cocaine can cause vasoconstriction by blocking reuptake of norepinephrine.

Central nervous system effects

Although local anesthesia usually produces no central effects, excessive absorption can cause restlessness, irritability, convulsions, and eventually respiratory depression. It is believed on the basis of animal experiments that the local anesthetics block inhibitory cortical activity. This leads to excitation. Larger doses that depress both inhibitory and facilitatory neurons produce general central nervous system depression.

Miscellaneous effects

Other than their effects on the cardiovascular and central nervous systems, local anesthetics cause few systemic responses. They may depress ganglionic and neuromuscular transmission. These actions are unimportant unless another agent that affects these systems is used concomitantly. For example, lidocaine may enhance the action of neuromuscular blocking agents.

Vasoconstrictors and local anesthetics

Vasoconstrictors, particularly epinephrine, are commonly added to local anesthetic solutions that are to be used for infiltration or nerve block. One purpose is to slow absorption of the drug, thereby prolonging the anesthetic action locally. The concentrations of epinephrine used for this purpose vary from 2 to 10 μg/ml, also referred to as 1:500,000 to 1:100,000. Vasoconstrictors can also enhance safety; delayed absorption depresses peak plasma concentration, thereby decreasing anesthetic toxicity. However, epinephrine used in this fashion may itself cause systemic effects such as anxiety, tachycardia, and hypertension. Although the addition of epinephrine to a drug such as procaine is useful, agents such as lidocaine, prilocaine, mepivacaine, and bupivacaine may be used without the addition of vasoconstrictors.

TOXICITY

The ester type of local anesthetics, such as procaine and tetracaine, may produce allergic reactions manifested as skin rashes or bronchospasm. Allergic reactions to the amides, such as lidocaine, are very rare if they occur at all, and there is no cross-reactivity with the esters. Consequently, allergy to an ester does not preclude use of an amide local anesthetic.

The majority of toxic reactions are a result of overdosage. Some local neurotoxicity can result from high concentrations of local anesthetics injected perineurally, but such reactions are rare.[3] The figures given in Table 37-4 refer to maximum dosages that can be administered safely to healthy adults, provided that inadvertent intravascular or subarachnoid injection is avoided.

In general the pharmacologic signs of toxicity from local anesthetics are central nervous system stimulation followed by depression and peripheral cardiovascular depression. Salivation, tremor, and convulsions, associated with hypertension and tachycardia followed by coma and hypotension, all occurring within a few minutes, characterize a full-blown episode.[4]

Treatment is symptomatic and essentially involves restoration of normal ventilation and circulation. Diazepam is used both for treatment and prevention of seizures.

CLINICAL CHARACTERISTICS

Cocaine

Cocaine is too toxic to be injected into tissues and is therefore used only topically. It produces excellent topical anesthesia and vasoconstriction, which shrinks mucous membranes. Absorption from the urinary mucous membranes is rapid, and cocaine

TABLE 37-4 Maximum safe dosages of local anesthetics administered to healthy adults

Anesthetic	mg/kg of body weight
4% cocaine	1 (topical)
1% procaine	10 (injection)
0.15% tetracaine	1 (injection)
1% lidocaine	1 (injection)
0.5% bupivacaine	2.5 (injection)

should not be used in this area. Some clinicians believe that vasoconstriction with 10% cocaine is better than that with a 4% solution and that toxicity will be less with the stronger preparation because the cocaine will be more slowly absorbed. This may be dangerous, however. The vasoconstrictor effect of cocaine and potentiation by this local anesthetic of the actions of catecholamines are most likely consequences of inhibition of catecholamine uptake by adrenergic nerve terminals. Cocaine abuse is discussed in Chapter 34.

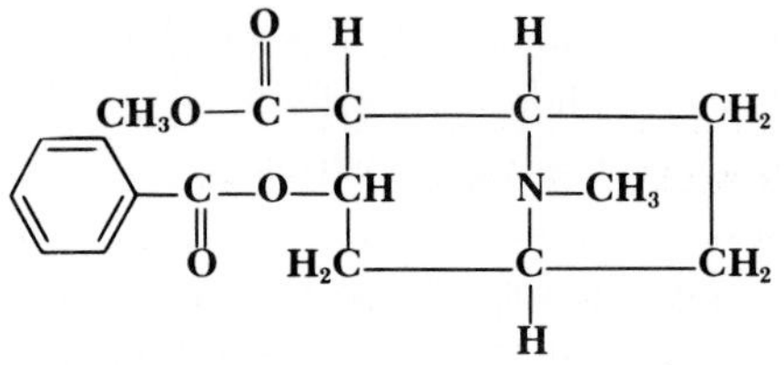

Cocaine

Benzocaine

Benzocaine (ethyl aminobenzoate) is so poorly soluble that it is not absorbed from mucous membranes. Ointments and other topical preparations containing 0.5% to 20% concentrations of the drug are available over-the-counter for topical anesthesia.

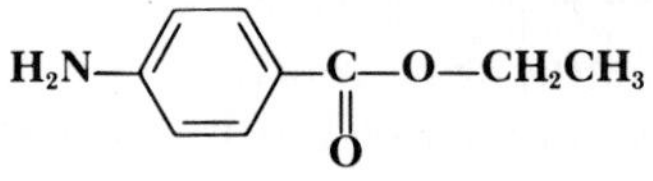

Benzocaine

Procaine

Procaine was once the standard to which all local anesthetics were compared. However, it is a poor topical anesthetic. Its duration of action is approximately 1 hour but can be significantly prolonged by the presence of epinephrine. Onset of anesthesia occurs rapidly. Procaine will block small to large nerve fibers in concentrations of 0.5% to 2%.

Chloroprocaine is a derivative of procaine that has a much shorter duration of action because of its more rapid hydrolysis.

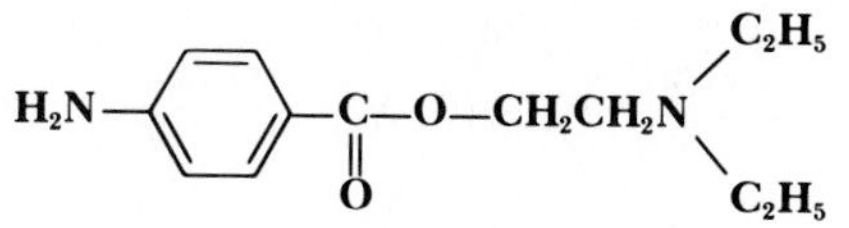

Procaine

Lidocaine

Lidocaine, in concentrations of 0.5% to 2%, has supplanted procaine as the standard of comparison for local anesthetics. It is twice as potent as procaine and is more versatile, being suitable not only for infiltration and nerve block but for surface anesthesia as well. It also has a rapid anesthetic action. Lidocaine has one other characteristic that distinguishes it from procaine and other local anesthetics—it very often produces sedation along with the anesthesia. Lidocaine is an amide rather than an ester. It is metabolized in the liver by N-dealkylation. Two of its metabolites retain activity and may contribute to toxic central nervous system reactions in patients with altered metabolism.

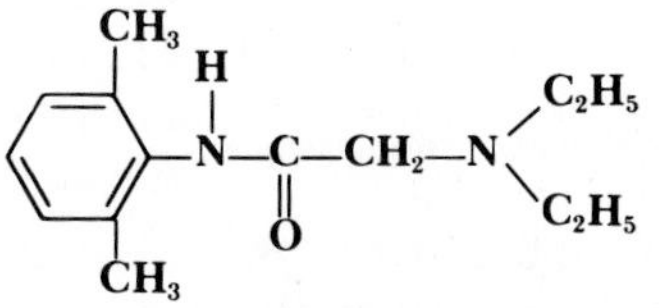

Lidocaine

Tetracaine

The chief differences between tetracaine and procaine or lidocaine are tetracaine's slower onset of maximal effect (10 minutes or more), approximately 50% longer duration of action, and greater potency. Tetracaine is available for injection in 0.2% to 1% solutions. For topical anesthesia it is used in 1% and 2% concentrations. Tetracaine should not be sprayed into the airway in concentrations greater than 2%. The total dose should be carefully calculated and probably should not, in this situation, exceed 0.5 mg/kg of body weight. The drug is rapidly absorbed topically and has resulted in several fatalities from topical misuse. The chief disadvantage of tetracaine is slowness in onset of action.

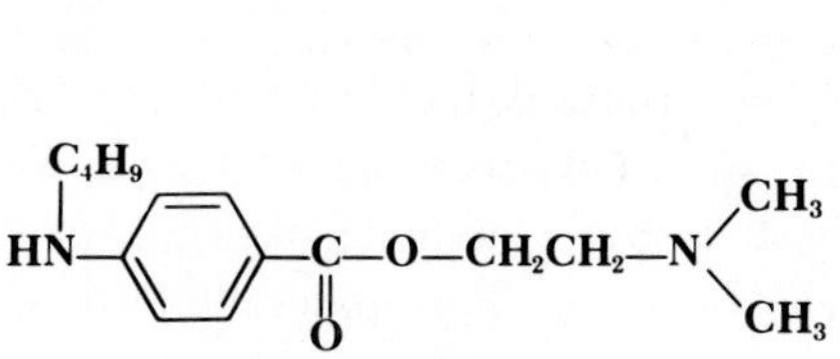

Tetracaine

Mepivacaine

Mepivacaine has essentially the same clinical activity as lidocaine, but it does not spread in the tissues quite so well, and its duration of action is longer.

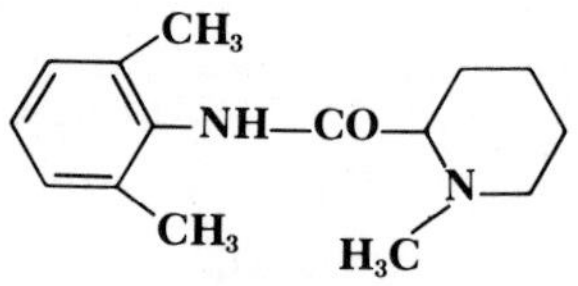

Mepivacaine

Bupivacaine

Bupivacaine is an amide chemically related to mepivacaine. It has a long duration of action, and its potency is four times greater than that of mepivacaine. Bupivacaine is used for infiltration, nerve block, and peridural anesthesia. Its adverse effects are similar to those produced by other local anesthetics. Bupivacaine is available in solutions containing 0.25% to 0.75% of the drug.

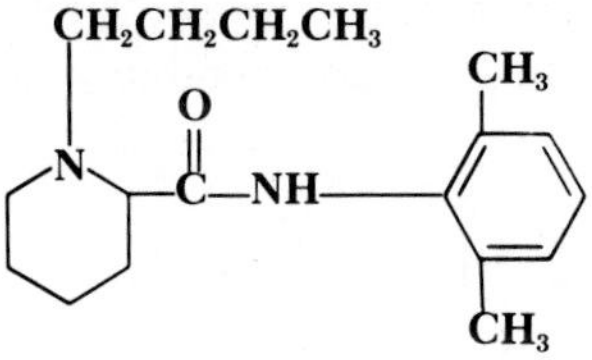

Bupivacaine

Dibucaine

Dibucaine is a potent local anesthetic with a long duration of action. It is from 10 to 20 times more potent than procaine. Dibucaine is available over-the-counter in 0.5% and 1% preparations for topical use.

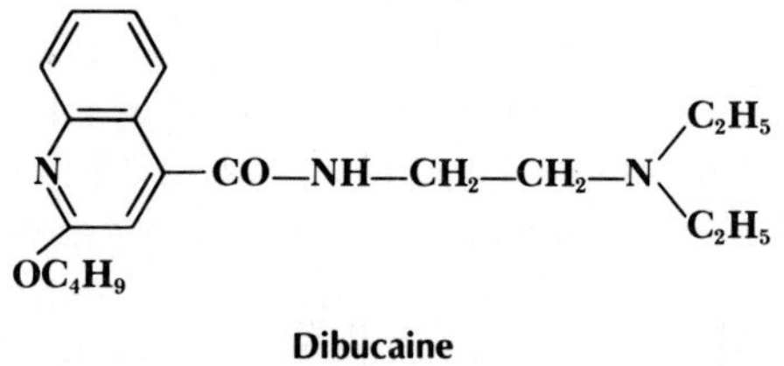

Dibucaine

CHOICE OF LOCAL ANESTHETICS

The needs of most physicians can be met by a few of the available local anesthetics. For infiltration lidocaine and bupivacaine are preferred. For spinal anesthesia tetracaine is one of the best. It has a duration of action of 2 hours or more and is hydrolyzed by plasma cholinesterase. For epidural anesthesia lidocaine (short duration) or bupivacaine (long duration) are often employed. Cocaine still has some use for topical anesthesia.

REFERENCES

1. Butterworth JF IV, Strichartz GR: Molecular mechanisms of local anesthesia: a review, *Anesthesiology* 72:711, 1990.
2. Gissen AJ, Covino BG, Gregus J: Differ-

ential sensitivities of mammalian nerve fibers to local anesthetic agents, *Anesthesiology* 53:467, 1980.
3. Reynolds F: Adverse effects of local anaesthetics, *Br J Anaesth* 59:78, 1987.
4. Scott DB: Toxicity caused by local anaesthetic drugs, *Br J Anaesth* 53:553, 1981.

ADDITIONAL READINGS

Cousins MJ, Brindenbaugh PO: *Neural blockade in clinical anesthesia and management of pain,* Philadelphia, 1980, JB Lippincott.

Stoelting RK: *Pharmacology and physiology in anesthetic practice,* Philadelphia, 1987, JB Lippincott.

section seven

Drugs used in cardiovascular disease

ALTHOUGH MANY DRUGS EXERT AN EFFECT ON THE HEART, FIVE GROUPS OF AGENTS ARE DISCUSSED IN THIS SECTION EITHER BECAUSE THEY ACT SELECTIVELY ON THE HEART OR BECAUSE THEY ARE PARTICULARLY USEFUL IN THE TREATMENT OF CARDIAC DISEASE: DIGITALIS GLYCOSIDES, ANTIARRHYTHMIC DRUGS, VASODILATOR DRUGS, ANTICOAGULANT DRUGS, AND DIURETIC DRUGS. IN ADDITION, THE HYPOCHOLESTEROLEMIC AGENTS ARE DISCUSSED. ANTIHYPERTENSIVE DRUGS ARE CONSIDERED IN CHAPTER 21.

Chapter 38

Digitalis

WILLIAM WITHERING, 1785 . . . *IT HAS A POWER OVER THE MOTION OF THE HEART, TO A DEGREE YET UNOBSERVED IN ANY OTHER MEDICINE, AND . . . THIS POWER MAY BE CONVERTED TO SALUTARY ENDS.*

GENERAL CONCEPT

Certain steroids and their glycosides have characteristic actions on contractility and electrophysiology of the heart. Most glycosides are obtained from leaves of the foxglove, *Digitalis purpurea* or *Digitalis lanata*, or from the seeds of *Strophanthus gratus*. These cardioactive steroids are used in treatment of heart failure and management of certain arrhythmias. They are collectively referred to as digitalis glycosides. Although catecholamines, methylxanthines, and glucagon also increase contractility of the myocardium, digitalis accomplishes its effect by a unique mechanism.

At the molecular level digitalis is a powerful inhibitor of sodium-potassium-adenosine triphosphatase (Na^+,K^+-ATPase). The resultant increase in Na^+ concentration within the cell enhances Ca^{++} availability to the contractile apparatus and thus increases contractility.[20]

Digitalis exerts striking actions on the *electrophysiology* of the heart. The effects are not the same in all portions of the organ. Most significant are more rapid repolarization of the ventricles (shortened electrical systole) and, in higher concentrations, increased automaticity or increased rate of diastolic depolarization with appearance of ectopic activity. The atrioventricular (AV) node is greatly affected by the glycosides. Digitalis slows conduction and prolongs the refractory period; these effects account for its use to slow transmission of impulses from the atria to the ventricles.

Digitalis toxicity is not uncommon in clinical practice.[2] However, with development of assays to monitor serum concentrations, and as changes in drug disposition in specific disease states have been characterized,[1,16] management has improved, and the occurrence of intoxication has decreased.[11]

HISTORY

The history of digitalis is an example of the discovery of an important drug from a folk remedy. William Withering,[24] having heard of a mixture of herbs that an old woman of Shropshire used successfully to treat dropsy (congestive heart failure), suspected that the beneficial properties of the mixture were attributable to the foxglove. In testing digitalis leaf, Withering was greatly impressed with its diuretic effect and believed that it probably acted on the kidney. However, he noted that the preparation had a remarkable "power over the . . . heart."

Over the years digitalis became the most important drug in treatment of congestive failure and atrial flutter and fibrillation. Now, it is used less frequently. Patients with heart failure are generally treated with diuretics and converting-enzyme inhibitors, and digitalis is added if they do not respond satisfactorily.[7] In atrial flutter and fibrillation digitalis is still used quite extensively, but some clinicians advocate use of the Ca^{++} antagonist verapamil for such patients.

EFFECTS ON THE HEART

The usefulness of digitalis in treatment of congestive failure is a consequence of its positive inotropic effect. In addition, some of its electrophysiologic actions make the drug highly useful for treatment of a variety of arrhythmias.

Contractility is enhanced by digitalis in both the normal and the failing heart. In a now classic study (Fig. 38-1), Braunwald and his co-workers demonstrated this effect in humans by attaching a Walton-Brodie strain gauge to the right ventricular myocardium of patients undergoing cardiac surgery. The effect of digitalis on contractility was also shown in the isolated heart. An idealized schema of the beneficial effect of digitalis in the failed heart is shown in Fig. 38-2. With heart failure the relationship between filling pressure and stroke work is shifted downward and to the right, that is, a greater pressure is required to generate the same cardiac output. Filling pressure

FIG. 38-1

Contractile force and arterial pressure recordings immediately and 20 minutes after injection of 1.4 mg of acetylstrophanthidin in a 28-year-old woman with an atrial septal defect. The lower tracings show contractile force recordings before injection and at intervals after acetylstrophanthidin. Notice that the drug augments the contractile force of the nonfailing human heart and constricts the systemic vascular bed as manifested by an increase in arterial pressure.

From Braunwald E, Bloodwell RD, Goldberg LI, Morrow AG: J Clin Invest 40:52, 1961.

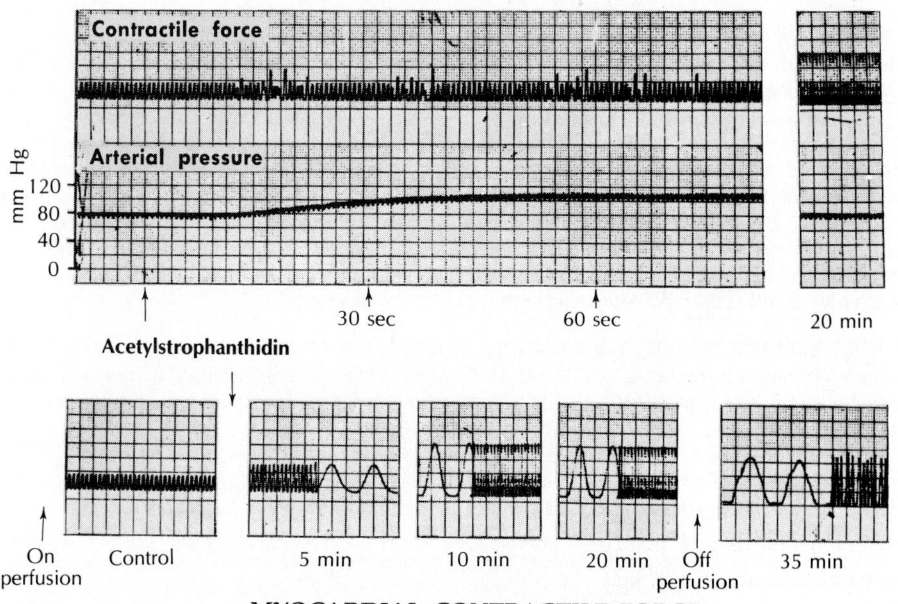

FIG. 38-2 *Effect of digitalis on left ventricular function curves. Left ventricular stroke work is a measure of ventricular performance. Notice that digitalis shifts the ventricular function curve upward and to the left; that is, myocardial contractility is increased.* CHF, *Congestive heart failure.*

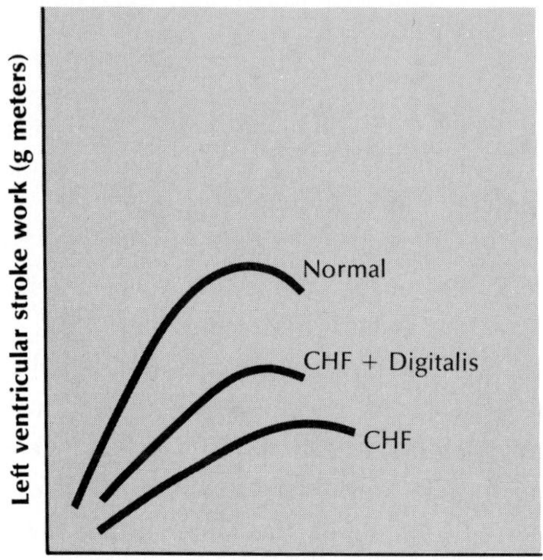

may be so great as to cause symptoms of congestive failure, including pulmonary edema. Administration of digitalis shifts this relationship toward normal.

Digitalis increases both the force and the velocity of myocardial contraction, and it shortens the duration of systole. It promotes more complete emptying of the ventricles and decreases the size of the failed heart. This reduction in heart size decreases cardiac wall tension.

PROBLEM 38-1. *Although digitalis increases the contractility of the normal as well as the failing heart, its effect on cardiac output is much greater in congestive failure. In fact, its ability to increase cardiac output in normal persons was questioned for many years.*

The explanation of this paradox is related to hemodynamic adjustments. In the normal person, digitalis not only increases cardiac contractility but also causes constriction of peripheral vessels. It may also decrease venous pressure and may slow the sinus rate. Under these circumstances no increase in cardiac output can be demonstrated despite the positive inotropic effect.

The situation is different in the failing heart. In patients with congestive failure, the peripheral resistance is already high because falling cardiac output increases sympathetic tone. Under these circumstances the positive inotropic effect of digitalis increases cardiac output because the tone of peripheral vessels is lowered as a result of decreased sympathetic tone.

PROBLEM 38-2. *Does digitalis increase the efficiency of the failing heart? It has been observed that digitalis will increase cardiac output in the failing heart without a corresponding increase in oxygen consumption. At first glance this could be interpreted as an increase in efficiency, since more work is performed by the heart per unit of oxygen consumed.*

The problem is much more complicated, however. Myocardial oxygen requirement is determined by heart rate, myocardial contractility, and wall tension, which is a function of ventricular size. In a patient with heart failure and a dilated heart, by improving cardiac function digitalis decreases sympathetic tone and heart rate. Similarly, the diuresis that occurs will decrease ventricular size. Hence overall there is a reduction in myocardial oxygen need even though contractility increased. In contrast, in a normal or nondilated heart there is no change in heart rate or ventricular size. In this setting the net result is an increase in oxygen need because of greater contractility.

Diagram of the effect of digitalis on isolated Purkinje fibers. Notice that digitalis decreases the duration of the action potential as it shortens the plateau. Refractory period is shortened. Increased rate of diastolic depolarization can result in the development of ectopic pacemaker activity. ***FIG. 38-3***

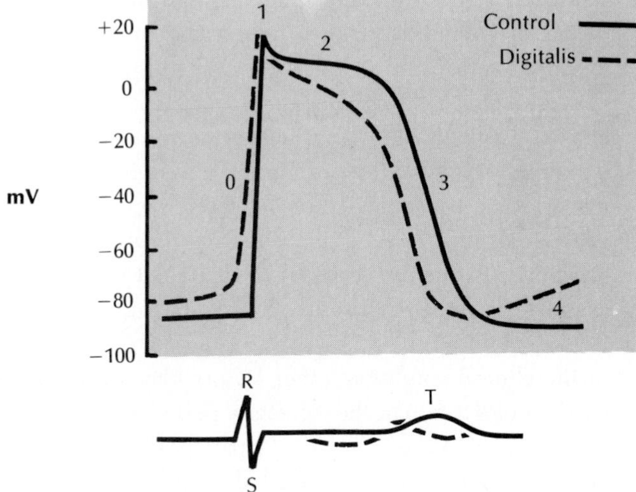

Electrophysiologic effects

The electrophysiologic effects of digitalis account for its actions on *conductivity*, *refractory period*, and *automaticity*. These effects differ among conducting tissue and ventricular and atrial muscle cells. The overall outcome of digitalis administration is complicated by the existence of both *autonomic* and *direct* actions of the glycosides and by differences in the sensitivity of normal and diseased heart to the electrophysiologic effects.

Conducting tissue

At low doses, digitalis slows AV conduction. Since this action is reversed by atropine, it is commonly referred to as a "vagal effect." The direct effect of the drug that is not reversed by atropine becomes evident with higher doses.

AV nodal conduction is prolonged by digitalis. Prolongation of the P-R interval and varying degrees of heart block are electrocardiographic manifestations of this action.

AV refractory period is also prolonged by digitalis. This action becomes important when the supraventricular rate is rapid, as in atrial flutter and fibrillation, when the purpose in using digitalis is to decrease the number of impulses reaching the ventricles.

Purkinje fibers and to a lesser extent ventricular muscle respond to digitalis with a shortening of the action potential, decreased refractory period, and the appearance of pacemaker activity as a result of increased rate of spontaneous diastolic depolarization (phase 4) (Fig. 38-3).

Ventricular and atrial muscle

By shortening the refractory period and the duration of the action potential, the Q-T interval shortens. Studies with isolated tissues imply that this effect may be dissociated from inotropy because low concentrations of digitalis increase contractility before a significant change in action potential occurs.

In the atrium, the actions of digitalis are complicated by vagal effects. Digitalis may increase release of acetylcholine and may also increase the sensitivity of the fibers to the released mediator.[20] In a normally innervated atrium, digitalis decreases the refractory period. On the other hand, in a denervated or atropine-treated atrium, digitalis may increase refractory period.

EFFECT ON HEART RATE

In normal persons, digitalis has little effect on heart rate. In congestive failure, digitalis slows the rapid sinus rhythm primarily by an indirect mechanism. The tachycardia in this case is a consequence of increased sympathetic activity brought about by decreased cardiac output. As digitalis improves cardiac output, sympathetic drive to the sinoatrial node is reduced. It should be apparent from this mechanism that digitalis is not useful in treatment of sinus tachycardia caused by fever and other conditions.

Depending on the clinical condition, other factors play a role in cardiac slowing caused by digitalis: (1) prolongation of the refractory period of the AV node when atrial rate is rapid; (2) slowing of AV conduction (a partial block may be converted to complete block); (3) reflex vagal stimulation elicited by digitalis. These mechanisms are discussed in Chapter 39.

Electrocardiographic effects

Electrocardiographic manifestations of the electrophysiologic effects are characterized by S-T segment depression, inversion of the T wave, shortened Q-T interval, and prolongation of the P-R interval. Toxic concentrations can cause AV dissociation and ventricular arrhythmias such as premature ventricular contractions, bigeminal rhythm, and ventricular fibrillation.

FUNDAMENTAL CELLULAR EFFECTS

Inhibition of Na^+,K^+-ATPase by digitalis increases intracellular Na^+. This Na^+ in turn exchanges with extracellular Ca^{++}.[20] Inhibition of the enzyme also decreases outward pumping of both Na^+ and Ca^{++}. The net effect is an increase in the Ca^{++} pool available for excitation-contraction coupling. This linkage of digitalis's effect with increased availability of intracellular Ca^{++} explains interactions observed clinically between the two. They are synergistic,[15] and Ca^{++} administration can be dangerous in digitalized patients. On the other hand, hypocalcemia causes insensitivity to digoxin.[5]

EXTRACARDIAC EFFECTS

Digitalis also has extracardiac effects that may aid recognition of impending cardiac toxicity. *Gastrointestinal effects* manifest as nausea and anorexia that are central in origin. With powdered digitalis or digitalis tincture, a local effect also contributes. *Neurologic effects* consist of blurred vision, paresthesias, and toxic psychosis. Classically described, though occurring rarely, patients may see objects with a yellow hue or see a yellow halo around objects. Toxic symptoms are often misdiagnosed, especially in elderly patients. *Endocrinologic changes* such as gynecomastia occur rarely. Allergic reactions are extremely uncommon.

Some evidence suggests that an action of digitalis on the central nervous system may contribute to arrhythmias and ventricular fibrillation.[10,22] In definitive experiments in cats, electrical activity was monitored in sympathetic, parasympathetic, and phrenic nerves before and after administration of ouabain, a short-acting digitalis compound.[10] Ouabain increased traffic in these nerves. Spinal transection prevented these effects and increased the dose of ouabain needed to elicit ventricular arrhythmias. It appears then that neural activation, probably at the level of the brainstem, plays a role in the development of digitalis-induced arrhythmias.

SOURCES AND CHEMISTRY

The cardioactive steroids and their glycosides are widely distributed in nature. Since their effects on the heart are qualitatively the same, it is sufficient to utilize only a few of them in therapeutics. The most important glycosides are as follows:

Digitalis purpurea	*Digitalis lanata*	*Strophanthus gratus*
Digitoxin	Digoxin	Ouabain
Digoxin	Lanatoside C	
Digitalis leaf	Deslanoside	

The structure of digitoxin is characterized by a steroid nucleus with an unsaturated lactone attached at the C-17 position. The three sugars attached to the C-3 position are unusual deoxyhexoses. The molecule without the sugars is called an *aglycone*, or *genin*. The steroidal structure and the unsaturated lactone are essential for cardioactivity. Removal of the sugars results in generally weaker and more evanescent activity.

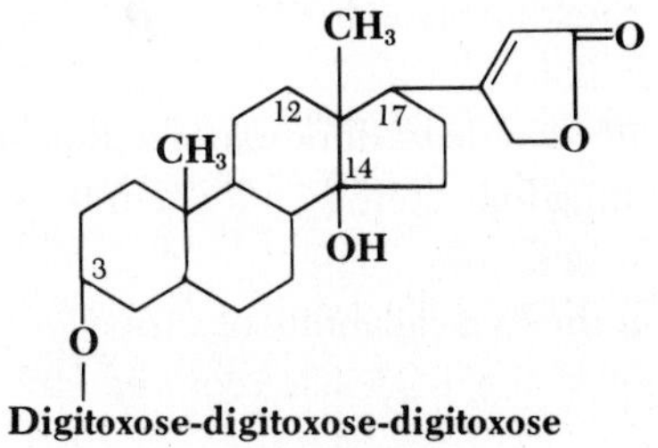

Digitoxose-digitoxose-digitoxose

Digitoxin

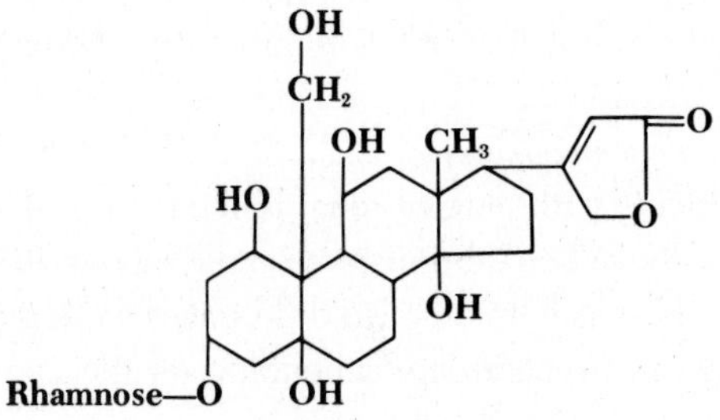

Rhamnose—O

Ouabain

Digoxin differs from digitoxin only in the presence of an OH group at the C-12 position. Lanatoside C is the parent compound of digoxin and differs from the latter in having an additional glucose molecule and an acetyl group on the oligosaccharide side chain. Removal of the acetyl group by alkaline hydrolysis yields deslanoside, and further removal of glucose by enzymatic hydrolysis gives digoxin.

Ouabain differs somewhat in its steroidal portion from the previously discussed compounds. Its aglycone is known as G-strophanthidin, and the sugar to which it is attached in the glycoside is rhamnose.

PHARMACOKINETICS AND DOSING

The clinically useful glycosides differ mainly in their kinetic characteristics, which are a reflection of their water or lipid solubility, gastrointestinal absorption, metabolism, and excretion. Digitoxin is highly lipid soluble; digoxin is less so, and ouabain is water soluble. As expected from their solubilities, digitoxin is completely absorbed from the gastrointestinal tract and persists in the body for a long time (Table 38-1). Ouabain, a highly polar compound, is not well absorbed from the gastrointestinal tract and has a relatively brief action. Digoxin is intermediate.

Digitoxin is highly bound to plasma proteins and is metabolized in the liver. In contrast, digoxin is eliminated mainly by the kidney, and renal insufficiency reduces its clearance. Therefore patients with diminished renal function require lower maintenance doses.

Elimination of the various digitalis compounds is first order. In a patient with normal renal function, the half-life of digoxin is 1.5 days. Because about a week is required to reach steady-state concentrations when maintenance dosing is instituted, a loading dose strategy is often applied to patients who need a more rapid effect. The loading dose is usually 0.75 to 1.5 mg divided into three doses several hours apart. Alternatively, a continuous infusion of the same dose can be given. In a comparative study,[19] infusion of 1.5 mg of digoxin over 6 hours provided greater efficacy and a quicker onset of effect (8 to 9 hours) than did giving 0.5 mg as an intravenous bolus on three separate occasions 8 hours apart (onset of effect 18 to 20 hours).

PREPARATIONS

Digoxin is the prototype digitalis glycoside. Physicians should usually limit themselves to this drug whenever a digitalis preparation is needed. For all digitalis glycosides the therapeutic to toxic ratios are the same, and the same caution should be exercised with all. Pure glycosides should be used rather than the older digitalis powdered leaf or other impure preparations, which must be standardized by bioassay.

DIGOXIN

Pharmacokinetics (Table 38-1). Digoxin has an intermediate duration of action in patients with normal renal function. The drug may be administered orally or intravenously. When administered orally about 75% is absorbed.

Because pronounced differences were reported in the bioavailability of various oral digoxin preparations depending on the manufacturer,[12] the FDA has required since

TABLE 38-1 Properties of digitalis preparations

Preparation	Gastro-intestinal absorption	Onset of action* (min)	Half-life†	Excretion or metabolism	Loading dose (mg)		Oral maintenance dose (mg)
					Oral	Intravenous	
Digoxin	75%	15-30	36 hr	Renal; some GI	1.25-1.5	0.75-1.0	0.25-0.5
Digitoxin	95%	25-120	5 days	Hepatic‡	0.7-1.2	1.0	0.1
Ouabain	Unreliable	5-10	21 hr	Renal; some GI	—	0.3-0.5	—
Deslanoside	Unreliable	10-30	33 hr	Renal	—	0.8	—

Modified from Smith TW: N Engl J Med 288:721, 1973.
*Intravenous administration.
†For normal subjects.
‡Enterohepatic circulation exists.
GI, Gastrointestinal.

1974 that manufacturers meet minimum specifications for tablet dissolution rate and content. As a result, all forms of digoxin marketed in the United States are essentially bioequivalent. A possible exception is an encapsulated form that appears to be consistently 80% bioavailable.

Gastrointestinal absorption of digoxin is influenced by several conditions. Decreased absorption can occur in patients with malabsorption syndromes or when cholestyramine and other resins that bind digoxin in the gut are given. Various antacids, kaolin, and pectin also reduce absorption of the glycoside.[4] In contrast, absorption can be increased by broad-spectrum antibiotics in the approximately 10% of patients who harbor digoxin-degrading bacteria in their intestinal tract. The antibiotic kills the intestinal flora and thereby decreases degradation and increases bioavailability.

Digoxin is excreted primarily by glomerular filtration but also has secretory and minor reabsorptive pathways in the renal tubules. The secretory component occurs in the distal nephron; it can be inhibited by drugs such as quinidine, verapamil, and spironolactone. The half-life of digoxin can increase to over 4 days in anuric patients.[8,13]

Oral preparations of digoxin (Lanoxin) include tablets of 0.125 to 0.5 mg, capsules (Lanoxicaps) of 0.05 to 0.2 mg, and an elixir of 0.05 mg/ml. It is also available in solution for injection, 0.1 and 0.25 mg/ml.

DIGITOXIN

Digitoxin is the main active glycoside in digitalis leaf. It is the least polar of the useful cardiac glycosides and is highly bound (97%) to plasma proteins. In contrast to digoxin, digitoxin is predominantly metabolized by the liver, and renal failure has little or no effect on elimination. Digitoxin undergoes enterohepatic circulation; if it is bound to compounds such as cholestyramine in the intestinal tract, this pathway is short circuited. Hence cholestyramine can be used to enhance its elimination, particularly in overdose settings. The half-life of digitoxin is about 5 days.

A patient receiving digitoxin therapy loses about 10% of the amount in the body each day. A loading dose is generally given to begin treatment, since on a daily maintenance dose approximately a month would be required for full digitalization. Because of its slow degradation, toxic effects persist for a long time after the drug is discontinued. This is the primary reason for the preference for digoxin. Metabolism of digitoxin is accelerated by drugs, such as phenobarbital, that induce hepatic microsomal enzymes.

Digitoxin (Crystodigin) is supplied as tablets containing 0.1 or 0.2 mg.

OUABAIN

Ouabain, a crystalline compound, is a highly polar glycoside that is suitable for intravenous injection only, because it is poorly absorbed from the gastrointestinal tract. It is commonly used in experimental work.

DESLANOSIDE

Deslanoside (Cedilanid-D), a derivative of lanatoside C, is available for injection, 0.2 mg/ml. It is poorly absorbed from the gastrointestinal tract and is rarely used.

THERAPEUTIC INDICATIONS

Digitalis is one of the principal drugs for treatment of congestive heart failure and certain arrhythmias.

Congestive heart failure

Congestive heart failure caused by a variety of underlying mechanisms responds to digitalis treatment. By increasing contractility, the drug increases cardiac output, which in turn reduces elevated ventricular end-diastolic pressure, pulmonary congestion, and venous pressure by way of a secondary diuresis.

Because digitalis has such a narrow margin of safety and because of the proven efficacy of converting-enzyme inhibitors to decrease mortality, most physicians usually initiate therapy for heart failure with an inhibitor plus a diuretic.[7] Digitalis is then added to this regimen if the patient's response is inadequate.

Arrhythmias

Atrial fibrillation, atrial flutter, and paroxysmal atrial tachycardia are important indications for the use of digitalis.

Atrial fibrillation

The main purpose of using digitalis in atrial fibrillation is to slow the ventricular rate. This is achieved by prolongation of the refractory period of the AV node, which allows fewer of the supraventricular impulses to be transmitted to the ventricle. Digitalis does not generally stop the fibrillation itself. The calcium antagonist verapamil has also been advocated for this purpose. Its advantage over digitalis is that it slows conduction through the AV node both at rest and during exercise. Digitalis is less efficacious during exercise. However, the negative inotropic effect of verapamil may be deleterious in some patients. The choice of drug should be tailored to each individual patient.

Atrial flutter

In flutter, the rapid atrial rate is accompanied by a 2:1 or 3:1 AV block. Digitalis further increases the magnitude of AV block, thus slowing the ventricular rate. As to the flutter itself, digitalis tends to convert it to fibrillation. This is probably attributable to a decrease in atrial refractory period.

Paroxysmal atrial tachycardia

Paroxysmal atrial tachycardia often responds to increased vagal activity, which can be elicited by pressure on the carotid sinus. Digitalis may act by its vagal effect. With the availability of newer drugs, digitalis is infrequently used to treat this condition.

Cor pulmonale

Digitalis should be used only rarely to treat persistent right-sided heart failure secondary to chronic obstructive lung disease. On the one hand, little beneficial effect can be demonstrated, and, on the other hand, toxicity is increased. The arterial hypoxemia of these patients increases digitalis toxicity. Other factors predisposing to toxicity include electrolyte imbalance, respiratory acidosis, and concomitant treatment with sympathomimetic agents, all of which are prevalent in such patients (see also box on the next page).

DIGITALIS POISONING

Intoxication with digitalis is relatively common and hazardous. In mild to moderate intoxication, anorexia, ventricular ectopic beats, and bradycardia may occur. These

Clinical factors modifying digitalis dosage
Clinical states that increase sensitivity to toxic effects
Acute myocardial infarction
Advanced ventricular failure
Latent disease of the AV node
Chronic pulmonary disease; hypoxemia
Hypokalemia
Hypothyroidism
Hypomagnesemia
Hypercalcemia
Clinical states that decrease sensitivity to toxic effects
Hyperthyroidism
Infancy
Hypocalcemia

Modified from Lucchesi BR: Inotropic agents and drugs used to support the failing heart. In Antonaccio M, editor: Cardiovascular pharmacology, New York, 1977, Raven Press, p 361.

may progress to nausea and vomiting, headache, malaise, and more complex ventricular arrhythmias. Severe intoxication is characterized by blurring of vision, disorientation, diarrhea, ventricular tachycardia or fibrillation, and sinoatrial and AV block.

There are several reasons for the frequency of digitalis intoxication relative to that of other drugs. Its margin of safety is low and highly variable in different patients. Furthermore, concomitant use of diuretics can cause K^+ and Mg^{++} depletion, which aggravate digitalis toxicity.

Development of methods to determine serum concentrations of digoxin and digitoxin has contributed to prevention of digitalis intoxication (Fig. 38-4). It should be stressed, however, that such determinations should not replace good clinical judgment because numerous factors influence the significance of a given serum concentration. Some of these factors are the underlying heart disease, the plasma concentrations of K^+ and Mg^{++}, and endocrine factors. When digoxin serum concentration is determined, the blood sample should be obtained at least 6 (and preferably 8) hours after an oral dose to avoid sampling during the distribution phase.

Drug interactions and digitalis intoxication

In addition to the interactions noted previously, there are other drug interactions of clinical significance (Table 38-2). Digoxin toxicity is enhanced by quinidine.[3] When therapeutic doses of quinidine are administered to patients maintained on digoxin, there is on average a doubling of the plasma digoxin concentration. The exact mechanism of this interaction remains controversial. However, in most of these patients renal clearance of digoxin decreases, and many exhibit a reduced volume of distribution.[3,13] If it is judged clinically necessary to administer digoxin and quinidine concomitantly, serum digoxin concentration should be monitored closely so that appropriate dosage adjustments can be made. Physicians should anticipate this interaction and halve the digoxin dose to maintain the same serum concentration.

FIG. 38-4 *Serum digoxin and digitoxin concentrations related in general to effects.*

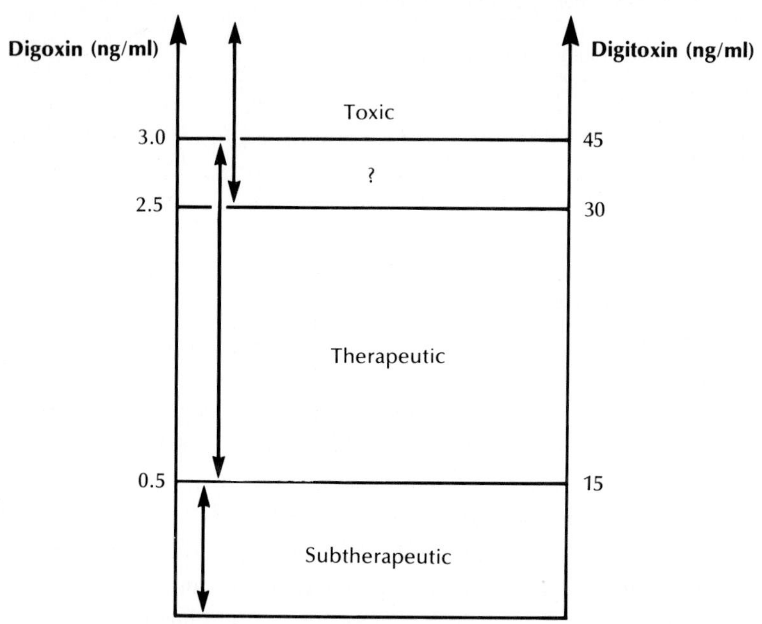

TABLE 38-2 Drug interactions with digoxin (see also Chapter 70)

Drug	Effect	Mechanism
Amphotericin B	↑	Induces hypokalemia
Cholestyramine, colestipol	↓	Binds digoxin in gastrointestinal tract; interferes with enterohepatic circulation
Quinidine	↑	Decreases renal clearance of digoxin
Spironolactone	↑	Inhibits tubular secretion of digoxin
Thiazides, furosemide, bumetanide	↑	Diuretic-induced hypokalemia and/or hypomagnesemia potentiate digitalis action
Verapamil, diltiazem	↑	Decreases renal clearance of digoxin

↑, Enhances digitalis effect; ↓, diminishes digitalis effect.

Treatment of digitalis poisoning

The most important measure in the treatment of digitalis poisoning is discontinuation of the drug. Potassium chloride by mouth or by slow intravenous infusion may be helpful in stopping ventricular arrhythmias. It should be remembered, however, that an elevated K^+ concentration may aggravate AV block, although K^+ may lessen the block if plasma K^+ is low. It is believed by many investigators that infusion of K^+ in a digitalized patient may produce an abnormally high plasma concentration because the effect of the glycosides on the membrane ATPase in various tissues prevents K^+ entry into cells. The antiarrhythmic drugs phenytoin and lidocaine are used occasionally in digitalis poisoning. Purified Fab fragments of digoxin-specific antibodies (digoxin immune Fab [ovine], Digibind) have been used successfully in patients with advanced, life-threatening digitalis toxicity.[21] The fragments bind digitalis and sequester it in plasma, away from tissue sites. Thus the toxic effects abate even though a very elevated concentration of the glycoside may be present in plasma (bound to Fab and thereby inactive). The Fab-digitalis is then excreted by the kidney. Hemoperfusion, a technique that passes the patient's blood over an adsorbing substance such as charcoal, has been used to accelerate digitalis elimination in patients poisoned with digoxin[18] and digitoxin.[9] With the availability of Fab fragments, such treatment should rarely be needed.

NEWER INOTROPIC AGENTS

Dobutamine (Dobutrex) hydrochloride is a derivative of isoproterenol. It increases myocardial contractility but causes less tachycardia or peripheral arterial effects.[14] Available in vials of 250 mg for reconstitution and administration by intravenous infusion, the drug may be useful in heart failure without severe hypotension. In cardiogenic shock with severe hypotension, dobutamine cannot elevate blood pressure adequately, since it does not increase peripheral resistance. Other vasoconstrictors are used concomitantly in this setting. Because the electrophysiologic effects of dobutamine are similar to those of isoproterenol, the drug may increase heart rate. In the presence of coronary artery disease ischemia may be aggravated.

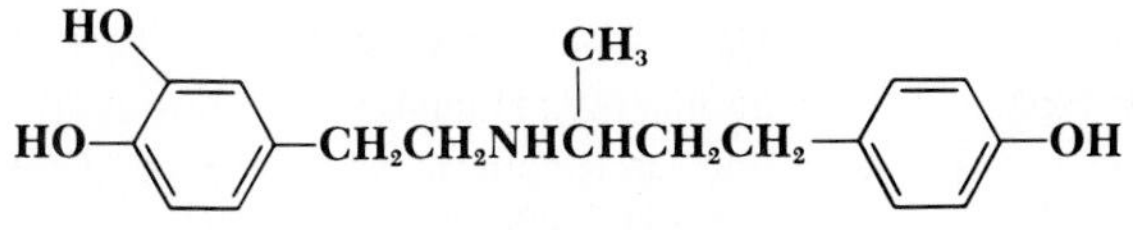

HO, HO–C$_6$H$_3$–$CH_2CH_2NHCH(CH_3)CH_2CH_2$–C$_6H_4$–OH

Dobutamine

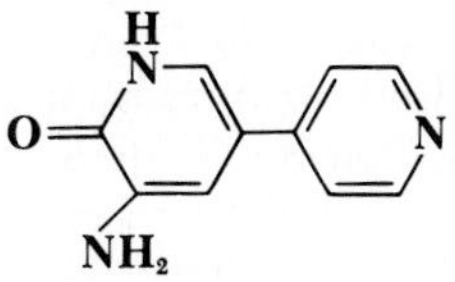

Amrinone

Amrinone lactate (Inocor) is the first of a new series of inotropic agents that differ in mode of action from digitalis and β-adrenergic receptor agonists.[23] These drugs appear to inhibit cardiac phosphodiesterase selectively.[6,17] They are bipyridine derivatives with positive inotropic activity in a variety of experimental preparations. In patients with congestive heart failure who have not responded adequately to digitalization, amrinone and milrinone (experimental) further increase resting cardiac output while decreasing left ventricular end-diastolic, pulmonary capillary wedge, and right atrial pressures as well as systemic vascular resistance. The exact mechanism of action of such compounds remains unclear, though they are believed to influence excitation-contraction coupling in cardiac muscle. Whether the increased inotropy in patients is direct or indirect as a result of decreased afterload is uncertain.

Amrinone, though efficacious, has considerable toxicity with chronic administration. As a result, only the intravenous formulation (5 mg/ml) has been marketed, to be used for short-term treatment of severe refractory heart failure. When used in this fashion, a loading dose of 0.75 mg/kg is administered, followed by a maintenance infusion of 5 to 10 μg/kg/min.[6,17]

REFERENCES

1. Aronson JK: Clinical pharmacokinetics of cardiac glycosides in patients with renal dysfunction, *Clin Pharmacokinet* 8:155, 1983.
2. Beller GA, Smith TW, Abelmann WH, et al: Digitalis intoxication: a prospective clinical study with serum level correlations, *N Engl J Med* 284:989, 1971.
3. Bigger JT, Jr, Leahey EB Jr: Quinidine and digoxin: an important interaction, *Drugs* 24:229, 1982.
4. Brown DD, Juhl RP: Decreased bioavailability of digoxin due to antacids and kaolin-pectin, *N Engl J Med* 295:1034, 1976.
5. Chopra D, Janson P, Sawin CT: Insensitivity to digoxin associated with hypocalcemia, *N Engl J Med* 296:917, 1977.
6. Colucci WS, Wright RF, Braunwald E: New positive inotropic agents in the treatment of congestive heart failure: mechanisms of action and recent clinical developments, *N Engl J Med* 314:290,349, 1986.
7. Deedwania PC: Angiotensin-converting enzyme inhibitors in congestive heart failure, *Arch Intern Med* 150:1798, 1990.
8. Doherty JE, de Soyza N, Kane JJ, et al: Clinical pharmacokinetics of digitalis glycosides, *Prog Cardiovasc Dis* 21:141, 1978.
9. Gilfrich H-J, Kasper W, Meinertz T, et al: Treatment of massive digitoxin overdose by charcoal haemoperfusion and cholestyramine, *Lancet* 1:505, 1978.
10. Gillis RA, Raines A, Sohn YJ, et al: Neuroexcitatory effects of digitalis and their role in the development of cardiac arrhythmias, *J Pharmacol Exp Ther* 183:154, 1972.
11. Henry DA, Lowe JM, Lawson DH, Whiting B: The changing pattern of toxicity to digoxin, *Postgrad Med J* 57:358, 1981.
12. Huffman DH, Azarnoff DL: Absorption of orally given digoxin preparations, *JAMA* 222:957, 1972.
13. Koren G: Clinical pharmacokinetic significance of the renal tubular secretion of digoxin, *Clin Pharmacokinet* 13:334, 1987.
14. Morgan DJ: Clinical pharmacokinetics of β-agonists, *Clin Pharmacokinet* 18:270, 1990.
15. Nola GT, Pope S, Harrison DC: Assessment of the synergistic relationship between serum calcium and digitalis, *Am Heart J* 79:499, 1970.
16. Ochs HR, Greenblatt DJ, Bodem G, Dengler HJ: Disease-related alterations in cardiac glycoside disposition, *Clin Pharmacokinet* 7:434, 1982.
17. Rocci ML Jr, Wilson H: The pharmacokinetics and pharmacodynamics of newer inotropic agents, *Clin Pharmacokinet* 13:91, 1987.
18. Smiley JW, March NM, Del Guercio ET: Hemoperfusion in the management of digoxin toxicity, *JAMA* 240:2736, 1978.
19. Smit AJ, Scaf AHJ, van Essen LH, et al: Digoxin infusion versus bolus injection in rapid atrial fibrillation: relation between serum level and response, *Eur J Clin Pharmacol* 38:335, 1990.
20. Smith TW: Digitalis: mechanisms of action and clinical use, *N Engl J Med* 318:358, 1988.
21. Smith TW, Butler VP Jr, Haber E, et al: Treatment of life-threatening digitalis intoxication with digoxin-specific Fab antibody fragments: experience in 26 cases, *N Engl J Med* 307:1357, 1982.
22. Somberg JC, Smith TW: Localization of the neurally mediated arrhythmogenic properties of digitalis, *Science* 204:321, 1979.
23. Ward A, Brogden RN, Heel RC, et al: Amrinone: a preliminary review of its pharmacological properties and therapeutic use, *Drugs* 26:468, 1983.
24. Withering W: An account of the foxglove, and some of its medicinal uses: with practical remarks on dropsy, and other diseases, London, 1785, CGJ and J Robinson; reprinted in *Medical Classics* 2:305, 1937.

Chapter 39

Antiarrhythmic drugs

GENERAL CONCEPTS

Antiarrhythmic drugs are used to prevent and treat disorders of cardiac rhythm that have high morbidity and mortality. Major advances have taken place in our understanding of cardiac electrophysiology and of the modes of action of antiarrhythmic compounds. In general, cardiac arrhythmias can be considered to arise from abnormal conduction, abnormal impulse initiation, or both.[27]

Antiarrhythmic agents have been placed into four groups on the basis of their electrophysiologic effects (Table 39-1). *Class I* drugs depress the fast inward Na^+ current in cardiac muscle, thereby prolonging the effective refractory period and reducing phase 4 depolarization. These agents have been further divided into subclasses. *Class II* drugs, the β-adrenergic blocking agents, reduce sympathetic stimulation of the heart and inhibit phase 4 depolarization, especially that augmented by catecholamines. *Class III* agents prolong the action potential and refractory period. Finally, *Class IV* drugs selectively block the slow Ca^{++} channel.

CARDIAC ELECTROPHYSIOLOGY

An understanding of the pharmacology of antiarrhythmic drugs requires some knowledge of cardiac electrophysiology. Fig. 39-1 depicts a normal cardiac action potential from a Purkinje fiber. The resting cell membrane potential is approximately -90 mV, with the inside of the cell electronegative relative to the outside. This negative potential results primarily from a transmembrane K^+ gradient maintained by Na^+,K^+-ATPase. If the cell is adequately stimulated, there is rapid influx of Na^+ through specific membrane channels. This rapid depolarization (phase 0) of ventricular

TABLE 39-1 Classification of antiarrhythmic drugs

Class I: blockade of fast sodium ion channel
- A. *Quinidine-like:* quinidine, procainamide, disopyramide, moricizine
- B. *Lidocaine-like:* lidocaine, mexiletine, tocainide
- C. *Flecainide-like:* flecainide, encainide, propafenone, indecainide, lorcainide*, aprindine*
- Phenytoin

Class II: β-adrenergic antagonists, propafenone

Class III: repolarization prolonging
- Bretylium, amiodarone, *N*-acetylprocainamide (acecainide),* sotalol*

Class IV: calcium ion-channel blockade
- Verapamil

*Investigational drug.

tissue corresponds to the QRS complex of the surface electrocardiogram. As Na^+ influx decreases, the cell membrane starts to repolarize (that is, becomes more negative), resulting in phase 1 of the action potential. In addition, a second inward current, arising primarily from movement of Ca^{++}, begins. This Ca^{++} influx maintains a depolarized state and is primarily responsible for phase 2 (the plateau) of the action potential. Finally, both inward Na^+ and Ca^{++} currents decline, and rapid repolarization (phase 3) occurs as a result of K^+ efflux. In essence, the action potential is a coordinated sequence of ion movements; initially Na^+ rapidly enters the cell, followed by Ca^{++} influx and finally K^+ efflux, which returns the cell to its resting state. Several antiarrhythmic drugs exert their effects by altering these ion fluxes.

ELECTROPHYSIOLOGIC BASIS OF ANTIARRHYTHMIC ACTION

Most tachyarrhythmias are consequences of two basic mechanisms:[27,35] ectopic focal activity and reentry. With ectopic focal activity a potential pacemaker fires independently, either because of an increase in the slope of diastolic depolarization, or because the threshold potential for discharge has become more negative, or because of a decrease in the maximum diastolic potential.[32] Myocardial ischemia, excessive catecholamine action, stretching of the myocardium, and cardiac glycoside toxicity can be causal.

The conditions necessary for reentry to occur are as follows:[35] (1) the conduction pathway must be blocked in a unidirectional fashion; (2) there must be slow conduction over an alternate route to a point beyond the block; and (3) there must be delayed excitation beyond the block. With a sufficient delay in excitation beyond the block, the

FIG. 39-1 *Cardiac action potential as recorded from a Purkinje fiber* (top) *and a ventricular fiber electrogram* (bottom). *Phases of the action potential are indicated by 0, 1, 2, 3, and 4. Major changes in transmembrane conductance* (g) *of the important ions are also indicated.*

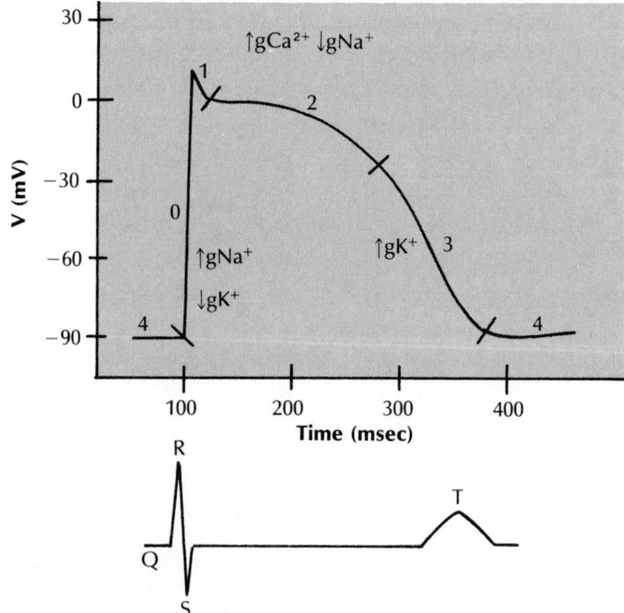

tissue proximal to the block can be excited from the opposite direction and a circular (reentry) circuit is then established. These principles are illustrated in Fig. 39-2.

The various classes of antiarrhythmic drugs have characteristic electrophysiologic effects on the myocardium, modified in some instances by extracardiac effects.

Class I antiarrhythmic drugs have local anesthetic properties. Their effects are depicted in Fig. 39-3, with quinidine as an example. They slow the fast inward Na^+ current and, by so doing, reduce the maximum rate of depolarization; this is manifest as a more shallow slope of phase 0 depolarization. These drugs also increase the threshold of excitability because resting membrane potential becomes more negative, as compared with an ectopic pacemaker. Conduction velocity is slowed, and the effective refractory period is prolonged. Spontaneous diastolic depolarization in pacemaker cells is decreased and manifests as a flattening of phase 4. The decrease in diastolic depolarization tends to suppress ectopic focal activity. Prolongation of the refractory period tends to abolish reentry. These drugs generally increase the duration of the action potential, but lidocaine, its derivatives, and phenytoin differ from other members of the class in shortening the action potential. Quinidine, procainamide, and disopyramide also have anticholinergic activity.

Class II antiarrhythmic drugs are the β-adrenergic receptor blocking agents such as propranolol. Their β-blocking action is much more important than any local anesthetic activity they may have. Their mode of action is related to depression of the slope of spontaneous diastolic depolarization (phase 4).

FIG. 39-2

Schema of reentry in the Purkinje system. Purkinje fiber (P) *in the distal ventricular conducting system divides into two branches* (a *and* b) *before making contact with ventricular muscle* (VM) *to form a loop. Panel A shows the sequence of activation under normal conditions; the sinus impulse descends via the main Purkinje bundle leading to the loop, conducts through both branches* (a *and* b) *into ventricular muscle, collides, and terminates. Panel B shows the pattern of activation when an area of unidirectional conduction block is present* (shaded area in branch b). *Conduction is blocked in the antegrade direction in b but not in the retrograde direction (from VM to b). The impulse in limb a conducts slowly around the loop and returns to the site of antegrade block in limb b. Because retrograde conduction can occur, this impulse is able to conduct. In panel* C *the impulse traveling retrogradely past the site of antegrade block into* b *conducts into* P *after the refractory period has passed so that depolarization can occur and give rise to a reciprocal beat. It may also continue the "circus" via limb* a, *to produce repetitive reciprocal beats. The rate of this reciprocal beating will be determined by the total conduction time around the loop.*

From Vera A, Mason DT: Am Heart J, 101:329, 1981.

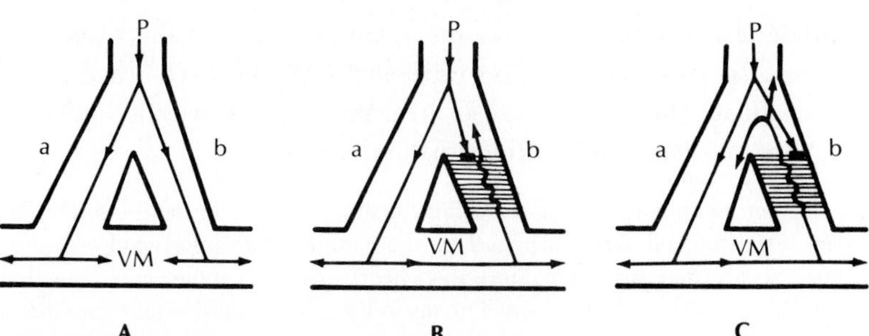

FIG. 39-3 *Diagram of the effect of quinidine on the transmembrane electrical potential of a spontaneously depolarizing conductive fiber in the ventricular myocardium.*

Modified from Mason DT et al: Clin Pharmacol Ther 11:460, 1970.

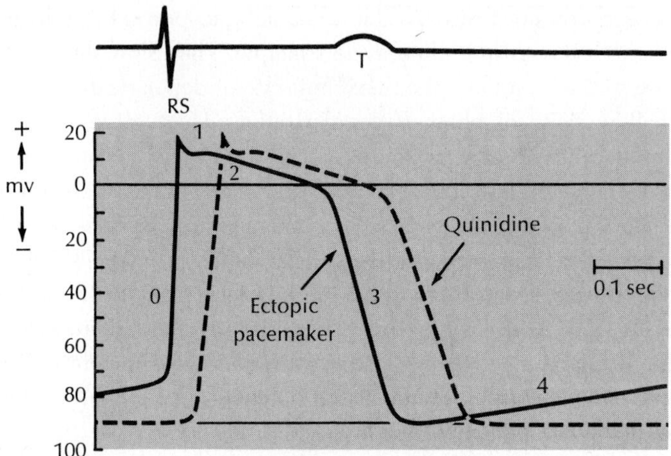

Class III antiarrhythmic drugs appear to act by prolonging the action potential, an effect associated with prolongation of the effective refractory period.

Class IV antiarrhythmic drugs selectively block the slow inward current (slow response) carried primarily by Ca^{++}.[1,24] Verapamil reduces the action potential amplitude in the upper- and mid-AV nodal regions and prolongs the time-dependent recovery of excitability and the effective refractory period of AV nodal fibers. These effects block conduction of premature impulses in the AV node.

CLASS I ANTIARRHYTHMIC DRUGS

Quinidine

Quinidine is the dextrorotatory isomer of quinine.

HOCH—CH—N—CH₂ / CH₂ / CH₂ / CH_3O / N / H_2C—CH—CHCH=CH_2

Quinidine

The introduction of quinidine into therapeutics is one of the classic stories of medical history. In 1914 the Viennese cardiologist Wenckebach[36] had a Dutch sea captain as a patient. The captain had an irregular pulse as a consequence of atrial fibrillation. Wenckebach described the situation in this way:

> He did not feel great discomfort during the attack but, as he said, being a Dutch merchant, used to good order in his affairs, he would like to have good order in his heart business also and asked why there were heart specialists if they could not abolish this very disagreeable phenomenon. On my telling him that I could promise him

> nothing, he told me that he knew himself how to get rid of his attacks, and as I did not believe him he promised to come back the next morning with a regular pulse, and he did. It happens that quinine in many countries, especially in countries where there is a good deal of malaria, is a sort of drug for everything, just as one takes acetylsalicylic acid today if one does not feel well or is afraid of having taken cold. Occasionally, taking the drug during an attack of fibrillation, the patient found that the attack was stopped within from twenty to twenty-five minutes, and later he found that a gram of quinine regularly abolished his irregularity.*
>
> *From Beckman H: Treatment in general practice, ed 2, Philadelphia, 1934, WB Saunders, p 516.

In 1918 Frey[12] tested drugs related to quinine in patients with atrial fibrillation and introduced quinidine into cardiac therapy. During the succeeding years the antifibrillatory effect of quinidine was confirmed, but its widespread use led to several sudden deaths. Eventually definite contraindications to use of the drug were recognized. In the presence of conduction defects it may produce cardiac standstill and should be avoided. Once its mode of action was understood and the contraindications were identified, quinidine reached its present position in cardiac therapy.

Cardiac effects

Quinidine is useful in both supraventricular and ventricular tachyarrhythmias. In many patients it converts atrial tachyarrhythmias to normal sinus rhythm.

A complicating factor in use of quinidine is its "vagolytic" or anticholinergic action, which tends to predominate at low plasma quinidine concentrations. This action increases conduction through the AV node and accounts for the paradoxical tachycardia seen in some patients during treatment of atrial flutter with AV block. At therapeutic plasma concentrations the direct electrophysiologic actions of quinidine predominate.

Electrocardiographic effects. Quinidine in higher doses prolongs the P-R, QRS, and Q-T intervals (Fig. 39-4). Widening of the QRS complex is related to slowed conduction in the His-Purkinje system and in ventricular muscle. Changes in the Q-T interval and alterations in T waves are related to changes in repolarization. The direct effect of the drug on AV conduction and refractoriness of the AV system explains the prolongation of the P-R interval.

Extracardiac and adverse effects

Quinidine tends to depress all muscle tissue, including vascular smooth muscle and skeletal muscle. When it is rapidly injected intravenously, sufficient vasodilatation can develop to cause profound hypotension and shock. The vasodilatation is at least partially caused by blockade of α-adrenergic receptors. The effect of quinidine on skeletal muscle becomes particularly evident in patients with myasthenia gravis, in whom it exacerbates weakness.

Cinchonism induced by quinidine is characterized by ringing of the ears and dizziness and is the same syndrome produced by quinine or salicylates. Quinidine commonly causes adverse gastrointestinal effects, particularly diarrhea, which is probably the most common reason patients cannot tolerate the drug.

Quinidine-induced thrombocytopenia appears to have an immune basis. Typically, a patient taking quinidine for several weeks notices the development of petechial

FIG. 39-4 *Effect of quinidine on electrocardiogram. Notice changes in P wave, QRS complex, and T wave at varying dose levels.*

From Burch GE, Winsor T: A primer of electrocardiography, Philadelphia, 1960, Lea & Febiger.

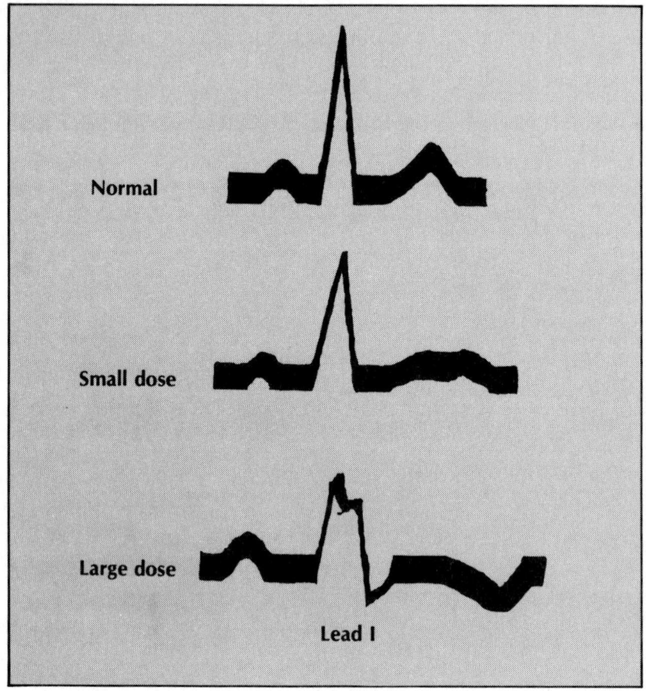

hemorrhages. The symptoms disappear when the drug is discontinued and reappear after reinstitution of therapy. This disorder is attributed to formation of a plasma protein-quinidine complex that evokes antibodies that destroy the platelets.[15]

Quinidine is a highly specific inhibitor of cytochrome P-450 IID6, the isoenzyme that metabolizes debrisoquin, sparteine, and many other drugs.[6] Thus patients taking quinidine are converted to the poor metabolizer phenotype for all drugs metabolized by this enzyme.

CARDIOTOXICITY

Quinidine can elicit effects termed "proarrhythmic" and may paradoxically cause ventricular arrhythmias and even ventricular fibrillation. So-called quinidine syncope is probably a consequence of the latter. Quinidine is particularly dangerous in patients with conduction defects. In such patients, when conduction is further impaired and automaticity of the Purkinje system is depressed, the ventricles may not take over when AV conduction fails, and cardiac standstill may ensue. Administration of the drug should be stopped when significant QRS widening or Q-T prolongation supervenes during treatment. In addition, patients who have Q-T prolongation for other reasons (for examples, genetic variants or tricyclic antidepressant overdose) are at risk of quinidine-induced ventricular arrhythmias. Quinidine and other Class I antiarrhythmics should be avoided in such patients.

PHARMACOKINETICS

When given orally, quinidine sulfate is rapidly absorbed, with the peak concentration occurring in about 1.5 hours. Quinidine gluconate is absorbed more slowly, reaching peak concentration about 4 hours after a dose.[14] The more prolonged absorption of the gluconate results in lower peak concentrations, but allows it to be administered less frequently than the sulfate. About 10% to 50% of administered quinidine is excreted unchanged. The amount is influenced by urinary pH, though at physiologic ranges of pH this effect is unlikely to be clinically important. The rest is hydroxylated in the liver. An important kinetic interaction of quinidine with digoxin is noted in Chapter 38.

ADMINISTRATION AND DOSAGE

The usual initial adult dosage of quinidine is 600 to 900 mg daily. The actual dose and dosage interval vary with the formulation, the effects of disease, and individual variations in kinetics. Optimum therapy requires monitoring of serum concentrations.

Quinidine gluconate is available for intramuscular injection. Intravenous administration requires caution; if used, the infusion should be very slow and careful monitoring must be employed. Additional information on preparations of antiarrhythmic drugs is given in Table 39-2.

Procainamide

DEVELOPMENT AS CARDIAC DRUG

The commonly used local anesthetic procaine was shown by Mautz[23] in 1936 to elevate the threshold to electrical stimulation when applied to the myocardium of animals. In subsequent years thoracic surgeons and anesthesiologists frequently used topical procaine to reduce premature ventricular and atrial contractions during surgery. Procaine was even administered intravenously for this purpose.

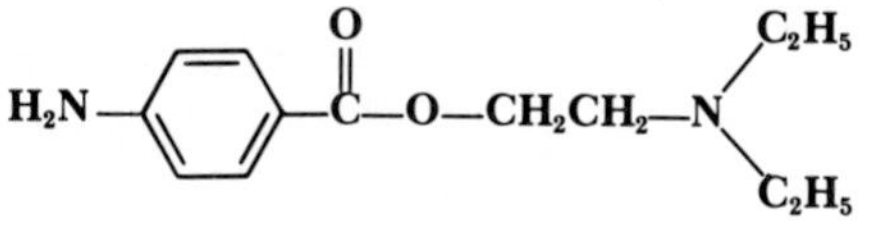

$H_2N-C_6H_4-C(=O)-O-CH_2CH_2-N(C_2H_5)_2$

Procaine

$H_2N-C_6H_4-CONH-CH_2CH_2-N(C_2H_5)_2$

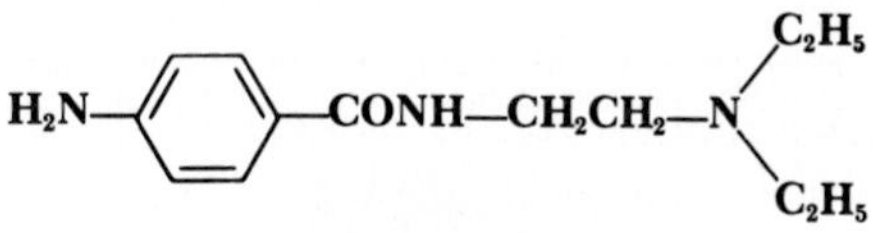

Procainamide

Encouraged by such results, investigators studied the antifibrillatory activities of compounds related to procaine and found that if the ester linkage in procaine was replaced by an amide linkage, the resulting compound had distinct advantages as an antiarrhythmic drug, that is, greater stability in the body and fewer central nervous system effects. Procainamide is so similar in its actions to quinidine that the two drugs can be used interchangeably in most patients.

EXTRACARDIAC EFFECTS AND TOXICITY

Large intravenous doses of procainamide may decrease blood pressure. This is probably a consequence of vascular smooth muscle relaxation and depressed myocardial contractility. Although the drug has local anesthetic properties, it is not useful for nerve block. Nausea, anorexia, mental confusion, hallucinations, skin rashes, agranulocytosis, chills, and fever have been reported after the use of procainamide.

Quinidine is preferred by some physicians for prolonged oral use because procainamide can cause a lupus erythematosus–like syndrome characterized by rheumatic

TABLE 39-2 Preparations of antiarrhythmic drugs

Drug	Dosage forms* (mg)
Class I	
Quinidine sulfate (Cin-Quin, others)	C: 200,300; T: 100-300; I: 200/ml
Quinidine gluconate (Quinaglute, others)	T: 324,330; I: 80/ml
Quinidine polygalacturonate (Cardioquin)	T: 275
Procainamide hydrochloride (Pronestyl, others)	C: 250-500; T: 250-1000; I: 100,500/ml
Disopyramide (Norpace, Napamide) phosphate	C: 100,150
Moricizine hydrochloride (Ethmozine)	T: 200-300
Lidocaine hydrochloride (Xylocaine)	I: 2-8/ml,† 10-200/ml
Mexiletine hydrochloride (Mexitil)	C: 150-250
Tocainide hydrochloride (Tonocard)	T: 400,600
Flecainide acetate (Tambocor)	T: 100
Encainide hydrochloride (Enkaid)	C: 25-50
Propafenone hydrochloride (Rythmol)	T: 150,300
Phenytoin (Dilantin)	S: 30,125/5ml; T: 50
Phenytoin sodium (Dilantin, Diphenylan)	C: 30,100; I: 50/ml
Class II	
Esmolol hydrochloride (Brevibloc)	I: 10, 250/ml
Class III	
Bretylium tosylate (Bretylol)	I: 50/ml
Amiodarone hydrochloride (Cordarone)	T: 200
Class IV	
Verapamil hydrochloride (Calan, Isoptin)	T: 40-240; I: 2.5/ml

**C*, Capsules; *I*, injection; *S*, suspension; *T*, tablets.
†Specifically for infusion.

symptoms, pleuropericardial inflammation, and antinuclear antibodies.[4] On the other hand, procainamide is safer than quinidine when used intravenously and has fewer gastrointestinal side effects.

PHARMACOKINETICS

Procainamide is absorbed well from the gastrointestinal tract and is 15% protein bound. The liver converts it to *N*-acetylprocainamide (see p. 435). The rate of acetylation is genetically determined, and patients may be fast or slow acetylators. The latter have an earlier onset of and a higher prevalence of procainamide-induced lupus, compared with rapid acetylators.[37] Renal disease decreases the clearance of procainamide to some degree but has a major effect on its metabolite, which is predominately excreted. Regular and sustained-release preparations of procainamide are available.

Disopyramide

Disopyramide resembles quinidine and procainamide in its actions.[5] However, its considerable anticholinergic and negative inotropic activities limit its use. The drug is absorbed well from the gastrointestinal tract. Renal impairment decreases its clearance.

Disopyramide may cause or worsen congestive heart failure or produce severe hypotension as a consequence of its negative inotropic property. This is most likely to occur in patients with marginally compensated underlying cardiac failure.[26] Disopyramide is administered as a racemic mixture, but its antiarrhythmic activity resides primarily, if not entirely, in the S-enantiomer.[21] Both the S- and R-stereoisomers are negative inotropes. Thus use of the racemic mixture enhances the adverse action on cardiac contractility with no gain in terms of arrhythmia suppression. It is unfortunate that the drug was not developed as the pure S-enantiomer. Because of its anticholinergic action disopyramide should not be given to patients with glaucoma, myasthenia gravis, or urinary retention. Disopyramide is administered every 6 hours to patients with normal renal function.

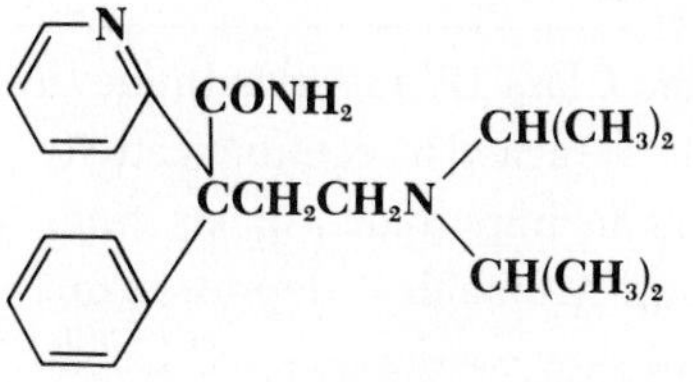

N
$CONH_2$
$CH(CH_3)_2$
CCH_2CH_2N
$CH(CH_3)_2$

Disopyramide

Moricizine

Moricizine, though a phenothiazine compound, does not affect brain dopaminergic activity in animal models.[11] In the heart it causes frequency-dependent inhibition of the fast Na^+ current during phase 0 of the action potential. It also slows conduction throughout the heart. Unlike disopyramide, moricizine does not appear to have negative inotropic activity and may therefore prove particularly useful in patients with impaired cardiac function.

The response to moricizine does not relate to its plasma concentration, and there is speculation that one or more of its numerous metabolites contribute to or account for its antiarrhythmic effects.

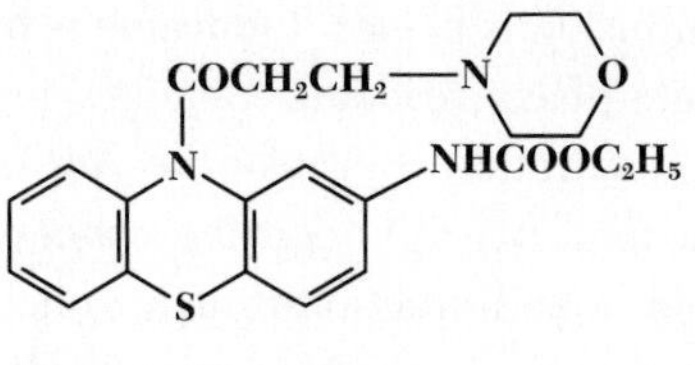

$COCH_2CH_2$—N O
N
$NHCOOC_2H_5$
S

Moricizine

ADVERSE EFFECTS

Moricizine infrequently causes gastrointestinal and central nervous system effects, including oral paresthesias, dizziness, and headache. The incidence of proarrhythmic effects with moricizine is low (about 3%) and may be less than with Class IC compounds.

Pharmacokinetics

Moricizine is extensively distributed to tissues (volume of distribution about 2.5 L/kg) despite marked protein binding (98%). It is rapidly converted by the liver (half-life = 2 to 4 hr) to numerous, as yet poorly characterized, metabolites. Pharmacologic activity is delayed relative to plasma concentration and persists after the drug is no longer detectable. These observations imply that efficacy is related to drug concentration in a "deep" compartment or that one or more metabolites account for activity, at least in part.

Dosing

Therapy of symptomatic or life-threatening arrhythmias is started with 600 mg per day in three divided doses. Total daily dosage can be increased by 150 mg increments to a maximum of 900 mg. Although thrice daily dosing is recommended, two doses per day are probably sufficient.

Lidocaine

Lidocaine, the prototypic Class IB antiarrhythmic drug, is the agent most widely used to treat and prevent ventricular ectopic activity associated with myocardial infarction. Lidocaine differs in important aspects from most other members of the Class I antiarrhythmic drugs. Although it depresses automaticity and diastolic depolarization, lidocaine does not slow conduction and has little effect on atrial function. It does not prolong the action potential or refractory period. Lidocaine must be injected intravenously or intramuscularly because when given orally the first-pass effect is so extensive that therapeutic systemic concentrations are not attained.

Pharmacokinetics

The distribution half-life of lidocaine is about 10 minutes. Its elimination half-life is 1.5 to 2 hours. The volume of distribution is about 500 ml/kg, and its clearance is 10 ml/kg/min. Clearance of lidocaine is reduced in patients with chronic liver disease or congestive heart failure (because of decreased hepatic blood flow), and dosage must be reduced to prevent toxicity.

Lidocaine is given as a loading dose followed by a continuous infusion designed to attain total plasma concentrations of 1.5 to 5 μg/ml. The loading dose is given as repeated bolus doses of 75 to 100 mg every 5 minutes. However, if a beneficial response develops before loading is complete, additional bolus administration is withheld and the maintenance infusion is begun. Lidocaine is bound (about 40%) to α_1-acid glycoprotein (AAG), an acute-phase reactant. Changes in AAG level can complicate monitoring of lidocaine concentration. Because the AAG concentration usually rises after myocardial infarction, total plasma lidocaine concentration also increases even though the free (non–protein bound) fraction remains unchanged.[31] Misinterpretation of the total concentration could lead to the incorrect conclusion that the dosage should be reduced. Short of measuring the concentration of free lidocaine, one must be guided by the clinical response of the patient.

Adverse effects

Central adverse effects of lidocaine include agitation, drowsiness, convulsions, and coma. In the heart very large doses can depress AV conduction and cause a negative inotropic effect.

Mexiletine

Mexiletine is very similar to lidocaine in its electrophysiologic effects, chemical structure, and clinical spectrum of antiarrhythmic actions.[7] It differs from lidocaine in its suitability for oral administration and its pharmacokinetics and side effects. Unlike lidocaine, mexiletine has high systemic availability (90%) after ingestion. Peak plasma concentration is obtained 2 to 4 hours after the dose is taken, and the drug is eliminated primarily by hepatic metabolism, with a minor component of urinary pH-dependent renal excretion.

Mexiletine has minimal hemodynamic effects and only a mild negative inotropic action. However, its myocardial depressant action can become clinically evident in patients with poorly compensated congestive heart failure. The major therapeutic indication for mexiletine is in long-term treatment of symptomatic or life-threatening ventricular arrhythmias, particularly those associated with previous myocardial infarction.

The major adverse effects of mexiletine are neurologic and include tremors, nystagmus, diplopia, ataxia, and confusion. Nausea and vomiting may also occur; the incidence of these diminishes when the medication is taken with food. The usual dosage of mexiletine is 600 to 1000 mg daily, divided every 8 to 12 hours.

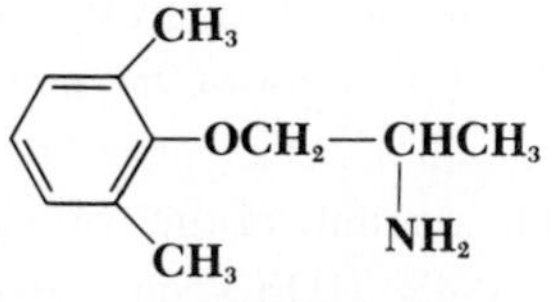

CH_3 / $-OCH_2-CHCH_3$ / NH_2 / CH_3

Mexiletine

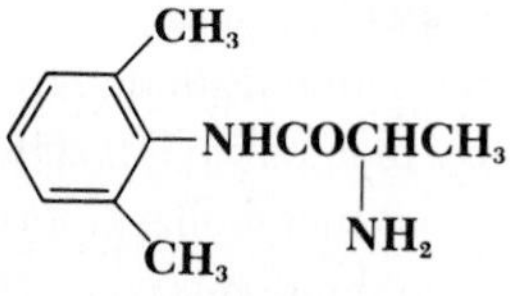

CH_3 / $-NHCOCHCH_3$ / NH_2 / CH_3

Tocainide

Tocainide

Tocainide is another lidocaine congener, similar to mexiletine in its electrophysiologic properties and antiarrhythmic action.[29] Tocainide is active after ingestion, with peak plasma concentration occurring within 60 to 90 minutes. Effective plasma concentrations can usually be achieved with a total oral daily dose between 400 and 1200 mg of the hydrochloride given in two or three divided doses. Tocainide can produce the same neurologic and gastrointestinal side effects as mexiletine. A low incidence of bone marrow depression has caused this drug to be used less frequently than mexiletine.

Flecainide

Flecainide represents a newer group of antiarrhythmic drugs (Class IC), which also includes encainide and propafenone.[28] Investigational compounds include lorcainide and aprindine. Although indecainide has been approved, it is not yet available. These drugs are characterized by a lack of effect on the duration of the action potential. They are effective in patients with ventricular tachyarrhythmias and are reserved for those in whom other drugs have failed or were poorly tolerated. Their proarrhythmic tendency to cause ventricular tachyarrhythmias and death precludes their use in other patients.[8] Other side effects include dizziness, visual disturbances, headache, and nausea.

Flecainide has a bioavailability of 90% to 95%. Approximately 60% of a dose is metabolized by cytochrome P-450 IID6.[25] Thus about 10% of Caucasians are poor metabolizers. Elimination in these persons is more dependent on renal function, and concomitant renal insufficiency mandates dosage reduction. Flecainide can be administered twice a day. At therapeutic concentrations, P-R intervals and QRS durations are increased approximately 25%.

Flecainide is available for oral administration. Dosing usually begins at 100 mg twice daily with average daily maintenance dosages from 200 to 600 mg.

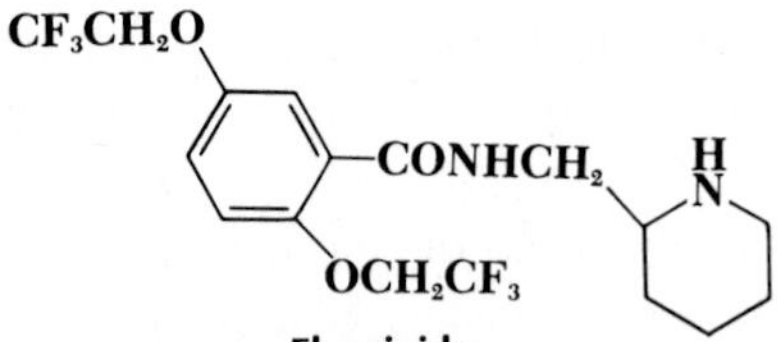

CF_3CH_2O — CONHCH$_2$ — H N — OCH_2CF_3

Flecainide

Encainide Encainide is similar pharmacologically to flecainide. Of interest, however, is that much of the activity of encainide is attributable to the *O*-desmethyl metabolite (ODE) and its 3-methoxy metabolite (MODE); the formation of both metabolites is genetically controlled.[30,38] Poor metabolizers form negligible amounts of the two metabolites and exhibit no antiarrhythmic response. Because the P-450 IID6 isoenzyme is responsible, this phenotype occurs in 10% of Caucasian patients. As with flecainide, therapeutic doses of encainide prolong P-R intervals and QRS durations (40% or more).

Dosing is started with 25 mg three times daily and can be doubled.

Propafenone Propafenone, another Class IC compound, exhibits extremely complex pharmacokinetics and pharmacodynamics and must be prescribed only by cardiologists expert in its use. Complexities include saturable protein binding and metabolism, genetically determined metabolism (by cytochrome P-450 IID6), active metabolites (5-hydroxypropafenone, *N*-desalkylpropafenone), and its administration as a racemic mixture wherein the R-enantiomer possesses the antiarrhythmic activity and the S-enantiomer is a nonselective β-adrenergic antagonist.[13,16] These features should appropriately frighten most clinicians from using the drug. Dosing begins with 150 mg three times a day and can gradually be increased to twice the starting dosage.

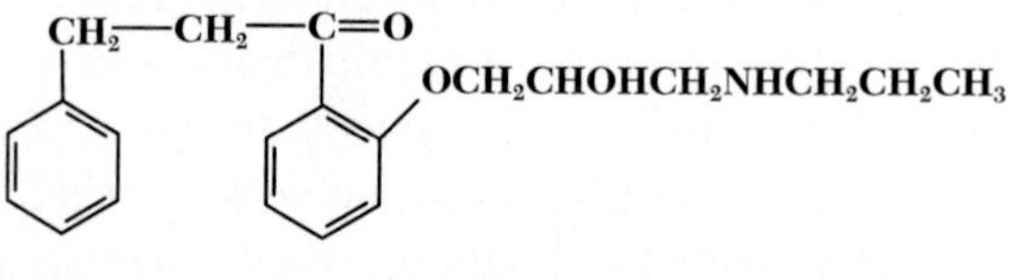

CH_2—CH_2—C=O $OCH_2CHOHCH_2NHCH_2CH_2CH_3$

Propafenone

Indecainide

Indecainide is structurally similar to aprindine (see below). It was approved for marketing by the Food and Drug Administration, but shortly thereafter results of CAST, a clinical trial, demonstrated considerable mortality associated with proarrhythmic effects of encainide, flecainide, and presumably all other Class IC antiarrhythmics.[8] As a result, the manufacturer has not yet marketed the drug and perhaps never will. The pharmacologic features of indecainide are similar to those of other agents in its class.

Lorcainide

Lorcainide is similar to other Class IC agents. Interestingly, it appears to cause a syndrome of inappropriate secretion of antidiuretic hormone, which results in hyponatremia in some patients.[34] The mechanism is unknown.

Aprindine

Aprindine (Fibocil) is a powerful Class I antiarrhythmic drug that may reverse both supraventricular and ventricular arrhythmias. It is orally active and has a very long half-life but may cause neurologic side effects in a small percentage of patients.

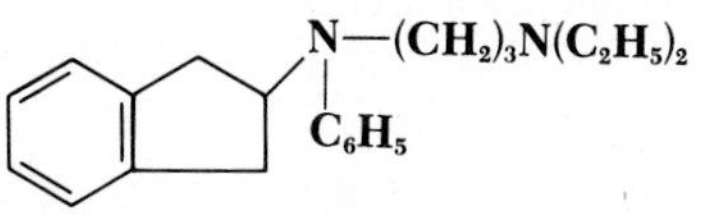

$N—(CH_2)_3N(C_2H_5)_2$, C_6H_5

Aprindine

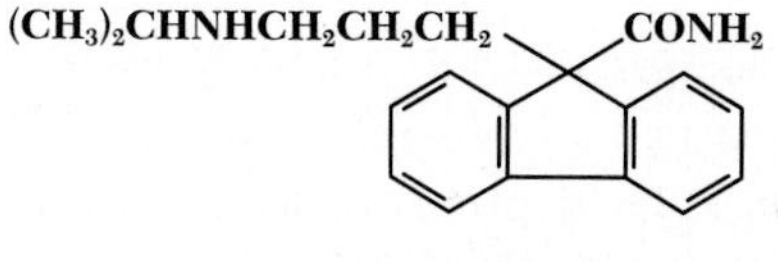

$(CH_3)_2CHNHCH_2CH_2CH_2$, $CONH_2$

Indecainide

Phenytoin

The antiepileptic drug phenytoin was found in 1950 to decrease ventricular arrhythmias after coronary ligation in dogs. More recently it has also been used as an antiarrhythmic drug, especially in digitalis-induced tachyarrhythmias, perhaps its only indication.

Phenytoin depresses automaticity in ventricular and atrial tissues and may actually improve AV conduction. It is not a generally useful antiarrhythmic drug, and even in digitalis toxicity lidocaine is usually preferred.

PHARMACOKINETICS

Ingested phenytoin is absorbed slowly, and peak concentration is not obtained for several hours. The drug should not be given intramuscularly, since its absorption is erratic. It is parahydroxylated by liver microsomal enzymes. The disappearance of phenytoin does not follow first-order kinetics because of saturation of the microsomal enzymes at therapeutic plasma concentrations. Within the usual therapeutic range, plasma concentration falls by one half in 18 to 24 hours.

DOSAGE

To obtain a prompt effect, one may administer phenytoin as an oral or intravenous loading dose of 1 g the first day, usually in three or four divided doses spread several hours apart, after which a maintenance oral dosage of 300 to 400 mg per day is appropriate, guided by measurement of serum concentration.

Phenytoin should be given by intravenous infusion only to severely ill patients. The infusion rate should be 25 to 50 mg/min. A total dose of 500 mg to 1 g should not be exceeded.

CLASS II ANTIARRHYTHMIC DRUGS

β-Receptor antagonists exert their antiarrhythmic activity through their β-blocking rather than membrane-stabilizing activity. The latter occurs only at very high plasma concentrations that are not achieved with conventional dosing.

β-Blockers depress automaticity, prolong AV conduction, reduce heart rate (unless they have intrinsic sympathomimetic activity), and also decrease contractility. These drugs are primarily effective in treatment of tachyarrhythmias caused by increased sympathetic activity and for slowing the ventricular response in patients with atrial flutter or fibrillation. They have been used to treat arrhythmias of digitalis toxicity, but lidocaine and phenytoin are preferred.

Adverse effects of β-blockers include bronchospasm and arteriolar vasoconstriction (less prevalent with cardioselective agents and those with intrinsic sympathomimetic activity) and congestive heart failure.

Dosage

β-Blockers that are primarily used in management of hypertension and angina are listed in Table 19-2, and specific information on dosage is given in Chapter 21. Esmolol is used primarily for supraventricular tachyarrhythmias in emergent settings.[2] It is particularly useful because its action is very brief (half-life 9 minutes); its effects can be easily titrated when it is administered as a continuous intravenous infusion. A loading dose of 500 μg/kg/min is infused over 1 minute, followed by a maintenance infusion of 50 μg/kg/min. If no response, or an inadequate one, occurs after 5 minutes, the loading procedure is repeated and followed by a new infusion rate of 100 μg/kg/min. This process can be continued until a maximum dosage of 300 μg/kg/min is reached.

CLASS III ANTIARRHYTHMIC DRUGS

Bretylium tosylate

Bretylium is an adrenergic neuronal blocking drug that was originally developed as an antihypertensive agent. Troublesome side effects made it useless as an antihypertensive drug, but its antiarrhythmic properties brought it back into clinical use.

Bretylium simultaneously prolongs the action potential and the effective refractory period. The drug is used to treat severe ventricular tachyarrhythmias that are unresponsive to other drugs. Even after intravenous injection, its effect may be delayed for several minutes or even hours. Initially, the drug causes norepinephrine release and an increase in blood pressure. This is followed by a fall in pressure. Other adverse effects include nausea, bradycardia, angina, diarrhea, and rash.

Bretylium, a quaternary ammonium compound, is eliminated unchanged by the kidney. It is administered intramuscularly or by slow intravenous infusion.

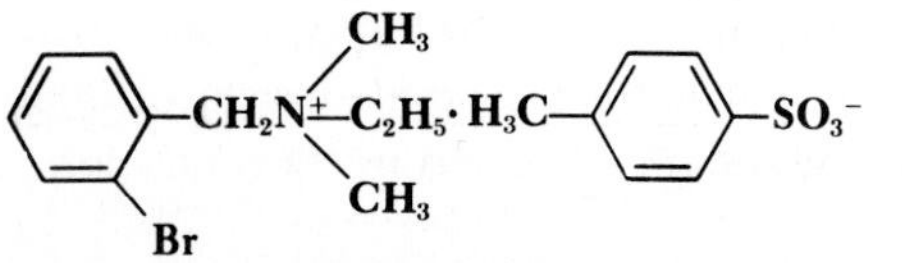

CH_3

(o-Br-phenyl)$-CH_2N^{+}(CH_3)_2-C_2H_5 \cdot H_3C-$(phenyl)$-SO_3^-$

CH_3

Br

Bretylium tosylate

Amiodarone

Amiodarone is useful for both supraventricular and ventricular tachyarrhythmias. Despite its proved efficacy, because of its extremely prolonged action and its profile of adverse effects, it has been reserved for patients refractory to other modes of therapy.[20] As many as 90% of patients receiving amiodarone will develop side effects. Photosensitivity is frequent. Some patients develop a gray skin discoloration ("gray man syndrome"). Most patients develop corneal microdeposits during prolonged therapy. Thyroid disorders, either hyperthyroidism or hypothyroidism, are related by unknown mechanisms to the iodine contained in the drug (0.375 μg of organic iodine per milligram of drug). Other toxicities include neuropathies, pulmonary fibrosis, and hepatotoxicity.

Bioavailability of amiodarone is highly variable, ranging from 22% to 86%. The drug is almost entirely eliminated by metabolism. Amiodarone can inhibit metabolism of other drugs, such as oral anticoagulants (see Chapter 70). Its half-life, as long as 100 days, makes dosing difficult. Most authorities agree on an average daily maintenance dose of 400 mg alternating with 600 mg. However, various loading regimens have been promulgated, the simplest of which may be 1200 mg daily for approximately 2 weeks.

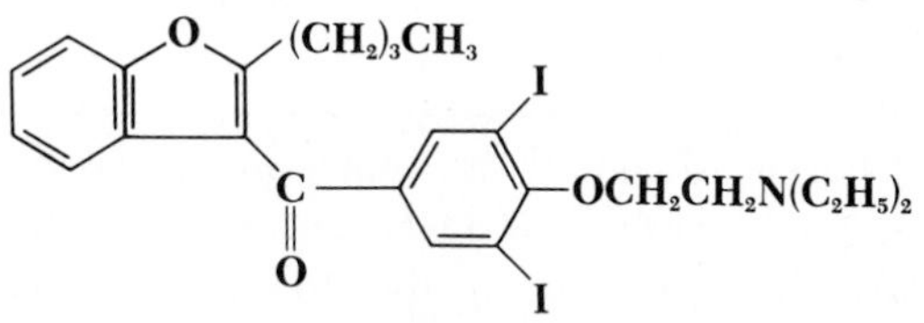

$(CH_2)_3CH_3$ I $OCH_2CH_2N(C_2H_5)_2$ I

Amiodarone

N-Acetylprocainamide

N-Acetylprocainamide (NAPA or acecainide) is the primary metabolite of procainamide, but it differs from the parent drug in having Class III antiarrhythmic activity and in being eliminated primarily by the kidney.[17] It is not yet marketed, but preliminary studies show it to be effective in suppressing a variety of ventricular arrhythmias. Interestingly, it lacks potential for the lupus-like syndrome associated with procainamide.[19]

Sotalol

Sotalol was initially studied as a β-adrenergic antagonist but was subsequently discovered to have potent Class III antiarrhythmic activity with efficacy against both supraventricular and ventricular arrhythmias.[33] Its long half-life (about 15 hours) allows twice daily dosing. The drug depends on the kidney for elimination; this mandates dosage adjustment in patients with renal insufficiency.

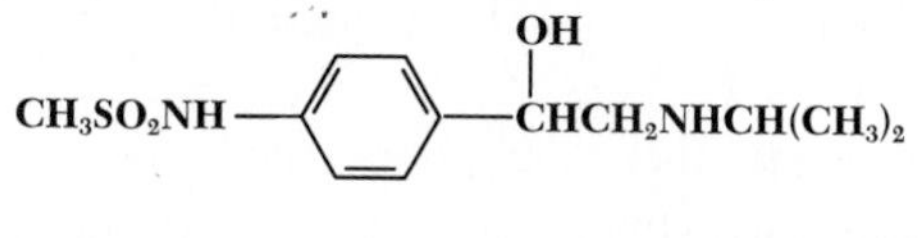

CH_3SO_2NH—C6H4—$CH(OH)CH_2NHCH(CH_3)_2$

Sotalol

CLASS IV ANTIARRHYTHMIC DRUGS

Verapamil

Verapamil is a *papaverine* derivative that is of value in certain atrial tachyarrhythmias and also in management of angina pectoris[1] (see Chapter 40). It inhibits the slow Ca^{++} flux (phase 2).[32] The drug suppresses firing of the sinoatrial (SA) node, prolongs AV refractoriness, and depresses the potential of latent pacemaker cells. Verapamil also produces vasodilatation, which accounts for its use as an antihypertensive agent.

Intravenous verapamil is effective in converting reentrant paroxysmal supraventricular tachycardia (PSVT) to normal sinus rhythm.[24] Long-term oral therapy with verapamil decreases the frequency and duration of PSVT and the severity of symptoms.[22] Because of its ability to slow AV conduction and hence ventricular response, verapamil is also useful for patients with atrial fibrillation. The slower heart rate is maintained with exercise (in contrast to use of cardiac glycosides for this same purpose), and many patients experience subjective improvement as manifested by increased effort tolerance and decreased palpitations during exertion.[18]

Verapamil is administered as a racemic mixture and exhibits the interesting property of stereoselective first-pass metabolism.[10] The active (-)-enantiomer is cleared more avidly by the liver during the first pass. Consequently, after ingestion only a small proportion of the active drug reaches the systemic circulation, and oral doses (up to 480 mg) are much greater than intravenous doses (10 mg) to achieve comparable plasma concentrations of active drug.

Dosing

For acute administration to control the ventricular response in atrial flutter or fibrillation, 5 to 10 mg is administered as a slow intravenous bolus over 2 minutes. If no response has occurred by 30 minutes, another 10 mg dose can be given. Daily oral dosage is 180 to 480 mg.

ADENOSINE

Adenosine is an endogenous nucleoside that inhibits sinus node automaticity and depresses AV nodal conduction and refractoriness. It does not "fit" into any of the categories of antiarrhythmics described above. The drug is used to treat paroxysmal supraventricular tachyarrhythmias, including those associated with accessory bypass pathways.[9] Its precise mechanism of action is not yet defined.

Like endogenous adenosine, the drug is actively transported into cells and disappears from plasma with a half-life of about 10 seconds. Caffeine and theophylline bind adenosine receptors and prevent the effects of the nucleoside; conversely, dipyridamole blocks adenosine uptake and potentiates its pharmacologic activity.

Adenosine causes multiple effects, but in antiarrhythmic doses they are usually mild and include flushing, headache, and occasionally hypotension. Shortness of breath, hyperventilation, and lightheadedness can also occur.

Adenosine (Adenocard) is available for injection (6 mg/2 ml) and is given as a 6 mg dose by rapid intravenous injection. If no response has occurred within 1 to 2 minutes, a 12 mg dose can be given and, if needed, repeated in another 1 to 2 minutes.

SELECTION OF DRUGS

There are certain principles that should be remembered before one selects a drug for treatment of a cardiac arrhythmia: (1) many arrhythmias do not require drug treatment; (2) most antiarrhythmic drugs can be dangerous; (3) cardioversion (DC countershock) is often easier and safer.

With these limitations, the use of antiarrhythmic drugs in various arrhythmias is briefly summarized below.

Supraventricular arrhythmias

PAROXYSMAL ATRIAL TACHYCARDIA

Paroxysmal atrial tachycardia can occur in otherwise normal persons. Spontaneous termination, but with recurrences, is common. It may also be a manifestation of digitalis toxicity.

Vagal maneuvers, such as carotid massage or administration of the anticholinesterase drugs edrophonium and neostigmine, can be used to end attacks. Vasoconstrictors, such as methoxamine or phenylephrine, may terminate an attack by eliciting reflex vagal activity as a consequence of blood pressure elevation. However, verapamil and adenosine (less frequently esmolol) have become the agents of choice for most supraventricular tachyarrhythmias and successfully convert at least 90% to normal sinus rhythm. Hence previous strategies are for the most part of historic interest. Verapamil should be avoided if there is suspicion of an accessory pathway.

Digitalis is also effective and is commonly used in atrial tachycardias in children. β-Blockers, as well as verapamil, may be of benefit for chronic therapy.

ATRIAL FLUTTER

Digitalis, verapamil, and esmolol are the most important drugs in treatment of atrial flutter. They act primarily by increasing the degree of AV block, thereby decreasing ventricular rate. As for the flutter itself, digitalis tends to convert it to fibrillation by shortening the refractory period in the atrial muscle. Occasionally quinidine is used to convert flutter to normal sinus rhythm. In this case digitalis, verapamil, or a β-blocker should be employed first to prevent excessive tachycardia, a consequence of the vagolytic action of quinidine. When quinidine is added to digoxin treatment, the plasma concentration of the glycoside doubles and may rise to a dangerous level.[3]

Intravenous verapamil converts atrial flutter to normal sinus rhythm in about 30% of cases.[24] As with digitalis, verapamil often converts flutter to atrial fibrillation, which, in turn, may convert to sinus rhythm.

ATRIAL FIBRILLATION

Digitalis and verapamil are also the most important drugs in management of atrial fibrillation. They do not convert atrial fibrillation to normal sinus rhythm, but they slow ventricular rate. Quinidine can convert atrial fibrillation to normal sinus rhythm. Cardioversion can also be employed. Even when DC countershock is employed, chronic therapy with quinidine may be helpful in preventing the recurrence of atrial fibrillation. Administration of quinidine is often started before cardioversion, and it may terminate the fibrillation by itself. Disopyramide may be used in the same manner.

Ventricular arrhythmias

The CAST results have demonstrated that ventricular arrhythmias should not be treated unless they are symptomatic or life threatening.[8] Although DC countershock is commonly used for stopping ventricular tachycardia, it should not be employed if the arrhythmia is caused by digitalis.

For acute treatment of ventricular tachyarrhythmias, lidocaine is the drug of choice, but procainamide can be used as well. For chronic treatment, quinidine, procainamide, or disopyramide are suitable. If they fail or toxicity supervenes, mexiletine or tocainide may be effective. If these drugs also fail, flecainide or other Class IC agents and finally amiodarone can be tried. Lastly, combinations are sometimes successful. Guiding the choice of antiarrhythmic agent by electrophysiologic testing is often helpful in difficult cases.

Digitalis-induced arrhythmias may be treated with lidocaine, phenytoin, or β-blockers. Antibody fractions that bind digitalis are also now available (see Chapter 38).

REFERENCES

1. Antman EM, Stone PH, Muller JE, Braunwald E: Calcium channel blocking agents in the treatment of cardiovascular disorders: Part I. Basic and clinical electrophysiologic effects, *Ann Intern Med* 93:875, 1980.
2. Benfield P, Sorkin EM: Esmolol: a preliminary review of its pharmacodynamic and pharmacokinetic properties, and therapeutic efficacy, *Drugs* 33:392, 1987.
3. Bigger JT Jr, Leahey EB Jr: Quinidine and digoxin: an important interaction, *Drugs* 24:229, 1982.
4. Blomgren SE, Condemi JJ, Vaughan JH: Procainamide-induced lupus erythematosus: clinical and laboratory observations, *Am J Med* 52:338, 1972.
5. Brogden RN, Todd, PA: Disopyramide: a reappraisal of its pharmacodynamic and pharmacokinetic properties, and therapeutic use in cardiac arrhythmias, *Drugs* 34:151, 1987.
6. Broly F, Libersa C, Lhermitte M, et al: Effect of quinidine on the dextromethorphan *O*-demethylase activity of microsomal fractions from human liver, *Br J Clin Pharmacol* 28:29, 1989.
7. Campbell RWF: Mexiletine, *N Engl J Med* 316:29, 1987.
8. The Cardiac Arrhythmia Suppression Trial (CAST) Investigators: Effect of encainide and flecainide on mortality in a randomized trial of arrhythmia suppression after myocardial infarction, *N Engl J Med* 321:406, 1989.
9. DiMarco JP, Miles W, Akhtar M, et al: Adenosine for paroxysmal supraventricular tachycardia: dose ranging and comparison with verapamil: assessment in placebo-controlled, multicenter trials, *Ann Intern Med* 113:104, 1990.
10. Eichelbaum M, Mikus G, Vogelgesang B: Pharmacokinetics of (+)-, (-)- and (±)-verapamil after intravenous administration, *Br J Clin Pharmacol* 17:453, 1984.
11. Fitton A, Buckley MM-T: Moricizine: a review of its pharmacological properties, and therapeutic efficacy in cardiac arrhythmias, *Drugs* 40:138, 1990.
12. Frey W: Weitere Erfahrungen mit Chinidin bei absoluter Herz unregelmässigkeit, *Klin Wochenschr* 55:849, 1918.
13. Funck-Brentano C, Kroemer HK, Lee JT, Roden DM: Propafenone, *N Engl J Med* 322:518, 1990.
14. Greenblatt DJ, Pfeifer HJ, Oches HR, et al: Pharmacokinetics of quinidine in humans after intravenous, intramuscular and oral administration, *J Pharmacol Exp Ther* 202:365, 1977.
15. Hackett T, Kelton JG, Powers P: Drug-induced platelet destruction, *Semin Thromb Hemostas* 8:116, 1982.
16. Haefeli EW, Vozeh S, Ha H-R, Follath F: Comparison of the pharmacodynamic effects of intravenous and oral propafenone, *Clin Pharmacol Ther* 48:245, 1990.
17. Harron DWG, Brogden RN: Acecainide (*N*-acetylprocainamide): a review of its pharmacodynamic and pharmacokinetic properties, and therapeutic potential in cardiac arrhythmias, *Drugs* 39:720, 1990.

18. Klein HO, Pauzner H, Di Segni E, et al: The beneficial effects of verapamil on chronic atrial fibrillation, *Arch Intern Med* 139:747, 1979.
19. Kluger J, Drayer DE, Reidenberg MM, Lahita R: Acetylprocainamide therapy in patients with previous procainamide-induced lupus syndrome, *Ann Intern Med* 95:18, 1981.
20. Latini R, Tognoni G, Kates RE: Clinical pharmacokinetics of amiodarone, *Clin Pharmacokinet* 9:136, 1984.
21. Lima JJ, Boudoulas H, Shields BJ: Stereoselective pharmacokinetics of disopyramide enantiomers in man, *Drug Metab Dispos* 13:572, 1985.
22. Mauritson DR, Winniford MD, Walker WS, et al: Oral verapamil for paroxysmal supraventricular tachycardia: a long-term, double-blind randomized trial, *Ann Intern Med* 96:409, 1982.
23. Mautz FR: Reduction of cardiac irritability by the epicardial and systemic administration of drugs as a protection in cardiac surgery, *J Thorac Surg* 5:612, 1936.
24. McGoon MD, Vlietstra RE, Holmes DR Jr, Osborn, JE: The clinical use of verapamil, *Mayo Clin Proc* 57:495, 1982.
25. Mikus G, Gross AS, Beckmann J, et al: The influence of the sparteine/debrisoquin phenotype on the disposition of flecainide, *Clin Pharmacol Ther* 45:562, 1989.
26. Podrid PJ, Schoeneberger A, Lown B: Congestive heart failure caused by oral disopyramide, *N Engl J Med* 302:614, 1980.
27. Reder RF, Rosen MR: Mechanisms of cardiac arrhythmias, *Cardiovasc Rev Rep* 2:1007, 1981.
28. Roden DM, Woosley RL: Flecainide, *N Engl J Med* 315:36, 1986.
29. Roden DM, Woosley RL: Tocainide, *N Engl J Med* 315:41, 1986.
30. Roden DM, Woosley RL: Clinical pharmacokinetics of encainide, *Clin Pharmacokinet* 14:141, 1988.
31. Routledge PA, Stargel WW, Wagner GS, Shand DG: Increased alpha-1-acid glycoprotein and lidocaine disposition in myocardial infarction, *Ann Intern Med* 93:701, 1980.
32. Singh BN, Collett JT, Chew CYC: New perspectives in the pharmacologic therapy of cardiac arrhythmias, *Prog Cardiovasc Dis* 22:243, 1980.
33. Singh BN, Deedwania P, Nademanee K, et al: Sotalol: a review of its pharmacodynamic and pharmacokinetic properties, and therapeutic use, *Drugs* 34:311, 1987.
34. Somani P, Temesy-Armos PN, Leighton RF, et al: Hyponatremia in patients treated with lorcainide, a new antiarrhythmic drug, *Am Heart J* 108:1443, 1984.
35. Vera Z, Mason DT: Reentry versus automaticity: role in tachyarrhythmia genesis and antiarrhythmic therapy, *Am Heart J* 101:329, 1981.
36. Wenckebach KF: *Die unregelmässige Herztätigkeit und ihre Klinische Bedeutung*, Leipzig, 1914, W Englemann.
37. Woosley RL, Drayer DE, Reidenberg MM, et al: Effect of acetylator phenotype on the rate at which procainamide induces antinuclear antibodies and the lupus syndrome, *N Engl J Med* 298:1157, 1978.
38. Woosley RL, Wood AJJ, Roden DM: Encainide, *N Engl J Med* 318:1107, 1988.

Chapter 40

Antianginal drugs

GENERAL CONCEPT

It is an old empiric observation that amyl nitrite (1867) and nitroglycerin (1879) relieve the pain of angina pectoris. Since nitrates and nitrites dilate blood vessels, including the coronary arteries, coronary vasodilatation has generally been assumed to provide relief of angina.

The pathophysiology and pharmacology are much more complex, however. Angina results from an imbalance between oxygen demand and supply in ischemic regions of the myocardium. Theoretically, drugs may improve angina by reducing the demand for or by increasing the supply of oxygen. In addition to increasing oxygen supply, nitrates reduce demand by a peripheral action to cause venodilatation, thereby decreasing cardiac preload and reducing myocardial wall tension, a major determinant of oxygen demand.[1] In addition to its use in angina pectoris, this same effect of nitrates is of benefit in management of patients with congestive heart failure. Use of nitrates has expanded because of recent availability of intravenous formulations and longer acting oral and topical preparations.

β-Adrenergic receptor antagonists are also used extensively to treat angina. They illustrate the importance of reduction of cardiac work.[6]

Ca^{++}-channel blocking drugs, such as verapamil, diltiazem, and the dihydropyridines, nifedipine and nicardipine, are additional effective antianginal agents. They dilate coronary arteries, decrease afterload (blood pressure), and are particularly useful in patients with Prinzmetals variant angina resulting from coronary artery spasm. It is now apparent that coronary spasm is an important component of unstable angina, acute myocardial infarction, stable effort-induced angina, and so-called silent ischemia.[2,4] Ca^{++} antagonists can therefore be of benefit in all myocardial ischemic syndromes.

NITRATES AND NITRITES

Chemistry

The effects of nitrates, Ca^{++}-channel blockers, and β-blockers on myocardial oxygen requirement and oxygen supply are shown in Table 40-1. Clinically useful nitrates and nitrites cause qualitatively similar effects. The formulas of the most interesting compounds in the group are shown on the next page.

Effects of nitroglycerin

If a patient suffering from an attack of angina pectoris places a tablet of nitroglycerin (glyceryl trinitrate) under the tongue, the attack frequently subsides within minutes. Furthermore, the drug provides protection if taken before performance of a task, such as an exercise tolerance test, that ordinarily induces angina.

The original interpretation of this effect of nitroglycerin was that it improves blood

TABLE 40-1 Effects of nitrates, Ca^{++}-channel blockers, and β-blockers on myocardial oxygen requirement and supply

	Nitrates	Ca^{++}-channel blockers			β-blockers
		DHP	DZ	VP	
Determinants of myocardial oxygen requirement					
Heart rate	↑	↑	↓ –	↓ –	↓ *
Left ventricular pressure	↓	↓	↓ –	↓	↓ *
Left ventricular volume/radius	↓ *	↓	↓	↑ –	↑
Velocity of contraction	↑	↑	–	↓	↓
Systolic ejection period	↓	↓	↑ –	–	↑
Determinants of myocardial oxygen supply					
Coronary vasodilatation	↑ *	↑ *	↑ *	↑ *	↓
Aortic diastolic pressure	↓	↓	↓	↓	↓
Diastolic perfusion time	↓	↓	↑	↑	↑

*Most significant effects.
–, No change; *DHP*, dihydropyridines (nifedipine, nicardipine); *DZ*, diltiazem; *VP*, verapamil.

Nitrates

$CH_2—O—NO_2$
$CH—O—NO_2$
$CH_2—O—NO_2$

Nitroglycerin

$CH_2—O—NO_2$
$O_2N—O—CH_2—C—CH_2—O—NO_2$
$CH_2—O—NO_2$

Pentaerythritol tetranitrate

H_2C
$HC—O—NO_2$
CH
HC
$O_2N—O—CH$
CH_2
O O

Isosorbide dinitrate

H_2C
$HC—O—H$
CH
HC
$O_2N—O—CH$
CH_2
O O

Isosorbide mononitrate

$CH_2—O—NO_2$
$CH—O—NO_2$
$CH—O—NO_2$
$CH_2—O—NO_2$

Erythrityl tetranitrate

Nitrites

$NaNO_2$

Sodium nitrite

H_3C
$CHCH_2CH_2NO_2$
H_3C

Amyl nitrite

flow to ischemic regions of myocardium by dilating coronary vessels. However, the antianginal effect of nitroglycerin is now believed to result primarily from reduction of venous tone with diminished venous return, decreased cardiac preload, decreased myocardial wall tension, and subsequently decreased oxygen demand.[1] In addition, some benefit is derived from peripheral arterial dilatation and from dilatation of coronary arteries. All nitrate esters produce the same effects as nitroglycerin.

In addition, certain specific vascular regions such as the cutaneous vessels of the face and neck, the so-called blush area, are susceptible to the action of nitrates. Dilatation of meningeal vessels is the likely cause of nitrate-induced headaches.

Effects of nitrates on other smooth muscles

Probably all smooth muscles are relaxed by nitrates. Sublingual nitroglycerin decreases biliary pressure. Nitrates also relax the ureter and the lower esophageal sphincter. Occasionally, relief of pain by nitrates is assumed to indicate a myocardial ischemic cause when, in fact, the salutary effect has occurred elsewhere. Although nitrates relax bronchial smooth muscle, more effective medications are available for this purpose.

Mechanism of cellular action

The action on smooth muscle of nitrates and other nitrosovasodilators such as nitroprusside involves a nitrosothiol intermediate formed within the smooth muscle itself by a reaction of the nitrate with glutathione. This intermediate, in turn, enhances formation of cyclic guanine nucleotides, which relax smooth muscle.

Preparations

Nitroglycerin is available in oral, sublingual, buccal, topical, and intravenous formulations.[3,7] A variety of oral and buccal sustained-release preparations, nitroglycerin ointment, and synthetic nitrate esters have been designed to provide a longer action (Table 40-2). Oral preparations are given in large doses to overcome extensive first-pass hepatic metabolism.

In addition to the ointment, a variety of transdermal nitroglycerin preparations are available. These adhesive bandages contain nitroglycerin on lactose in a viscous silicone fluid (Transderm) or nitroglycerin microsealed in a solid silicone polymer (Nitrodisc). Such delivery systems are intended to release nitroglycerin continuously over a 24-hour period. Pharmacokinetic studies show that in most patients once-a-day application of these patches produces a stable plasma concentration of nitroglycerin over 24 hours. Unfortunately, a stable concentration is now known to cause tolerance. Current usage entails removal of the patch at night to allow plasma concentration to decline; responsiveness is then restored.

Tolerance to the vascular action of nitrosovasodilators

Tolerance develops to the headache produced by nitrates. Thus munitions workers when first exposed to nitrates complain of headache, but they become tolerant in a few days. Not much attention was given to this phenomenon until transdermal delivery systems became available. With maintenance of stable nitroglycerin concentrations, it was discovered that efficacy persisted up to 6 hours after placement of a patch but had disappeared at 24 hours. A similar phenomenon occurs with continuous intravenous

TABLE 40-2 Nitrates: preparations, routes, recommended dosage, and duration of action

Drug	Dosage	Duration of action (hr)
Nitroglycerin		
Buccal	1-3 mg every 3-5 hr	3-5
Oral	6.5-19.5 mg every 4-6 hr*	4-6
Spray	1 spray every 5 min, 3 times	0.5-1
Sublingual	0.15 mg every 5 min, 3 times	0.5-1
2% Ointment	½-2 in (1.3-5 cm; 7.5-30 mg) every 4-8 hr	3-6
Patches	1-2 patches every 24 hr	24
Isosorbide dinitrate		
Sublingual	2.5-10 mg every 2-3 hr	2-3†
Oral	5-60 mg every 4-6 hr*	4-6
Chewable	5-10 mg every 2-4 hr	2-3
Isosorbide 5-mononitrate		
Oral	20-50 mg three times daily	6-8
Pentaerythritol tetranitrate		
Oral	40-80 mg every 4-6 hr*	3-5
Erythrityl tetranitrate		
Sublingual	5-10 mg	3
Oral	10 mg four times daily	6

*Large doses, often greater than manufacturers recommend, may be necessary to produce a therapeutic effect.
†Most studies indicate a duration of action for sublingual isosorbide dinitrate of 90 to 120 minutes; some indicate activity for 4 hours.

infusion of nitroglycerin and with frequent dosing of longer-acting nitrate preparations, for example, isosorbide dinitrate every 6 hours. In contrast, the response is maintained by intermittent dosing that allows decline of plasma concentration. Thus dosing of isosorbide dinitrate every 8 hours or removal of patches at night will maintain efficacy. It is postulated that a period of low or negligible plasma nitrate concentration permits regeneration of cellular glutathione so that subsequent nitrate administration results in generation of the active nitrosothiol intermediate.

Nitrites

Amyl nitrite is a volatile liquid available in small glass pearls containing 0.2 ml. These are crushed in a handkerchief by the patient, and the vapor is inhaled. Amyl nitrite acts within 1 minute, but its duration of action does not exceed 10 minutes. It is particularly prone to cause cutaneous vasodilatation, pronounced lowering of systemic blood pressure, and even syncope and tachycardia. In addition, its odor is objectionable. Thus nitroglycerin is preferred.

Sodium nitrite has more toxicologic (see p. 743) than therapeutic importance. Although its action on smooth muscle is similar to that of other nitrites, irritation of the gastric mucosa and its tendency to produce methemoglobin, by oxidizing the iron of hemoglobin from the ferrous to the ferric state, make it unsuitable as a coronary vasodilator.

Toxic effects of nitrites and nitrates

Any of the nitrates can cause a severe decrease in blood pressure with syncope, particularly if the patient is volume depleted. Headache, glaucoma, and elevated intracranial pressure can result from excessive dosage or unusual susceptibility.

Nitrite poisoning may be acute or chronic. It can follow therapeutic or accidental intake of nitrites or ingestion of a nitrate that is converted to a nitrite by intestinal bacteria. This has occurred after ingestion of bismuth subnitrate. Well water in some rural areas may contain enough nitrate to cause chronic methemoglobinemia. Chronic poisoning from nitrates and nitrites is an industrial hazard, particularly in the explosives industry.

There is also concern about the addition of nitrites and nitrates to meat products. The nitrites may be converted in the stomach to nitrosamines, which are carcinogenic.

Therapeutic aims in use of nitrites and nitrates

The most important indication for use of these compounds is management of angina pectoris. If necessary, nitrates can be used in combination with β-adrenergic antagonists or Ca^{++}-channel antagonists.

Nitrates are also used in management of congestive heart failure, in which the benefit derives primarily from venodilatation (which decreases preload) and to a lesser extent from arteriolar dilatation (which decreases afterload).

Continuous intravenous nitroglycerin infusions have been used for unstable angina, acute myocardial infarction, refractory congestive heart failure, perioperative control of blood pressure in patients undergoing coronary artery bypass surgery, and controlled hypotension during noncardiac surgery.[7] Because nitroglycerin can be absorbed by various plastics, care must be taken to use approved infusion sets for intravenous administration. The infusion is generally begun at a rate of 5 μg/min, and the dose is titrated to the clinically desired end point (that is, the desired blood pressure, cessation of chest pain, or the appropriate reduction in the pulmonary capillary wedge pressure).

β-ADRENERGIC RECEPTOR BLOCKING AGENTS

β-Receptor antagonists are widely used in management of angina pectoris.[6] The general pharmacology of this class of drugs is discussed in Chapter 19. They are effective in angina because they reduce myocardial oxygen demand as a result of their negative chronotropic and inotropic effects, their ability to reduce blood pressure, and blockade of catecholamine-induced increments in heart rate (see Table 19-1). These agents must be used cautiously because of their ability to precipitate congestive heart failure or bronchospasm in susceptible patients.

CA^{++}-CHANNEL BLOCKERS

Variant, or Prinzmetals, angina is characterized by chest pain at rest rather than during exercise. Coronary artery spasm appears to be the cause of the pain and S-T segment elevation. Attacks may be precipitated by administration of epinephrine, norepinephrine, and sympathomimetic drugs in general. Ergonovine maleate, a constrictor of vascular smooth muscle, has been used as a diagnostic agent for variant angina. However, this drug is not without danger, since it can cause prolonged spasm.

Coronary artery spasm can be treated effectively with Ca^{++}-channel blocking agents.[2,4,12] These drugs interfere with Ca^{++} entry into vascular smooth muscle and cause coronary vasodilatation. Spasm was recently recognized to be important in other anginal syndromes. In unstable angina and acute myocardial infarction, coronary spasm is prevalent and may be caused by platelet plugging at sites of atheromatous lesions, associated with release of vasoconstrictors such as thromboxane and serotonin. Although Ca^{++} antagonists do not affect platelet aggregation, they can blunt or block the secondary vasoconstriction. Spasm may also play a role in stable angina and in silent ischemia—painless and therefore asymptomatic ischemic episodes in patients with coronary artery disease.

Vasodilatation by these agents also occurs in the peripheral vasculature and decreases afterload. This additional mechanism contributes to the antianginal activity of Ca^{++} antagonists and to their efficacy in chronic effort-induced angina. Because of vasodilatation these drugs have proved effective in treatment of hypertension as well.

The use of verapamil as an antiarrhythmic agent is discussed in Chapter 39. Although these drugs are classified together as Ca^{++} antagonists, there are considerable differences in their pharmacology as indicated in Table 40-3. Their side effects and dosages are summarized in Tables 40-4 and 40-5 respectively. It should be noted that these agents, particularly verapamil, can induce left ventricular dysfunction. For this reason the Ca^{++}-channel blockers should be used cautiously in patients with myocardial disease, especially if given in combination with β-blocking agents.

Verapamil

Because verapamil slows conduction through the AV node, it is the agent of choice to treat many cases of supraventricular tachyarrhythmias. In addition, it has been used successfully in all forms of angina and is an effective antihypertensive drug. In the latter settings, its effects on cardiac conduction may be unwanted.

Verapamil is eliminated by the liver and has a substantial first-pass effect; bioavailability is only about 20%.[9] Its half-life of 3 to 5 hours mandates dosing 3 to 4 times per day or use of a sustained-release preparation that can be taken once daily. Interestingly, the stereoisomers of verapamil have different efficacies. After oral dosing the more active isomer is selectively metabolized during the first pass through the liver.

TABLE 40-3 Pharmacologic activities of calcium antagonists

	Coronary vasodilatation	Peripheral vasodilatation	Negative inotropy	Slowed AV conduction
Verapamil	+ + +	+ +	+	+ +
Dihydropyridines	+ + +	+ + +	−	−
Diltiazem	+ + +	+	±	+

+, Mild; + +, moderate; + + +, pronounced; −, negligible.

TABLE 40-4 Side effects of antianginal drugs*

	Hypotension, flushing, headache	Left ventricular dysfunction	Decreased heart rate, atrioventricular block†	Gastrointestinal symptoms	Broncho-constriction‡
β-blockers	0	+ +	+ + +	+	+ + +
Nitrates	+ + +	0	0	0	0
Diltiazem	+	+	+	0	0
Dihydropyridines	+ + +	0	0	0	0
Verapamil	+	+	+ +	+ +	0

From Braunwald E: N Engl J Med 307:1618, 1982. Reprinted by permission of the New England Journal of Medicine.
*0, Absent; +, mild; + +, moderate; + + +, sometimes severe.
†In patients with sick-sinus-node syndrome or conduction-system disease.
‡In patients with obstructive lung disease.

TABLE 40-5 Dosages and preparations of Ca^{++}-channel blockers

Drug	Initial dosage* (mg)	Maximum daily dosage (mg)	Oral dosage forms (mg)
Verapamil hydrochloride (Calan, Isoptin, Verelan)	80	480	T: 40-120, 180†; C†: 120, 240; CL†: 180, 240
Nifedipine (Adalat, Procardia)	10	120	C: 10, 20; T†: 30-90
Nicardipine hydrochloride (Cardene)	20	120	C: 20, 30
Diltiazem hydrochloride (Cardizem)	30	240	T: 30-120; C†: 60-120

C, Capsules; *CL,* caplets; *T,* tablets.
*Given three times daily unless sustained-release preparation.
†Sustained-release preparation.

Therefore, the active isomer in blood after oral administration is a smaller fraction of the total than after intravenous dosing. The result is that after ingestion a *total* plasma concentration three times higher than after intravenous dosing is needed to cause the same effect.

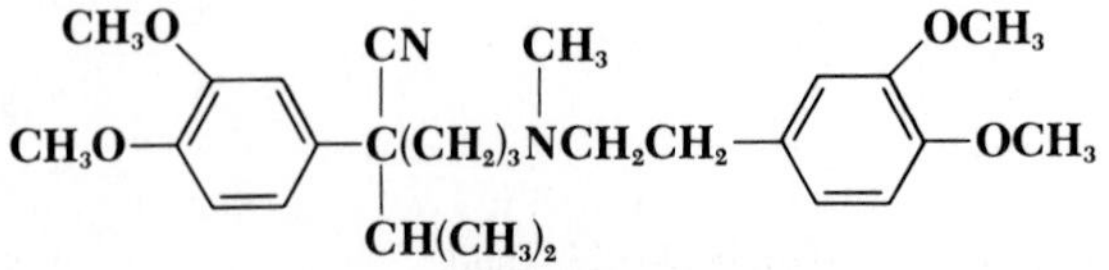

CH_3O, CH_3O, CN, CH_3, $C(CH_2)_3NCH_2CH_2$, $CH(CH_3)_2$, OCH_3, OCH_3

Verapamil

S, OCH_3, N, $OOCCH_3$, O, $CH_2CH_2N(CH_3)_2$

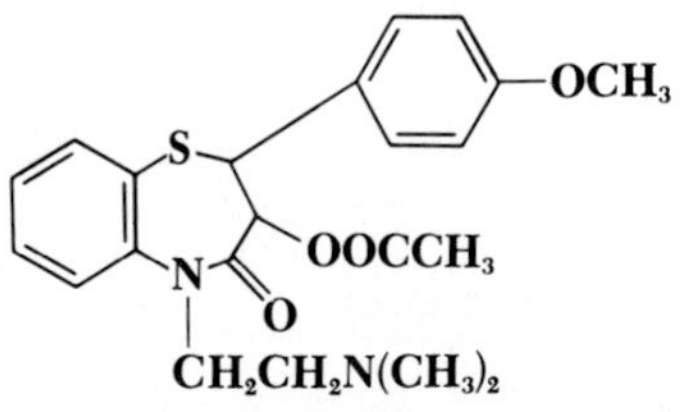

Diltiazem

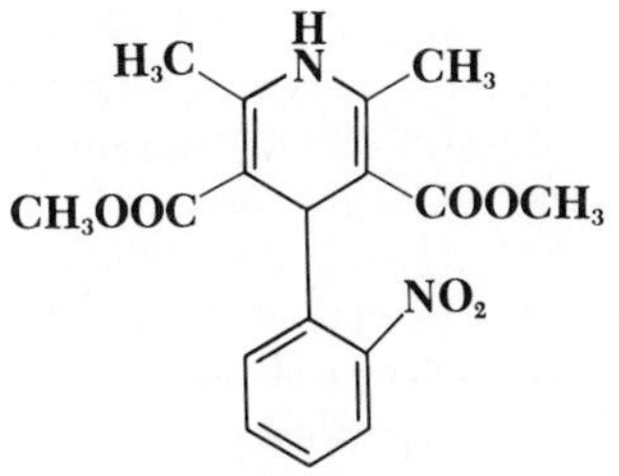

Nifedipine

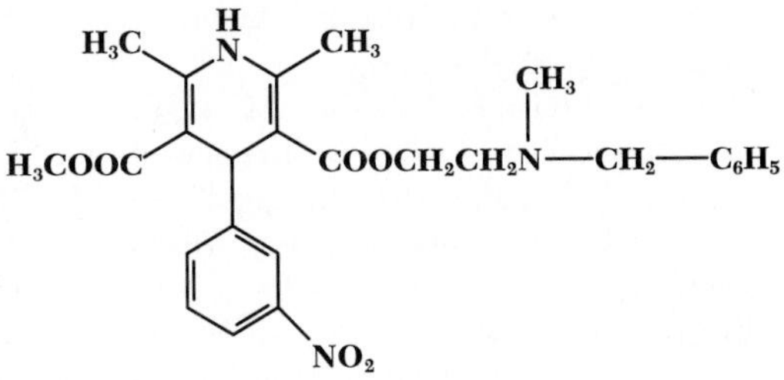

Nicardipine

Diltiazem

Diltiazem has pharmacologic properties intermediate between those of verapamil and dihydropyridine Ca^{++} antagonists. It has less activity on cardiac conduction than verapamil and less activity on the vasculature than the dihydropyridines.

Diltiazem is eliminated by the liver, with a half-life of about 4 hours.[5] A sustained-release preparation allows twice daily dosing. The drug has an active metabolite, but this probably contributes little to its effects.

Dihydropyridine Ca^{++} antagonists

In contrast to verapamil, dihydropyridine Ca^{++} antagonists cause negligible changes in cardiac conduction but can markedly lower peripheral vascular resistance. Hence, in addition to decreasing coronary spasm, they may be used to decrease afterload and to lower blood pressure. Because of their pronounced vasodilating activity, their use is associated with a higher incidence of headache, reflex tachycardia, and fluid retention than occurs with verapamil or diltiazem. A sustained-release preparation of nifedipine allows once daily dosing. In addition, it avoids the high peak concentration that occurs shortly after dosing with conventional formulations of nifedipine and with nicardipine. Sustained release thus diminishes the incidence of acute side effects such as headache and flushing, but the incidence of peripheral edema (about 15%) is unchanged.

Nifedipine and nicardipine are eliminated by the liver; nifedipine has a bioavailability approaching 90%, whereas that for nicardipine is dose dependent and varies from 6% at low doses (10 mg) to 30% at high doses (40 mg).[8,10,11] The half-life of both drugs is 1 to 2 hours. Thus, without a sustained-release preparation, dosing must be frequent, every 6 to 8 hours.

REFERENCES

1. Abrams J: Nitroglycerin and long-acting nitrates, *N Engl J Med* 302:1234, 1980.
2. Antman EM, Stone PH, Muller JE, Braunwald E: Calcium channel blocking agents in the treatment of cardiovascular disorders: Part I, Basic and clinical electrophysiologic effects, *Ann Intern Med* 93:875, 1980.
3. Bogaert MG: Clinical pharmacokinetics of glyceryl trinitrate following the use of systemic and topical preparations, *Clin Pharmacokinet* 12:1, 1987.
4. Braunwald E: Mechanisms of action of calcium-channel-blocking agents, *N Engl J Med* 307:1618, 1982.
5. Buckley MM-T, Grant SM, Goa KL, et al: Diltiazem: a reappraisal of its pharmacological properties and therapeutic use, *Drugs* 39:757, 1990.
6. Frishman WH: β-Adrenoceptor antago-

nists: new drugs and new indications, *N Engl J Med* 305:500, 1981.

7. Hill NS, Antman EM, Green LH, Alpert JS: Intravenous nitroglycerin: a review of pharmacology, indications, therapeutic effects and complications, *Chest* 79:69, 1981.
8. Kleinbloesem CH, van Brummelen P, Breimer DD: Nifedipine: relationship between pharmacokinetics and pharmacodynamics, *Clin Pharmacokinet* 12:12, 1987.
9. McTavish D, Sorkin EM: Verapamil: an updated review of its pharmacodynamic and pharmacokinetic properties, and therapeutic use in hypertension, *Drugs* 38:19, 1989.
10. Sorkin EM, Clissold SP: Nicardipine: a review of its pharmacodynamic and pharmacokinetic properties, and therapeutic efficacy, in the treatment of angina pectoris, hypertension and related cardiovascular disorders, *Drugs* 33:296, 1987.
11. Sorkin EM, Clissold SP, Brogden RN: Nifedipine: a review of its pharmacodynamic and pharmacokinetic properties, and therapeutic efficacy, in ischaemic heart disease, hypertension and related cardiovascular disorders, *Drugs* 30:182, 1985.
12. Stone PH, Antman EM, Muller JE, Braunwald E: Calcium channel blocking agents in the treatment of cardiovascular disorders: Part II. Hemodynamic effects and clinical applications, *Ann Intern Med* 93:886, 1980.

Chapter 41

Drugs that affect hemostasis

GENERAL CONCEPT

Hemostatic mechanisms that prevent excessive bleeding are normally activated by tissue injury. A carefully regulated cascade of biochemical reactions promotes aggregation of platelets, blood coagulation, and the eventual resolution of the clot by fibrinolysis. These events involve reactions on cellular surfaces and in the fluid phase of blood. Generation of thrombin usually occurs on the surface of activated platelets, whereas the conversion of fibrinogen to fibrin occurs within the fluid phase. The vascular endothelium also provides a surface for binding of coagulation proteins and produces various regulator molecules, such as prostacyclin and plasminogen activator.[23]

Coagulation may occur inappropriately as a complication of cardiovascular disease, vascular injury, neoplasms, sickle cell anemia, or tissue trauma and may cause significant morbidity and mortality, particularly in patients who must remain immobilized for extended periods. An exaggerated platelet response is believed to contribute to the pathogenesis of stroke, myocardial infarction, and atherosclerosis.

The judicious use of *anticoagulants*, *platelet inhibitors*, and *thrombolytic agents* requires an understanding of how they affect primary hemostasis, blood coagulation, and thrombolysis.

Anticoagulant drugs prevent progression of coagulation by interference with one or more clotting factors or their controlling proteins. For example, binding of heparin to the plasma protein antithrombin III enhances the affinity of this inhibitor for thrombin (factor II) and for factor X, a pivotal protein in the coagulation cascade. Warfarin decreases hepatic synthesis of several vitamin K–dependent protein coagulation factors and thereby lowers the rate of coagulation.

Platelet inhibitors interfere with platelet adhesion and aggregation and with release of platelet-derived vasoactive mediators. This group of compounds includes nonsteroidal anti-inflammatory drugs, such as aspirin and indomethacin, which block platelet cyclooxygenase and prevent conversion of arachidonic acid to thromboxane A_2, a potent platelet aggregator. Other platelet inhibitory drugs, such as dipyridamole and ticlopidine, modulate activation of platelets.

Thrombolytic agents include activators of *plasmin*, a fibrinolytic enzyme that stimulates the lysis and removal of an existing clot. Streptokinase causes a nonenzymatic alteration of the conformation of plasminogen to generate plasmin; urokinase and tissue plasminogen activator activate plasmin through an enzymatic mechanism. Activation of fibrinolysis by these agents enhances digestion of fibrin and other components of a clot.

THE CLOTTING PROCESS AND DRUG ACTION

A complex integration of control mechanisms maintains fluidity of the blood or promotes coagulation in response to imbalances within the system. Various factors, including diet, hormones, or the presence of disease, influence the normal balance. Coagulation is a surface-oriented phenomenon that integrates interaction of enzymes, cofactors, and substrates within a specific environment. The process is limited by specific inhibitors and inactivators, including antithrombin III, an inhibitor of serine proteases, and protein C, a protease that inactivates factors V and VIII. Deficiencies of these regulatory proteins result in recurrent thromboses, pulmonary emboli, and occlusive arterial complications.[3]

Coagulation and clot resolution proceed through discrete stages, each of which may involve several enzymatic steps. These are outlined in simplified form below.

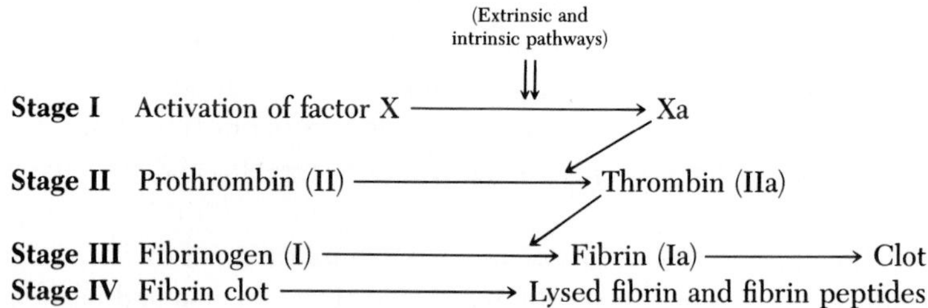

In stage I factor X is activated by a series of enzymatic steps. Next, thrombin (IIa) is formed by interaction of activated factor X (Xa) and additional coagulation factors. Fibrin (Ia), the basic component of a clot, is generated from fibrinogen, a soluble plasma protein, by the proteolytic action of thrombin. Insoluble fibrin forms a mechanical barrier to blood flow and provides the surface upon which additional coagulation and platelet activation reactions can occur. Finally, lysis of fibrin by plasmin results in dissolution of the clot and restoration of flow.

There are two converging pathways of thrombin formation, the *intrinsic* and *extrinsic* pathways (Fig. 41-1). Both involve complex formation between coagulation factors, cofactors, and Ca^{++} on a phospholipid surface, such as cell membranes. Both pathways require vitamin K–dependent coagulation factors, and activation of either pathway results in formation of activated factor X (Xa).[22]

Contact with a negatively charged surface, such as glass or collagen, triggers activation of Hageman factor (XII) to start the intrinsic pathway cascade. In addition, Hageman factor can be activated by proteases, such as kallikrein. Coagulation requires complex formation between activated factor IX (IXa) and factor VIII and cell-membrane phospholipids. This complex activates factor X.

The extrinsic pathway bypasses several steps of the intrinsic pathway but depends on the proteolytic action of factors from the intrinsic pathway. The calcium ion–dependent binding of factor VII to cell membrane–associated tissue factor (thromboplastin) on a phospholipid-containing surface is probably the most important physiologic mechanism for initiation of coagulation. Injury to the vessel wall exposes tissue factor

FIG. 41-1

Compartmentalization of blood coagulation into the intrinsic and extrinsic system is useful in the diagnostic laboratory. The intrinsic system is evaluated with the activated partial thromboplastin time and the extrinsic system with the prothrombin time. HMK, *High molecular weight kininogen;* KAL, *kallikrein;* PF_3, *platelet factor 3.*

From Triplett DA: Clin Lab Med 4:221, 1984.

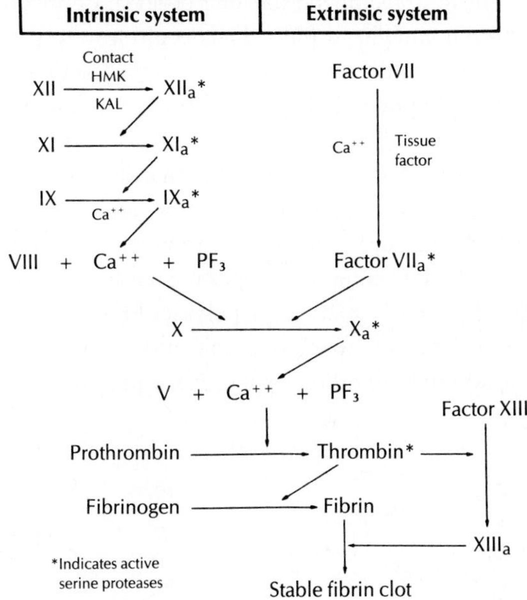

on damaged cell membranes. Tissue factor complexes with factor VII to form an enzymatically active complex that activates factor X; the reaction then proceeds to the generation of thrombin through assembly of the prothrombinase complex composed of factor Xa, Va, and Ca^{++} on an appropriate surface. Although platelets usually provide this surface, the prothrombinase complex may also form on the endothelium or on negatively charged phospholipids, such as plasma lipoproteins.[20]

Thrombin has other important enzymatic actions that can amplify or attenuate coagulation. It can activate factor XIII to XIIIa, which promotes cross-linking and stabilization of the fibrin clot. Thrombin aggregates platelets, and it activates factors V and VIII to further enhance coagulation. In addition, thrombin plays a role in limiting coagulation. It forms an enzymatically active complex with thrombomodulin, derived either from platelets or the vessel wall. This complex converts a zymogen, protein C, to an active protease that then inactivates factors Va and VIIIa, the major cofactors of the coagulation cascade.[12]

ANTICOAGULANTS

Thrombus formation results from an imbalance of promoting and controlling factors within the normal hemostatic process. Thrombi can form in either arteries or veins, but the triggering mechanisms are quite different. Thrombi that occur within small arterioles are composed primarily of platelet aggregates, whereas venous thrombi result from fibrin formation within vessels. Accordingly, antiplatelet agents (see p. 459) are used in management of arterial thrombi, and anticoagulants are employed to minimize venous thrombi. The latter can result from cardiac disease, surgery, neoplasm, or trauma. Extended inhibition of coagulation is desirable in patients who must remain immobilized for long periods. Formation of thrombi within deep leg veins in these immobilized individuals could lead to potentially fatal pulmonary embolism. Anticoagulant drugs do not dissolve clots, but they reduce formation of new ones and decrease the possibility of embolism to the lung and other organs.

Heparin

Heparin is a negatively charged mucopolysaccharide composed of repeating units of sulfated glucosamine and glucuronic acid. The numerous sulfate and carboxyl groups interact with several different blood proteins, including certain coagulation proteins and control factors. Commercial heparin from bovine lung or porcine intestinal mucosa is a heterogeneous mixture of polymers ranging from 6000 to approximately 25,000 daltons. The different size molecules vary in anticoagulant activity, probably because of different affinities for coagulant proteins.

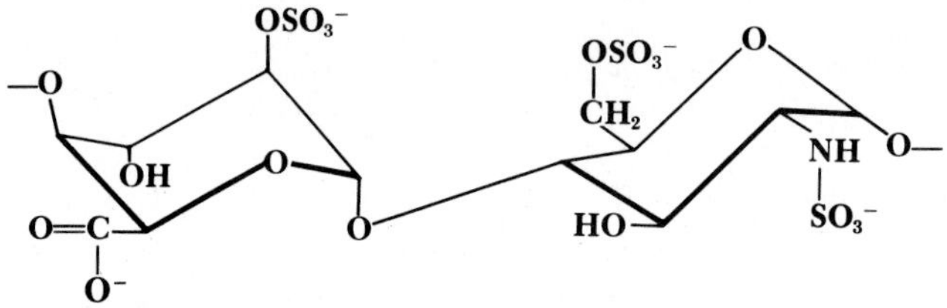

Configuration of disaccharides in heparin

Heparin accelerates complex formation between antithrombin III and factors IXa, Xa, XIa, XIIa, and thrombin (IIa). Antithrombin III, an α_2-globulin, neutralizes thrombin and other serine proteases through binding to an arginine-containing active site[17] (Fig. 41-2). In the absence of heparin this complex forms slowly. Heparin binds to lysyl residues on antithrombin III and, through a conformational change in the molecule, accelerates complex formation approximately a thousandfold. The heterogeneity of heparin is important because high and low molecular weight species have different spectra of activity, and multiple functional domains are involved in their interactions.[17] Low molecular weight heparin has the most potent action on factor Xa binding, whereas high molecular weight heparin is most active on thrombin binding.[3]

Because of its concentrated anionic charge, heparin also inhibits the actions of factors II and X directly, by disrupting formation of protein complexes between the coagulation protein and proactivator. However, this mechanism contributes minimally to the overall anticoagulant activity of heparin.

The vascular endothelial surface contains heparin-like proteoglycans that also accelerate complex formation between activated serine proteases and antithrombin

Effect of heparin on antithrombin III. Heparin will accelerate the inactivation of active serine proteases by antithrombin III. *FIG. 41-2*

From McGann MA, Triplett DA: Lab Med 13:742, 1982.

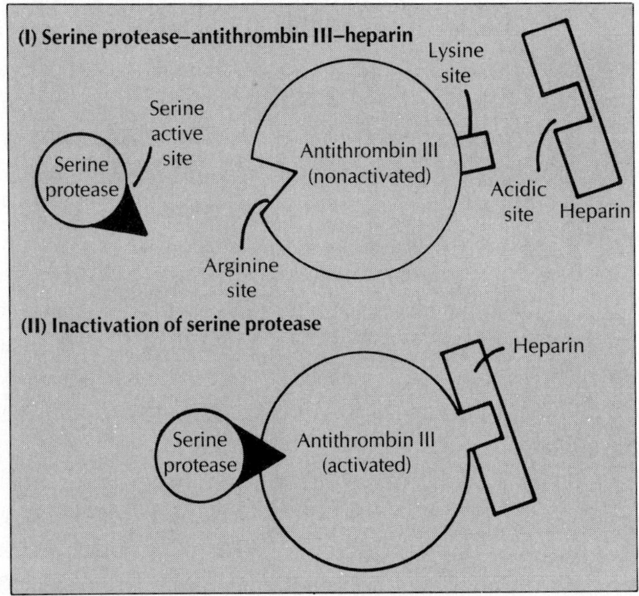

III. Formation of these protease-antithrombin III complexes is probably one mechanism through which the endothelium maintains its antithrombotic surface.[17] In addition, circulating heparin is taken up by the endothelium where it increases the electronegative potential of the vessel wall.

ADMINISTRATION AND DOSAGE

Heparin is not absorbed from the gastrointestinal tract. Because its action depends on the large number of anionic groups, enteric sulfatases, which remove these groups, inactivate it. However, heparin administered either intravenously or subcutaneously is readily absorbed and retains its activity. Intramuscular administration should be avoided because of risk of bleeding at the injection site. Approximately 80% of the heparin in circulation is inactivated by the liver, and the metabolites and residual heparin are excreted by the kidneys.

Heparin is usually the first drug administered when anticoagulation is desired. It is immediately effective after intravenous administration and is effective within hours after subcutaneous injection. Its duration of action is short, however, and it must be administered by continuous infusion or by frequent intermittent (4 to 6 hours) injection. Because heparin requires parenteral administration and its effect must be rigorously monitored, it is usually not used outside of a hospital setting.

Commercial heparin is standardized by its activity, which is expressed in units rather than by weight. One hundred USP units corresponds to approximately 1 mg of heparin.

USE

Heparin is administered when there is an acute need for anticoagulation, as in individuals with suspected or verified pulmonary emboli or deep vein thrombosis.[5] The dose can be adjusted to the predicted rate of thrombin formation. Small doses are usually adequate for prevention of thrombosis in patients at risk, such as those undergoing surgery, but higher doses will be required for those who have already formed deep venous thrombi.[23] Doses on the order of 30,000 units per day will usually prevent extension of clots and lessen the chance for embolization from a leg to the lungs or from the heart to the brain. Low-dose heparin (5000 units) may be administered subcutaneously every 8 to 12 hours to patients at risk for thromboembolism from various surgical procedures. Low-dose heparin imposes only a slight risk of bleeding because the anticoagulant effect is slight.

Heparin is also used to prevent coagulation in vitro, for example, in solutions for extracorporeal circulation and dialysis. One technique is to add heparin to the patient's blood before it enters the extracorporeal device and then to neutralize the heparin with protamine before returning the blood to the patient. Because the blood is anticoagulated only within the extracorporeal circulation, the patient avoids the risk of systemic anticoagulation.

Laboratory monitoring of the degree of anticoagulation is essential because the response to heparin varies from one patient to another and sometimes even within the same patient over time. Close control achieves a greater antithrombotic effect with less risk of hemorrhage. The activated partial thromboplastin time (APTT or PTT) is generally used to monitor heparin-induced anticoagulation. Plasma concentrations of about 0.3 to 0.4 units/ml will extend the APTT to approximately twice control values, which will usually prevent extension of a thrombus.

TOXICITY AND COMPLICATIONS OF THERAPY

Except for anticoagulation, heparin causes few important effects. Even with standard anticoagulant dosage, however, heparin may promote bleeding from open wounds and mucous membranes. Cerebral hemorrhage or retroperitoneal bleeding can be catastrophic. Fortunately, these complications are rare. Alcoholics, elderly individuals (over 60 years of age), and persons with altered hemostasis are at greater risk for hemorrhagic complications. Heparin therapy during pregnancy appears relatively safe. In a recent study 77 women treated with anticoagulant doses of heparin during pregnancy experienced negligible risk of bleeding and no more than the expected incidence of fetal abnormalities or prematurity.[8]

The acute effects of heparin are relatively short lived because the drug is rapidly metabolized. Its half-life is about 1 hour; overdosage can be rapidly corrected by cessation of administration. **Protamine sulfate**, a positively charged polymer, will chemically neutralize heparin.

Heparin does not usually affect platelet function, but a mild thrombocytopenia sometimes occurs after 2 to 3 days of treatment. The effect is slight, and platelet count generally returns to normal even with continued therapy. An immune-mediated thrombocytopenia associated with intravascular thrombosis is a rare complication of heparin therapy. Since commercial heparin contains some impurities, allergic reactions may occur at sites of subcutaneous injection.

Prolonged administration of heparin (more than 6 months) has been linked to osteoporosis. This phenomenon, which likely results from inhibition of osteoblasts, is of little importance with short-term anticoagulation in most patients. For patients at particular risk of osteoporosis or those with bone disorders, it may be more significant. Chronic therapy also diminishes aldosterone secretion, a change that can manifest clinically as hyperkalemia.

Orally effective anticoagulant drugs

A hemorrhagic disorder in cattle fed spoiled sweet clover hay led to discovery of orally effective agents for anticoagulation. The observation that the bleeding was caused by a low prothrombin concentration prompted Link and associates at the University of Wisconsin to isolate from the hay a *coumarin* compound that suppressed prothrombin synthesis.[11]

Synthesis of **dicumarol** (bishydroxycoumarin) provided a compound for use in clinical medicine. Related drugs were synthesized by modification of the dicumarol molecule. One of these, **warfarin,** was originally used as a rodent poison because it was believed too toxic for use in patients. Warfarin is still the active ingredient in various rodenticides, but it is now the drug of choice for maintaining an extended anticoagulated state in humans, in part because it is readily absorbed from the gastrointestinal tract. Coumarin anticoagulants are widely used to manage thromboembolic vascular disease. Although the various compounds differ in structure, potency, and duration of action, they all act by the same basic mechanism.

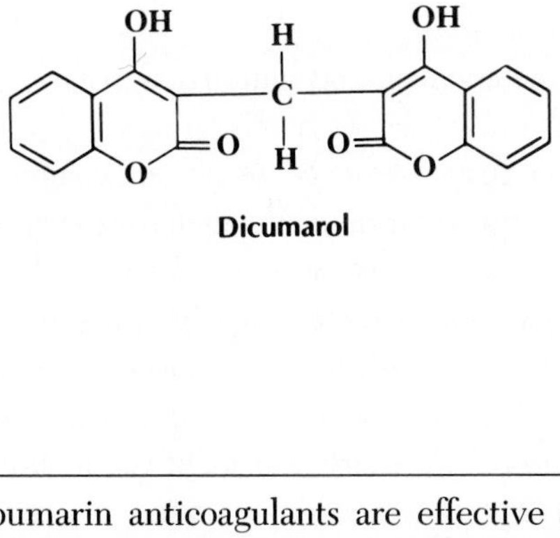

Dicumarol

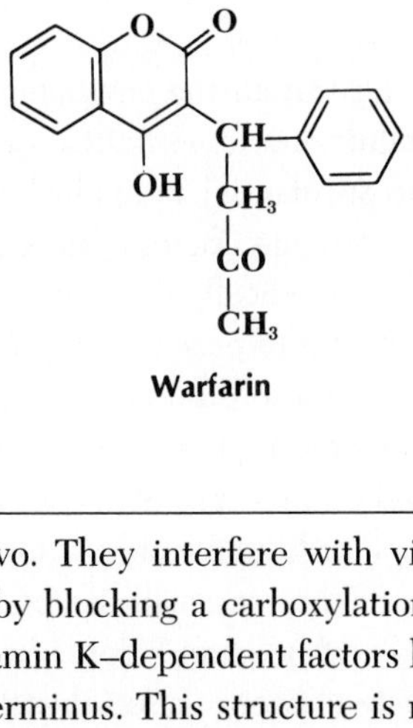

Warfarin

MECHANISM OF ACTION

Coumarin anticoagulants are effective *only* in vivo. They interfere with vitamin K–dependent synthesis of factors II, VII, IX, and X by blocking a carboxylation step required to produce the active factors. Each of the vitamin K–dependent factors has 10 to 12 γ-carboxyglutamic acid residues at the amino terminus. This structure is necessary for binding of the proteins to charged phospholipid membranes during the coagulation process; if binding is inadequate they cannot function either as enzymes or substrates within the assembled complex. Coumarin anticoagulants prevent postribosomal incorporation of the γ-carboxyglutamate residues and thus prevent synthesis of functional factors (Fig. 41-3). Factor VII, the first protein affected, decreases to less than 10% of its original activity within 12 hours. However, a clinically observable anticoagulant effect does not appear this rapidly. Active vitamin K–dependent clotting

FIG. 41-3 *Mechanism of coumarin action. Drugs of the coumarin type interfere with the vitamin K cycle by blocking the enzyme that reduces vitamin K epoxide to vitamin K. Carboxylation of the glutamic acid residues of factors II, VII, IX, and X* (left) *is prevented, thereby inhibiting the activation of these factors.*

Modified from Walsh PN: Hosp Pract 18(1):101, 1983.

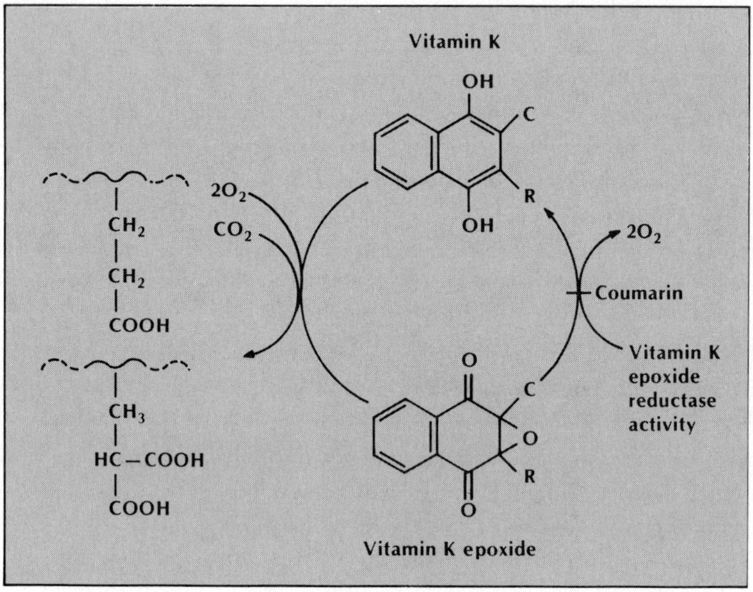

factors already in the circulation must be metabolized and eliminated, a process that may require up to 48 hours.

The substantial individual variability in response to coumarin anticoagulants is caused by many factors, including rate of absorption and metabolic transformation, diet, and genetically determined resistance to the drugs. Because coumarin drugs are highly bound to plasma proteins, other drugs or clinical conditions that affect concentrations of these proteins (particularly albumin) or their binding capacities may influence the efficacy of therapy.

Warfarin, the prototype coumarin anticoagulant, exerts a peak effect within 36 to 72 hours, and the effect lasts for 2 to 5 days. The time needed to attain a plateau effect is due to the long half-life of warfarin. This also accounts for the need to initiate therapy with a loading dose. As Table 41-1 indicates, a much higher dose is required to initiate anticoagulation than to maintain it.

USE Warfarin and related drugs are used in patients with pulmonary embolism or deep venous thrombosis and to prevent thrombosis in those with artificial heart valves or who must remain immobilized for long periods. Warfarin is used in patients undergoing orthopedic surgery as well.[16]

Because the effect of coumarin drugs is delayed, anticoagulation is often initiated with heparin. Coumarin drugs are then administered to sustain the effect. As the

TABLE 41-1 Daily doses and tablet strengths of oral anticoagulants

Preparation	Initial (mg)	Maintenance (mg)	Oral tablet forms (mg)
Dicumarol	200-300	25-200	25, 50
Warfarin sodium (Coumadin, others)	10-15	2-15	2-10
Anisindione (Miradon)	300	25-250	50

anticoagulant effect of the coumarin drug increases, the dosage of heparin may be gradually reduced. Once the desired degree of anticoagulation is achieved, the oral anticoagulant may be continued for as long as 3 to 6 months or more in ambulatory patients.

The use of anticoagulants in acute myocardial infarction remains controversial. Long-term anticoagulation after infarction offers little benefit, but the judicious use of heparin or coumarin drugs for the hospitalized, immobile patient may prevent thrombotic sequelae.[5] Anticoagulant drugs are generally contraindicated in stroke victims because of the potential danger associated with cerebrovascular damage and uncontrolled bleeding into the brain.

Laboratory control

Control of the anticoagulant effect is very important to prevent bleeding complications. The effect of warfarin is monitored at regular intervals by the one-stage *prothrombin time*, which is the time required for clotting in the presence of standardized tissue thromboplastin. Dosage is adjusted to achieve a prothrombin time between one and a half to twice that of normal plasma. Control of coagulation requires accurate and frequent testing under standardized laboratory conditions, particularly when therapy is first initiated. Severe depression of prothrombin concentration may result in bleeding, which may vary from microscopic hematuria to gastrointestinal or cerebral hemorrhage.

If serious bleeding occurs, withdrawal of the drug is insufficient to reverse its action immediately because time is required to synthesize new coagulation factors; furthermore, the coumarin drugs are eliminated slowly. Transfusion of fresh plasma or whole fresh blood can supply the depleted factors, and phytonadione (vitamin K_1, AquaMEPHYTON) can be administered intravenously to promote synthesis of new factors. Because anaphylactic reactions have occurred with phytonadione, this preparation is used only in the event of severe bleeding. Furthermore, treatment with vitamin K may interfere with subsequent coumarin therapy for as long as 2 weeks.

Contraindications

Contraindications to warfarin therapy stem from the possibility of severe bleeding. Major contraindications include a history of recent bleeding, known hemorrhagic disease, gastrointestinal bleeding or disorders that increase risk of hemorrhage, unexplained anemia, central nervous system trauma or surgery, malignant hypertension, and pregnancy. Anticoagulant therapy should be avoided in unreliable persons or when adequate laboratory facilities for continued monitoring are lacking.

CLINICAL PHARMACOLOGY AND DRUG INTERACTIONS

Drug interactions are an important consideration in anticoagulant therapy. Although interactions with the short-lived heparin are few, the coumarin anticoagulants can interact with many other agents. Table 41-2 lists some prominent interactions and probable mechanisms (see also Chapter 70).

Warfarin and other coumarin drugs in circulation are largely bound to albumin (in excess of 99%). Factors such as other drugs can dramatically affect binding, but any increased risk of bleeding from addition of another drug should be temporary. Changes in binding cause a transient, rather than persistent, alteration of the amount of *unbound* drug, and thus there is no prolonged increase in anticoagulant activity.

Drug interactions with anticoagulants involve several mechanisms in addition to changes in protein binding. Because warfarin interferes with vitamin K–dependent synthesis of coagulation factors, its action is enhanced by drugs or conditions that interfere with absorption of vitamin K. Some antibiotics affect the normal flora of the intestine and thereby the endogenous production of vitamin K. Drugs that alter hepatic synthesis of coagulation proteins or affect their catabolism will interact with warfarin. Agents that affect hepatic microsomal enzymes will alter the metabolism and activity of warfarin and related drugs. For example, induction of these enzymes by barbiturates increases warfarin metabolism, and larger doses are required to achieve the desired anticoagulant effect. Cimetidine inhibits hepatic metabolism of many drugs and might be expected to prolong the anticoagulant effect of warfarin. Indeed, cimetidine inhibits warfarin metabolism, but it affects only the inactive stereoisomer; the active stereoisomer and thus the therapeutic effect are unaffected.

Their significant potential for drug interactions is yet another reason for monitoring the prothrombin time of patients taking coumarin drugs. Disruption of the stabilized

TABLE 41-2 Interactions of warfarin with other drugs

Drugs that potentiate warfarin action	**Probable mechanism**
Antibiotics (some)	Decreased production of vitamin K
Cholestyramine, colestipol	Decreased absorption of vitamin K
Aspirin, clofibrate, diazoxide, mefenamic acid, nalidixic acid, phenylbutazone	Competition with warfarin for binding to plasma proteins (transient)
Chloramphenicol, disulfiram, ethyl alcohol (acute), phenylbutazone, propafenone	Inhibition of warfarin degradation
Drugs that inhibit warfarin action	**Probable mechanism**
Cholestyramine, colestipol	Decreased absorption of warfarin
Carbamazepine, ethyl alcohol (chronic), griseofulvin, phenobarbital, phenytoin, rifampin	Enhanced metabolism of warfarin by liver microsomal enzymes
Potentiation of other drugs by warfarin	**Probable mechanism**
Phenytoin, tolbutamide	Competition with warfarin for binding to plasma proteins (transient)

anticoagulated state by drug interactions is both dangerous and costly, as it may take some time to stabilize the dosage again.

ANTIPLATELET DRUGS

Platelet activation is an essential component of hemostasis. When tissue is damaged, vasoconstriction initially decreases blood flow from severed vessels and reduces the area to be occluded by a hemostatic plug. Platelets adhere to damaged cell surfaces or collagen and release proaggregatory and vasoconstrictive substances, such as ADP, thromboxane A_2, and serotonin. As platelets aggregate at the wound site, they form a plug that occludes the severed vessel. Tissue factor (thromboplastin) from injured tissues in combination with factor VII produces thrombin, which stimulates further platelet aggregation to produce a network of fibrin that stabilizes the plug.[7] The reactions between platelets, coagulation factors, and the vessel are shown in Fig. 41-4.

Platelets contribute to cardiovascular disease by aggregating and occluding vessels and by release of vasoactive agents, such as thromboxane, that cause spasm of cerebral and coronary arteries. In addition, platelet activation may promote atherogenesis through release of a growth factor for smooth muscle cells. Because smooth muscle proliferation occurs early in the atherosclerotic process, platelet activation is believed to play a pivotal role in the pathogenesis of stroke, myocardial infarction, and atherosclerosis. Platelets from persons with these disease states appear more easily activated by physiologic stimuli. Platelet hyperreactivity has been associated with cigarette smoking, elevated plasma catecholamines, hypertension, atherosclerotic heart disease, and the presence of artificial surfaces, as in heart valve replacement. A recent study showed that spontaneous platelet aggregation in vitro is a useful predictor for coronary events and mortality of survivors of myocardial infarction.[21]

Drugs can affect platelet activation and response by several different mechanisms. Some decrease adherence of platelets to the vascular wall; others prevent production of thromboxane A_2 to block aggregation. Still other agents affect platelet survival in the circulation through mechanisms that remain obscure.[7] Anticoagulants neither block platelet aggregation nor prevent formation of arterial thrombi. Table 41-3 lists several platelet-inhibitory agents and their mechanisms of action.

Aspirin and other nonsteroidal anti-inflammatory agents

Aspirin is the most commonly used antiplatelet drug. It is inexpensive, effective, and usually well tolerated in low doses. It appears to increase survival after myocardial infarction,[18] to prevent reinfarction, to prevent transient cerebral ischemia, and to decrease the incidence of strokes. It has also proved effective in maintaining patency of bypass grafts.[6]

Aspirin and other nonsteroidal anti-inflammatory agents, such as indomethacin, inhibit platelet function by blocking formation of thromboxane A_2. Aspirin irreversibly inhibits platelet cyclooxygenase through acetylation. (Salicylates that lack an acetyl group do not act by this mechanism.) Since the platelet is unable to synthesize new cyclooxygenase, the effect persists for the life of the cell. The effect of aspirin is cumulative, and even doses as low as 1 mg per day can inhibit platelet activation. Indomethacin, ibuprofen, and other nonsteroidal anti-inflammatory drugs inhibit cyclooxygenase reversibly.

FIG. 41-4 *In arterial thrombus formation, platelet adhesion is initiated by exposure of collagen fibers on injured endothelial surface, and platelets spread by pseudopodia* (top). *Platelets aggregate; discharge of ADP and generation of thromboxane A_2 enhance aggregation* (middle). *Last, the clotting mechanism is activated, generating thrombin, and the action of thrombin on fibrinogen yields fibrin polymers, which stabilize the thrombus.*

From Frishman WH: Hosp Pract 17(5):73, 1982; this illustration drawn by Nancy Lou Makris, Wilton, Conn.

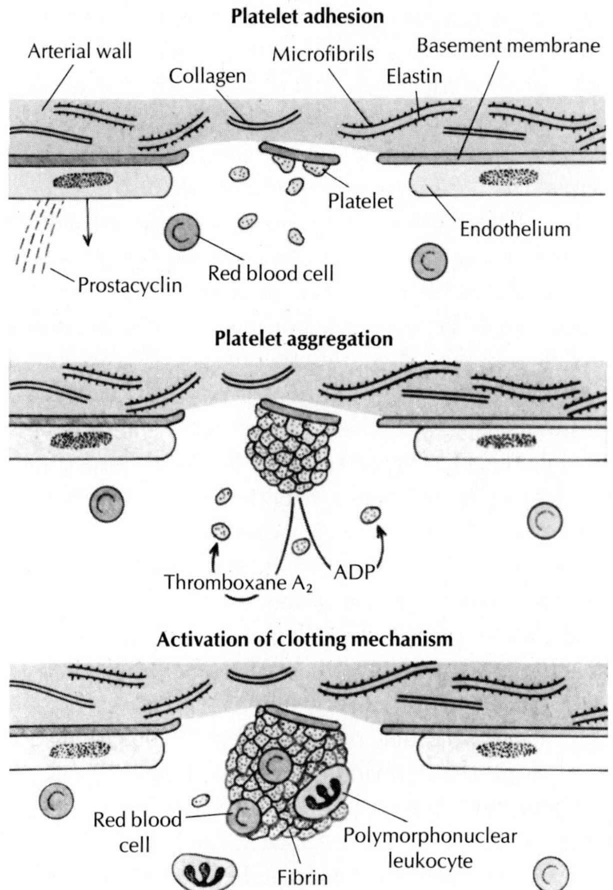

Dipyridamole

Cyclic AMP decreases in platelets undergoing activation and aggregation, and agents that increase platelet cyclic AMP inhibit activation and the release reaction. When circulating platelets contact the vascular endothelium, prostacyclin from the endothelium stimulates platelet adenylyl cyclase to increase formation of cyclic AMP. The transient action of prostacyclin renders it ineffective as a drug for prevention of platelet thrombi, but its continuous production by the endothelium helps to maintain the fluidity of blood.

TABLE 41-3 Platelet-inhibiting agents

Mechanism	Examples
Inhibition of thromboxane formation	Glucocorticoids, aspirin, indomethacin, sulfinpyrazone
Inhibition of ADP-induced aggregation	Ticlopidine
Thromboxane receptor antagonist	Sulotroban*
Thromboxane synthase inhibitor	Pirmagrel,* Dazoxiben*
Increased cyclic AMP; inhibition of activation and aggregation	Prostacyclin, propranolol, dipyridamole
Integrin receptor antagonist	Monoclonal antibody*
Inhibition of thrombin formation	Heparin, oral anticoagulants
Coated surfaces block interactions	Dextran

*Experimental.

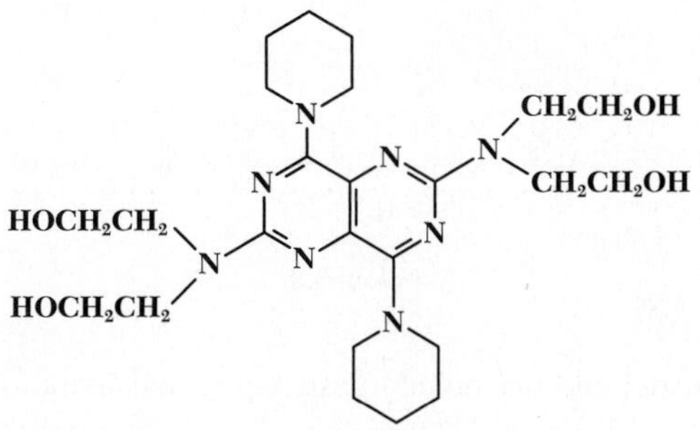

CH_2CH_2OH CH_2CH_2OH $HOCH_2CH_2$ $HOCH_2CH_2$ N N N N N N N N

Dipyridamole

Animal models and early clinical studies indicated that dipyridamole effectively inhibits platelet activation, and several mechanisms were proposed for its actions. One mechanism is inhibition of platelet phosphodiesterase. Inhibition of this enzyme, coupled with enhancement of adenylyl cyclase activity by endogenous prostacyclin, increases platelet cyclic AMP and decreases activation. Dipyridamole also inhibits the cellular uptake and metabolism of adenosine, increasing its concentration locally within the vessel.[6] Because dipyridamole inhibits adhesion of platelets to damaged endothelium or to artificial surfaces, it was used to prevent emboli in patients with artificial heart valves. Most studies using this drug in combination with aspirin, however, show no benefit over aspirin alone, and its use is declining.

Sulfinpyrazone

Sulfinpyrazone inhibits platelet cyclooxygenase, but it is a competitive and reversible inhibitor. Unlike aspirin, sulfinpyrazone neither prolongs bleeding time nor affects platelet aggregation in normal persons. Sulfinpyrazone increases platelet survival within the circulation, but the mechanism of this effect is unknown.

Certain subgroups of patients who have chronically elevated concentrations of plasma catecholamines appear to be at risk for thrombosis, even when aspirin is given to inhibit platelet thromboxane formation. These persons may be better protected with sulfinpyrazone or other drugs that affect catecholamine-induced aggregation.

Ticlopidine

Ticlopidine inhibits platelet aggregation by ADP. Although its mechanism is still unknown, it probably affects an early step common to platelet activation by many agents. It decreases platelet adherence to atheromatous plaques,[13] possibly by decreasing exposure of the platelet *integrin* receptor that is involved in platelet adherence.[4]

In large multicenter clinical trials ticlopidine was superior to aspirin or placebo in reducing the incidence of stroke and myocardial infarction. The drug also appears to prevent transient ischemic attacks, intermittent claudication, and angina. It may also prove useful in preventing progression of nonproliferating diabetic retinopathy.[13]

Ticlopidine is much more effective in vivo than in vitro. It is rapidly metabolized and requires several days to produce maximal benefit. At least one metabolite is more active than the parent drug.[13]

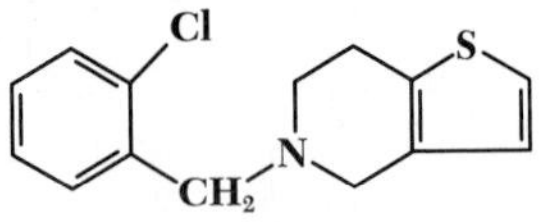

Ticlopidine

Adverse effects of ticlopidine include gastrointestinal irritation, diarrhea, and skin reactions. Leukopenia and thrombocytopenia are less common.[13]

Other agents

Selective inhibition of thromboxane synthesis or blockade of thromboxane receptors has theoretical advantages over aspirin therapy, particularly for patients with peptic ulcer. However, limited trials of reversible thromboxane synthase inhibitors indicate that these compounds are no more effective than low-dose aspirin for inhibition of platelet function. Thromboxane receptor antagonists could benefit individuals with thromboxane-dependent vascular occlusion but would be of little value in thromboxane-independent pathways of platelet activation.[15] Alternate strategies, still in the experimental stage, involve antibody blockade of the integrin receptor.[4]

Use

Antiplatelet drugs help prevent recurrent cerebral ischemic events and stroke, coronary heart disease, and systemic arterial embolism in persons with prosthetic heart valves. They are also used in patients who have arteriovenous shunts and in those with peripheral arterial disease. Because platelet aggregation may contribute to the vasospasm of unstable angina, antiplatelet drugs are a rational choice for treatment of this condition as well.

There have been numerous clinical trials of antiplatelet drugs in patients with cardiovascular disease. These agents are now an integral part of the management of myocardial infarction and stroke. Prevention of recurrence is a major goal for patients who have had a myocardial infarction. Obvious control measures include treatment of hypertension, reduction of abnormally high lipid levels, and cessation of smoking. Prophylactic aspirin therapy reduces initial cardiac events. It also provides effective secondary prophylaxis; it decreases cardiovascular mortality and recurrence of nonfatal myocardial infarction.[14] Aspirin is now suggested as routine therapy after a first myocardial infarction in patients without contraindications.[14,18]

FIBRINOLYTIC AGENTS

The fibrinolytic system is normally activated simultaneously with coagulation. Fibrin strands form the structural matrix of a thrombus that will be lysed subsequently by plasmin. Dissolution of a formed clot stimulates repair of damaged tissues as the fibrinolytic system clears fibrin deposits that form within small vessels. Plasmin, or fibrinolysin, is a serine protease generated from plasminogen, a precursor molecule. Plasmin is activated by two biochemically distinct activators, tissue (tPA) and urokinase (UPA) *plasminogen activators*. Plasmin can cleave various proteins, but it has a particular affinity for fibrin. Degradation of insoluble fibrin dissolves the clot.

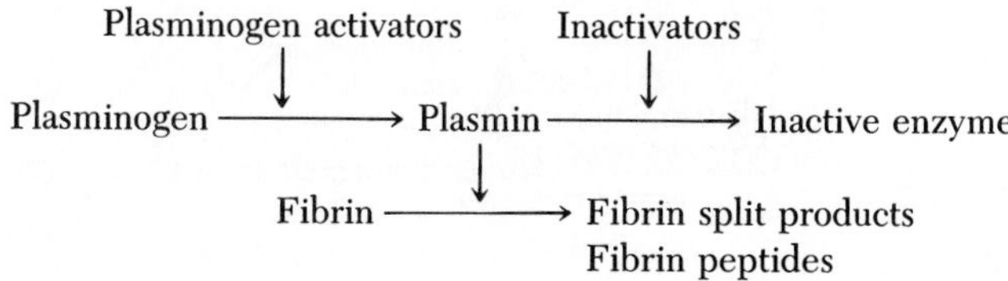

Control mechanisms for fibrinolysis are important for both limitation of clot formation and their removal. One mechanism is the expression of tissue-type plasminogen activator on the endothelial surface and on circulating blood cells (Fig. 41-5). Several naturally occurring inhibitors of plasminogen activator in blood and tissues prevent inappropriate action of plasminogen. tPA, the principal mediator of fibrinolysis, becomes effective when it contacts fibrin within a clot or along the vessel wall. The proteolytic activity of tPA is, in turn, regulated by inhibitors in blood. Plasmin is thus usually activated within a thrombus where tPA is enhanced and concentrations of inhibitors are low. Plasmin released into the circulation is immediately neutralized by circulating inactivators.

Thrombolytic therapy is based on the need for rapid dissolution of clots that can cause significant morbidity or mortality. Administration of either streptokinase or urokinase activates the fibrinolytic system by stimulating conversion of plasminogen to plasmin. Two other agents, alteplase and anistreplase, are approved for intravenous thrombolytic therapy of coronary thrombosis.[1] Thrombolytic therapy with any of these agents, although originally controversial, has proved effective in early treatment of myocardial infarction when lysis of clots helps to salvage ischemic regions of myocardium. Thrombolytic therapy decreases morbidity and mortality in carefully selected patients.

Streptokinase

Streptokinase (Kabikinase, Streptase) is an enzyme produced by certain strains of streptococci. It activates plasminogen in blood or in a clot by a nonenzymatic alteration

FIG. 41-5 *Fibrinolysis is localized in consolidating thrombus. There plasminogen, bound to fibrin and to platelets, is activated by fibrin-bound tissue plasminogen activator, with local release of plasmin.*

From Del Zoppo GJ, Harker LA: Hosp Pract 19(5):163, 1984.

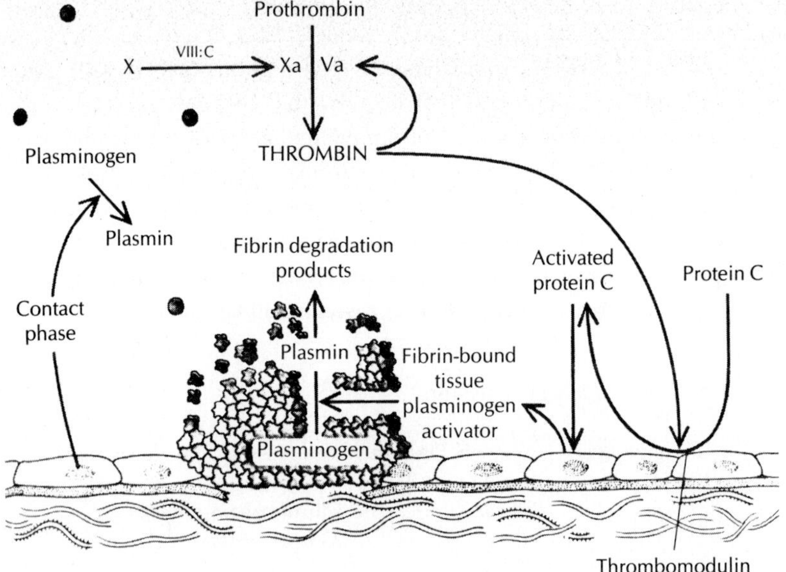

in the conformation of the molecule, which results in an active proteolytic moiety. Streptokinase is a foreign protein, and most problems with this agent, other than bleeding, result from its antigenicity. Many people have antibodies to streptokinase from previous streptococcal infections. These antibodies can cause hypersensitivity reactions ranging from skin rashes to anaphylaxis. Antibody neutralization of infused streptokinase greatly diminishes its fibrinolytic effect.

Anistreplase (APSAC)

Anistreplase (Eminase) is an anisoylated, inactivated complex of streptokinase and plasminogen that acts as a slow release form of plasminogen activator. Coupling of the streptokinase-plasminogen complex to *p*-amidinophenyl-*p*-anisate blocks the catalytic center of the complex, but allows it to bind to fibrin. As the anisoyl group is slowly hydrolyzed at the site of the clot, the activity of the plasminogen activator is regenerated. Although anistreplase is less fibrin specific than tPA, it offers some advantages over streptokinase: principally that it is less inhibited by streptokinase antibodies, it has a longer half-life, and it can be given as a single injection. Anistreplase causes fibrinogen depletion, however, and the rate of bleeding complications is comparable to that with streptokinase therapy.[2]

Urokinase

Urokinase (Abbokinase) was originally isolated from human urine and was the first naturally occurring plasminogen activator used therapeutically. It has been used for intravenous therapy of coronary thrombosis, but, because of the high cost, alternative agents are preferred.

Urokinase is produced by the human kidney and is thus not antigenic in man. However, some preparations may be pyrogenic because of contaminating substances. Urokinase activates plasminogen either in circulation or within a fibrin-containing thrombus by an enzymatic mechanism. Like streptokinase, urokinase has a twofold action. It activates plasmin that is adsorbed to fibrin to cause fibrinolysis. It also converts plasminogen to plasmin within the circulation. Even though free plasmin is readily bound by plasmin inhibitors, urokinase therapy can cause a decrease in both plasminogen and plasmin inhibitors, with potentially serious consequences. One form of urokinase that consists of a single rather than double chain is reported to have greater affinity for fibrin and thus increased specificity.[2]

Urokinase is highly effective but very expensive. It is now obtained from cultures of human kidney cells, but the cost of therapy remains high.

Tissue plasminogen activator (tPA)

tPA was isolated from blood and various tissues, but the amounts that could be purified were sparse. Alteplase (Activase), recombinant tPA produced by genetically engineered cells, is identical to the naturally occurring enzyme. It was introduced as an alternative to streptokinase in therapy of evolving myocardial infarction, and it was recently approved for treatment of massive pulmonary embolism. Its action occurs primarily within the thrombus and is more selective than either streptokinase or urokinase. Such specificity was presumed to confer lower risk of bleeding, but this has not proved true in clinical trials. tPA forms a complex with fibrin, and the complex converts inactive plasminogen into plasmin within the confines of the clot.

There are some drawbacks to therapy with tPA. Its duration of action is very short and continuous infusion for 1 to 3 hours is required to maintain thrombolytic activity, in contrast to anistreplase. Treatment is approximately 10 times as expensive as streptokinase therapy. The rate of bleeding complications is high, particularly if tPA is used in combination with anticoagulants such as heparin. tPA use in coronary occlusion is reportedly associated with a high incidence of reocclusion, but it appears that aspirin can help prevent this.[19] A recent multicenter trial indicated that streptokinase and tPA are equally effective, with or without added heparin, in patients with no complications.[9] However, noncardiac complications, including stroke, were greater with tPA.[10]

Use

The decision to use a fibrinolytic agent is based on definitive diagnosis of thrombotic or thromboembolic disease and a careful determination of its severity. Early thrombolytic therapy in acute myocardial infarction affects reperfusion of ischemic myocardium, limits infarct size, and decreases mortality. Thrombolysis is indicated in diseases such as acute pulmonary embolism with hemodynamic instability, extensive deep venous thrombosis, and arterial thrombosis. It is also used to reverse occlusion of access shunts and catheters. Because streptokinase and urokinase act only on newly formed clots, therapy must be prompt. It is believed that most thrombus dissolution by these agents occurs within the first 12 hours of therapy. Thrombi composed primarily of platelets, however, will resist lysis. The action of tPA is less influenced by the age of the clot. Even so, the use of tPA in myocardial infarction is limited to the first 24 to 48 hours, the major consideration being the extent to which myocardium deprived of blood can be salvaged.

Studies comparing different strategies for thrombolysis are often difficult to interpret because of differences in protocols, patient selection, and endpoints from one study to another. However, when thrombolytic therapy was administered early there was generally a reduction of infarct damage, preservation of left ventricular function, and an improved prognosis.[19]

Contraindications to use of fibrinolytic agents include active internal bleeding, cerebrovascular injury or disease, bleeding disorders, and recent surgery or the need for further invasive procedures. Fibrinolytic agents should be avoided during pregnancy and the postpartum period. Their use in pulmonary embolism requires confirmation of the diagnosis by angiography.

Adverse effects and complications. Therapy with any of the fibrinolytic agents can result in bleeding. Fibrinolysis will occur not only at the target site but also wherever hemostatic plugs have formed, and hematomas frequently occur where intravenous or intraarterial catheters are inserted.

Allergic reactions may occur as complications of streptokinase therapy and, less commonly, with urokinase therapy. Recombinant tPA avoids such complications but may introduce others, such as an increased incidence of reocclusion.[2]

Reocclusion. Data from animal studies indicate that platelets play a major role in reocclusion after thrombolysis has been successfully completed. This could explain why, even when heparin is administered along with a thrombolytic drug, the therapy is ineffective in as many as 20% to 30% of treated patients. It also explains why aspirin can help to prevent reocclusion.[2] Large scale studies of survival after myocardial infarction indicate that a combination of aspirin and streptokinase is more effective than either agent alone in reduction of cardiovascular sequelae and death.[4]

Vasodilating prostaglandins have been given via intracoronary perfusion along with thrombolytic agents. Their lack of specificity for platelets, however, limits their usefulness. A goal of future thrombolytic regimens is to utilize agents that are platelet- or fibrin-specific and that lack systemic effects.

REFERENCES

1. Anistreplase for acute coronary thrombosis, *Med Lett Drugs Ther* 31:15, 1990.
2. Bang NU, Wilhelm OG, Clayman MD: Thrombolytic therapy in acute myocardial infarction, *Annu Rev Pharmacol Toxicol* 29:323, 1989.
3. Brandt JT: The role of natural coagulation inhibitors in homeostasis, *Clin Lab Med* 4:245, 1984.
4. Coller BS: Platelets and thrombolytic therapy, *N Engl J Med* 322:33, 1990.
5. Collins R, Scrimgeour A, Yusuf S, Peto R: Reduction in fatal pulmonary embolism and venous thrombosis by perioperative administration of subcutaneous heparin: overview of results of randomized trials in general, orthopedic, and urologic surgery, *N Engl J Med* 318:1162, 1988.
6. FitzGerald GA: Dipyridamole, *N Engl J Med* 316:1247, 1987.

7. Frishman WH: Antiplatelet therapy in coronary heart disease, *Hosp Pract* 17(5):73, 1982.
8. Ginsberg JS, Kowalchuk G, Hirsh J, et al: Heparin therapy during pregnancy: risks to the fetus and mother, *Arch Intern Med* 149:2233, 1989.
9. Gruppo Italiano per lo Studio della Sopravvivenza nell'Infarto Miocardico: GISSI-2: a factorial randomised trial of alteplase versus streptokinase and heparin versus no heparin among 12 490 patients with acute myocardial infarction, *Lancet* 336:65, 1990.
10. International Study Group: In-hospital mortality and clinical course of 20 891 patients with suspected acute myocardial infarction randomised between alteplase and streptokinase with or without heparin, *Lancet* 336:71, 1990.
11. Link KP: The anticoagulant from spoiled sweet clover hay, *Harvey Lect* 39:162, 1944.
12. Mann KG: The biochemistry of coagulation, *Clin Lab Med* 4:207, 1984.
13. McTavish D, Faulds D, Goa KL: Ticlopidine: an updated review of its pharmacology and therapeutic use in platelet-dependent disorders, *Drugs* 40:238, 1990.
14. Moss AJ, Benhorin J: Prognosis and management after a first myocardial infarction, *N Engl J Med* 322:743, 1990.
15. Oates JA, FitzGerald GA, Branch RA, et al: Clinical implications of prostaglandin and thromboxane A_2 formation, *N Engl J Med* 319:689, 1988.
16. Powers PJ, Gent M, Jay RM, et al: A randomized trial of less intense postoperative warfarin or aspirin therapy in the prevention of venous thromboembolism after surgery for fractured hip, *Arch Intern Med* 149:771, 1989.
17. Rosenberg RD: The biochemistry and pathophysiology of the prethrombotic state, *Annu Rev Med* 38:493, 1987.
18. Schreiber TL: Aspirin and thrombolytic therapy for acute myocardial infarction: should the combination now be a routine therapy? *Drugs* 38:180, 1989.
19. Simoons ML: Thrombolytic therapy in acute myocardial infarction, *Annu Rev Med* 40:181, 1989.
20. Tracy PB: Regulation of thrombin generation at cell surfaces, *Semin Thromb Hemost* 14:227, 1988.
21. Trip MD, Cats VM, van Capelle FJL, Vreeken J: Platelet hyperreactivity and prognosis in survivors of myocardial infarction, *N Engl J Med* 322:1549, 1990.
22. Triplett DA: The extrinsic system, *Clin Lab Med* 4:221, 1984.
23. Wu KK: New pharmacologic approaches to thromboembolic disorders, *Hosp Pract* 20(7):101, 1985.

Chapter 42

Diuretic drugs

GENERAL CONCEPT

Diuretic agents increase renal excretion of solutes and water, for the most part by decreasing renal tubular reabsorption of solutes (usually $Na^+ \pm Cl^-$) and secondarily water. Excretion of K^+, HCO_3^- and, to a much lesser extent, divalent cations such as Ca^{++} and Mg^{++} may also be increased. Diuretics do not affect either glomerular filtration rate (GFR) or the action of antidiuretic hormone (ADH) on the distal portion of the nephron. Atrial natriuretic peptide (ANP) is an endogenous hormone that does cause natriuresis by increasing GFR.[7] It is released by the cardiac atrium in response to stretch such as occurs with volume expansion. It is being studied as a potential diuretic agent but is not yet available for clinical use. Similarly, aquaretics that inhibit the effects of antidiuretic hormone (ADH) are being evaluated but are not yet marketed.

Reduction in water reabsorption by diuretic drugs depends on their ability to decrease solute reabsorption. This reduction in solute and secondarily water reabsorption can be accomplished either by glomerular ultrafiltration of a substance that the tubules have limited or no ability to reabsorb (an osmotic diuretic) or by a drug that decreases reabsorption of Na^+ and preferably Cl^- (a saluretic agent). The electrolyte tends to keep with it in the urine an osmotic equivalent of water, depending on how and where the drug acts. The types of diuretics to be considered include (1) osmotic diuretics, (2) carbonic anhydrase inhibitors that act predominantly in the proximal segment of the nephron, (3) diuretics that act on the ascending limb of the loop of Henle, (4) diuretics that inhibit solute reabsorption in the distal tubule, and (5) antikaliuretic or K^+-retaining diuretics, which decrease exchange of Na^+ (reabsorption) for K^+ (secretion) in the distal segment of the nephron.

To use a diuretic drug effectively, the status of both renal and extrarenal factors involved in diuresis must be understood.[8] For instance, if glomerular filtration is decreased by disease or by a reduction in systemic blood pressure, the amount of filtered Na^+ may be limiting, and diuresis will be lessened. On the other hand, a diuretic agent may induce only limited diuresis by normal kidneys if the patient's disease results in avid reabsorption of solute at a site in the tubules either prior to or distal to the site of diuretic action.

EXTRARENAL ASPECTS

The use of diuretic drugs for relief of edema (extravascular accumulation of fluid in tissues) requires an understanding of the factors that influence movement of plasma water from the vascular system to the extravascular space and its return. Salient features of these factors follow:

1. The site of action of a diuretic agent on the renal tubules may be remote to the site at which edema is evident. However, as the drug inhibits the reabsorption of salt and water, it reduces commensurately the volume of extracellular fluid and ultimately total body water. In other words, the diuresis derives from the intravascular and then the extracellular fluid space.
2. Even slight changes in the relationship between cardiac output and peripheral vascular resistance can profoundly alter the action of diuretics. For instance, simple bed rest and salt restriction in an edematous patient may be sufficient to cause an impressive loss of edema fluid as reflected by a decline in body weight (Fig. 42-1).
3. Either an improvement in the function of a failing heart induced by a cardiotonic agent such as digitalis or inhibition of electrolyte and water reabsorption by a diuretic may increase urine volume and reduce edema. Employed together, these two mechanisms have greater efficacy than either alone.

INTRARENAL ASPECTS

The rate of glomerular ultrafiltration can be increased by plasma volume expansion (at least in part mediated by ANP) or increased systemic blood pressure, or both. It can be reduced by decreased systemic arterial pressure or renal afferent arteriolar constriction. Diuretic agents do not affect glomerular filtration directly, though they can have indirect effects. Diuretic-induced volume depletion can increase concentrations of angiotensin II and catecholamines, vasoconstrictors that in turn decrease glomerular filtration rate and limit diuresis.

The proximal portion of the renal tubules is responsible for reabsorption of 70% or more of filtered monovalent electrolytes; isosmotic water reabsorption occurs passively.[16,18,28] At the initial portions of the proximal tubule, filtered organic solutes, including amino acids and glucose, are actively reabsorbed with salt and water following passively.[28] The only diuretics (osmotic) that block this pathway do so indirectly. In addition, the proximal tubules actively reabsorb Na^+ in exchange for H^+ (Fig. 42-2) via the Na^+-H^+ antiporter. The H^+ becomes available on dissociation of $H_2CO_3 \rightleftharpoons H^+ + HCO_3^-$ under the influence of an enzyme, carbonic anhydrase, located on the luminal side of the cell membrane. The H^+ that enters the lumen combines with filtered HCO_3^-:

$$H^+ + HCO_3^- \rightarrow H^+ + OH^- + CO_2$$

The CO_2 then diffuses into the cell where the reverse reaction occurs. The net result is reabsorption of $NaHCO_3$. This exchange can be blocked by inhibiting carbonic anhydrase as occurs with compounds having a characteristic NH_2SO_2–R structure. Removal of $NaHCO_3$ leaves a favorable concentration gradient for passive Cl^- reabsorption with accompanying Na^+ and water to maintain charge and osmotic neutrality.[1,16] Finally, there also appears to be additional active Na^+ reabsorption in the proximal tubule. Osmotic diuretics indirectly inhibit all these pathways.

Na^+ and K^+ balance within the cells is sustained by the action of Na^+,K^+-dependent ATPase located at the peritubular border of the cell.[12]

The permeability and physical characteristics of the loop of Henle combine with

FIG. 42-1 *Effect of bed rest and low sodium diet on loss of weight (edema) and sodium in a cirrhotic patient.*

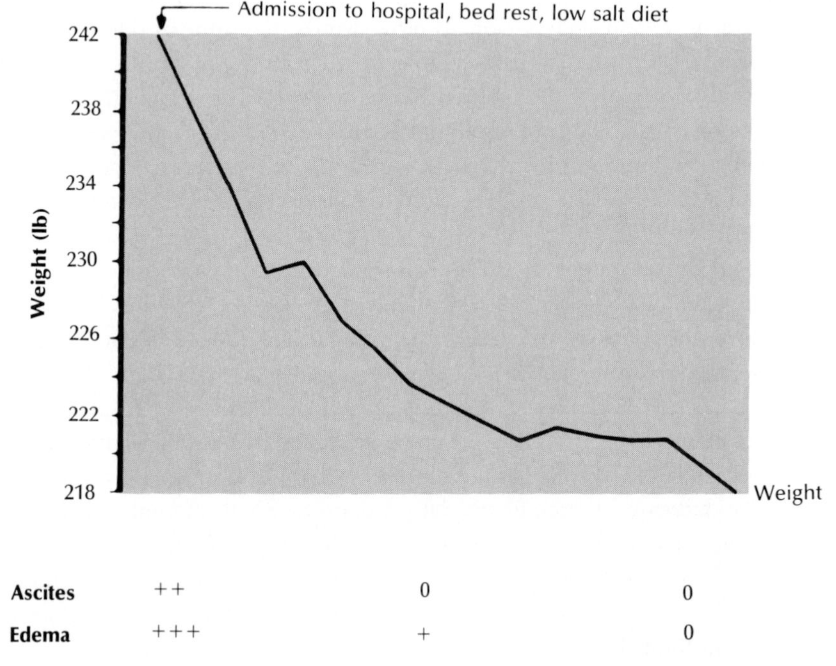

Ascites	++	0	0
Edema	+++	+	0

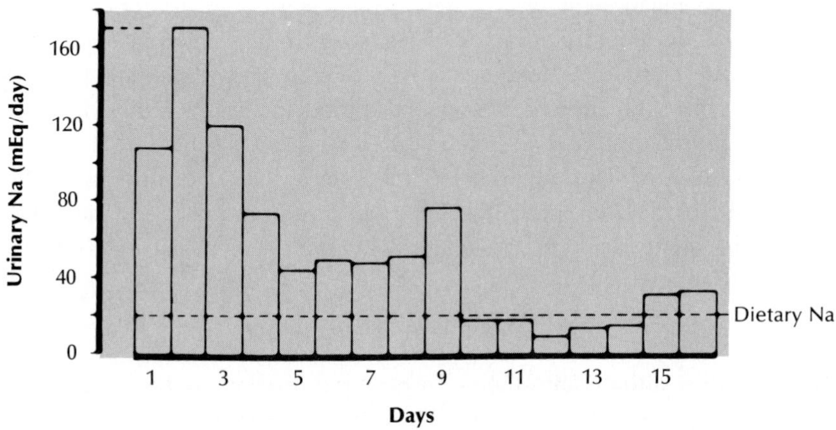

those of the vasa recta to sustain, through countercurrent exchange, an increasing concentration gradient of Na^+, Cl^-, and urea from the cortex to the papilla of the medulla[10] (Fig. 42-2). Critical to this concentration gradient is solute reabsorption by the thick segment of the ascending limb of the loop, which is impermeable to water. Because of this impermeability to water, selective removal of solute occurs, resulting in hypotonic luminal contents; hence this segment is also called the diluting segment. The loop is permeable to diffusion of urea into the interstitium in such a manner that

Diagram of a nephron to illustrate electrolyte and water transport across the cells and the site or sites of action of some diuretic agents. *FIG. 42-2*

Tubule

	Proximal	Loop	Distal	Collecting
Mannitol	+	+	+	+
Thiazides	±		+ +	
Acetazolamide	+ +			
Loop diuretics	+	+ + +		
Mercurial	+	+ +		
Spironolactone			+	
Triamterene			+	
Amiloride			+	
ADH				+

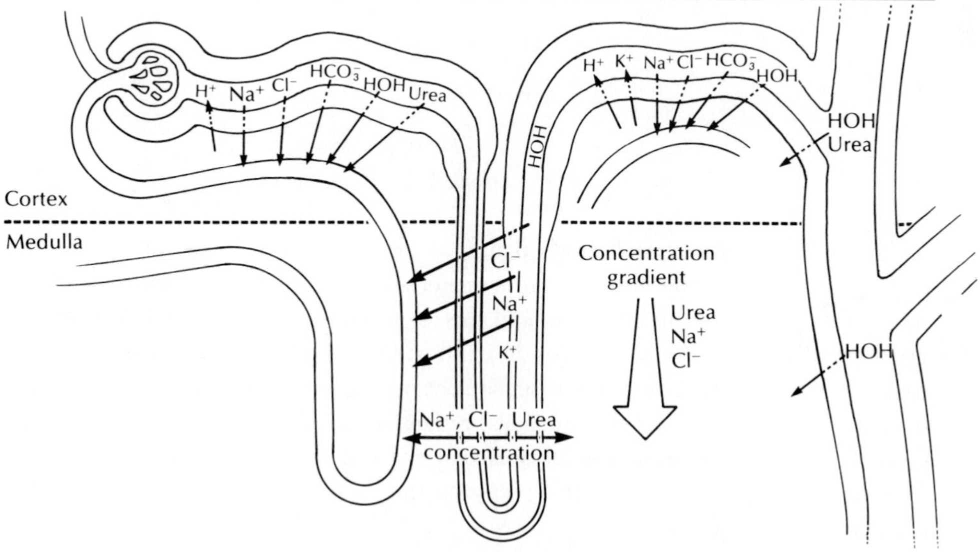

the countercurrent mechanism sustains the increasing gradient from cortex to inner medulla. This tubular segment reabsorbs 25% to 30% of filtered Na^+. Reabsorption of electrolyte occurs as two Cl^- coupled to one Na^+ and one K^+.[10] This transporter is inhibited by loop diuretics.

In the distal portion of the tubule, the remaining 5% or less of Na^+ is reabsorbed. Na^+ and Cl^- are absorbed electroneutrally by a pump that is inhibited by thiazide diuretics.[23] Active reabsorption of Na^+ by exchange with H^+ also occurs and is made possible by the action of carbonic anhydrase. The H^+ contributes to urine acidification so that little or no HCO_3^- escapes reabsorption, and Cl^- remains the principal anion excreted. In addition, active reabsorption of Na^+ is facilitated by the action of aldosterone, the hormone of the adrenal cortex that also causes K^+ secretion.

Antidiuretic hormone (ADH) acts in the collecting tubules to facilitate reabsorption of urea and water to the extent of some 99% of the amount filtered. This diffusion of water is driven by the high osmotic gradient of Na^+ and Cl^- in the medulla, to which urea also contributes. If secretion of ADH by the hypothalamus is depressed by a high consumption of water, water reabsorption is prevented and urine flow increases.

OSMOTIC DIURETICS

Mannitol is the prototype osmotic diuretic.[26] Its chemical structure resembles that of glucose. The compound is eliminated completely by filtration at the glomeruli. Mannitol is not absorbed when given orally; its distribution in the body is limited to extracellular fluid; and, when filtered, it is not reabsorbed by the renal tubules. Consequently an osmotic equivalent of water passes along the renal tubules with mannitol to increase the volume of urine excreted.

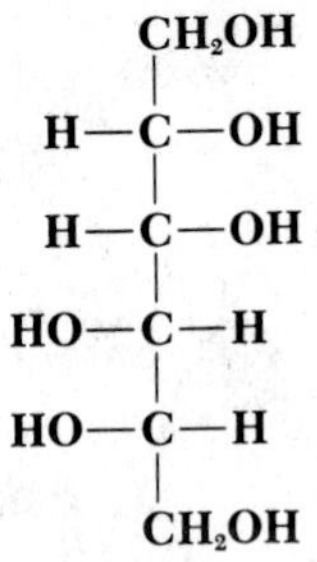

$$
\begin{array}{c}
CH_2OH \\
| \\
H-C-OH \\
| \\
H-C-OH \\
| \\
HO-C-H \\
| \\
HO-C-H \\
| \\
CH_2OH
\end{array}
$$

Mannitol

The main use of mannitol, rather than as a diuretic, is to decrease intracranial and intraocular pressure. Because mannitol increases extracellular osmolality, water is drawn from the intracellular space, and this is useful for treating cerebral edema.[26] However, this intervention, by expanding intravascular volume or by causing hyponatremia (by drawing water into the vascular space), can also be hazardous. For example, mannitol is not ordinarily employed for reduction of edema associated with heart failure because expansion of the intravascular space in this setting can be disastrous. In such cases a diuretic that acts directly on the tubules to increase salt and water excretion is more desirable.

Mannitol (Osmitrol) is administered intravenously in hypertonic concentrations, greater than 5% and up to 25%, in from 50 to 1000 ml of distilled water. Its duration of action is short (2 or 3 hours) if glomerular filtration rate is normal.

ORGANOMERCURIAL DIURETICS

In 1920 Saxl and Heilig[19] reported that when syphilitic patients were injected with the antisyphilitic (organomercurial) drug merbaphen, they tended to excrete more urine. Until the 1950s, the organomercurials were the only diuretics that could be relied upon. Today these agents are no longer used.

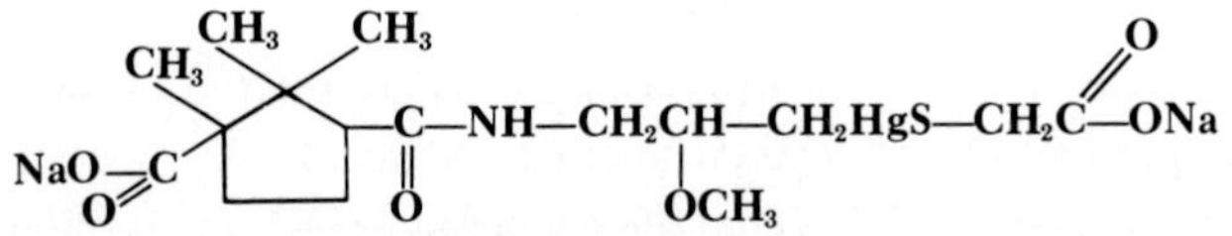

CH_3 CH_3 CH_3 O

NaO—C(=O)— [ring] —C(=O)—NH—CH_2CH(OCH_3)—CH_2HgS—CH_2C(=O)—ONa

Mercaptomerin sodium

Typically, organomercurials increased excretion (inhibited reabsorption) of Na^+ and Cl^-. Their effect on K^+ was variable. Water excretion was in excess of electrolyte, an increased *free water clearance* consistent with their effect on the thick segment of the loop of Henle.

The propensity of these compounds to cause renal tubular damage to the point of necrosis, if administered in too high a dosage or too frequently, limited their utility. Fortunately, there are safer potent diuretics today that are more convenient to use.

CARBONIC ANHYDRASE INHIBITORS

Shortly after sulfanilamide introduced the modern era of antimicrobial chemotherapy (see Chapter 56), it was noted to cause alkaline urine and a metabolic acidosis.[22] Mann and Keilin[14] showed that sulfanilamide inhibits carbonic anhydrase. Schwartz[20] in 1949 then reported the clinical use of sulfanilamide for relief of edema in decompensated cardiac patients, though increased excretion of HCO_3^- limited its utility. The stage for modern diuretic therapy was set by this report and by Krebs' publication[13] on chemical structure-activity relationships demonstrating that (1) substitution of the sulfamoyl-nitrogen of sulfanilamide destroyed activity, (2) heterocyclic sulfonamides were more active, and (3) acetylation of the *p*-amino group enhanced activity of sulfanilamide.

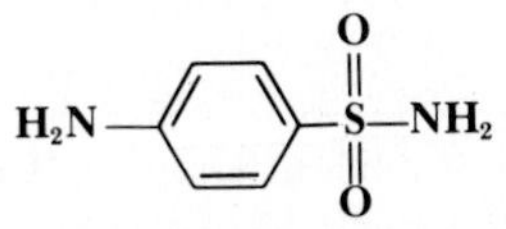

Sulfanilamide

The development of diuretics based on carbonic anhydrase inhibition then took two directions: (1) the search for more potent carbonic anhydrase inhibitors as such and (2) the search for compounds that would increase Cl^- rather than HCO_3^- excretion as the predominant anion with Na^+.

The search for more potent carbonic anhydrase inhibitors culminated in **acetazolamide**,[15] the clinical utility of which was reported in 1953. Its in vitro activity is about 1000 times greater than that of sulfanilamide; their pharmacodynamic profiles are otherwise similar.

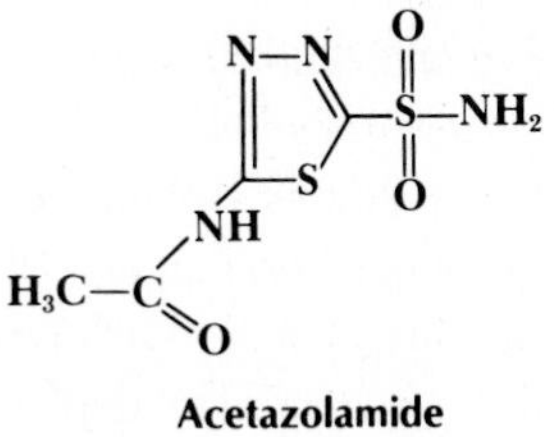

Acetazolamide

Acetazolamide was the first diuretic to be well absorbed and well tolerated when administered orally. It is filtered at the glomeruli, actively secreted by the proximal renal tubules, and is also reabsorbed; reabsorption is least at alkaline urinary pH.

Typically, acetazolamide increases urinary pH and excretion of Na^+, K^+, HCO_3^-, and water. Little or no Cl^- appears in the urine. The increase in K^+ excretion is a compensatory effort by the nephron to conserve (reabsorb) Na^+ more distally in the nephron where Na^+ reabsorption occurs in exchange for K^+. In addition, the increased HCO_3^- in the tubular lumen establishes an electronegative charge that facilitates K^+ secretion.

Acetazolamide (Diamox, others) is available as tablets of 125 and 250 mg and as a 500 mg sustained-release formulation. It is also available for parenteral use in vials containing 500 mg of the cryodesiccated sodium powder.

When acetazolamide is administered as a diuretic, it should be given intermittently to permit recovery of plasma HCO_3^- concentration between doses. Otherwise, continuous therapy soon induces a metabolic (hyperchloremic) acidosis, in which condition acetazolamide becomes ineffective.

In present practice, reduction of intraocular tension in glaucoma is the main indication for carbonic anhydrase inhibitors (see Table 14-1) because more useful diuretics have been developed. The drug is also effective treatment for altitude sickness.

Because of the ubiquitous distribution of carbonic anhydrase in the nervous system, side effects of drugs of this type may include paresthesias, which are reversible on withdrawal of the agent.

THIAZIDES AND RELATED DIURETICS

Early research on sulfanilamide analogs showed that its *p*-carboxy congener was weakly chloruretic. A search ensued with the description in 1957 of **chlorothiazide**, which predominantly increases excretion of Na^+, Cl^-, and water.[4]

Chlorothiazide and related compounds act from the tubular lumen. They reach this site by secretion at the proximal tubules, and to the extent that they are not bound to plasma albumin they are also filtered at the glomeruli. These agents retain a mild activity to decrease solute reabsorption in the proximal nephron, presumably by inhibiting carbonic anhydrase. However, their predominant effect is a reduction in solute reabsorption in the distal convoluted tubule by inhibiting an electroneutral Na^+-Cl^- reabsorption pump that serves as a receptor for thiazide diuretics.[23]

In general, thiazides induce the same maximum natriuretic response regardless of drug (Fig. 42-3), and their activity is not sensitive to urine pH.

Hypokalemia may result from increased K^+ excretion. It is more likely with larger doses; in contrast, antihypertensive and diuretic effects can usually be attained at low doses. Thus low doses of the drugs maximize efficiency and minimize toxicity, whereas high doses primarily increase adverse effects without additional benefit. Hypokalemia may manifest as complaints of weakness or fatigue. Patients receiving digitalis are likely to be more sensitive to digitalis toxicity. Ordinarily, patients with good renal function on a normal diet should not become K^+ depleted. In some settings, such as the secondary hyperaldosteronism of heart failure or cirrhosis, more pronounced K^+ loss may require treatment.

Hyperuricemia and increased BUN may ensue from volume depletion. Impaired glucose tolerance can result from unknown mechanisms and is not necessarily indicative of diabetes.

Single-dose response curves for trichlormethiazide, hydrochlorothiazide, and chlorothiazide showing differences in potency but identity of efficacy (upper plateau). *FIG. 42-3*

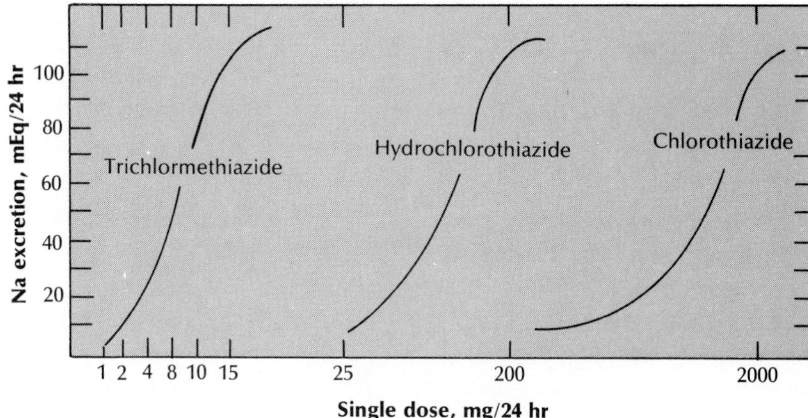

Since the development of chlorothiazide, numerous analogs have been marketed that differ only in dose administered and duration of action[27] (Table 42-1). **Chlorthalidone** and some other agents, though structurally distinct, are pharmacologically indistinguishable from the thiazides.

The thiazides are well tolerated and effective when administered orally or parenterally to edematous patients with normal or moderate impairment of renal function. They are also useful alone or as adjuncts to other antihypertensive medications.

LOOP DIURETICS

Currently used loop diuretics derive from two structural types: (1) sulfonamides in the instance of **furosemide**[24] and **bumetanide**[25] and (2) a sulfhydryl-reactive agent **ethacrynic acid.**[6] Both types have severalfold greater efficacy than the thiazides at optimum dosage; loop diuretics can elicit excretion of about 20% of filtered Na^+, in contrast to 5% for thiazides. All three loop diuretics are well absorbed and active when administered by mouth or intravenously.

Ethacrynic acid

Furosemide

Bumetanide

TABLE 42-1 Thiazide diuretics

Name	Structure	Formulation (mg)	Adult daily dose (mg)	Duration of action (hours)
Chlorothiazide (Diuril, others)	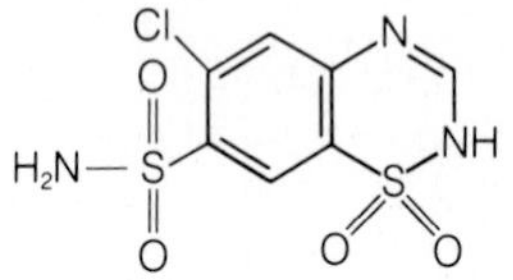	T: 250, 500; S: 250/5 ml	250-1000	6-12
Chlorothiazide sodium (Diuril sodium)		I: 500		
Hydrochlorothiazide (HydroDIURIL, others)	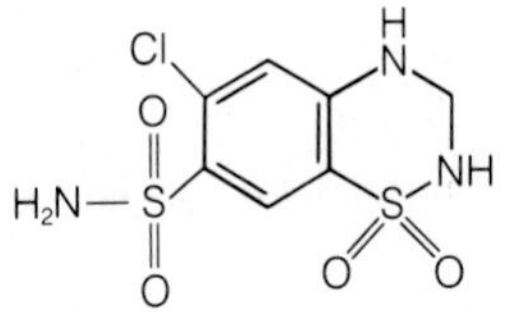	T: 25-100; S: 50/5 ml, 100/ml	25-100	6-12
Bendroflumethiazide (Naturetin)	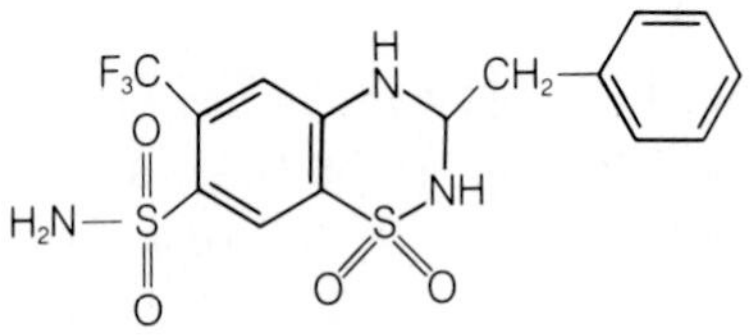	T: 5-10	2.5-15	18-24
Benzthiazide (Aquatag, others)	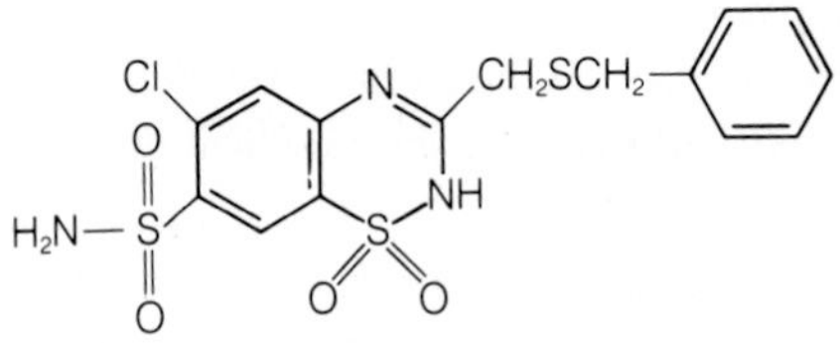	T: 50	50-200	12-18
Cyclothiazide (Anhydron)	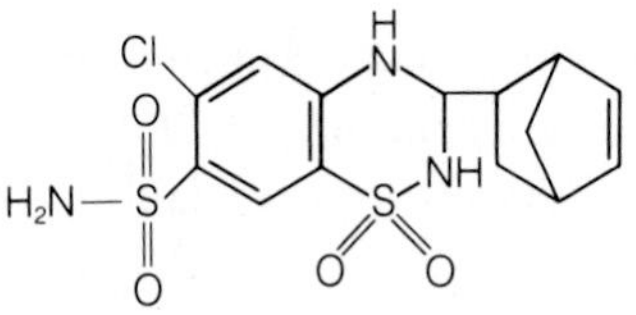	T: 2	1-2	18-24
Hydroflumethiazide (Diucardin, Saluron)	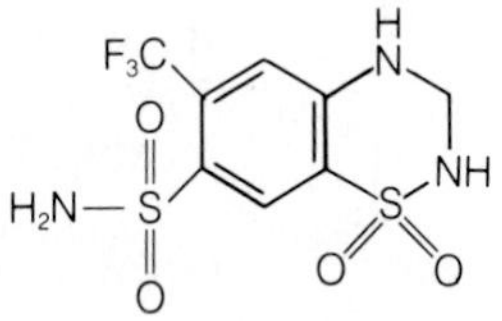	T: 50	25-200	18-24
Methyclothiazide (Aquatensen, others)	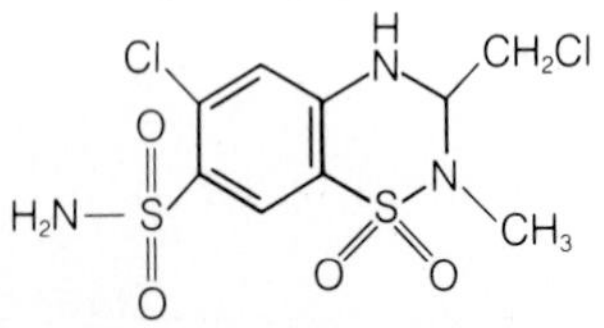	T: 2.5, 5	2.5-10	24-28

I, Injection (powder for reconstitution); *S*, suspension or solution (oral); *T*, tablets.
*Structurally not thiazides but with virtually identical pharmacology.

TABLE 42-1 Thiazide diuretics—cont'd

Name	Structure	Formulation (mg)	Adult daily dose (mg)	Duration of action (hours)
Polythiazide (Renese)	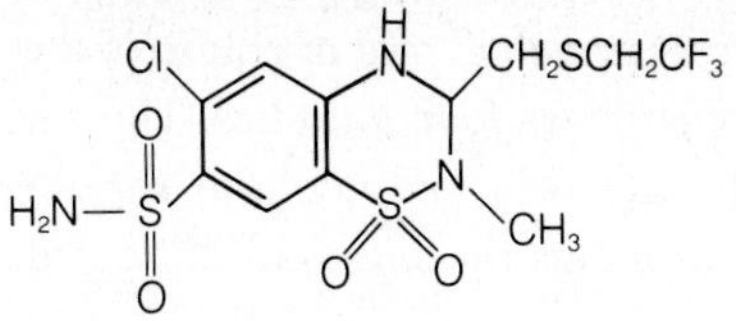	T: 1-4	1-4	24-48
Trichlormethiazide (Metahydrin, others)	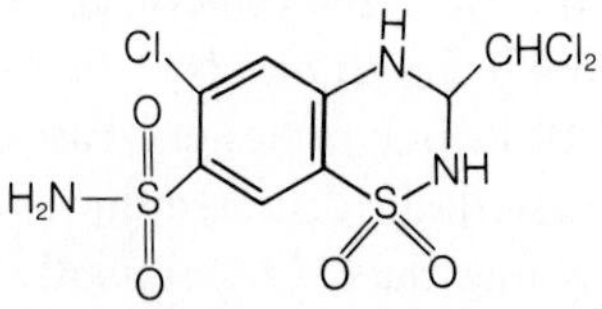	T: 2, 4	2-4	24
Chlorthalidone* (Hygroton, others)	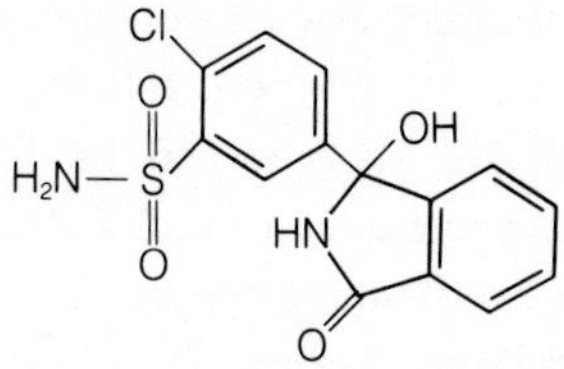	T: 25-100	25-100	24-72
Quinethezone* (Hydromox)	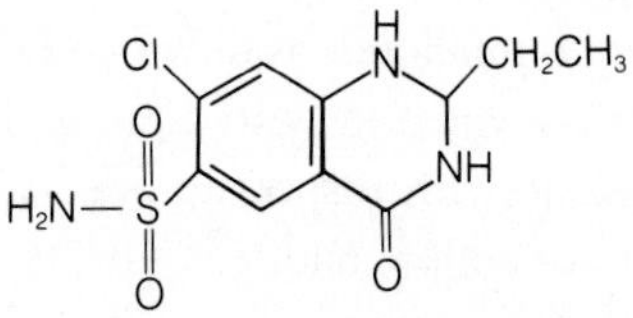	T: 50	2.5-20	12-24
Metolazone* (Diulo, others)	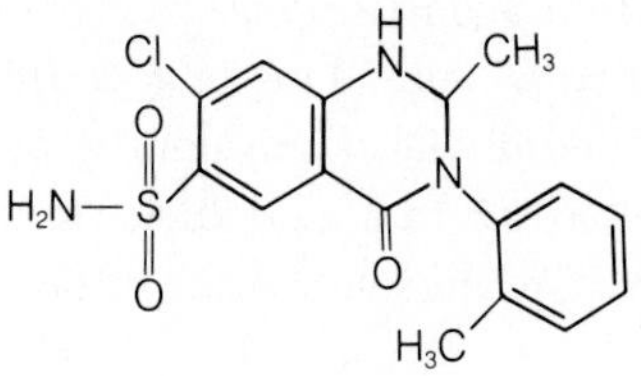	T: 0.5-10	2.5-20	12-24
Indapamide* (Lozol)	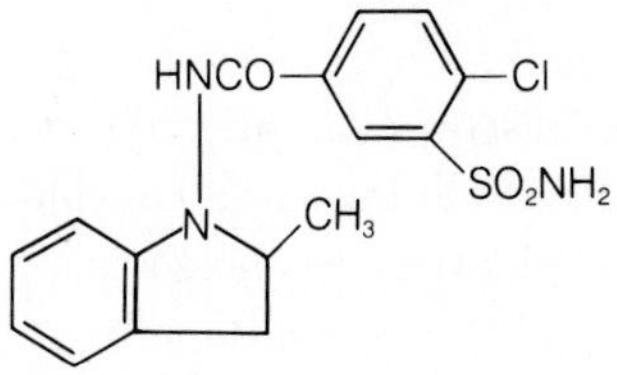	T: 2.5	2.5-5	to 36

They cause a NaCl diuresis as do thiazides, but urine volume is likely to be greater and specific gravity less after administration of the loop diuretics. These drugs extend therapy to edematous patients who may not be adequately controlled by thiazides.[8]

Since more than 95% of drug in the plasma is bound to albumin, their glomerular filtration is negligible. The principal site of action is the thick segment of the loop of Henle, hence their designation as *loop diuretics*. They act from the luminal side of the tubule; thus secretion by the proximal nephron is essential for their effectiveness.[17] Reduced renal function prolongs the action of these drugs by slowing their entry into the lumen of the tubule.

Loop diuretics reduce or abolish the osmotic gradient of the medulla by inhibiting reabsorption of two Cl^- coupled with one Na^+ and one K^+ at the thick segment of the ascending limb.[3,5,10,11] All loop diuretics decrease Na^+, Cl^-, and urea gradients in the medulla. In so doing, these drugs decrease the osmotic force responsible for water reabsorption from the collecting duct. Consequently these compounds decrease the ability to concentrate urine. Since the thiazides do not affect the medullary concentration gradient, they do not affect urinary concentrating ability.

Because of their pronounced natriuretic activity, loop diuretics can be life saving, as in acute pulmonary edema, or they can be life threatening if misused. Like thiazides, they cause hyperuricemia. Furosemide can alter glucose tolerance, but this seems less well established for ethacrynic acid. When employed at high dosage, as in an attempt to prevent acute renal failure, loop diuretics may induce vestibular dysfunction or loss of hearing.

An equivalent dosage of bumetanide is only one fortieth that of furosemide, and its bioavailability is about 80% compared with 40% for furosemide. Otherwise, the two drugs are essentially the same with respect to effects on electrolyte and water excretion, oral efficacy, duration of action, and side effects.[9]

Furosemide (Lasix, others) is supplied as 20 to 80 mg tablets (500 mg in some countries) and as oral and intravenous solutions containing 8 or 10 mg/ml. Ethacrynic acid (Edecrin) is available as 25 and 50 mg tablets. Intravenous ethacrynate sodium is a dry white powder supplied in vials equivalent to 50 mg of ethacrynic acid. Bumetanide (Bumex) is supplied as 0.5 to 2 mg tablets. It is also available in 2 ml ampules containing 0.25 mg/ml in a sterile solution for intravenous or intramuscular administration.

ANTIKALIURETIC (POTASSIUM-SPARING) AGENTS

The saluretic diuretic agents discussed to this point cause a concomitant increase in K^+ excretion. Efforts to discover diuretics that would increase Na^+ excretion by inhibiting its exchange with K^+ in the distal convoluted tubule produced two classes of antikaliuretic agents: (1) aldosterone antagonists and (2) agents that inhibit Na^+ reabsorption and secondary K^+ secretion directly.

Aldosterone antagonists

Spironolactone is the only available antagonist of aldosterone.

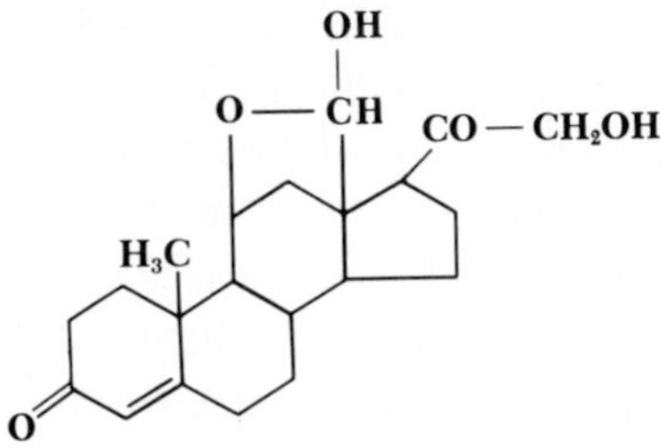

Aldosterone 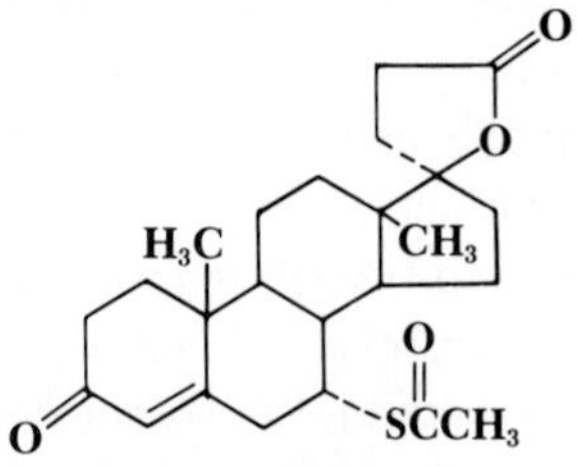 **Spironolactone**

As an aldosterone antagonist, spironolactone is most effective in settings in which enhancement of Na^+ reabsorption and increased K^+ excretion induced by aldosterone are greatest, namely, cirrhosis of the liver, aldosterone-secreting tumors, and high-renin hypertension. Spironolactone is not active in adrenalectomized animals.[21] The effect of the drug is sustained but slow to develop and is not so great as that for other categories of saluretic agents. The spectrum of saluretic effect is one of increased Na^+ and Cl^- and reduced K^+ excretion. Water excretion is isotonic.

Side effects relate both to mode of action and to the chemistry of progestational hormones from which spironolactone was developed. Perhaps the most common undesirable effect is hyperkalemia from excessive K^+ retention. Although spironolactone is at most very weakly progestational, it can cause gynecomastia, which may or may not be reversible. Spironolactone has been reported to be tumorigenic in chronic toxicity studies in rats.

Spironolactone (Aldactone) is supplied as 25 to 100 mg tablets. A parenteral dosage form is not marketed in the United States.

Directly acting antikaliuretic agents

Presently, two directly acting antikaliuretic agents are available: **triamterene** and **amiloride**. They are administered orally.

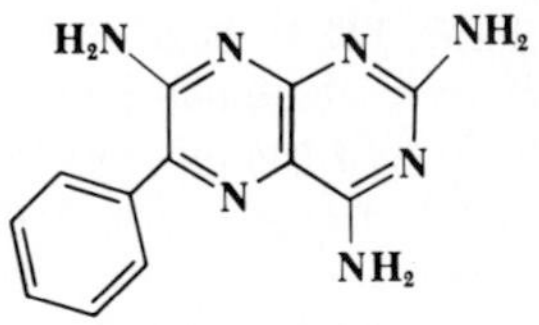

Triamterene 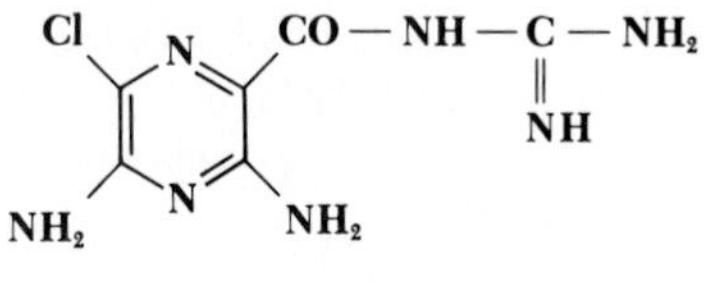 **Amiloride**

Unlike spironolactone, these basic compounds promptly inhibit Na^+ reabsorption and K^+ secretion in the distal cortical segment of the nephron. They are effective regardless of aldosterone status and thus are more reliable than spironolactone.

These diuretics are filtered at the glomeruli and are secreted by the organic base transport system of the proximal convoluted tubules. Access to the tubular lumen is essential to their activity.

Amiloride is the more potent of these compounds.[2] Both are inherently less active than thiazides because they act at a more distal site in the nephron.

Triamterene and amiloride are well tolerated except that their propensity to retain K^+ can result in hyperkalemia. Their saluretic, antikaliuretic characteristics make them seemingly natural adjuncts to thiazide therapy. The different modes of action of the antikaliuretic agents and the thiazides make their combined saluretic effects additive or even synergistic, whereas their qualitatively opposite actions on K^+ excretion offset each other. There are several formulations that combine a thiazide with amiloride, triamterene, or spironolactone. It has not been established that such formulations provide better therapy than does concurrent use of the individual components.

Triamterene (Dyrenium) is supplied as 50 and 100 mg capsules. Amiloride hydrochloride (Midamor) is available in 5 mg tablets.

REFERENCES

1. Alpern RJ, Howlin KJ, Preisig PA: Active and passive components of chloride transport in the rat proximal convoluted tubule, *J Clin Invest* 76:1360, 1985.
2. Baer JE, Jones CB, Spitzer SA, Russo HF: The potassium-sparing and natriuretic activity of N-amidino-3,5-diamino-6-chloropyrazinecarboxamide hydrochloride dihydrate (amiloride hydrochloride), *J Pharmacol Exp Ther* 157:472, 1967.
3. Beermann B, Groschinsky-Grind M: Clinical pharmacokinetics of diuretics, *Clin Pharmacokinet* 5:221, 1980.
4. Beyer KH Jr, Baer JE: The site and mode of action of some sulfonamide-derived diuretics, *Med Clin North Am* 59:735, 1975.
5. Burg MB: Tubular chloride transport and the mode of action of some diuretics, *Kidney Int* 9:189, 1976.
6. Burg M, Green N: Effect of ethacrynic acid on the thick ascending limb of Henle's loop, *Kidney Int* 4:301, 1973.
7. Cogan MG: Atrial natriuretic peptide, *Kidney Int* 37:1148, 1990.
8. Frazier HS, Yager H: The clinical use of diuretics, *N Engl J Med* 288: 246 and 455, 1973.
9. Hammarlund-Udenaes M, Benet LZ: Furosemide pharmacokinetics and pharmacodynamics in health and disease—an update, *J Pharmacokinet Biopharm* 17:1, 1989.
10. Hebert SC, Andreoli TE: Control of NaCl transport in the thick ascending limb, *Am J Physiol* 246:F745, 1984.
11. Jacobson HR, Kokko JP: Diuretics: sites and mechanisms of action, *Annu Rev Pharmacol Toxicol* 16:201, 1976.
12. Katz AI: Renal Na-K-ATPase: its role in tubular sodium and potassium transport, *Am J Physiol* 242:F207, 1982.
13. Krebs HA: Inhibition of carbonic anhydrase by sulphonamides, *Biochem J* 43:525, 1948.
14. Mann T, Keilin D: Sulphanilamide as a specific inhibitor of carbonic anhydrase, *Nature* 146:164, 1940.
15. Maren TH: Carbonic anhydrase: chemistry, physiology, and inhibition, *Physiol Rev* 47:595, 1967.
16. Neumann KH, Rector FC Jr: Mechanism of NaCl and water reabsorption in the proximal convoluted tubule of rat kidney: role of chloride concentration gradients, *J Clin Invest* 58:1110, 1976.
17. Odlind B: Relation between renal tubular secretion and effects of five loop diuretics, *J Pharmacol Exp Ther* 211:238, 1979.
18. Rector FC Jr: Sodium, bicarbonate, and chloride absorption by the proximal tubule, *Am J Physiol* 244:F461, 1983.
19. Saxl P, Heilig R: Ueber die diuretische Wirkung von Novasurol-undanderen Quecksilberinjektionen, *Wien Klin Wochenschr* 33:943, 1920.
20. Schwartz WB: The effect of sulfanilamide on salt and water excretion in congestive heart failure, *N Engl J Med* 240:173, 1949.
21. Seller RH, Swartz CD, Ramirez-Muxo O, et al: Aldosterone antagonists in diuretic therapy: their effect on the refractory phase, *Arch Intern Med* 113:350, 1964.
22. Southworth H: Acidosis associated with the administration of para-amino-benzene-sulfonamide (Prontylin), *Proc Soc Exp Biol Med* 36:58, 1937.

23. Stokes JB: Electroneutral NaCl transport in the distal tubule, *Kidney Int* 36:427, 1989.

24. Suki W, Rector FC Jr, Seldin DW: The site of action of furosemide and other sulfonamide diuretics in the dog, *J Clin Invest* 44:1458, 1965.

25. Ward A, Heel RC: Bumetanide: a review of its pharmacodynamic and pharmacokinetic properties and therapeutic use, *Drugs* 28:426, 1984

26. Warren SE, Blantz RC: Mannitol, *Arch Intern Med* 141:493, 1981.

27. Welling PG: Pharmacokinetics of the thiazide diuretics, *Biopharm Drug Dispos* 7:501, 1986.

28. Windhager EE, Giebisch G: Proximal sodium and fluid transport, *Kidney Int* 9:121, 1976.

Chapter 43

Pharmacologic treatment of atherosclerosis

GENERAL CONCEPTS

Both clinical and experimental research indicate a probable causal relationship between hyperlipidemia and arterial disease. The incorporation of lipids from blood (triglycerides, phospholipids, and cholesterol) into the arterial wall to form the lesions of *atherosclerosis* can lead to coronary artery disease, myocardial infarction, and occlusion of cerebral and peripheral arteries. Although it is recognized that other factors, such as vessel wall injury, also contribute to the pathologic process, the rationale for reducing concentrations of circulating lipids is that high concentrations of cholesterol-rich lipoproteins can accelerate atherosclerosis.

There are several drugs that lower abnormally elevated plasma lipoproteins by reducing their production or enhancing their removal. The most commonly used are the fibric acids, *clofibrate* and *gemfibrozil*; these agents inhibit release of lipoproteins from the liver, and they also inhibit cholesterol synthesis. *Cholestyramine* and *colestipol* are resins that bind bile acids and prevent their absorption. *Nicotinic acid* decreases secretion of very–low-density lipoprotein (VLDL) and consequently formation of low-density lipoprotein (LDL) cholesterol. *Probucol* reduces LDL, high-density lipoprotein (HDL) cholesterol, and apolipoprotein A-I by enhancing their clearance. Inhibitors of 3-hydroxy-3-methylglutaryl (HMG) coenzyme A reductase are a new class of cholesterol-lowering compounds that increase expression of LDL receptors to reduce circulating concentrations of LDL-cholesterol. These agents have considerable promise for management of certain types of severe hypercholesterolemia.[7]

None of the lipid-lowering drugs is completely satisfactory. However, when used in combination with dietary control of lipid intake, treatment of concomitant disease (hypertension, diabetes, hypothyroidism), and elimination of other significant risk factors (smoking, high alcohol intake), they may reduce development of atherosclerotic lesions.

Pathogenesis of atherosclerosis

Many factors are believed to contribute to development of atherosclerosis. One concept is that atherosclerotic lesions develop subsequent to an inflammatory insult. It has also been proposed that factors from adherent platelets stimulate growth of smooth muscle cells. The exact mechanisms are still not clear, but formation of atherosclerotic plaques probably involves both inflammatory cells and growth factors.[21] The rationale for lowering plasma lipids is that some of the cellular events appear to be influenced by high concentrations of plasma cholesterol, specifically by LDL.

FIG. 43-1

All plasma lipoproteins are spherical particles consisting of a disorganized core of triglycerides and cholesterol esters surrounded by a thin lipid monolayer of cholesterol and phospholipid. Apolipoproteins are embedded in the surface lipid shell, with their hydrophobic domains oriented toward the core and their hydrophilic domains oriented outward. This configuration is highly stable and facilitates the solubilization of these microdroplets of nonpolar lipids.

From Weinberg RB: Lipoprotein metabolism: hormonal regulation, Hosp Pract 22(6):223, 1987; this illustration was drawn by Alan Iselin, New York, N.Y.

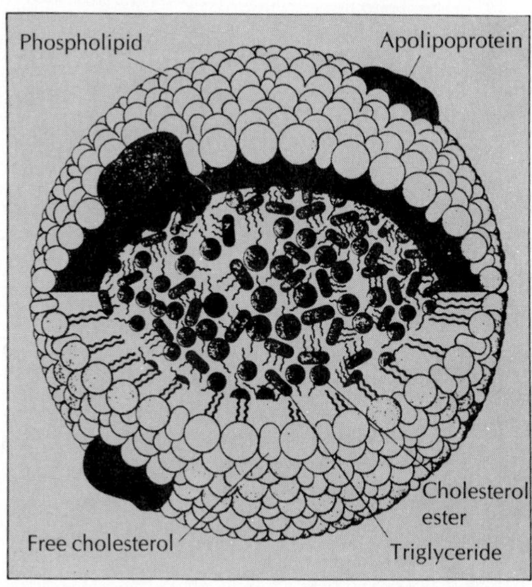

Lipoproteins and lipid transport

The two major indices used to assess hyperlipoproteinemias are blood cholesterol and triglyceride concentrations.[12] These lipids are transported in blood in *lipoproteins*, macromolecular assemblies of lipids and specialized *apolipoproteins* that act as recognition sites for interactions of lipoproteins with tissues.[24] Lipoproteins vary in size and density, but all are spherical particles with a lipid core. The apoproteins and phospholipids that surround the core control the interactions and eventual fate of the particle (Fig. 43-1).

When dietary fat is absorbed from the intestine, it is incorporated into the largest of the lipoprotein particles, the *chylomicrons*, which are formed in intestinal mucosal cells. Chylomicrons are composed primarily of triglycerides and apoproteins A, B, C, and E. Once in the circulation, they are catabolized by the action of *lipoprotein lipase* associated with vessel walls. Free fatty acids released from the triglycerides enter the metabolic pool or are stored as fat.[19] The chylomicron *remnants* are then taken up by cells in the liver, broken down further, and used for synthesis of triglycerides.

Classes of lipoproteins can be separated by analytic methods on the basis of size and density. They range in diameter from 5 nm (50Å) to more than 500 nm (5,000Å). The larger the particle, the greater is its lipid content and the lower its density.[18] Fig. 43-2 shows relative sizes and densities of the lipoproteins. The progressive removal of

FIG. 43-2 *Relative densities of the lipoproteins as they would appear on ultracentrifugation, along with their physical dimensions. The largest are the least dense because they have the highest lipid content, which weighs less than protein.*

From Kreisberg RA: Consultant 23:197, Oct. 1983.

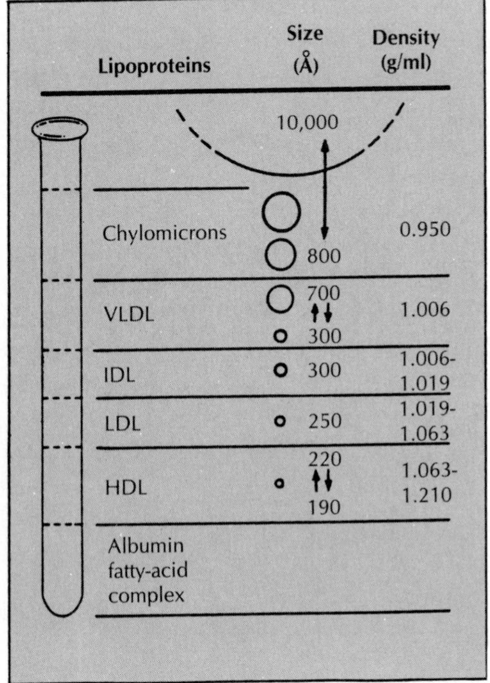

free fatty acids from the triglyceride core results in an increasingly dense particle.

VLDL consists of triglyceride-rich particles formed in the liver. These particles, which are smaller than chylomicrons, are the major form of transport for endogenously synthesized triglycerides. They contain some cholesterol as well. As VLDL circulates it is degraded by lipoprotein lipase, and triglycerides are removed. The remaining apoproteins, phospholipids, and cholesterol form a particle of intermediate density, the IDL. As more triglycerides are removed, the smaller, cholesterol-rich LDL is formed. These particles are destined for peripheral tissues and the liver. HDL comprises small lipoproteins, formed in the intestine, liver, and vascular tissue, that transport cholesterol from peripheral tissues to the liver where it is either excreted or processed into bile salts. Fig. 43-3 shows the schema for removal and transport of fats in lipoproteins. Table 43-1 summarizes the classes and functions of the plasma lipoproteins.

LDL contains the major portion of plasma cholesterol and is believed to be the most harmful lipoprotein because risk of coronary disease correlates directly with high concentrations of LDL.[18]

The apolipoproteins associated with circulating lipoproteins are particularly important. Many of the apolipoproteins affect lipoprotein metabolism by acting as enzyme cofactors, inhibitors, or receptors.[11] For example, apo C-II is an activator of lipoprotein

Schema for origin and removal of lipids and lipoproteins. *FIG. 43-3*

From Kuske TT, Feldman EB: Arch Intern Med 147:357, copyright 1987, American Medical Association.

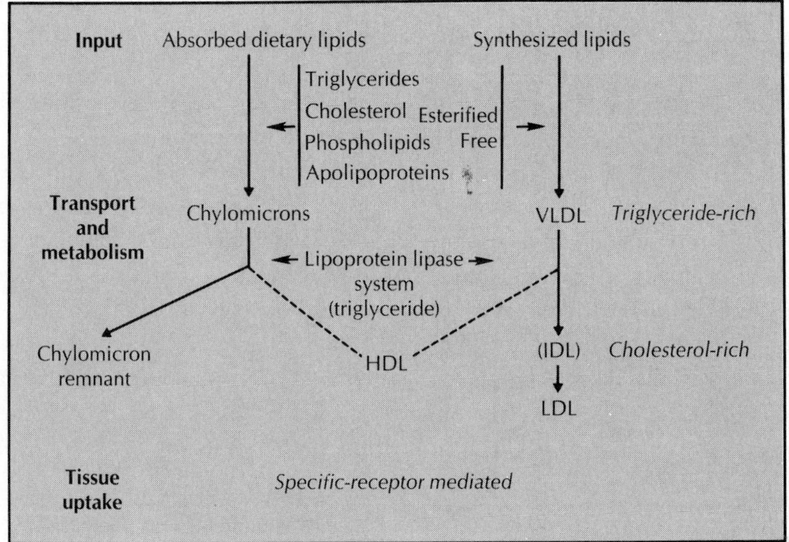

TABLE 43-1 Classes of plasma lipoproteins

	Origin	Major apolipoproteins	Core lipids	Function	Destination
Chylomicrons	Intestine	Apo B, apo C, apo E	Triglycerides	Transport of dietary tryglyceride	Triglyceride storage cells, triglyceride metabolizing cells, liver
Very–low-density lipoproteins (VLDL)	Liver (intestine)	Apo B, apo C, apo E	Triglycerides (cholesterol esters)	Transport of endogenously synthesized triglyceride (and some cholesterol)	Triglyceride storage cells, triglyceride metabolizing cells
Low-density lipoproteins (LDL)	Intravascular metabolism of VLDL	Apo B	Cholesterol esters	Transport of cholesterol esters of hepatic and intravascular origin	Peripheral cells (liver)
High-density lipoproteins (HDL)	Intestine, liver, intravascular metabolic reactions	Apo A-1, apo A-II	Cholesterol esters	"Reverse" transport of cholesterol of peripheral origin	Liver, steroidogenic tissues

Modified from Weinberg RB: Lipoprotein metabolism: hormonal regulation, Hosp Pract 22(6):223, 1987.

lipase.[19] Apolipoproteins also function as ligands for cell receptors, directing uptake of lipoprotein particles by the liver and other tissues. Genetic deficiencies of apolipoproteins have been described and related to disorders of lipid metabolism. A defect in apolipoprotein E that renders it incapable of binding lipoproteins causes a type of familial hypercholesterolemia. Apolipoprotein E appears to be involved in functions, such as immunoregulation and cell growth, that are unrelated to lipid transport.[20]

Regulation of cholesterol through LDL receptors

The regulation of cholesterol in blood depends largely on the disposition of LDL; elevation of plasma cholesterol is usually attributable to increased LDL.[2] LDL receptors in tissues intercept circulating LDL and carry it into cells by receptor-mediated endocytosis (Fig. 43-4). Cholesterol, in the form of cholesteryl esters, is then utilized for synthesis of plasma membranes, bile acids, or steroid hormones. The liver contains the greatest number of LDL receptors, but they are found on many types of cells.

The number of LDL receptors expressed at the cell surface is a key control mechanism for plasma cholesterol. When LDL receptors are saturated, the removal of LDL is proportional to the number of receptors. LDL receptors are continuously recycled. Once the complex is taken into the cell, LDL dissociates from its receptor,

FIG. 43-4 *Route of the low-density-lipoprotein (LDL) receptor in mammalian cells. The receptor begins life in the endoplasmic reticulum from which it travels to the Golgi complex, cell surface, coated pit, and endosome and back to the surface.* Vertical arrows, *Direction of regulatory effects.*

From Brown MS, Goldstein JL: Curr Top Cell Regul 26:3, 1985.

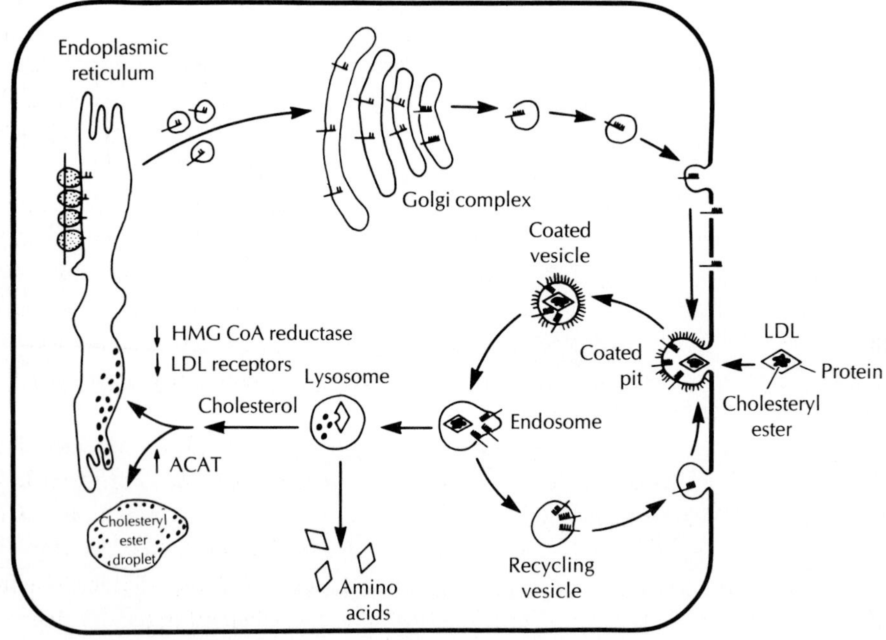

and the receptor returns to the cell surface. A reduced number of receptors results in elevated plasma LDL. A second important function of LDL receptors is suppression of cholesterol synthesis in the liver. After LDL is internalized, the core cholesteryl esters are hydrolyzed by an acid lipase. The free cholesterol inhibits activity of HMG-CoA reductase, the rate-limiting enzyme in cholesterol synthesis, and suppresses the expression of LDL receptors at the cell surface. Thus the LDL receptor controls not only uptake of cholesterol in the form of LDL but also its synthesis. LDL-receptor binding of IDL, the precursor of LDL, also helps to control the amount of circulating LDL.[2]

An increased risk for atherosclerosis is clearly associated with a deficit of LDL receptors, as demonstrated in familial hypercholesterolemia. Individuals with this genetic disease have a very high concentration of circulating cholesterol and a dramatically increased incidence of myocardial infarction. There are four subgroups of this genetic defect, and several different mutations have been defined. All result in diminished binding of LDL to cells.[2] Because of the importance of LDL receptors in determining circulating LDL concentration, modulation of receptor number has become a major focus of therapy of hypercholesterolemia (see the next page).

High-density lipoproteins

HDL plays an important role in both metabolism of lipoproteins and their transport. These heterogeneous particles consist of a core of apolar cholesterol ester and triglyceride enveloped by a shell of specific apoproteins and phospholipids. One important function of HDL is to bind free cholesterol. Its role is opposite to that of LDL—LDL transports cholesterol from the liver and gastrointestinal tract to peripheral tissues, whereas HDL removes cholesterol from cells and transports it back to the liver, which is the only organ that can efficiently catabolize and excrete cholesterol. The antiatherogenic actions ascribed to HDL depend, at least in part, on this "reverse transport" of cholesterol.[6]

Apoprotein C-II is a minor component of HDL, but it activates lipoprotein lipase, which breaks down VLDL and chylomicrons. Apoprotein A-I is also important for the role of HDL by activating lecithin cholesterol acetyl transferase (LCAT), which is required for esterification of cholesterol and transport by HDL.

DIETARY MODIFICATION AND EXERCISE

It is well recognized that a diet rich in fats can promote development of atherosclerosis. Sustained elevation of triglycerides and cholesterol in the blood indicates a need for dietary modification and possibly for drug therapy. Alteration of a traditionally atherogenic diet is, however, a first step in therapy of hyperlipidemia. Other measures include the correction of ongoing metabolic defects; for example, hyperlipidemia is a common accompaniment of diabetes.

Although most epidemiologic studies emphasize the need to reduce LDL-cholesterol concentration, reduced HDL-cholesterol may also constitute a risk for coronary heart disease.[6,8] Several factors that decrease HDL, such as cigarette smoking, obesity, and lack of exercise, can be readily corrected without drug therapy.

Saturated animal fats contain large amounts of cholesterol. A diet rich in these fats will increase blood cholesterol, whereas substitution by polyunsaturated fats tends to lower cholesterol and triglyceride concentrations. A recent study with normal volunteers showed that a decrease in the percentage of dietary calories in the form of fat caused significant reduction of plasma LDL-cholesterol without changing HDL concentration.[4] Others have reported that increased dietary intake of cholesterol elevated LDL-cholesterol and apolipoprotein B, even in healthy individuals who exercised regularly and consumed restricted amounts of saturated fats.[13] This indicates that restriction of cholesterol intake is an important dietary modification in any regimen.

Removal of refined sugars from the diet and substitution of complex carbohydrates is also beneficial. Some studies indicate that increased dietary fiber aids in lipid reduction, possibly by trapping and eliminating cholesterol (in the form of bile acids) within the intestinal contents.[19] Another mechanism may be inhibition of cholesterol synthesis by short-chain fatty acids produced by fermentation of soluble fiber.[1]

The first goal of any dietary regimen is maintenance of ideal body weight. Obesity is an additional risk factor for cardiovascular disease. To this end, exercise combined with caloric restriction tends to shift the ratio of LDL to HDL to a more favorable setting (reduced LDL and increased HDL). Even when combined with drug therapy, dietary counseling and supervision play a vital role in management of hyperlipidemia.

DRUG THERAPY OF HYPERLIPIDEMIA

Therapeutic implications for receptor regulation

Regulation of LDL is the goal in therapy of hyperlipidemias. One way to lower plasma cholesterol is to indirectly increase LDL receptors by inhibiting intestinal absorption of bile acids. Because the liver must continually synthesize bile acids from cholesterol to maintain sufficient body pools, sequestration of these acids increases the need for cholesterol. Thus the demand for cholesterol uptake, and the need for LDL receptors, increases. An increase in LDL receptors in the liver will decrease plasma cholesterol.

Diet can also be used to influence LDL receptors. A diet high in fat reduces the number of LDL receptors; conversely, decreased fat intake aids in maintaining LDL-receptor number.[2] Another strategy for increasing LDL receptors is to inhibit HMG-CoA reductase, the rate-limiting enzyme in cholesterol synthesis. The regulatory adjustment to this inhibition involves synthesis of new LDL receptors.

HMG-CoA reductase inhibitors

Lovastatin (mevinolin), a competitive inhibitor of HMG-CoA reductase, was originally used in patients heterozygous for familial hypercholesterolemia, but it is now used in hypercholesterolemia of many causes when dietary modification has not succeeded in controlling plasma LDL concentration. When administered with inhibitors of bile acid reabsorption, it is even more effective in reducing plasma cholesterol. Most patients are helped by this combined therapy. Neither of these therapeutic interventions works with homozygotes because they lack LDL receptors and the attendant regulatory mechanisms controlled by LDL receptors.

HMG-CoA reductase inhibitors also reduce LDL-cholesterol in individuals with primary hypercholesterolemia, possibly by correcting metabolic suppression of LDL receptors. These agents also appear promising for dyslipidemias in non-insulin-dependent diabetes, in nephrotic syndrome, and in patients with renal insufficiency maintained by dialysis, many of whom develop lipid abnormalities.[7]

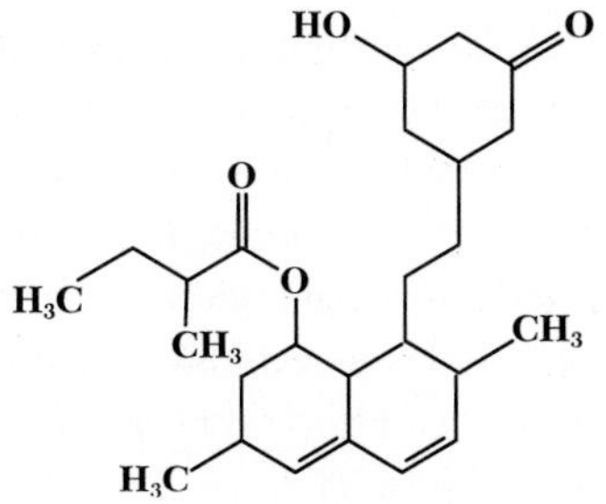

Lovastatin

Clinical experience with lovastatin and related drugs thus far indicates few adverse effects. A small number of patients experienced myositis, particularly when the drug was used with fibric acid derivatives, and in some, plasma concentrations of hepatic enzymes increased. There have also been a few reports of cataract development, but HMG-CoA reductase inhibitors, in general, appear free of major side effects. These drugs are expensive, however, and patients must continue to take them to maintain the reduction in cholesterol.

Lovastatin (Mevacor) is available as tablets, 20 mg. The drug itself is inactive but is rapidly converted to the active β-hydroxyacid in the liver. It is excreted into bile and eliminated through the intestinal tract.

Clofibrate and gemfibrozil

The fibric acids are effective in treatment of familial dysbetalipoproteinemia (hyperlipidemia, type III) and may reduce LDL concentration in mild hypercholesterolemia. Clofibrate, the oldest of the fibric acids, is hydrolyzed during gastrointestinal absorption to the active compound chlorophenoxyisobutyric acid (CPIB), which is transported in plasma largely bound to albumin. Clofibrate is particularly effective in lowering plasma triglycerides, presumably by enhancing activity of lipoprotein lipase, which increases clearance of VLDL.[10] It is less effective in lowering plasma cholesterol.

Although clofibrate significantly improves lipid profiles, it also increases the incidence of gallstone formation and can cause myositis. Consequently gemfibrozil, a newer, nonhalogenated derivative, is preferred.[9] Gemfibrozil also inhibits secretion of VLDL from the liver.[16]

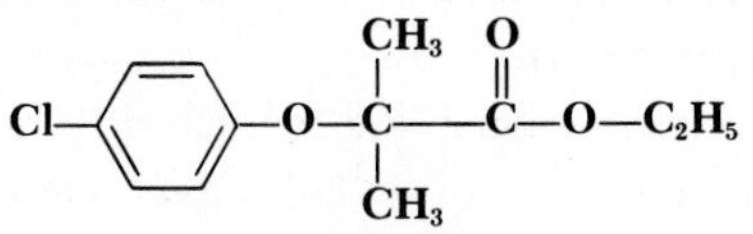

Clofibrate

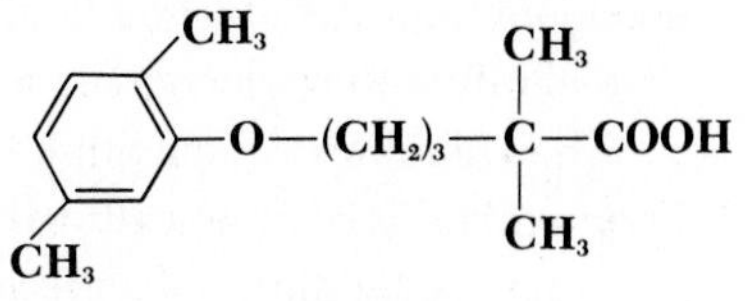

Gemfibrozil

Primary prevention trials with clofibrate produced equivocal results and indicated an increased risk of cholelithiasis and pancreatitis.[14] Recent studies with gemfibrozil have been more encouraging. Gemfibrozil lowers plasma triglycerides and VLDL and increases HDL-cholesterol. In a 5-year trial in patients with hypercholesterolemia, gemfibrozil decreased the incidence of myocardial infarction in parallel with beneficial changes in blood lipids.[22]

Clofibrate decreases clearance of coumarin anticoagulants and requires downward adjustment of anticoagulant dosage. Other side effects of clofibrate include myopathy, gastrointestinal disturbances, and decreased libido. Because of its potential for myalgia and its elimination by the kidney, clofibrate is not used in patients with impaired renal function.

Clofibrate (Atromid-S) is available as 500 mg capsules, gemfibrozil (Lopid) as 300 mg capsules and 600 mg tablets.

Bile acid–binding resins

Cholestyramine and colestipol are anion-exchange resins that bind bile acids in the intestinal lumen, in exchange for chloride ion. Since the resin is not absorbed, it promotes fecal excretion of bile acids. The liver then increases bile acid synthesis to replace the lost acids. Because cholesterol is the precursor for bile acids, the net result is increased utilization of cholesterol and, usually, a lowering of its plasma concentration. The effectiveness of bile acid–binding resins in lowering plasma LDL-cholesterol concentration appears to depend on the ability of the liver to increase the population of LDL receptors that supply cholesterol.[15]

Cholestyramine (Questran) and colestipol hydrochloride (Colestid) are powder and granular preparations, respectively, that should be mixed with juice or other liquid, allowed to hydrate for a few minutes, and then taken with meals. They are available in bulk or in individual packets containing 4 g of cholestyramine or 5 g of colestipol. One packet of the former is taken up to six times a day; the daily dose of 15 to 30 g of the latter is divided over two to four doses. Cholestyramine (Cholybar) is also available as a bar to be chewed and taken with fluids. Common side effects of these agents are constipation and abdominal pain, perhaps with nausea and bloating. They also interfere with absorption of fat-soluble vitamins and numerous drugs (see Table 70-1).

Nicotinic acid

Nicotinic acid (niacin) acts primarily by inhibiting secretion of VLDL without accumulation of triglycerides in the liver. This in turn decreases production of LDL. The drug also inhibits lipolysis in adipose tissue, but this effect may not be sustained with chronic administration.[14] Another effect of nicotinic acid is a decrease in the fractional catabolic rate of HDL, which results in higher concentrations of HDL and apolipoprotein A-I. In one large-scale clinical trial, nicotinic acid was the only agent that significantly reduced the incidence of coronary events.[15]

The usefulness of nicotinic acid is limited by troublesome side effects. Flushing occurs initially in practically all patients and may persist in some. This effect appears to be prostaglandin mediated and can be blocked, at least partially, by pretreatment with aspirin. Activation of peptic ulcer and hepatic dysfunction are toxic effects that can occur with large doses. Although nicotinic acid is available in tablets of 20 to 500 mg and in timed-release capsules of 125 to 500 mg, only the larger sizes are useful for treating hyperlipidemia; the usual dosage is 1 to 2 g three times daily. To minimize side effects, patients begin taking small doses and gradually increase the amount. Occasionally nicotinic acid is used in combination with bile acid–binding resins.[10]

Probucol

Probucol is a cholesterol-lowering agent that is unrelated chemically to other lipid-lowering drugs. It is believed to increase uptake of LDL by receptor-*independent* pathways.[23] It reduces plasma cholesterol concentration in laboratory animals by inhibiting cholesterol synthesis.[5] Probucol is also thought to have an antioxidant effect that may help to prevent atherogenic injury. In experimental animals probucol inhibits LDL degradation by macrophages and retards development of atherosclerosis.[17] It was also shown to increase fecal excretion of bile acids in some clinical studies. Concurrent use of probucol and a resin (colestipol) was more effective than either agent alone.[3]

One problem with probucol is that it reduces both LDL- and HDL-cholesterol. Since HDL is believed to protect against development of atherosclerotic disease, a reduced concentration may be detrimental. Additionally, animal studies indicate that probucol can cause serious cardiotoxicity,[14] limiting its potential for treatment of hypercholesterolemia. Probucol (Lorelco) is available in 250 and 500 mg tablets.

$(CH_3)_3C$ CH_3 $C(CH_3)_3$
HO—[ring]—S—C—S—[ring]—OH
$(CH_3)_3C$ CH_3 $C(CH_3)_3$

Probucol

Combined drug regimens

Certain combinations of drugs are more effective than the individual agents, indicative of complementary mechanisms. For example, nicotinic acid administered with cholestyramine or colestipol is more effective than either agent alone. The combination of a bile acid–binding resin with an HMG-CoA reductase inhibitor lowers LDL concentration into the normal range in patients with heterozygous familial hypercholesterolemia or familial multiple hyperlipidemia.[14]

REFERENCES

1. Anderson JW, Gustafson NJ: Hypocholesterolemic effects of oat and bean products, *Am J Clin Nutr* 48:749, 1988.
2. Brown MS, Goldstein JL: A receptor-mediated pathway for cholesterol homeostasis, *Science* 232:34, 1986.
3. Choice of cholesterol-lowering drugs, *Med Lett Drugs Ther* 30:85, 1988.
4. Ginsberg HN, Barr SL, Gilbert A, et al: Reduction of plasma cholesterol levels in normal men on an American Heart Association Step 1 diet or a Step 1 diet with added monounsaturated fat, *N Engl J Med* 322:574, 1990.
5. Glueck CJ: Colestipol and probucol: treatment of primary and familial hypercholesterolemia and amelioration of atherosclerosis, *Ann Intern Med* 96:475, 1982.
6. Gordon DJ, Rifkind BM: High-density lipoprotein—the clinical implications of recent studies, *N Engl J Med* 321:1311, 1989.
7. Grundy SM: HMG-CoA reductase inhibitors for treatment of hypercholesterolemia, *N Engl J Med* 319:24, 1988.
8. Grundy SM, Goodman DS, Rifkind BM, Cleeman JI: The place of HDL in cholesterol management: a perspective from the

National Cholesterol Education Program, *Arch Intern Med* 149:505, 1989.

9. Gwynne JT, Lawrence MK: Current concepts in the evaluation and treatment of hypercholesterolemia, *Mod Med* 57:126, 1989.
10. Havel RJ, Kane JP: Therapy of hyperlipidemic states, *Annu Rev Med* 33:417, 1982.
11. Hoeg JM, Gregg RE, Brewer HB Jr: An approach to the management of hyperlipoproteinemia, *JAMA* 255:512, 1986.
12. Illingworth DR: Lipid-lowering drugs: an overview of indications and optimum therapeutic use, *Drugs* 33:259, 1987.
13. Johnson C, Greenland P: Effects of exercise, dietary cholesterol, and dietary fat on blood lipids, *Arch Intern Med* 150:137, 1990.
14. Kane JP, Havel RJ: Treatment of hypercholesterolemia, *Annu Rev Med* 37:427, 1986.
15. Kane JP, Malloy MJ: Treatment of hypercholesterolemia, *Med Clin North Am* 66:537, 1982.
16. Kesäniemi YA, Grundy SM: Influence of gemfibrozil and clofibrate on metabolism of cholesterol and plasma triglycerides in man, *JAMA* 251:2241, 1984.
17. Kita T, Nagano Y, Yokode M, et al: Probucol prevents the progression of atherosclerosis in Watanabe heritable hyperlipidemic rabbit, an animal model for familial hypercholesterolemia, *Proc Natl Acad Sci USA* 84:5928, 1987.
18. Kreisberg RA: High-density lipoproteins: a 'delicate balance' helps the HDL help us to prevent CHD, *Consultant* 23:197, Oct 1983.
19. Kuske TT, Feldman EB: Hyperlipoproteinemia, atherosclerosis risk, and dietary management, *Arch Intern Med* 147:357, 1987.
20. Mahley RW: Apolipoprotein E: cholesterol transport protein with expanding role in cell biology, *Science* 240:622, 1988.
21. Majno G, Zand T, Nunnari JJ, Joris I: The diet/atherosclerosis connection: new insights, *J Cardiovasc Med* 9:21, 1984.
22. Manninen V, Elo MO, Frick MH, et al: Lipid alterations and decline in the incidence of coronary heart disease in the Helsinki Heart Study, *JAMA* 260:641, 1988.
23. Naruszewicz M, Carew TE, Pittman RC, et al: A novel mechanism by which probucol lowers low density lipoprotein levels demonstrated in the LDL receptor-deficient rabbit, *J Lipid Res* 25:1206, 1984.
24. Weinberg RB: Lipoprotein metabolism: hormonal regulation, *Hosp Pract* 22(6):223, 1987.

section eight

Drug effects on the respiratory and gastrointestinal tracts

Chapter 44

Drug effects on the respiratory tract

GENERAL CONCEPT

The respiratory system includes the nasal cavities, pharynx, trachea, bronchi, bronchioles, and the alveoli, the terminal airspaces of the lungs. Pulmonary disease may result from an acute injury, such as an infection or hypersensitivity reaction, from genetic causes, such as cystic fibrosis, or from chronic exposure to an injurious agent, as occurs with smoking or occupational exposure to chemicals and dusts.

Drug therapy of pulmonary disorders is generally directed toward altering a specific physiologic function. As examples, *bronchodilators* relax constricted bronchiolar smooth muscle and open blocked airways; *mucolytic agents* alter the characteristics of respiratory tract fluids; *antibiotics* combat infections; *glucocorticoids* reduce inflammation within the respiratory tract. Various agents may be used in combination, particularly with persistent infection or chronic airway disease. In addition, *nasal decongestants*, which constrict dilated vessels in the nasal mucosa, and *antitussives*, which reduce coughing, are over-the-counter preparations used by many people to relieve symptoms of the common cold.

DRUGS THAT AFFECT UPPER AIRWAYS

Nasal decongestants

Air entering the nasal passages is warmed and humidified before reaching the lungs. Resistance to airflow within the upper airways is regulated by autonomic control of smooth muscle within mucosal blood vessels. Nasal congestion from dilatation of these vessels is a common feature of allergic, viral, and inflammatory conditions. Vasoconstrictors reduce congestion but do not influence the underlying cause. All of the numerous, over-the-counter nasal decongestants act by the same mechanism but vary in duration of action. Direct application to engorged membranes of the nasal passages relieves stuffiness by constricting the mucosal vessels through α-adrenergic mechanisms. Some of the commonly used drugs are phenylephrine, oxymetazoline, ephedrine, and xylometazoline. The pharmacology of this class of drugs is discussed in detail in Chapter 18.

USE

Decongestants provide temporary relief of nasal stuffiness associated with acute rhinitis of viral or allergic origin. Addition of antihistamines or anticholinergic drugs is a common practice, but of questionable additional efficacy. Antihistamines of the H_1 class relieve symptoms of allergic rhinitis but not those of the common cold. Anticholinergic agents are sometimes included to diminish nasal secretions, but these dry the nasal mucosa and may be absorbed systemically.

Nasal decongestants may be applied topically or taken in an oral preparation. Although the topical form, usually administered as drops or a spray, is convenient and acts rapidly, frequent use can cause rebound vasodilatation. This condition is characterized by chronic swelling of the nasal mucosa and a need to increase the frequency of decongestant application. Timed-release forms of decongestant taken orally offer prolonged action but may cause unwanted cardiovascular or central nervous system effects.

Cough remedies

Coughing is a protective mechanism through which foreign materials, irritants, and secretions are cleared from the respiratory tract. Complete suppression of coughing is undesirable, but severe and prolonged coughing can be painful and exhausting. Cough suppressants depress the cough reflex that arises from irritated pharyngeal tissues. Mechanical or chemical stimulation of receptors within these tissues initiates impulses that are carried by vagal and glossopharyngeal afferent pathways to a region within the medulla. Efferent pathways pass from this central cough center through peripheral nerves to the abdomen, thoracic muscles, and the diaphragm.

MECHANISMS OF ANTITUSSIVE ACTION

Coughing may be diminished by reducing respiratory secretion, eliminating a source of irritation, or decreasing the sensitivity of irritant receptors within the respiratory tract. Some drugs act at one or more sites within the respiratory tract; others act at the medullary cough center to inhibit activation of the efferent limb of the response.

The volume of respiratory secretions can be reduced by anticholinergic agents, such as atropine or scopolamine. This property is sometimes useful before surgery, but these drugs are not generally used to treat cough due to irritants. Drying of secretions causes retention and impaction of viscous material that can worsen asthma or infectious bronchitis. However, **ipratropium**, a quaternary derivative of atropine, is sometimes beneficial in chronic bronchitis and as adjunctive therapy in asthma.

Some antitussive agents have a local anesthetic action. **Benzonatate** (Tessalon) is chemically related to tetracaine. It is believed to act by two mechanisms: the selective anesthesia of stretch receptors within the lungs and central suppression of cough.

Other antitussives act primarily through central mechanisms. Dextromethorphan, a synthetic nonopioid compound, and the opioids codeine and hydrocodone act on the medullary cough center to suppress the efferent limb of the cough response. The pharmacology of opioid compounds is discussed in Chapter 33.

Interventions that decrease bronchoconstriction and drying of respiratory secretions help to reduce the frequency and severity of coughing. For example, *mists* and *vapors*, which moisturize airways, blunt reactivity to irritant stimuli. *Bronchodilators*, by dilating reactive airways, help to mobilize dried or impacted secretions and ultimately to relieve a dry, unproductive cough. *Expectorants* and *mucolytic agents* facilitate removal of irritant material from the lower respiratory tract toward the pharynx by increasing the volume and reducing the viscosity of respiratory secretions. Their mode of action is not clearly understood, but some expectorants stimulate secretion reflexly through vagal pathways. **Guaifenesin** (glyceryl guaiacolate) and **potassium iodide** solutions are examples of expectorant drugs.

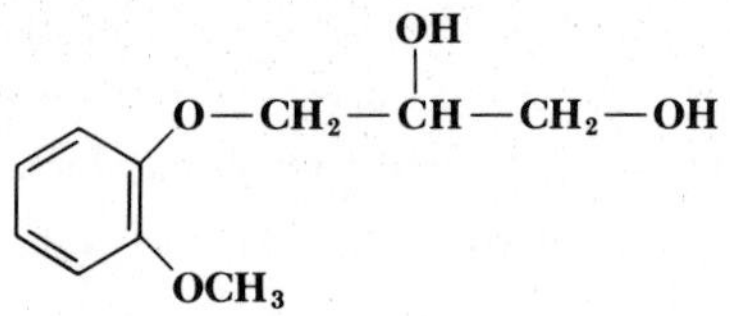

$$\text{C}_6\text{H}_4(\text{OCH}_3)-\text{O}-\text{CH}_2-\underset{|}{\overset{\text{OH}}{\text{CH}}}-\text{CH}_2-\text{OH}$$

Guaifenesin

MUCOLYTIC AGENTS

Mucolytic agents help to reduce the viscosity of sputum by depolymerizing mucopolysaccharides into smaller, more soluble molecules. **Acetylcysteine** (Mucomyst, Mucosol), a widely used mucolytic drug, is an important adjunctive therapy in asthma and other diseases when viscous secretions compromise air exchange. The free sulfhydryl group of this thiol compound reacts with disulfide bonds in mucoproteins and breaks them into less viscous compounds. Acetylcysteine is a free radical scavenger that protects the airways against oxidant damage. In addition, it may be a mucoregulator; prolonged use in patients with abnormal respiratory tract secretions helps to return the amount and quality of secretions toward normal.[16]

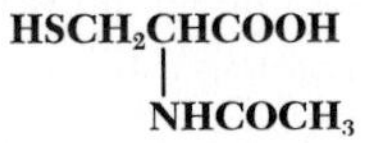

$$HSCH_2\underset{\displaystyle NHCOCH_3}{\underset{|}{C}H}COOH$$

Acetylcysteine

Acetylcysteine may be given orally or by nebulization. Because it releases hydrogen sulfide, it can react with rubber and certain metals and nebulization produces an unpleasant odor. Nebulization may also irritate the airways and cause rhinorrhea and, possibly, bronchospasm in susceptible persons.

USE

Antitussive agents help to suppress coughing when the cough is disturbing or debilitating rather than productive. They are frequently used to blunt airway irritation in the common cold or in other acute upper respiratory infections. Individuals with acute bronchial asthma should avoid antitussives because inspissation of mucus may worsen the disease. Often a combination of mucolytic, vapor, and expectorant therapy will suppress coughing in asthmatics, though pulmonary function may not improve. Agents such as codeine or dextromethorphan are indicated for continued unproductive coughing. Codeine is sometimes administered in an elixir of terpin hydrate, a volatile oil that acts on bronchial secretory cells. The alcohol vehicle is also an expectorant.

DRUGS THAT AFFECT LOWER AIRWAYS

Bronchoconstriction is a prominent feature of diseases that affect the lower airways. Bronchoreactivity in conditions such as bronchial asthma, acute and chronic bronchitis, viral infections, and bacterial respiratory infections is intimately linked to autonomic innervation and secretory activity of cells along the tracheobronchial tree.[9] Primary therapeutic modalities are bronchodilator drugs and anti-inflammatory steroids, though mucolytic and expectorant agents can facilitate removal of secretions.

When release of proinflammatory mediators from lung mast cells is likely, as in hypersensitivity reactions, cromolyn sodium may help to *prevent* bronchoconstriction and inflammation, but it does not affect contraction of bronchial smooth muscle once it has occurred.

Asthma

The pathophysiologic changes of asthma involve pharmacologically reversible airway obstruction, airway inflammation, and increased airway responsiveness to endogenous and exogenous stimuli. Although bronchodilators remain the mainstay of therapy, inflammation is increasingly recognized as an important component of this condition. It is believed to underlie bronchial hyperresponsiveness and to cause the bronchoconstriction, though there is still uncertainty about the specific inflammatory cells and mediators involved. Recognition of asthma as an inflammatory disease has an important implication for therapy, namely that treatment should be directed toward reduction of inflammation, as well as to management of bronchoconstriction.[2]

Bronchodilator compounds may have additional beneficial properties. For example, β-adrenergic agonists, by increasing mast cell cyclic AMP, blunt mediator release, and theophylline appears to have an uncharacterized anti-inflammatory action. Ketotifen, an antihistamine, inhibits airway inflammation in experimental animals, although it has not proved generally useful in therapy of asthma.[2]

Pharmacology of bronchial smooth muscle

The entire tracheobronchial tree is invested with smooth muscle to a greater or lessor degree. In humans bronchial smooth muscle is innervated exclusively by parasympathetic fibers.[1] Parasympathetic stimulation causes bronchoconstriction, whereas circulating adrenergic agonists generally exert a relaxing action through β_2-adrenergic receptors. There are α-adrenergic receptors, however, that mediate contraction of bronchial smooth muscle. At the molecular level, activation of either cholinergic or α-adrenergic receptors increases the concentration of cyclic guanosine 3',5'-monophosphate (cyclic GMP) via a calcium ion-dependent cyclase system. These events stimulate muscle contraction through a series of phosphorylation and dephosphorylation steps. By a similar mechanism, enhanced formation of cyclic AMP within bronchial smooth muscle by β_2-adrenergic receptor stimulation promotes relaxation.[13]

Various drugs and proinflammatory mediators cause contraction or relaxation of bronchial smooth muscle. The most important ones are listed in Table 44-1.

Agents that cause bronchoconstriction are of no therapeutic value but are important as mediators of allergic, inflammatory, or infectious processes. Interactions can occur among various mediators, neurons, smooth muscle, and mast cells.[8] *Slow-reacting substance* (SRS-A), a combination of leukotrienes C_4 and D_4 formed by lung mast cells, probably plays a major role in acute asthmatic episodes. Because asthmatics are unusually sensitive to histamine and kinins, release of these mediators may also contribute to the process. Some drugs, such as the α-adrenergic receptor agonists or β-adrenergic receptor antagonists, also cause bronchoconstriction. Although these drugs have valid therapeutic uses, as a general rule persons with asthma should avoid them.

TABLE 44-1 Drugs that act on bronchial smooth muscle

Cause contraction	Cause relaxation or block contraction
Muscarinic agonists	Muscarinic antagonists
Histamine	H_1 antagonists
β-Adrenergic receptor antagonists	β-Adrenergic receptor agonists
α-Adrenergic receptor agonists	Methylxanthines (theophylline)
Leukotrienes (SRS-A)	Prostaglandin E_2
Prostaglandins D_2 and $F_{2\alpha}$	Prostacyclin (prostaglandin I_2)
Thromboxane A_2	
Kinins	

Bronchodilators

The major drugs used to treat bronchospasm are the β-adrenergic receptor agonists and the methylxanthines. Drugs of either class relax bronchial smooth muscle. The mechanism of relaxation caused by β_2-receptor agonists is believed to be related to changes in cyclic nucleotides. Within the cell membrane these agonists activate adenylyl cyclase, which in the presence of Mg^{++} catalyzes formation of cyclic AMP from cytoplasmic ATP. Catabolism of cyclic AMP depends on phosphodiesterase, an enzyme that is inhibited in vitro by high concentrations of methylxanthines. However, methylxanthines are now believed to cause bronchodilatation by some other mechanism.

β-ADRENERGIC RECEPTOR AGONISTS

The effectiveness of epinephrine and other sympathomimetic drugs in treatment of bronchial asthma is well recognized. Use of ephedrine in respiratory disease dates back many centuries. As described in Chapter 18, sympathomimetic drugs exhibit profiles of activity that are attributed to activation of α, β_1, and β_2 classes of receptors. Bronchodilatation is the major effect of β_2-agonists in the lung, though some studies indicate that these agonists also promote ciliary movement and diminish release of mediators from mast cells.[13]

The chemical structure affects the selectivity of β-adrenergic receptor agonists for bronchial smooth muscle. The basic structure is that of a catecholamine (epinephrine, isoproterenol) or phenethylamine (ephedrine). Other compounds developed with substitutions along the ethanolamine side chain or on the aromatic ring have greater selectivity for β_2-receptors (terbutaline, albuterol). Table 44-2 lists the commonly used drugs and their selectivity for β_2-receptors.

Side effects and complications of therapy with these agents stem primarily from actions on β_1-receptors. Their unwanted effects are predictable from their adrenergic pharmacology. Agonists with both β_1 and β_2 activity can cause tachycardia; some clinicians suspected that they could provoke arrhythmias in susceptible patients, but a connection between inhaled β-adrenergic agents and arrhythmia has never been established. The most limiting effect of β_2-agonists is muscle tremor, especially when

TABLE 44-2 β_2-Adrenergic receptor agonist selectivity and dosage forms

Drug	β_2-Receptor selectivity	Dosage forms
Epinephrine, ephedrine	0	See Chapter 18
Isoproterenol hydrochloride (Isuprel)	0	See Chapter 18
Isoetharine hydrochloride (Dey-Lute, others)	+ +	A: 340 μg; SN: 0.062-1%
Metaproterenol sulfate (Alupent, Metaprel)	+ +	A: 225 mg as powder; S: 10; SN: 0.6,5%; T: 10,20
Terbutaline sulfate (Brethine, others)	+ + +	A: 200 μg, I: 1; T: 2.5,5
Albuterol (Proventil, Ventolin)	+ + +	A: 90 μg; S: 2 as sulfate; T: 2,4 as sulfate
Bitolterol mesylate (Tornalate)	+ + +	A: 370 μg
Pirbuterol acetate (Maxair)	+ + +	A: 200 μg

A, Aerosol, dose per actuation except for metaproterenol; *I*, injection, mg/ml; *S*, syrup, mg/5ml; *SN*, solution for nebulization; *T*, tablets, mg.

the drugs are taken orally. Inhalation, however, provides a more local action and usually avoids systemic adverse effects. Tremor may occur with extended use of metaproterenol or terbutaline but is infrequent with albuterol. The tolerance and refractoriness to further administration that occur with frequent use of epinephrine and isoproterenol is less pronounced with β_2-selective agents. Excessive use of inhalers containing any of the β_2-adrenergic drugs may dry mucous membranes and irritate the airways. Drugs with α-adrenergic actions cause vasoconstriction and sometimes also central nervous system stimulation.

Specific agents. **Epinephrine** is a highly effective bronchodilator widely used in emergencies to relieve acute bronchoconstriction. Epinephrine is not selective for β_2-receptors, however, and it is not effective by mouth. The α-adrenergic component causes vasoconstriction, which reduces edema within the airways and thus improves airflow. Epinephrine has a short duration of action (approximately 20 minutes) when injected or administered by inhalation, and tachyphylaxis develops with repeated use. Mechanisms for terminating the action of epinephrine are discussed in Chapter 13.

Ephedrine, the oldest of the adrenergic agents used to treat asthma, is seldom used anymore because the amounts available in over-the-counter preparations are usually insufficient and larger doses commonly cause side effects. Although active by either oral or parenteral routes and long lasting, ephedrine is not so effective as epinephrine for acute attacks of asthma. In addition, tachyphylaxis develops with continued use.

Isoproterenol was introduced in the 1940s as a pure β-agonist, and it was widely used as a bronchodilator. Administration by inhalation contributed to its popularity. Disadvantages are stimulation of the heart by its action on β_1-receptors and its short-lived bronchodilatory effect.

Isoetharine was the first of the β_2-selective drugs. Like isoproterenol, it is a catecholamine with a short duration of action. Isoetharine is used in aerosol form, but its brief action makes it less popular than other selective agents.

Metaproterenol is an analog of isoproterenol with a moderately long duration of action. The placement of hydroxyl groups in the *meta* positions on the benzene ring provides resistance to degradation by catechol-*O*-methyltransferase and conveys enhanced β_2-receptor selectivity. The drug can be administered orally or by inhalation, and its action lasts up to 4 hours.

Terbutaline has a slightly greater selectivity for β_2-receptors. It is slower in onset of action than metaproterenol, but with oral administration the bronchodilator action persists for as long as 8 hours. Terbutaline appears to have little or no action on β_1-receptors. Some degree of tolerance to the β_2 activity may develop, but less than that with either isoproterenol or epinephrine.

Albuterol is also a relatively selective β_2-adrenergic agent. Modification of the catecholamine structure makes it resistant to degradation and prolongs its action. In equieffective bronchodilator doses, albuterol causes fewer cardiac effects than isoproterenol, and the bronchodilator action persists for 4 to 8 hours.

Use. β_2-agonists are safer and more useful in therapy of acute obstructive airway disease than drugs that stimulate both β_1- and β_2-receptors. Currently β_2-receptor agonists administered by inhalation are the first-line therapy for asthma. Inhalation is the preferred route because the onset of action is rapid (within minutes) and the drug is delivered directly to the target organ. Oral administration of β_2-agonists is indicated only in chronic asthma and is frequently limited by side effects, such as tremor. β_2-agonists are also used in conjunction with ipratropium bromide (see p. 504) in treatment of chronic bronchitis and emphysema.[7]

METHYLXANTHINES

The methylxanthine group (see Chapter 31) includes caffeine, theophylline, and theobromine. Their pharmacologic effects include relaxation of smooth muscle, cardiac stimulation, central nervous system stimulation, and diuresis. Of these compounds only **theophylline**, its salts **aminophylline** and **oxtriphylline**, and **dyphylline**, an analog, are used as bronchodilators.

Mechanism of action. For many years the mechanism of bronchodilatation by theophylline was believed to be inhibition of phosphodiesterase, which would permit accumulation of cyclic AMP within bronchial smooth muscle. However, several potent theophylline derivatives that inhibit phosphodiesterase have little efficacy as bronchodilators. The possibility that theophylline acts by competitive antagonism of adenosine, a bronchoconstrictor, is discounted by observations that **enprophylline**, a methylxanthine bronchodilator more potent than theophylline, does not bind to adenosine receptors. Additional mechanisms for bronchodilatation, such as prostaglandin antagonism and stimulation of endogenous catecholamine release, have been proposed but not proved.

One way that theophylline can improve respiration is by enhancing diaphragmatic contraction. A clinical trial of theophylline in patients with severe, chronic obstructive lung disease showed that the drug improved pulmonary gas exchange, stimulated diaphragmatic contraction, and reduced muscle fatigue, thus improving respiratory function and decreasing dyspnea.[12] The positive inotropic effect of theophylline, which enhances both right and left heart systolic function while decreasing pulmonary arterial pressure, is also beneficial in patients with obstructive lung disease who have increased pulmonary arterial pressure.[3]

Two other actions of theophylline may benefit patients with asthma or chronic obstructive pulmonary disease. Therapeutic concentrations are reported to inhibit airway inflammation by allergic or nonallergic stimuli and to improve mucociliary transport.[3]

Use. Theophylline is used to treat moderate to severe airway obstruction in both acute and chronic situations. By reversing bronchospasm and alleviating diaphragmatic fatigue that accompanies chronic respiratory disease, it relieves dyspnea and can significantly improve the quality of life for pulmonary patients. Theophylline is used primarily in asthma, but it also improves respiratory function in patients with severe chronic obstructive lung disease.[12] In addition, aminophylline combats diaphragmatic fatigue in patients after upper abdominal surgery.[5] Because of its central nervous system stimulating activity theophylline, as well as caffeine, is used to treat apneic episodes in neonates.

Pharmacokinetics and metabolism. Clearance of theophylline and related methylxanthines varies widely among individuals and can be affected by many different factors. Theophylline undergoes biotransformation in the liver where it is hydroxylated and demethylated. Diseases or drugs that affect hepatic enzymes would be expected to alter the plasma concentration of theophylline and its duration of action. For example, clearance of theophylline and related compounds is increased by smoking and by phenytoin, both of which induce hepatic microsomal enzymes. The action of theophylline is prolonged in patients with congestive heart failure, liver disease, or alcoholism. Similarly, concomitant therapy with drugs that inhibit biotransformation, such as erythromycin, cimetidine, ciprofloxacin, or omeprazole, will decrease clearance of theophylline. Because of the narrow therapeutic range of theophylline, these conditions can induce toxicity.

Administration and dosage. Theophylline is effective after either oral or parenteral administration, as is its congener dyphylline (Dilor, Lufyllin, others). Salts of theophylline, aminophylline and oxtriphylline (Choledyl), are slightly more soluble but have no major therapeutic advantage. These salts, in which theophylline is combined with ethylenediamine or choline respectively, contain about 85% theophylline. Aminophylline can be given intravenously, but caution must be used to avoid acute toxicity associated with too rapid elevation of the plasma concentration.

Theophylline is well absorbed after oral administration, with onset of activity from 45 to 60 minutes; its duration of action is about 5 to 6 hours. Because both efficacy and toxicity are related to its plasma concentration, monitoring is an integral part of therapy. Salutary effects on diaphragmatic function occur at concentrations of 5 to 10 μg/ml, bronchodilatation is generally achieved between 10 and 20 μg/ml, and toxic effects begin to appear above 20 μg/ml. The dosage required to reach a therapeutic concentration varies greatly among individuals and must be carefully determined for each patient. A common target concentration when initiating therapy is about 12 μg/ml. Once a maintenance regimen is established, however, sustained-release oral preparations (Theo-Dur, Slo-Phyllin, others) are effective and well tolerated, and they generally improve compliance. In most patients these can be given twice a day. Such preparations result in greater variability in plasma concentration, and absorption is influenced more by meals than for the shorter acting forms of the drug.[6]

Theophylline is available in a variety of forms for oral administration: capsules, 100 to 250 mg; tablets, 100 to 300 mg; elixirs, solutions, syrups, and suspensions, 80 to 300 mg in 15 ml; timed-release capsules, 50 to 300 mg; and timed-release tablets, 100 to 500 mg.

Toxicity and adverse effects. Therapeutic and toxic doses of theophylline vary considerably with the individual. Because theophylline is metabolized by hepatic microsomal enzymes, numerous factors that influence its metabolism will alter its duration of action and the potential for toxic effects. Even at therapeutic concentrations, the drug may cause some gastrointestinal distress, which is believed to be central in origin. Many persons experience central nervous system stimulation, manifested by irritability and insomnia, and headache. Other side effects include tachycardia, hypotension, and diuresis. Most of these effects can be avoided by starting therapy at low doses and increasing the dose gradually to attain desired plasma concentrations.

Serious toxicities involving the central nervous and cardiovascular systems can occur at only twice the usual therapeutic concentrations. Increasing irritability and hyperexcitability can extend to generalized convulsions. These seizures are especially dangerous because they often occur without warning signs and may be refractory to standard anticonvulsant therapy.[3] Cardiac toxicity includes arrhythmias and, in extreme cases, circulatory collapse. A pronounced increase in body temperature may also develop.

Anti-inflammatory steroids

Glucocorticoids are used to reduce inflammation in certain types of pulmonary disease. The basic pharmacology of these agents is discussed in Chapter 47. Because of the involvement of inflammation in the pathogenesis of chronic asthma,[3] administration of glucocorticoids can reduce the frequency and severity of attacks. However, they do not cause their effects rapidly, and they do not directly cause bronchodilatation. Since systemic preparations have potential for serious side effects with extended use, glucocorticoids are usually used systemically only after other measures have proved ineffective. Unfortunately, not all forms of asthma and not all persons respond adequately to glucocorticoid therapy.

All the available glucocorticoids have the same actions and the same potential for adverse effects. A local anti-inflammatory action can be achieved with minimal side effects by selection of the appropriate route of administration.

Mechanisms of action. As described in Chapter 47, the glucocorticoid agents have similar actions that depend on chemical substitution onto the four-ring steroid structure.

Glucocorticoids have several biologic actions that affect the inflammatory process. They reduce microvascular leakage, inhibit influx of inflammatory cells into the lungs, and block the late response to allergens.[2] It is still not clear how glucocorticoids reduce bronchoreactivity. Two possibilities have been suggested. First, there is some indication that they enhance the action of adrenergic agonists on bronchial β_2-receptors, either through modification of receptors or by an influence on signaling events between receptor stimulation and muscle contraction. A second mechanism may be modulation of eicosanoid production. Glucocorticoids suppress arachidonate release, thereby reducing synthesis of prostaglandins and leukotrienes. Decreased synthesis of the potent bronchoconstrictor leukotrienes C_4 and D_4 would clearly be beneficial in asthma. Additional mechanisms may involve inhibition of release of mediators from mast cells or leukocytes within the lung and modification of the immune response.[15]

Specific agents. **Prednisone** (Deltasone, others) is commonly used for oral administration. It is converted in the liver to prednisolone, an active congener, and it has a relatively slow onset of action. As with any steroid therapy, continued use may result in side effects, some of which are not reversed by cessation of therapy. These include the development of osteoporosis, cataract formation, and stunting of growth in children.

Methylprednisolone (Solu-Medrol, others) is used for intravenous administration in emergency treatment of status asthmaticus, a life-threatening exacerbation of asthma with persistent, unrelieved bronchospasm. Methylprednisolone is also available in oral form, and its effects may persist for as long as 24 hours.

Beclomethasone (Beclovent, Vanceril) is a topically active glucocorticoid that can be administered as an aerosol. This helps to limit its action to the airways. Beclomethasone aerosol appears to control asthma without causing systemic effects. Therapy with this agent usually enables patients to minimize or discontinue oral steroids.

Flunisolide (AeroBid) can also be used by inhalation. It has a longer duration of action than beclomethasone, but greater systemic absorption occurs. **Triamcinolone** and **dexamethasone** are also available as aerosols.

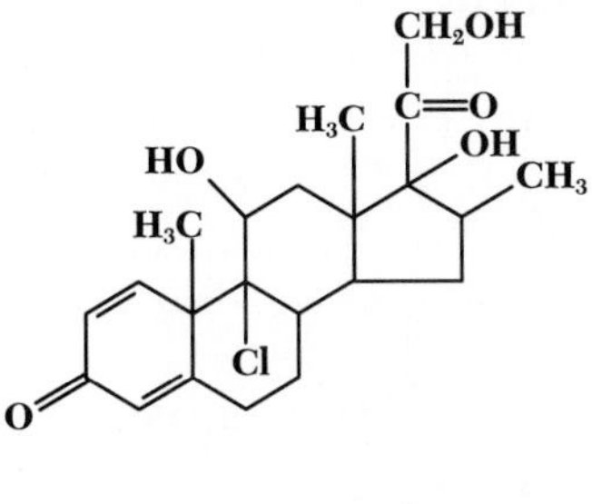

CH_2OH, H_3C, C=O, OH, CH_3, HO, H_3C, Cl, O

Beclomethasone

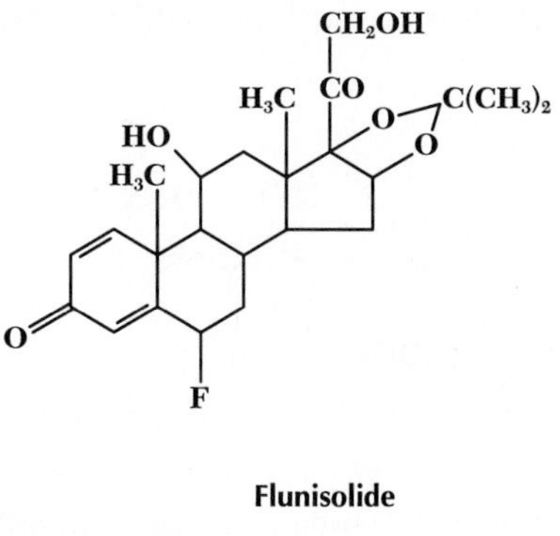

CH_2OH, H_3C, CO, O, $C(CH_3)_2$, O, HO, H_3C, O, F

Flunisolide

See Table 47-2 for preparations of glucocorticoids.

Use. The major use of glucocorticoids in respiratory disease is in management of serious, chronic asthma. Bronchitis, hypersensitivity alveolitis, and allergic rhinitis may be relieved by glucocorticoids if there is an associated asthmatic component, but they are of little use in chronic obstructive pulmonary disease. Steroid therapy is contraindicated in pulmonary infections.

Adverse effects and toxicity. Short-term use of glucocorticoids in asthma usually avoids serious systemic side effects. Extended use or high doses, however, can produce a spectrum of unpleasant and potentially dangerous effects. Steroid toxicity is discussed in more detail in Chapter 47.

Common side effects in adults include weight gain, capillary fragility (easy bruising), osteoporosis, and development of cataracts. With prolonged use, steroids may cause immune suppression, psychologic depression, and a variety of endocrine and metabolic disturbances. In addition, users of inhalers experience dryness of the mouth and throat and are at increased risk of oral candidiasis (thrush). Inhalant forms may trigger asthmatic attacks in some persons, probably by irritating airways.

Alternative therapy of asthma

Although bronchodilators and steroids remain basic therapeutic modalities for management of asthma, some patients, particularly those with exercise-induced asthma, are helped by prophylactic therapy. Since inflammatory mediators presumably contribute to bronchoconstriction, inhibition of mediator release may reduce the severity of the response. Cromolyn and related drugs act through this mechanism. Cromolyn does not relax bronchial smooth muscle, nor does it block histamine or kinin receptors. By inhibiting release of histamine and SRS-A (leukotrienes C_4 and D_4) from mast cells within the airway mucosa and along bronchial blood vessels, it blunts both immediate and late asthmatic reactions to inhaled or absorbed antigens.

Cromolyn sodium (disodium cromoglycate, Intal) is inhaled in the form of a dry powder, is nebulized in an aqueous spray, or is administered as an aerosol. The nebulized form is recommended for young children who may not be able to use an inhaler. Cromolyn is available also in an ophthalmic solution (Opticrom), a nasal solution (Nasalcrom), and in capsules for oral use (Gastrocrom).

For effective prevention of asthmatic attacks, cromolyn must be used several times a day; poor patient compliance will limit its effectiveness. In addition, there is no means of predicting which patients will respond to the drug.

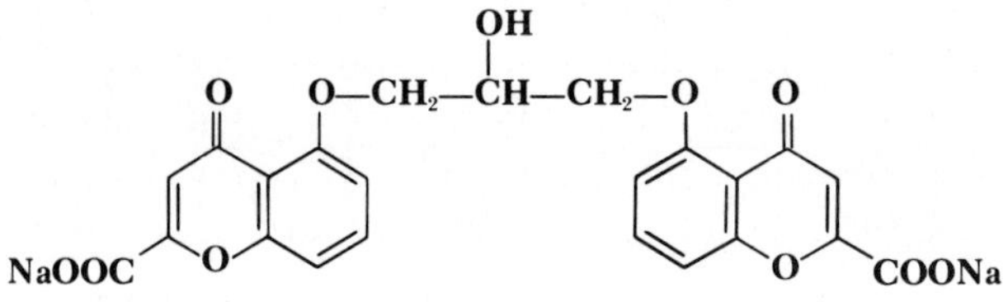

Cromolyn sodium

Ipratropium bromide (Atrovent), an anticholinergic drug, has been more widely used in Europe than in the United States to treat asthma. It acts primarily on larger, central airways, rather than on smaller, peripheral airways, and is thus not as effective as β_2-adrenergic receptor agonists against stimulus-induced bronchospasm.[11] Ipratropium depresses mucociliary function less than atropine does,[14] however, and it is useful in situations in which β-agonists and theophylline are undesirable. Ipratropium may also be used in combination with β-agonists if additional bronchodilatation is needed.

```
H2C————CH————————CH2
 |      |               |         CH2OH
 |      |    CH3        |           |
 |      |   /           |           |
 |  CH3—N+—CH           CH—O—CO—CH · Br−
 |      |   \           |           |
 |      |    CH3        |          C6H5
 |      |               |
H2C————CH————————CH2
```

Ipratropium bromide

Nonsteroidal anti-inflammatory drugs, such as aspirin and ibuprofen, may prove useful, particularly when inflammation is a contributing factor; one must remember, however, that these agents will precipitate bronchoconstriction in intolerant asthmatics.

ELABORATION AND METABOLISM OF MEDIATORS WITHIN THE LUNGS

In addition to its primary function of gas exchange, the lung also processes many different biologically active substances from blood or tissues. The lung is a rich source of *autacoids*, including histamine, prostaglandins, thromboxane, leukotrienes, and peptides. Histamine released from mast cells of the lung probably contributes to asthmatic bronchospasm, and the mixture of leukotrienes (SRS-A) formed during the release response appears to be a key mediator in both allergic and intrinsic asthma. Histamine release from mast cells of the nasal mucosa is clearly involved in allergic rhinitis and possibly in other inflammatory reactions involving the upper airways. Peptides such as substance P, neurotensin, bradykinin, and the complement-derived C5a may also contribute to inflammatory reactions within the lungs. Influx of neutrophils in response to chemotactic factors further amplifies the reaction.

The lung exercises several protective mechanisms to regulate formation and circulation of inflammatory mediators. Serotonin and epinephrine are rapidly removed from the pulmonary circulation by active uptake. Prostaglandins E_2 and $F_{2\alpha}$ and bradykinin are completely inactivated during a single passage through the pulmonary vascular bed. Angiotensin I converting enzyme on the luminal surface of the pulmonary endothelium both activates angiotensin I to angiotensin II and inactivates circulating kinins. Substance P, a bronchoconstrictor peptide, is inactivated within the airways by neutral endopeptidase on the pulmonary epithelium and subepithelial tissues.[10]

GENETIC DISEASES AND THE LUNG

Certain diseases with a genetic basis, such as cystic fibrosis and deficiency of α_1-antitrypsin, cause major pulmonary complications. The recent discovery of the gene defect in cystic fibrosis may lead to improved interventions through gene therapy.

α_1-Antitrypsin is an antiprotease that inhibits elastase released from neutrophils. A deficiency of α_1-antitrypsin, due to faulty synthesis in the liver, can result in progressive destruction of alveoli. Unless corrected, an imbalance between circulating elastase and the protease inhibitor causes emphysema. Therapy is directed toward restoring the balance. This has been accomplished by intravenous administration of purified human α_1-antitrypsin (α_1-proteinase inhibitor; Prolastin). Such *augmentation therapy* appears safe, and if started early enough it may prevent the irreversible changes of emphysema.[4] Ultimately, gene replacement therapy should be applicable to this deficiency disease as well.

REFERENCES

1. Andersson RGG, Grundström N: Innervation of airway smooth muscle: efferent mechanisms, *Pharmacol Ther* 32:107, 1987.
2. Barnes PJ: A new approach to the treatment of asthma, *N Engl J Med* 321:1517, 1989.
3. Bukowskyj M: Theophylline: an overview, *Ration Drug Ther* 22(1), 1988.
4. Crystal RG: α1-Antitrypsin deficiency, emphysema, and liver disease: genetic basis and strategies for therapy, *J Clin Invest* 85:1343, 1990.
5. Dureuil B, Desmonts JM, Mankikian B, Prokocimer P: Effects of aminophylline on diaphragmatic dysfunction after upper abdominal surgery, *Anesthesiology* 62:242, 1985.
6. Jonkman JHG: Food interactions with sustained-release theophylline preparations: a review, *Clin Pharmacokinet* 16:162, 1989.
7. Kesten S, Rebuck AS: Management of chronic obstructive pulmonary disease, *Drugs* 38:160, 1989.
8. Leff AR: Endogenous regulation of bronchomotor tone, *Am Rev Respir Dis* 137:1198, 1988.
9. Marin MG: Pharmacology of airway secretion, *Pharmacol Rev* 38:273, 1986.
10. Martins MA, Shore SA, Gerard NP, et al: Peptidase modulation of the pulmonary effects of tachykinins in tracheal superfused guinea pig lungs, *J Clin Invest* 85:170, 1990.
11. Morris HG: Review of ipratropium bromide in induced bronchospasm in patients with asthma, *Am J Med* 81(suppl 5A):36, 1986.
12. Murciano D, Auclair M-H, Pariente R, Aubier M: A randomized, controlled trial of theophylline in patients with severe chronic obstructive pulmonary disease, *N Engl J Med* 320:1521, 1989.
13. Popa V: Beta-adrenergic drugs, *Clin Chest Med* 7:313, 1986.
14. Wanner A: Effect of ipratropium bromide on airway mucociliary functions, *Am J Med* 81(suppl 5A):23, 1986.
15. Ziment I: Steroids, *Clin Chest Med* 7:341, 1986.
16. Ziment I: Acetylcysteine: a drug that is much more than a mucokinetic, *Biomed Pharmacother* 42:513, 1988.

Chapter 45

Drug effects on the gastrointestinal tract

GENERAL CONCEPT

Disorders of the gastrointestinal tract are among the most common of medical problems. Approximately 4 to 5 million persons suffer from peptic ulcer disease, and many more suffer from minor disturbances. Drugs for management of such disorders are discussed below according to their therapeutic indications. *Antispasmodics* and *antisecretory agents*, as well as *antacids*, are used to correct esophageal dysfunction and to treat peptic ulcer. *Sucralfate* and prostaglandin analogs such as *misoprostol* aid ulcer healing. *Metoclopramide* promotes gastric emptying in reflux disorders and gastroparesis. Important adjunctive measures include avoidance of agents that increase gastric acid secretion (alcohol and caffeine) or that alter normal protective properties of the gastric mucosa (glucocorticoids and nonsteroidal anti-inflammatory drugs).

Laxatives, *antidiarrheal agents*, and *antispasmodics* are used to treat lower gastrointestinal tract problems. Because diarrhea or spasm can be a manifestation of many different disorders, every effort should be made to identify the underlying cause and to determine if further therapy is indicated. Additional treatment includes eradication of infectious agents, correction of malabsorption, or reversal of inflammatory disorders, such as ulcerative colitis or Crohns disease (regional enteritis).

THE BALANCE BETWEEN MUCOSAL DEFENSE AND INJURY

Mucosal defense mechanisms

Various endogenous defense mechanisms normally prevent damage to the gastric mucosa by acid and pepsin. The epithelial layer of the mucosa is composed of tightly adjoined cells that are specialized for existence in an acid medium. Their tight junctions, synthesis of prostaglandins, and secretion of mucus and bicarbonate all contribute to maintenance of the epithelial barrier. Fig. 45-1 is a schematic representation of some of these factors.

Continued renewal of the mucosal cell layer is an important part of the defense mechanism. Gastric prostaglandins are thought to enhance resistance to injury, at least in part, by maintaining blood flow to the mucosa. This provides a continuous supply of nutrients and removes acid that may penetrate the mucosa at sites of minor injury.[1] Animal experiments indicate that polypeptide growth factors, such as epidermal growth factor and transforming growth factor α, are also important in renewal of the gastric mucosa.[2]

Factors that predispose to peptic ulceration

SMOKING

Experimental and epidemiologic evidence clearly indicates that cigarette smoking can promote peptic ulceration and slow ulcer healing (Fig. 45-2). Combinations of impaired mucosal defense, inhibited pancreatic bicarbonate secretion, and enhanced gastric acid and pepsin secretion probably contribute.[17] Smoking also aggra-

FIG. 45-1 *Illustration of the mucus/bicarbonate barrier that protects the gastric mucosa. Bicarbonate is produced by the gastric surface epithelium. Bicarbonate ions diffuse into the mucus layer from the epithelial side, and hydrogen ions from the other side, to create a pH gradient within the mucus layer.*

From Aase S: Scand J Gastroenterol 24(suppl 163):17, 1989.

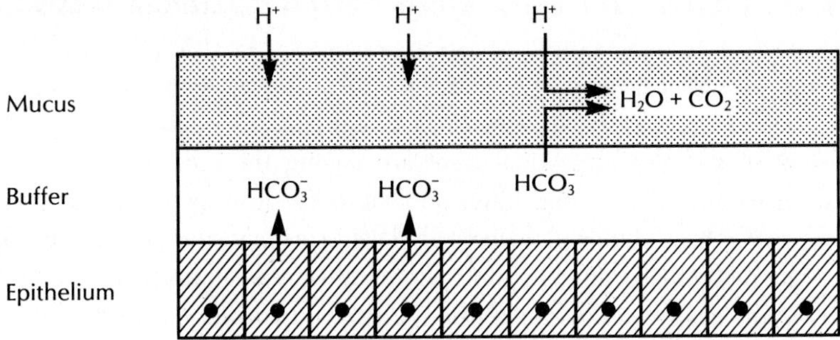

FIG. 45-2 *Model of the pathogenesis of peptic ulcer. Acid and peptic activity overpower mucosal defence to cause ulcers most commonly when defense is impaired by exogenous factors. Two factors, nonsteroidal anti-inflammatory drugs (NSAIDs) and* H. pylori *infection, appear linked to impairment of mucosal defense. Hypersecretion of gastric acid in the Zollinger-Ellison syndrome* (Z-E) *is an exception in which ulcers occur in the absence of* H. pylori *infection. In ordinary peptic ulcer disease, smoking, genetic factors, and psychological stress are also important, but the evidence is conflicting about whether these factors impair mucosal defense, modulate secretion of acid, or both.*

From Soll AH: Reprinted by permission of the New England Journal of Medicine 322:909, 1990.

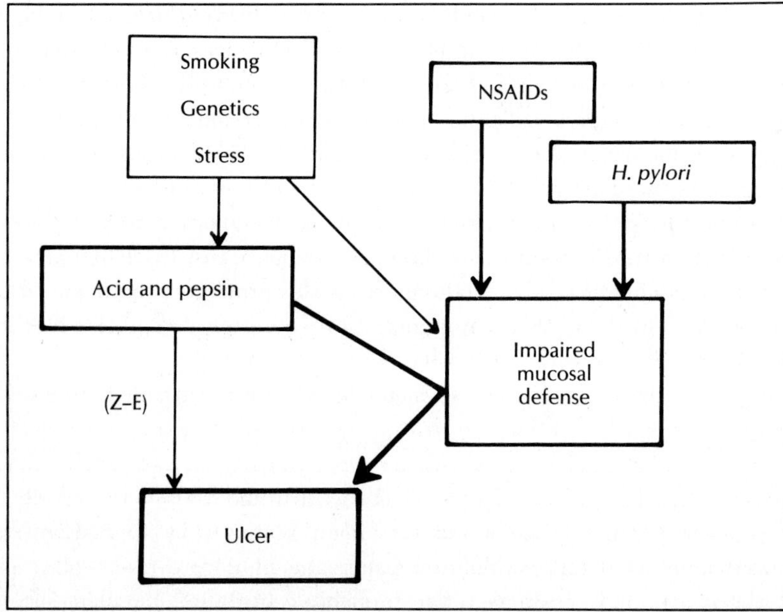

vates gastroesophageal reflux disease by decreasing esophageal sphincter pressure.[7]

Helicobacter pylori infection

Recognition of *H. pylori* (formerly *Campylobacter pyloridis*) as a potential cause of gastritis and peptic ulcer disease prompted a number of clinical studies. Some investigators estimate that the organism is found in 75% to 90% of patients with duodenal or gastric ulcers. Electron microscopy of biopsy material shows that the bacilli adhere to the epithelial surface and cause loss of microvilli, depletion of mucus granules, and other degenerative changes.[8] Once infection is established, antibiotic therapy is indicated.

Nonsteroidal anti-inflammatory drugs

Nonsteroidal anti-inflammatory drugs (NSAIDs) are directly irritating to the gastric mucosa. Taken in large doses they may cause erosion and bleeding. However, their ulcerogenic effect is more likely due to systemic inhibition of prostaglandin production. Epidemiologic studies indicate that NSAIDs increase the morbidity associated with ulcer complications and severe bleeding, particularly in elderly patients or those who smoke.[17]

Several drugs can prevent or delay gastric complications of NSAID therapy. Coadministration of H_2-antagonists or sucralfate is one approach, but the prostaglandin analog, misoprostol, reportedly provides better protection (see p. 512).

DRUGS USED IN DISORDERS OF THE UPPER GASTROINTESTINAL TRACT

The general management of acid-peptic disorders involves (1) agents that inhibit secretion of gastric acid and pepsin, (2) those that neutralize secreted acid, and (3) those that enhance mucosal resistance to erosion. Because they are much more effective with fewer side effects, the histamine (H_2) antagonists have essentially replaced anticholinergic agents for reducing volume and acidity of gastric secretions. Omeprazole, a new drug that suppresses acid secretion, is reported to heal gastric ulcers that do not respond to conventional therapy. Antacids neutralize secreted acid, whereas prostaglandins and sucralfate enhance mucosal resistance. If infection with *H. pylori* is present, its eradication is an integral part of therapy.[6]

Agents that inhibit gastric secretion of acid and pepsin

Histamine antagonists

Antagonists at H_2-receptors reduce the volume and acidity of gastric secretions in both the resting state and after stimulation by food, histamine, or pentagastrin. Competitive antagonism of histamine at H_2-receptors within parietal cells of the gastric mucosa reduces secretion of acid and intrinsic factor. Concomitant reduction of gastric secretory volume decreases secretion of pepsin from chief cells. These agents are highly effective and widely used to treat peptic ulcer and reflux esophagitis. They are available as oral preparations, and serious side effects are uncommon. Cimetidine (Tagamet) has been used extensively, and much is known about its pharmacology (see Chapter 22). Ranitidine (Zantac) is more potent and can be taken less frequently. Famotidine (Pepcid) is more potent and longer acting than either cimetidine or ranitidine. Nizatidine (Axid), the newest member of this class, has essentially the same actions as its predecessors. Neither ranitidine, famotidine, nor nizatidine inhibits hepatic metabolism of other drugs to the extent that cimetidine does (see Table 70-3).

OMEPRAZOLE

Omeprazole (Losec) inhibits secretion of acid by irreversibly blocking H^+,K^+-ATPase, the enzyme that initiates acid secretion. It is used for short-term treatment of reflux esophagitis and for various hypersecretory syndromes.[11] Omeprazole was judged to be superior to ranitidine in a double-blind study comparing the two drugs for healing of gastric ulcers and relief of symptoms.[18] However, little is known about long-term effects of the drug on acid secretion. It inhibits hepatic mixed-function oxygenases, however, much like cimetidine. Omeprazole is available as 20 mg sustained-release capsules.

ANTICHOLINERGIC AGENTS

Before development of H_2-receptor antagonists, atropine-like drugs (see Chapter 15) were used to suppress gastric secretion and motility. In sufficient doses such compounds decrease by 30% to 50% both nocturnal (unstimulated) acid secretion and secretion stimulated by histamine, pentagastrin, or food. Their use is limited by their other antimuscarinic effects at the doses required to inhibit gastric secretion. Contraindications to these drugs include glaucoma, prostatic hypertrophy, and gastric retention.

Agents that neutralize acid

Antacids provide immediate relief from hyperacidity, and adequate dosing promotes healing of ulcers. Acid alone is not the primary cause of ulceration, but an acid environment activates pepsin. To maintain gastric contents within a pH range of 3.5 to 4.5, at which pepsin activity is greatly diminished, large doses of antacids must be taken frequently. This regimen is often difficult to maintain, and antacids are frequently used concurrently with H_2-blockers.

The buffering action of the various antacid preparations depends on their composition. Effectiveness can be predicted by measuring neutralizing capacity. Table 45-1 shows that acid-neutralizing capacity varies considerably among preparations, as does their sodium content.

Effective doses of antacids contain at least 75 to 150 mEq of buffer; patients with hypersecretion of acid, as in duodenal ulcer, may need larger quantities than those with gastric ulcer or esophageal reflux. In addition to excessive production of acid, patients with duodenal ulcers are reported to have rapid gastric emptying, which results in loss of buffering by food.[5]

Antacid preparations are weakly basic and consist of metal salts, most commonly aluminum hydroxide or magnesium hydroxide. These salts dissociate to neutralize gastric acid and form neutral salts.

Long-term use of antacids may cause systemic effects. For example, chronic use of aluminum-containing antacids by patients with renal insufficiency can lead to aluminum accumulation, central nervous system toxicity, and osteomalacia. Hypermagnesemia with central effects can also occur in patients with impaired renal function. Antacids may also cause electrolyte imbalances via absorption of Na^+.

INDIVIDUAL PREPARATIONS

Sodium bicarbonate (baking soda) is a popular agent used (and misused) for self-medication by the lay public. Although it is effective and rapidly acting, absorption can cause metabolic alkalosis; it should not be taken repeatedly. This antacid is found

TABLE 45-1 Characteristics of various antacids

Antacid	Composition	Buffering capacity* (mEq of hydrochloric acid per ml)	Sodium content (mg/5 ml)
Aludrox	Magnesium and aluminum hydroxides, simethicone	2.81	4.5
Amphojel	Aluminum hydroxide gel	1.93	8.1
Gelusil	Aluminum hydroxide gel, magnesium trisilicate	1.33	6.5
Gelusil M	Aluminum hydroxide gel, magnesium hydroxide, magnesium trisilicate	2.23	5.7
Maalox	Aluminum hydroxide gel, magnesium hydroxide	2.58	2.5
Magaldrate (Riopan)	Magnesium and aluminum hydroxides	2.21	0.7
Mylanta	Magnesium and aluminum hydroxides, simethicone	2.38	3.9
WinGel	Aluminum hydroxide gel, magnesium hydroxide, stabilized with hexitol	2.25	1.25

*From Fordtran JS, Morawski SG, and Richardson CT: N Engl J Med 288:923, 1973.

in several over-the-counter medications, such as Alka Seltzer. Because of its systemic effects, it is not prescribed for acid-peptic disease.

Aluminum salts, such as aluminum hydroxide or aluminum hydroxide gel, are found in many preparations. The gel forms aluminum chloride after interaction with gastric acid. Because the chloride is reabsorbed within the intestine, there is no alteration in systemic acid-base balance. Aluminum salts are relatively insoluble and can cause constipation. They may deplete phosphate with excessive use; in fact, they are administered to patients with renal insufficiency to prevent phosphate absorption. In addition, aluminum salts can impair absorption of other drugs.

Magnesium salts, such as the hydroxide or trisilicate, can retain water within the gut by an osmotic effect and cause diarrhea. Bowel disturbances are minimized when they are combined with aluminum salts. Magnesium trisilicate is changed in the stomach to magnesium chloride and silicon dioxide. The chloride is absorbed in the intestine, and magnesium carbonate is formed. Magnesium salts can elevate the pH of the stomach contents to 7 or higher. An 8% aqueous suspension of magnesium hydroxide (milk of magnesia) is one of the most effective antacids available. In normal persons the small amount of Mg^{++} that is absorbed is rapidly cleared by the kidney. However, in patients with poor renal function, retention of Mg^{++} may cause neurologic, cardiovascular, and neuromuscular toxicity.

MIXTURES

Combinations of aluminum and magnesium hydroxides have less neutralizing power than the magnesium salt alone. Such mixtures minimize the disadvantages of the individual agents, however, increase the duration of buffering, and improve palatability.

Simethicone, a defoaming agent sometimes combined with antacids, is said to relieve painful distention caused by formation of gas in the gastrointestinal tract.

Agents that protect the mucosa or augment mucosal defense

SUCRALFATE

Sucralfate (Carafate) is a complex of sulfated sucrose and aluminum hydroxide. This disaccharide does not alter gastric acid or pepsin secretion. Its action is limited to the ulcer surface where it becomes hydrated by the gastric fluid and forms complexes with albumin, fibrinogen, and globulin. These complexes create a protective barrier to acid and pepsin. The rate of ulcer healing with the drug is similar to that with H_2-antagonists.[13] Sucralfate may also be used with antacids; it must be taken four times daily. Mild constipation may occur with continued use. Sufficient aluminum can be absorbed to be hazardous in patients with renal insufficiency. In addition, sucralfate can interact with a variety of other drugs, including tetracyclines, phenytoin, warfarin, and digoxin.

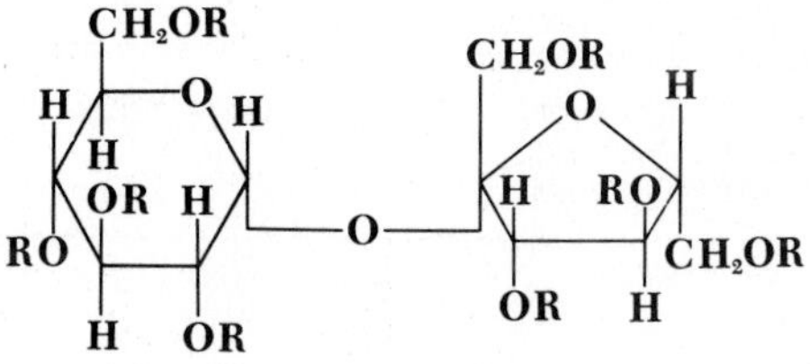

$$R = SO_3[Al_2(OH)_5]$$

Sucralfate

PROSTAGLANDINS

Endogenous prostaglandins play an important role in protecting gastric and duodenal mucosa from acid and pepsin. Prostaglandins produced by the gastric mucosa inhibit acid secretion and help maintain the cellular integrity of the mucosa, probably by promoting secretion of mucus and bicarbonate.[1] Prostaglandins also increase blood flow to the gastric mucosa and facilitate tissue repair. Although PGE_2 is readily destroyed when taken orally, several analogs appear promising as therapy for peptic ulcers. Misoprostol and enprostil were effective in clinical trials. Misoprostol (Cytotec), a synthetic methyl analog of PGE_1, is reported to be highly effective in healing aspirin-induced ulcers in patients taking high doses for rheumatoid arthritis.[9,14] It is also effective in prophylaxis against NSAID-induced gastropathy. It is provided as tablets, 200 μg. Because the prostaglandin derivatives stimulate smooth muscle contraction in the intestine and uterus, however, their adverse effects (that is, diarrhea and risk of abortion) may outweigh their beneficial effects. They are also expensive.

COLLOIDAL BISMUTH SUSPENSIONS

Colloidal bismuth suspensions and bismuth subsalicylate, the active ingredient in Pepto-Bismol, appear to promote ulcer healing, possibly by inhibiting the action of pepsin or by binding to proteins within the ulcer itself. In addition colloidal bismuth may prevent degradation of peptide growth factors that aid in mucosal repair.[16] It also helps to clear *H. pylori* from the upper gastrointestinal tract.

METOCLOPRAMIDE

Metoclopramide is a dopamine antagonist that enhances motility of the upper gastrointestinal tract, an effect antagonized by anticholinergic drugs. The drug is used in therapy of reflux esophagitis, in disorders of intestinal motility, such as diabetic gastroparesis, and as an antiemetic (see p. 248). Metoclopramide elevates lower esophageal sphincter pressure, increases resting esophageal tone, and hastens gastric emptying. It facilitates procedures such as endoscopy and intubation and is used in radiologic examination of gastrointestinal motility.

Adverse reactions to metoclopramide include drowsiness, fatigue, insomnia, dizziness, and bowel disturbances. It can also cause movement disorders and other forms of neurotoxicity in some patients.[10] The drug is contraindicated in patients with pheochromocytoma in whom it may cause hypertension.

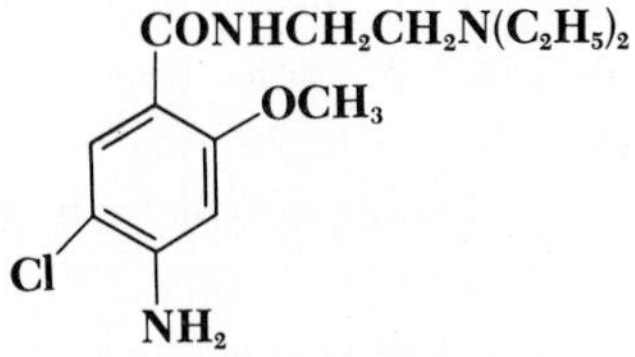

$CONHCH_2CH_2N(C_2H_5)_2$

OCH_3

Cl

NH_2

Metoclopramide

Metoclopramide hydrochloride (Reglan, others) is available in tablets containing 10 mg of the base, as a syrup (5 mg/5 ml), and in vials for injection (5 mg/ml).

CISAPRIDE

Cholinomimetic agents may also prove useful for stimulating gastrointestinal motor function. Cisapride, an experimental compound, acts indirectly by stimulating release of acetylcholine from neurons in the stomach and intestine. In experimental models it has been more effective than metoclopramide in overcoming delayed gastric emptying and has also stimulated smooth muscle of the colon.[15] Because cisapride does not block dopamine receptors, it might be useful in hypomotility disorders.

DRUGS USED IN DISORDERS OF THE LOWER GASTROINTESTINAL TRACT

Most disorders of the lower gastrointestinal tract involve abnormalities of fluid and electrolyte transport or smooth muscle responsiveness. Diarrhea may have many causes, including infection with bacteria or parasites, toxins, inflammation, and malabsorption.

Constipation is sometimes caused by organic disease, such as tumors of the bowel, and sometimes by drugs, such as aluminum hydroxide, opioid analgesics, and tricyclic antidepressants or other anticholinergic agents. Otherwise, it is generally due to poor dietary habits, lack of bulk-producing foods, and inattention to the stimulus for defecation. A sedentary life style and lack of regular exercise also promote constipation. Correction of such factors will often relieve chronic constipation without the need for laxative treatment.

Antidiarrheal agents

Severe diarrhea causes water and electrolyte depletion, which may progress to dehydration and electrolyte imbalance. Even mild, chronic diarrhea can cause hypokalemia. Basic management is directed toward elimination of the cause, if possible, and replacement of fluid and electrolytes. The cytoprotective action of bismuth salts can prevent or decrease diarrhea. Small doses of opioids decrease intestinal motility. Opioid analgesics and anticholinergic drugs reduce pain and diarrhea associated with inflammatory bowel disease.

SPECIFIC AGENTS

Adsorbents coat the lining of the gastrointestinal tract to adsorb bacteria and toxic products, which are then eliminated in the feces. *Bismuth subsalicylate* binds toxins produced by *Vibrio cholerae* and *Escherichia coli* and reduces intestinal inflammation and hypermotility. This agent is now preferred over antibiotics for prevention of travelers' diarrhea because it avoids the side effects of antibiotics as well as acquisition of resistant intestinal flora.[4] However, large amounts must be ingested for efficacy.

Bismuth is essentially insoluble in the gastrointestinal tract, but the salicylate moiety is nearly completely absorbed. A single adult dose of Pepto-Bismol in liquid or tablet form provides approximately 200 to 250 mg of salicylate. Unless taken excessively or with other salicylate-containing products, there is no danger of salicylate toxicity.[3]

Other agents such as kaolin, activated charcoal, and pectin are also adsorbent. Unfortunately, these adsorbents can bind other drugs, and they may cause constipation after counteracting the diarrhea.

Cholestyramine (Questran, Cholybar) and *colestipol hydrochloride* (Colestid) are affinity resins that bind acidic materials. Although they also bind toxins from bacterial organisms, their main action in the gastrointestinal tract is to control diarrhea caused by malabsorption of bile acids, as after ileal resection. The resins also reduce some types of hyperlipidemia (see Chapter 43). Constipation is a major problem, and the drugs also adsorb vitamins and other nutrients.

Opioids are the most effective agents for relief of diarrhea. They enhance the tone and segmenting activity of both the large and small intestine; this increases resistance to transit of fecal material. In addition, they reduce propulsive motility of the bowel, increase sphincter tone, and decrease secretory activity along the gastrointestinal tract. Decreased motility enhances fluid reabsorption and decreases the volume of intestinal material.

Paregoric (camphorated tincture of opium) is a schedule III drug because it has potential for misuse and addiction. Codeine is an effective antidiarrheal agent, but it too may be abused. The opiate-like drug **diphenoxylate** in combination with atropine (Lomotil, others) is recommended for treating chronic diarrhea; in this case the more addictive opiate compounds are undesirable. Diphenoxylate is unlikely to cause physical dependence, but it can enhance the effects of other central nervous system depressants.

Loperamide hydrochloride (Imodium) is an antiperistaltic, antidiarrheal agent. It has a structure similar to that of haloperidol, and it can affect opiate receptors. Loperamide is very effective in reducing diarrhea, but, as with any of the opioid compounds, it should not be used in infectious diarrhea because retention of organisms might result in bacterial invasion of the intestinal wall.

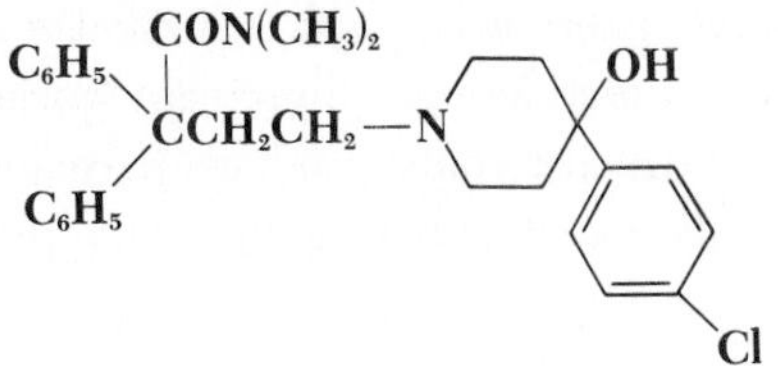

Loperamide

Psyllium hydrophilic mucilloid (Metamucil, others) is a powder that swells in water to form a bland, nonirritating bulk. It is used to treat irritable bowel syndrome, one of the most common causes of diarrhea. Paradoxically, this substance is also used as a bulk laxative to relieve constipation (see Table 45-2).

Drugs used in inflammatory bowel disease

Severe inflammatory bowel disease is usually treated with anti-inflammatory steroids (Chapter 47). Sulfasalazine (Azulfidine, Azaline), a combination of a sulfonamide and an analog of aspirin, is also widely prescribed for patients with this problem. This agent is a *prodrug* that delivers active **mesalamine** (5-aminosalicylic acid) to the lower gastrointestinal tract. Mesalamine as such is not effective orally because it is completely absorbed in the proximal small intestine. A preparation was approved recently for rectal administration (Rowana Suspension Enema). This route of administration is not satisfactory for extended treatment, however, and the drug is ineffective in patients with small bowel inflammation. Currently, research is directed toward developing a stable, orally effective form of 5-aminosalicylate for inflammatory bowel disease.[12]

TABLE 45-2 Common laxative-cathartics

Agent	Mechanism
Hydrophilic agents	
Dietary fiber (bran) Carboxymethylcellulose Psyllium colloid	Absorb water to form softened but formed stools by increasing bulk of intestinal contents; decrease intestinal transit time
Osmotic laxatives	
Magnesium salts	Hypertonic solutions draw fluid into intestinal lumen by osmosis
Lactulose	Low molecular weight metabolites have an osmotic action within the intestinal lumen
Contact laxatives	
Bisacodyl Phenolphthalein	Decrease fluid and electrolyte absorption in small intestine
Cascara sagrada	Stimulates peristalsis
Castor oil	Lipolysis in intestine liberates ricinoleic acid
Lubricant-emollients	
Mineral oil Glycerin	Coat fecal mass, soften stool, and facilitate passage
Wetting agents	
Docusate salts	Allow entry of water and lipids to soften stool

Other agents that have been used with varying degrees of success include immunosuppressants, such as azathioprine, 6-mercaptopurine, and cyclosporine. Neither aminosalicylates nor corticosteroids produce permanent remission of Crohns disease; immunosuppressants may thus have a legitimate place in management of this inflammatory disorder.

Cathartics and laxatives

Laxatives are agents that produce a soft, but formed, stool, whereas cathartics are those that produce a fluid or semifluid stool. Both increase accumulation of water and electrolytes in the lumen of the small bowel and promote defecation. The terminology reflects a difference in the intensity and latency of the effect.

Laxatives promote and ease defecation by influencing the consistency of the stool. Soft stools and lack of straining during defecation are especially desirable in some clinical settings, as in postsurgical patients or those with diseases of coronary or cerebral vessels. Cathartics are used to speed elimination of toxic materials or parasites after treatment with anthelmintics and to prepare the bowel for radiologic or surgical procedures. A technique involving ingestion of a large volume (4 liters) of a solution containing nonabsorbable polyethylene glycol with sodium sulfate and other salts (CoLyte, GoLYTELY) appears to be a superior means of cleansing the bowel.

Mechanisms

The various laxative-cathartics act by several mechanisms (Table 45-2). There is some overlap among the various groups. In general, hydrophilic and osmotic agents increase the bulk of the intestinal contents and the rate of transit. Agents that stimulate motility also expand intestinal contents, in this case by decreasing absorption of electrolytes and fluids. Contact laxative-cathartics have a direct action on intestinal mucosa. They inhibit cyclic AMP–mediated absorption of fluid and electrolytes. Other drugs act as emollients or stool softeners. There is no indication for combinations of laxative preparations, since individual agents are just as effective.

Specific agents

Bulk laxatives are not absorbed from the intestine. Some dietary components, such as bran fiber, aid normal bowel function by adding bulk to the stool. *Carboxymethylcellulose*, when mixed with water, forms a hydrophilic colloid that, by retaining a large quantity of water, softens the stool, distends the colon, and stimulates evacuation. Bulk laxatives are generally safe but sometimes cause obstruction of a narrowed intestinal lumen.

Osmotic laxatives include such diverse substances as magnesium salts, hypertonic saline, and lactulose. By increasing water content in the intestinal lumen, osmotic laxatives also increase bulk. Magnesium sulfate is widely used, as is magnesium in the form of milk of magnesia.

Lactulose (Chronulac, Cephulac) is a semisynthetic disaccharide that is not hydrolyzed in the small intestine but is metabolized, by bacteria in the large bowel, to lactate and other compounds that are not well absorbed. Because it acts within the large bowel, its onset of action is slow. Lactulose is administered in the form of a syrup. Excessive dosage can produce diarrhea, cramps, and flatulence. Lactulose is also used in portal systemic encephalopathy, in which it reduces blood ammonia.

Glycerin suppositories, which are useful in children and elderly or debilitated persons, promote defecation by stimulating evacuation reflexly through a hyperosmotic action on the rectal mucosa. Glycerin also lubricates hardened fecal material.

Contact agents stimulate vigorous intestinal motility. They promote formation of watery stools and can cause cramping and pain. An exception is *bisacodyl* (Dulcolax, others), which produces a soft stool and minimal colic. This agent stimulates the large intestine, and it is useful in preparing patients for proctoscopic or colonoscopic procedures. Preparations of bisacodyl include enteric-coated tablets and suppositories. The latter should not be used in patients with a fissure or ulcerations because systemic absorption may occur.

Another contact agent, *phenolphthalein*, is found in various nonproprietary preparations. This substance acts primarily in the large intestine, and it will color alkaline feces. It is partially absorbed and can cause undesirable skin eruptions and prolonged discoloration. The phenomenon of fixed eruption by phenolphthalein probably has an allergic mechanism because even small doses cause the dermal response in sensitive persons.

Surface-active agents include *docusate* (dioctyl sulfosuccinate) salts (Colace, others). They are mild laxatives because of a surface effect on the intestinal contents. They act as dispersing or wetting agents that permit water and lipids to enter the mass and soften it. Wetting agents are otherwise inert. They are slow in onset; the full effect may require as long as 2 days to develop. Diarrhea is an occasional adverse reaction.

REFERENCES

1. Aase S: Disturbances in the balance between aggressive and protective factors in the gastric and duodenal mucosa, *Scand J Gastroenterol* 24(suppl 163):17, 1989.
2. Beauchamp RD, Barnard JA, McCutchen CM, et al: Localization of transforming growth factor α and its receptor in gastric mucosal cells: implications for a regulatory role in acid secretion and mucosal renewal, *J Clin Invest* 84:1017, 1989.
3. Bierer DW: Bismuth subsalicylate: history, chemistry, and safety, *Rev Infect Dis* 12(suppl 1):S3, 1990.
4. DuPont HL, Ericsson CD, Johnson PC, et al: Prevention of travelers' diarrhea by the tablet formulation of bismuth subsalicylate, *JAMA* 257:1347, 1987.
5. Fordtran JS, Walsh JH: Gastric acid secretion rate and buffer content of the stomach after eating: results in normal subjects and in patients with duodenal ulcer, *J Clin Invest* 52:645, 1973.
6. Goodwin CS, Armstrong JA, Marshall BJ: *Campylobacter pyloridis*, gastritis, and peptic ulceration, *J Clin Pathol* 39:353, 1986.
7. Kahrilas PJ, Gupta RR: Mechanisms of acid reflux associated with cigarette smoking, *Gut* 31:4, 1990.
8. Kazi JL, Sinniah R, Zaman V, et al: Ultrastructural study of *Helicobacter pylori*-associated gastritis, *J Pathol* 161:65, 1990.
9. Lanza FL: A review of mucosal protection by synthetic prostaglandin E analogs against injury by non-steroidal anti-inflammatory agents, *Scand J Gastroenterol* 24(suppl 163):36, 1989.
10. Miller LG, Jankovic J: Metoclopramide-induced movement disorders: clinical findings with a review of the literature, *Arch Intern Med* 149:2486, 1989.
11. Omeprazole, *Med Lett Drugs Ther* 32:19, 1990.
12. Peppercorn MA: Advances in drug therapy for inflammatory bowel disease, *Ann Intern Med* 112:50, 1990.
13. Richardson CT: Sucralfate, *Ann Intern Med* 97:269, 1982.

14. Roth S, Agrawal N, Mahowald M, et al: Misoprostol heals gastroduodenal injury in patients with rheumatoid arthritis receiving aspirin, *Arch Intern Med* 149:775, 1989.
15. Schuurkes JAJ, Van Nueten JM: Stimulation of myenteric cholinergic nerves and gastrointestinal motility, *Prog Pharmacol* 7:83, 1988.
16. Slomiany BL, Nishikawa H, Bilski J, Slomiany A: Colloidal bismuth subcitrate inhibits peptic degradation of gastric mucus and epidermal growth factor in vitro, *Am J Gastroenterol* 85:390, 1990.
17. Soll AH: Pathogenesis of peptic ulcer and implications for therapy, *N Engl J Med* 322:909, 1990.
18. Walan A, Bader J-P, Classen M, et al: Effect of omeprazole and ranitidine on ulcer healing and relapse rates in patients with benign gastric ulcer, *N Engl J Med* 320:69, 1989.

section nine

Drugs that influence metabolic and endocrine functions

Chapter 46

Hypothalamic releasing factors and growth hormone

GENERAL CONCEPT

The anterior pituitary produces hormones that regulate the activity of other endocrine glands. These hormones include peptides such as somatotropin (growth hormone), prolactin, and ACTH (corticotropin), as well as glycoproteins such as TSH (thyrotropin), LH (luteinizing hormone), and FSH (follicle-stimulating hormone). Secretion of these regulatory hormones is controlled by a multimessenger neuroendocrine system that includes hormones from target organs and neurotransmitters from the hypothalamus and the median eminence.[18]

Neuroendocrine regulation of anterior pituitary secretion is functionally and anatomically different from that of the posterior pituitary. Secretion of hormones from the anterior pituitary is stimulated by polypeptide releasing-factors that originate in the hypothalamus and play both neurotransmitter and neuroendocrine roles.

The releasing factors are secreted by neural cells in the ventral hypothalamus in response to neural or humoral signals. They are transported via a capillary plexus to the venous portal system of the pituitary stalk where they reach cells in which thyrotropin, gonadotropin, ACTH, somatotropin, and prolactin are stored. The hormones are secreted from five different types of pituitary cells: thyrotrophs, gonadotrophs, corticotrophs, somatotrophs, and lactotrophs. Additional regulation occurs at the level of adrenergic, dopaminergic, tryptaminergic, and peptidergic transmitters in the hypothalamus. Drugs that affect the concentrations of these transmitters within the hypothalamus are expected to influence hormone secretion as well.

NEUROPHARMACOLOGIC AGENTS AND HYPOTHALAMIC RELEASING FACTORS

Many different peptides have been identified and mapped within the central nervous system, and several are established as neurotransmitters or neuromodulators. The isolation, characterization, and synthesis of hormone-releasing factors firmly established their role in the physiology of endocrine secretion but also unveiled additional complexities. Some of these peptides (TRH and GnRH) release more than one hormone; others inhibit release (PIF, somatostatin). In addition, these peptide hormones influence behavior and affect neuronal excitability within the hypothalamus. Synthetic peptide releasing-factors provided important research tools, as well as the possibility of therapeutic intervention in various endocrine disorders.[17]

TRH (thyrotropin-releasing hormone)

TRH was the first hypothalamic releasing hormone to be isolated, fully characterized, and synthesized, through the independent efforts of Drs. R. Guillemin and A.V. Schally, who shared a Nobel prize in medicine for their work on the hypothalamic regulation of the pituitary gland.[14]

Thyroid-stimulating hormone (TSH), the primary regulator of the thyroid gland, is secreted in response to TRH. TRH stimulates thyrotrophs and lactotrophs to release TSH and prolactin respectively, through an adenylyl cyclase–dependent mechanism. Thyroid hormone inhibits this effect at the thyrotropin-producing cell, but only partially decreases the effect on prolactin secretion. Somatostatin also blocks TRH-induced secretion of TSH, but not that of prolactin, indicative of differential regulation of the two target cells. In some types of pituitary abnormalities, for example, in acromegaly or in certain tumors, TRH also stimulates release of growth hormone.

Neuronal cell bodies and fibers throughout the brain contain TRH and TRH receptors, but these are most common in regions concerned with cardiorespiratory control. When TRH is administered to experimental animals or humans it elicits an increase in plasma norepinephrine and a potent pressor response, probably through adrenergic mechanisms in the central nervous system.[15]

The structure of TRH was determined by amino acid sequencing. This facilitated synthesis of TRH, as well as various structural analogs. **Protirelin** (Relefact TRH, Thypinone) is a synthetic tripeptide, 5-oxo-L-prolyl-L-histidyl-L-proline amide, identical to naturally occurring TRH. It is available in solution, 0.5 mg/ml. TRH has a short half-life and requires continuous intravenous infusion. Protirelin is used in diagnosis of thyroid and pituitary disorders, and it stimulates prolactin secretion in experimental studies. TRH also appears promising as treatment for amyotrophic lateral sclerosis[17] and for spinal cord injury.[6] Studies in experimental animals and in man suggest that TRH may be a trophic substance for motor neurons.[6] Despite its potent pressor effect, the use of TRH in shock remains controversial. Results differ according to the type of shock and the animal species studied.[15]

CRF (corticotropin-releasing factor)

CRF, a polypeptide of 41 residues, is a potent stimulant of pituitary secretion of ACTH and other pro-opiomelanocortin products.[12,19] It is the predominant regulator of ACTH formation and release (see Chapter 47). CRF has been identified in multiple sites in the central nervous system and also in peripheral tissues and some tumors. Its colocalization with other hormones in certain areas of the hypothalamus suggests additional functions. As with other regulators of hormone secretion, CRF acts through intracellular messengers that promote protein phosphorylation by cyclic AMP-dependent kinase. Extrapituitary receptors also appear to be coupled to adenylyl cyclase, but their functions are unknown. CRF mediates the response of an individual to stress through activation of the pituitary-adrenal axis; it may also serve as a central integrating signal to coordinate other physiologic responses.[16]

CRF is used clinically to test for abnormalities of the hypothalamic-pituitary-adrenal axis. Patients with Cushings disease exhibit a normal or exaggerated release of ACTH in response to exogenous CRF, in contrast to those with ectopic ACTH secretion who fail to respond. CRF is also used to evaluate ACTH release in depressed persons and in patients with anorexia nervosa. These individuals have a blunted ACTH response to CRF injection, presumably because of an elevated concentration of hydrocortisone.[3] A similar response occurs in individuals who have undergone strenuous exercise or other types of physiologic stress.

Dextroamphetamine releases CRF, and this response is blocked by α-adrenergic receptor antagonists. Reserpine transiently increases basal secretion. Phenothiazines reduce secretion of CRF in response to hypoglycemia, metyrapone, and pyrogens, perhaps through blockade of amine receptors. An interesting development is that certain lymphokines from the immune system augment some actions of CRF.[16] Synthesis of CRF receptor antagonists should help define the multiple actions of CRF and stimulate exploration of additional interactions between neuroendocrine and immune functions.

Gn-RH (gonadotropin-releasing hormone)

Gn-RH, or luteinizing hormone–releasing hormone (LH-RH), is a decapeptide that stimulates release of the pituitary gonadotropins FSH and LH. Although Gn-RH causes secretion of both glycoproteins and their common α-subunit, use of Gn-RH antagonists in normal women determined that the hormones were differentially regulated. Secretion of LH appears to be more controlled by Gn-RH than is secretion of FSH.[8]

Neuronal regulation of Gn-RH secretion is important in controlling onset of puberty, as well as in determining reproductive potential in the adult. Neural signals from the arcuate nucleus in the hypothalamus stimulate the oscillatory release of Gn-RH from neurons in the median eminence. Dopamine stimulates release of Gn-RH, whereas serotonin inhibits secretion, as reflected by changes in plasma gonadotropins. Dopaminergic agonists, such as bromocriptine, can also release Gn-RH.

In addition to its potential for regulation of conception and steroidogenesis,[4] Gn-RH is used to treat hypothalamic amenorrhea, isolated gonadotropin deficiency, and carcinoma of the prostate.[5] Intermittent administration of the hormone, which mimics the pulsatile nature of endogenous release, causes sustained secretion of both FSH and LH. Subcutaneous administration of Gn-RH, with a peristaltic infusion pump, to men with primary Gn-RH deficiency resulted in growth of the testes and increased sperm counts over a period of two years.[20]

Analogs of Gn-RH that are more potent and longer lasting than the parent molecule can desensitize the pituitary and thus reduce gonadotropin and sex steroid concentrations in men with prostatic carcinoma. This technique avoids use of estrogens and may obviate the need for orchiectomy. **Leuprolide acetate** (Lupron) is available for subcutaneous injection, 5 mg/ml. The usual dose is 1 mg daily. A depot suspension, 7.5 mg/ml, can be diluted for monthly intramuscular injection.

Prolactin-inhibiting factor (PIF) and prolactin-releasing factors (PRF)

Prolactin secretion is regulated by both releasing and inhibiting factors from the hypothalamus. The major inhibiting factor is probably dopamine or a second mediator controlled by dopamine. There are at least two releasing factors, TRH and VIP (vasoactive intestinal polypeptide). In experimental animals suckling increases TRH concentration in plasma from the hypophyseal stalk, and antibodies to VIP block the suckling-induced rise in prolactin.

Dopaminergic neurons from the tuberoinfundibular region complete a negative feedback loop to the anterior pituitary to provide a stable, low basal concentration of circulating prolactin. Alterations of dopamine release probably account for the effects of various drugs on prolactin secretion. For instance, neuroleptic agents can cause pseudopregnancy and lactation in experimental animals and menstrual disorders in women. Dopamine inhibits prolactin synthesis and release from pituitary cells in vitro, and there is some indication that neuroleptics cause a delayed increase in dopamine turnover in hypothalamic neurons.[18]

Hyperprolactinemia is associated with a syndrome of gonadal dysfunction, galactorrhea, hirsutism, and obesity. Excessive prolactin secretion also interferes with release of Gn-RH and may lower concentrations of gonadotropins and the sex hormones estradiol and testosterone. Galactorrhea can be a side effect of some psychotropic drugs, presumably by effects on dopamine release or dopamine receptors. Conversely, the semisynthetic ergot alkaloid bromocriptine, a dopamine agonist, has been used to control galactorrhea, as well as other manifestations of abnormal pituitary hormone secretion. Bromocriptine mesylate (Parlodel) is available in 2.5 mg tablets and 5 mg capsules.

GRF (growth hormone–releasing factor, GH-RF)

Secretion of growth hormone (GH) from the anterior pituitary is under dual control by the stimulatory GRF and the inhibitory factor somatostatin (see below). A peptide of 40 to 44 amino acids first isolated from pancreatic tumors in patients with acromegaly was later recognized as identical to GRF from the hypothalamus. Synthesis of several derivatives showed that the first 29 amino acids of the amino terminal contain full biologic activity. GRF is also found in some normal tissues and in certain other tumors, but its function in these extrapituitary sites is not known.[10] Although several other hypothalamic peptides, such as TRH, Gn-RH, neurotensin, substance P, and opioid peptides, stimulate release of GH under certain conditions, GRF from the pituitary appears to be the primary physiologic stimulus for secretion.

Release of GRF is regulated by a complex interaction with somatostatin. Secretion of somatostatin correlates inversely with GRF release. Dopaminergic stimulation enhances basal GH secretion, probably at the level of the pituitary somatotroph, but drugs that affect dopaminergic receptors also influence GRF. Additional evidence indicates adrenergic control of GRF secretion. For example, dextroamphetamine stimulates GRF secretion; this effect is enhanced by propranolol. In general, GRF secretion is stimulated by α-adrenergic mechanisms and inhibited by β-adrenergic mechanisms.

Somatostatin

The hypothalamus has a tonic stimulatory effect on GH production; hypothalamic lesions decrease GH production and retard growth. Early research on control of GH secretion by GRF led to isolation and purification of somatostatin, a tetradecapeptide that inhibits GH release. This peptide has an extensive distribution within the nervous system and in many peripheral tissues, including the gastrointestinal tract and endocrine and exocrine glands.[11] Like many other regulatory factors, somatostatin is synthesized in a longer form that is also active.

Somatostatin is a potent suppressor of GH release both in vitro and in vivo. It blocks the GH response to exercise, insulin-induced hypoglycemia, and levodopa injection. Neurotransmitters and neuropeptides that modify somatostatin release also affect GH concentration.

Somatostatin is also found in many cells that have nothing to do with GH, and it inhibits secretion of several other pituitary and peripheral hormones, such as TSH, prolactin, ACTH, glucagon, insulin, and gastrin. Inhibition of hormone secretion and also secretion of peptides from cancer cells may depend on a common mechanism such as interaction with a guanine nucleotide regulatory protein that inhibits adenylyl cyclase.[9] Furthermore, somatostatin is believed to be involved in virtually all sensory systems.[11]

Octreotide, a somatostatin analog, can decrease GH secretion from pituitary adenomas. It has produced both biochemical and clinical improvement of acromegaly due to tumor-derived GH.[1] **Octreotide acetate** (Sandostatin), 50 to 500 μg/ml, is usually injected subcutaneously.

GROWTH HORMONE

Growth hormone (GH), *somatotropin*, is the most abundant hormone of the anterior pituitary. It constitutes approximately 10% of the weight of the gland in the human and has several different functions. Some actions of GH are probably mediated by *somatomedin C* (insulin-like growth factor), which is derived from the liver and stimulates bone and peripheral tissue growth.[17] GH has important effects on metabolism. By decreasing glucose utilization, antagonizing insulin, increasing amino acid transport and protein synthesis, GH promotes protein synthesis at the expense of carbohydrate and fat.

Glucocorticoids oppose the anabolic actions of GH. GH release is stimulated by hypoglycemia and by exercise. Release also increases during REM sleep and is enhanced by dopaminergic stimulation.[18] In humans GH and gonadal steroid secretion occur in unison throughout the life cycle. During childhood GH secretion is much lower than during puberty, when both GH and gonadal hormone concentrations increase dramatically.

Human GH, extracted from pituitaries or prepared by recombinant DNA technology, provides a means of treating GH deficiency. Because several persons who received the pituitary extract developed a fatal neurologic disorder (Creutzfeldt-Jakob disease),[2] that preparation was withdrawn. However, recombinant forms are available as powders, 5 mg per vial, for reconstitution and subcutaneous or intramuscular injection. Somatrem (Protropin) contains an extra methionine group; somatropin (Humatrope) is identical to the native hormone. Dosage of somatropin is 0.06 mg/kg three times per week; somatrem is given at 0.1 mg/kg three times a week.

The only approved indication for GH therapy is for replacement of deficient endogenous hormone. Recombinant GH administration has been remarkably free of side effects. Hyperglycemia and glycosuria were reported with high doses. Neutralizing antibodies decreased the beneficial effect in some persons, but the major limitation is epiphyseal fusion. Treatment with GH at an early age is necessary for accelerated growth[7] because no significant growth occurs in persons who have achieved mature bone age.

Because GH accelerates growth of children and increases mobilization of fat in obese persons, there is considerable interest in this hormone for its cosmetic effects. A decline of GH secretion may also be important in aging. A study in elderly men showed that short-term administration of the recombinant hormone increased lean body mass, decreased adipose tissue, and increased lumbar vertebral bone density. These findings suggest that GH may attenuate loss of bone and muscle in the elderly.[13]

REFERENCES

1. Barakat S, Melmed S: Reversible shrinkage of a growth hormone-secreting pituitary adenoma by a long-acting somatostatin analogue, octreotide, *Arch Intern Med* 149:1443, 1989.
2. Brown P, Gajdusek DC, Gibbs CJ, Asher DM: "Epidemic" Creutzfeldt-Jakob disease from human growth hormone therapy, *N Engl J Med* 313:728, 1985.
3. Chrousos GP, Schuermeyer TH, Doppman J, et al: Clinical applications of corticotropin-releasing factor, *Ann Intern Med* 102:344, 1985.
4. Conn PM, Staley D, Harris C, et al: Mechanism of action of gonadotropin releasing hormone, *Annu Rev Physiol* 48:495, 1986.
5. Cutler GB Jr, Hoffman AR, Swerdloff RS, et al: Therapeutic applications of luteinizing-hormone-releasing hormone and its analogs, *Ann Intern Med* 102:643, 1985.
6. Faden AI: Pharmacotherapy in spinal cord injury: a critical review of recent developments, *Clin Neuropharmacol* 10:193, 1987.
7. Frasier SD: Human pituitary growth hormone (hGH) therapy in growth hormone deficiency, *Endocrine Rev* 4:155, 1983.
8. Hall JE, Whitcomb RW, Rivier JE, et al: Differential regulation of luteinizing hormone, follicle-stimulating hormone, and free α-subunit secretion from the gonadotrope by gonadotropin-releasing hormone (GnRH): evidence from the use of two GnRH antagonists, *J Clin Endocrinol Metab* 70:328, 1990.
9. Kee KA, Finan TM, Korman LY, Moody TW: Somatostatin inhibits the secretion of bombesin-like peptides from small cell lung cancer cells, *Peptides* 9(suppl 1):257, 1988.
10. Losa M, Wolfram G, Mojto J, et al: Presence of growth hormone-releasing hormone-like immunoreactivity in human tumors: characterization of immunological and biological properties, *J Clin Endocrinol Metab* 70:62, 1990.
11. Reichlin S: Somatostatin, *N Engl J Med* 309:1495 and 1564, 1983.
12. Rivier C, Vale W: Effects of corticotropin-releasing factor, neurohypophyseal peptides, and catecholamines on pituitary function, *Fed Proc* 44:189, 1985.
13. Rudman D, Feller AG, Nagraj HS, et al: Effects of human growth hormone in men over 60 years old, *N Engl J Med* 323:1, 1990.
14. Schally AV: Aspects of hypothalamic regulation of the pituitary gland: its implications for the control of reproductive processes, *Science* 202:18, 1978.
15. Sirén A-L: Cardiovascular pharmacology of thyrotropin releasing hormone, *Peptides* 9(suppl l):69, 1988.
16. Taylor AL, Fishman LM: Corticotropin-releasing hormone, *N Engl J Med* 319:213, 1988.

17. Thorner MO: Hypothalamic releasing hormones: clinical possibilities, *Hosp Pract* 21(12):63, 1986.
18. Tuomisto J, Männistö P: Neurotransmitter regulation of anterior pituitary hormones, *Pharmacol Rev* 37:249, 1985.
19. Vale W, Greer M: Corticotropin-releasing factor, *Fed Proc* 44:145, 1985.
20. Whitcomb RW, Crowley WF Jr: Clinical Review 4: diagnosis and treatment of isolated gonadotropin-releasing hormone deficiency in men, *J Clin Endocrinol Metab* 70:3, 1990.

Chapter 47

Adrenal corticosteroids

GENERAL CONCEPTS

Since the observation by Hench in 1949 of a dramatic response to *cortisone* in patients with rheumatoid arthritis, adrenal steroids and synthetic *glucocorticoids* have become widely used in medicine. They owe their popularity to their anti-inflammatory and immunosuppressive effects. More rarely, these drugs are used for substitution therapy in adrenal insufficiency, which is often iatrogenic.

Aldosterone, the main *mineralocorticoid* of the adrenal gland, stimulates Na^+ reabsorption and K^+ and H^+ secretion by the distal tubules and collecting ducts of the kidney. It is not used therapeutically, but a synthetic derivative is occasionally administered to patients with autonomic insufficiency and orthostatic hypotension. On the other hand, spironolactone, an aldosterone antagonist, has important therapeutic applications.

DEVELOPMENT OF IDEAS

During the 1940s there was an intense search for the active principles responsible for the life-sustaining role of the adrenal glands. Reichstein and von Euw synthesized desoxycorticosterone in 1937 and later demonstrated its presence in the gland.[9] Although this steroid powerfully affects salt reabsorption by the kidney and became useful in management of Addisons disease, it was obvious that extracts of adrenal cortex contained other compounds that had a greater influence on metabolism of carbohydrates and proteins.

Hench observed that patients with rheumatoid arthritis tended to improve when jaundiced or when pregnant. He attributed this improvement to an "antirheumatic" factor from the adrenal gland. Subsequently, Kendall at the Mayo Clinic isolated *hydrocortisone* (cortisol). A milestone in the history of adrenal steroids was the report of Hench and co-workers[8] on the remarkable effectiveness of cortisone in rheumatoid arthritis.

Results of clinical trials in rheumatoid arthritis were dramatic, and soon cortisone was found to cause symptomatic improvement in a large number of disease conditions. It was also recognized that cortisone did not cure these many diseases. Rather, it seemed "to provide the susceptible tissues with a shieldlike buffer against the irritant."[7]

Although hydrocortisone was largely responsible for the glucocorticoid activity of adrenal extracts, it was suspected that the extracts also contained a material with much greater mineralocorticoid activity than that of desoxycorticosterone. This compound, aldosterone, was isolated in 1953.

Subsequent research on glucocorticoids led to development of many new steroids with significantly greater anti-inflammatory potency than cortisone. Their influence on carbohydrate metabolism generally parallels their anti-inflammatory activity. An important advantage of steroids such as prednisone, methylprednisolone, triamcinolone, and dexamethasone is that they exert little effect on renal Na^+ reabsorption while possessing potent anti-inflammatory activity.

PITUITARY-ADRENAL RELATIONSHIPS

ACTH

ACTH (adrenocorticotropic hormone, corticotropin), a polypeptide released from the anterior pituitary gland, stimulates adrenal steroid synthesis. Its release (Fig. 47-1) is promoted by the hypothalamic polypeptide CRF (corticotropin-releasing factor, see p. 521).

ACTH release is regulated largely through a negative feedback on CRF production that is related to the blood hydrocortisone concentration. Stressful stimuli, including epinephrine release or administration, can override the feedback inhibition, release CRF and ACTH, and elevate plasma hydrocortisone concentration. In addition to these important influences, there is diurnal variation in ACTH release.

Human ACTH consists of 39 amino acids, not all of which are essential for biologic activity. The first 19 N-terminal amino acids are sufficient for stimulating hydrocortisone production. The first 13 amino acids in ACTH constitute α-melanocyte–stimulating hormone (α-MSH); thus it is not surprising that ACTH acts on melanocytes.

ACTH promotes synthesis of hydrocortisone by stimulating conversion of cholesterol to pregnenolone. This activity of ACTH is mediated by cyclic AMP (adenosine 3',5'-monophosphate), which acts similarly to ACTH both in vitro and on the perfused dog adrenal gland. Other compounds, such as forskolin and cholera toxin, that increase intracellular cyclic AMP also promote synthesis of hydrocortisone.

Oral administration of ACTH is ineffective because the polypeptide is broken down in the gastrointestinal tract. When injected intravenously, ACTH is destroyed in minutes. For this reason, the hormone is administered either by intravenous infusion

FIG. 47-1 *Diagrammatic summary of the principle factors regulating ACTH secretion.* Dashed arrows *indicate inhibitory influences.*

From Ganong WF, Alpert LC, Lee TC: Review of medical physiology, ed 6, Los Altos, Calif, 1973, Mange Medical Publications.

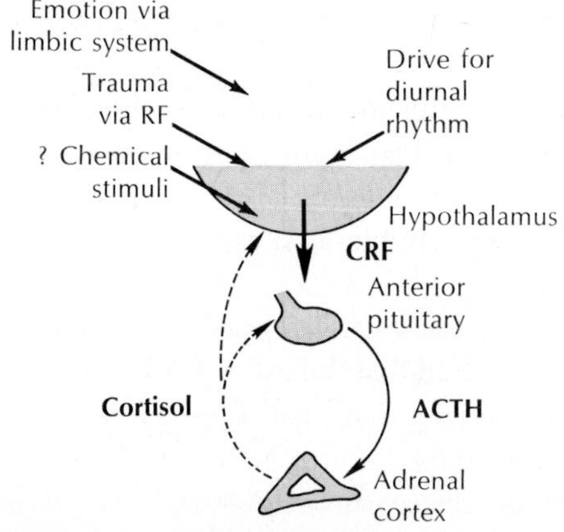

or as a repository injection (Cortrophin Gel, others) by intramuscular or subcutaneous routes. Corticotropin zinc hydroxide suspension is also given intramuscularly.

ACTH is used to diagnose disturbed adrenocortical function. Intravenous infusion of the hormone will increase urinary excretion of hydrocortisone metabolites if the adrenal glands are normal or hyperplastic.

BIOSYNTHESIS OF ADRENAL STEROIDS

Adrenal corticosteroids are not stored but are synthesized as needed. In the zona fasciculata and zona reticularis, cholesterol is changed to pregnenolone, which is metabolized to progesterone, to desoxyhydrocortisone, and then to hydrocortisone. Another product of pregnenolone is androstenedione, the precursor of testosterone. In the zona glomerulosa, the sequence of events is cholesterol → pregnenolone → progesterone → desoxycorticosterone → aldosterone.

Inhibitors of corticosteroid synthesis

Certain toxic compounds such as amphenone B and the insecticide tetrachlorodiphenylethane (DDD) may damage the adrenal cortex. Amphenone B blocks several hydroxylation steps, whereas DDD is believed to inhibit cholesterol esterase. Aminoglutethimide also blocks steroidogenesis, by interfering with cholesterol side-chain cleavage and the conversion of cholesterol to pregnenolone. Trilostane and cyanoketone, an experimental drug, block synthesis of hydrocortisone and aldosterone by inhibiting the conversion of pregnenolone to progesterone. Aminoglutethimide (Cytadren) and trilostane (Modrastane) are used to treat hypersecretion of the adrenal gland when surgical removal is not possible.

Metyrapone (Metopirone) is used as a diagnostic tool in patients with disorders of adrenal function. It inhibits 11β hydroxylation and blocks biosynthesis of hydrocortisone, corticosterone, and aldosterone. The 11-desoxycorticosteroids that accumulate after blockade by metyrapone do not inhibit ACTH release. Thus the decrease in hydrocortisone and corticosterone enhances ACTH release from the anterior pituitary gland in normal persons. In this circumstance, ACTH stimulates production of 11-desoxyhydrocortisone and 11-desoxycorticosterone. The metabolites of these steroids, 17-hydroxycorticosteroids and 17-ketosteroids, can be measured in the urine (Fig. 47-2). If anterior pituitary function is deficient, metyrapone administration will not increase excretion of these metabolites. Hence metyrapone can be used to identify adrenal insufficiency that arises from pituitary, as opposed to adrenal, dysfunction. As would be predicted, however, the metyrapone test is useless if adrenocortical function is defective. This is assessed beforehand by determining the influence of an ACTH infusion on urinary steroid output.

In adults, metyrapone is administered orally in doses of 750 mg every 4 hours for six doses. Urinary steroids are determined over the next 24 hours.

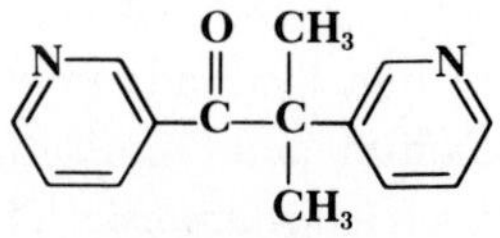

O CH$_3$
N C C N
CH$_3$

Metyrapone

FIG. 47-2 *Pituitary-adrenal feedback system and its inhibition by metyrapone.*

Modified from Coppage WS Jr, Island D, Smith M, Liddle GW: J Clin Invest 38:2101, 1959.

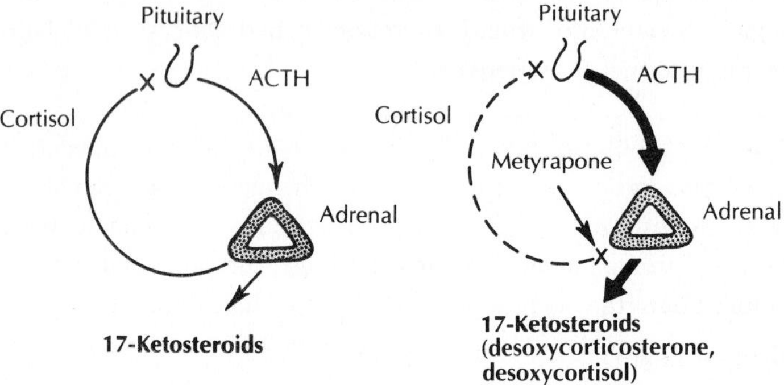

GLUCOCORTICOIDS

Hydrocortisone and corticosterone

Hydrocortisone is the principle glucocorticoid of the human adrenal cortex. Human adrenal glands contain 2 to 6 μg of hydrocortisone per gram of wet tissue. In the plasma of normal persons its concentration is about 80 ng/ml. The rate of secretion follows a characteristic rhythm or diurnal variation. Secretion increases in the early morning hours, before the person awakens, and gradually declines toward late evening.

Hydrocortisone **Corticosterone**

PHARMACOLOGIC EFFECTS

Glucocorticoids control the rate of protein synthesis (Fig. 47-3).[1,10] The steroid diffuses into the cell and binds to a cytosolic receptor. The steroid-receptor complex undergoes a conformational change and is translocated to the nucleus. In the nucleus, the complex binds to chromatin and stimulates transcription of certain messenger RNAs that code for synthesis of specific proteins. These proteins mediate the biologic effect of the steroids. In addition, glucocorticoids may alter post-translational processing of proteins.

The three major influences of adrenal steroids are on (1) carbohydrate, protein, and fat metabolism, (2) mineral metabolism, and (3) inflammation.

Effects on carbohydrate and protein metabolism. The primary effects of hydrocortisone on carbohydrate and protein metabolism are summarized below and in Fig. 47-4.

Steps in glucocorticoid action. St, *Steroid;* R, *specific glucocorticoid receptor; the dissimilar shapes of R are intended to represent different conformations of this protein.* ***FIG. 47-3***

From Baxter JD, Forsham PH: Am J Med 53:573, 1972.

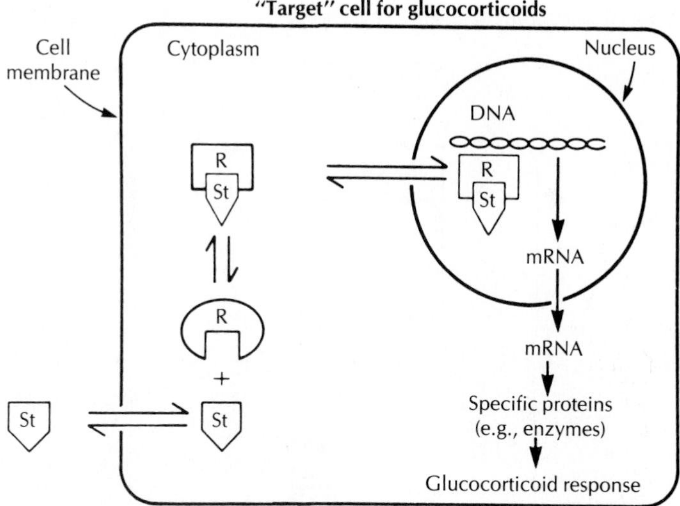

1. Carbohydrate metabolism
   a. An increase in gluconeogenesis (synthesis of glucose from protein)
   b. An increase in liver glycogen
   c. An increase in plasma glucose concentration
   d. A decrease in peripheral glucose utilization
2. Protein metabolism
   a. Mobilization of amino acids from tissues, mainly skeletal muscle
   b. An increase in nitrogen excretion in the urine because of protein metabolism

Little is known about the basic action of hydrocortisone on fat metabolism. Unusual accumulations of fat occur in the patient treated with glucocorticoids.[1,12] Fat is redistributed from the periphery to the face to produce a "moon face," to the back of the neck to cause a "buffalo hump," and to the supraclavicular region. The glucocorticoids promote fat mobilization and exert complex effects on ketone metabolism. For example, hydrocortisone has a *permissive* effect on free fatty acid release from adipose tissue by catecholamines.

Effects on electrolyte and water metabolism. Glucocorticoids have much less effect on renal handling of electrolytes than desoxycorticosterone and aldosterone do; nevertheless, administration of hydrocortisone or cortisone increases Na^+ retention and K^+ excretion and, if prolonged, can cause hypokalemic alkalosis. On the other hand, patients with Addisons disease cannot be maintained in electrolyte balance with glucocorticoids alone. Adrenalectomized animals cannot excrete a large water load, but cortisone will restore this particular function.

The cardiovascular effects of glucocorticoids and mineralocorticoids can be accounted for by their actions on salt and water balance. For example, patients with

FIG. 47-4 *Glucocorticoid action on carbohydrate, lipid, and protein metabolism.* Arrows, *General flow of substrate in response to the catabolic and anabolic actions of glucocorticoids when unopposed by secondary secretions of other hormones. Not shown is increased gluconeogenesis by kidney. + or −, Stimulation or inhibition respectively.*

From Baxter JD, Forsham PH: Am J Med 53:573, 1972.

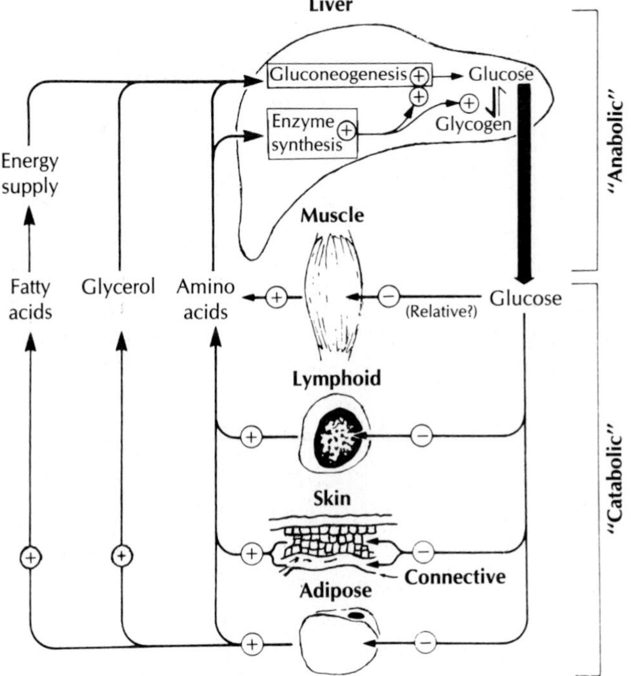

Cushings syndrome or primary aldosteronism retain Na^+ and have hypokalemia and hypertension. In contrast, patients with Addisons disease excrete an excess of Na^+ and have hyperkalemia, and cardiovascular collapse may develop because of volume depletion (Table 47-1).

Calcium ion metabolism is also affected by hydrocortisone.[12] It promotes renal excretion of Ca^{++}, and it may reduce Ca^{++} absorption from the intestine. Osteoporosis develops in patients with Cushings syndrome and with glucocorticoid therapy. Cessation of long-bone growth is a problem in children who receive a glucocorticoid; final adult height may be reduced in those treated for longer than 6 months.

Anti-inflammatory action. Most clinical use of glucocorticoids and ACTH may be attributed to the remarkable ability of the steroids to inhibit inflammatory and immune processes. The mechanisms responsible are numerous and varied.[2,3,4,11] The effects of glucocorticoids that contribute to their therapeutic benefit include the following:

Lymphocytopenia, eosinophilia, and monocytopenia. Glucocorticoids promote sequestration of lymphocytes and monocytes in the spleen, lymph nodes, and bone marrow. This reduces the number of these cells that reach the site of inflammation and thereby inhibits cell-mediated immunity and inflammation (Fig. 47-5).

TABLE 47-1	Effects of bilateral adrenalectomy
Circulatory	Decreased blood pressure Decreased blood volume Hyponatremia, hypochloremia, hypoglycemia, and hyperkalemia Increased nonprotein nitrogen
Renal	Increased excretion of Na^+ and Cl^- Decreased excretion of K^+
Digestive	Loss of appetite, nausea, and vomiting
Muscular	Weakness Decreased Na^+ and increased K^+ and water in muscle
Miscellaneous	Decreased resistance to all forms of stress Hypertrophy of lymphoid tissue and thymus Death unless treatment is instituted

Effect of hydrocortisone administration on circulating lymphocytes and monocytes. Hydrocortisone, 400 mg, was administered intravenously in a single dose to a normal volunteer. *FIG. 47-5*

From Fauci AS, Dale DC, Balow JE: Ann Intern Med 84:304-315, copyright 1976; reproduced with permission from American Medical Association.

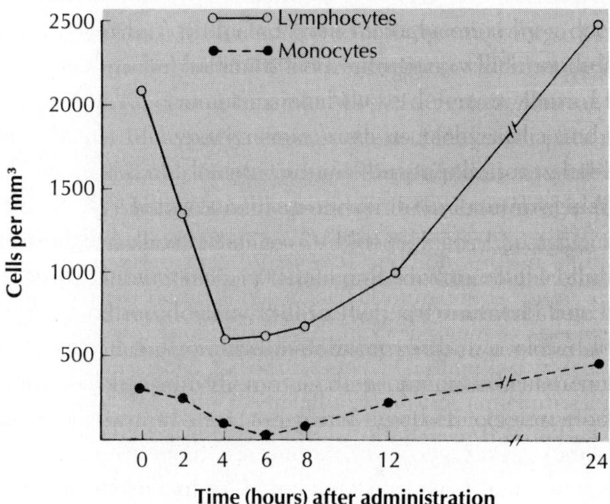

A decrease in migration of polymorphonuclear leukocytes. Glucocorticoids inhibit adherence of neutrophils to vascular endothelium and thereby reduce their movement from the vasculature into the site of inflammation.

Inhibition of macrophage processing of antigens. Antigens must be modified or processed before they can stimulate T- or B-lymphocytes. Glucocorticoids inhibit the ability of macrophages to perform this function.

Inhibition of the actions of lymphokines. Lymphocytes release *lymphokines,* proteins that are chemotactic, mitogenic, and cytotoxic (see Chapter 68). Glucocorticoids may modify synthesis of some cytokines or lymphokines, such as interleukin 1, and inhibit the actions of others, for example interleukin 2.

Inhibition of antibody-dependent cell-mediated cytotoxicity. Antibodies directed against a target cell will bind to the cell surface and coat it. Macrophages have receptors to the F_c portion of the antibody. This allows the macrophage to attach to the target cell by an antibody bridge that facilitates phagocytosis. Glucocorticoids prevent this process by inhibiting attachment of the antibodies to the F_c receptor.

Inhibition of arachidonic acid metabolism. Prostaglandins are vasodilators and promote pain, whereas leukotrienes promote leukocyte chemotaxis and increase capillary permeability (see Chapter 25). Thus these arachidonic acid metabolites are believed to be mediators of inflammation. Glucocorticoids promote synthesis of lipomodulin, a protein that inhibits phospholipase A_2.[4,11] Inhibition of phospholipase A_2 prevents release of arachidonic acid and synthesis of prostaglandins, leukotrienes, and related compounds. Furthermore, glucocorticoids inhibit the induction of cyclooxygenase by cytokines and thereby block cytokine enhancement of prostaglandin synthesis.

Miscellaneous effects. There is little doubt that glucocorticoids can act on the central nervous system.[1,12] Treated individuals may experience euphoria and other behavioral abnormalities that cannot be explained by improvement of the primary disease. They may also develop psychoses. In addition, there is evidence that glucocorticoid treatment can lower convulsive thresholds.

On the one hand, glucocorticoids improve muscle strength in adrenalectomized animals. On the other, they can cause weakness with prolonged treatment, perhaps because of K^+ loss or mobilization of muscle protein.[12]

Adverse effects. Glucocorticoid treatment increases the risk of infection.[12,13] After prolonged steroid therapy, varicella and herpes can disseminate, herpes of the eye may be more severe, tuberculosis may be reactivated, and fungal diseases may develop. Infection is an added factor to consider, rather than an absolute contraindication, when risks of using glucocorticoids are appraised.

Excessive doses of glucocorticoids over a prolonged period produce the various manifestations of Cushings disease. The most serious systemic complications that result from clinical use of high doses of steroids are: diabetogenic effects; dissolution of supporting tissues such as bone, muscle, and skin; hypertension; and impairment of defense mechanisms against serious infections.

Prolonged therapy with glucocorticoids may produce a long-term suppression of the pituitary-adrenal axis (Fig. 47-6).[5,6,12] Suppression may occur when high dosages, equivalent to 15 to 20 mg per day of prednisone, are given for periods as short as 2 weeks; lower dosages require a longer period. The time necessary for pituitary-adrenal recovery after discontinuation likewise depends on the dosage and duration of treatment. Pituitary and adrenal function may not return to normal for 9 to 12 months; patients may not respond normally to stress for up to 2 years. Thus, after long-term therapy, abrupt withdrawal of a glucocorticoid can cause adrenal insufficiency because the pituitary or adrenal cannot respond normally. Pituitary-adrenal suppression can be avoided by using intermediate-acting glucocorticoids at the lowest possible dose, by

Pattern of plasma ACTH and hydrocortisone values in patients recovering from prior long-term daily glucocorticoid therapy that resulted in suppression of the pituitary-adrenal axis. *FIG. 47-6*

From Ney RL: In Thorn GW, editor: Steroid therapy, New York, 1971, Medcom, Inc (presently 12601 Industry St, Garden Grove, CA 92641).

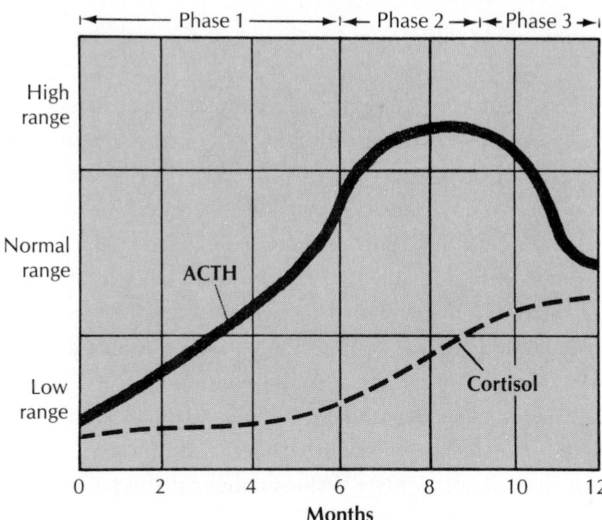

giving the entire daily dose in the early morning to coincide with the diurnal peak of adrenal secretion, by using alternate-day administration, and by limiting the duration of therapy.[6]

Glucocorticoids increase the incidence of cataracts,[12] which are usually bilateral and occur more frequently in children than in adults. Cataracts may develop with either brief or prolonged treatment.

METABOLISM

Cortisone and synthetic glucocorticoids are absorbed rapidly and completely from the gastrointestinal tract. After oral administration, maximum plasma concentration is reached in 1 to 2 hours. Hepatic degradation of glucocorticoids reduces plasma concentration fairly rapidly; after 8 hours only 25% of the peak value remains, and the active drug disappears completely in about 12 hours.

Drugs that promote the activity of microsomal enzymes in the liver tend to accelerate metabolism of glucocorticoids. These drugs, which include phenobarbital and phenytoin, may necessitate an increase in glucocorticoid dosage.

GLUCOCORTICOID ANTAGONISTS

Glucocorticoid antagonists bind to the cytosolic receptor; however, the antagonist-receptor complex does not undergo transformation or translocation.[10] Mesylates of glucocorticoids, such as cortisol mesylate, behave as antagonists. Mifepristone (RU 486) is an antagonist at both glucocorticoid and progesterone receptors and has been used to treat Cushings disease. Inhibition of progesterone accounts for its use to induce abortion (see Chapter 48).

GLUCOCORTICOID PREPARATIONS AND CLINICAL USAGE

Hydrocortisone is available in tablets; in lotions, creams, and ointments for topical application; and in preparations for injection by various routes.

Cortisone is used almost entirely in tablet form or in suspension for intramuscular injection.

Certain principles concerning therapeutic use of adrenal steroids can be stated, as follows:

1. These drugs do not cure any disease. They are used predominantly for their anti-inflammatory properties and provide only symptomatic relief. They do not represent replacement therapy, as insulin does in diabetes, except in the rare conditions of Addisons disease or hypoadrenocorticism.
2. Adrenal steroid therapy is particularly useful in disease processes that occur episodically and therefore do not require extended treatment. They are also very useful in conditions in which topical application is sufficient.
3. Every effort should be made to use other drugs or procedures before prolonged steroid treatment is undertaken. With continued use, hyperadrenocorticism resembling Cushings syndrome may be inevitable. Cessation of treatment with these steroids may acutely exacerbate various diseases. Suppression of the pituitary-adrenal axis presents a serious danger if the patient encounters stressful situations.
4. Despite their many disadvantages, adrenal glucocorticoids provide great benefit in self-limiting diseases and in chronic disabling processes that fail to respond to any other treatment. The systemic use of these drugs is a calculated risk that is often worth taking in the presence of incapacitating and otherwise unresponsive disease.

Comparison of various glucocorticoids

Several glucocorticoids have been introduced into therapeutics because they have greater anti-inflammatory potency than hydrocortisone without a corresponding increase in their tendency to retain salt.

The chemical relationships among these newer glucocorticoids may be summarized in comparison with the structural formula of cortisone:

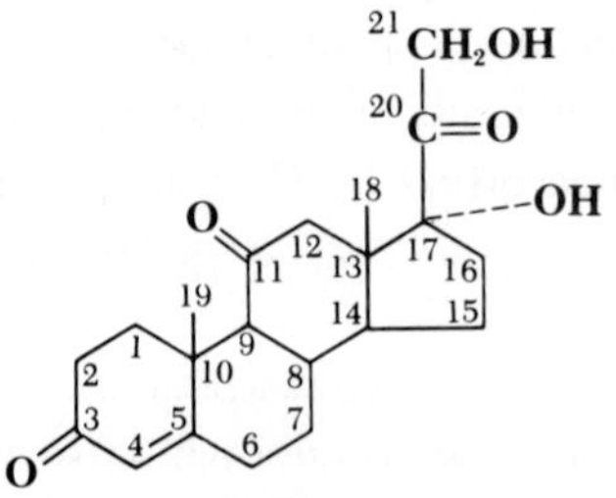

Cortisone

Hydrocortisone has the same structural formula as cortisone except that OH is in position 11.

Prednisone is the same as cortisone except that there is a double bond between positions 1 and 2. It is therefore 1,2-dehydrocortisone.

Prednisolone is the same as hydrocortisone except for a double bond between positions 1 and 2. It is therefore 1,2-dehydro-hydrocortisone. It and prednisone are interconverted in the body.

Methylprednisolone is the same as prednisolone except that an α-CH_3 is in position 6.

Triamcinolone is the same as prednisolone except that an α-F is in position 9 and there is an additional α-OH in position 16. It is therefore 9α-fluoro-16α-hydroxyprednisolone.

Dexamethasone is the same as prednisolone except for an α-F in position 9 and an α-CH_3 in position 16. It is therefore 9α-fluoro-16α-methylprednisolone.

Paramethasone is the same as dexamethasone except that the α-F is in position 6 rather than position 9. It is 6α-fluoro-16α-methylprednisolone.

Betamethasone is the same as dexamethasone except that the CH_3 in position 16 is a β substitution instead of α. It is therefore 9α-fluoro-16β-methylprednisolone.

Fludrocortisone is the same as hydrocortisone except that an α-F is in position 9. It is 9α-fluorohydrocortisone.

Halcinonide (Halog) differs from triamcinolone by substitution of a chlorine for the hydroxyl group in position 21 and reduction of the double bond at positions 1 and 2.

The introduction of prednisone and prednisolone into therapeutics was of great practical importance because their high anti-inflammatory activity is not coupled with a correspondingly high Na^+-retaining potency. This separation of activities allows the physician to use these compounds without special salt-free diets and K^+ supplementation. Glucocorticoids also differ in their duration of action (Table 47-2). Suppression of the adrenal-pituitary axis is more pronounced with the long-acting steroids.[6]

The synthetic analogs of hydrocortisone (Table 47-2) are usually administered orally in the form of tablets. Suspensions of some of the drugs are available for intramuscular and intra-articular administration. Although they are of low solubility, water-soluble preparations of some of the steroids, such as succinates or phosphates, are available for intravenous use. In addition, some preparations can be inhaled into the sinus cavities or into the lungs to relieve rhinitis or asthma.

Dermatologic and other topical applications

Topical treatment of dermatologic, ophthalmologic, and otologic diseases has been revolutionized by the introduction of the anti-inflammatory glucocorticoids. The percutaneous absorption, particle size, and vehicle composition of these preparations are important determinants of their topical activity. Excessive use of these preparations over a large surface area may cause systemic effects.

MINERALOCORTICOIDS

Aldosterone and desoxycorticosterone

Aldosterone is the main mineralocorticoid of the adrenal cortex. *Primary aldosteronism,* characterized by hypertension and K^+ depletion, results from its excessive secretion. Aldosterone itself is not used therapeutically. Instead, fludrocortisone is used clinically to correct electrolyte abnormalities in adrenal insufficiency. Fludrocortisone is occasionally used to treat patients with autonomic insufficiency accompanied by severe orthostatic hypotension.

TABLE 47-2 Comparison and dosage forms of various steroids

Steroid	Anti-inflammatory potency	Sodium retention	Daily dose (mg)	Dosage forms (mg)
Glucocorticoids				
Short-acting				
Cortisone (Cortone)	0.8	0.8	50-100	T: 5-25; I: 25,50
Hydrocortisone (Cortef, Hydrocortone)	1	1	50-100	T: 5-20; I: 25,50*
Intermediate-acting				
Prednisone (Orasone, others)	4	0.8	10-20	T: 1-50; S: 5
Prednisolone (Delta-Cortef, others)	4	0.8	10-20	T: 5; S: 15; I:*
Methylprednisolone (Medrol, Meprolone)	5	0.5	10-20	T: 2-32; I:*
Triamcinolone (Aristocort, others)	5	0	5-20	T: 1-8; S: 2,4; I:*
Long-acting				
Dexamethasone (Decadron, others)	30	0	0.75-3	T: 0.25-6; S: 0.5,5; I:*
Paramethasone acetate (Haldrone)	10	0	4-6	T: 1,2
Betamethasone (Celestone)	30	0	0.6-3	T: 0.6; S: 0.6; I:*
For oral inhalation				
Beclomethasone dipropionate (Beclovent, Vanceril)				A: 0.042
Dexamethasone sodium phosphate (Decadron)				A: 0.084
Flunisolide (AeroBid)				A: 0.250
Triamcinolone acetonide (Azmacort)				A: 0.100
For nasal inhalation				
Beclomethasone diproprionate (Beconase, Vancenase)				A: 0.042
Dexamethasone sodium phosphate (Decadron)				A: 0.084
Flunisolide (Nasalide)				A: 0.025
Mineralocorticoids				
Fludrocortisone acetate (Florinef)	12	100	0.1	T: 0.1
Aldosterone	0.2	250		

A, Aerosol or spray (approximate dose per actuation); *I*, injection (per milliliter); *P*, pellets for subcutaneous implantation; *RI*, repository injection (per milliliter); *S*, syrup, elixir, or oral solution (per 5 ml); *T*, tablet.
*Various salts are available for injection by various routes.

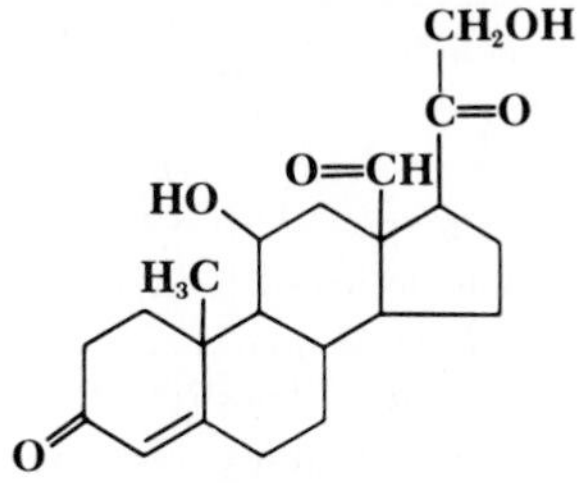

Aldosterone 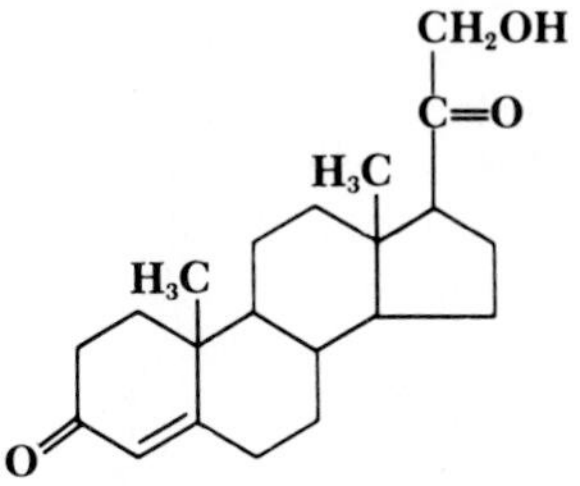 **Desoxycorticosterone**

Although aldosterone can affect carbohydrate metabolism, its salt-retaining potency is so great and its concentration in blood is so low in relation to hydrocortisone that it has no effect on carbohydrate metabolism in physiologic concentrations. Release of aldosterone is regulated mainly by three factors: ACTH, the renin-angiotensin system, and the plasma concentration of K^+. All three stimulate zona glomerulosa cells to synthesize aldosterone. A reduction in blood pressure or extracellular fluid volume is sensed by the kidney and promotes release of renin (see Chapter 21). Renin causes synthesis of angiotensin and, in turn, aldosterone release. By enhancing retention of Na^+ and water, aldosterone may then indirectly feed back to suppress renin release.

Aldosterone production is increased in either "primary" or "secondary" hyperaldosteronism. The former may be caused by adenoma or hyperplasia of the adrenal glands. Secondary hyperaldosteronism occurs with renal artery constriction, malignant hypertension, pregnancy and toxemia of pregnancy, cirrhosis of the liver, nephrotic edema, and, in some patients, congestive heart failure.

ALDOSTERONE ANTAGONIST

Spironolactone (Aldactone, Alatone) antagonizes aldosterone at the level of the renal tubules (see Chapter 42). Spironolactone is a synthetic steroid that competes with aldosterone for its receptor in the distal tubule and collecting duct. By blocking the action of aldosterone, it increases Na^+ excretion and diminishes K^+ secretion.

Desoxycorticosterone and fludrocortisone

Desoxycorticosterone and fludrocortisone are mineralocorticoids with little or no glucocorticoid activity. Their main action is exerted on the renal tubules. Like aldosterone, they increase reabsorption of Na^+ and loss of K^+; these effects are believed responsible for the hypertension and necrotic changes in the heart and skeletal muscle of experimental animals given prolonged, intensive treatment with desoxycorticosterone. Fludrocortisone has replaced desoxycorticosterone in therapeutic usage.

ANDROGENS

In addition to glucocorticoids and aldosterone, the adrenal cortex produces androgenic steroids such as dehydroepiandrosterone. The production of androgenic steroids is greatly increased in the *adrenogenital syndrome* in which an enzymatic defect channels much of the adrenal steroid production toward androgens. Glucocorticoid therapy tends to depress the androgen output of the adrenal gland through inhibition at the level of the pituitary gland.

REFERENCES

1. Baxter JD, Forsham PH: Tissue effects of glucocorticoids, *Am J Med* 53:573, 1972.
2. Claman HN: Corticosteroids and lymphoid cells, *N Engl J Med* 287:388, 1972.
3. Fauci AS, Dale DC, Balow JE: Glucocorticosteroid therapy: mechanisms of action and clinical considerations, *Ann Intern Med* 84:304, 1976.
4. Flower RJ, Blackwell GJ: Anti-inflammatory steroids induce biosynthesis of a phospholipase A_2 inhibitor which prevents prostaglandin generation, *Nature* 278:456, 1979.
5. Graber AL, Ney RL, Nicholson WE, et al: Natural history of pituitary-adrenal recovery following long-term suppression with corticosteroids, *J Clin Endocrinol* 25:11, 1965.
6. Helfer EL, Rose LI: Corticosteroids and adrenal suppression: characterizing and avoiding the problem, *Drugs* 38:838, 1989.
7. Hench PS: Introduction: cortisone and ACTH in clinical medicine, *Proc Staff Meet Mayo Clin* 25:474, 1950.
8. Hench PS, Slocumb CH, Barnes AR, et al: The effects of the adrenal cortical hormone 17-hydroxy-11-dehydrocorticosterone (compound E) on the acute phase of rheumatic fever: preliminary report, *Proc Staff Meet Mayo Clin* 24:277, 1949.
9. Reichstein T, von Euw J: Constituents of the adrenal cortex: isolation of substance Q (desoxy-corticosterone) and R with other materials, *Helv Chim Acta* 21:1197, 1938.
10. Rousseau GG: Control of gene expression by glucocorticoid hormones, *Biochem J* 224:1, 1984.
11. Schleimer RP: The mechanisms of antiinflammatory steroid action in allergic diseases, *Annu Rev Pharmacol Toxicol* 25:381, 1985.
12. Truhan AP, Ahmed AR: Corticosteroids: a review with emphasis on complications of prolonged systemic therapy, *Ann Allergy* 62:375, 1989.
13. Weiss MM: Corticosteroids in rheumatoid arthritis, *Semin Arthritis Rheum* 19:9, 1989.

Chapter 48

Sex hormones

GENERAL CONCEPT

Gonadotropins from the anterior pituitary control synthesis and secretion of steroid hormones in specific target cells in the ovaries, testes, and adrenal cortex. Secretion of gonadotropins is, in turn, regulated by hypothalamic centers that communicate with the anterior pituitary via release of Gn-RH (see Chapter 46) and by the concentrations of sex steroids in circulation. FSH (follicle-stimulating hormone) and LH (luteinizing hormone), also known as interstitial cell–stimulating hormone (ICSH) of the testes, are found in the placenta and urine, as well as in the pituitary.

GONADOTROPINS

In the female, FSH and LH act in concert to regulate hormone production during the ovarian cycle and during pregnancy. FSH promotes growth of the ovarian follicle and stimulates secretion of estrogen. LH promotes ovulation and stimulates secretion of progesterone from the corpus luteum after ovulation. Mechanisms that control de novo synthesis of steroid hormones in the ovary are almost exclusively regulated by LH and human chorionic gonadotropin, a hormone with actions similar to LH that is produced by the implanting blastocyst. By activation of protein kinases to phosphorylate regulatory proteins, these gonadotropins facilitate conversion of cholesterol to pregnenolone, and thereby increase synthesis of the sex hormones estradiol and progesterone.

In the male, testosterone secretion and spermatogenesis are also under control of pituitary gonadotropins. FSH secretion in men is controlled by two mechanisms: negative feedback by sex steroids and inhibition by a nonsteroidal factor (inhibin) produced by Sertoli cells in the testes. Both FSH and testosterone act directly on the seminiferous tubular epithelium to promote spermatogenesis. FSH also regulates the number of LH receptors expressed by the Leydig (interstitial) cells and thus indirectly influences LH-stimulated androgen synthesis from cholesterol. Although androgen synthesis involves several enzymatic steps, expression of LH receptors is a crucial control mechanism. The control of LH receptors by the gonadotropin concentration and regulation of LH secretion by testosterone maintain a relatively constant secretion of testosterone.

Puberty

Dramatic physical and functional changes accompany sexual maturation in both males and females. These changes depend primarily on an integrated action of the hypothalamus, the anterior pituitary, and the gonads.[13] Before puberty the low, basal secretion of Gn-RH results in low concentrations of FSH and LH. Pulsatile secretion of Gn-RH governs the functional status of the system, and in both sexes the approach of puberty coincides with an increasing amplitude of Gn-RH pulses. The pituitary responds by secreting sufficient LH and FSH to stimulate gametogenesis. Both sexes experience a growth spurt and development of secondary sexual characteristics in response to rising levels of sex steroids. Cyclic secretion of estrogen and progesterone in the female induces the onset of menstruation, and continued sequential action of both hormones is required for normal menstrual cycles.

Ovarian cycle

Neural signals from the hypothalamus and feedback signaling of ovarian steroids to the hypothalamic-pituitary axis regulate the cyclic formation and secretion of estrogen and progesterone in a precisely timed manner.

Gonadotropin secretion is both tonic and cyclic. Tonic or basal secretion is regulated by inhibitory mechanisms, such as changes in circulating sex steroids. Cyclic secretion involves stimulatory feedback mechanisms. For example, elevation of circulating estrogens to a critical concentration initiates a synchronous, pulsatile burst of LH and FSH secretion during the ovarian cycle.[13]

The ovarian cycle in the mature female reflects changes in gonadotropins, in steroid synthesis, and in the histology of the ovaries and endometrium. The underlying mechanism that coordinates these events is the acquisition of specific hormone receptors that enable cells to respond to the circulating hormones. The traditional schema for these changes is shown in Fig. 48-1, whereas the actual measurements of serum hormone concentrations are depicted in Fig. 48-2.

FIG. 48-1 *Hormonal control of menstruation.*

From Riley GM: Gynecologic endocrinology, New York, 1959, Harper & Row, Publishers, Inc.

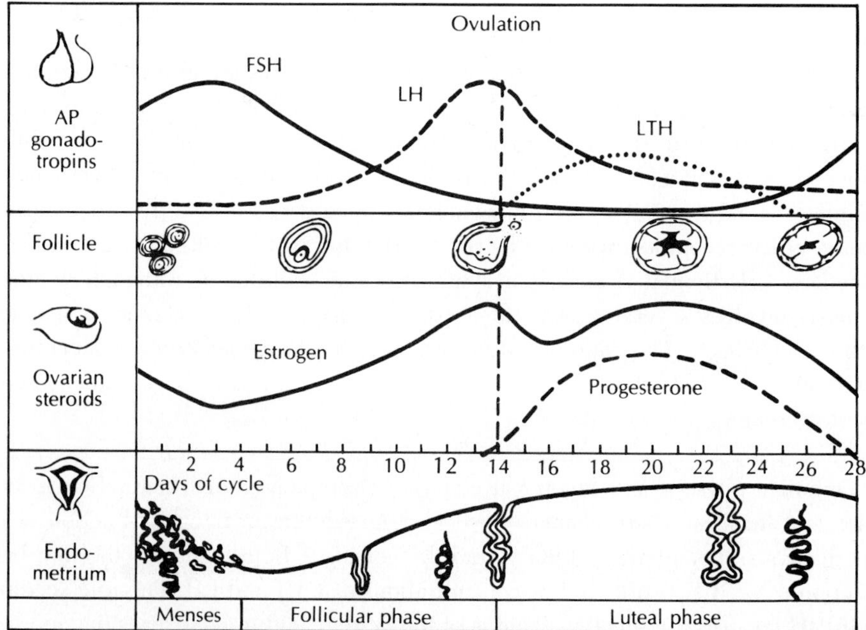

Follicular phase. Release of FSH and LH in the early (follicular) phase of the cycle is believed responsible for the growth and development of ovarian follicles. Maturation of the oocyte then influences hormone synthesis within the ovary. The follicle contains two major populations of endocrine cells, granulosa and thecal (interstitial) cells. FSH initially induces differentiation and proliferation of the granulosa cells and induces an aromatizing enzyme that converts androgens to estradiol. It also induces ovarian receptors for LH, a mechanism that is essential for ovulation.

Ovulation. Episodic or pulsatile release of LH is characteristic of the adult pattern

Serum concentrations of progesterone plotted against mean concentrations of FSH and LH determined in normal women. Centered according to day of LH peak (day 0). *FIG. 48-2*

From Yen SSC, Vela P, Rankin J, Littell, AS: JAMA 211:1513, 1970.

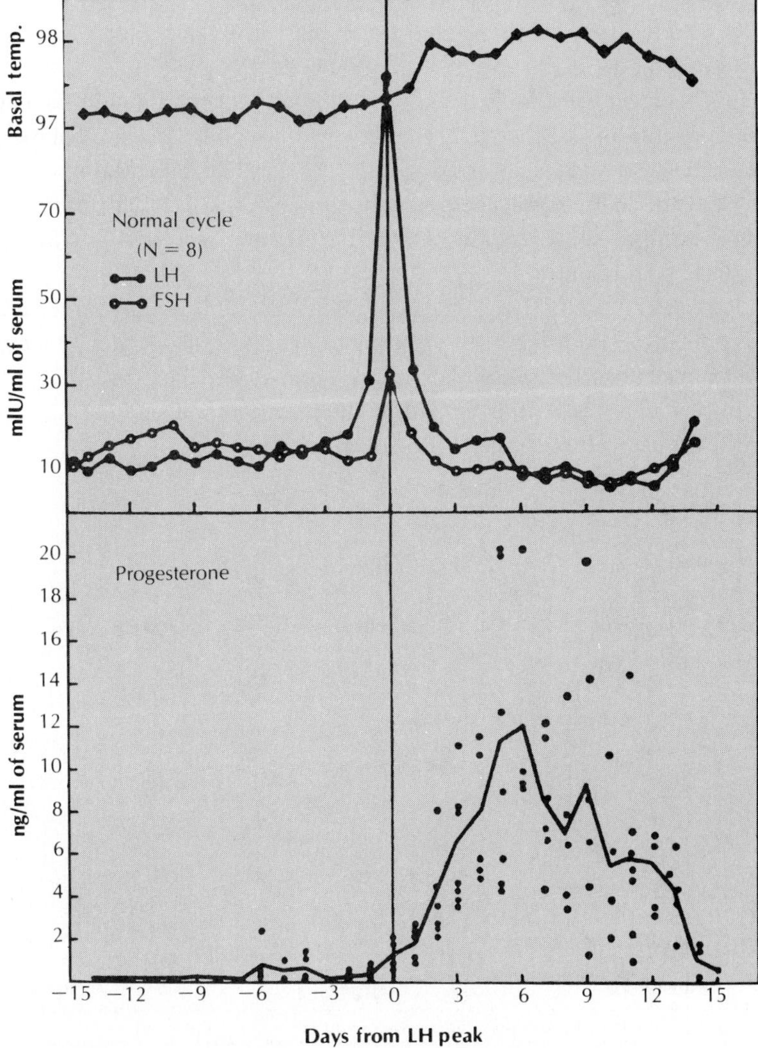

of gonadotropin secretion. The simultaneous increase (midcycle surge) in LH and FSH necessary for ovulation requires positive feedback of increased estrogen during the latter part of the follicular phase. Estrogen influences gonadotropin-secreting cells of the pituitary, which are also exposed to Gn-RH. The granulosa cells in the mature follicle, bearing a large number of LH receptors, are now primed to respond to the LH surge by secreting progesterone. Although the molecular mechanisms of LH-induced ovulation are still unclear, increased synthesis of progesterone is important. Prostaglandin production may promote release or activation of hydrolytic enzymes required for expulsion of the developed oocyte.

Luteal phase. After ovulation the ovarian follicle undergoes significant changes, and progesterone synthesized from the corpus luteum dominates in the latter part of the cycle. Although progesterone secretion begins before ovulation, the rising concentration of LH at ovulation greatly enhances progesterone synthesis. Despite the limited life-span of the corpus luteum, if pregnancy occurs, LH-like activity remains high. HCG secreted from the implanted trophoblast maintains a high rate of progesterone synthesis by the ovary until placentation occurs.

Menses. The decline of estrogen and progesterone concentrations at the end of the luteal phase results in degenerative changes in the spiral arteries that supply the endometrium. These vessels undergo spasm, possibly attributable to prostaglandin formation, and the subsequent necrosis and desquamation cause menstruation. The decreased circulating concentration of estrogen permits secretion of FSH, and the follicular phase begins anew.

Biosynthesis of steroids

One action of gonadotropins is to promote synthesis of enzymes that catalyze various steps in synthesis of steroid hormones. Androstenedione, the common precursor of androgens and estrogens, is formed by the same mechanism in testis, ovary, and adrenal cortex. The synthetic schema is shown below:

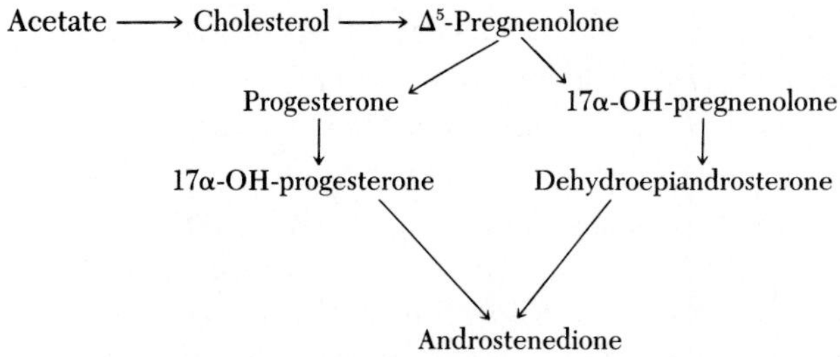

Acetate ⟶ Cholesterol ⟶ Δ^5-Pregnenolone

Progesterone | 17α-OH-pregnenolone

17α-OH-progesterone | Dehydroepiandrosterone

Androstenedione

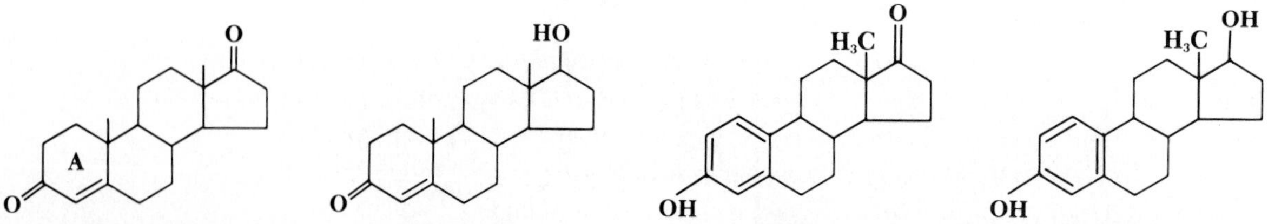

O, A, O — **Androstenedione**

HO, O — **Testosterone**

O, H_3C, OH — **Estrone**

OH, H_3C, OH — **Estradiol**

Clinical use

Gonadotropins can be used therapeutically to induce ovulation in women with ovarian failure. Extracts (menotropins) prepared from urine of menopausal women are highly effective. These extracts contain large amounts of both FSH and LH, and continued therapy results in ovarian enlargement, often with multiple follicles. Multiple births may occur in as many as 20% of patients treated with menotropins.

Human chorionic gonadotropin (HCG) is a glycoprotein extracted from the urine of pregnant women. It has some structural homology with LH, but it has slight FSH activity in addition to its LH-like activity. HCG stimulates androgen production in testes and progesterone production by ovaries. It is used to replace LH in prepubertal cryptorchism, hypogonadotropic hypogonadism, and failure of ovulation.

A synthetic analog of Gn-RH, nafarelin acetate (Synarel), may be used to treat endometriosis. Continuous (nonpulsatile) administration of this analog, after a transient increase in FSH and LH, suppresses gonadotropin production and thus estrogen production.[10]

ESTROGENS

Chemistry

Estrogens are formed from the androgenic precursors androstenedione and testosterone. Androstenedione is converted by the ovary to testosterone, which is then aromatized and demethylated to estrogens. Aromatization of the A ring of the steroid is required for estrogenic activity. If this reaction is defective, circulating androgenic precursors can cause virilization.

The major product of the ovary and the most potent estrogen is estradiol-17β. This compound is also synthesized by the placenta. A less potent estrogenic compound, estrone, may be formed directly from androstenedione in adipose tissue and other extragonadal sites or from oxidation of estradiol by the liver. Estriol, a metabolite of estrone, also has limited estrogenic activity. All three of these estrogens are excreted in urine as glucuronides and sulfates.

Actions

Estrogens are the growth hormones of reproductive tissues in the female. In addition, they share some actions of androgens on the skeleton and other tissues. The ovarian steroids, like androgens and glucocorticoids, control the timing and magnitude of gene expression in responsive tissues. These changes in gene expression, in turn, result in specific physiologic changes. For example, increased estrogen synthesis at puberty acts in concert with androgens and progesterone to establish the changes of puberty: the molding of body contours caused by redistribution of fat, growth of breast tissue, growth and shaping of the skeleton, and maturation of the sexual organs. Estrogen is the dominant hormone both in the earliest part of reproductive life and at the approach of menopause.

In the early part of the ovarian cycle (follicular or proliferative phase) estrogen stimulates protein synthesis in uterine tissues to increase the myometrial mass and vascularity. There is a simultaneous increase in contractile activity of both the uterus and the fallopian tubes. This proliferative phase is dedicated to rebuilding the endometrium that was sloughed during the previous menstrual period.

In the breast, estrogens stimulate proliferation of ductal epithelium and fibrous stroma. They promote elasticity of the skin by an effect on connective tissues, and they enhance deposition of calcium in bone. Like androgens, they are anabolic agents, and they stimulate rapid skeletal growth at puberty. Similarly, estrogens can promote closure of the epiphyses, but they are less potent than androgens.

Estrogen receptors. The actions of estrogens on target tissues are mediated through specific tissue receptors. High concentrations of estrogen-binding protein are found in the uterus, vagina, and mammary glands, but estrogen receptors are also found in many other tissues. These receptors, like those for androgens and glucocorticoids, belong to a superfamily of proteins, all of which are regulators of gene transcription. As shown in Fig. 48-3, steroids from the circulation diffuse into the cells, but only target cells have the appropriate intranuclear receptors to retain them.

The steroid hormone binds to the receptor and induces a conformational change (activation) that allows the complex to bind with high affinity to nuclear chromatin. Binding of the steroid-receptor complex to a specific nuclear acceptor site alters gene transcription and sometimes posttranslational steps as well.[14]

Although nuclear binding of the complex occurs within a few minutes after the steroid contacts the target cell, changes in amounts of specific gene products are observed only 12 to 24 hours later.

Estrogen receptors are quantified in certain forms of metastatic carcinoma to estimate the patient's response to hormone therapy. Without estrogen receptors, metastases will not respond to treatment with an estrogen antagonist such as tamoxifen. Approximately 60% of patients with metastatic breast cancer have tumors that

FIG. 48-3 *Radioactive estradiol injected into a female rat is retained by estrogen-responsive target tissue (uterus) but is rapidly lost by nontarget tissues (blood, spleen). Such results indicate that the target tissue contains estrogen receptors.*

From Harrison RW III, Lippman SS: Hosp Pract 24(9):63-76, 1989. Illustration by Albert Miller. Modified with permission.

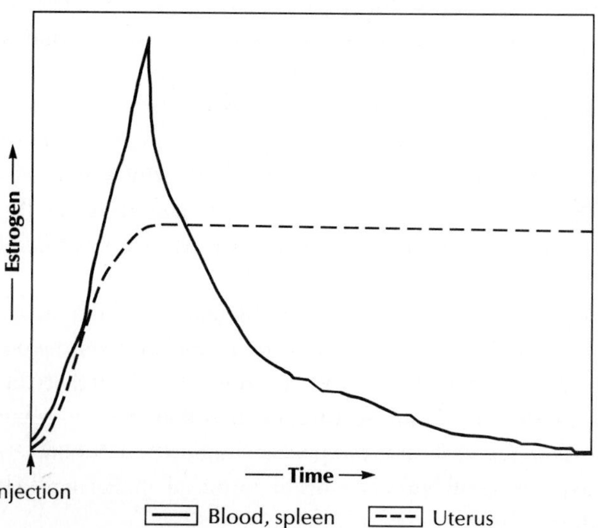

express estrogen receptors. Tamoxifen competes with estrogens for nuclear binding receptors and prevents estrogen-induced growth of the tumor. This therapy is beneficial in approximately 30% of patients with hormone-dependent tumors.[6] Tamoxifen citrate (Nolvadex) is marketed as tablets, 10 mg.

Metabolism

The naturally occurring estrogens, estradiol and estrone, are rapidly inactivated by the liver and are not effective orally. Semisynthetic and totally synthetic estrogens are less readily metabolized and can be taken by mouth. The attachment of an ethinyl group at the 17α position of estradiol (ethinyl estradiol) slows hepatic metabolism and produces a derivative highly effective for oral administration.

Therapeutic uses

All estrogenic compounds elicit the same responses, even though not all are steroids. The choice of an estrogenic agent depends on its convenience and cost.

The most prevalent use of estrogens is in combination with progestins in oral contraceptive preparations. The constant concentrations of circulating hormones suppresses basal secretion of FSH and LH and also the midcycle surge of LH just before ovulation. As a consequence, follicle maturation is retarded and the stimulus for ovulation is suppressed. Estrogens are also used in combination with progestins to treat menstrual disorders. Endometriosis often responds favorably to combined steroid therapy, and there is regression of tissues that are stimulated by naturally cycling hormones.

Estrogens are used as replacement therapy in ovarian failure or at menopause to prevent osteoporosis and to relieve symptoms of estrogen deficiency.[2] When estrogen secretion decreases at menopause, estrogen-responsive target tissues atrophy, causing a variety of symptoms including vasomotor instability ("hot flashes"), drying and atrophy of the vaginal mucosa, insomnia, irritability, and other mood changes. As ovarian function declines with age, androstenedione from the adrenal cortex becomes the primary source of estrogen, in the form of estrone. Because the naturally occurring concentration of androstenedione and the efficiency of its conversion may vary considerably among persons, estrogen replacement therapy is frequently provided to ease the transition into menopause.

Estrogens are commonly used to prevent or treat osteoporosis, a reduction of bone mass with resultant fragility and risk of fracture. There is, however, still some controversy about the ultimate benefits of estrogen therapy and how long it should be continued. In a double-blind study of oophorectomized women, estrogen prevented bone loss during a year of continuous therapy.[15] Estrogen is also effective in retarding bone loss in menopausal women. However, the studies up to now indicate that estrogen is effective only with continued administration; cessation of therapy results in accelerated bone loss. Estrogen is believed to retard bone resorption by influencing the action of parathyroid hormone, possibly through calcitonin (see Chapter 51), but it does not reverse bone loss once osteoporosis is established.[15]

Estrogens are used as androgen antagonists in certain androgen-sensitive cancers. The doses required are much higher than those needed for hormone replacement, and adverse effects are limiting.

Adverse effects of estrogen therapy

All compounds with estrogenic activity have virtually the same side effects and risks. Preparations differ in their duration of action and route of administration. Side effects are usually minimal but can decrease patient acceptance. Nausea is the most prominent. Other undesirable effects include fluid retention and breast tenderness. The severity of the symptoms, which usually subside with continued use, is related to the potency of the compound used.

Several recent studies indicate an increase in the relative risk for endometrial or breast cancer in women who take estrogens as hormone replacement.[1,12] However, addition of progestins to the therapeutic regimen essentially eliminates the risk of estrogen-induced neoplasia.[15] Other serious risks of estrogen therapy include an increased tendency toward thromboembolic disease, and there is a link to hypertension in a small number of persons. Interestingly, women who undergo early menopause or loss of ovulatory function have an increased incidence of cardiovascular disease.

Contraindications to estrogen therapy include estrogen-dependent neoplasia, prior or active thromboembolic disease, coronary or cerebral arterial disease, active liver disease, or severe liver damage. Relative contraindications include hypertension, fibrocystic breast disease, cholecystitis, uterine leiomyoma, and familial hyperlipoproteinemia. Diethylstilbestrol is absolutely contraindicated in pregnancy because maternal therapy with this compound is associated with later development of adenocarcinoma in the offspring.

Specific agents

Estradiol-17β can be administered in a variety of forms (Table 48-1), including a polyester form (Estradurin) that is injected intramuscularly for therapy of prostatic carcinoma. A transdermal form (Estraderm) is used to treat postmenopausal symptoms. Advantages of this preparation, which is applied in a skin patch, is that estradiol is absorbed directly into the circulation, avoiding first-pass hepatic metabolism and effects on hepatic enzymes, and plasma concentrations more closely resemble those found before menopause.[19]

Conjugated estrogens are a mixture of estrone sulfate and equine estrogens (equilin sulfate) derived from the urine of pregnant mares. They are water soluble and can be taken orally. **Esterified estrogens** are similar to conjugated estrogens.

Ethinyl estradiol, a semisynthetic compound, is the most potent estrogen available. Ethinyl estradiol and its 3-methyl ether derivative, **mestranol**, are commonly used in oral contraceptive combinations. Mestranol is metabolized to ethinyl estradiol.

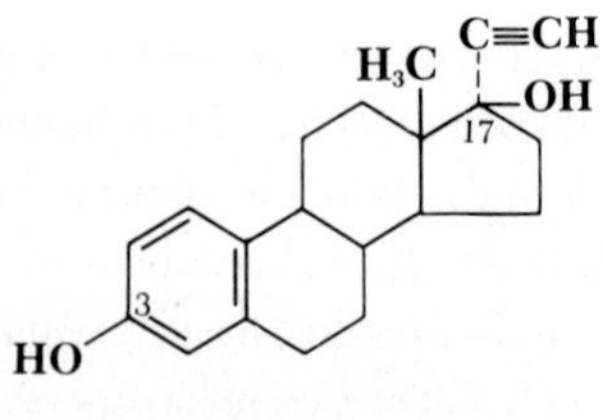

H_3C C≡CH OH 17 3 HO

Ethinyl estradiol

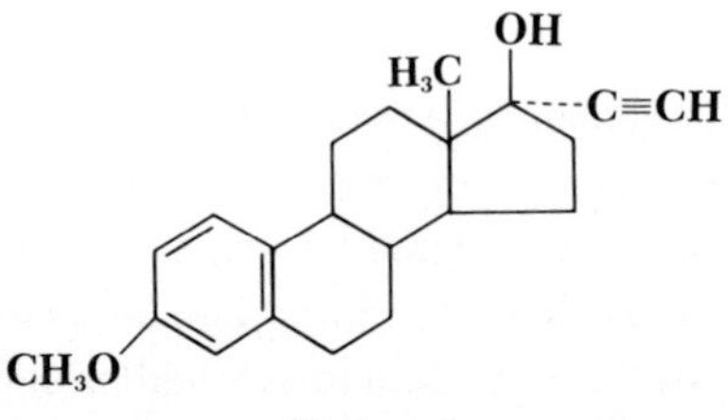

OH H_3C C≡CH CH_3O

Mestranol

TABLE 48-1 Estrogen preparations

Preparation	Dosage forms (mg)
Estradiol (Estrace)	T: 1,2; V: 0.1/g of cream
Polyestradiol phosphate (Estradurin)	I: 40 as powder
Estradiol cypionate (Depogen, others)	I: 1,5/ml
Estradiol valerate (Delestrogen, others)	I: 10-40/ml
Conjugated estrogens (Premarin)	T: 0.3-2.5; V: 0.625/g of cream
Esterified estrogens (Menest, Estratab)	T: 0.3-2.5
Ethinyl estradiol (Estinyl, Feminone)	T: 0.02-0.5
Diethylstilbestrol	T: 1-5
Diethylstilbestrol diphosphate (Stilphostrol)	I: 250/5 ml; T: 50
Chlorotrianisene (Tace)	C: 12-72
Dienestrol (DV)	V: 0.01%
Estrone (Kestrone, others)	I: 2,5/ml
Estropipate (Ogen)	T: 0.75-6; V: 1.5/g of cream
Quinestrol (Estrovis)	T: 0.1

C, Capsules; *I*, injection; *T*, tablets; *V*, vaginal cream.

Diethylstilbestrol is a potent nonsteroidal compound with estrogenic actions. It is active on oral administration and is also available for intravenous injection.

Chlorotrianisene has a very long duration of action, probably because it is stored in fat. It is an inactive compound that is metabolized to an active estrogen.

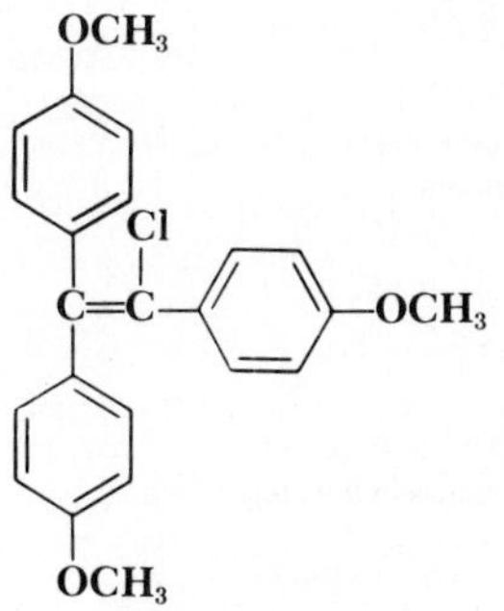

Chlorotrianisene

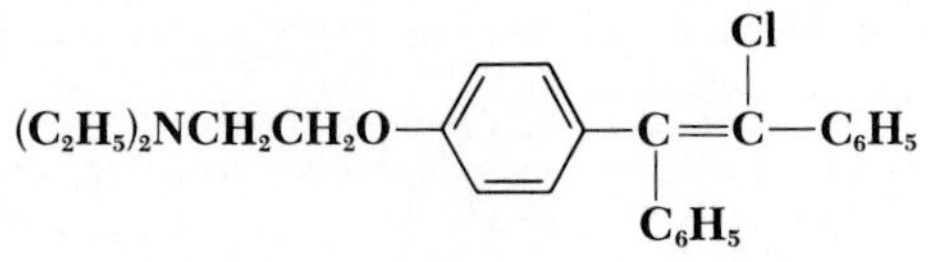

Clomiphene

Clomiphene citrate (Clomid, Serophene) is structurally related to chlorotrianisene but has an antiestrogenic action. It blocks the negative feedback action of estrogen at the level of the hypothalamus and thus promotes pituitary gonadotropin secretion. It has been used to induce ovulation in women who are infertile because they fail to ovulate. A high incidence of multiple births accompanies the use of clomiphene. It can also cause adverse effects related to estrogen blockade, including hot flashes, enlargement of the ovaries, and atrophy of vaginal mucosal cells. The recommended initial course is one 50 mg tablet each day for 5 days.

PROGESTINS

Progesterone is formed from steroid precursors in the ovary, testis, placenta, and adrenal cortex. It is the hormone produced in the corpus luteum that stimulates development of a secretory endometrium in the latter part of the ovarian cycle. Progesterone is essential for maintenance of pregnancy, and once implantation and placentation occur, the luteal function is assumed by the placenta.

Semisynthetic derivatives, *progestins*, are used in oral contraceptives and as replacement for the naturally occurring hormone in conditions of ovarian failure or dysfunction.

Chemistry

The synthetic oral progestins are derivatives of testosterone. Removal of the 19-methyl group of testosterone greatly reduces its androgenic properties and unmasks progestational activity. Acetylation at the 17α position also conveys progestational activity and produces compounds that are less rapidly metabolized by the liver. Acetylation at the 17β position further enhances progestational activity. These orally active progestins are 19-norsteroids; they are primarily used in oral contraceptive preparations. Some chemical modifications are shown in Fig. 48-4.

FIG. 48-4 *Chemical structures of important progestins related to testosterone and 19-nortestosterone that are used as progestational agents.* Arrows, *Points where the basic norethindrone structure has been modified to produce new compounds.*

From Batzer FR: J Reprod Med 29(suppl):503, 1984; adapted with permission from Edgren RA: Progestagens. In Given JR, editor: Clinical use of sex steroids. Chicago, copyright 1980, Mosby–Year Book, Inc.

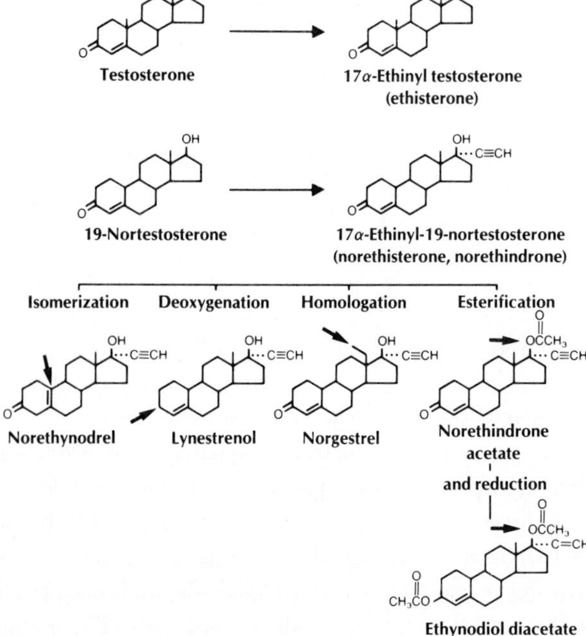

Actions

Progesterone and progestins act on specific receptors in estrogen-primed target tissues. Their effects are generally opposite to those of estrogens. They decrease myometrial contractions, increase glandular development of the breast and endometrium, and promote secretion of a viscous mucus from cervical glands. Priming with estrogen is essential for development of an adequate secretory endometrium.

Progestins, like estrogens, inhibit LH secretion through a negative feedback on the hypothalamic-anterior pituitary axis. This is one way by which these synthetic hormones prevent conception. However, other activities may be equally important for contraception. First, alteration of cervical mucus from a watery, nonviscous secretion to a viscous, cellular secretion physically blocks sperm penetration. In addition, progestational stimulation early in the ovarian cycle causes premature development of endometrial glands and endometrial involution. The estrogen component of the preparation stimulates stromal development, and the resulting endometrium is unsuitable for implantation.

Use

Progestins are primarily used in oral contraceptive formulations, and they are administered along with estrogens for treatment of menopausal symptoms. In most oral contraceptive combinations, progestins are combined with a semisynthetic estrogen. Some compounds can be used alone, but oral contraceptives containing only a progestin have a higher failure rate and may cause irregular bleeding. Progestins are also used to treat menstrual dysfunction, such as irregular cycles, protracted uterine bleeding, dysmenorrhea, amenorrhea, and endometriosis. Poorly cycling estrogens are believed to promote hypertrophy of the endometrium. The addition of a progestin can help repair the necrotic endometrium, which permits natural shedding once the hormone is withdrawn. Progestins alone will not cause menstrual bleeding, but in patients who have endogenous estrogen or are treated first with estrogen, the cyclic treatment with progestin will help restore normal cycling.

Androgenic actions of some progestins are useful in other diseases. For example, megestrol acetate (Megace) is used to treat hormone-sensitive breast cancer, and in a limited study it improved appetite and stimulated weight gain in 14 patients with AIDS-induced cachexia.[21] The compound is available in tablets, 20 and 40 mg.

Adverse effects

Many minor side effects associated with use of oral contraceptives or progestational agents are similar to symptoms associated with pregnancy. Effects generally attributed to the progestational component include weight gain, depression, fatigue, acne, and hirsutism. These are probably due to its androgenic action, and, in contrast to the nausea caused by estrogens, the symptoms do not usually subside with continued use. One of the more annoying side effects attributable to progestins is development of candidiasis due to changes in the vaginal environment.

Although reports of increased risk of neoplasia in long-term progestin users continue to appear, there is no convincing evidence linking these hormones to cancer. In fact, oral contraceptives appear to prevent some forms of cancer. A review of this issue[17] indicated that blockade of ovulation by pregnancy, lactation, or hormonal suppression may protect against endometrial and ovarian cancer. The case for cervical cancer is, however, less clear.

Oral contraceptive preparations, as well as individual hormones, can affect measurements of plasma lipids, but there is, as yet, no clear link between these drugs and atherosclerotic disease. In fact, a prospective study of more than 100,000 subjects between 30 and 55 years of age revealed no evidence of increased risk of cardiovascular diseases among oral contraceptive users.[16]

Specific agents

There are many compounds with progestational activity. Semisynthetic derivatives of progesterone include **medroxyprogesterone** (Depo-Provera, 100 and 400 mg/ml) and **hydroxyprogesterone caproate** (Delalutin, others; 125 and 250 mg/ml). These have little estrogenic or androgenic activity and can be injected intramuscularly in depot form. Medroxyprogesterone acetate (Provera, others) is available in tablets, 2.5 to 10 mg.

The 19-norsteroids have slight estrogenic potency, probably because of metabolism to estrogenic compounds. Some also have androgenic actions. The most commonly used agents are those included in oral contraceptives: **ethynodiol diacetate**, **norethindrone**, **norethynodrel**, **norgestrel**, and **levonorgestrel**. Table 48-2 gives the composition of some oral contraceptives.

At least one preparation (Ovral) has been used to prevent pregnancy following unprotected intercourse. This combination (50 μg of ethinyl estradiol and 0.5 mg of norgestrel) was effective for postcoital prevention of pregnancy if given within 72 hours.[11]

Progesterone antagonists

Because continued exposure to progesterone is required to maintain pregnancy, antagonism of progesterone receptors early in pregnancy can cause abortion. Mifepris-

TABLE 48-2 Formulations of combined oral contraceptives containing less than 50 μg of estrogen, by brand

	Estrogen (μg)	Progesterone (mg)
Ortho-Novum 1/35	Ethinyl estradiol, 35	Norethindrone, 1.0
Norinyl 1+35		Norethindrone, 1.0
Demulen 1/35		Ethynodiol diacetate, 1.0
Brevicon		Norethindrone, 0.5
Modicon		Norethindrone, 0.5
Ovcon-35		Norethindrone, 0.4
Ortho-Novum 10/11		Norethindrone, 0.5/1.0
Ortho-Novum 7/7/7		Norethindrone, 0.5/0.75/1.0
Tri-Norinyl		Norethindrone, 0.5/1.0/0.5
Nordette	Ethinyl estradiol, 30	Levonorgestrel, 0.15
Loestrin 21 1.5/30		Norethindrone acetate, 1.5
Lo-Ovral		Norgestrel, 0.3 (0.15 D-norgestrel)
Loestrin 21 1/20	Ethinyl estradiol, 20	Norethindrone, 1.0

Modified from Batzer FR: *J Reprod Med* 29 (suppl):503, 1984.

tone, also known as RU 486, is an antagonist at progesterone and glucocorticoid receptors. It is used in France and other countries to terminate early pregnancy but has not been approved in the United States. In a recent study, a single dose of RU 486 combined with prostaglandin terminated pregnancy in 96% of the cases treated.[20]

Another drug, epostane, terminates pregnancy through an effect on progesterone synthesis. Conversion of pregnenolone to progesterone requires 3β-hydroxysteroid dehydrogenase; inhibition of this enzyme results in termination of pregnancy. In a clinical trial orally administered epostane, an inhibitor of the enzyme, terminated early pregnancy in 84% of subjects.[3]

ANDROGENS

The principle androgen of the testes, testosterone, is formed in the Leydig (interstitial) cells under control of a highly integrated system involving the hypothalamus and pituitary. Release of LH dictated by Gn-RH (see Chapter 46) and subsequent binding of LH by Leydig cell receptors is the first step in androgen production. Interaction of LH with its receptor triggers a cascade of events that increase testosterone synthesis. The process appears to be regulated, in part, by the number of LH receptors expressed on the Leydig cells. Exposure to high levels of androgen reduces the number of receptors and downregulates further androgen production.

Testosterone is not stored in the Leydig cells but is continually synthesized and released into the circulation, where it is complexed with a specific β-globulin. Testosterone is also synthesized in the ovaries and adrenal cortex, but plasma testosterone concentrations in males are approximately 10 times higher than those in females.

Chemistry

Testosterone, formed from pregnenolone, is the precursor of both estradiol and the 5α reduced androgen dihydrotestosterone. De novo synthesis of cholesterol from acetate in the Leydig cells or uptake of plasma cholesterol provides the substrate for steroidogenesis. Dihydrotestosterone is more potent than testosterone and mediates most of the androgenic effects attributed to testosterone. Orally effective derivatives of testosterone include methyltestosterone, fluoxymesterone, and methandrostenolone.

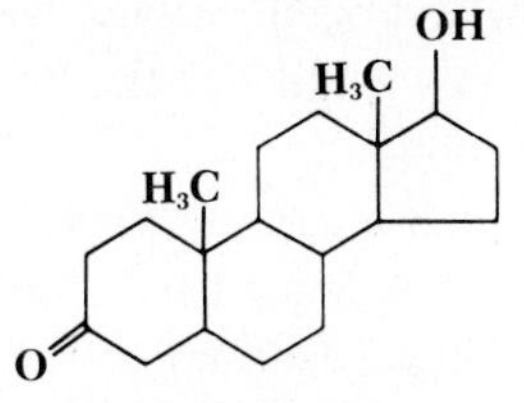

OH H_3C H_3C O

Dihydrotestosterone

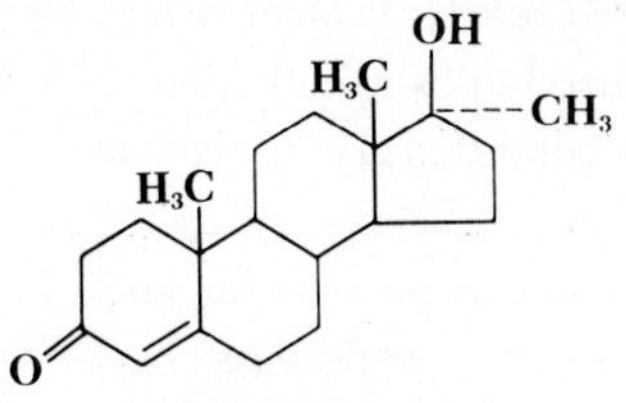

OH H_3C CH_3 H_3C O

Methyltestosterone

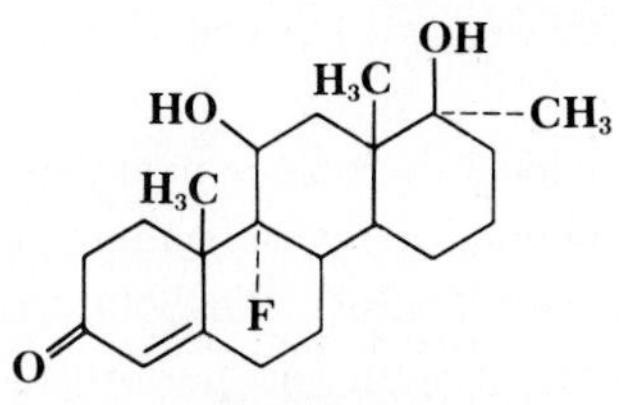

OH HO H_3C CH_3 H_3C F O

Fluoxymesterone

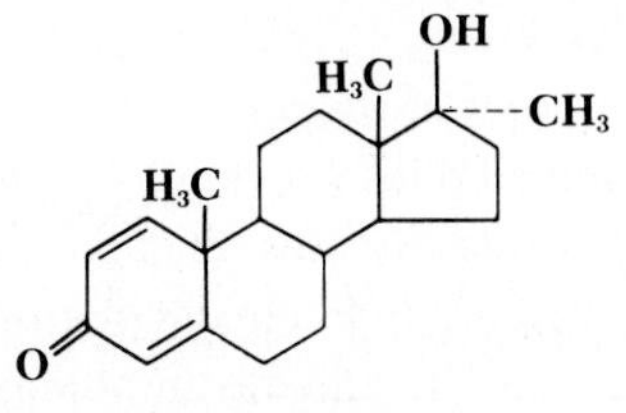

OH H_3C CH_3 H_3C O

Methandrostenolone

Testosterone is metabolized in the liver, and the metabolites, androsterone and etiocholanolone, are excreted in the urine. 17-Methyl—substituted compounds such as methyltestosterone and fluoxymesterone are not readily inactivated by the liver and are effective orally. Esters of testosterone, such as the propionate, must be administered parenterally and are slowly absorbed.

Actions

Androgenic steroids can affect all tissues. Testosterone exerts its hormonal actions through a sequence of events similar to those described for other steroid hormones. After attachment to a specific receptor, the receptor-hormone complex binds to chromatin in the nucleus and initiates a series of transcriptional and post-transcriptional events, resulting in synthesis of specific proteins.

Feminization can occur in males who lack androgen receptors, despite a high concentration of circulating testosterone. This occurs because the testosterone provides sufficient estradiol to result in a female phenotype.

Testosterone and active derivatives have basically two general actions: androgenic and anabolic. All natural and synthetic androgens have both types of activity to some degree. The androgenic actions are responsible for changes associated with sexual maturation and for stimulation of spermatogenesis. Early in embryonic life, androgens promote development of the male phenotype. They are also responsible for the growth spurt at puberty and for the increase in muscle mass that accompanies maturation of the male. In addition, androgens stimulate growth and secretion of sebaceous glands and growth of facial hair.

A recent study reported the effects of chronic androgen treatment in normal males. When 51 normal men were treated with testosterone enanthate weekly for 6 months, their concentrations of serum LH and FSH were reduced and sperm production was suppressed; otherwise they suffered no major adverse effects.[8]

The anabolic steroids that cause nitrogen retention and enhance protein synthesis are of particular interest. It has not been possible to dissociate completely the anabolic and androgenic actions, but some steroids, such as nandrolone, have a greater action on nitrogen retention than would be predicted by androgenic assays. Nandrolone was recently used to treat osteoporotic bone loss in women; although the steroid increased vertebral bone density, it also caused masculinization.[9]

Use

The major indication for androgen therapy is deficiency because of testicular or pituitary failure. Androgens have been used in hypogonadism in the male and in certain types of infertility with some degree of success. Testosterone propionate is also used as an estrogen antagonist in estrogen-sensitive tumors, such as metastatic carcinoma of the breast. Its virilizing action, however, makes this hormone less acceptable than other types of therapy.

Anabolic steroids are used in conditions in which there is a negative nitrogen balance: wasting diseases, malnutrition, severe anemia, or severe trauma. They also have a limited use in treatment of growth deficits or osteoporosis. Anabolic steroids are widely misused by athletes in attempts to improve strength and performance or by body builders who want to increase muscle weight. Such misuse can result in hepatic abnormalities, an elevated concentration of LDL, and coronary artery disease.[5] In some individuals, misuse produces psychotic and sociopathic symptoms.[7] A syndrome of "addiction" with features of opioid dependence was described in one individual who took large doses of anabolic steroids over a period of three years.[18]

Androgen antagonists are sometimes used to treat hormone-sensitive tumors. For example, flutamide (Eulexin) is used to treat metastatic prostatic cancer.[4] Side effects include gynecomastia, nausea, and sometimes hepatitis.

Adverse effects

Androgen use in the female can cause virilization, acne, and symptoms of estrogen deficiency. Androgen administration to the immature male can cause precocious puberty and all the structural changes of the mature male phenotype. Premature closure of long-bone epiphyses may occur in children who receive androgens. Retention of water and Na^+ can worsen hypertension in athletes who misuse anabolic steroids, and cholestatic jaundice has occurred in patients treated with compounds containing a 17α-alkyl substitution. In addition, androgenic actions may worsen hormone-sensitive neoplasms, such as carcinoma of the prostate.

Specific agents

Testosterone (Table 48-3) is used for correction of male hypogonadism and for palliative treatment of breast carcinoma. It is administered by intramuscular injection. **Methyltestosterone** is quite similar but is also administered as regular or buccal tablets.

Fluoxymesterone is a synthetic halogenated derivative of methyltestosterone. It is more potent with respect to both androgenic and anabolic actions. It is used for androgen replacement and for its nitrogen-retaining effect.

Nandrolone has greater anabolic than androgenic activity and is used when nitrogen retention is desirable.

TABLE 48-3 Androgen preparations

Preparation	Dosage forms (mg)
Testosterone (Histerone, others)	I: 25-100/ml
Testosterone cypionate (Duratest, others)	I: 50-200/ml
Testosterone enanthate (Everone, others)	I: 100,200/ml
Testosterone proprionate (Testex)	I: 25-100/ml
Methyltestosterone (Oreton Methyl, others)	BT: 5,10; C: 10; T: 10,25
Fluoxymesterone (Halotestin, others)	T: 2-10
Nandrolone phenpropionate (Durabolin, others)	I: 25,50/ml
Nandrolone decanoate (Neo-Durabolic, others)	I: 50-200/ml
Ethylestrenol (Maxibolin)	E: 2/5 ml; T: 2
Methandrostenolone	T: 2.5,5
Oxandrolone (Anavar)	T: 2.5
Oxymetholone (Anadrol-50)	T: 50
Stanozolol (Winstrol)	T: 2

BT, Buccal tablet; *E*, elixir; *I*, injection; *T*, tablet.

Nandrolone phenpropionate

REFERENCES

1. Bergkvist L, Adami HO, Persson I, et al: Breast cancer: does hormone replacement increase risk? *N Engl J Med* 321:293, 1989.
2. Carr BR, MacDonald PC: Estrogen treatment of postmenopausal women, *Adv Intern Med* 28:491, 1983.
3. Crooij MJ, de Nooyer CCA, Rao BR, et al: Termination of early pregnancy by the 3β-hydroxysteroid dehydrogenase inhibitor epostane, *N Engl J Med* 319:813, 1988.
4. Flutamide for prostate cancer, *Med Lett Drugs Ther* 31:72, 1989.
5. Holden SC, Calvo RD, Sterling JC: Anabolic steroids in athletics, *Texas Med* 86(3):32, 1990.
6. Legha SS: Tamoxifen in the treatment of breast cancer, *Ann Intern Med* 109:219, 1988.
7. Marshall E: The drug of champions, *Science* 242:183, 1988.
8. Matsumoto AM: Effects of chronic testosterone administration in normal men: safety and efficacy of high dosage testosterone and parallel dose-dependent suppression of luteinizing hormone, follicle-stimulating hormone, and sperm production, *J Clin Endocrinol Metab* 70:282, 1990.
9. Need AG, Horowitz M, Bridges A, et al: Effects of nandrolone decanoate and antiresorptive therapy on vertebral density in osteoporotic postmenopausal women, *Arch Intern Med* 149:57, 1989.
10. Nafarelin for endometriosis, *Med Lett Drugs Ther* 32:81, 1990.
11. *Ovral* as a "morning-after" contraceptive, *Med Lett Drugs Ther* 31:93, 1989.
12. Persson I, Adami H-O, Bergkvist L, et al: Risk of endometrial cancer after treatment with oestrogens alone or in conjunction with progestogens: results of a prospective study, *Br Med J* 298:147, 1989.
13. Reiter EO, Grumbach MM: Neuroendocrine control mechanisms and the onset of puberty, *Annu Rev Physiol* 44:595, 1982.
14. Rories C, Spelsberg TC: Ovarian steroid action on gene expression: mechanisms and models, *Annu Rev Physiol* 51:653, 1989.
15. Ryan KJ: Postmenopausal estrogen use, *Annu Rev Med* 33:171, 1982.
16. Stampfer MJ, Willett WC, Colditz GA, et al: A prospective study of past use of oral contraceptive agents and risk of cardiovascular diseases, *N Engl J Med* 319:1313, 1988.
17. Stubblefield PG: Oral contraceptives and neoplasia, *J Reprod Med* 29(suppl):524, 1984.
18. Tennant F, Black DL, Voy RO: Anabolic steroid dependence with opioid-type features, *N Engl J Med* 319:578, 1988.
19. Transdermal estrogen, *Med Lett Drugs Ther* 28:119, 1986.
20. Ulmann A, Teutsch G, Philibert D: RU 486, *Sci Am* 262(6):42, 1990.
21. Von Roenn JH, Murphy RL, Weber KM, et al: Megestrol acetate for treatment of cachexia associated with human immunodeficiency virus (HIV) infection, *Ann Intern Med* 109:840, 1988.

Chapter 49

Insulin, glucagon, and oral hypoglycemic agents

GENERAL CONCEPT

Insulin, the hormone elaborated by the β cells of the pancreas, is a key regulator of metabolic processes. Insulin stimulates glucose transport and metabolism, enhances glycogen synthesis, and stimulates lipogenesis to promote storage of fuel for energy. It also has important growth-promoting actions in a variety of tissues. Although its action on carbohydrate metabolism has received the most attention, an absolute or relative deficiency of insulin results in other serious metabolic changes. The insulin receptor has been isolated and cloned. *Glucagon*, the hormone produced by the α cells of pancreatic islets, opposes the anabolic effects of insulin by stimulating glycogenolysis and causing hyperglycemia. The ratio of these two hormones thus determines the overall metabolic effect. Control of their release by somatostatin is also an important physiologic mechanism. Orally active *sulfonylurea* compounds, which promote insulin release from β cells and improve peripheral utilization of glucose, are useful only in patients with functional β cells.

INSULIN

Current concepts

Diabetes mellitus is among the most common metabolic diseases. In 1889 surgical removal of the pancreas from dogs was shown to cause diabetes. Approximately 30 years later insulin was isolated from the canine pancreas. In the 1960s, after its amino acid sequence was established, the hormone was synthesized.

The introduction of insulin as replacement therapy in diabetes mellitus revolutionized management of this disease and has greatly prolonged the lives of many diabetic patients. Various techniques have been used to produce forms of the hormone with an extended duration of action, and it recently became possible to produce human insulin through genetic engineering. Finally, with the development of programmable continuous-delivery systems, the normal hormone release in response to meals or exercise can be approximated in highly motivated and compliant patients.

Biosynthesis and release of insulin

Insulin is formed in the β cells of the pancreatic islets as part of a larger protein, *proinsulin* (Fig. 49-1). This precursor, approximately 1.5 times the molecular weight of insulin, is one of a family of peptides that includes the somatomedins or insulin-like growth factors. Proinsulin is processed, within acidified secretory vesicles of the islet cells, to insulin and a C-peptide (connecting peptide).[15] Insulin consists of two polypeptide chains joined by disulfide linkages. It is secreted into the portal system of normal adults at a basal rate of about 1 U/hr; intake of food increases secretion five- to

FIG. 49-1 *Structure of bovine proinsulin showing A and B chains and C-peptide. Human proinsulin differs in three amino acids in the chains and several amino acids in the C-peptide.*

From Steiner DF: TRIANGLE, the Sandoz Journal of Medical Science 2(2):52, 1972.

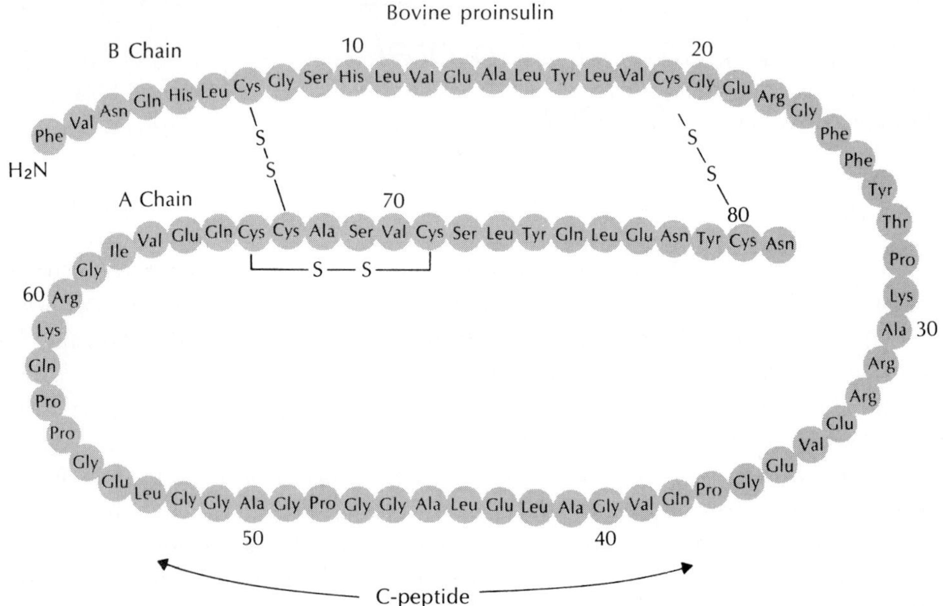

tenfold.[24] Insulin circulates as free hormone, is degraded in the liver and kidneys, and has a half-life of approximately 9 minutes.

Proinsulin is also released to some extent into the circulation. Normally about 6% to 8% of plasma insulin is in the form of this precursor; in some islet adenomas the percentage is higher. The C-peptide released from proinsulin has no biologic activity, but it can be used to assess insulin secretion in persons who may have decreased insulin activity attributable to circulating antibodies.

Regulation of blood glucose

Regulation of blood glucose is a complex process that integrates hormonal and neural mechanisms in the central nervous system, the pancreas, and the autonomic nervous system.[4] Early experimental studies showed that insulin deficiency caused the metabolic derangements in diabetes and that replacement of insulin alleviated the symptoms and changes associated with the disease. Neural stimuli and secretion of counterregulatory hormones influence insulin secretion, as well as target cell response.

Two regions in the hypothalamus regulate glucose production in the liver independently of pancreatic or adrenal hormones. Stimulation of the *ventromedial* hypothalamus rapidly increases glycogenolysis, whereas stimulation of the *ventrolateral* region leads to hepatic glycogenesis; it is believed that the former pathways involve β-adrenergic receptor mechanisms and that the latter pathways are primarily cholinergic.

Neural regulation of insulin secretion from the pancreas is also mediated by both sympathetic and parasympathetic pathways. Islet β cells contain both α- and β-adrenergic, as well as muscarinic, cholinergic receptors. Vagal stimulation and stimulation of β-receptors increase insulin secretion, whereas sympathetic nerve activity and circulating catecholamines inhibit secretion through α-adrenergic receptors.

The primary physiologic stimulus for insulin secretion is glucose, but certain amino acids, gastrointestinal hormones, ketone bodies, α-adrenergic receptor antagonists, and sulfonylureas also enhance insulin release. Inhibitors of insulin release include muscarinic antagonists, α-adrenergic receptor agonists, β-receptor antagonists, and diazoxide.

The α cell is much more sensitive to glucose than the β cell, and a normal concentration of glucose suppresses stimulated glucagon release. As glucose concentration increases, insulin release is stimulated. It has long been proposed that β cells contain a glucose sensor that promotes insulin release. Although this sensor might be a membrane-associated receptor, some investigators propose that glucokinase (ATP-glucose 6-phosphotransferase) serves this function. An extension of this hypothesis is that different, possibly aberrant, isoforms of glucokinase might account for defects in the sensitivity of the β cell to glucose.[14]

Somatostatin, a polypeptide found in the central nervous system, the gastrointestinal tract, and the pancreas, also plays a role in glucoregulation. Its primary effects are inhibition of glucagon and insulin secretion by a paracrine mechanism that involves inhibition of a cyclic AMP-mediated process; however, it also affects glucose absorption from the gut and production by the liver. Somatostatin is synthesized in D cells, which constitute about 10% of the pancreatic islet cells. Excessive production of somatostatin from pancreatic tumors is associated with mild carbohydrate intolerance and relative hypoinsulinemia.[4]

Growth hormone from the anterior pituitary gland (Chapter 46) has complex effects on carbohydrate and lipid metabolism. By promoting lipolysis and utilization of fats rather than carbohydrates as a source of fuel, an excess of growth hormone worsens hyperglycemia and ketosis in diabetic patients.

Insulin receptors

Like other receptors, the insulin receptor serves two functions: recognition and binding and transmission of a signal, which in the case of insulin alters intracellular metabolic pathways. These functions are carried out by a plasma membrane glycoprotein composed of two α subunits and two β subunits that are generated by proteolytic processing of a single-chain proreceptor. This processing is essential for normal functioning of the receptor.[23] Based on its protein sequence, the insulin receptor appears similar to certain other growth factors and viral oncogenes.[10]

Binding of insulin to the α subunits stimulates the tyrosine kinase of the β subunits to cause autophosphorylation of the receptor and conformational changes. Rapid phosphorylation and dephosphorylation of intermediary tyrosine-containing substrates modulate metabolic enzymes within the cell, promote release of secondary mediators of insulin action, and alter gene expression.[11]

Because the insulin receptor plays a crucial role in signal transmission, alterations of its structure could lead to defective insulin action. Some forms of insulin-resistant diabetes are thought to result from genetic defects of the receptor.[20,23] A model of the insulin receptor is shown in Fig. 49-2.

How the insulin-receptor complex mediates the biologic effects of the hormone is still unclear, but it is probably linked to the tyrosine-specific protein kinase of the β subunit. Observations that insulin receptors from adipocytes of non–insulin-dependent diabetic subjects have less tyrosine kinase activity than those of normal subjects support this idea.[3] Tyrosine kinase is also associated with proteins that participate in cell growth.

Another possible mechanism is that insulin-receptor activation generates a second messenger. However, in contrast to glucagon, insulin does not appear to act through formation of cyclic AMP. In fact, insulin may inhibit cyclic AMP-dependent protein kinase.[21]

Actions of insulin

Insulin affects carbohydrate, lipid, and protein metabolism. Effects such as increased glucose transport, phospholipid turnover, and activation of intracellular enzymes occur within minutes of hormone-receptor interaction and are evoked by relatively low concentrations of the hormone. Growth-promoting effects, including enhanced protein, lipid, and nucleotide synthesis, are expressed over hours or days and require higher insulin concentrations. These anabolic effects appear to be particularly important during fetal growth and organogenesis, as well as in tissue repair and regeneration.[10]

When insulin is injected into a normal or diabetic person, it causes several changes in blood chemistry: (1) a reduction in glucose, (2) increased pyruvate and lactate, (3) decreased inorganic phosphate, and (4) decreased K^+. In diabetics insulin also lowers

FIG. 49-2 *Insulin receptor.*

From Kahn CR: Annu Rev Med 36:429, copyright 1985; reproduced with permission from Annual Reviews, Inc.

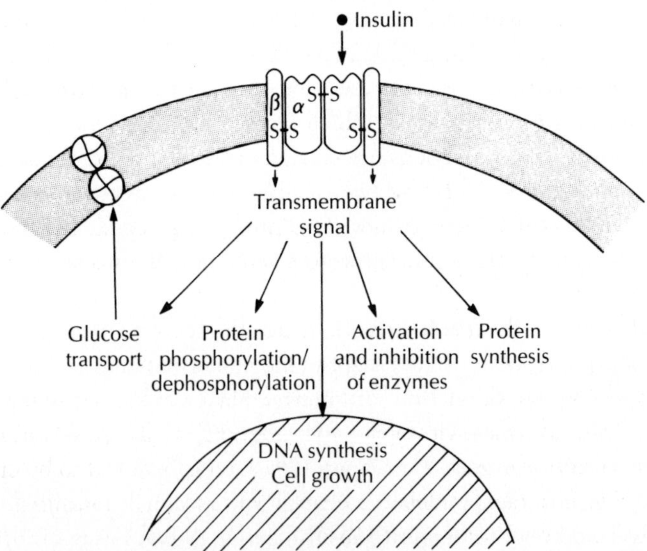

circulating amino acid concentrations by promoting uptake and incorporation into protein. The effect on blood glucose may be explained by enhanced uptake by tissues such as muscle and fat. Insulin also inhibits glycogenolysis in the liver. The changes in pyruvate and lactate concentration are generally attributed to greater glucose utilization. As more glucose 6-phosphate is produced, more metabolic products accumulate. The fall in phosphate concentration is believed to reflect increased glucose phosphorylation. The decrease in K^+ concentration accompanies glycogen deposition in the liver.

Insulin deficiency

When insulin availability is inadequate, as in insulin-dependent diabetes, and glucose uptake is severely decreased, other hormones act to provide alternate sources of fuel. Epinephrine, glucagon, growth hormone, and hydrocortisone mobilize free fatty acids, which are converted into ketone bodies by the liver. These agents also accelerate gluconeogenesis in the liver. Major problems arise when these counterregulatory mechanisms are inadequate or when they produce large amounts of harmful metabolites. When glucose is not available, enhanced conversion of protein to glucose increases urea and ammonia. Increased lipolysis leads to elevation of fatty acids, formation of ketones, and eventually to the development of metabolic acidosis.

Insulin resistance

Insulin resistance is a prominent feature in obese individuals and in non–insulin-dependent diabetes. Some resistance may be caused by defects in binding of insulin. Other possible mechanisms include secretion of an abnormal β-cell secretory product or the presence of circulating insulin antagonists. Patients with familial hyperproinsulinemia fail to convert proinsulin to insulin within the secretory granules. In other individuals, circulating hormones such as glucocorticoids, growth hormone, or glucagon counteract the actions of insulin. Insulin resistance in obese individuals may be due, in part, to decreased blood flow to insulin-sensitive tissues.[12]

Almost all patients who take animal-derived insulin eventually develop antibodies to the injected insulin. Although antibodies alone do not usually produce an insulin-resistant state, they can alter the pharmacokinetics of injected insulin or, by binding it, act as a reservoir for insulin. Antibodies are less of a problem with semisynthetic or recombinant forms of human insulin.

GLUCAGON

The hyperglycemic effect of pancreatic extracts was noted by Banting and Best at the time of their signal studies on insulin. Later, a hyperglycemic factor was separated from such extracts and named "glucagon," the mobilizer of glucose. It was only many years later that its contribution to the physiology of the pancreas was recognized.

Synthesis and secretion

Glucagon is synthesized as a prohormone in pancreatic α cells and converted proteolytically to a polypeptide of 29 amino acids. In contrast to insulin, glucagon is a single chain with no disulfide linkages. It is degraded by liver and kidney and has a plasma half-life of approximately 5 minutes. Glucagon is believed to be one of a family of peptide hormones that includes secretin, VIP (vasoactive intestinal polypeptide), and gastrointestinal inhibitory peptide (GIP).

Actions and relation to diabetes

The actions of glucagon generally oppose those of insulin, but the coordinated secretion of both hormones prevents significant fluctuations in blood glucose concentration. The pattern of coordination is complex and involves paracrine regulation of insulin secretion by both glucagon from the α cells and somatostatin from D cells. Neural signals also control glucagon secretion, probably through release of somatostatin and other regulatory hormones.

Glucagon promotes production of glucose through both hepatic glycogenolysis and gluconeogenesis, and it stimulates lipolysis. When there is a relative or absolute decrease in circulating insulin, hyperglycemia and ketosis develop. The metabolic actions of glucagon are mediated by cellular receptors that activate adenylyl cyclase and thus cyclic AMP-dependent protein kinases.[22] There is also evidence that glucagon increases cytoplasmic Ca^{++} via metabolism of PIP_2 to IP_3 (see Chapter 3). These effects mobilize fuels to meet energy requirements of the brain and other tissues in the absence of circulating glucose.

Normally, glucagon secretion is suppressed by insulin, whereas insulin secretion is stimulated by a small increase in glucagon concentration. Insulin also antagonizes the actions of glucagon by stimulating phosphodiesterase activity.[22] Development of diabetes depends on a shift in the balance between these opposing hormones; because of the insulin deficiency in insulin-dependent diabetes mellitus the normal suppression of glucagon is lost. However, insulin deficiency in the absence of glucagon does not cause increased production of glucose and ketones.

Somatostatin, which suppresses both insulin and glucagon secretion, has been used experimentally to decrease glucagon concentration in insulin-dependent diabetes. Unfortunately, both the hyperglycemia and the ketonemia characteristic of glucagon excess reappear on cessation of somatostatin infusion.[21] A long-acting and more specific somatostatin analog that improves metabolic profiles in patients with insulin-dependent diabetes may prove more useful.[8]

DRUG THERAPY OF DIABETES

Diabetes mellitus is a heterogeneous group of hyperglycemic disorders. Hyperglycemia can result from a relative or absolute insulin deficiency when there is a relative excess of glucagon. Prolonged elevation of blood glucose in an uncontrolled manner leads to complications that involve the retina, kidney, nerves, and blood vessels.

Classification of diabetes

Diabetes is divided into two major categories based on whether endogenous insulin secretion is sufficient to prevent ketoacidosis. The type 1 diabetic, the patient with insulin-dependent diabetes mellitus (IDDM), lacks β-cell function and requires insulin therapy to prevent ketoacidosis. The common form of IDDM is believed to have a genetic basis, and over 90% of affected persons express particular major histocompatibility (MHC) antigens. The development of the disease, however, appears to require both the genetic background of susceptibility and certain environmental factors, such as viral infection. Hyperexpression of MHC antigens by B cells, stimulated by viral infection, probably precedes an autoimmune response. The clinical onset of the disease is generally sudden. Studies in animals indicate that T cells contribute to destruction of islet cells and rejection of islet implants.[9] It is still unclear whether the circulating anti-islet antibodies found in experimental or clinical diabetes are a cause or a result of the disease process.[21]

Type 2 diabetes, in which there are functional β cells, is generally referred to as non–insulin-dependent diabetes mellitus (NIDDM). This more common hyperglycemic disorder occurs in 70% to 80% of patients with diabetes.[13] These persons do not usually require exogenous insulin to prevent ketosis, and their symptoms usually appear gradually during adult life. They are, however, at high risk for the same complications that affect patients with IDDM. Although a genetic basis for NIDDM appears likely, the mode of inheritance in most cases remains unknown.

Controversy still remains as to whether a defect in insulin secretion or in insulin action at the target cell is more important in NIDDM. Impaired islet function manifested by a disproportionate release of proinsulin to insulin is thought by some to reflect an intrinsic β-cell defect.[17] Another mechanism may involve desensitization of the β cell to glucose under conditions of chronic hyperglycemia.[18]

The therapeutic objectives are the same for IDDM and NIDDM, but there are several subcategories of NIDDM with a broad spectrum of islet cell function. Comparison of the secretory responses in normal and diabetic individuals given a meal or glucose showed that non–insulin-dependent diabetics have significant blunting of both amount and rate of insulin secretion.[16] Although insulin may not be required to prevent life-threatening ketoacidosis in these patients, it is a necessary part of the therapeutic regimen for some of them. Others can be maintained by dietary restrictions and weight loss. Only patients with functional β cells can be treated with oral antihyperglycemic agents, the sulfonylureas (see pp. 565 to 568).

Rationale for metabolic control

Therapy in either IDDM or NIDDM is based on the assumption that the degenerative processes of long-term diabetes are caused, either directly or indirectly, by hyperglycemia. Benefits of glycemic control include a return toward normal of blood glucose, amino acid, free fatty acid, triglyceride, cholesterol, lactate, and pyruvate concentrations; plasma glucagon concentration is normalized, and most patients experience an improved sense of well-being. Healing of foot ulcers is accelerated, and gastroparesis may improve. Meticulous control during pregnancy is required to protect the fetus from metabolic abnormalities associated with diabetes and to minimize maternal complications.

Microvascular disease is a major cause of morbidity and mortality in diabetes. Because many patients with NIDDM have abnormal lipid concentrations, correction of these abnormalities is an important goal. Reduction of other risk factors such as smoking, obesity, and hypertension aids in long range management of the disease.

Insulin therapy

Insulin therapy of diabetes is more than simply replacement of a deficient hormone. First, the half-life of insulin is short; it is readily metabolized and removed from circulation. Second, the intricate pattern of insulin secretion under neural, endocrine, and paracrine influences is difficult to mimic with exogenous hormone. Third, administration of insulin by injection differs from the normal secretion from the pancreas into the portal circulation. Finally, institution of insulin therapy in NIDDM requires a commitment to implement the therapeutic regimen because control of hyperglycemia involves at least some inconvenience to the patient; in IDDM there is no choice.[1]

PREPARATIONS AND CLINICAL USE

Optimal use of insulin requires knowledge of factors that affect its rate of absorption, onset of action, and elimination. The choice of an insulin preparation for chronic therapy depends on the individual's metabolic needs, response to insulin, and motivation to achieve optimum glycemic control.

Insulin preparations differ mainly in their rate of absorption after subcutaneous injection. The rapidly absorbed and short-acting *regular insulin* is the only preparation that can be given intravenously. It has been modified by two methods to form less readily absorbed suspensions. First, protamine, a basic compound, has been added to raise the isoelectric point of the acidic insulin peptide. This combination produces protamine insulin. A second approach is to use high concentrations of zinc and acetate buffer to prepare insulin with various particle sizes. Aside from regular insulin, the most widely used insulins are isophane insulin suspension (NPH insulin) and insulin zinc suspension (lente insulin), which are intermediate in onset and duration. All insulin preparations are available in strengths of 40 and 100 units/ml. Other properties of the various insulin preparations are listed in Table 49-1.

In addition to USP insulins, which contain up to 25 parts per million proinsulin, single-component insulins are available that are less likely to elicit antibody formation.

Both human insulin and proinsulin have been produced by recombinant DNA technology. The biologic activity and pharmacokinetics of human insulin are similar to those of the porcine hormone, but the human form is less antigenic and more rapidly absorbed after subcutaneous injection.[24] Human proinsulin, which is more active in suppressing hepatic production of glucose than in increasing its peripheral uptake, was proposed as a potential treatment for patients with NIDDM. However, an increased incidence of myocardial infarction in patients treated with proinsulin prevented further trials.[24]

Most insulins are administered two or three times daily, often in combinations of regular and intermediate-acting forms. More precise glucoregulation is achieved by

TABLE 49-1 Insulin preparations

Action	Preparation	Hours after subcutaneous injection	
		Peak action	Duration of action
Rapid	Insulin injection (regular, crystalline zinc)	2.5-5	6-8
	Prompt insulin zinc suspension (semilente)	5-10	12-16
Intermediate	Isophane insulin suspension (NPH)	4-12	24
	Insulin zinc suspension (lente)	7-15	24
Long	Protamine zinc insulin suspension (PZI)	14-24	36
	Extended insulin zinc suspension (ultralente)	10-30	>36

continuous infusion. Infusion devices provide the most flexible form of therapy; they can be programmed to provide insulin at a constant basal rate with boluses administered just before meals.[21] Because of the constant monitoring necessary and the potential for hypoglycemia during nighttime fasting, these devices should be used only by highly motivated and adequately trained persons.

MONITORING

Although the degree of glycemic control needed to prevent complications is still not established, most clinicians expect that maintenance of blood glucose within a normal range will retard progression of neuropathic and vascular sequelae. Close monitoring of blood glucose can be done at home with kits that use capillary blood and a glucose oxidase–coated paper strip. Other means of control that can be used in an office or hospital setting include biochemical assays of blood glucose[13] and determination of the degree of glycosylation of hemoglobin.

ADVERSE EFFECTS OF INSULIN

Adverse effects of insulin include hypoglycemia, local or systemic allergic reactions, lipoatrophy, and visual disturbances. Hypoglycemia is the most serious problem for patients with diabetes because it can cause permanent brain damage or death. Patients with IDDM are vulnerable to insulin-induced hypoglycemia during exercise or fasting. Normal persons are protected from hypoglycemia by a decrease in insulin and a rise in glucagon or catecholamine concentration, which modulate further islet hormone secretion. Diabetics cannot marshal these defenses. During sleep they may be unaware of symptoms of hypoglycemia, such as tachycardia and sweating. Thus continuous insulin infusion and long-acting insulin preparations should be used with great caution in patients who are unable to generate a counterregulatory response to hypoglycemia.[13] Fig. 49-3 shows changes in blood glucose in subjects who lack this response. Implantable glucose sensors that monitor extracellular glucose might help prevent hypoglycemia. These devices, still in the experimental stage, can be inserted in an infusion pump to control insulin delivery within a closed-loop system. An additional complication of insulin therapy is development of cutaneous abscesses.

Oral hypoglycemic agents

The introduction of sulfonylurea compounds was a notable development in management of diabetes. Loubatières observed in 1942 that some sulfonamides, administered to patients suffering from typhoid fever, produced symptoms and signs of hypoglycemia. Extensive investigation then established that certain sulfonylureas cause hypoglycemia in normal animals but not in animals made diabetic by administration of alloxan. Since most diabetics have NIDDM without loss of β cells, the search for additional hypoglycemic agents has been extensive. At present, the only drugs available in the United States are sulfonylureas.

These orally effective agents are widely used. Second-generation compounds are more potent but provide no substantive improvement in efficacy or differences in mechanism of action. Their major advantage is that they expand the range of options, and some cause fewer side effects. In addition, some patients who do not respond to first-generation sulfonylureas may respond to the newer agents. The structures of the available drugs are given on p. 567.

FIG. 49-3 *Recovery from insulin-induced hypoglycemia.* 1, *Control;* 2, *glucagon and epinephrine deficiency;* 3, *glucagon deficiency with α- and β-adrenergic receptor blockade. Hypoglycemia counterregulation is governed by glucagon and epinephrine. Plasma glucose in controls with normal glucagon and epinephrine concentrations rebounds quickly after moderate drop. Glucose concentrations in glucagon- and epinephrine-deficient subjects plunge dangerously low; adrenergic blockade in glucagon-deficient subjects causes significant fall with early partial recovery.*

Data of Cryer PE, Gerich JE; modified from Levin PA, McLaughlin J, Kowarski AA: Hosp Pract 19(10):137, 1984.

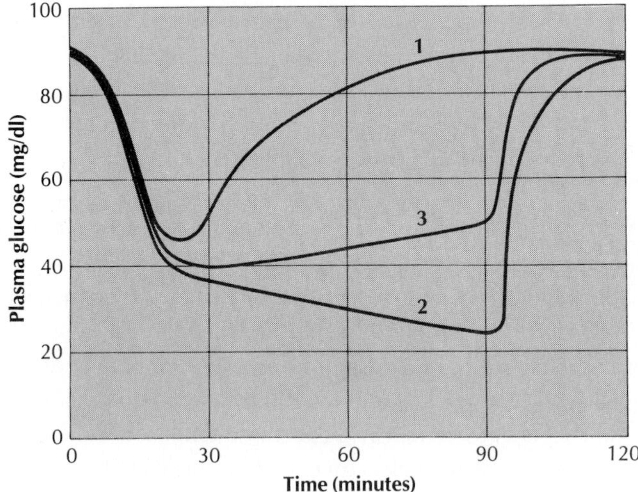

FIG. 49-4 *Proposed mechanism for the action of sulfonylureas on insulin secretion.* ADP, *Adenosine diphosphate;* cAMP, *cyclic AMP.*

From Gerich JE: Reprinted by permission of the New England Journal of Medicine 321:1231, 1989.

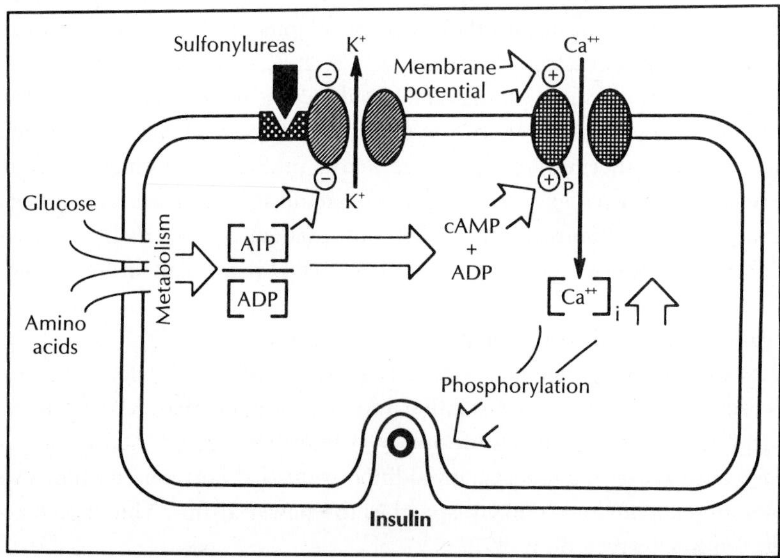

First generation

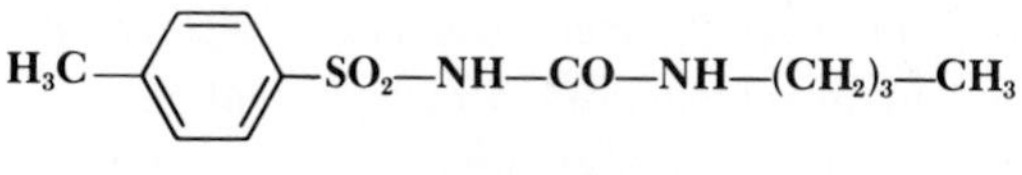

$H_3C-C_6H_4-SO_2-NH-CO-NH-(CH_2)_3-CH_3$

Tolbutamide

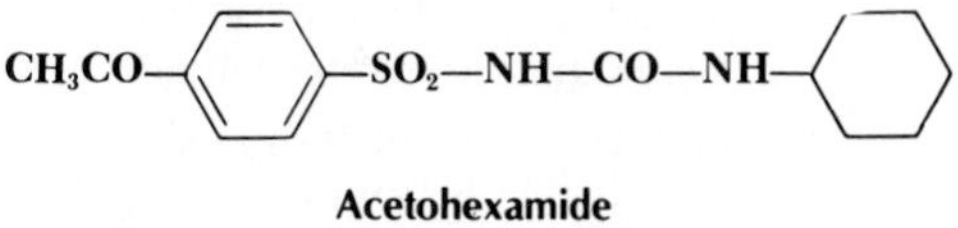

$CH_3CO-C_6H_4-SO_2-NH-CO-NH-C_6H_{11}$

Acetohexamide

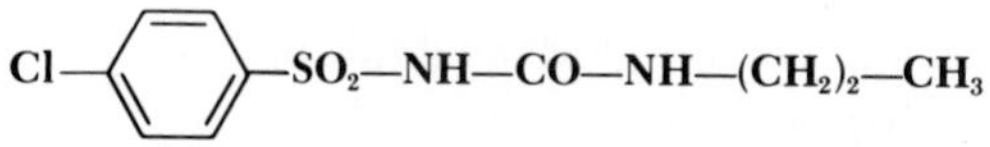

$Cl-C_6H_4-SO_2-NH-CO-NH-(CH_2)_2-CH_3$

Chlorpropamide

$CH_3-C_6H_4-SO_2-NH-\overset{O}{\overset{\|}{C}}-NH-N(CH_2)_6$

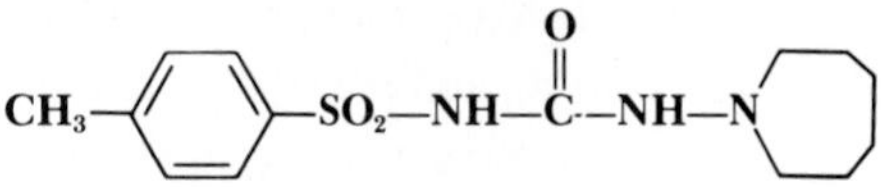

Tolazamide

Second generation

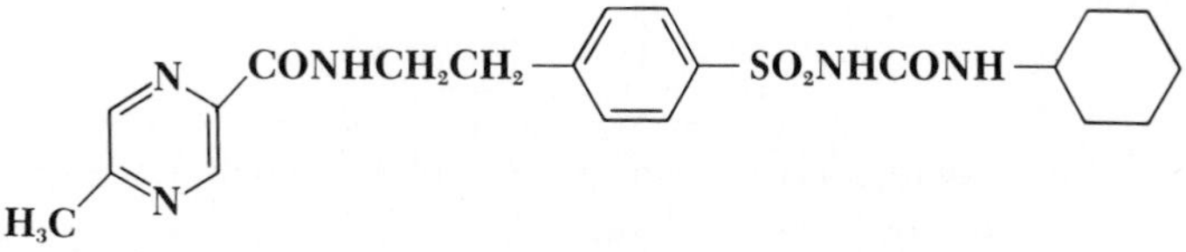

H_3C–pyrazine–$CONHCH_2CH_2-C_6H_4-SO_2NHCONH-C_6H_{11}$

Glipizide

(Cl, OCH_3)–$C_6H_3-CONHCH_2CH_2-C_6H_4-SO_2NHCONH-C_6H_{11}$

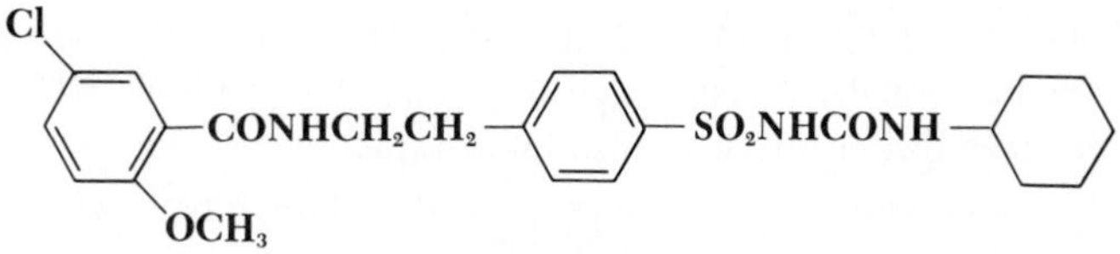

Glyburide

MECHANISM OF ACTION

Despite earlier arguments to the contrary, intact pancreatic β cells are essential for the hypoglycemic action of sulfonylureas. Acute administration of these drugs stimulates insulin release, which correlates with degranulation in the β cells. Their major action is to lower the glycemic threshold for the β-cell secretory response; more insulin is released for a given increment of blood glucose. Sulfonylureas do not affect the synthesis of insulin.[7] β Cells contain sulfonylurea receptors that appear to be linked to an ATPase-sensitive K^+ channel. The model in Fig. 49-4 suggests that inhibition of K^+ efflux leads to depolarization of the β-cell membrane and opens voltage-dependent Ca^{++} channels. Increased entry of Ca^{++} and intracellular binding to calmodulin could activate kinases involved in exocytosis of secretory granules.

Additional mechanisms of lowering of blood glucose include release of somatostatin, which suppresses glucagon secretion, and enhanced binding of insulin to target-cell receptors. In addition, sulfonylureas appear to act synergistically with insulin, possibly by increasing insulin sensitivity at a postreceptor level.[7]

In general, patients with a fasting glucose concentration above 330 mg/100 ml do not respond to sulfonylurea drugs. Those with a lower glucose concentration exhibit at least a partial response, though as many as 25% eventually become unresponsive. Loss of responsiveness may be caused by infection or stress. Failure of dietary control and weight gain may also contribute.[21]

Preparations and Clinical Use

The characteristics of oral hypoglycemic drugs are listed in Table 49-2. The major differences in half-life and duration of action are determined by their fate in the body. Tolbutamide and tolazamide are rapidly metabolized. Acetohexamide is also rapidly metabolized, but its principal metabolite, hydroxyheximide, is more potent than the original drug. Chlorpropamide, the longest acting sulfonylurea, is less completely metabolized than the previous drugs. As with other sulfonylureas, metabolites of chlorpropamide are eliminated by the kidney, and impaired renal function may lead to accumulation and an increased chance of hypoglycemia.[7]

Glipizide and glyburide, the second-generation compounds, are approximately 100 to 150 times as potent as tolbutamide. Like other sulfonylureas they are metabolized by the liver and excreted in urine. Metabolites of glyburide have some hypoglycemic activity; thus glipizide is preferred for patients with renal insufficiency. Both drugs have an extended action, up to 24 hours, which makes once daily dosing feasible.

Adverse Effects

Sulfonylurea compounds are usually well tolerated with few side effects. Hypoglycemia is generally not so great a danger as with insulin, but occasionally it may be serious and of long duration in elderly patients and in those with impaired renal function. Chlorpropamide causes an intolerance to alcohol similar to the disulfiram reaction, and it may also cause hyponatremia. Gastrointestinal and allergic skin reactions occur infrequently. Weight gain is common in patients who achieve glycemic control, but this also occurs with insulin therapy.[7]

Drug interactions complicate therapy with sulfonylureas. The metabolism of tolbutamide can be inhibited by several drugs (see Chapter 70). Most sulfonylureas are highly protein bound and may therefore be susceptible to displacement interactions. Glipizide and glyburide appear to bind by nonionic interactions, which should minimize their interactions with other drugs that bind to plasma proteins.[7] Thiazide diuretics reduce the activity of sulfonylureas through an independent effect on glucose.

TABLE 49-2 Characteristics of oral sulfonylurea drugs

Name	Half-life (hours)	Duration of action (hours)	Tablet size (mg)
First generation			
Tolbutamide (Orinase, Oramide)	4-6	6-12	250, 500
Acetohexamide (Dymelor)	6-8*	12-24	250, 500
Chlorpropamide (Diabenese)	24-42	24-60	100, 250
Tolazamide (Tolamide, Tolinase)	7	10-14	100-500
Second generation			
Glipizide (Glucotrol)	3-7	24	5, 10
Glyburide (DiaBeta, Micronase)	10	24	1.25-5

*Including active metabolite.

ALTERNATIVE THERAPIES AND NEW APPROACHES

Other aspects of diabetes management, such as diet, have been reevaluated in recent years. Some patients with NIDDM can be controlled by dietary measures alone, particularly if obesity is corrected. Although for many years a low-carbohydrate diet was considered mandatory for diabetic control, a diet containing up to 60% total calories in carbohydrates is acceptable, provided that simple sugars are avoided. Fat intake should be limited. However, a recent study of patients with NIDDM showed that partial replacement of complex carbohydrates with monounsaturated fatty acids did not increase the concentration of LDL-cholesterol and improved glycemic control.[6] Foods with a high fiber content are recommended.

An intestinal glycosidase inhibitor, acarbose, may provide a means to delay absorption of complex carbohydrates, which would improve the effectiveness of insulin therapy in patients with IDDM. It might partially compensate for delayed insulin secretion in those individuals with NIDDM treated by diet modification alone or with oral hypoglycemic agents.

Other potential means of control include inhibitors of gluconeogenesis and inhibitors of counterregulatory hormones. For example, some analogs of somatostatin and glucagon appear promising as inhibitors of glucagon secretion. Another means of altering blood glucose is to use insulin-mimetic agents. Vanadate ions, which are low molecular weight phosphate analogs, mimic many of insulin's metabolic actions in animals. Vanadate appears to activate glucose metabolism by insulin-independent mechanisms and thus may be particularly useful in conditions that involve insulin resistance.[19]

Aldose reductase inhibition

Despite recent advances in therapy, patients with diabetes mellitus continue to develop complications that cause significant morbidity and mortality. Ample evidence indicates an association between chronic hyperglycemia and development of microvascular and neurologic complications. Because the underlying mechanism of diabetic retinopathy and neuropathy is believed to involve accumulation of sorbitol, a potential means of controlling these complications is the use of *aldose reductase inhibitors*.[5] The tissues that bear the brunt of diabetic complications, the lens, retina, nerves, kidney, and blood vessels, do not require insulin for glucose uptake as muscle and adipose tissues do. With continual exposure to high concentrations of glucose, which is converted by aldose reductase to sorbitol and subsequently to fructose, the products accumulate within such tissues (Fig. 49-5). Galactose is an even better substrate for aldose reductase, and the product, galactitol, is not further metabolized. Because sorbitol and other polyols do not readily pass through cell membranes, they cause osmotic swelling and eventual cell disruption. Increased glycosylation of proteins may also contribute to thickening of basement membranes and further compromise of vascular perfusion.

Studies of experimental diabetes in animals and clinical disease in humans implicate aldose reductase in cataract formation, retinopathy, and diabetic neuropathy. The first clinical trial of an aldose reductase inhibitor, in 1982, indicated that both motor and sensory nerve conduction were improved in patients treated with *sorbinil*. Subsequent studies provided further evidence that sorbinil decreased endoneural levels of

FIG. 49-5 Pathway of sorbitol in the lens.

From Kinoshita JH: Ann Intern Med 101:83, copyright 1984; reproduced with permission from the American Medical Association.

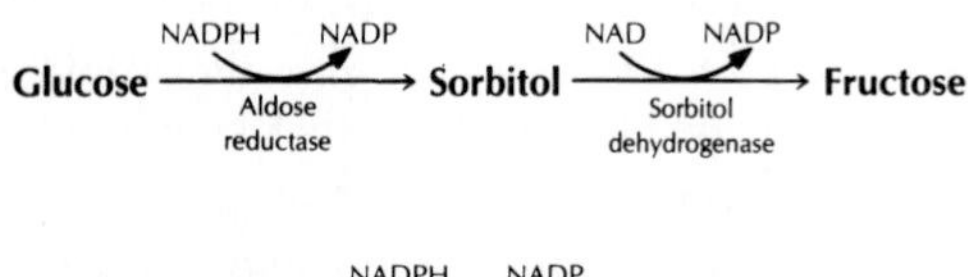

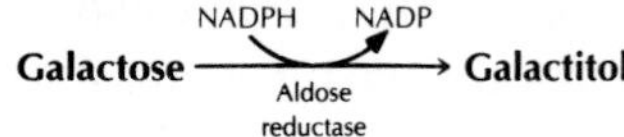

sorbital and fructose.[2] Aldose reductase inhibitors may prove valuable for long-term management of diabetes and its complications.

REFERENCES

1. Dupré J: Insulin therapy: progress and prospects, *Hosp Pract* 18(11):171, 1983.
2. Dyck PJ, Zimmerman BR, Vilen TH, et al: Nerve glucose, fructose, sorbitol, *myo*-inositol, and fiber degeneration and regeneration in diabetic neuropathy, *N Engl J Med* 319:542, 1988.
3. Freidenberg GR, Henry RR, Klein HH, et al: Decreased kinase activity of insulin receptors from adipocytes of non–insulin-dependent diabetic subjects, *J Clin Invest* 79:240, 1987.
4. Frohman LA: CNS peptides and glucoregulation, *Annu Rev Physiol* 45:95, 1983.
5. Gabbay KH: The sorbitol pathway and the complications of diabetes, *N Engl J Med* 288:831, 1973.
6. Garg A, Bonanome A, Grundy SM, et al: Comparison of a high-carbohydrate diet with a high-monounsaturated-fat diet in patients with non-insulin-dependent diabetes mellitus, *N Engl J Med* 319:829, 1988.
7. Gerich JE: Oral hypoglycemic agents, *N Engl J Med* 321:1231, 1989.
8. Grossman LD, Shumak SL, George SR, et al: The effects of SMS 201-995 (Sandostatin) on metabolic profiles in insulin-dependent diabetes mellitus, *J Clin Endocrinol Metab* 68:63, 1989.
9. Janeway C: The immune destruction of pancreatic β cells, *Immunol Today* 6:229, 1985.
10. Kahn CR: The molecular mechanism of insulin action, *Annu Rev Med* 36:429, 1985.
11. Kahn CR, White MF: The insulin receptor and the molecular mechanism of insulin action, *J Clin Invest* 82:1151, 1988.
12. Laakso M, Edelman SV, Brechtel G, Baron AD: Decreased effect of insulin to stimulate skeletal muscle blood flow in obese man: a novel mechanism for insulin resistance, *J Clin Invest* 85:1844, 1990.
13. Levin PA, McLaughlin J, Kowarski AA: Diabetes mellitus: customizing management, *Hosp Pract* 19(10):137, 1984.
14. Matschinsky FM: Glucokinase as glucose sensor and metabolic signal generator in pancreatic β-cells and hepatocytes, *Diabetes* 39:647, 1990.
15. Orci L, Ravazzola M, Storch M-J, et al: Proteolytic maturation of insulin is a post-golgi event which occurs in acidifying clathrin-coated secretory vesicles, *Cell* 49:865, 1987.
16. Polonsky KS, Given BD, Hirsch LJ, et al: Abnormal patterns of insulin secretion in non-insulin-dependent diabetes mellitus, *N Engl J Med* 318:1231, 1988.
17. Porte D Jr, Kahn SE: Hyperproinsulinemia and amyloid in NIDDM: clues to etiology of islet β-cell dysfunction? *Diabetes* 38:1333, 1989.
18. Robertson RP: Type II diabetes, glucose "non-sense," and islet desensitization, *Diabetes* 38:1501, 1989.
19. Shechter Y: Insulin-mimetic effects of vanadate: possible implications for future treatment of diabetes, *Diabetes* 39:1, 1990.
20. Taira M, Taira M, Hashimoto N, et al:

Human diabetes associated with a deletion of the tyrosine kinase domain of the insulin receptor, *Science* 245:63, 1989.

21. Unger RH, Foster DW: Diabetes mellitus. In Wilson JD, Foster DW, editors: *William's textbook of endocrinology*, ed 7, Philadelphia, 1985, WB Saunders Co, p 1018.
22. Unger RH, Orci L: Glucagon. In Rifkin H, Porte D Jr, editors: *Ellenberg and Rifkin's diabetes mellitus: theory and practice,* ed 4, New York, 1989, Elsevier, p 104.
23. Yoshimasa Y, Seino S, Whittaker J, et al: Insulin-resistant diabetes due to a point mutation that prevents insulin proreceptor processing, *Science* 240:784, 1988.
24. Zinman B: The physiologic replacement of insulin: an elusive goal, *N Engl J Med* 321:363, 1989.

Chapter 50

Thyroid hormones and antithyroid drugs

BASIC BIOCHEMISTRY AND PHYSIOLOGY

Biosynthesis of thyroid hormones

The structural formulas of the various organic iodine compounds in the thyroid are shown below:

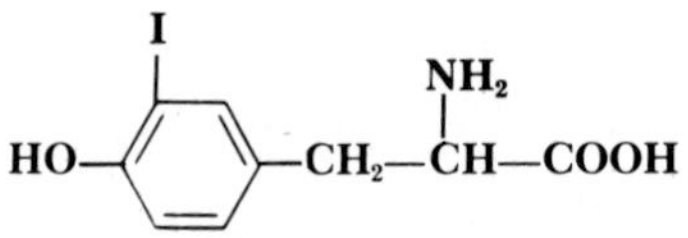

Monoiodotyrosine

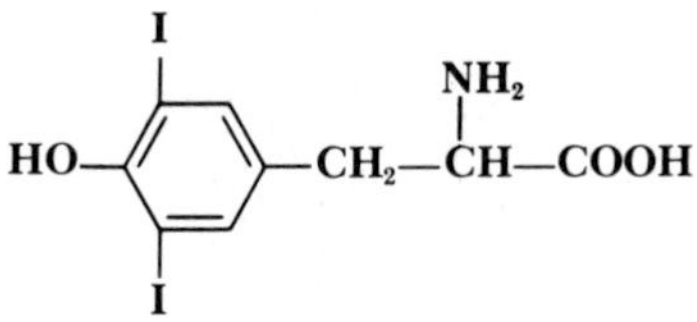

Diiodotyrosine

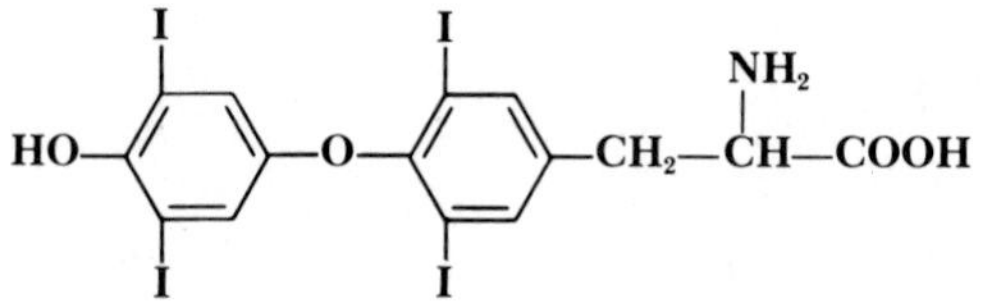

Thyroxine (T_4): 3,5,3′,5′-tetraiodothyronine

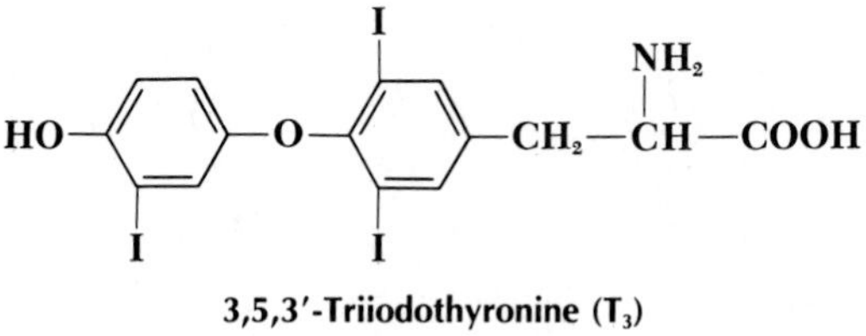

3,5,3′-Triiodothyronine (T_3)

These compounds occur primarily as peptide-linked amino acids within thyroglobulin, a large (660,000-dalton) protein unique to the thyroid gland. T_4 and T_3 are the active hormones secreted by the gland. DIT (diiodotyrosine) and MIT (monoiodotyrosine) are hormonally inactive precursors for T_4 and T_3.

Iodine enters the thyroid follicular cells as inorganic I^- and is transformed through a series of metabolic steps into the thyroid hormones, as illustrated in Fig. 50-1. The steps in this sequence are (1) active transport of I^-, resulting in an intracellular concentration of I^- in the gland 20 to 40 times greater than that in plasma; (2) iodination of tyrosyl residues of thyroglobulin catalyzed by thyroid peroxidase, a membrane-bound hemoprotein that, in the presence of H_2O_2, oxidizes I^- to an active iodinating form, presumably I^+; and (3) conversion of DIT and MIT to T_4 and T_3

FIG. 50-1 *Schema depicting some of the more important steps in thyroid hormone biosynthesis, secretion, and metabolism.* ALB, *Albumin;* DIT, *diiodotyrosine;* I, *iodine;* MIT, *monoiodotyrosine;* PA, *prealbumin;* PBI, *protein-bound iodine;* rT_3, *3,3',5'-triiodothyronine, or reverse* T_3; T_3, *3,5,3'-triiodothyronine;* T_4, *thyroxine;* TBG, *thyroxine-binding globulin;* Tg, *thyroglobulin;* TPO, *thyroid peroxidase.*

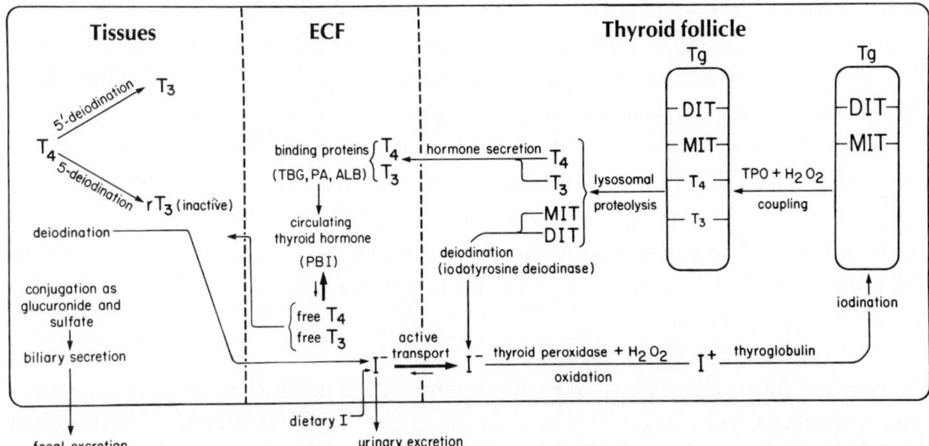

within the matrix of thyroglobulin. Coupling of two molecules of DIT forms T_4, whereas T_3 is formed by coupling one molecule of DIT with a molecule of MIT. Thyroid peroxidase catalyzes coupling as well as iodination. In the normal human thyroid the ratio of T_4 to T_3 in thyroglobulin is about 10:1.

Thyroglobulin contains the bulk of the iodine in the normal thyroid. In a typical human thyroid, about 60% of thyroglobulin iodine is in the form of DIT and MIT and less than 40% as T_4 and T_3. Only two to four residues of T_4 are normally present per molecule of thyroglobulin. Inorganic I^- generally represents less than 1% of total glandular iodine.

Secretion of thyroid hormones

Thyroglobulin must be hydrolyzed to release T_4 and T_3 for secretion into the circulation. As illustrated in Fig. 50-1, this is accomplished by lysosomal proteases. Digestion of thyroglobulin presumably releases all the iodoamino acids in the free form. The iodotyrosines DIT and MIT are deiodinated by an iodotyrosine deiodinase, which removes the bound iodine as I^- and preserves it for reutilization within the gland. T_4 and T_3 are not substrates for the deiodinase and are free to diffuse into the blood. Thyroglobulin itself normally enters the circulation only in small amounts, but increased concentrations of thyroglobulin are found in sera from persons with various thyroid disorders.

Hypothalamic-pituitary-thyroid interrelationships

In normal subjects, activity of the thyroid is largely controlled by thyrotropin (thyroid-stimulating hormone, TSH), a glycoprotein secreted by the anterior pituitary. In hypophysectomized rats all steps in thyroid hormone biosynthesis and secretion are greatly reduced. TSH acts at the level of the thyroid cell membrane, primarily by activating the adenylyl cyclase system. Many of the effects of TSH on the thyroid can be duplicated by dibutyryl cyclic AMP or by forskolin, a potent activator of adenylyl cyclase. There is also evidence that some effects of TSH are mediated by another major cell-signaling system, the Ca^{++}-phosphoinositide system.

TSH secretion is controlled by two major factors: (1) thyrotropin-releasing hormone (TRH), a tripeptide produced in the hypothalamus, which stimulates TSH secretion, and (2) feedback inhibition on the pituitary and hypothalamus by circulating T_4 and T_3. Excessive thyroid hormone concentrations in the circulation inhibit secretion of TSH, whereas deficient concentrations increase TSH secretion.

In the hyperthyroidism of Graves disease, the thyroid gland secretes excessive amounts of T_4 and T_3. In this condition, circulating TSH concentration becomes very low, and pituitary secretion of TSH becomes unresponsive to TRH. Graves disease is an autoimmune disease in which the thyroid gland is stimulated by a circulating abnormal immunoglobulin instead of by TSH, bypassing the normal feedback control by circulating T_4 and T_3.

Thyroid hormones in the circulation

T_4 is the major circulating thyroid hormone with a mean concentration in normal human serum of 80 to 90 ng/ml. Even though the mean concentration of T_3 is only 1 to 1.5 ng/ml, most of the hormone action at the receptor level is mediated by T_3. Both T_4 and T_3 are transported in plasma largely bound to protein (>99%). Three proteins are involved: thyroxine-binding globulin (TBG), prealbumin, and albumin. Approximately two thirds of plasma T_4 is carried by TBG, even though it is the least abundant of the three proteins. This can be attributed to its extremely high affinity for T_4 (association constant = $1 \times 10^{10} M^{-1}$). TBG is also the major carrier for T_3, though the association constant is about one twentieth that for T_4. Association constants are intermediate for prealbumin and lowest for albumin. However, because of the high concentration of albumin in plasma, an appreciable fraction of T_4 and T_3 is bound to this protein.

There is good reason to believe that it is the free hormone fraction in plasma that is available to tissues; the bound form is primarily an inert reservoir. Measurement of free T_4 and T_3 concentrations is best performed by equilibrium dialysis, though this is not a readily available clinical procedure. Results of such measurements, combined with measurements of total T_4 and T_3 concentrations by routine radioimmunoassay procedures, indicate that free T_4 is only about 0.03% of the total T_4 in serum. For T_3 the corresponding value, though significantly higher, is still only about 0.3%.

The high degree of binding of T_4 and T_3 to protein shields these hormones from elimination processes and accounts for their long half-lives in plasma. The half-life for plasma T_4 in humans is about 6 days, whereas that for T_3 is about 1 day. These half-lives are much longer than those for other hormones.

Indirect procedures have been developed for estimating free T_4 and T_3 concentrations. One such method makes use of a T_3 resin-uptake test that measures the distribution of $^{125}I\text{-}T_3$ between serum proteins and a specially prepared resin. From this procedure one can derive a free thyroxine index that, in many cases, correlates fairly well with free T_4 concentrations measured by equilibrium dialysis.

Peripheral metabolism of thyroid hormones

T_4 is produced exclusively in the thyroid gland. T_3 is also secreted but only to the extent of about one tenth the secretion of T_4. In peripheral tissues a major pathway for T_4 metabolism is deiodination, in both the 5′ and 5 positions (see Fig. 50-1). 5′-Deiodination forms T_3, which displays 5 to 10 times the potency of T_4 in most tests of thyroid hormone activity. About 80% of the total T_3 in the human body arises from peripheral deiodination of T_4. Since T_3 is responsible for most of the hormonal activity, it is obvious that factors controlling T_4 to T_3 conversion are of major interest in studies of thyroid function. Deiodination of T_4 in the 5 position yields the isomer of T_3, 3,3′,5′-triiodothyronine, known as reverse T_3 (rT_3). Reverse T_3 displays little or no hormonal activity and is thus a pathway of T_4 inactivation. Measurement of rT_3 concentration has proved useful in the study of factors controlling T_4 conversion to T_3.

Estimates of mean serum concentrations, metabolic clearances, and production rates for a 70 kg human are listed below.* The production rate of approximately 100 μg of T_4 per day is important in determining the replacement dose for treatment of hypothyroidism.

COMPOUND	SERUM CONCENTRATION (NG/ML)	METABOLIC CLEARANCE (LITERS/DAY)	PRODUCTION RATE (μG/DAY)
T_4	86	1.2	103
T_3	1.35	23.6	32
rT_3	0.38	111	42

Deiodination of T_4 also releases I^-, which is then available for reentry into the thyroid. Similarly, further deiodination of T_3 and rT_3 makes additional I^- available for recycling. Such metabolism conserves iodine, which is a trace element available in short supply in many areas of the world. The optimum iodine requirement for adults is 150 to 300 μg/day.

T_4 and T_3 also undergo conjugation with glucuronic acid and sulfate, primarily in the liver. The conjugates are secreted into the bile. Conjugation of T_3 with sulfate greatly facilitates deiodination.

Physiologic effects of thyroid hormones

Thyroid hormones do not have discrete target organs. Their effects are manifest throughout the body, as shown by the following list of responsive organ systems and physiologic functions:

1. Growth and differentiation
2. Calorigenesis and thermoregulation
3. Cardiovascular system
4. Neuromuscular system
5. Endocrine and reproductive systems
6. Carbohydrate, protein, and lipid metabolism
7. Enzyme synthesis
8. Vitamin metabolism
9. Bone metabolism

Deficiency or excess of thyroid hormones may affect any or all of these.

*Data modified from Chopra IJ. In Ingbar SH, Braverman LE, editors: *Werner's the thyroid: a fundamental and clinical text*, ed 5, Philadelphia, 1986, JB Lippincott.

Much effort has been expended in recent years to determine the molecular basis for thyroid hormone activity. The area that has received the most attention is the cell nucleus. There is good evidence that binding of T_3 to specific receptors in the nucleus initiates hormone action through control of gene expression.[4] The good correlation between the biologic potency of various thyroid hormone analogs and their binding affinity for nuclear receptors supports this view. The thyroid hormone nuclear receptor is now recognized as a member of a superfamily of receptors that includes steroid hormone receptors, as well as the receptor for retinoic acid.[2] These receptors are encoded by different forms of the cellular proto-oncogene c-erb A. Multiple forms of the nuclear thyroid hormone receptor have been described. It has also been proposed that specific receptors for T_3 exist in mitochondria and in the plasma membrane and that these are additional sites for initiation of thyroid hormone action.

PHARMACOLOGY

Drugs that affect thyroid hormone concentrations

The most commonly used thyroid function test is measurement of serum T_4 concentration by radioimmunoassay. It is important to recognize that the results of this test may be affected by some commonly used drugs.[3] In patients receiving these drugs, alterations in serum T_4 and T_3 concentrations may not reflect thyroid dysfunction. The most widespread drugs of this type are those that alter plasma protein binding of T_4 and T_3. This may occur by two mechanisms: (1) by changing the plasma concentration of TBG and (2) by competing with T_4 and T_3 for binding sites on TBG.

Increased concentrations of TBG are seen most often in pregnancy and in women receiving exogenous estrogens, including birth control pills. In this situation plasma T_4 and T_3 concentrations may be above the normal range. However, the proportion of free T_4 and T_3 is reduced, and the net effect is that the free hormone concentrations remain essentially unchanged. Since it is the free hormone concentration available to tissues that determines the distribution and fractional turnover rate of the hormones, the subject remains euthyroid despite elevated concentrations of total plasma T_4 and T_3.

Decreased TBG may occur in subjects receiving androgens or glucocorticoids in pharmacologic doses. The consequences are the converse of those associated with increased TBG. Plasma concentrations of T_4 and T_3 are reduced, accompanied by an increase in the proportion of free hormone. The concentration of free hormone is essentially unchanged, and the subject is euthyroid.

Several drugs inhibit binding of T_4 and T_3 to TBG. This occurs in patients taking large doses of salicylates, for example, in rheumatoid arthritis. The effect is an increase in the proportion of free hormone and a decrease in total plasma hormone concentration. Free hormone concentrations remain essentially unchanged, and the patients are euthyroid. Phenytoin also inhibits binding of T_4 to TBG and lowers total plasma T_4. However, in this case the plasma free T_4 fraction remains unchanged so that the free T_4 concentration is also reduced. Plasma T_3 concentration, in contrast, is in the normal range. Patients with a low plasma T_4 concentration while receiving phenytoin are not hypothyroid, as indicated by normal basal and TRH-stimulated serum TSH concentrations. Phenytoin probably alters thyroid hormone economy in vivo by multiple mechanisms. The predominant effect may be an acceleration of some of the pathways of intracellular T_4 metabolism, possibly leading to an increase in T_4 conversion to T_3. These effects of phenytoin probably involve induction of enzymes in the smooth endoplasmic reticulum.

As indicated for phenytoin, an important site of drug action, in addition to effects on plasma binding proteins, is on peripheral conversion of T_4 to T_3. Drugs reported to reduce peripheral T_4 to T_3 conversion include iopanoic acid and ipodate (oral cholecystographic agents), amiodarone, propranolol, and propylthiouracil. In general, such drugs initially decrease plasma concentration of T_3 and increase concentrations of T_4 and rT_3. The metabolic consequences may be quite complex, especially in the case of amiodarone.

Changes in circulating thyroid hormone concentrations are also observed in severe nonthyroid illness, in surgical stress, and in caloric deprivation. Under these conditions both total and free T_3 concentrations are reduced, whereas total and free T_4 concentrations may be increased, unchanged, or decreased. Total and free rT_3 concentrations increase. This condition is referred to as the "low T_3 syndrome," or the "euthyroid sick syndrome." The decrease in T_3 and the increase in rT_3 occur primarily because of slower peripheral 5′-deiodination of T_4. There is generally a diminished or absent TSH response to decreased thyroid hormone concentrations and to TRH. In the presence of severe nonthyroidal illness therefore the task of diagnosing intrinsic disease of the pituitary-thyroid axis is particularly challenging and requires a clear understanding of the limitations of thyroid function tests and of the assumptions underlying their use.

Clinical preparations and diagnostic tests

Replacement therapy

Several preparations are available when treatment with thyroid hormone is indicated for hypothyroidism:

Thyroid tablets and **capsules** (16 to 325 mg), derived from porcine thyroid glands, contain both T_4 and T_3, in a molar ratio of approximately 4:1. Most adult patients require 60 to 120 mg once daily. **Liotrix** (Euthyroid, Thyrolar) is a 4:1 mixture by weight of synthetic T_4 and T_3.

Thyroglobulin tablets (Proloid), obtained from a purified extract of hog thyroid, contain both T_4 and T_3 in a molar ratio similar to that in thyroid tablets. The usual dose should be about half that for thyroid tablets.

Levothyroxine sodium (Synthroid, Levothroid, others), a synthetic salt of l-T_4, is chemically identical to the major form of circulating thyroid hormone. The usual adult dosage is 100 to 200 μg once daily.

Liothyronine sodium (Cytomel, Cyronine), a synthetic salt of l-T_3, is more rapidly acting than l-T_4 and may be injected intravenously in myxedema coma, for which it is the drug of choice.

Even though liothyronine is several times more potent than levothyroxine, most thyroidologists recommend levothyroxine for replacement therapy in hypothyroidism. Levothyroxine is also preferred over the crude preparations, which contain both T_4 and T_3 and may vary in composition and potency.

THYROTROPIN-RELEASING HORMONE (TRH)

This hypothalamic tripeptide (pyroglutamyl-histidyl-prolinamide) stimulates release of TSH and prolactin from the anterior pituitary. Intravenous administration of TRH to normal subjects promptly increases plasma TSH concentration. This response is exaggerated in hypothyroidism and greatly blunted in hyperthyroidism. The TRH stimulation test is useful in diagnosis of mild cases of decreased or increased thyroid function and also in differential diagnosis of primary, hypothalamic, and pituitary hypothyroidism.

SENSITIVE SERUM TSH ASSAY

Plasma TSH is elevated in patients with primary hypothyroidism, and measurement of serum concentration by radioimmunoassay has been used for more than 20 years for diagnosis and management of hypothyroidism. However, this test cannot distinguish reliably between euthyroid and hyperthyroid patients. Recently, serum TSH assays have been developed that are an order of magnitude more sensitive than conventional radioimmunoassays. These depend on non-competitive "sandwich" immunometric assays, the principle of which is illustrated in Fig. 50-2. Immunometric assays make it possible to measure serum TSH concentrations that are one-tenth the normal values, thus enabling the lower concentrations associated with hyperthyroidism to be reliably distinguished from normal concentrations. This has led some investigators to propose that the sensitive TSH assay should be the first-line test of thyroid function, replacing the commonly used combination of serum T_4 and T_3 resin

FIG. 50-2 *Diagram of principles involved in immunoradiometric assay for thyroid-stimulating hormone (TSH). In the immunoradiometric assay, in contrast to the conventional radioimmunoassay, the antigen (TSH) is not labeled. In place of labeled antigen, a monoclonal antibody against TSH is labeled with ^{125}I. Also in contrast to immunoassays, the labeled antibody is generally added in excess, permitting all the TSH in the sample to be bound by the antibodies. Separation of bound antigen-antibody complexes from nonspecifically bound ^{125}I is accomplished with the aid of a second monoclonal antibody linked to a solid plase support. The two monoclonal antibodies used in the assay recognize different epitopes on the TSH molecule. This minimizes cross reaction with other human glycoprotein hormones (chorionic gonadotropin, LH, FSH).*

From Ridgway EC: Mayo Clin Proc 63:1028, 1988. With permission from Celltech Ltd, Celltech Research, Berkshire, UK.

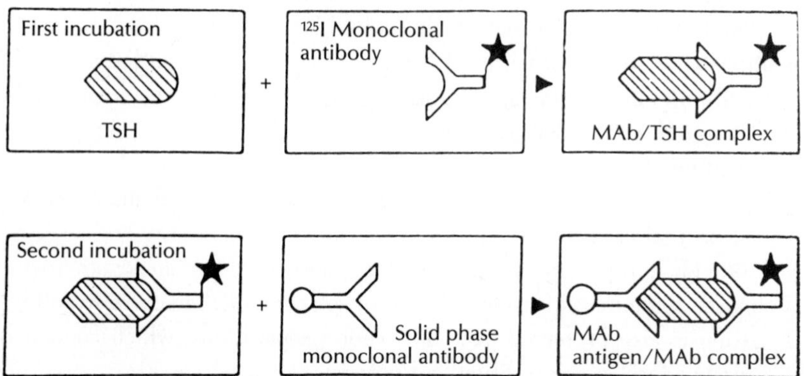

uptake. If the results of the sensitive TSH test are normal, no further testing is necessary. A potential strategy for the use of the sensitive serum TSH assay for laboratory investigation of thyroid function is shown in Fig. 50-3.

The sensitive serum TSH test can generally replace the TRH test and is much more convenient to perform. Another major use of the sensitive serum TSH test is to monitor the T_4-replacement dose in patients treated for hypothyroidism. Evidence of tissue hyperthyroidism has been reported in hypothyroid patients receiving T_4-replacement therapy. The optimal T_4 dosage is that which reduces the serum TSH concentration to the normal range, not below.

General aspects of antithyroid agents

There are several classes of drugs that act directly on the thyroid gland to depress function.

INHIBITORS OF ORGANIC IODINE FORMATION

The most important drugs in this class are the thioureylenes (propylthiouracil, methimazole, and carbimazole) that are used clinically to treat Graves disease and are discussed in detail below. Miscellaneous agents that inhibit organic iodine formation when administered in vivo include resorcinol, *p*-aminosalicylic acid, aminotriazole, and derivatives of sulfanilamide.

INHIBITORS OF IODIDE TRANSPORT

Perchlorate and thiocyanate inhibit I^- concentration by the thyroid, as well as by other tissues that actively concentrate I^- (salivary and mammary glands, gastric mucosa).

FIG. 50-3 *Potential strategy for use of sensitive thyrotropin (TSH) immunoradiometric assay (IRMA) for laboratory investigation of thyroid function.*

From Klee GG, Hay ID: Mayo Clin Proc 63:1123, 1988.

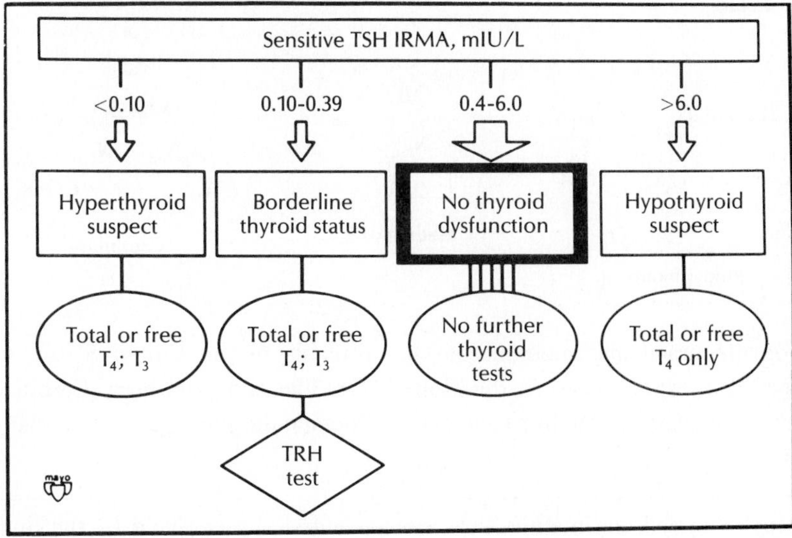

IODIDE

In large doses, I^- inhibits hormone release from the thyroid, especially in patients with Graves disease. This effect is believed to involve inhibition of thyroglobulin endocytosis, possibly through an influence on the adenylyl cyclase system. Pharmacologic doses of I^- may also greatly decrease the rate of thyroid hormone synthesis, possibly through inhibition of peroxidase-catalyzed iodination. The antithyroid effects of I^- are somewhat paradoxical in view of the fact that a smaller intake of I^- is essential for thyroid hormone biosynthesis. In patients with Graves disease who are undergoing treatment with large doses of I^-, the combined effects of iodide-mediated inhibition of hormone synthesis and secretion usually lead to an abrupt and striking improvement in symptoms. Within a few weeks, however, these beneficial effects disappear, and so I^- alone is not generally used for long-term therapy. It is very useful, however, in preparation of patients for surgical removal of the thyroid (see p. 582).

RADIO-LABELED IODINE

Because I^- is so greatly concentrated in the thyroid, large doses of $^{131}I^-$ can provide sufficient internal radiation to destroy thyroid tissue. This procedure is widely used to treat Graves disease. Smaller doses of $^{131}I^-$, or preferably of the more short-lived $^{123}I^-$, can be used diagnostically for thyroid uptake tests or for thyroid scintiscans.

Thioureylene drugs

STRUCTURE

The development of the thioureylene drugs in the 1940s was based on earlier studies of naturally occurring antithyroid substances in plants. The first drug to receive clinical trials for treatment of Graves disease was thiourea. More extensive tests were soon performed with thiouracil, but its use led to a significant incidence of agranulocytosis. The continued search for antithyroid compounds with high clinical effectiveness but minimal side effects led to development of **propylthiouracil** and soon thereafter to **methimazole** (1-methyl-2-mercaptoimidazole) and its carbethoxy derivative, **carbimazole**.

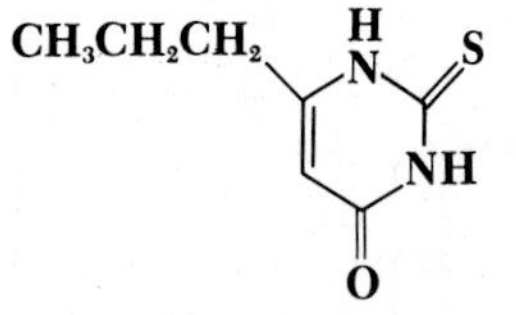

$CH_3CH_2CH_2$ H N S NH O

Propylthiouracil

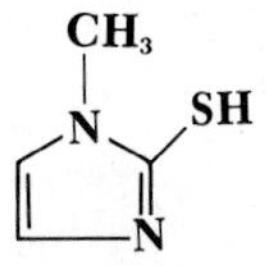

CH_3 N SH N

Methimazole

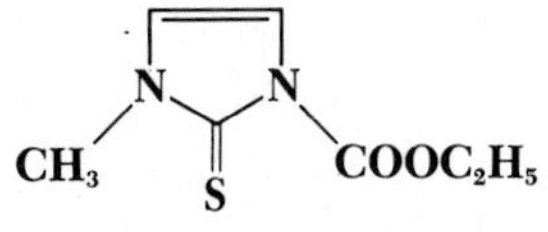

N N CH_3 S $COOC_2H_5$

Carbimazole

Propylthiouracil and methimazole are available in the United States, whereas carbimazole is widely used in the United Kingdom and elsewhere. Carbimazole is rapidly metabolized to methimazole and for therapeutic purposes is essentially identical to it.

MECHANISM OF ACTION

Propylthiouracil and methimazole are concentrated severalfold by the thyroid, in which they inhibit thyroid peroxidase-catalyzed iodination of thyroglobulin. They compete with tyrosyl residues of thyroglobulin for the active iodinating agent I^+ (see Fig. 50-1), which is also a potent drug oxidant. Additional inhibitory mechanisms may involve inactivation of thyroid peroxidase and direct inhibition of the coupling reaction. The thioureylene drugs, unlike perchlorate and thiocyanate, do not inhibit active I^- transport.

When given in sufficient doses, thioureylene drugs may completely prevent hormone formation in the thyroid. These drugs therefore are commonly used in the research laboratory to produce "chemical thyroidectomy" in rats; plasma T_4 and T_3 are reduced to very low concentrations, thus greatly increasing TSH secretion by the pituitary. This causes considerable enlargement of the thyroid, but the goitrous gland remains essentially unable to secrete hormones as long as the drug is continued. The therapeutic aim in humans, of course, is not to eliminate hormone secretion but to reduce it to a normal rate. Overtreatment and undertreatment are both to be avoided.

CLINICAL PHARMACOLOGY

Methimazole is approximately 10 times more potent than propylthiouracil. The usual starting dose for methimazole (Tapazole) is 30 to 60 mg per day, whereas that for propylthiouracil is 300 to 600 mg daily. The average dosage required to maintain the euthyroid state is 5 to 20 mg daily for methimazole and 50 to 200 mg per day for propylthiouracil. The choice of drug and dosage depend on several factors. Propylthiouracil, but not methimazole, inhibits T_4 to T_3 conversion in peripheral tissues and may be selected for patients with more severe hyperthyroidism, in whom more rapid improvement is sought. With both drugs several weeks are usually required to reach a euthyroid state. It has generally been recommended that propylthiouracil and methimazole be given in divided doses (3 or 4 times daily) based on their short half-lives in plasma. However, it is the half-life in the thyroid that determines the biologic effect of these agents, and it is now accepted that a majority of patients can be well controlled with once-a-day therapy, especially with methimazole.

Propylthiouracil is about 75% bound to protein in plasma, whereas methimazole displays little or no binding. This explains, at least partly, why propylthiouracil crosses the placenta less readily and is less readily secreted into maternal milk. Based on these observations, propylthiouracil has been favored over methimazole in the management of Graves disease in pregnancy and, though best avoided, during lactation.[1]

Although thioureylene drugs are definitive therapy for Graves disease, only 40% to 50% of patients so treated remain in remission when the drug is withdrawn after a 12- to 18-month course of treatment. To explain this observation, it has been proposed that, in addition to the mechanism described above, thioureylene drugs exert an immunosuppressive action localized to thyroid gland lymphocytes and that successful long-range treatment depends on this action. Many tests have been used at the end of treatment (including suppression tests, TRH stimulation tests, and measurement of TSH antibodies in serum) to try to predict which patients will relapse; so far these have met with only limited success. For patients who relapse, subtotal thyroidectomy or treatment with $^{131}I^-$ may be used. Indeed, many thyroidologists prefer primary treatment with $^{131}I^-$ or surgery. Many factors, beyond the scope of this chapter, enter into the choice of antithyroid drugs, $^{131}I^-$, or surgery as the primary mode of therapy for a given patient with Graves disease.

In addition to their use for definitive therapy, thioureylene drugs are frequently used to prepare hyperthyroid patients for surgical removal of the gland. After the patient is made euthyroid by the drugs, iodine in the form of Lugols solution is administered daily for 1 to 2 weeks before surgery. The addition of iodine reduces the vascularity and friability of the gland and facilitates the surgical procedure.

β-Adrenergic antagonists

It has been recognized for many years that some of the abnormalities of hyperthyroidism bear a resemblance to overstimulation of the sympathetic nervous system; these include tachycardia, palpitations, tremor, sweating, nervousness, and irritability. It is a common belief that the myocardium in patients with hyperthyroidism is hypersensitive to catecholamines.

When sympatholytic agents were introduced into medicine, they were tested for their effects in hyperthyroid patients. Reserpine was first used, then guanethidine, and most recently more specific β-adrenergic antagonists. Clinically, propranolol and other β-blockers produce prompt and pronounced improvement in symptoms of hyperthyroidism. These drugs are generally used as adjuncts to more definitive therapy, such as thioureylenes, to provide symptomatic relief until the patient reaches a euthyroid state.

Propranolol has no direct action on the thyroid, and its inhibitory effect on T_4 to T_3 conversion requires larger doses than those that are effective in relieving symptoms of hyperthyroidism. The mechanism of its action is still under investigation. There is evidence that excess thyroid hormone increases the number of β-adrenergic receptors in the myocardium. This could account for amelioration of cardiac symptoms by propranolol in hyperthyroid patients. However, in liver and in adipose tissue, thyroid hormones act in some other manner to modulate the effects of β-receptor activation.

Perchlorate

Perchlorate is a potent inhibitor of the iodide-concentrating mechanism of the thyroid. It has been tested as treatment of Graves disease. Although perchlorate is very effective in decreasing excessive hormone production, its therapeutic use has been limited by rare but serious side effects, including aplastic anemia.

Perchlorate discharges inorganic I^- previously accumulated by the thyroid. This property makes it useful for diagnosis of defects in organic iodine formation in the thyroid. In such conditions, radioiodine accumulated by the thyroid remains largely in the form of inorganic I^-, whereas ordinarily radioiodide is rapidly bound to thyroglobulin (see Fig. 50-1). Discharge by perchlorate of an appreciable fraction of the radioiodine previously accumulated in the gland is diagnostic for an iodination defect.

Lithium

Lithium carbonate has been used successfully to treat manic-depressive psychosis. It inhibits thyroid-hormone release, probably through inhibition of the adenylyl cyclase system, and chronic use may lead to hypothyroidism.

REFERENCES

1. Cooper DS: Antithyroid drugs, *N Engl J Med* 311:1353, 1984.
2. Evans RM: The steroid and thyroid hormone receptor family, *Science* 240:889, 1988.
3. Kaplan MM, Hamburger JI: Nonthyroidal causes of abnormal thyroid function test data, *J Clin Immunoassay* 12:90, 1989.
4. Samuels HH, Forman BM, Horowitz ZD, Ye Z-S: Regulation of gene expression by thyroid hormone, *J Clin Invest* 81:957, 1988.

GENERAL REFERENCES

Braverman LE, Utiger RD, editors: *Werner's the thyroid: a fundamental and clinical text*, ed 6, Philadelphia, JB Lippincott Co, in press.

DeGroot LJ, Besser GM, Cahill GF Jr, et al, editors: *Endocrinology*, ed 2, vol 1, part III: Thyroid gland, Philadelphia, 1989, WB Saunders Co, p 505.

Larsen PR: The thyroid gland. In Wilson JD, Foster DW, editors: *Williams textbook of endocrinology*, ed 8, Philadelphia, WB Saunders Co, in press.

Chapter 51

Parathyroid hormone and vitamin D

GENERAL CONCEPT

The concentration of ionized calcium in plasma is maintained by several mechanisms, including absorption from the intestine, rapid exchange with bone calcium, and excretion by the kidney. Parathyroid hormone and vitamin D have major roles in calcium homeostasis. A fall in plasma Ca^{++} concentration promotes parathyroid secretion, whereas a rise in the concentration inhibits secretion.

Control of Ca^{++} concentration in blood is important for many physiologic processes, and abnormal concentrations occur in malignancies, hyperparathyroidism, and several other disease states. Hypercalcemia can be treated with furosemide and saline, phosphate, calcitonin, plicamycin, or glucocorticoids. Hypocalcemia is treated with calcium salts or with vitamin D and related agents.

Several important discoveries led to understanding of the role of vitamin D in bone metabolism. The first was the discovery that rickets, a disease associated with abnormalities of calcium homeostasis and skeletal deformities, could be prevented by a component of cod liver oil. This component was later discovered to be cholecalciferol, or vitamin D_3. A second discovery was that rickets could be reversed or prevented by exposure to ultraviolet light; this led to the concept that the active vitamin was formed by ultraviolet irradiation of a precursor found in skin and in certain foods.[5] Finally, it was noted that patients with kidney failure could not adequately regulate blood Ca^{++} or utilize calcium from the diet. It is now established that vitamin D must be hydroxylated in both the liver and kidney and that *calcitriol*, the active form, then circulates to bone and other target cells.

PARATHYROID HORMONE

Parathyroid hormone (PTH) is an 84 amino acid polypeptide that, like insulin, is derived from a prohormone (proparathyroid hormone), which in turn is produced by proteolytic cleavage of a *pre*prohormone.[8] The preprohormone and prohormone forms have little or no activity. Secretion of the active hormone by the parathyroid gland is under negative-feedback regulation by plasma Ca^{++} concentration and possibly by activated vitamin D_3.

Functions

Parathyroid hormone has three primary actions that regulate mineral homeostasis: it (1) promotes renal reabsorption of Ca^{++} and decreases reabsorption of phosphate, thereby regulating plasma concentrations of these ions, (2) stimulates conversion of vitamin D_3 to calcitriol, the major regulator of intestinal absorption of Ca^{++} and phosphate,[1,3] and (3) mobilizes calcium and phosphate from bone. The last action does not require the kidney; it is promoted by parathyroid extract in nephrectomized animals. Furthermore, parathyroid transplants can cause local bone resorption. Hyperparathyroidism in humans results in loss of bone density and an increased prevalence of vertebral fractures.

Calcium ion homeostasis

A variety of factors act in concert to maintain extracellular Ca^{++} concentration within narrow limits. Approximately 1 g of calcium is ingested daily with a normal diet. Absorption of dietary calcium is enhanced by calcitriol and is affected indirectly by formation of calcitriol by parathyroid hormone. Ca^{++} homeostasis is directed toward prevention of hypocalcemia, which can cause life-threatening tetany. Thus, when dietary calcium is insufficient or intestinal absorption is depressed, the combination of parathyroid hormone release with its independent effects in concert with increased formation of activated vitamin D mobilizes bone calcium. Antacids containing aluminum promote Ca^{++} absorption indirectly, by binding and reducing absorption of phosphate from the intestine; hypophosphatemia then enhances formation of calcitriol. In contrast, dietary phosphate, oxalate, and phytate form nonabsorbable salts with Ca^{++}.

Extracellular Ca^{++} is in equilibrium with the exchangeable calcium of bone. When the extracellular concentration falls, release of exchangeable bone calcium helps to return it toward normal. In addition, renal reabsorption of Ca^{++} and excretion of phosphate help to buffer the hypocalcemia.

Hypercalcemia is frequently associated with malignant disease, and it can occur in primary hyperparathyroidism as well. The discovery of a tumor-derived polypeptide of 36 amino acids with significant homology to parathyroid hormone suggests that the humoral hypercalcemia of many malignancies and that of hyperparathyroidism may be produced by similar mechanisms involving kidney and bone.[14]

CALCITONIN

Calcitonin (thyrocalcitonin) is a second peptide hormone that affects calcium homeostasis, but a physiologic role in adult mammals has not been demonstrated. Calcitonin is a 32 amino acid polypeptide secreted by the parafollicular (C) cells of the thyroid. By directly inhibiting bone resorption calcitonin produces hypocalcemia, an effect more apparent in children and in patients treated with calcitonin for Pagets disease than in normal adults.

Calcitonin is normally present in blood, and its concentration increases when Ca^{++} concentration is excessive (>90 μg/ml), for example, after eating or when calcium salts are administered. Calcitonin release by Ca^{++} is greatly enhanced in patients with medullary carcinoma of the thyroid.

Synthetic salmon calcitonin (Calcimar, Miacalcin) is used clinically to treat Pagets disease[7] and hypercalcemia, and it has been tried unsuccessfully in postmenopausal osteoporosis. Resistance may develop with continued administration, especially in patients who have a high antibody titer to the polypeptide. Adverse reactions include allergic responses, nausea, vomiting, and inflammation at injection sites. This preparation is available for subcutaneous or intramuscular administration, 100 or 200 IU/ml. Depending on the indication, injections are given at 6- to 48-hour intervals. Synthetic human calcitonin (Cibacalcin) is now available (in vials containing 0.5 mg with mannitol) for subcutaneous administration to patients with Pagets disease. Hypersensitivity reactions and loss of effectiveness due to formation of antibodies are not usually a problem with the synthetic peptide.

VITAMIN D

Current Nomenclature

It was discovered more than 40 years ago that irradiation of plant sterols formed antirachitic compounds. What was originally called "vitamin D_1" was a mixture of products. The active sterol produced by irradiation of ergosterol became known as "vitamin D_2," or *ergocalciferol.* The vitamin produced in skin by irradiation of 7-dehydrocholesterol[9] was named "vitamin D_3," or *cholecalciferol.* Fish liver oils, eggs, and milk also contain this form. Vitamin D must be activated by metabolism, and most of the vitamin in circulation is in the form of metabolites. Vitamin D_2, found in yeast, differs from vitamin D_3 only in having a double bond between C-22 and C-23 and a methyl group at position 24.

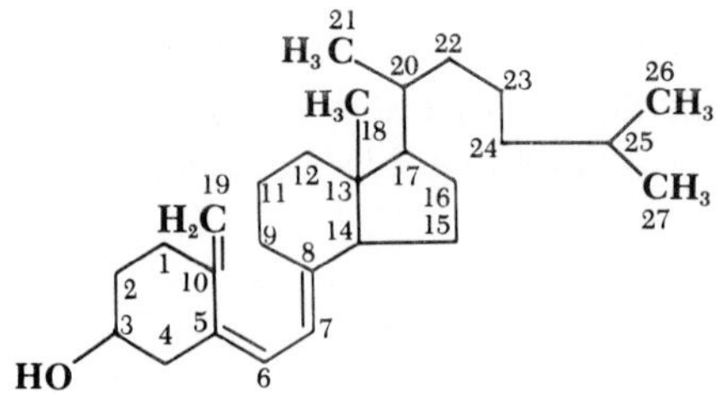

Vitamin D_3

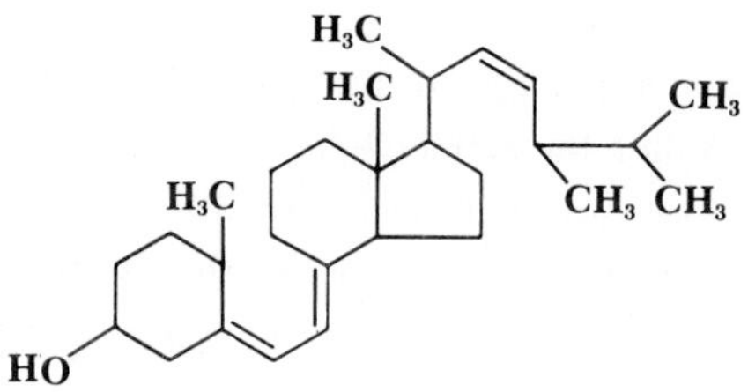

Dihydrotachysterol

Metabolic activation

Vitamin D_3 is hydroxylated in the C-25 position by microsomal and, in higher doses, mitochondrial enzymes in the liver. The former, but not the latter, metabolic pathway is under feedback inhibition by the product, 25-hydroxycholecalciferol, or *calcifediol,* which is bound in the circulation to a specific α-globulin. A second activating step occurs in the kidney where 25-hydroxycholecalciferol is hydroxylated to 1,25-dihydroxycholecalciferol, or calcitriol; this is the step stimulated by parathyroid hormone. Calcitriol, the most active form of vitamin D_3, can act on receptors in a wide variety of organs.[6] It has a half-life in plasma of 2 to 4 hours.[4] Vitamin D is now considered to be a true hormone that affects a number of different tissues, including the pituitary, skin, reproductive organs, and pancreas.[11]

Vitamin D_2 and **dihydrotachysterol**, a vitamin D analog, are also hydroxylated in the liver. The 25-hydroxy derivative of dihydrotachysterol, the active form, does not require further activation in the kidney. This drug, given in high doses, is much more effective than cholecalciferol in promoting bone resorption and is commonly used to treat hypoparathyroidism.

Functions

The classic function of vitamin D_3 is to promote absorption of Ca^{++} and phosphate from the intestine. Binding of the vitamin to intestinal receptors is believed to cause formation of calcium- and phosphate-binding proteins, which transport these ions across the intestinal mucosal cells.[4,12] In severe renal disease administration of calcitriol bypasses its lack of production by the failing kidney.

Vitamin D_3 potentiates the action of parathyroid hormone on release of calcium from bone,[4] and it may act in concert with parathyroid hormone to facilitate Ca^{++} reabsorption by the kidney. Its effects are depicted in Fig. 51-1. In the presence of sufficient plasma concentrations of Ca^{++} and phosphate, mineralization of bone proceeds without a direct influence of vitamin D_3.[4]

Additional roles for vitamin D_3 are assumed because it is found in keratinocytes of the skin and in bone marrow cells. It may play a role in insulin secretion, immunoregulation, and differentiation.[11] Several studies with malignant cells in culture indicate that the activated form of vitamin D_3 suppresses malignant growth and promotes differentiation into a benign phenotype.[5] In addition, some evidence suggests that activated vitamin D_3 modulates endocrine processes related to seasonal and daily biorhythms.[13]

The biologic actions of vitamin D_3 are mediated through a hormone-receptor complex that regulates gene expression in a manner similar to that of steroid hormones, such as estrogens, androgens, and glucocorticoids. As shown in Fig. 51-2, the steroid (S) is taken up by target cells where it interacts with a receptor (R); the

FIG. 51-1 *Hypercalcemic and hyperphosphatemic effects of calcitriol. The vitamin (1) mobilizes mineral from bone, (2) enhances intestinal absorption of Ca^{++} and phosphate, and (3) also augments renal tubular reabsorption of these ions. Maintenance of normal plasma Ca^{++} and phosphate concentrations allows mineralization of bone.*

From Popovtzer MM, Knochel JP. In Schrier RW, editor: Renal and electrolyte disorders, ed 3, Boston, 1986, Little, Brown & Co, p 251.

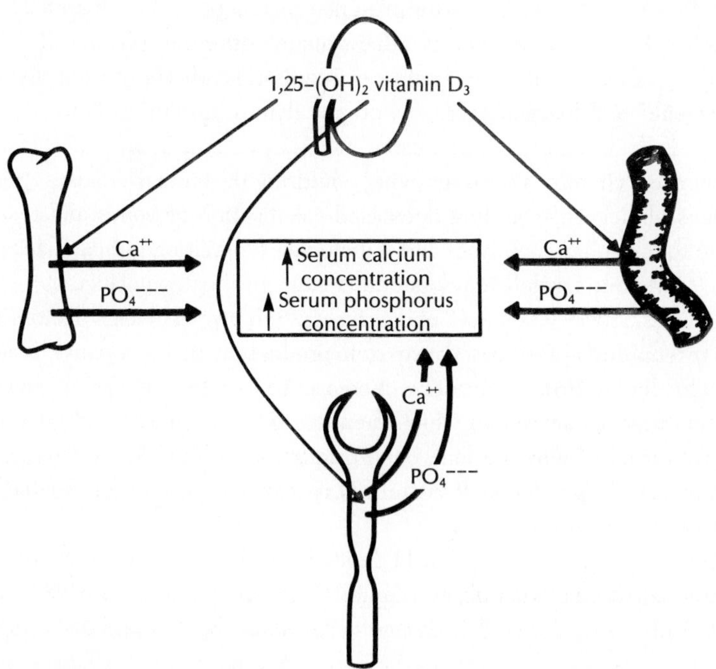

FIG. 51-2 From Norman AW: Physiologist 28:219, 1985.

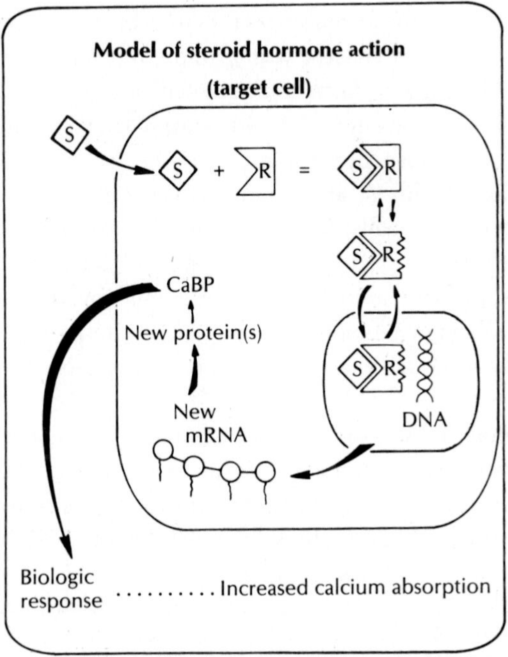

complex promotes DNA-directed synthesis of messenger RNA and synthesis of calcium-binding proteins (CaBP). The presence of receptors for vitamin D on many different cell types suggests that it affects many different physiologic processes. Recent studies indicate that the vitamin can regulate synthesis of such diverse products as oncogenes and lymphokines, as well as calcium-binding proteins.[11]

Vitamin D deficiency

Deficiency of vitamin D_3 in growing children or animals causes the various manifestations of rickets, including decreased calcification of bones and teeth. Bones may become soft; swollen epiphyses and radiologic examination indicate lack of normal calcification.[2] Vitamin D_3 deficiency in adults can cause osteomalacia.[10]

Abnormalities of the vitamin D endocrine system are suspected factors in development of osteoporosis. Decreased estrogen production in menopause is associated with loss of calcium from bone. The increase in circulating Ca^{++} concentration suppresses parathyroid secretion, which then decreases production of vitamin D_3. As Ca^{++} absorption falls below normal, bone calcium is utilized for soft tissue requirements. A defect in hydroxylation of vitamin D is suspected in the age-related decrease in Ca^{++} absorption and osteoporosis.[5]

The daily requirement for vitamin D depends on the calcium needs of the person. The international unit is 0.025 μg of vitamin D_3. Normal adults over 25 years of age require 200 units daily. Twice this dosage is recommended for infants, children, and

TABLE 51-1 Vitamin D preparations

Vitamin or product	Alternative name	Dosage forms (μg)
D_2 (Calciferol, Drisdol)	Ergocalciferol	C: 1250 (50,000 IU) I: 12500/ml (500,000 IU) S: 200/ml (8000 IU/ml) T: 1250 (50,000 IU)
D_3	Cholecalciferol	T: 10, 25 (400, 1000 IU)
Calcifediol (Calderol)	25-Hydroxycholecalciferol (25-hydroxy-vitamin D_3)	C: 20, 50
Calcitrol (Rocaltrol, Calcijex)	1,25-Dihydroxycholecalciferol (1,25-dihydroxy-vitamin D_3)	C: 0.25, 0.5; I: 1,2/ml
Dihydrotachysterol (DHT, Hytakerol)		C: 125; S: 40-250/ml T: 125-400

C, Capsules; *I*, injection; *IU*, international units; *S*, solution; *T*, tablets.

also pregnant or lactating women, to enhance Ca^{++} absorption. In treatment of hypoparathyroidism or refractory rickets, vitamin D_2 may be administered in very large doses (12,000 to 500,000 IU). Dihydrotachysterol may be given initially in doses of 0.8 to 2.4 mg (compared with 10 mg or more of vitamin D_2); for maintenance a dose of 0.2 to 1 mg/day is usually sufficient. The vitamin may be administered in the form of fish liver oils or as the preparations listed in Table 51-1. Vitamin D_2 and calcitriol are also formulated for injection.

Drug Interactions

Phenobarbital and phenytoin can increase microsomal hydroxylase activity in the liver. Development of rickets or osteomalacia in patients taking anticonvulsants may be a consequence of increased enzymatic transformation of vitamin D_2 or D_3 to inactive metabolites or, alternatively, of direct inhibition of Ca^{++} absorption or decreased tissue sensitivity to the vitamin.[8]

TOXIC EFFECTS OF PARATHYROID HORMONE AND VITAMIN D

Toxic effects of parathyroid injection and of vitamin D are manifested as (1) hypercalcemia with numerous clinical consequences, (2) demineralization of bone, and (3) renal calculi and metastatic calcifications of soft tissue.

Clinical indications of hypercalcemia include anorexia, vomiting, diarrhea, fatigue, and lack of muscle tone. Electrocardiographic changes can occur, as shown in Fig. 51-3. Serious toxic manifestations may be seen at a concentration of 150 μg/ml (15 mg/dl). Signs of hypocalcemia are tetany, cataracts, and mental lethargy.

OTHER DRUGS THAT INFLUENCE PLASMA CALCIUM ION CONCENTRATION

Phosphates, sodium sulfate, sodium citrate, and **edetate disodium** (Endrate, others), when given by intravenous infusion, lower blood Ca^{++} concentration. Their administration should not be undertaken without consideration of potential adverse effects.

Glucocorticoids antagonize the effects of vitamin D on Ca^{++} absorption in the intestine. They are useful in hypercalcemia caused by sarcoidosis, certain neoplastic

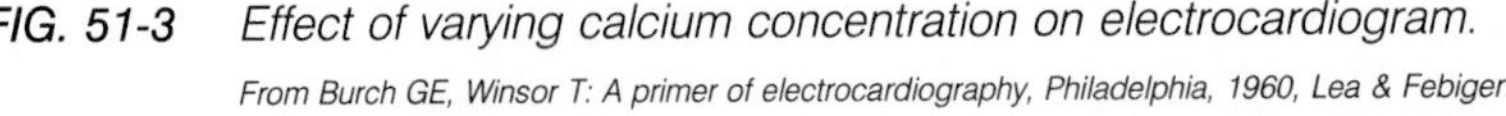

FIG. 51-3 *Effect of varying calcium concentration on electrocardiogram.*
From Burch GE, Winsor T: A primer of electrocardiography, Philadelphia, 1960, Lea & Febiger.

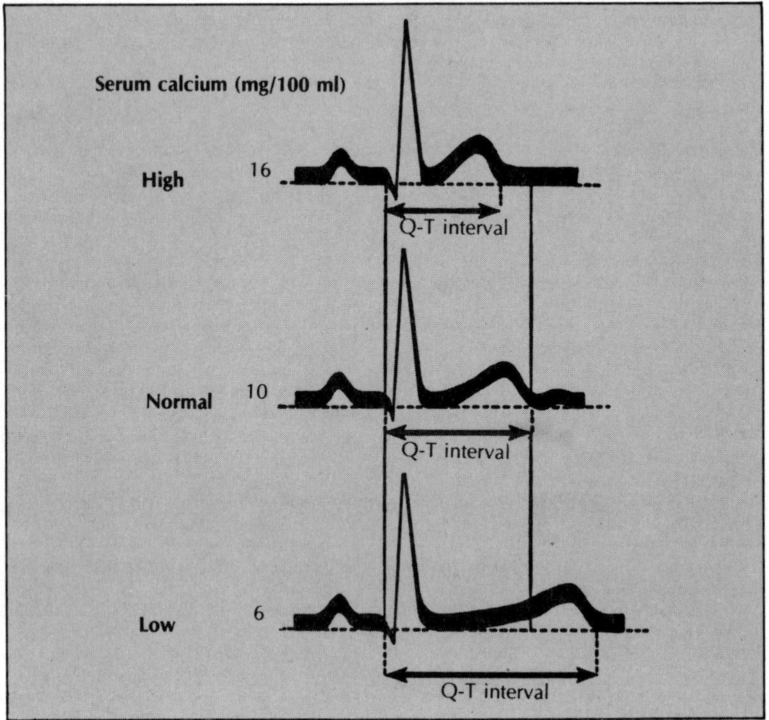

diseases such as lymphomas and myelomas, and hypervitaminosis D.

Etidronate is a diphosphonate used in treatment of Pagets disease and more recently in control of hypercalcemia secondary to malignancy.[15] It seems to slow both osteoclastic and osteoblastic activity. The drug can cause hyperphosphatemia and diarrhea and may increase arthalgia. Etidronate disodium (EHDP, Didronel) is available in tablets of 200 and 400 mg and in 6 ml ampules containing 300 mg for dilution and intravenous injection.

Loop diuretics, such as **furosemide**, tend to promote Ca^{++} excretion, whereas **thiazides** have the opposite effect and may cause hypercalcemia.

Plicamycin (mithromycin, Mithracin), an antibiotic used to treat testicular neoplasms, lowers Ca^{++} concentration, perhaps by a toxic effect on osteoclasts. It has been used successfully to treat Pagets disease and for chronic management of the hypercalcemia of malignancy.

For the initial treatment of *hypocalcemia*, an intravenous infusion of a 10% solution of **calcium gluconate** (Kalcinate) is highly effective. **Calcium gluceptate** may also be given, intramuscularly as well as intravenously. Salts used orally include calcium gluconate, glubionate, lactate, citrate, carbonate, and dibasic and tribasic calcium phosphate.

REFERENCES

1. Agus ZS, Wasserstein A, Goldfarb S: PTH, calcitonin, cyclic nucleotides and the kidney, *Annu Rev Physiol* 43:583, 1981.
2. Anast CS, Carpenter TO, Key LL: Rickets. In Krieger DT, Bardin CW, editors: *Current therapy in endocrinology and metabolism*, 1985-1986, St Louis, 1985, Mosby–Year Book, p 310.
3. Cohn DV, Kumarasamy R, Ramp WK: Intracellular processing and secretion of parathyroid gland proteins, *Vitam Horm* 43:283, 1986.
4. DeLuca HF: The metabolism, physiology, and function of vitamin D. In Kumar R, editor: *Vitamin D: basic and clinical aspects*, Boston, 1984, Martinus Nijhoff Publishing, p 1.
5. DeLuca HF: The vitamin D story: a collaborative effort of basic science and clinical medicine, *FASEB J* 2:224, 1988.
6. Haussler MR: Vitamin D receptors: nature and function, *Annu Rev Nutr* 6:527, 1985.
7. Horwith M: Paget's disease of bone. In Krieger DT, Bardin CW, editors: *Current therapy in endocrinology and metabolism,* 1985-1986, St Louis, Mosby–Year Book Co, p 350.
8. Kronenberg HM, Igarashi T, Freeman MW, et al: Structure and expression of the human parathyroid hormone gene, *Recent Prog Horm Res* 42:641, 1986.
9. Lawson DEM, Davie M: Aspects of the metabolism and function of vitamin D, *Vitam Horm* 37:1, 1979.
10. Marks J: *The vitamins: their role in medical practice*, Lancaster, 1985, MTP Press Ltd.
11. Minghetti PP, Norman AW: 1,25$(OH)_2$-Vitamin D_3 receptors: gene regulation and genetic circuitry, *FASEB J* 2:3043, 1988.
12. Norman AW: The vitamin D endocrine system, *Physiologist* 28:219, 1985.
13. Stumpf WE, Privette TH: Light, vitamin D and psychiatry: role of 1,25 dihydroxyvitamin D_3 (soltriol) in etiology and therapy of seasonal affective disorder and other mental processes, *Psychopharmacology* 97:285, 1989.
14. Suva LJ, Winslow GA, Wettenhall REH, et al: A parathyroid hormone–related protein implicated in malignant hypercalcemia: cloning and expression, *Science* 237:893, 1987.
15. Symposium: Etidronate disodium: a new therapy for hypercalcemia of malignancy, *Am J Med* 82(2A), 1987.

Chapter 52

Posterior pituitary hormones—vasopressin and oxytocin

The posterior lobe of the pituitary gland, the neurohypophysis, contains hormones with vasoactive, antidiuretic, and oxytocic properties. Based on these activities, neurohypophyseal extracts were originally separated into two fractions; one contained most of the vasoactive and antidiuretic activities, and the other was predominantly oxytocic. Later, two peptide hormones were isolated: vasopressin (antidiuretic hormone) was responsible for the vasoactive and antidiuretic actions, and oxytocin caused uterine contractions.

The posterior pituitary probably contains other peptide hormones as well. A peptide similar to oxytocin is released by administration of estrogen in humans,[1] and endothelin, a potent vasoconstrictor originally isolated from vascular endothelial cells, has been identified in the posterior pituitary by histochemical methods.[14] The roles of these peptides in normal physiology and their relation to the more well known hormones vasopressin and oxytocin remains uncertain.

CHEMISTRY

Vasopressin and oxytocin are nonapeptides composed of a six-member disulfide ring with a tripeptide tail, amidated at the carboxyl end. As shown below, they have similar amino acid sequences. The hormones from most other animal species are identical, but vasopressin from hog pituitary has lysine instead of arginine in the tripeptide tail.

Cys-Tyr-Phe-Gln-Asn-Cys-Pro-Arg-GlyNH_2

Vasopressin (human)

Cys-Tyr-Ile-Gln-Asn-Cys-Pro-Leu-GlyNH_2

Oxytocin

Various synthetic derivatives of these hormones made it possible to identify their tissue receptors and to define their biologic actions. Some of them also have clinical application.[13]

SYNTHESIS AND SECRETION

Vasopressin and oxytocin are synthesized in hypothalamic structures, in separate cells of the supraoptic and paraventricular nuclei. They form insoluble complexes with carrier proteins (neurophysins) and are transported to the neurohypophysis via axons from the hypothalamus. They are stored in nerve terminals until released by an appropriate stimulus. Both hormones are produced in a larger (prohormone) form that is cleaved by proteolytic enzymes in neurosecretory granules of the pituitary cells. Secretion is thought to involve a Ca^{++}-dependent exocytotic process.[13]

VASOPRESSIN

The hormone responsible for decreasing urine output was originally purified from the posterior pituitary with use of a bioassay on rat blood pressure. Because it increased blood pressure, it was named *vasopressin*. Studies with various synthetic analogs of vasopressin showed that the pressor and antidiuretic actions can be altered independently and are mediated by two different types of receptors.[13]

Stimulus for secretion

Vasopressin secretion is influenced by a number of factors. Osmolarity of the extracellular fluid, which affects receptors in certain areas of the hypothalamus, is a primary determinant of secretion.[2] Dilution of extracellular fluid inhibits vasopressin secretion; hyperosmolarity promotes its secretion.

Hemodynamic variables such as change in blood pressure or volume influence vasopressin secretion, presumably through neurogenic mechanisms. Exercise, pain, and emotional excitement also inhibit water diuresis, probably by affecting central control of vasopressin release. The release of vasopressin that contributes to hyponatremia in diseases such as congestive heart failure, cirrhosis, or the nephrotic syndrome appears to be mediated by the autonomic nervous system.

Nausea is a potent stimulus for vasopressin secretion. Because drugs such as apomorphine, morphine, and nicotine can cause a similar response, the pathway probably includes the chemoreceptor trigger zone in the medulla. Vasopressin release also occurs in motion sickness.[13]

A cholinergic mechanism for vasopressin release was indicated by the demonstration that release followed injection of acetylcholine or isoflurophate (DFP) into supraoptic nuclei. There is considerable interest in the regulatory role of endogenous opioid peptides and other mediators in vasopressin secretion.[4] Antidiuresis after general anesthesia or injection of histamine, morphine, or barbiturates (but not thiopental) has been attributed to release of vasopressin.

Alcohol inhibits release of vasopressin in response to dehydration and produces inappropriate water diuresis in a dehydrated individual. Alcohol does not block the action of nicotine on vasopressin release. Phenytoin can also block release of vasopressin and has been used therapeutically in cases of inappropriate hormone secretion.

Receptors

Synthetic analogs of vasopressin were used to define biologic activities of the peptide and to identify its specific receptors. Receptors on blood vessels, platelets, and liver cells were classified as V_1-receptors. Enhancement of phosphatidylinositol metabolism through stimulation of these receptors may explain such diverse actions as vascular contraction, platelet aggregation, and glycogenolysis. Other effects of vasopressin, the increase in water reabsorption and release of coagulation factor VIII, are mediated by cyclic AMP-dependent V_2-receptors. *Desmopressin*, an analog of arginine vasopressin, is a highly selective agonist for V_2-receptors and is used clinically to treat diabetes insipidus and bleeding disorders.[13] As predicted from the structural similarities, oxytocin is an agonist for vasopressin receptors, but it is much less potent than vasopressin.[6]

Physiologic and pharmacologic effects

The only clearly established physiologic function of vasopressin is its action on the kidney. The hormone conserves body water by reducing the output of urine. This antidiuretic action occurs through an increase in the size or number of channels for flow of water along osmotic gradients in the distal tubules and collecting ducts to increase reabsorption of water. In isolated systems, such as the toad urinary bladder, vasopressin acts through V_2-receptors to activate adenylyl cyclase in the serosal membrane of epithelial cells.[8] In physiologic doses, however, the hormone does not influence electrolyte absorption. Fig. 52-1 shows how vasopressin (ADH) controls reabsorption of water in epithelia.

Vasopressin has a potent action on vascular smooth muscle, but for many years its diuretic action overshadowed the vascular effects. This was due in part to the fact that much higher doses of injected vasopressin are required to raise blood pressure than to enhance water reabsorption. Later studies indicated that sufficient circulating hormone can affect blood pressure as well as urine output.[7]

FIG. 52-1 *View of a collecting duct cell or an amphibian bladder granular cell. ADH (vasopressin) activates adenylyl cyclase,* AD Cyc, *at the basolateral membrane. The cyclic AMP generated stimulates a protein kinase. Ultimately, cytoplasmic tubules fuse with the luminal membrane and deliver particles to the membrane* (A, B, *and* C). *These particles are believed to conduct water. Elements of the terminal web and tight junction are included, as well as a large subluminal granule,* Gr.

Modified from Hays RM, Sasaki J, Tilles SM, et al: In Schrier RW, editor: Vasopressin, New York, 1985, Raven Press.

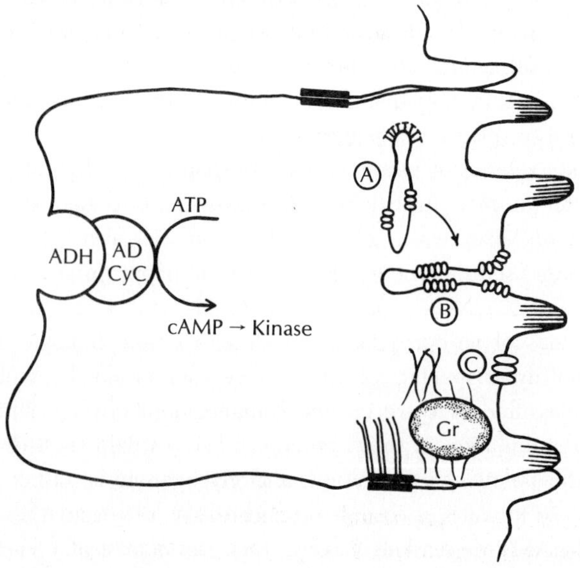

Vasoconstriction via V_1-receptors does not involve cyclic AMP but appears linked to increases in phosphatidylinositol turnover and intracellular Ca^{++} concentration (see Chapter 3). This vasoconstrictive action is used therapeutically to decrease gastrointestinal bleeding, particularly in patients with esophageal varices.

There is considerable interest in the role of vasopressin in neurotransmission.[3] Studies with the Brattleboro rat, a strain genetically deficient in vasopressin, have been useful in exploring this possibility.

Vasopressin increases the concentration of circulating factor VIII in patients with hemophilia A or with von Willebrands disease,[11] provided that the concentration of factor VIII is at least 5% of normal before treatment.

Pathologic conditions involving vasopressin

A lack of vasopressin produces *diabetes insipidus*, which is characterized by failure of water reabsorption in the collecting duct. In the absence of vasopressin this distal tubular epithelium resists diffusion of water as well as solutes, and the hypotonic filtrate from more proximal nephron sites is excreted unchanged. Persons with this condition excrete copious amounts of dilute urine (polyuria) and drink large quantities of fluids (polydipsia).

Chlorpropamide (see p. 568) is used to increase the potency of vasopressin in diabetes insipidus of central origin.[12] Because chlorpropamide increases the response of the nephron to vasopressin, it is more likely to be useful in moderate forms of the disease. Thiazide diuretics, in contrast, are effective treatment in *nephrogenic* diabetes insipidus, in which the kidney is unresponsive to circulating vasopressin. The thiazides act, in part, by reducing the dilution of tubular fluid that normally occurs in the distal portion of the nephron (see Chapter 42). As a result, a less hypotonic urine is excreted. The mild degree of volume depletion that occurs causes a greater proportion of water to be reabsorbed with salt at more proximal sites, and urinary volume decreases. Na^+ intake must be concurrently restricted with thiazide therapy.

Certain hyponatremic syndromes are associated with inappropriately increased secretion of vasopressin. These conditions are characterized by primary water retention unassociated with Na^+ retention or edema. Underlying causes include a variety of cancers, neurologic disorders, and drugs.

The effect of vasopressin can be blocked at the level of the distal tubule and collecting duct. Lithium carbonate, in particular, and demeclocycline have been used to treat patients with hyponatremia and inappropriate release of vasopressin. Li^+ therapy may be associated with reversible nephrogenic diabetes insipidus (see p. 261). Development of specific antagonists to vasopressin might improve therapy for patients with hyponatremia.[9]

Antidiuretic preparations

The treatment of choice for diabetes insipidus is **desmopressin acetate** (1-desamino-8-D-arginine vasopressin, DDAVP), an analog with a longer action than the native peptide. It is highly selective for V_2-receptors and has much less effect on smooth muscle of the intestine, uterus, or blood vessels than vasopressin. Because desmopressin also induces release of factor VIII, it can be used for bleeding disorders as well.[13] For example, parenteral desmopressin may be administered before tooth extraction to minimize bleeding in patients with von Willebrands disease or hemophilia A.

Desmopressin is more resistant than vasopressin to degradation by peptidases. It is usually taken intranasally with a calibrated spray dispenser, as a solution containing 100 μg/ml. Its antidiuretic effect lasts 8 to 20 hours. The drug is also available for subcutaneous or intravenous injection (DDAVP; 4 μg/ml) for patients who are unable to take the drug intranasally. The parenteral route is preferable for prophylaxis in bleeding disorders, since higher doses are required for factor VIII release than for the antidiuretic effect.

Synthetic **lypressin** (8-lysine-vasopressin, Diapid) is administered by intranasal spray up to six times daily. It can cause adverse vasoconstriction even in therapeutic doses.

Vasopressin (8-arginine-vasopressin, Pitressin) is a synthetic preparation that produces an antidiuretic effect lasting 2 to 8 hours when administered subcutaneously or by intramuscular injection. The solution may also be applied intranasally. Vasopressin may cause fluid retention, hypertension, myocardial ischemia, gastrointestinal and uterine contraction, and allergic reactions. The solution available for injection contains 20 pressor units/ml.

Other vasopressin analogs. There are several other analogs of vasopressin. **Terlipressin** (Glypressin) is activated in the body to release 8-lysine-vasopressin. It has a slower onset of action than the native peptide and is used principally to control esophageal bleeding. It has the same effects as vasopressin on water reabsorption and on uterine and intestinal smooth muscle.

Felypressin is an analog with five times the vasopressor potency of vasopressin but with greatly reduced antidiuretic potency. It may have use as a local vasoconstrictor, particularly as an adjuvant to local anesthetics. One advantage of vasopressin analogs for this use is that, unlike epinephrine, they do not affect the autonomic nervous system.[13]

OXYTOCIN

Oxytocin is the peptide hormone responsible for the uterine smooth muscle–stimulating property of posterior pituitary extracts. It differs from vasopressin structurally only by substitution of isoleucine and leucine for phenylalanine and arginine, respectively, but it has several important functional differences. It is a potent stimulant of the gravid uterus at term and postpartum (Fig. 52-2). It also contracts myoepithelial cells of lacteal glands to produce milk letdown during nursing.[10]

Oxytocin has a weaker antidiuretic action than vasopressin but can cause water intoxication when given parenterally in a large volume of fluid.[5] It does not cause vasoconstriction, however, and may even lower blood pressure. In contrast to vasopressin, oxytocin has little effect on intestinal smooth muscle and coronary arteries.

Factors that regulate synthesis and release of oxytocin are less well defined than those for vasopressin. Because of its potent uterine stimulating action, various investigators have suggested a role for oxytocin in the onset of labor. Nursing is a postpartum stimulus for its release. Although some activities of oxytocin appear related to

Comparison of the uterine sensitivity of oxytocin throughout pregnancy in different species. *FIG. 52-2*

From Dawood MY: In Amico JA, Robinson AG, editors: Oxytocin: clinical and laboratory studies, Amsterdam, 1985, Excerpta Medica (Elsevier Science Publishers BV), p 391.

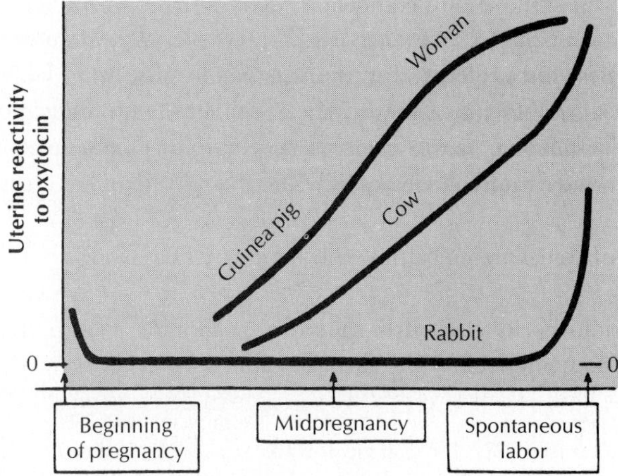

female reproduction, it probably has other, more general functions because males synthesize it as well.

Preparations

Oxytocin injection (Pitocin, Syntocinon; 10 units/ml) is a synthetic preparation infused intravenously to induce or enhance uterine contractions in labor. It may be administered intramuscularly, 10 units, or infused to control postpartum bleeding. For intravenous infusion, oxytocin, 10 to 40 units, is added to a liter of normal saline. To facilitate milk ejection, a nasal spray (Syntocinon; 40 units/ml) can be administered into one or both nostrils 2 to 3 minutes before nursing.

OTHER DRUGS THAT STIMULATE THE UTERUS

The uterus receives sympathetic and parasympathetic innervation. α_1-Adrenergic receptors mediate stimulation; β_2-receptors mediate inhibition. In addition, muscarinic receptors are stimulatory. Estrogens enhance uterine responsiveness, whereas progesterone decreases uterine tone and contraction.

In addition to oxytocin, drugs used to enhance uterine contractions include ergot compounds and prostaglandins. **Ergonovine** (Ergotrate) **maleate** and **methylergonovine maleate** (Methergine) decrease postpartum uterine bleeding. Administered after delivery of the placenta they stimulate uterine contraction, which clamps off the multiple sites of bleeding.

Prostaglandins are used to induce abortion by stimulation of uterine contractions. **Carboprost tromethamine** (Prostin/15 M; 250 μg/ml) is the 15-methyl derivative of prostaglandin $F_{2\alpha}$. It is injected intramuscularly and is effective from the thirteenth to the twentieth week of pregnancy. **Dinoprostone** (Prostin E2) is available in 20 mg vaginal suppositories. Frequent adverse reactions to these agents include nausea, vomiting, diarrhea, and fever.

UTERINE RELAXANTS

β-Adrenergic receptor agonists and prostaglandin synthesis inhibitors, such as indomethacin, promote relaxation of contracting uterine smooth muscle. The latter agents are widely used to treat dysmenorrhea, whereas β-receptor agonists are used to prevent premature delivery.

Ritodrine hydrochloride (Yutopar), which preferentially stimulates β_2-adrenergic receptors, is currently a preferred uterine relaxant in premature labor. The drug can cause such adverse effects as tachycardia and tremor. Contraindications include maternal eclampsia, cardiovascular problems, hyperthyroidism, and uncontrolled diabetes mellitus. Ritodrine is available in tablets of 10 mg and in an injectable form (10 mg/ml).

REFERENCES

1. Amico JA, Ervin MG, Leake RD, et al: A novel oxytocin-like and vasotocin-like peptide in human plasma after administration of estrogen, *J Clin Endocrinol Metab* 60:5, 1985.
2. Baylis PH, Robertson GL: Physiological control of vasopressin secretion. In Baylis PH, Padfield PL, editors: *The posterior pituitary: hormone secretion in health and disease*, New York, 1985, Marcel Dekker, Inc, p 119.
3. Buijs RM: Vasopressin and oxytocin: their role in neurotransmission, *Pharmacol Ther* 22:127, 1983.
4. Carter DA, Lightman SL: Neuroendocrine control of vasopressin secretion. In Baylis PH, Padfield PL, editors: *The posterior pituitary: hormone secretion in health and disease*, New York, 1985, Marcel Dekker, Inc, p 53.
5. Dawood MY: *Oxytocin*, vol 2, Montreal, 1984, Eden Press.
6. Fox AW: Vascular vasopressin receptors, *Gen Pharmacol* 19:639, 1988.
7. Goldsmith SR: Vasopressin as vasopressor, *Am J Med* 82:1213, 1987.
8. Goodman DBP, Davis W: The mode of action of antidiuretic hormone: membrane reorganization, recycling, and intracellular transport. In Reichlin S, editor: *The neurohypophysis: physiological and clinical aspects*, New York, 1984, Plenum Medical Book Co, p 51.
9. Kinter LB, Huffman WF, Stassen FL: Antagonists of the antidiuretic activity of vasopressin, *Am J Physiol* 254:F165, 1988.
10. Leake RD, Fisher DA: Oxytocin secretion and milk ejection in the human. In Amico JA, Robinson AG, editors: *Oxytocin: clinical and laboratory studies*, Amsterdam, 1985, Excerpta Medica (Elsevier Science Publishers BV), p 200.
11. Lusher JM, Warrier AI: dDAVP in von Hillebrand's disease and in moderately severe hemophilia A. In Reichlin S, editor: *The neurohypophysis: physiological and clinical aspects*, New York, 1984, Plenum Medical Book Co, p 201.
12. Moses AM: Drug-induced states of impaired water excretion. In Baylis PH, Padfield PL, editors: *The posterior pituitary: hormone secretion in health and disease*, New York, 1985, Marcel Dekker, Inc, p 227.
13. Robertson GL, Harris A: Clinical use of vasopressin analogues, *Hosp Pract* 24(10):114, 1989.
14. Yoshizawa T, Shinmi O, Giaid A, et al: Endothelin: a novel peptide in the posterior pituitary system, *Science* 247:462, 1990.

Chapter 53

Pharmacologic approaches to gout

GENERAL CONCEPTS

Gout is characterized by hyperuricemia and arthritis. The disease may be *primary*—caused by either overproduction or defective renal excretion of uric acid. The *secondary* form develops during some other disease such as leukemia, which results in overproduction, or is caused by drugs such as thiazide diuretics, which diminish excretion of uric acid. The thiazides interfere with secretion of uric acid and decrease its glomerular filtration consequent to volume depletion.

In general, patients with gout may be divided into those who overproduce uric acid and those who underexcrete it.[2,8] Daily excretion of more than 750 mg indicates overproduction.[8] Although the body pool of uric acid is only moderately increased in underexcretors, it is greatly increased in overproducers.

The pharmacologic approach to an acute attack of gout is different from management of the chronic disease. The acute attack is a form of arthritis that traditionally has been treated with *colchicine*. More recently, it has become apparent that virtually any of the nonsteroidal anti-inflammatory drugs (NSAIDs) can be used effectively.[2,4,9]

The aim of management of the chronic form of the disease is to reduce the uric acid content of the body. This can be accomplished with uricosuric drugs such as *probenecid* and *sulfinpyrazone* or by use of *allopurinol*, a xanthine oxidase inhibitor.[2] The latter may have advantages over the uricosuric drugs in some cases. It is important to realize that one treats *gout* and not *hyperuricemia*. For a patient who has gout, the concentration of uric acid in serum can be used as a guide in therapy. In contrast, an asymptomatic increase in plasma uric acid concentration that occurs in patients receiving thiazide diuretics or in those with diminished renal function is not an indication for therapy. Although a small number of patients with hyperuricemia from these causes will develop gout and need treatment, most will have no symptoms; data have shown that the elevated uric acid concentration presents no long-term risk such as urate nephropathy.[1,5-7]

COLCHICINE

Colchicine is an alkaloid obtained from *Colchicum autumnale*, the meadow saffron, a plant belonging to the lily family. *Colchicum* has been used for centuries for arthralgia that is presumably of gouty origin.

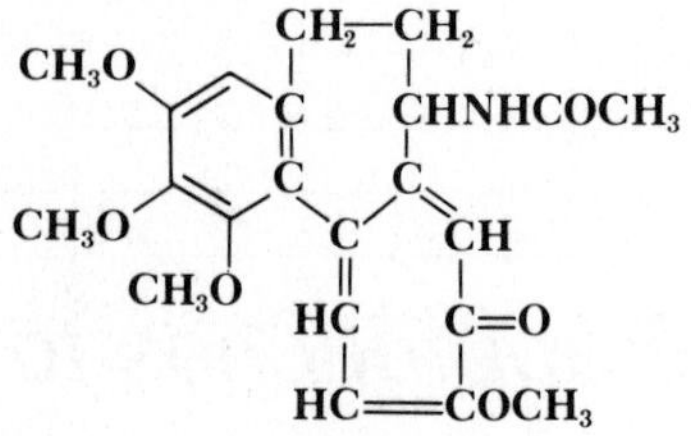

Colchicine

Colchicine is well absorbed from the gastrointestinal tract and has a short half-life in plasma. However, it may be retained in cells such as leukocytes. Also, since the kidney is an important route of elimination of this drug, patients with renal disease eliminate colchicine more slowly than normal persons do.

When colchicine is given in doses of 0.5 to 1 mg every hour to a patient having an attack of acute gouty arthritis, relief occurs in 2 to 3 hours. In severe attacks a somewhat longer period may be required. It is quite common for disturbances such as anorexia, nausea, vomiting, diarrhea, and abdominal pain to appear with about the same dosage as that required for relief. As a consequence, colchicine is administered every hour until relief is obtained or until significant gastrointestinal symptoms develop. Colchicine may also cause, though rarely, fever, alopecia, liver damage, and neural and hematopoietic complications.

Colchicine interferes with the microtubular system of cells.[3] In gout, it is believed that this action is exerted on leukocytes, which accumulate in affected joints and ingest the sharp urate crystals. It is quite possible, however, that the action of colchicine is also exerted on synovial cells.

In chronic gout the administration of colchicine has prophylactic value to reduce the incidence of acute exacerbations.[10] Colchicine is available as tablets, 0.5 or 0.6 mg, and for injection, 1 mg/2 ml.

NONSTEROIDAL ANTI-INFLAMMATORY DRUGS

NSAIDs (see Chapter 35) are replacing colchicine in management of acute gouty arthritis.[2,4,8,9] Phenylbutazone was first shown to be beneficial; four doses of 150 mg every 6 hours are usually sufficient. This drug currently is used infrequently, however, because it has been associated with bone marrow depression. It is important to note that this adverse effect is unlikely to occur with short-duration therapy of gout. Indomethacin can also be used, as an initial dose of 75 to 100 mg followed by 50 mg every 6 to 8 hours. After resolution of symptoms, the dose is tapered over 3 to 4 days. These doses of indomethacin can cause headache, light-headedness, and, less frequently, confusion and fluid retention.

Efficacy has also been demonstrated with other NSAIDs, and it is likely that all can be used. It is important to realize that NSAIDs with a short half-life will have a quicker onset and offset of action and may be preferable to longer-acting agents.

PROBENECID

Even if colchicine is taken chronically for prophylaxis of acute gouty arthritis, it is generally accepted that promotion of uric acid excretion through the use of uricosuric drugs or reduction in synthesis with allopurinol is beneficial in the gouty patient. The most effective uricosuric agents are probenecid and sulfinpyrazone.

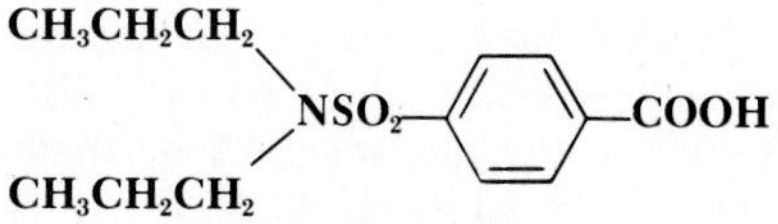

$$(CH_3CH_2CH_2)_2NSO_2-C_6H_4-COOH$$

Probenecid

Renal handling of uric acid involves glomerular filtration, tubular reabsorption, and tubular secretion (Fig. 53-1). Low doses of organic anions such as probenecid itself, salicylates, or other NSAIDs cause retention of uric acid. It is likely that in small doses these anions compete with uric acid for secretion, thereby decreasing excretion and increasing plasma concentration; in contrast, with high doses of salicylates or probenecid, blockade of reabsorption predominates to increase uric acid excretion and decrease plasma concentration.

The effect of probenecid on transport of uric acid reflects its general action on organic acid transport. Many other drugs used clinically are organic acids, and their renal excretion can be affected by probenecid. In contrast to uric acid, however, transport of organic acid drugs is predominantly in the secretory direction. Hence probenecid decreases excretion of these drugs, and a reduction of their dosage may be necessary. Examples include the penicillins, many cephalosporins, methotrexate, and many NSAIDs.

Large doses of probenecid greatly increase excretion of uric acid in gouty patients and thereby lower plasma uric acid. Unfortunately, the associated increase in urinary concentration of uric acid incurs risk of formation of urate stones (urolithiasis). This risk is lessened if patients drink large volumes of fluid to maintain low urinary urate concentrations or if they alkalinize their urine by ingesting bicarbonate or potassium citrate. The latter not only increases urate solubility but also enhances citrate excretion, and the citrate itself inhibits stone formation.

Probenecid (Benemid, others) is rapidly absorbed from the stomach and reaches peak plasma concentration in 4 hours. Treatment should begin with small doses, 250 mg twice a day, to decrease the potential for renal stone formation. Dosage is then gradually increased to a 1 or 1.5 g daily maintenance level; ultimate dosage is guided by serum uric acid determinations. The drug is available in tablets, 500 mg. Colchicine is often administered concurrently with probenecid to decrease the likelihood of acute gouty attacks; combination products are available.

Probenecid may cause adverse effects in a small percentage of patients. The figure generally given is less than 2%, but in some series adverse reactions have developed in 8% of patients. Nausea and vomiting, skin rash, and drug fever may occur. Urate stones may cause renal colic.

SULFINPYRAZONE

Sulfinpyrazone (Anturane, Aprazone), which is structurally related to phenylbutazone, also prevents tubular reabsorption of uric acid. Its action is antagonized by

FIG. 53-1 *Schema of the effects of drugs on uric acid excretion.* 1, *Below normal;* 2, *normal;* 3, *above normal. By decreasing secretion of uric acid, thiazide diuretics, relatively low doses of salicylates, other nonsteroidal anti-inflammatory drugs (NSAIDs), and probenecid can exacerbate preexisting hyperuricemia or may actually be the initiating cause of hyperuricemia. Filtration of uric acid will return to normal as hyperuricemia is resolved by "high" doses of probenecid (or another uricosuric agent).*

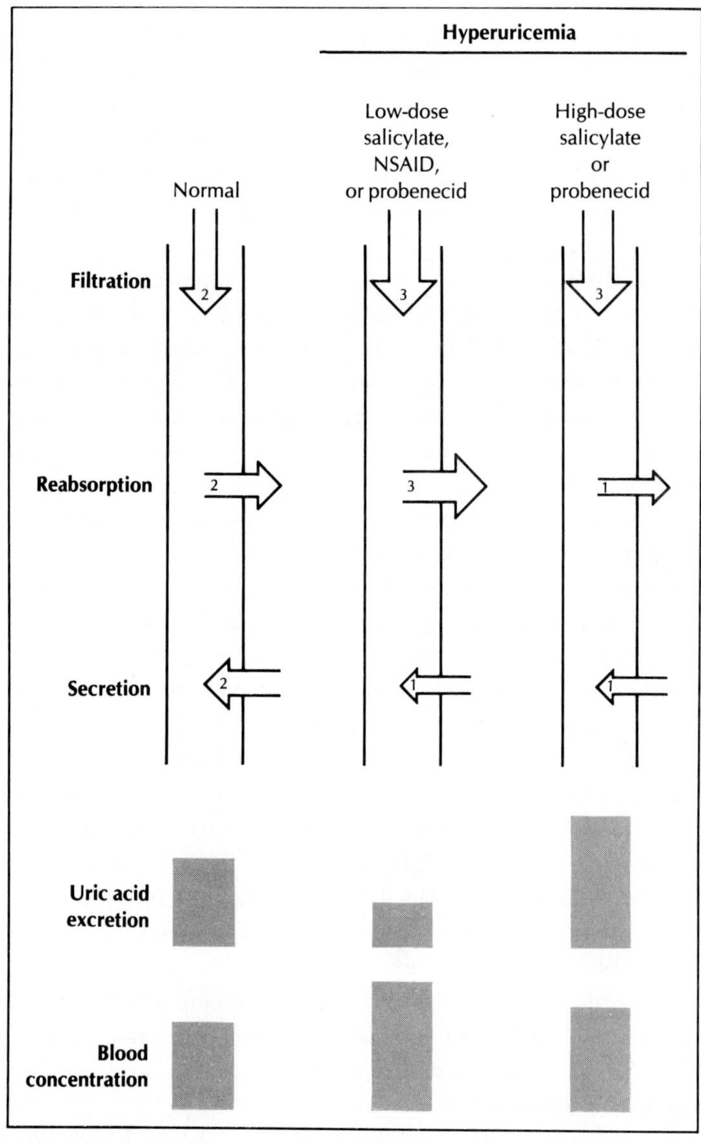

salicylates but not by probenecid. As with probenecid the sharp increase in urate excretion may predispose to urolithiasis. An acute gouty attack may occur at the beginning of treatment, and epigastric distress has been reported. The dosage is initially 50 to 100 mg four times daily; maximum daily dosage is 400 mg. Sulfinpyrazone can be taken in tablets, 100 mg, or in capsules, 200 mg.

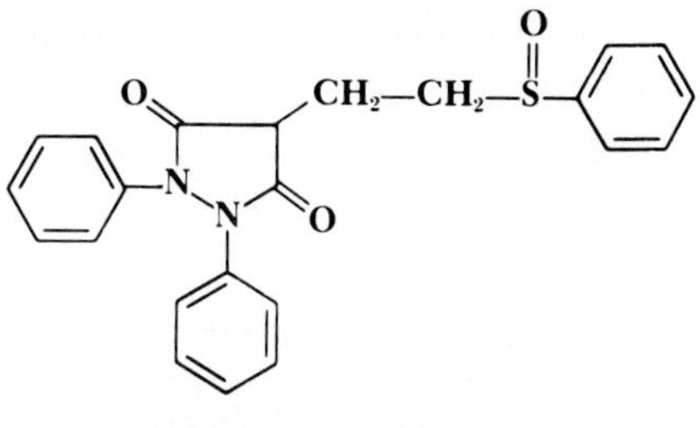

O
CH$_2$—CH$_2$—S
N
N
O
O

Sulfinpyrazone

ALLOPURINOL

Another approach to treatment of gout is to use an inhibitor of *xanthine oxidase*, an enzyme that converts hypoxanthine to uric acid. Allopurinol (Zyloprim, others) was originally developed to protect 6-mercaptopurine (a cancer chemotherapeutic agent) from rapid inactivation by this enzyme. Allopurinol causes a sharp decrease in both plasma uric acid concentration and in urinary uric acid excretion. As a result, the metabolic precursors xanthine and hypoxanthine replace uric acid in the urine.

Allopurinol is rapidly metabolized to oxypurinol, which also inhibits xanthine oxidase and is excreted by the kidney. Patients with renal insufficiency retain this metabolite, which can be toxic.

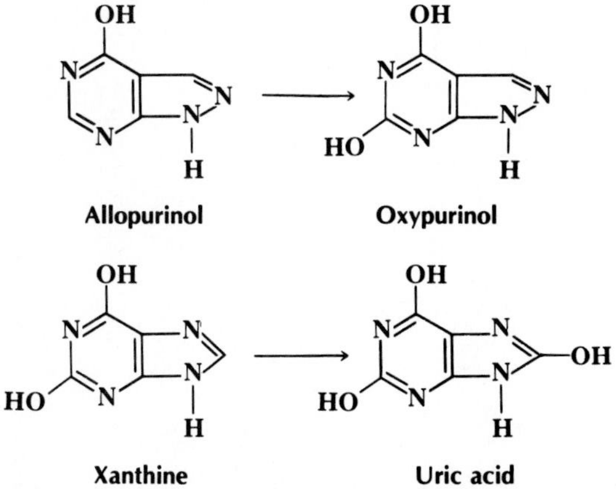

OH N N N N H → OH N N N N HO H

Allopurinol **Oxypurinol**

OH N N N N HO H → OH N N N N HO H OH

Xanthine **Uric acid**

In gouty patients intolerant or unresponsive to uricosuric agents, normal plasma urate concentrations are achieved with 200 to 600 mg/day of allopurinol. Tablets contain 100 or 300 mg of the drug.

Although uricosuric agents are effective in controlling hyperuricemia in most gouty patients, allopurinol may be more useful for a number of reasons. Gouty nephropathy and formation of urate stones are theoretically less likely with allopurinol therapy because the drug *reduces* the amount of uric acid excreted. In patients with impaired renal function or with urate stones, allopurinol is the agent of choice. It is also the best option in patients with lymphoma or leukemia. Therapy of the malignancy kills many cells, and consequent uric acid formation can be sufficient to cause acute urate nephropathy. This adverse effect can be prevented by allopurinol.

Reactions to allopurinol have been mild or moderate, though about 3% of patients taking the drug may develop skin eruptions, fever, hepatomegaly, leukopenia, gastrointestinal distress, diarrhea, pruritus, rash, headache, or alterations of liver function.

REFERENCES

1. Berger L, Yü T-F: Renal function in gout. IV. An analysis of 524 gouty subjects including long-term follow-up studies, *Am J Med* 59:605, 1975.
2. Boss GR, Seegmiller JE: Hyperuricemia and gout: classification, complications and management, *N Engl J Med* 300:1459, 1979.
3. Bryan J: Biochemical properties of microtubules, *Fed Proc* 33:152, 1974.
4. Emmerson BT: Drug control of gout and hyperuricaemia, *Drugs* 16:158, 1978.
5. Fessel WJ: Renal outcomes of gout and hyperuricemia, *Am J Med* 67:74, 1979.
6. Langford HG, Blaufox MD, Borhani NO, et al: Is thiazide-produced uric acid elevation harmful? Analysis of data from the Hypertension Detection and Follow-up Program, *Arch Intern Med* 147:645, 1987.
7. Liang MH, Fries JF: Asymptomatic hyperuricemia: the case for conservative management, *Ann Intern Med* 88:666, 1978.
8. Rastegar A, Thier SO: The treatment of hyperuricemia in gout, *Ration Drug Ther* 8(3), 1974.
9. Simkin PA: Management of gout, *Ann Intern Med* 90:812, 1979.
10. Yü T-F: The efficacy of colchicine prophylaxis in articular gout: a reappraisal after 20 years, *Semin Arthritis Rheum* 12:256, 1982.

Chapter 54

Antianemic drugs

GENERAL CONCEPT

The normal oxygen-carrying capacity of blood depends on maintenance of an adequate number of erythrocytes, as well as continual synthesis of hemoglobin and stromal (structural) proteins. Synthesis of these essential components normally adjusts to accommodate physiologic loss of blood elements. Anemia results when there is excessive loss or diminished replacement of erythrocytes or when the newly formed erythrocytes have inadequate hemoglobin. Anemia is a sign of disease. It can result from chronic blood loss, abnormal shape or size of erythrocytes, nutritional deficiency, chronic disease, or malignancy. Differential diagnosis to determine the underlying cause of the anemia is essential. For example, although nutritional deficiency of iron is a common cause of hypochromic, microcytic anemia in growing children and pregnant women, the development of a similar defect in adult males usually signals bleeding from an occult source. Nutritional deficiency of either vitamin B_{12} or folic acid can cause megaloblastic anemia. However, vitamin B_{12} deficiency may also cause serious neuronal damage. Correcting the deficiency will ameliorate this damage if an early and accurate diagnosis is made.

Erythrocytes

The mature erythrocyte is a biconcave disk with a diameter of approximately 8 μm. Its large surface-to-volume ratio facilitates gas exchange, and its flexibility enables it to pass easily through capillaries. The normal life-span is about 120 days; aging cells are replaced by maturation of reticulocytes from the bone marrow. Erythropoietin, which is produced in the kidney in response to decreased oxygenation of blood, circulates to the bone marrow to stimulate erythropoiesis, the process of differentiation of stem cells into mature erythrocytes.

Erythrocyte maturation requires multiple nutritional factors, including vitamins B_{12} and folic acid. These vitamins are required by the immature erythrocyte for synthesis of nuclear DNA. They are also necessary for replication of the immature erythrocyte and synthesis of heme, the porphyrin that combines with globin to form hemoglobin.

Many anemias are attributable to nutritional deficiency of iron, folate, or vitamin B_{12}. Diagnosis and therapy may be confounded by the interdependence of these factors for erythrocyte maturation and replication. The nutritional anemias are, however, generally treatable with replacement of the deficient factors. Often, inadequate intake of vitamins coupled with increased body demand produces a relative deficit. Pregnancy, for example, increases the need for iron severalfold.

IRON

Distribution

Approximately 70% of the iron in the body is functional; it has an essential role in the actions of hemoglobin, myoglobin, and other enzymes. Hemoglobin constitutes the bulk of erythrocyte mass. Normal blood contains approximately 130 to 150 mg of hemoglobin per milliliter, and each gram of hemoglobin contains 3.4 mg of iron. Myoglobin and cytochrome enzymes also contain minute quantities of iron. Although most of the iron in the body is in the form of hemoglobin, iron is also stored in tissues as *hemosiderin* and *ferritin*, and in blood it is bound to *transferrin*, a carrier protein. In conditions in which hemoglobin is depleted, enough iron can be mobilized from tissue stores to replace as much as half of the circulating hemoglobin.[7]

Total body iron amounts to approximately 35 mg/kg of body weight. Increased iron stores have been linked to increased risk of cancer in men,[12] possibly because it can catalyze production of oxygen radicals.[6]

Absorption, metabolism, and excretion

The intestine is the primary site for both absorption and excretion of iron. Iron is absorbed by a carefully regulated transport process (Fig. 54-1). The mucosal cells of the duodenum and proximal jejunum take up iron but transfer only a small amount to blood. The remainder is stored as ferritin and excreted when mucosal cells are sloughed. Iron is absorbed in the ferrous (Fe^{++}) form; the rate of absorption is influenced by gastric acidity, the presence of reducing substances, such as ascorbic acid, and food intake. Antacids and phosphates decrease absorption. Excessive iron intake or decreased marrow activity reduces absorption. In contrast, mucosal absorption is stimulated in iron deficiency and when erythropoiesis increases.

Iron is rigidly conserved in the body. Most iron released from degradation of hemoglobin in the liver is recycled. The daily requirement for normal adults, approximately 1 mg, is readily available in a normal diet, although only 10% of ingested iron is absorbed. Increased demand for iron during periods of growth, menstruation, or pregnancy, however, may result in a deficiency if dietary intake is inadequate. Once

FIG. 54-1 *Metabolism of iron.*

Courtesy Lederle Laboratories, American Cyanamid Co, Pearl River NY.

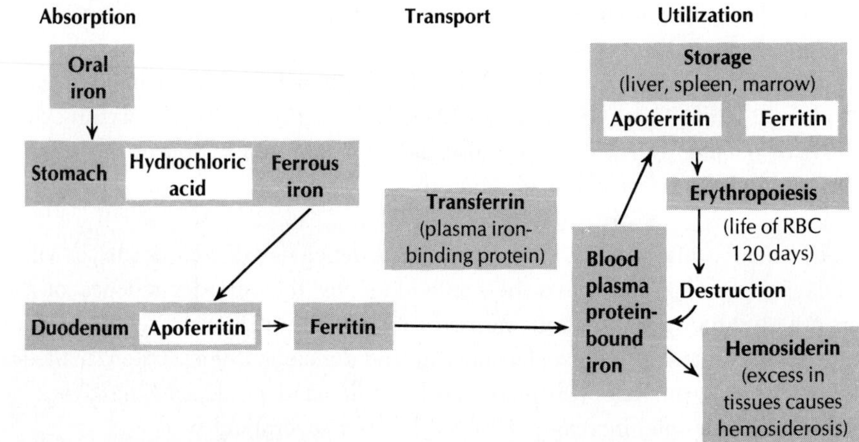

iron deficiency develops and iron stores are depleted, a normal diet no longer suffices to replenish iron stores.

Transferrin, the protein that transports iron to sites of hemoglobin synthesis, is usually incompletely saturated with iron. As the amount of iron bound to transferrin decreases, iron is mobilized from tissues and more is absorbed from the intestine. As tissue stores become depleted, erythrocytes change in size and hemoglobin content to produce the characteristic microcytic, hypochromic anemia of iron deficiency. Fig. 54-2 shows the progression of biochemical and hematologic events in iron-deficiency anemia.

Iron-deficiency anemia

Iron deficiency develops when the amount of iron in the body is less than that required for formation of hemoglobin and other essential compounds. It is by far the most common of the nutritional anemias and occurs in about 25% of infants, 6% of young children, 15% of menstruating women, and 30% of pregnant women in the United States.[7] Women athletes appear particularly susceptible because they must offset not only menstrual blood loss but also increased destruction of erythrocytes.

Iron-deficiency anemia differs from anemias of certain chronic diseases in which, despite sufficient iron, the number of erythrocytes is deficient. In iron deficiency the amount of available iron falls short of that needed to maintain adequate erythropoiesis.[1] Usually iron deficiency due to inadequate intake develops only in infants and growing children. Once body growth is completed the need for iron decreases, and the

FIG. 54-2

From Herbert V: Hosp Pract 15(3):75, 1980. Illustration by Irwin Kuperberg; data from Hillman, Bothwell, Finch, 1962 and 1974.

Biochemical and hematologic sequence of events in iron deficiency

Iron stores
Serum iron
Red blood cell iron

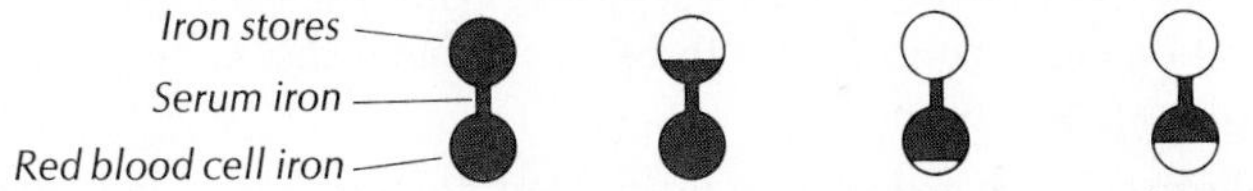

	Normal	Iron depletion	Iron-deficient erythropoiesis	Iron-deficiency anemia
RE marrow iron	2-3 +	0-1 +	0	0
Transferrin iron-binding capacity (μg/100 ml)	330±30	360	390	410
Plasma ferritin (ng/ml)	100±60	20	10	<10
Iron absorption (%)	5-10	10-15	10-20	10-20
Plasma iron (μg/100 ml)	115±50	115	<60	<40
Transferrin saturation (%)	35±15	30	<15	<10
Sideroblasts (%)	40-60	40-60	<10	<10
RBC protoporphyrin (μg/100 ml of RBC)	30	30	100	200
Erythrocyte morphology	Normal	Normal	Normal	Microcytic/ hypochromic

Abnormal (shaded)

small amount lost daily is replaced from dietary intake. The primary cause of iron deficiency in adults is an increased need for iron imposed by pregnancy or by blood loss. In males or postmenopausal females the most common cause of iron-deficiency anemia is chronic blood loss, usually from the gastrointestinal tract. The deficiency may be compounded by an inadequate diet or by drugs that irritate the gastric mucosa, such as aspirin or other NSAIDs. Likewise, the gastrointestinal irritation and nutritional deficiency associated with chronic alcoholism may promote iron-deficiency anemia.

The hallmark of severe iron-deficiency anemia is the microcytic, hypochromic erythrocyte that contains less than a normal complement of hemoglobin. In mild deficiency erythrocytes are often of normal size, but they can usually be distinguished from normal erythrocytes by variations in size and shape.[1] Physical signs of anemia include pallor of the skin and mucous membranes, and patients complain of fatigue and loss of appetite. The circulating concentration of iron is low, iron binding by transferrin is increased, and plasma ferritin concentration is decreased.[11]

TREATMENT

Iron-deficiency anemia responds readily to supplementation with appropriate ferrous iron salts. The goal is to provide immediately available iron for synthesis of hemoglobin and to replenish tissue stores. Because iron stores are replaced only slowly, therapy may be required for 6 months to a year. Many laboratory tests, however, may become normal within a few weeks.[7] On the average, erythrocytic hemoglobin concentration will increase approximately 10 mg/ml (1 g/dl) per week.

Although many different preparations of iron are available, there is little indication that any are better than orally administered ferrous salts. The ferrous salts differ only in their rate of absorption from the gastrointestinal tract. Dosage usually provides excess iron, but no more than 15% will be absorbed, even in deficiency. Recommended adult doses are tailored to provide daily absorption of 15 to 25 mg. The most popular preparations are listed in Table 54-1. All have the same mode of action and cause similar side effects.

Injectable forms of iron are seldom used. Iron-dextran injection (Imferon, others) is a complex of ferric hydroxide with dextrans, used in patients who are unable to take oral medication. The iron is released only after the complex is taken up by cells in the reticuloendothelial system. Parenteral administration of iron can readily restore tissue depots because absorption is no longer limiting.

TABLE 54-1 Oral iron preparations

Preparation	Dosage
Ferrous sulfate (Feosol, others)	300 mg three times a day
Ferrous gluconate (Fergon, others)	600 mg three times a day
Ferrous fumarate (Feostat, others)	500 mg three times a day

Side effects and toxicity

Both the therapeutic and adverse effects of iron therapy depend on the amount of elemental iron released. Oral iron preparations frequently irritate the gastrointestinal tract and may be poorly tolerated by debilitated patients. The most common complaints are abdominal cramping and diarrhea. Nausea, gastric pain, and headache are not uncommon. Gastrointestinal irritation can be reduced by administration of iron salts after meals.

Parenteral administration of iron can cause serious reactions including iron overload and anaphylactic shock, particularly if oral iron is administered concurrently. Saturation of transferrin elevates the blood concentration of unbound metal, and there is no adequate means of excretion. Excess iron is deposited in tissues where it can cause hemochromatosis. Acute overdose may result in cardiovascular collapse. Adults rarely experience serious toxicity from oral iron preparations because an overdose usually promotes vomiting. However, children who ingest large amounts of iron are at definite risk.

Deferoxamine

The potent iron-chelating agent deferoxamine (Desferal) is a water-soluble compound used to treat acute toxic reactions to iron or to remove iron from tissues of patients with an overload. As shown below, one molecule of deferoxamine binds one molecule of ferric iron. This removes iron from ferritin and blocks further absorption from the gastrointestinal tract.

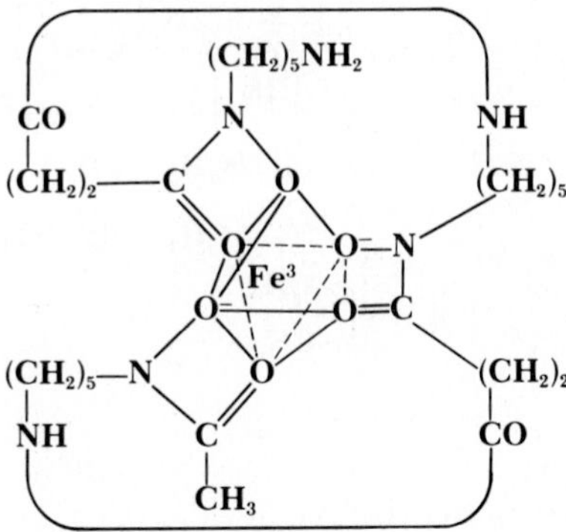

Deferoxamine (in combination with iron)

Deferoxamine can be administered by gastric tube to patients with acute iron poisoning, or it may be injected intramuscularly or intravenously. Pediatric patients may require repeated doses.

Thalassemia

The thalassemias result from hereditary defects in the rate of hemoglobin synthesis. Severe forms are relatively rare; the milder forms present as a microcytic anemia similar to that in iron-deficiency anemia.[1] The microcytic anemia of thalassemia, however, does not respond to iron therapy.

MEGALOBLASTIC ANEMIAS

Nutritional anemias due to a deficiency of either vitamin B_{12} or folate are much less common than iron-deficiency anemia.[7] Either deficiency impairs DNA synthesis and erythropoiesis and causes an anemia characterized by functional abnormalities of erythrocytes as well as a distinctive cytologic appearance. Because of the interrelationship of replicative and synthetic processes, a deficiency of folate may cause vitamin B_{12} deficiency and vice versa. Furthermore, anemia from a deficiency of either factor responds to treatment with the other. To compound the problem further, cells with slower DNA synthesis use iron inefficiently for hemoglobin synthesis.[7] Thus a compound anemia may present with iron overload. Because an untreated deficiency of vitamin B_{12} can cause progressive neurologic damage, it is essential to establish the cause of the megaloblastic anemia before treatment.

Vitamin B_{12}

Vitamin B_{12} is the collective name for cyanocobalamins, cobalt-containing compounds that are synthesized by microorganisms and ingested through animal products in the food chain.[3] Unlike many other vitamins, B_{12} is not found in plants.

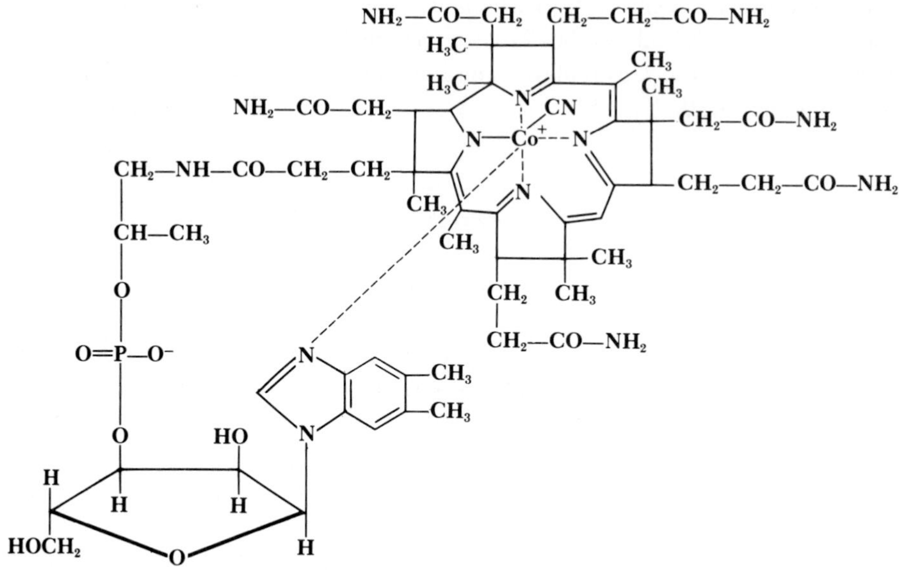

Vitamin B_{12}

Although neurologic symptoms usually occur after development of anemia in cobalamin deficiency, some patients develop a neurologic disorder in the absence of anemia or macrocytosis.[10] Hereditary disorders of cobalamin metabolism can also cause neurologic dysfunction and megaloblastic anemia. These conditions can be discriminated from dietary cobalamin deficiency by urinary excretion of large amounts of methylmalonic acid or homocysteine.[4]

To become biologically active, cyanocobalamin must be converted to methylcobalamin or adenosylcobalamin. Methylcobalamin is an essential cofactor in conversion of homocysteine to methionine. Adenosylcobalamin is involved in conversion of methylmalonyl coenzyme A to succinyl coenzyme A. Both active forms of the vitamin are required for erythropoiesis, and a defect in production of succinyl coenzyme A is believed to cause the neurologic complications of vitamin B_{12} deficiency.[3] The primary defect found only in vitamin B_{12} deficiency and not in folate deficiency is the inability to synthesize myelin, which results in a demyelinating neuropathy that eventually causes nerve deterioration. The process is partially reversible, if replacement therapy begins before deterioration occurs.

The isolation of vitamin B_{12} from liver and its identification as the missing extrinsic factor in pernicious anemia were major discoveries. Pernicious anemia is characterized by megaloblastic anemia, a sharp reduction in gastric secretions, and neurologic damage. This condition was once incurable and inevitably fatal. It was recognized by Castle that the gastric mucosa is the source of an *intrinsic factor* needed for absorption of the extrinsic factor supplied by meats and that liver is a rich source of this extrinsic factor. It was subsequently established that both intrinsic factor and extrinsic factor are needed for erythropoiesis.[5] Isolation of folic acid in 1943 led to the suggestion that a deficiency of this compound might cause pernicious anemia. However, even though folic acid can correct the hematologic manifestations of the disease, it does not improve, and even aggravates, the neurologic symptoms. Since liver extract corrects both defects in patients with pernicious anemia, it is clear that folic acid deficiency is not involved.

The picture was clarified when it was shown that oral synthetic vitamin B_{12} corrected both hematologic and neurologic defects provided that intrinsic factor was available. It was later established that intrinsic factor, a thermolabile glycoprotein isolated from gastric mucosa, is essential for adequate absorption of vitamin B_{12}.

ABSORPTION AND FATE

A normal diet contains a sufficient quantity of vitamin B_{12}. This water-soluble vitamin is conserved through enterohepatic recycling, and only about 1 μg is lost each day. Since the body normally stores about l mg, it takes a long time for a deficiency to develop, even after gastrectomy.

Absorption of vitamin B_{12} from dietary sources or from oral supplements requires intrinsic factor from the gastric mucosa. This thermolabile glycoprotein binds to vitamin B_{12} in the stomach and remains bound to it until the complex reaches the lower ileum where the vitamin is absorbed. Several conditions can reduce absorption. Loss of gastric mucosal cells from gastric resection or malignancy reduces available intrinsic factor and hence absorption. Histamine H_2-receptor antagonists, such as cimetidine and ranitidine, decrease secretion of intrinsic factor,[2] but this effect is probably not clinically relevant. Malabsorption syndromes, such as tropical sprue, celiac disease, or regional enteritis, limit absorption in the intestine. Competition for uptake by intestinal parasites such as the fish tapeworm (*Diphyllobothrium latum*) is another cause. Finally, coadministration of other drugs or vitamins can affect absorption and utilization of vitamin B_{12}. Megadoses of vitamin C, for example, can destroy vitamin B_{12} during transit through the gastrointestinal tract.[8]

MECHANISM OF ACTION

The characteristic delayed nuclear maturation in megaloblastosis results from inadequate DNA synthesis, which can be corrected by vitamin B_{12} and folic acid. The pathway affected by these vitamins involves synthesis of thymidine from deoxyuridylate (dUMP):

$$\text{Deoxyuridine} \rightarrow \text{Deoxyuridylate} \rightarrow \text{Thymidylate} \rightarrow \text{Thymidine}$$

The methylation of deoxyuridylate to thymidylate requires 5,10-methylenetetrahydrofolic acid (Fig. 54-3). This explains the folate requirement in DNA synthesis. Vitamin B_{12} is also a cofactor in regeneration of tetrahydrofolate from the 5-methylated form. This reaction is responsible for conversion of homocysteine to methionine. Additional transfers of one-carbon fragments include conversion of serine to glycine, a reaction that utilizes pyridoxal phosphate as a cofactor.

THERAPEUTIC USE

Vitamin B_{12} is indicated for treatment of megaloblastic anemia caused by nutritional deficiency. This condition usually results from defective absorption rather than inadequate intake. *Pernicious anemia,* in which patients cannot make intrinsic factor, is the most prevalent cause of vitamin B_{12} deficiency, but gastrectomy, damage to the gastric mucosa, and malabsorption can also cause it.

Treatment of pernicious anemia must be parenteral because absorption is negligible without added intrinsic factor. The vitamin is injected intramuscularly (or subcutaneously) in a dosage of 100 μg, repeated daily for a week, then every other day for 2 weeks, and then twice weekly for an additional 2 or 3 weeks. Dosage must be continued monthly throughout life to prevent progression of neurologic damage. Individuals who suffer from malnutrition or a correctable disorder may be treated with oral forms of the vitamin.

Injections of vitamin B_{12} have been used to treat fatique and other complaints, but such therapy is likely of little value unless there is an established deficiency. When cyanocobalamin and liver extracts were used together in a double-blind trial to treat chronic fatigue syndrome in 15 patients, they were no more effective than placebo.[9]

Folic acid

Folic acid (pteroylglutamic acid) is a combination of pteridine, *p*-aminobenzoic acid, and glutamic acid.

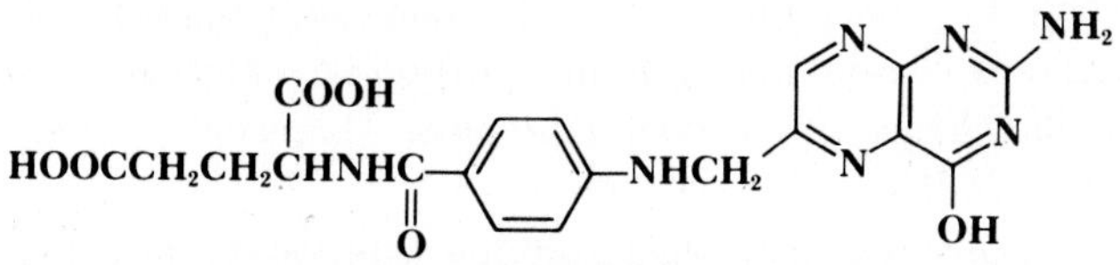

Folic acid

FUNCTIONS

Folic acid participates in reactions important for synthesis of DNA (Fig. 54-3). It is essential when DNA synthesis and turnover is rapid, as in hematopoietic tissues, the mucosa of the gastrointestinal tract, and the developing embryo.

Pathways for DNA thymine synthesis. *FIG. 54-3*

From Waxman S, Corcino J, Herbert V: JAMA 214:101, copyright 1970; reproduced with permission from American Medical Association.

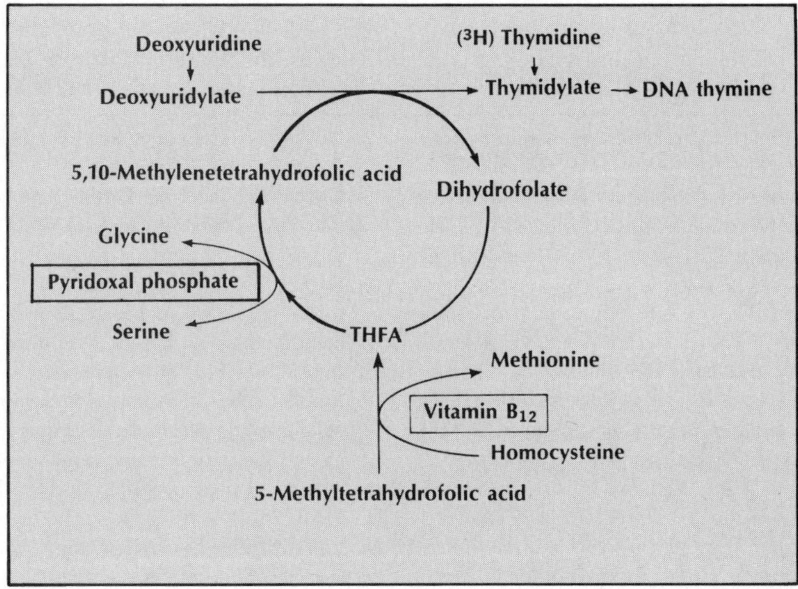

Pteroylglutamic acid is the pharmaceutical form of folic acid, but folates in foods are conjugated to six additional glutamic acid residues and are stored as polyglutamates. These naturally occurring folates are destroyed by prolonged cooking. Folates are cleaved to a monoglutamate form during absorption and are converted to several coenzymes that differ structurally in substitution on the pteridine moiety and in the number of glutamate residues. Each of these forms has a specific action in metabolic processes. For example, the interrelationship with vitamin B_{12} involves 5-methyltetrahydrofolic acid as a methyl donor in conversion of homocysteine to methionine.

Absorption, metabolism, and excretion

Folic acid is well absorbed from the proximal intestine. Injectable forms are seldom used except in parenteral alimentation. Like vitamin B_{12}, folic acid is conserved by enterohepatic recycling, and conditions that produce malabsorption in the intestine also decrease absorption of folic acid. Liver damage from various diseases also compromises enterohepatic recycling of folate.

Therapeutic use

Folic acid is used as a dietary supplement when there is clearly a nutritional deficiency. Conditions such as chronic alcoholism, pregnancy, lactation, sprue, and ileal disease are indications for supplementation. Conditions in which there is a need for increased erythropoiesis, such as hemolytic anemia or malnutrition, may be treated with folic acid. Long-term use of drugs such as anticonvulsants, antimalarial compounds, and steroids also predisposes to folate deficiency. Folic acid should not be included in multivitamin preparations because it may obscure underlying pernicious anemia. The danger is that folic acid can improve the megaloblastic anemia without affecting the demyelinating defect. Incorrect diagnosis may then permit undetected progression of neurologic damage to an irreversible stage. Even if folic acid is administered with vitamin B_{12} to a person with pernicious anemia, neurologic defects will not be prevented because vitamin B_{12} is still not absorbed without intrinsic factor.

REFERENCES

1. Beutler E: The common anemias, *JAMA* 259:2433, 1988.
2. Binder HJ, Donaldson RM Jr: Effect of cimetidine on intrinsic factor and pepsin secretion in man, *Gastroenterology* 74:371, 1978.
3. Bunn HF, Lee GR, Wintrobe MM: Pernicious anemia and other megaloblastic anemias. In Thorn GW, Adams RD, Braunwald E, et al, editors: *Harrison's principles of internal medicine*, ed 8, New York, 1977, McGraw-Hill, p 1656.
4. Carmel R, Watkins D, Goodman SI, Rosenblatt DS: Hereditary defect of cobalamin metabolism (*cblG* mutation) presenting as a neurologic disorder in adulthood, *N Engl J Med* 318:1738, 1988.
5. Castle WB: Current concepts of pernicious anemia, *Am J Med* 48:541, 1970.
6. Halliwell B, Gutteridge JMC: Oxygen free radicals and iron in relation to biology and medicine: some problems and concepts, *Arch Biochem Biophys* 246:501, 1986.
7. Herbert V: The nutritional anemias, *Hosp Pract* 15(3):65, 1980.
8. Herbert V, Jacob E: Destruction of vitamin B_{12} by ascorbic acid, *JAMA* 230:241, 1974.
9. Kaslow JE, Rucker L, Onishi R: Liver extract—folic acid—cyanocobalamin vs placebo for chronic fatigue syndrome, *Arch Intern Med* 149:2501, 1989.
10. Lindenbaum J, Healton EB, Savage DG, et al: Neuropsychiatric disorders caused by cobalamin deficiency in the absence of anemia or macrocytosis, *N Engl J Med* 318:1720, 1988.
11. Lipschitz DA, Cook JD, Finch CA: A clinical evaluation of serum ferritin as an index of iron stores, *N Engl J Med* 290:1213, 1974.
12. Stevens RG, Jones DY, Micozzi MS, Taylor PR: Body iron stores and the risk of cancer, *N Engl J Med* 316:1047, 1988.

Chapter 55

Vitamins

GENERAL CONCEPT

Observations that certain naturally occurring diseases such as scurvy and beriberi improved with dietary modification led astute clinicians to surmise that a nutritional deficiency caused the pathologic process. Feeding experiments with animals later established that small amounts of certain organic nutrients are essential for health. The term "vitamine" was coined to describe the trace nutrient that prevented beriberi. Subsequent discoveries that vitamins are involved in vital enzymatic reactions focused attention on the relationship of nutrition to growth and development as well as to maintenance of general well-being.

Although individual vitamins vary considerably with respect to chemistry and metabolism, there are two general classes, water soluble and fat soluble. Fat-soluble vitamins can be stored within body fat for long periods of time, but water-soluble vitamins must be continuously replaced through the diet. Many water-soluble vitamins are coenzymes that have essential metabolic functions.[9]

WATER-SOLUBLE VITAMINS

The B vitamins (thiamine, niacin, riboflavin, pyridoxine, cyanocobalamin, and folic acid) as well as pantothenic acid, ascorbic acid (vitamin C), and biotin are water-soluble substances. Only very small amounts of these compounds are required for adequate nutrition, but, as carriers of oxygen, hydrogen, or reactive chemical groups, they are essential for life.

Historically, short-term deficiencies of thiamine, niacin, and vitamin C resulted in diseases that were linked to lack of an adequate diet; beriberi, pellagra, and scurvy are relatively rare in the developed world. However, because water-soluble vitamins are not stored, deficiencies may occur with chronic alcoholism, anorexia, and other conditions involving malnutrition.

Thiamine

Thiamine (vitamin B_1) in the form of thiamine pyrophosphate participates in decarboxylation of α-keto acids and in transketolation reactions involved in carbohydrate oxidation by mammalian cells.

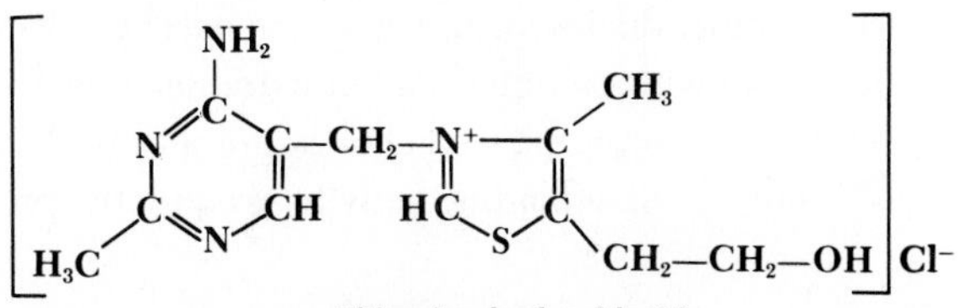

Thiamine hydrochloride

DEFICIENCY

Severe deficiency results in the disease beriberi, which is characterized by peripheral neuritis, high-output heart failure, or cerebral involvement with Wernickes encephalopathy. Symptoms include paresthesia, muscle weakness, depression, confusion, and memory deficit. Alcoholism is a major cause of thiamine deficiency. As such, alcoholic patients who present to an emergency room in a stuporous or comatose condition are given thiamine intravenously, in case their central impairment is due to this deficiency.

OCCURRENCE

Foods such as yeast, wheat germ, and pork contain sufficient thiamine for most dietary needs. Young children and pregnant women have an increased requirement, but ingestion of approximately 1 mg/day will prevent deficiency.

Niacin

Niacin (nicotinic acid, B_3) is an integral part of at least two important coenzymes, nicotinamide-adenine dinucleotide (NAD) and nicotinamide-adenine dinucleotide phosphate (NADP).[6]

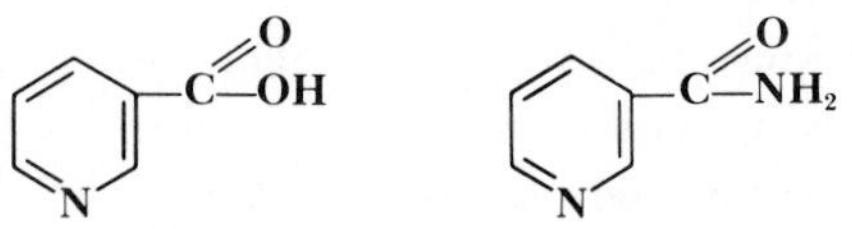

C—OH, O, N
Niacin

C—NH$_2$, O, N
Niacinamide

Because NAD and NADP can be in either an oxidized or a reduced state, they act as hydrogen acceptors or donors in many reactions of intermediary metabolism. The requirement for NADP of some microsomal enzymes of drug metabolism is one example of the importance of nicotinic acid.

DEFICIENCY

A deficiency of niacin causes pellagra, a disease characterized by increased pigmentation and lesions of exposed skin and by gastrointestinal mucosal changes resulting in glossitis, stomatitis, anorexia, and diarrhea. Individuals with niacin deficiency often suffer mental symptoms similar to those with thiamine deficiency.

OCCURRENCE

Yeast, cereals, nuts, liver, and other meats contain significant amounts of niacin. Mammals can synthesize niacin from tryptophan, but much larger amounts of tryptophan than of niacin are needed to meet the daily requirement. Pellagra can develop in patients with carcinoid tumor, even when tryptophan intake is normal, because tryptophan is shunted to synthesis of serotonin (5-hydroxytryptamine).

PHARMACOLOGY

Niacin, but not nicotinamide, dilates small vessels, apparent as facial flushing. This transient effect may be severe with parenteral administration. Niacin is also effective, on a purely empiric basis, in lowering plasma cholesterol and triglyceride concentrations (see Chapter 43), but its vasodilating activity frequently precludes patients' ability to take it.

Riboflavin

Riboflavin (vitamin B_2) is a component of flavin-adenine dinucleotide (FAD), a coenzyme of flavoproteins involved in hydrogen transfer in oxidation-reduction reactions. FAD and a mononucleotide form, FMN, serve as carriers for hydrogen atoms.

DEFICIENCY

Deficiency of riboflavin causes a symptom complex of cheilosis, stomatitis, dermatitis, photophobia, and anemia.

OCCURRENCE

Riboflavin is found in green vegetables, liver, eggs, and milk.

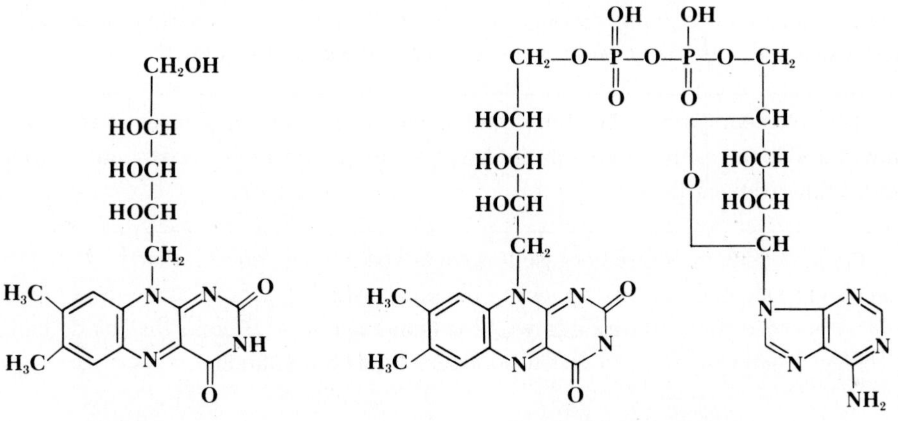

Riboflavin

Flavin-adenine dinucleotide

Pyridoxine

Pyridoxine, pyridoxal, and pyridoxamine are various forms of vitamin B_6.[7] Pyridoxal 5′-phosphate functions in many different reactions, including transamination between amino acids and keto acids. It is involved in synthesis of carbohydrates, amino acids, and such diverse molecules as sphingolipids and heme. It is also a cofactor for formation of the amines dopamine, serotonin, and histamine by decarboxylation of their precursor amino acids levodopa, tryptophan, and histidine, respectively.[10]

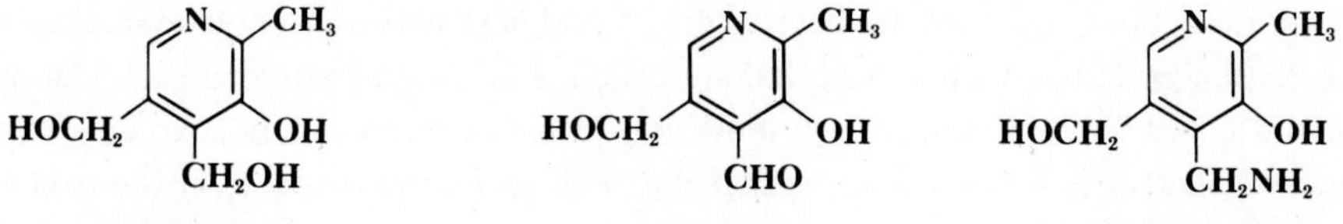

Pyridoxine **Pyridoxal** **Pyridoxamine**

DEFICIENCY

Deficiency of pyridoxine is generally manifest by central or peripheral nervous system symptoms, including convulsions in infants. Pyridoxal 5′-phosphate is bound by apoenzymes and by albumin. These interactions can alter the effective concentration of the vitamin. For example, complex formation with albumin can contribute to deficiency.[10] Patients who take isoniazid, a drug used to treat *Mycobacterium* infections, may experience peripheral neuritis because isoniazide increases urinary excretion of pyridoxal phosphate. Levels of pyridoxal 5‘-phosphate may be reduced in pregnancy, and individuals with celiac disease do not adequately absorb the vitamin.

Occurrence

Pyridoxine in all three forms is found in a variety of foods, including yeast, liver, rice, bran, and wheat germ.

Toxicity

Pyridoxine supplementation, generally believed to be nontoxic, has been used with limited success to treat premenstrual edema and carpal tunnel syndrome. However, self-administration of doses ranging from 2 to 6 gm per day has caused megavitaminosis associated with ataxia and severe sensory nervous dysfunction.[15]

Biotin

As a transient carrier of carboxyl groups, biotin in the form of biocytin is involved in carboxylation reactions. It is an integral part of certain biotin-dependent enzymes, such as pyruvate carboxylase.

Deficiency

Biotin deficiency is rare because it is contained in many different foods. Deficiency can occur in alcoholics, however, or in individuals who ingest large amounts of raw egg whites because undenatured egg white contains avidin, a protein that binds biotin. Cooking denatures avidin so that it no longer binds the vitamin.

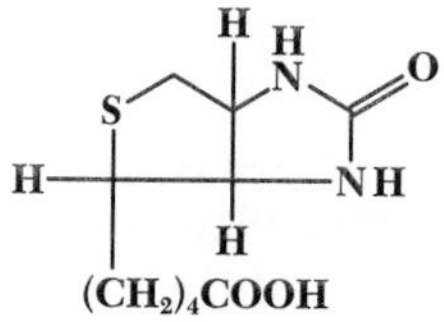

Biotin

Pantothenic acid

Pantothenic acid is a constituent of coenzyme A, the coenzyme required in many different reactions involving transfer of acetyl and acyl groups. Acetyl coenzyme A is essential for reactions such as acetylation of choline to acetylcholine and acetylation of *p*-amino compounds. Coenzyme A initiates the first reaction of the Krebs cycle in which citric acid is formed from oxaloacetic acid, and it participates in the oxidative metabolism of fatty acids.

Deficiency

Pantothenic acid deficiency in animals is associated with dermatitis, adrenal degeneration, and central nervous symptoms, but it is rare in humans. In a few clinical cases, the deficiency was reported to cause a burning sensation in the feet. In vitro studies indicate that turnover of pantothenic acid in the brain is slow; this may account for the lack of central symptoms in man.[12]

Occurrence

Pantothenic acid is found in yeast, bran, egg yolk, and liver.

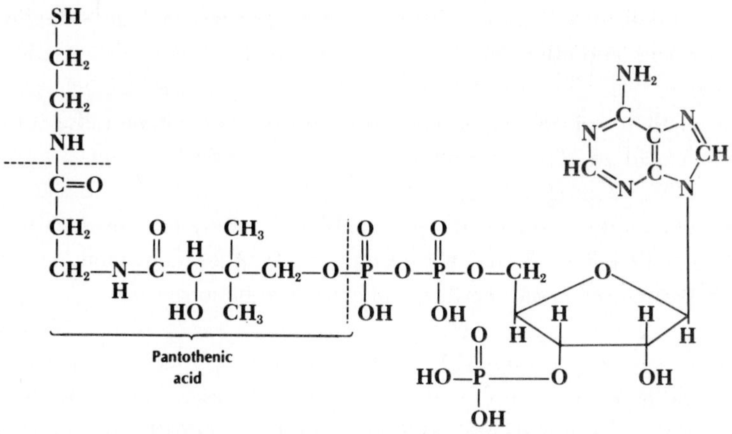

Pantothenic acid

Coenzyme A

Vitamin C

Vitamin C (ascorbic acid) is a reducing agent. Humans and a few other animal species require a dietary source of vitamin C; many animals and most plants synthesize it from glucose. Vitamin C has been implicated as a free-radical scavenger as well as a cofactor for transformation of folic to folinic acid, for dopamine β-hydroxylase, and for glucocorticoid formation. By acting as a cofactor for enzymatic hydroxylation of proline in the synthesis of collagen, it aids in formation and maintenance of normal connective tissue.[8,9]

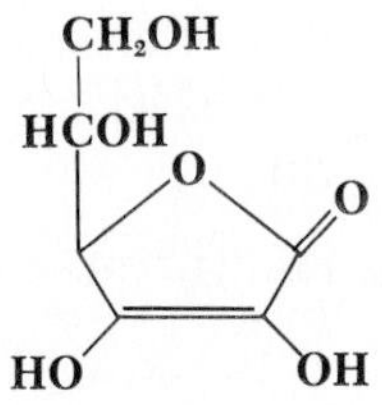

Vitamin C

Deficiency

Scurvy is the classic outcome of vitamin C deficiency. It is characterized by abnormalities in connective tissue. Bleeding gums and loose teeth result from defects in microvessels of the oral cavity. Hemorrhage can occur in skin and other tissues, and blood loss may cause anemia.

Occurrence

Citrus fruits and vegetables such as green peppers, lettuce, and tomatoes contain high concentrations of ascorbic acid.

Toxicity

Reduction of transition metals such as iron or copper by ascorbic acid can promote generation of reactive oxygen species; it has been suggested that this mechanism contributes to aging of human lens protein,[14] but it is not clear that this is a general phenomenon. Large doses of ascorbic acid can cause falsely high values in serum bilirubin, uric acid, and other laboratory tests that involve reduction reactions.

Vitamin B_{12} and folic acid

Because of their central importance in erythropoiesis, vitamin B_{12} (cyanocobalamin) and folic acid are discussed separately in Chapter 54.

FAT-SOLUBLE VITAMINS

The lipid solubility of some vitamins enables the body to concentrate and store them, and a dietary deficiency may not become apparent for many months. Vitamins A, D, E, and K participate in various metabolic and synthetic reactions.

Vitamin A

Vitamin A (retinol) has several functions in normal physiology. It is part of the visual purple of the retina and is essential for dark adaptation. Retinol is also involved in normal cellular growth and differentiation, and it maintains the structural integrity of various epithelial structures, possibly through an effect on glycoprotein synthesis. Research with both animals and humans suggests that β-carotene, a precursor of vitamin A, helps to prevent certain forms of cancer, possibly because it is an effective radical trapping antioxidant.[2] Several animal studies indicate that retinoids delay the onset of tumor appearance, slow tumor growth, and increase survival rate.

Retinoids are used to treat skin conditions such as acne and psoriasis, and they are effective against some types of dermal malignancies.[5]

DEFICIENCY

Vitamin A deficiency produces night blindness, dryness and thickening of the conjunctiva (xerosis), and ulcerations of the cornea (keratomalacia).[18] Hyperkeratosis results in dry and roughened skin. The deficiency can cause retarded growth and sterility in experimental animals.

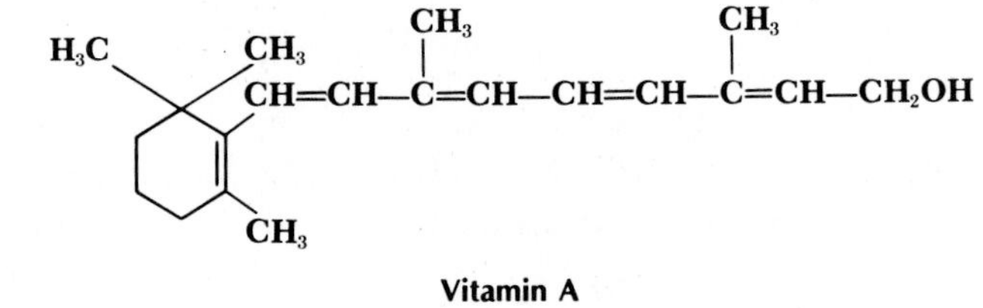

Vitamin A

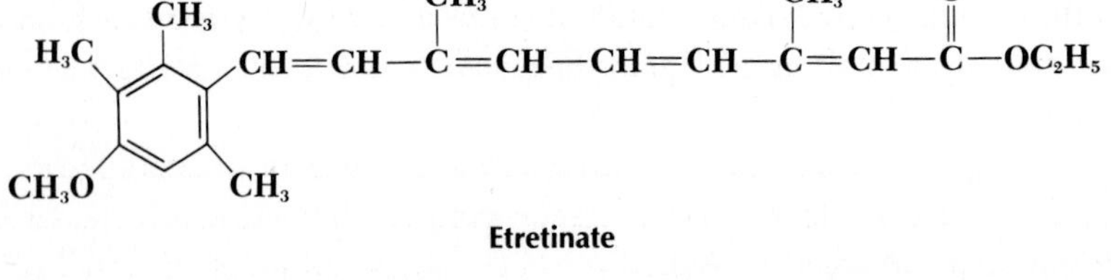

Etretinate

OCCURRENCE

Vitamin A in the form of retinol is found in fish liver, eggs, and milk. β-Carotene, the precursor form found in vegetables such as carrots, yams, and broccoli, is converted to retinol in the intestine.

Toxicity

Vitamin A is stored in the liver. Excessive accumulation is manifest as dryness of the skin and mucous membranes, cheilosis, dermatitis, joint pain, and occasionally central effects such as photophobia, anorexia, depression, and confusion. Toxicity can also develop in patients with jaundice. **Isotretinoin** (Accutane) and **etretinate** (Tegison), which are related to retinol, are used to treat severe acne, psoriasis, and disorders of keratinization. **Tretinoin** (Retin-A) is used to treat less severe acne. The teratogenic effects of excess vitamin A are well documented; pregnancy must be avoided for years after therapy with these *retinoids* is stopped.[4] Etretinate can persist in plasma for over 2 years after treatment and in tissues even longer.

Vitamin E

Vitamin E comprises several species of tocopherols. α-Tocopherol, the major component of commercial preparations, accounts for most of the activity. The vitamin is important for reproduction in laboratory animals, and it has immunostimulatory actions when administered in excess of established dietary requirements. Its antioxidant action helps to prevent free radical-catalyzed lipid peroxidation in tissues.[16] High doses of vitamin E appear to minimize the severity of retrolental fibroplasia in premature infants receiving oxygen.[9] Contrary to claims in the popular press, there is no evidence that vitamin E prevents cancer or delays aging in man.

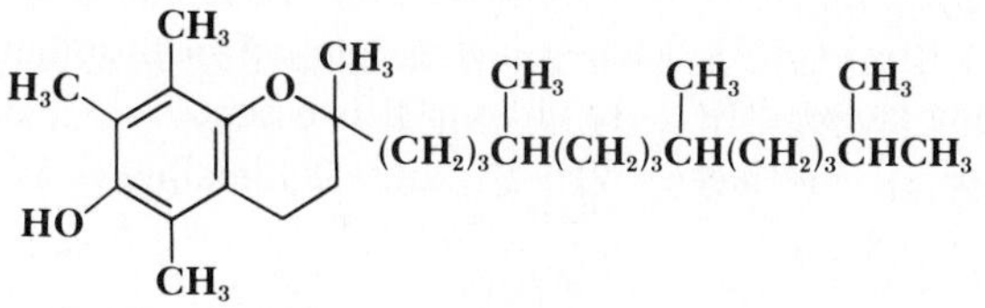

CH_3, H_3C, HO, CH_3, O, CH_3, $(CH_2)_3CH(CH_3)(CH_2)_3CH(CH_3)(CH_2)_3CH(CH_3)CH_3$

α-**Tocopherol**

Deficiency

Clinical signs of deficiency in laboratory animals usually involve impaired integrity of cell membranes; experimental evidence suggests that peroxidation of cell membranes and enzymes is responsible for many of the pathologic changes. Vitamin E deficiency in rats causes spontaneous abortion and degeneration of the germinal epithelium of the testes. Muscular dystrophy also develops in deficient animals.

Vitamin E deficiency is not likely to develop in humans with normal dietary intake and normal gastrointestinal function. Individuals who absorb fats poorly, such as those with cystic fibrosis, celiac disease, or pancreatic insufficiency, are more likely to become deficient. Deficiency after gastrectomy or another cause of malabsorption is manifested by muscle weakness, skin rash, and increased platelet adherence.

Occurrence

Vitamin E is found in leafy vegetables, whole grains, and vegetable oils. Additional sources are dairy products, fish, peanuts, and wheat germ.

Vitamin D

Vitamin D is necessary for adequate calcium and phosphorus metabolism. Because of its involvement in bone metabolism, this vitamin is discussed in Chapter 51.

Vitamin K

Two naphthoquinone compounds, vitamin K_1 (phytonadione) and vitamin K_2, are essential for production of prothrombin and other coagulation factors by the liver.[11] They are coenzymes in posttranslational carboxylation of glutamyl residues in newly synthesized coagulation factors. Carboxylation of γ-glutamyl residues is required for interaction with calcium and phospholipids in the coagulation cascade.

Various 1,4-naphthoquinones have similar activities. All are very insoluble in water and would generally be given orally. Emulsions of vitamin K_1, however, can be injected cautiously intravenously to reverse hemorrhage due to hypoprothrombinemia caused by warfarin-type anticoagulants.

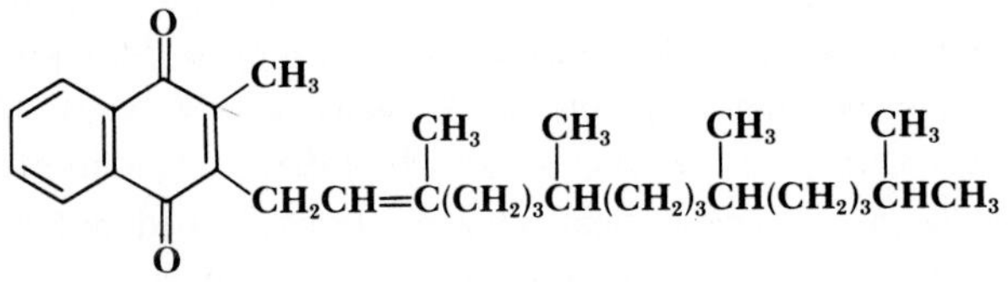

$$CH_2CH{=}\overset{CH_3}{\overset{|}{C}}(CH_2)_3\overset{CH_3}{\overset{|}{C}}H(CH_2)_3\overset{CH_3}{\overset{|}{C}}H(CH_2)_3\overset{CH_3}{\overset{|}{C}}HCH_3$$

(2-methyl-1,4-naphthoquinone ring, O, O, CH_3)

Vitamin K_1

DEFICIENCY

Vitamin K is synthesized by the bacterial flora of the intestine, and dietary deficiency is unlikely. However, deficiency has developed in hospitalized patients with various complicating factors.[1] Because vitamin K is essential for adequate synthesis of prothrombin (factor II) and factors VII, IX, and X, bleeding is associated with prolonged prothrombin time.

OCCURRENCE

Vitamin K is found in leafy green vegetables, and bacteria that normally inhabit the small intestine synthesize it. The relative contribution of dietary intake and intestinal synthesis is not established, but probably both are important in man.

PHARMACOLOGY

Vitamin K preparations are used to control bleeding due to hypoprothrombinemia. This may be secondary to severe liver disease, biliary obstruction, malabsorption syndromes, warfarin-like drugs, or to inadequate synthesis of the vitamin after reduction of intestinal flora by antibiotics or in the absence of intestinal bacteria in premature or newborn infants.[11]

Vitamin K_1 (AquaMEPHYTON, Konakion, Mephyton) and menadiol sodium diphosphate (vitamin K_4, Synkayvite) are currently available. The latter, a water-soluble naphthoquinone derivative that can be given parenterally, is converted to menadione (vitamin K_3) after absorption. It is not effective for reversal of hypoprothrombinemia caused by oral anticoagulants; furthermore, it should not be given to pregnant women near term or in labor or to newborns because it is more likely than vitamin K_1 to cause hyperbilirubinemia and hemolytic anemia in these infants. Individuals who are subject to primaquine-sensitive anemia may develop hemolysis in response to large doses of menadiol.

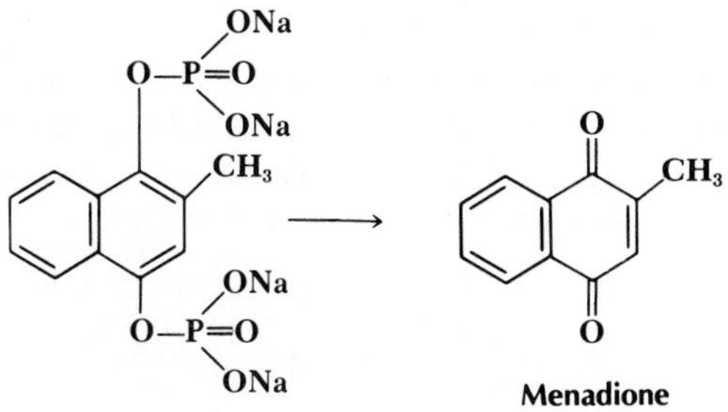

Menadiol sodium diphosphate → Menadione

Menadiol sodium diphosphate

Menadione

MEDICAL USES OF VITAMINS

Although exorbitant claims have been made for the curative powers of vitamins, which are often misused by the public, there are legitimate indications for vitamin therapy. Patients with poor dietary intake, deficiency diseases, or other relevant disease states, such as malabsorption syndromes, can benefit from vitamin supplementation; certain genetically determined conditions may also increase individual requirements for specific vitamins.

The minimum daily allowances (MDA) for vitamins are designed to avoid development of deficiency syndromes by healthy individuals; the recommended daily allowances (RDA) are two to six times higher. Table 55-1 lists vitamin requirements for males over 10 years of age and for pregnant or lactating women.

Specific vitamin requirements vary with the metabolic state of the individual and with diet. A strictly vegetarian diet lacking in dairy products or a diet lacking fruits and vegetables could cause specific deficiencies. Infants and pregnant women have predictably higher requirements and may benefit from vitamin therapy. Lactating women have increased requirements for ascorbic acid, thiamine, pyridoxine, folate, and riboflavin. Infants fed cow's milk should receive supplementary ascorbic acid daily, and low birth weight newborns may also need supplementation with vitamins C, D, E, folic acid, and pryidoxine.[9] Infants born to mothers who are taking phenytoin or phenobarbital may be deficient in vitamin K–dependent clotting factors and should be treated prophylactically with vitamin K_1.[11]

Vitamin deficiencies are attributable not only to poor dietary habits but also to concomitant disease. Alcoholism, pernicious anemia, total or partial gastrectomy, chronic pancreatitis, celiac disease (nontropical sprue), tropical sprue, and the short bowel syndrome can cause deficiencies of more than one vitamin and are usually associated with malnutrition.[17] Infection with *Diphyllobothrium latum*, hypoparathyroidism, and the carcinoid syndrome impose specific requirements for vitamins B_{12}, B_2, and niacin respectively.

There are a few genetically determined deficiency states in which failure of the apoenzyme to react normally with its coenzyme increases severalfold the requirement for a particular vitamin.[13] For example, an inborn error in the apoenzyme pyruvate carboxylase can produce lactic acidosis; this condition can be treated with 20 mg of thiamine daily. Disorders of this sort are rare, however, and, despite claims to the

TABLE 55-1 Recommended daily dietary allowances and therapeutic doses of vitamins

Vitamin	Adult requirement[3] Males (mg)	Adult requirement[3] Pregnant or lactating females (mg)	Daily oral therapeutic dose[9] (mg)
Water soluble			
Biotin	0.03-0.1	0.03-0.1	
Folic acid	0.15-0.2	0.26-0.4	5-10
Niacin	15-20	17-20	10-100
Pantothenic acid	4-7	4-7	100-200
Pyridoxine	1.7-2	2.1-2.2	20-50
Riboflavin	1.4-1.8	1.6-1.8	5-10
Thiamine	1.2-1.5	1.5-1.6	10-100
Vitamin B_{12}	0.002	0.0022-0.0026	0.1-0.25*
Vitamin C	50-60	70-90	100-200
Fat soluble			
Vitamin A	1.0	0.8-1.3	3-18
Vitamin D	0.005-0.01	0.01	0.125
Vitamin E	10	10-12	10-100
Vitamin K	0.045-0.08	0.065	5-10

*Weekly by intramuscular injection.

contrary, there is no adequate justification for megavitamin therapy. Vitamin megadosing has been promoted for improving the response to stress, correcting central nervous system disorders, preventing senility, and curing viral infections. Clinical documentation for such claims is lacking, and megadoses of vitamins can have harmful effects.

Other chemical compounds alleged to cure various ailments are frequently mislabeled as vitamins. The bioflavinoids, *p*-aminobenzoic acid, laetrile, and pangamic acid are widely touted as nutritional supplements, but none of these agents has any documented beneficial effect on human disease, and none have established functions in human nutrition.

TOXICITY

Doses of water-soluble vitamins above the recommended daily allowance are generally more wasteful than harmful. However, excessive intake of vitamin B_6 can cause peripheral neuropathy,[15] and injected thiamine can cause a shocklike state, similar to an anaphylactic reaction. Large doses of niacin cause vasodilatation and itching, and prolonged use can lead to liver damage. Ascorbic acid, originally considered to be harmless, can cause hyperoxaluria, uricosuria, and calculi formation when consumed in doses greater than 1 gm per day.

The fat-soluble vitamins A and D, which are stored in the body, have harmful effects at doses only 10 times greater than the recommended daily allowance. Hypervitaminosis A, from doses of 100,000 units or more per day, changes skeletal development in children and causes hepatomegaly, jaundice, anemia, and hair loss. Excess vitamin D can disturb calcium metabolism. Large parenteral doses of vitamin K can cause hemolytic anemia and jaundice; even death has occurred.

REFERENCES

1. Alperin JB: Coagulopathy caused by vitamin K deficiency in critically ill, hospitalized patients, *JAMA* 258:1916, 1987.
2. Burton GW, Ingold KU: β-Carotene: an unusual type of lipid antioxidant, *Science* 224:569, 1984.
3. *Drug Facts and Comparisons*, St Louis, 1990, JP Lippincott, p 2a.
4. Etretinate for psoriasis, *Med Lett Drugs Ther* 29:9, 1987.
5. Halter SA: Vitamin A: its role in the chemoprevention and chemotherapy of cancer, *Hum Pathol* 20:205, 1989.
6. Henderson LM: Niacin, *Annu Rev Nutr* 3:289, 1983.
7. Ink SL, Henderson LM: Vitamin B_6 metabolism, *Annu Rev Nutr* 4:455, 1984.
8. Levine M, Morita K: Ascorbic acid in endocrine systems, *Vitam Horm* 42:1, 1985.
9. Marks J: *The vitamins: their role in medical practice*, Lancaster, 1985, MTP Press.
10. Merrill AH Jr, Henderson JM: Diseases associated with defects in vitamin B_6 metabolism or utilization, *Annu Rev Nutr* 7:137, 1987.
11. Olson RE: The function and metabolism of vitamin K, *Annu Rev Nutr* 4:281, 1984.
12. Rose RC, McCormick DB, Li T-K, et al: Transport and metabolism of vitamins, *Fed Proc* 45:30, 1986.
13. Rudman D, Williams PJ: Megadose vitamins: use and misuse, *N Engl J Med* 309:488, 1983.
14. Russell P, Garland D, Zigler JS Jr, et al: Aging effects of vitamin C on a human lens protein produced in vitro, *FASEB J* 1:32, 1987.
15. Schaumburg H, Kaplan J, Windebank A, et al: Sensory neuropathy from pyridoxine abuse: a new megavitamin syndrome, *N Engl J Med* 309:445, 1983.
16. Sheffy BE, Schultz RD: Influence of vitamin E and selenium on immune response mechanisms, *Fed Proc* 38:2139, 1979.
17. Taylor KB: Uses and abuse of vitamin therapy, *Ration Drug Ther* 9(10):1, 1975.
18. Wittpenn J, Sommer A: Clinical aspects of vitamin A deficiency. In Bauernfeind JC, editor: *Vitamin A deficiency and its control*, Orlando Florida, 1986, Academic Press, p 177.

section ten

Chemotherapy

Chapter 56

Introduction to chemotherapy; mechanisms of antimicrobial action

HISTORIC DEVELOPMENT

The year 1935 was an important one in chemotherapy of systemic bacterial infections. In that year the red azo dye **Prontosil** was shown to protect mice against systemic streptococcal infection and to cure patients suffering from such infections. The chemotherapeutic activity of Prontosil was attributable to a metabolite, **sulfanilamide**. Although neither of these compounds is currently used therapeutically, these observations initiated a new era in medicine, as numerous derivatives of sulfanilamide were synthesized and systemic infections were controlled by them.

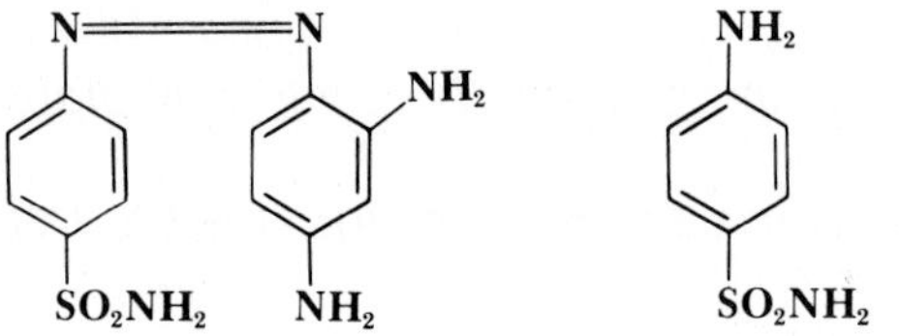

N=N NH$_2$ SO_2NH_2 NH_2

Prontosil

NH_2 SO_2NH_2

Sulfanilamide

Compounds produced by microorganisms (*antibiotics*) were also discovered to inhibit the growth of other microorganisms. Fleming found that a mold of the genus *Penicillium* prevented multiplication of staphylococci and that filtrates of cultures of this mold had similar properties.[4] A concentrate of this antibacterial factor was eventually prepared, and its remarkable activity and lack of toxicity were demonstrated by Florey and colleagues at Oxford.[7] A few years earlier, Dubos had reported on a bacteria-attacking microbe that contained gramicidin.[3] This compound was used successfully in animals (the Borden cow herd at the 1939 World's Fair) but was too toxic for use in humans. The discovery of the antimicrobial activity of penicillin turned the attention of investigators to antibiotics as potentially useful chemotherapeutic compounds. In the 1940s and 1950s streptomycin, the tetracyclines, chloramphenicol, polymyxin, bacitracin, and neomycin greatly increased the range of effectiveness of antibacterial chemotherapy. However, toxicity was a significant hazard, and organisms developed resistance to many of these agents. The continued search for effective antimicrobial drugs with less toxicity led to newer antibiotics of many classes, including semisynthetic penicillins, cephalosporins, and quinolones.

GENERAL CONCEPTS

Proper use of the large number of effective antimicrobial agents requires that several principles guide the physician in selecting the most appropriate drug and in using optimal dosage for a given patient. The choice of drug class may depend principally on the clinical situation, based on probabilities of bacteriologic diagnosis, but the specific compound and dosage relate to such host factors as renal function, age, and disease state. For instance, a patient with a bacterial infection who is receiving antineoplastic chemotherapy for leukemia has requirements different from those of an elderly person with pneumonia. Susceptibility tests do not automatically dictate which agent to use, but laboratories now report *minimal inhibitory concentrations* (MIC), which are more useful than just susceptibilities.

Several important concepts have been derived from extensive studies on antibacterial chemotherapy.[7]

Antibacterial spectrum refers to the range of activity of a compound. A broad-spectrum antimicrobial drug can affect a wide variety of microorganisms, usually including both gram-positive and gram-negative bacteria.

Antimicrobial or *bacteriostatic activity* of a chemotherapeutic agent is usually expressed as the lowest concentration (the MIC) at which the drug inhibits multiplication of the susceptible microorganism.[7]

Bactericidal activity refers to the ability to kill the microorganism, expressed as *minimal bactericidal concentration* (MBC). This requires tests beyond the usual plate or tube-dilution methods used to determine MIC. In certain clinical situations, as in treating bacterial endocarditis or the aforementioned leukemic patient, one must be certain that the agents are bactericidal for the organism. Antibacterial substances, such as penicillin or vancomycin, that bind to proteins in the microbial cell wall to disturb its synthesis or function, are usually bactericidal. In contrast, drugs, such as tetracyclines, that inhibit protein synthesis by attachment to ribosomal binding sites do not kill and are bacteriostatic.

Antibiotic synergism and *antibiotic antagonism* characterize the activity of combinations of antibiotics. Bacteriostatic combinations are indifferent (no more effective than either drug alone) or additive. However, if two antibiotics, such as penicillin and streptomycin, exert enhanced bactericidal activity in vitro when tested in combination relative to either alone, as occurs with *Enterococcus fecalis*, they are said to be synergistic.[8] If, on the other hand, a bacteriostatic antibiotic interferes with the killing action of a bactericidal agent, *antibiotic antagonism* has occurred. Clinical situations illustrating this latter phenomenon are infrequent, but a combination of penicillin with tetracycline was shown to be clinically less effective than penicillin alone in treatment of bacterial meningitis.[8] The following indications for combinations of antibiotics are justified: (1) to prevent emergence of resistant organisms during therapy, (2) to enhance the antimicrobial effect, especially for synergistic killing, and (3) to broaden the antibacterial spectrum in presumed mixed infections pending bacteriologic diagnosis.[1]

There are also many disadvantages to the combined use of antibiotics.[8] Combinations expose the patient to adverse effects of multiple drugs including drug interactions, and in rare instances antibiotic antagonism occurs. Furthermore, enhanced cost is incurred for multiple drug administration sets and for additional nursing time.

TABLE 56-1 Mechanisms of antimicrobial action

Action	Examples	Mechanism
1. Competitive antagonism	Sulfonamides	Competition with PABA interferes with synthesis of precursors of folic acid
2. Inhibition of cell-wall synthesis	β-lactams (penicillins)	Binding to PBPs and inhibition of cross-linking, with subsequent autolysis
3. Alteration of cell-membrane permeability	Amphotericin B	Binding to ergosterol results in loss of cations and fungal cell death
4. Inhibition of protein synthesis	Tetracyclines	Inhibition of binding of tRNA to 30S ribosomal subunit
5. Inhibition of nucleic acid synthesis	Acyclovir	Blockade of viral DNA replication after phosphorylation by viral thymidine kinase

Hence the search continues for single agents that can deliver broader antimicrobial activity at lower cost.

ANTIBACTERIAL CHEMOTHERAPEUTIC AGENTS—MECHANISMS OF ACTION

Most of the commonly used antimicrobial compounds act by one of five basic mechanisms (Table 56-1).

Competitive antagonism

Some antibacterial compounds act as antimetabolites (Fig. 56-1). Certain bacteria require *p*-aminobenzoic acid (PABA) for synthesis of folic acid precursors. Sulfonamide antimicrobials compete with PABA for binding to the appropriate microbial enzyme, an action that prevents synthesis of folic acid. Since mammalian organisms do not synthesize folic acid but require it as a vitamin, sulfonamides do not interfere with metabolism of mammalian cells.

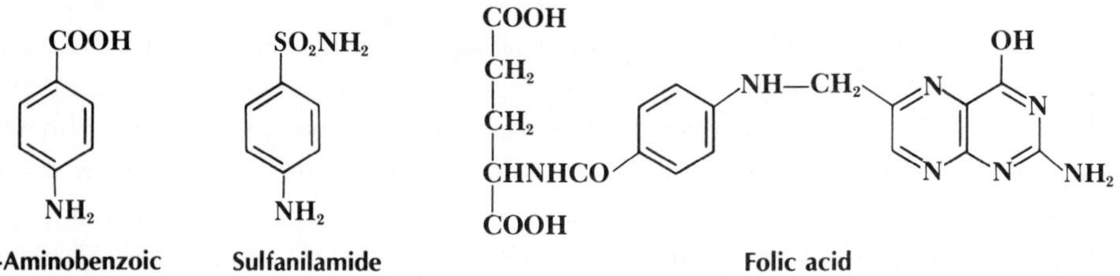

_p_-Aminobenzoic acid **Sulfanilamide** **Folic acid**

Another example of competitive antagonism in antibacterial chemotherapy involves the infrequently administered drug *p*-aminosalicylate, which also competes with PABA to produce its effect against mycobacteria.

Biosynthetic reactions blocked by sulfonamides and trimethoprim. *FIG. 56-1*

(Hydroxymethyl) dihydropteridine + *p*-Aminobenzoic acid (PABA)

Sulfonamides ⟶ Dihydropteroate synthase

Dihydropteroic acid

↓ plus glutamic acid

Dihydrofolic acid

Trimethoprim ⟶ Dihydrofolate reductase

Tetrahydrofolic acid

Inhibition of bacterial cell-wall synthesis

Several antibiotics inhibit synthesis of the bacterial cell wall.[7] This cell wall, in contrast to mammalian cell membranes, is rigid, so that bacteria can maintain a very high internal osmotic pressure. The structural element of the cell wall is known as *murein*. Cross-linkage of murein precursors is catalyzed by specific regulatory proteins, for example, transpeptidases and carboxypeptidases. These enzymes also bind β-lactam antibiotics, so they are called penicillin-binding proteins (PBPs)[10] (Fig. 56-2). After antibiotic binding to PBPs, autolytic enzymes that degrade the preformed cell wall are released. Cell-wall synthesis is inhibited and the bacteria die.

Action on cell membranes

Some antibiotics, such as polymyxins and antifungal polyenes, exert a detergent-like action that alters the permeability of cell membranes (Fig. 56-3).[7] Although antibiotics that act on cell membranes have some selective toxicity for microorganisms, they may also be toxic for mammalian cells. For this reason, polymyxins are rarely used clinically except in topical preparations. Interaction of the polyene antibiotics amphotericin B and nystatin with ergosterol (a cell-membrane lipid important for maintaining membrane integrity) causes loss of cations and, consequently, fungal cell death (Fig. 56-3, *D*).[7] Unfortunately, these polyenes also bind to mammalian cell sterols and are quite toxic, particularly for red blood cell and kidney tubular membranes. The detergent-like activity is prevented if the antimicrobial agent is unable to penetrate through the outer cell wall to reach the inner cytoplasmic membrane.

Inhibition of protein synthesis

Antibiotics such as the tetracyclines and aminoglycosides inhibit protein synthesis (Fig. 56-4). After these antibiotics traverse the cell membrane and enter the cell, they bind to ribosomal subunits.[7] Chloramphenicol inhibits mitochondrial protein synthesis. Other agents stop elongation of protein or lead to protein deformation. Highly toxic drugs like cycloheximide are potent inhibitors of protein synthesis in both microorganisms and mammals.

Inhibition of nucleic acid synthesis

Some antimicrobial or antiviral agents selectively inhibit nucleic acid synthesis by: (1) acting as nucleoside analogs (antiviral agents), (2) binding to RNA polymerase (rifampin), or (3) inhibiting DNA gyrase (quinolones) (Fig. 56-5).[6,9]

FIG. 56-2 *Inhibition of cell-wall synthesis.* ***A****, Precursors are cross-linked by penicillin-binding protein (PBP) and then added to the cell wall.* ***B****, Penicillin enters the cell through porins and binds to PBP.* ***C****, Binding leads to release of autolysins, which break down preformed cell wall.* ***D****, After penicillin binds to PBP, PBP can no longer synthesize proteins essential to cell-wall integrity.* ***E****, Cell wall loses integrity and can no longer preserve osmotic pressure.*

From Smith JW. In Murray PR, Drew WL, Kobayashi GS, Thompson JH Jr, editors: Medical microbiology, St Louis, 1990, Mosby–Year Book, p 37.

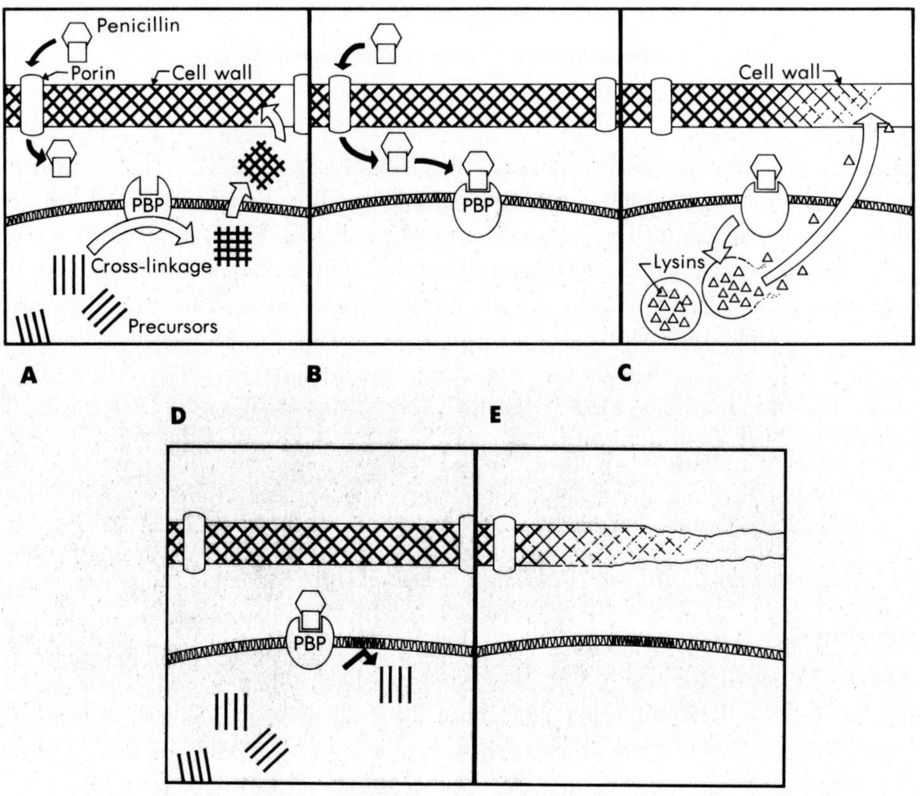

RESISTANCE

Bacterial resistance to antibiotics may have a *nongenetic* basis, or it may develop by genetic changes.[7] Nongenetic resistance is most frequently attributable to the absence of targets for the drug in the bacteria. If the bacteria have no receptors that bind to the drug or lack a metabolic pathway necessary for drug activity, they are intrinsically insensitive (for example, gram-negative bacilli and vancomycin). Inadequate permeability to a compound (Fig. 56-6, *A*) may also account for its ineffectiveness against gram-negative bacteria or fungi (for example, tetracycline for some gram-negative bacilli). Certain microorganisms can escape the consequences of drug action by synthesizing an enzyme that destroys or modifies the antibiotic (Fig. 56-6, *B*, *D*) or by altering the macromolecules to which the antibiotic binds (Fig. 56-6, *C*).

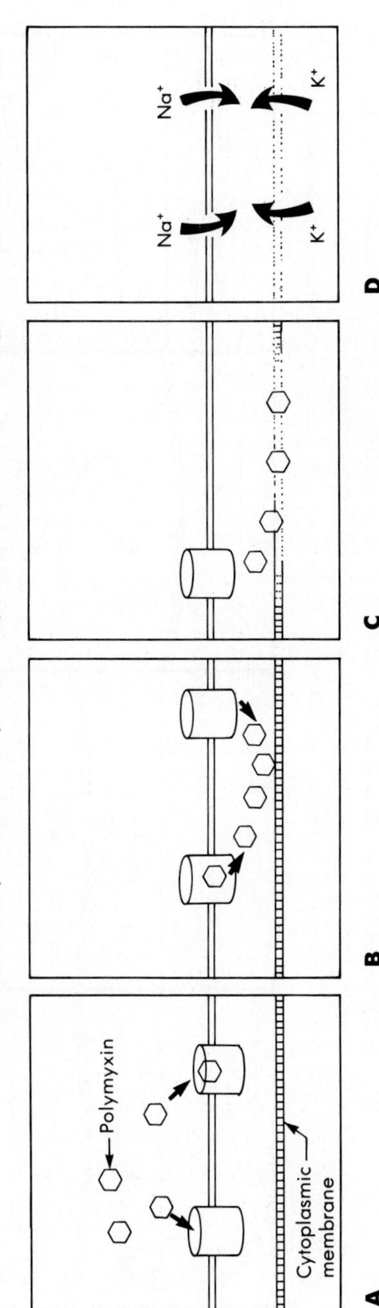

FIG. 56-3 Alterations of cell membranes. ***A***, Bacterial cell. ***B***, Penetration of polymyxin to inner cytoplasmic membrane. ***C***, Detergent-like disruption of cytoplasmic membrane. ***D***, Loss of cell integrity with subsequent cell death.

From Smith JW. In Murray PR, Drew WL, Kobayashi GS, Thompson JH Jr, editors: Medical microbiology, St Louis, 1990, Mosby–Year Book, p. 37.

FIG. 56-4 *Inhibition of protein synthesis.* ***A***, *Aminoglycoside (AG) enters bacterium through porins.* ***B***, *AG is actively transported across cytoplasmic membrane.* ***C***, *AG binds to 30 S ribosomal subunit.* ***D***, *As a consequence of binding there is: (1) failure to initiate protein synthesis; (2) failure of elongation of protein; and (3) misreading of tRNA, leading to deformed proteins.*

From Smith JW. In Murray PR, Drew WL, Kobayashi GS, Thompson JH Jr, editors: Medical microbiology, St Louis, 1990, Mosby–Year Book, p 37.

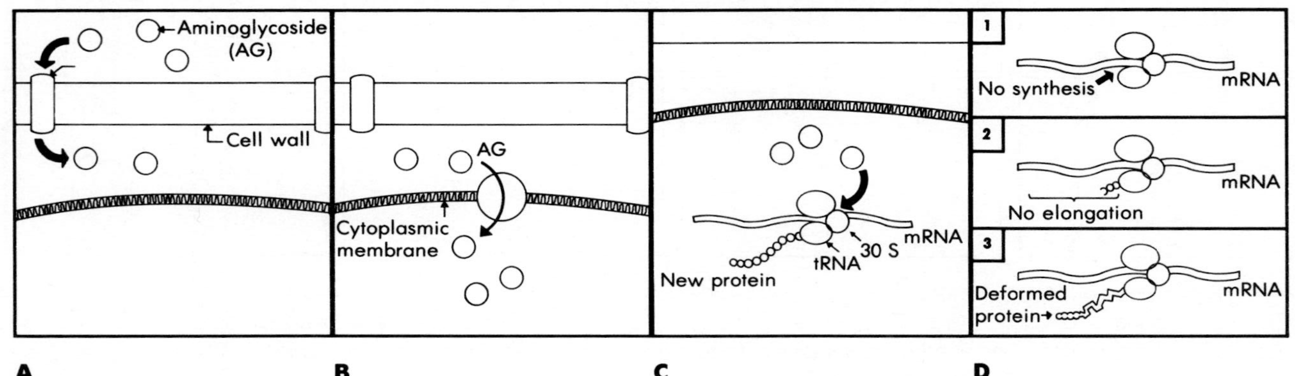

Inhibition of nucleic acid synthesis. 1, Rifampin (R) binds to DNA-dependent RNA polymerase and inhibits RNA synthesis. 2, Quinolone (Q) inhibits DNA gyrase to prevent supercoiling of DNA. **FIG. 56-5**

From Smith JW. In Murray PR, Drew WL, Kobayashi GS, Thompson JH Jr, editors: Medical microbiology, St Louis, 1990, Mosby–Year Book, p 37.

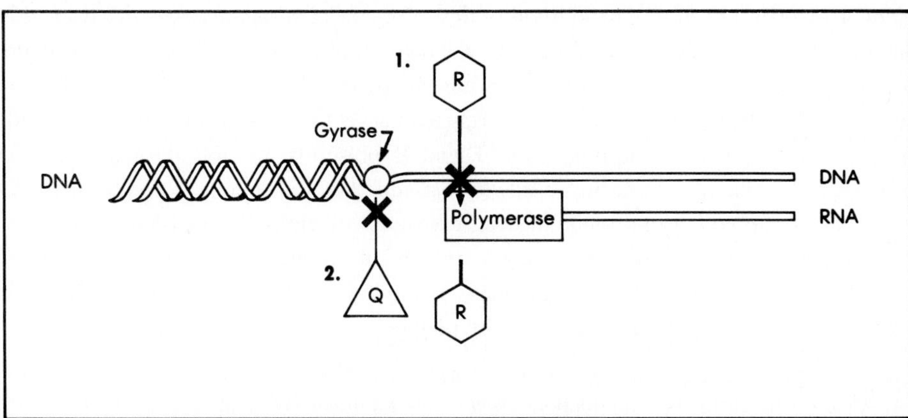

Bacterial development of resistance to antibiotics. ***A**, Change in porin so bacterium is impermeable to drug.* ***B**, Enzyme inactivates penicillin by opening β-lactam ring, so penicillin cannot bind to PBP.* ***C**, There is a decrease in the affinity of the target site on the ribosome for streptomycin (S).* ***D**, The enzyme acetylates gentamicin (Gm) so that gentamicin will not bind to the ribosome.* **FIG. 56-6**

From Smith JW. In Murray PR, Drew WL, Kobayashi GS, Thompson JH Jr, editors: Medical microbiology, St Louis, 1990, Mosby–Year Book, 37.

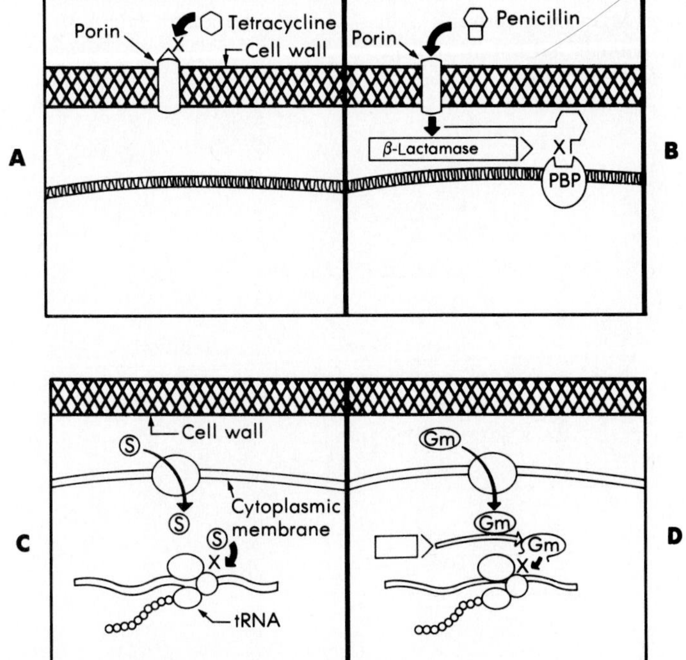

Genetic drug resistance

Genetic resistance may be of chromosomal origin or may be transmitted by extrachromosomal *plasmids*.[2] Chromosomal resistance can arise from spontaneous mutations. However, an important method of development of resistance was discovered by Japanese investigators in the 1950s. They showed that resistance to several unrelated antibiotics can be transferred to susceptible organisms by cell-to-cell contact or conjugation. The bacteria contain extrachromosomal DNA or resistance (R) plasmids, which act like viruses without coats. These R plasmids are found in a variety of gram-negative bacilli, including *Shigella*, *Salmonella*, *Klebsiella*, *Vibrio*, *Pasteurella*, and *Escherichia coli*. Emergence of drug-resistant enteric pathogens has been attributed to the feeding of subtherapeutic amounts of antimicrobial compounds to animals.[5] In addition to gram-negative organisms, staphylococci may also contain plasmids, which are transferred from cell to cell by phages, a form of *transduction*.[7]

REFERENCES

1. Allan JD Jr: Antibiotic combinations, *Med Clin North Am* 71:1079, 1987.
2. Benveniste R, Davies J: Mechanisms of antibiotic resistance in bacteria, *Annu Rev Biochem* 42:471, 1973.
3. Crease RP: Righting the antibiotic record, *Science* 246:883, 1989.
4. Fleming A: On antibacterial action of cultures of penicillium, with special reference to their use in isolation of *B. influenzae*, *Br J Exp Pathol* 10:226, 1929.
5. Holmberg SD, Osterholm MT, Senger KA, Cohen ML: Drug-resistant salmonella from animals fed antimicrobials, *N Engl J Med* 311:617, 1984.
6. Kaufman HE: Antiviral drugs, *Int J Dermatol* 16:464, 1977.
7. Pratt WB, Fekety R: *The antimicrobial drugs*, New York, 1986, Oxford University Press.
8. Rahal JJ Jr: Antibiotic combinations: the clinical relevance of synergy and antagonism, *Medicine* (Baltimore) 57:179, 1978.
9. Schinazi RF, Prusoff WH: Antiviral drugs: modes of action and strategies for therapy, *Hosp Pract* 16(6):113, 1981.
10. Tomasz A: Penicillin-binding proteins in bacteria, *Ann Intern Med* 96:502, 1982.

Chapter 57

Antimicrobial agents: sulfonamides and quinolones

GENERAL CONCEPT

The discovery of the antibacterial action of sulfanilamide and initial clinical trials in the 1930s are landmarks in the use of pharmacologic agents to treat infections. Sulfonamides (sulfas) are true *antimetabolites*; they block a specific step in the biosynthetic pathway of folic acid. Sulfonamides still have important applications, particularly as the trimethoprim-sulfamethoxazole combination. This chapter also discusses the quinolones and other nonsulfonamide drugs used to treat urinary tract infections.

SULFONAMIDE DRUGS

Chemistry

Nearly all currently used sulfonamides are derivatives of sulfanilamide. A free amino group is required in the *para* position—sulfonamides substituted in this amino group become active only if the substituent is removed in vivo. Substitution on the R_2 amide group influences the absorption, distribution, and solubility of the various compounds.

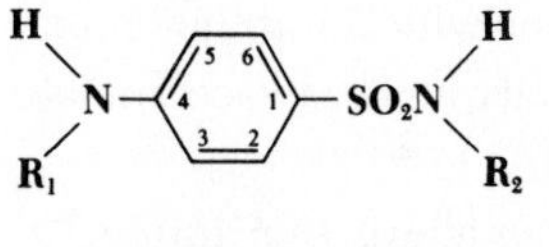

Sulfanilamide ($R_1 = R_2 = H$) 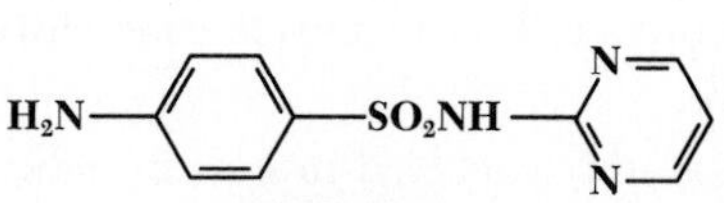 Sulfadiazine 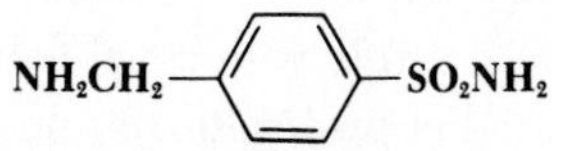 Mafenide

Antibacterial spectrum

Sulfonamides are effective against a broad range of microorganisms.[14] *Streptococcus pyogenes, Streptococcus pneumoniae*, and *Listeria monocytogenes* are sensitive gram-positive organisms. Susceptible gram-negative organisms include *Escherichia coli, Proteus, Salmonella* species, and some strains of meningococcus and *Vibrio cholerae*. The sulfonamides are also active against *Actinomyces, Nocardia, Chlamydia*, and some protozoa. However, because their efficacy is not comparable to that of newer agents, their usage has declined.

Sulfonamides such as sulfisoxazole (Gantrisin) have been used to treat acute urinary tract infections, but bacteria such as *Escherichia coli* are less susceptible than to other agents. Sulfonamides are presently useful in treatment of nocardiosis, trachoma, toxoplasmosis, and chancroid. In treating otitis media and lower respiratory infections, the sulfonamide is combined with an antibiotic such as erythromycin.[2]

Derivatives that are poorly absorbed from the gastrointestinal tract were once used for preoperative bowel "sterilization."

Mode of action

Sulfonamides are competitive inhibitors of the enzyme (dihydropteroate synthase) responsible for synthesis of dihydropteroic acid, a precursor of folic acid (see Fig. 56-1). The drugs are structurally similar to PABA, which combines with a dihydropteridine to form dihydropteroic acid, but they have a greater affinity for the microbial enzyme than PABA does. With decreased folic acid synthesis, there is a reduction in bacterial nucleotides and inhibition of growth. Mammalian cells require preformed folic acid and therefore are not affected by sulfonamides.[14]

Resistance

Organisms such as *Staphylococcus*, some species of the family *Enterobacter*, and all *Pseudomonas* strains are resistant to sulfonamides. The mechanism of resistance may be related to the ability of the bacteria to lower the affinity of their synthase for the drug or to overproduce dihydrofolate reductase, which may compensate for reduced dihydrofolate substrate. Resistance can also be mediated by plasmids (R factors).

Pharmacokinetics

Short-acting sulfonamides (**sulfisoxazole** and **sulfadiazine**) are absorbed rapidly from the gastrointestinal tract. They are given in oral doses of 2 to 4 g initially, followed by about 1 g every 4 to 6 hours to maintain a plasma concentration of approximately 100 μg/ml.[14] Pediatric maintenance dosage is 150 mg/kg/day. The half-life of the shorter-acting agents varies from 5 to 9 hours. **Sulfamethoxazole** (Gantanol, Urobak), an intermediate-duration drug, has a half-life of up to 12 hours. Serum concentrations of sulfonamides can be determined to monitor therapy in serious infections requiring intravenous administration or for patients with renal failure.

Acetylation of the free *p*-amino group produces a product with no antimicrobial activity, but the metabolite retains the capacity to cause toxicity and may accumulate in patients with renal failure.

Because sulfisoxazole is readily excreted in human milk, an alternative antimicrobial should be used for the lactating mother during an infant's first several weeks of life and also during the last month of pregnancy. Sulfonamides bind to plasma proteins and compete for bilirubin-binding sites; in infants this displacement of bilirubin increases its free concentration and the risk of kernicterus.[14]

Unbound sulfonamides are filtered through renal glomeruli, and the tubules reabsorb a portion of the filtered drug. The urinary concentration of sulfonamides may be 25 to 50 times higher than that in plasma, a circumstance that contributes to their usefulness as urinary antimicrobials.

Toxicity and hypersensitivity

Virtually every organ system has been involved in toxic reactions to sulfonamides. Gastrointestinal effects (nausea, vomiting, and loss of appetite) are fairly common. Hepatitis and bone marrow depression occur infrequently as do hemolytic anemia and other blood dyscrasias. Moreover, patients who are deficient in *glucose-6-phosphate dehydrogenase*, such as one third of American black males, are at risk for hemolysis.

Sulfonamides behave as weak acids because of dissociation of the sulfamyl group ($-SO_2NH-$). The molecular (acid) form of early sulfonamides is poorly soluble and can precipitate in urine. Because the salts (ions) formed at higher pH are much more soluble, alkalinization of the urine was used to decrease precipitation. However, the high solubility of newer derivatives such as sulfisoxazole eliminates the need to alkalinize the urine.

Hypersensitivity reactions are rare but of great clinical import. These include syndromes that resemble arteritis and lupus erythematosus. Skin eruptions may range from a diffuse morbilliform rash or erythema multiforme to exfoliative dermatitis (Stevens-Johnson syndrome). This latter complication is especially dreaded because of its high mortality. Some longer-acting sulfonamides were removed from the market because the Stevens-Johnson syndrome was associated with their use. Recent implication of sulfadoxine, a long-acting agent used in prophylaxis and treatment of chloroquine-resistant malaria, in Stevens-Johnson syndrome has also limited its use. Other serious hypersensitivity reactions include urticaria, a serum sickness–like syndrome, and frank anaphylaxis.

Trimethoprim-sulfamethoxazole

The trimethoprim-sulfamethoxazole preparation (co-trimoxazole) has truly synergistic actions on bacteria. It inhibits two steps in bacterial metabolism: the sulfonamide inhibits PABA utilization in folic acid synthesis, whereas trimethoprim is a competitive inhibitor of dihydrofolate reductase, another enzyme important in folic acid synthesis[11] (see Fig. 56-1). For 50% inhibition the mammalian enzyme requires 50,000 times the trimethoprim concentration needed for the bacterial enzyme. This most likely explains the relative lack of toxicity of trimethoprim.

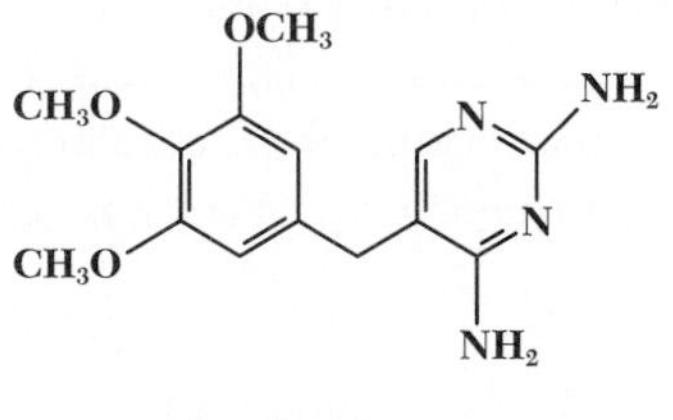

Trimethoprim

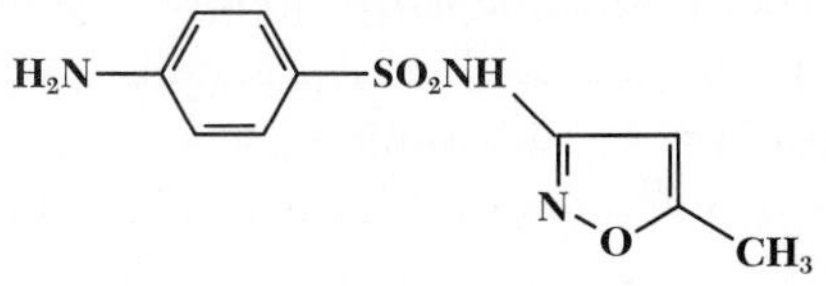

Sulfamethoxazole

Trimethoprim-sulfamethoxazole has replaced most sulfonamides in therapy because the combination covers a large variety of gram-positive and gram-negative microorganisms.[2] Acute and chronic urinary tract infections are prime indications. The combination is the drug of choice for infections caused by *Shigella* and *Pneumocystis carinii* and is also effective treatment for typhoid or paratyphoid fever, bacterial infections of the lower respiratory tract, otitis media, uncomplicated gonorrhea, and vivax and falciparum malaria. A parenteral preparation is available for severe infections, such as severe *Pneumocystis carinii* pneumonia.[2]

Absorption of trimethoprim-sulfamethoxazole is rapid. Effective concentrations may be present in plasma for 6 to 8 hours.[11] Trimethoprim is excreted mostly unchanged in the urine, while sulfamethoxazole is acetylated.

The adverse effects of sulfonamides have also been seen with trimethoprim-sulfamethoxazole. Crystalluria is rare. Trimethoprim alone can cause skin rashes and bone-marrow toxicity. Patients with blood dyscrasias, hepatic damage, and severe renal impairment are predisposed to aberrant changes in blood elements. The combination enhances the anticoagulant effect of warfarin and prolongs the half-life of phenytoin.

Trimethoprim-sulfamethoxazole is available in single-strength tablets containing trimethoprim, 80 mg, and sulfamethoxazole, 400 mg, as double-strength tablets with twice as much of each, and for intravenous infusion as 16/80 mg/ml. Pediatric suspensions contain 40 mg of trimethoprim and 200 mg sulfamethoxazole per 5 ml. The 1:5 ratio produces a concentration ratio of 1:20 trimethoprim to sulfamethoxazole in plasma.[11]

MISCELLANEOUS SULFONAMIDES

Mafenide (Sulfamylon) was widely used as a topical agent in seriously burned patients to prevent wound contamination, especially by *Pseudomonas* species. Currently, mafenide has been replaced by silver sulfadiazine (Silvadene, Flint SSD), which is painless and appears to have very low systemic toxicity. Bacterial resistance to silver sulfadiazine is not yet the problem that it is with mafenide.

Sodium sulfacetamide (AK-Sulf, others) is available in ophthalmic preparations (10% to 30%) to treat bacterial conjunctivitis. The pH of the solution is 7.4, thereby producing minimal conjunctival irritation.

Some sulfonamide compounds are used only for purposes other than antimicrobial therapy. Sulfasalazine, used to treat inflammatory bowel disease, is discussed in Chapter 45. Dermatitis herpetiformis is an indication for sulfapyridine.

OTHER ANTIBACTERIAL AGENTS FOR URINARY TRACT INFECTIONS

In addition to sulfonamides, several antimicrobial agents are used almost exclusively to treat urinary tract infections.[12] Their major characteristics are summarized in Table 57-1.

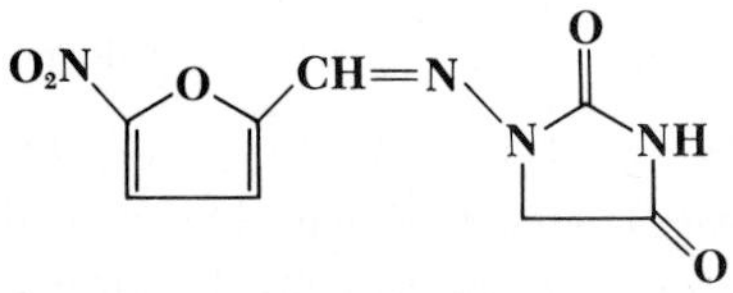

Nitrofurantoin

Nitrofurantoin, one of a series of nitrofurans, is absorbed rapidly, and much of it is excreted unchanged in the urine. Its mechanism of action is unknown, but it may inhibit a variety of enzyme systems in bacteria. It has a wide antibacterial spectrum; both gram-positive and gram-negative bacteria can be inhibited at concentrations attained in urine after daily oral administration of 5 to 7 mg/kg. Its use is limited to short-term treatment or low-dose suppression of urinary tract infection.[12] Nitrofuran-

TABLE 57-1 Antimicrobial agents used principally for urinary tract infections

Drug	Oral dosage	Activity
Sulfonamides	1 g every 4 to 6 hours	First-time infections in the young; resistance develops in fecal organisms, and so recurrent infections are likely resistant
Trimethroprim-sulfamethoxazole (Bactrim, Septra, others)	160/800 mg	First time, as 3-day course for lower or as 14-day course for upper tract infection; to prevent recurrences in women use 80/400 mg after sexual intercourse or three times weekly for 6 to 12 months; in men alternate daily tablet every 6 months with nitrofurantoin
Nitrofurantoin (Furadantin, others)	50 to 100 mg every 6 hours	Best as preventive or for recurrent lower tract infection (ineffective for upper tract); use to prevent recurrence in bacteriuric pregnant, or for 6-month periods in non-pregnant, women; do not use longer than 6 months because of toxicity; to prevent recurrence, it can be given on a full stomach to women the morning after intercourse
Methenamine mandelate (Mandelamine, Mandemeth)	1 g every 6 hours	Rarely used since must have very acid urine; toxic in renal insufficiency
Quinolones		
Nalidixic acid (NegGram)	1 g every 6 hours	Rarely used since resistance develops rapidly; difficult to swallow; replaced by other quinolones
Norfloxacin (Noroxin)	400 mg twice daily	Resistant infections; especially recurrent
Cinoxacin (Cinobac)	500 mg twice daily	Treat again, if recurs after initial course
Ciprofloxacin (Cipro)	250-750 mg twice daily	

toin can cause numerous adverse reactions. Nausea and vomiting are common; the frequency is lessened by concomitant administration with food or milk. Skin sensitization, peripheral neuritis, and cholestatic jaundice also occur. Hemolytic anemia can develop in patients deficient in glucose-6-phosphate dehydrogenase. Rarely, individuals develop an acute, dramatic pulmonary reaction. Interstitial fibrosis can develop with chronic therapy and is a reason for limiting even low-dose suppression to 6 months of administration. The drug can accumulate if renal function is impaired and is to be avoided in this setting.[4]

Preparations of nitrofurantoin include tablets and capsules, 50 and 100 mg, and a suspension, 25 mg/5 ml. A macrocrystalline preparation (Macrodantin), which may be less nauseating, is available in capsules, 25 to 100 mg.

Nitrofurazone (Furacin, 0.2%) is used topically for infections of the skin, but it may cause sensitization.

Methenamine mandelate is a combination of two old urinary antiseptics, methenamine and mandelic acid.

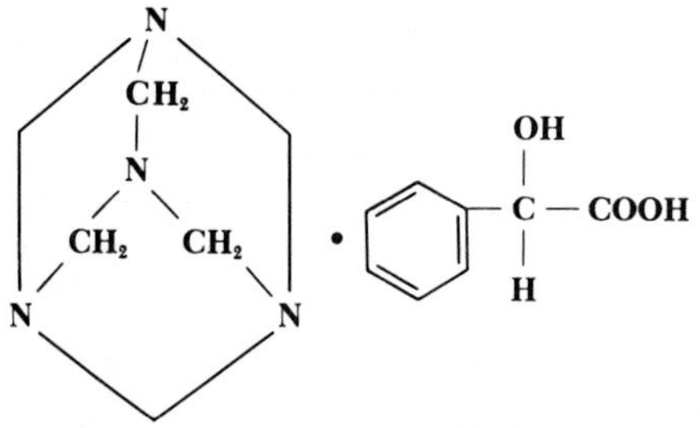

Methenamine mandelate

In acid urine methenamine liberates formaldehyde. If the pH of the urine is low, mandelic acid is bactericidal. If urinary pH is higher than 6, ascorbic acid or ammonium chloride must be taken in amounts of 0.5 to 1 g three or four times daily to acidify the urine.

Methenamine mandelate is relatively nontoxic, but gastric irritation can occur, probably as a result of formaldehyde production in the stomach. Because of bladder irritation, urinary frequency may develop. A variety of dosage forms containing from 0.25 to 1 g of the compound are available for oral administration. The usual dosage is 0.5 to 1 g four times a day. The drug is used primarily as a suppressive agent, though clinical efficacy has been difficult to establish.[13] In addition to methenamine mandelate, the hippurate salt of methenamine (Hiprex, Urex) is also available in tablets, 1 g.

QUINOLONES

The quinolones are synthetic chemotherapeutic agents that inhibit bacterial DNA gyrases. The gyrases, or topoisomerases, are required to supercoil strands of bacterial DNA into the bacterial cell.[5] Several compounds were recently approved that supersede nalidixic acid, to which resistance developed too readily. **Norfloxacin**, **cinoxacin**, and **ciprofloxacin** are presently approved for use in urinary tract infections.[8] Ciprofloxacin is effective for skin and soft tissue infections, bacterial gastroenteritis, and against some agents that cause respiratory tract infections.[1,3] Although these drugs are effective against virtually all gram-negative bacilli and staphylococci, they are not universally effective for streptococcal species.[7] Recently, rapid emergence of resistance has been noted with methicillin-resistant staphylococci, the strain found commonly in hospitals.[6]

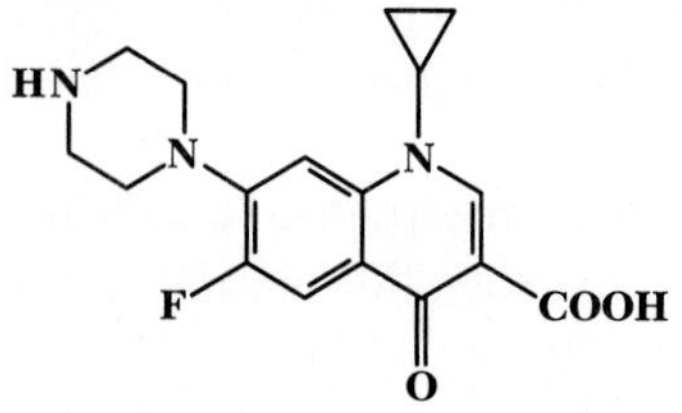

Ciprofloxacin 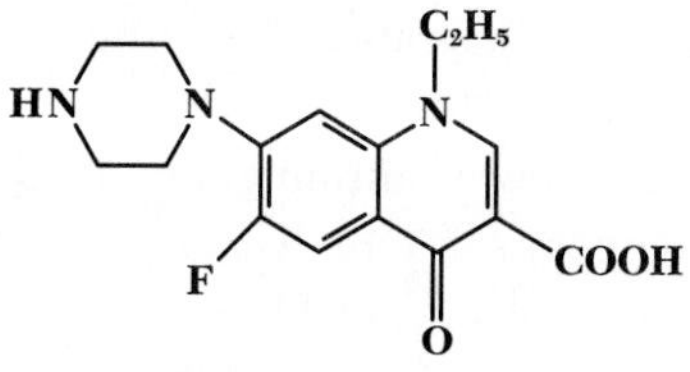 **Norfloxacin**

All of the quinolones are absorbed from the gastrointestinal tract to some degree; norfloxacin is the least well absorbed. Absorption is impaired by antacids.[9] A therapeutic plasma concentration persists for 8 to 12 hours but may be delayed in elderly patients. The quinolones are widely distributed in body tissues and fluids. They undergo metabolic conversion to compounds with reduced activity. All are also excreted in urine, even in patients with impaired renal function (see Appendix B); however, their dosage should be halved in such patients.

Nausea, vomiting, diarrhea, allergic reactions, and neurologic disturbances may occur after administration of quinolones.[1] The drugs may cause increased intracranial pressure in children and central nervous system reactions, including dizziness, headache, insomnia, and somnolence. Seizures while taking the drugs have been reported in patients with a previous convulsive disorder and focal neurologic deficits.[1] However, the incidence of toxicity with the new quinolones is quite low, in the range of 5%.[10] Because the drugs caused articular damage in tests on immature animals, they are not recommended for use in children. Patients who take quinolones along with theophylline should be closely monitored to prevent an excessive plasma concentration of theophylline.[1]

Preparations of nalidixic acid include tablets of 0.25 to 1 g. A pediatric suspension contains 250 mg/5 ml. Capsules of cinoxacin contain 250 or 500 mg, norfloxacin is available as tablets of 400 mg, and ciprofloxacin is available as 250 to 750 mg tablets.

REFERENCES

1. Campoli-Richards DM, Monk JP, Price A, et al: Ciprofloxacin: a review of its antibacterial activity, pharmacokinetic properties and therapeutic use, *Drugs* 35:373, 1988.
2. Foltzer MA, Reese RE: Trimethoprim-sulfamethoxazole and other sulfonamides, *Med Clin North Am* 71:1177, 1987.
3. Goodman LJ, Trenholme GM, Kaplan RL, et al: Empiric antimicrobial therapy of domestically acquired acute diarrhea in urban adults, *Arch Intern Med* 150:541, 1990.
4. Holmberg L, Boman G, Böttiger LE, et al: Adverse reactions to nitrofurantoin: analysis of 921 reports *Am J Med* 69:733, 1980.
5. Hooper DC, Wolfson JS: Mode of action of the quinolone antimicrobial agents: review of recent information, *Rev Infect Dis* 11(suppl 5):S902, 1989.
6. Isaacs RD, Kunke PJ, Cohen RL, Smith JW: Ciprofloxacin resistance in epidemic methicillin-resistant *Staphylococcus aureus*, *Lancet* 2:843, 1988.
7. Mazzulli T, Simor AE, Jaeger R, et al: Comparative in vitro activities of several new fluoroquinolones and β-lactam antimicrobial agents against community isolates of *Streptococcus pneumoniae*, *Antimicrob Agents Chemother* 34:467, 1990.
8. Neu HC: Quinolones: a new class of antimicrobial agents with wide potential uses, *Med Clin North Am* 72:623, 1988.
9. Nix DE, Wilton JH, Ronald B, et al: Inhibition of norfloxacin absorption by antacids, *Antimicrob Agents Chemother* 34:432, 1990.
10. Ramirez CA, Bran JL, Mejia CR, Garcia JF: Open, prospective study of the clinical efficacy of ciprofloxacin, *Antimicrob Agents Chemother* 28:128, 1985.
11. Rubin RH, Swartz MN: Trimethoprim-sulfamethoxazole, *N Engl J Med* 303:426, 1980.
12. Smith JW: Prognosis in pyelonephritis:

promise or progress? *Am J Med Sci* 297:53, 1989.

13. Vainrub B, Musher DM: Lack of effect of methenamine in suppression of, or prophylaxis against, chronic urinary infection, *Antimicrob Agents Chemother* 12:625, 1977.

14. Weinstein L, Madoff MA, Samet CM: The sulfonamides, *N Engl J Med* 263:793 and 842, 1960.

Chapter 58

Antibiotics: penicillin and other drugs used to treat gram-positive infections

A. FLEMING, 1929 While working with staphylococcus variants a number of culture-plates were set aside on the laboratory bench and examined from time to time. In the examinations these plates were necessarily exposed to the air and they became contaminated with various micro-organisms. It was noticed that around a large colony of a contaminating mould the staphylococcus colonies became transparent and were obviously undergoing lysis.

PENICILLIN

Penicillin is a highly effective antibiotic with an extremely wide margin of safety. Many derivatives have been synthesized by manipulations of its basic structure. The story of penicillin's discovery is both a scientific classic and a model for biomedical progress. It exemplifies Pasteur's dictum: "In research chance favors only the prepared mind." After the discovery of its antibiotic properties by Fleming,[7] the compound lay dormant for a decade awaiting biochemical studies by Florey and his group in England.[14] These studies built on Fleming's monumental observation and ushered in the modern age of chemotherapy.

Penicillin is an organic acid obtained from cultures of the mold *Penicillium chrysogenum*. If the mold is grown by a deep fermentation process, large amounts of the key intermediate, 6-aminopenicillanic acid, are produced. Newer derivatives are prepared by addition of side groups at the R position. Consequences of these substitutions include (1) decreased acid lability and thus increased gastrointestinal absorption, (2) resistance to destruction by penicillinase (also called β-lactamase), and (3) a widening of the spectrum of organisms susceptible to the compound.

Penicillin G (benzylpenicillin), as various salts, is the prototype drug. Bacteria that have *penicillinase*, an enzyme that breaks the lactam ring (ring A) in the penicillin structure (on next page), are resistant to penicillin G. Substitution of more bulky groups at the R site, as in methicillin and oxacillin, protects the lactam ring through steric hindrance. Other substitutions at the R site expand the antimicrobial spectrum to gram-negative organisms. These "broad-spectrum" penicillins such as ampicillin and ticarcillin are, however, sensitive to destruction by penicillinase; because resistance can develop if used alone, they are frequently combined with another antibiotic, such as an aminoglycoside.[19] In addition, synergism is often noted with combinations of these drugs.

Potency

Penicillin preparations are standardized on the basis of their capacity to inhibit growth of test organisms such as *Bacillus subtilis* or sensitive staphylococci. Activity was initially expressed in units and measured in comparison with a standard preparation. One milligram of penicillin G potassium equals 1600 units; conversely 1 unit is equivalent to 0.625 μg of penicillin G. The dose of penicillins is usually indicated in milligrams (or grams). Microorganisms inhibited by less than 1 μg of penicillin per milliliter may be considered moderately susceptible, since in clinical practice blood concentrations exceeding 1 μg/ml can be readily achieved. Highly susceptible microorganisms are usually inhibited by less than 0.1 μg/ml.

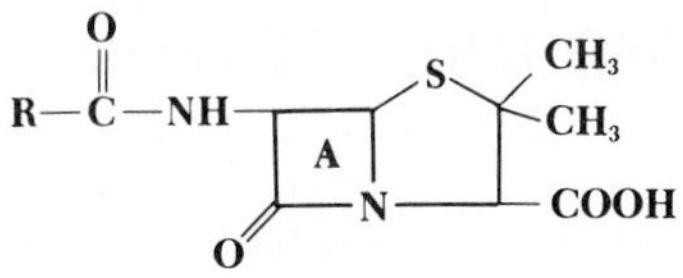

O
R—C—NH— A S CH_3 CH_3 N COOH O

Basic penicillin structure

R side chain

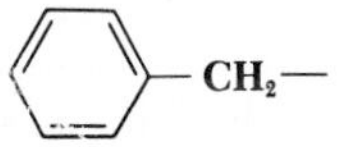

CH_2— **Penicillin G (benzylpenicillin)**

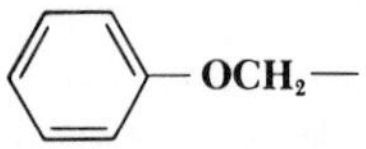

OCH_2— **Penicillin V (phenoxymethylpenicillin)**

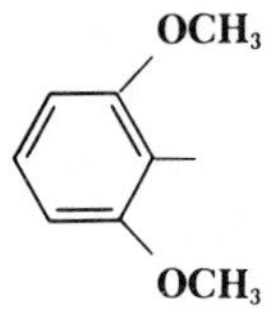

OCH_3 OCH_3 **Methicillin (Staphcillin)**

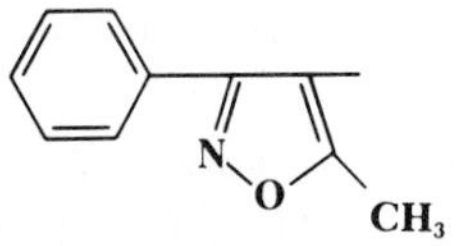

N O CH_3 **Oxacillin (Bactocill, Prostaphlin)**

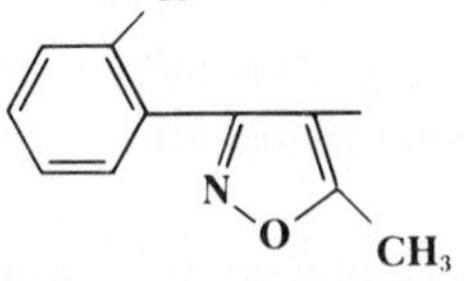

Cl N O CH_3 **Cloxacillin (Cloxapen, Tegopen)**

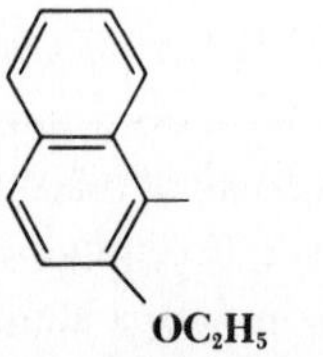

OC_2H_5 **Nafcillin (Nafcil, others)**

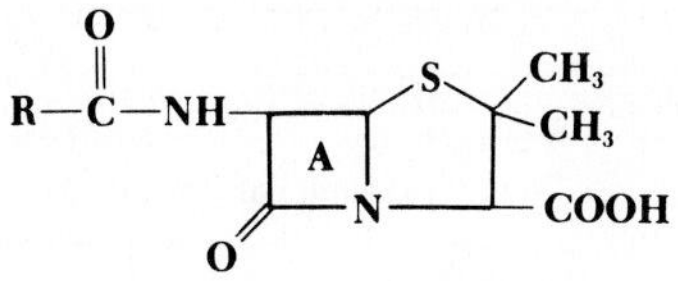

O
‖
R—C—NH— [β-lactam ring A]—N— COOH, S, CH_3, CH_3 **Basic penicillin structure**

R side chain

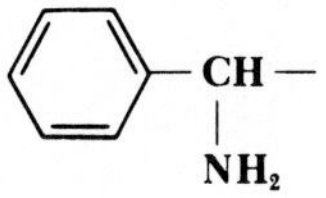

R side chain	Drug
C_6H_5—CH(—NH_2)—	**Ampicillin (Polycillin, Omnipen, others)**
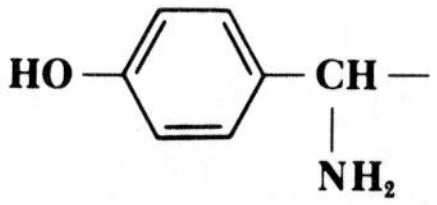 HO—C_6H_4—CH(—NH_2)—	**Amoxicillin (Amoxil, Polymox, others)**
C_6H_5—CH(—COOH)—	**Carbenicillin (Geopen, others)**
thienyl—CH(—COOH)—	**Ticarcillin (Ticar)**
C_6H_5—CH(—NHCO—[4-ethyl-2,3-dioxopiperazin-1-yl], N—C_2H_5)—	**Piperacillin (Pipracil)**

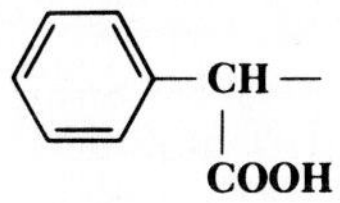

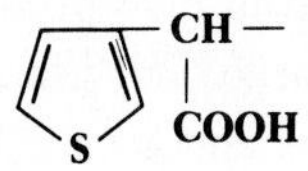

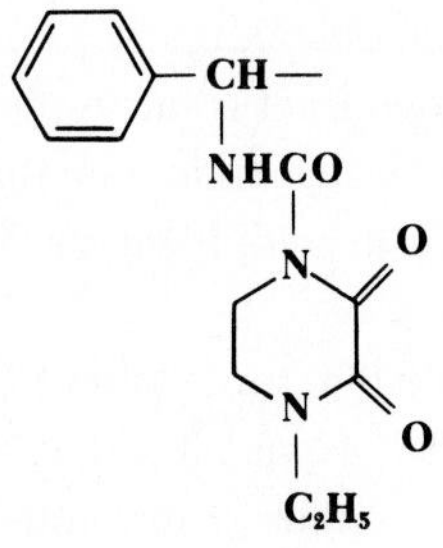

Mode of action

Several clinically useful antibiotics inhibit various enzymatic steps in cell-wall synthesis. Penicillins are bactericidal drugs that interfere with synthesis after attaching to penicillin-binding proteins (PBPs),[16] as illustrated in Fig. 56-2. Cross-linking of linear peptidoglycans is done by a transpeptidase PBP that also cleaves a terminal D-alanine. When penicillins and cephalosporins bind to a PBP, they act as competitive inhibitors. In addition, changes in the cellular shape of bacteria occur after binding of penicillins to various PBPs. Finally, cell lysis occurs after release of murein hydrolases, which degrade preformed cell wall.[28] The activity of these hydrolases is normally suppressed. Mutant organisms deficient in this autolytic capacity are inhibited, but not

TABLE 58-1 Pharmacologic properties of penicillins

Drug	Oral absorption	Therapeutic concentration (μg/ml)	Plasma half-life (hr)		Dosage reduction with renal failure
			Normal	Renal failure	
Oral					
G	Fair	2	0.5	10	Yes
V	Good	4	1	4	Slight
Nafcillin	Fair	1	1	1.5	None
Cloxacillin, dicloxacillin	Good	10	0.5	1	None
Ampicillin	Good	3	1	8	Yes
Amoxicillin	Excellent	7	1	8	Yes
Parenteral					
G		5-10	0.5	10	Yes
Ampicillin		10	1	8	Yes
Nafcillin		20	1	2	Slight
Carbenicillin, ticarcillin		100+	1	15	Yes
Piperacillin, mezlocillin		250-300	1	4	Yes

killed, by penicillins. Lysis by antibiotics also depends on pH and on components in the medium, such as Mg^{++}. Hence penicillin derivatives may produce a variety of changes in bacteria, such as swelling, elongation, and "large body" formation or, under optimal conditions, lysis and death. These morphologic changes may depend on which PBP binds to the β-lactam antibiotic, since these proteins determine a variety of activities.

Pharmacokinetics

Absorption of penicillin G from the gastrointestinal tract is incomplete and variable (Table 58-1). Also, penicillin G is inactivated by gastric juice so that penicillin V (Veetids, Pen-Vee K, others), which is more resistant to acid, is the preferred oral form against streptococcal organisms.

Serum concentrations after administration of 100,000 units (about 60 mg) of penicillin G by various routes are illustrated in Fig. 58-1. Concentrations reaching 2 to 4 units/ml (1.25 to 2.5 μg/ml) can be obtained by intravenous or intramuscular injection, but the same dose given orally produces a concentration of only about 0.4 units/ml. Since intramuscular injection of penicillin of any type is painful, only one or two injections a day are given to treat streptococcal pharyngitis or pneumococcal pneumonia. Seriously ill patients should receive penicillin compounds intravenously because absorption of oral preparations is less reliable.

Penicillin is eliminated from the body primarily by rapid renal clearance. With severe renal failure ($Cl_{Cr} < 10$ ml/min) the half-life increases (Table 58-1) so that the dosage interval must be extended. Penicillin is actively secreted by renal tubules. Probenecid, which blocks the tubular secretory mechanism, is occasionally used with penicillin to prolong its action after intramuscular or oral administration. Because the half-life of penicillin in patients with normal renal function is approximately 30

Relative serum concentrations of penicillin after intravenous, intramuscular, and oral administration of 100,000 units of crystalline sodium penicillin G. *FIG. 58-1*

From Welch H, et al: Principles and practice of antibiotic therapy, New York, 1954, Medical Encyclopedia, Inc.

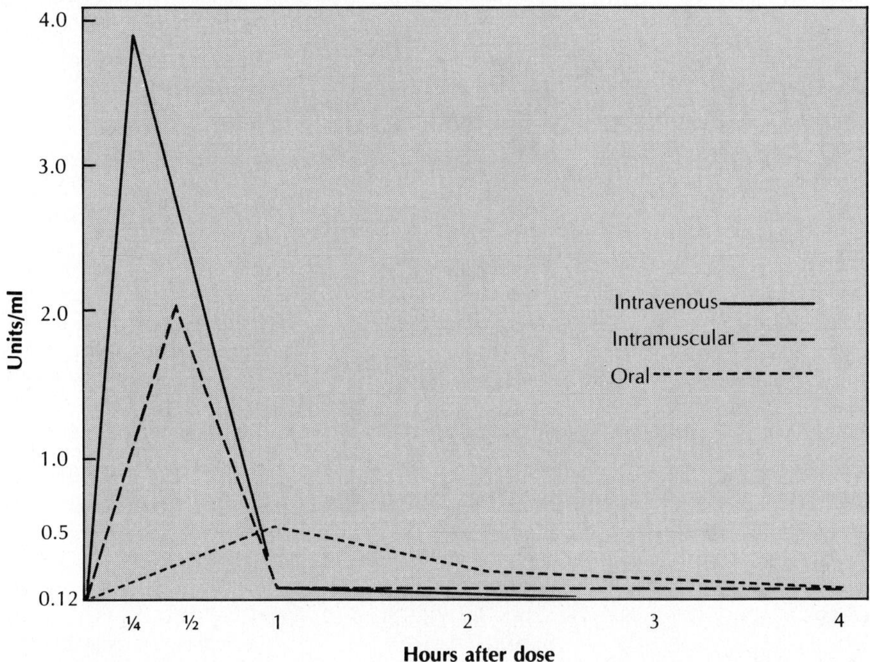

minutes, dosing every 2 to 4 hours is indicated for bacteremia or serious infections.

Repository preparations, such as penicillin G procaine (Wycillin, others) and penicillin G benzathine (Bicillin L-A, Permapen) can be used when sustained blood concentrations, in the range of 0.03 μg/ml or so, are required for 10 days or longer. This concentration is sufficient to treat streptococcal infections or syphilis and to prevent recurrent streptococcal infections in high-risk patients (as with rheumatic fever).

Penicillin is considerably bound to plasma proteins and is not uniformly distributed to most regions of the body. It achieves adequate concentrations in pleural and synovial spaces but penetrates poorly into cerebrospinal fluid and aqueous humor. However, inflammation increases meningeal permeability so that concentrations effective for treatment of meningitis can be achieved within 24 hours of administration.

Table 58-1 indicates the extent of absorption after ingestion, the elimination half-life, and the effect of renal failure on elimination of the penicillins.

Toxicity and hypersensitivity

The toxicity of penicillin G is extremely low, but very high doses can cause myoclonic seizures or platelet dysfunction with bleeding (Table 58-2). This is most likely to occur when doses greater than 20 million units are given to persons with impaired renal function. The percentage of patients who develop hypersensitivity to penicillin varies from 1% to 8% in the general population, but reactions actually occur

TABLE 58-2 Toxicity and hypersensitivity of penicillins

Type of reaction	Frequency of reaction	Most frequently seen with:
Hypersensitivity		
Anaphylaxis	<0.1%	Penicllin G, all others
Serum sickness	Rare	Penicillin G
Skin rash	Common	All
Idiopathic		
Skin rash	Common	Ampicillin
Fever	Rare	All
Gastrointestinal		
Diarrhea	Common	Ampicillin
Enterocolitis	Infrequent	All
Hematologic		
Neutropenia	Infrequent	Nafcillin, piperacillin
Platelet dysfunction	Infrequent	Carbenicillin (all, high doses)
Hemolytic anemia	Rare	Penicillin G
Electrolyte		
Hypokalemia	Infrequent	Carbenicillin, piperacillin
Liver function		
Elevated enzyme	Infrequent	Cloxacillin
Renal function		
Interstitial nephritis	Infrequent	Methicillin
Neurologic		
Seizures	Rare	Penicillin G (in renal failure)

in fewer than 1% of all treatments.[22] The reactions are diverse, ranging from immediate anaphylactic reactions (<0.1%) to late manifestations of the serum sickness type. These reactions are mediated by antibodies that develop to "minor" penicillin determinants, which combine with proteins to form haptens. After sensitization to the hapten-protein complex, administration of the parent compound can then induce a reaction.

Although skin tests with a mixture of penicillin, penicilloate, and other "minor" determinants can be done by allergists, clinicians must rely primarily on a history of previous penicillin reaction. It is best to be prepared for an anaphylactic reaction whenever the antibiotic is injected. Patients allergic to one penicillin must be assumed to be allergic to all since cross-reactions occur frequently between compounds with varied side-chains. If penicillin is required in an allergic patient, desensitization can be performed successfully by beginning with small quantities given orally.[27]

Other adverse effects are much more likely with the newer penicillins. These include leukopenia, hepatitis (oxacillin), interstitial nephritis (methicillin), diarrhea (oral preparations of ampicillin and amoxicillin), and platelet dysfunction (carbenicillin, ticarcillin, and methicillin). Penicillins are irritating to tissue and even to endothelial surfaces so that care must be taken during intravenous therapy. Certain penicillins, such as nafcillin, are particularly prone to elicit phlebitis.

Broad-spectrum penicillins susceptible to penicillinase

Ampicillin is more acid resistant and has a broader antimicrobial spectrum than penicillin G. It is effective against many gram-negative microorganisms. **Amoxicillin trihydrate** is a congener of ampicillin that reaches higher plasma concentrations on a milligram for milligram basis. Ampicillin is used to treat respiratory and urinary tract infections caused by susceptible organisms and intravenously for meningitis caused by *Listeria monocytogenes* and susceptible strains of *Haemophilus influenzae*. Ampicillin causes rash, by unknown mechanisms, with a very high frequency in patients with infectious mononucleosis.

Ampicillin and amoxicillin are available in 250 and 500 mg capsules and as powders for oral suspensions. The sodium salt of ampicillin is available for parenteral administration.

Carbenicillin disodium and **ticarcillin disodium** have greater activity than ampicillin against *Pseudomonas aeruginosa*, *Enterobacter*, *Serratia*, and *Proteus* organisms. Carbenicillin and ticarcillin are usually used in combination with an aminoglycoside to treat serious gram-negative infections,[19] particularly in leukopenic patients, since resistance develops if the penicillins are used alone. Since carbenicillin has a high sodium content (1 g of carbenicillin disodium powder, for injection, contains about 5 mEq of sodium), care must be observed to avoid overload. The drug is excreted as a nonreabsorbable anion that enhances K^+ excretion, and so hypokalemia can also develop.[6] Platelet function may be adversely affected with resultant bleeding if high doses are given to patients with renal failure; consequently, dosage must be altered.

Carbenicillin indanyl sodium (Geocillin) is available in tablets of 382 mg for oral treatment of urinary tract infections and prostatitis. Resistance frequently develops during therapy.

Piperacillin sodium is an acylureidopenicillin with a wider spectrum of activity than carbenicillin for gram-negative bacilli, including *Pseudomonas*, *Serratia*, *Enterobacter*, and *Klebsiella* species.[6] It is best given in combination with an aminoglycoside, since resistance or relapse, or both, can occur when piperacillin is used alone.

Mezlocillin sodium (Mezlin) and **azlocillin sodium** (Azlin) resemble piperacillin in clinical activity and use. Of the two, azlocillin is the more active against *Pseudomonas* species.[6] All of these drugs cause adverse effects similar to those of carbenicillin.

Penicillins resistant to penicillinase

Penicillinase-resistant penicillins are needed to treat infections caused by many organisms, especially staphylococci. Although these drugs are resistant to penicillinase, strains of "methicillin-resistant" (not based on inactivation by penicillinase) *Staphylococcus aureus* have appeared.[25] Most staphylococcal infections are resistant to treatment by penicillin G or V.

Methicillin sodium is administered intramuscularly or intravenously and is unstable in solution. Its only use is in treating infections caused by penicillin G–resistant staphylococci. The drug may cause interstitial nephritis.[11]

Nafcillin sodium can be administered orally, intramuscularly, or intravenously. Nafcillin passes into the spinal fluid and is largely excreted in the bile.

Oxacillin sodium is very similar to nafcillin. It is given orally or parenterally.

TABLE 58-3 Antimicrobial spectrum and dosage of penicillins and relatives

Penicillin	Susceptible organisms	Route: dosage
G	*Streptococcus* (aerobic and anaerobic)	IV: 4-10 million U/day
	Gonococcus	IM: 4.8 million U (single dose)
V	*Streptococcus* (aerobic only)	PO: 250-500 mg 4 × daily
Ampicillin	*Streptococcus*, *Haemophilus* species	IV: 1-2 g 6 × daily
	Listeria, some *Escherichia coli*	PO: 500 mg 4 × daily
Amoxicillin	Same as above	PO: 250-500 mg 3-4 × daily
Nafcillin, cloxacillin, dicloxacillin	*Staphylococcus aureus*	IV: 1-2 g 4-6 × daily, PO: 1-2 g daily
Carbenicillin	*Streptococcus*, anaerobic bacilli (facultative and obligate), *E. coli*, *Enterobacter*, *Pseudomonas*	IV: 5 g 6 × daily
Ticarcillin	Same as above	IV: 3 g 6 × daily
Piperacillin, mezlocillin	Same as above	IV: 3-4 g 4 × daily
Ticarcillin-clavulanate	Same as above	IV: 3.1 g 4 × daily
Ampicillin-sulbactam	Same as above (except *Pseudomonas*)	IV: 1 g 4 × daily
Imipenem-cilastatin	Same as above	PO: 1 g 4 × daily
Aztreonam	Gram-negative only	PO: 2 g 4 × daily

IM, Intramuscularly; *IV*, intravenously; *PO*, by mouth; *U*, units.

Cloxacillin sodium and **dicloxacillin sodium** (Dynapen, others) resemble oxacillin and are preferred for oral therapy of staphylococcal infections.

Uses of penicillins

Penicillins are the standard of therapy in both outpatient and inpatient treatment of infections. For many infectious agents, they remain medications of choice (see Table 58-3).[19] For serious infections they must be combined with other antibiotics, since their activity is not universal and resistance can develop. A perusal of guide-to-therapy booklets (for example, Sanford JB; *Guide to Antimicrobial Therapy*, West Bethesda, Maryland, 1990, Antimicrobial Therapy, Inc) illustrates the usefulness of penicillin for many conditions.

CEPHALOSPORINS

The cephalosporins are β-lactam antibiotics obtained originally from a *Cephalosporium* mold. These antibiotics have the same mechanism of action as penicillins but differ in antibacterial spectrum, resistance to β-lactamase, and pharmacokinetics.[8] Whereas penicillins are derivatives of 6-aminopenicillanic acid, cephalosporins are derivatives of 7-aminocephalosporanic acid. Many cephalosporins are presently available and offer certain advantages in range of activity, pharmacokinetics, and penetration into cerebrospinal fluid. However, they also retain certain limitations, and several are extremely costly.

The antibacterial spectrum of the original, so-called first generation, cephalosporins (Table 58-4) is similar to that of the penicillinase-resistant penicillins, with slightly

TABLE 58-4 Selected cephalosporins and dosage

	Proprietary name	Adult dose for serious infection
First generation		
Parenteral		
Cefazolin sodium	Ancef, Kefzol	1-2 g q6-8h
Cephalothin sodium	Keflin	2 g q4h
Cephapirin sodium	Cefadyl	2 g q4h
Cephradine	Velosef	0.5-1 g q6h
Oral		
Cefadroxil	Duricef, Ultracef	0.5-1 g q12h
Cephalexin monohydrate	Keflex, Keflet	0.5-1 g q6h
Cephradine	Anspor, Velosef	0.5-1 g q6h
Second generation		
Parenteral		
Cefamandole nafate	Mandol	2 g q4h
Cefonicid sodium	Monicid	2 g q24h
Cefoxitin sodium	Mefoxin	2 g q4h
Cefuroxime sodium	Kefurox, Zinacef	3 g q8h
Cefotetan disodium	Cefotan	2 g q12h
Oral		
Cefaclor	Ceclor	0.5-1 g q8h
Cefuroxime axetil	Ceftin	0.25-0.5 g q12h
Third generation		
Parenteral		
Cefoperazone sodium	Cefobid	3 g q6h
Cefotaxime sodium	Claforan	2 g q4h
Ceftazidime	Fortaz, others	2 g q6h
Ceftizoxime sodium	Cefizox	4 g q8h
Ceftriaxone sodium	Rocephin	1 g q12h
Moxalactam disodium	Moxam	2 g q4h
Oral		
Cefixime	Suprax	0.4 g q24h

greater gram-negative coverage. Cefaclor, cefuroxime (second generation), and cefixime are active against *Haemophilus influenzae*, an important pathogen in children.[4] The most recently developed, third-generation cephalosporins are active against a wide spectrum of gram-negative organisms, including *Escherichia coli* and species of *Proteus, Klebsiella, Serratia*, and *Enterobacter*.[8] Cephalosporins such as cefoxitin, cefotetan, and moxalactam are also active against *Bacteroides fragilis*.[5,18] Some second- and third-generation cephalosporins attain sufficient concentrations in cerebrospinal fluid to treat meningitis caused by the Lyme disease agent and gram-negative organisms.[13,23] However, cephalosporins are ineffective against penicillin-resistant *Streptococcus pneumoniae*, methicillin-resistant *Staphylococcus aureus, Listeria monocytogenes, Streptococcus fecalis, Legionella pneumophila, Clostridium difficile, Pylobacter jejuni*, and certain *Pseudomonas* species.[8] Furthermore, organisms such as *Enterobac-*

ter, *Serratia*, and *Pseudomonas* species can develop resistance; they then display resistance to all β-lactam therapy.[21]

Most cephalosporins are eliminated by glomerular filtration and tubular secretion. Their elimination half-lives are variably prolonged with renal failure; individual drugs require specific alterations in dosage (see Appendix B). Some of the newer cephalosporins are excreted in bile; some may need dosage adjustment with hepatic disease (for example, cefoperazone in patients with cirrhosis).

Toxicity

Cephalosporins share all the toxicities of the penicillins. Although fewer than 5% of patients with a history of reaction to penicillin will react to cephalosporins with hives, rash, or anaphylaxis, cephalosporins should be used with caution in such persons.[20] Certain cephalosporins may cause specific toxic reactions; for example, a disulfiram-like reaction and bleeding abnormalities attributable to hypoprothrombinemia can occur with drugs that have the "methylthiotetrazole-leaving" group (moxalactam, cefamandole, cefoperazone).[8] These agents have fallen out of favor because of the finite possibility of such life-threatening complications.

Uses of cephalosporins

Cephalosporins are commonly used in many clinical situations because they offer a lower frequency of toxicity than other antibiotics such as the aminoglycosides. Orally administered members of the group (Table 58-4) are indicated for respiratory tract, skin, or bone infections when gram-negative coverage is necessary (proved by culture) or for persons allergic to cloxacillin. Parenteral cephalosporins are useful in the following clinical settings:

1. As therapy for persons allergic to penicillin. However, one must proceed with caution in this situation.
2. For treatment of patients with gram-negative infections, such as the elderly with pneumonia or for hospital-acquired bacteremia caused by *Klebsiella* species (cefotaxime or ceftriaxone) or *Pseudomonas* infections (ceftazidime).
3. For therapy of mixed infections or initial treatment of certain infections of unknown causes (cefoxitin or cefotetan for postoperative abdominal infections).
4. For prophylaxis before surgery, especially for gastrointestinal, pelvic, or orthopedic surgery (the latter involving plastic or metal implants). Here, the least expensive drug, such as cefazolin, given preoperatively is as effective as more expensive ones.[8]
5. For meningitis potentially caused by either gram-positive or gram-negative organisms (cefotaxime or ceftriaxone).
6. For treatment of *N. gonorrhoeae* infections, because the organisms frequently produce penicillinase (a high probability at present).

Use of these antibiotics should be gauged by sensitivity testing of the microorganism isolated from the patient. Presently, testing shows that second- and third-generation cephalosporins are effective for a majority of gram-negative bacilli (see Table 59-2). Although cefoxitin, moxalactam, and cefotetan are satisfactory for obligate anaerobes, other drugs, such as metronidazole, are even more effective and less

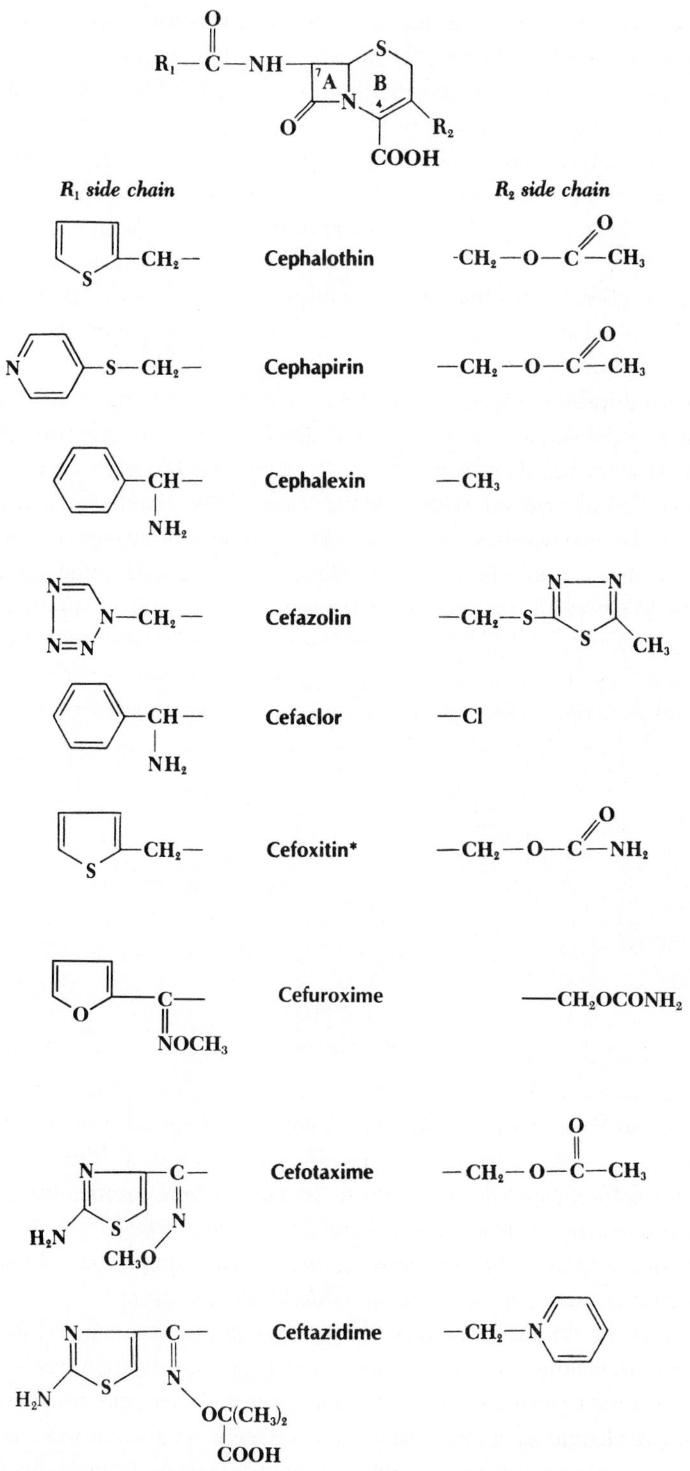

$R_1-\overset{O}{\overset{\|}{C}}-NH-$ (7, A, B, 4, N, S) R_2, COOH

R_1 *side chain*		R_2 *side chain*
(thiophene, S) $-CH_2-$	**Cephalothin**	$-CH_2-O-\overset{O}{\overset{\|}{C}}-CH_3$
N (pyridine) $-S-CH_2-$	**Cephapirin**	$-CH_2-O-\overset{O}{\overset{\|}{C}}-CH_3$
(benzene) $-\underset{NH_2}{\underset{\|}{CH}}-$	**Cephalexin**	$-CH_3$
(tetrazole: N=, N=N) $N-CH_2-$	**Cefazolin**	$-CH_2-S-$ (thiadiazole: N—N, S) CH_3
(benzene) $-\underset{NH_2}{\underset{\|}{CH}}-$	**Cefaclor**	$-Cl$
(thiophene, S) $-CH_2-$	**Cefoxitin***	$-CH_2-O-\overset{O}{\overset{\|}{C}}-NH_2$
(furan, O) $-\underset{NOCH_3}{\underset{\|\|}{C}}-$	**Cefuroxime**	$-CH_2OCONH_2$
(thiazole: N, S) H_2N; $-\underset{\|\|}{C}-$, N, CH_3O	**Cefotaxime**	$-CH_2-O-\overset{O}{\overset{\|}{C}}-CH_3$
(thiazole: N, S) H_2N; $-\underset{\|\|}{C}-$, N, $OC(CH_3)_2$, $COOH$	**Ceftazidime**	$-CH_2-N$ (pyridinium)

*Cefoxitin has a methoxy group at position 7 of the beta lactam ring.

expensive. In general, the greater the gram-negative spectrum, the less satisfactory the efficacy against staphylococci. Hence use of these agents must be accompanied by microbiologic evaluation, with consideration given to the likelihood of infection with organisms that are not susceptible to them.

Several newer β-lactam drugs differ slightly from penicillin and cephalosporins. Because of their great cost, they are reserved for special circumstances. **Imipenem** (Primaxin) is a carbapenem with excellent in vitro and in vivo activity for gram-positive and gram-negative (facultative and obligate) bacilli.[12] To prevent destruction in the kidney, it is combined with the enzyme inhibitor cilastatin. Side effects are similar to those of other β-lactams. Seizures may occur in patients with renal failure if dosage is not adjusted. Although the agent is useful for serious aerobic and anaerobic infections, resistance can develop, especially with *Pseudomonas* infections.[26] Monobactams, such as **aztreonam** (Azactam), have activity only for *Enterobacteriaceae* and *Pseudomonas* species. Aztreonam has been used to treat serious infections, particularly in patients with abnormal renal function, with good success and low toxicity.[17] Persons allergic to penicillin can be given aztreonam with little likelihood of allergic reactions. Finally, certain β-lactamase inhibitors, such as **clavulanic acid** and **sulbactam**, have been combined with amoxicillin (Augmentin), ticarcillin (Timentin), and ampicillin (Unasyn) with therapeutic benefit.[18,19] These combinations are more effective than the parent antibiotic, but they are still not uniformly effective for all gram-negative organisms; the combinations are expensive, and their use remains to be established.

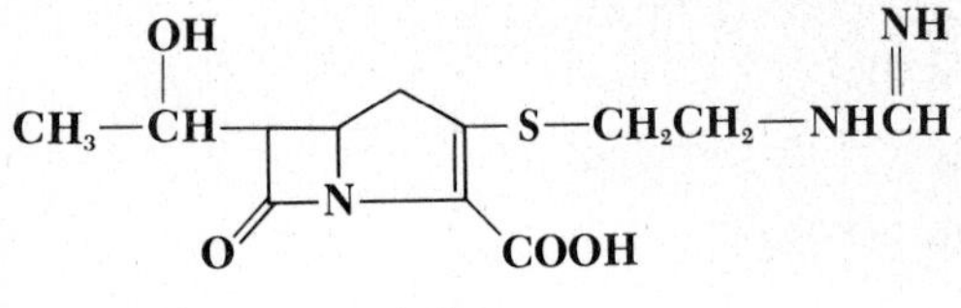

Imipenem

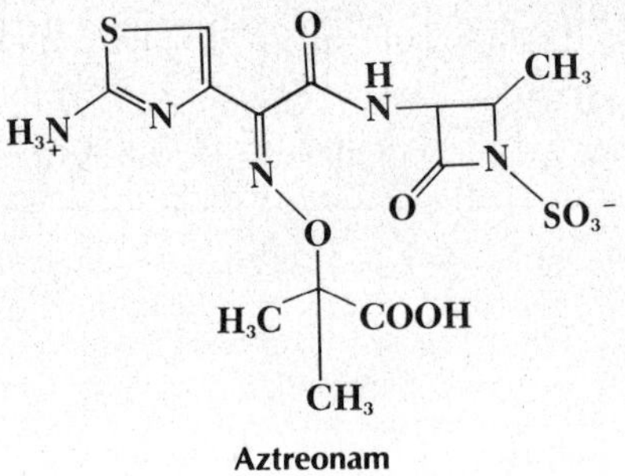

Aztreonam

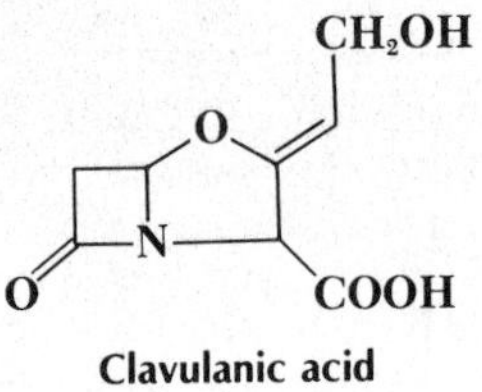

Clavulanic acid

OTHER ANTIBIOTICS THAT INHIBIT CELL-WALL SYNTHESIS

Vancomycin

Vancomycin (Vancocin, Vancoled) is a complex glycopeptide obtained from an actinomycete. It is bactericidal against gram-positive bacteria.[10] Vancomycin is poorly absorbed when administered orally but can be used to treat enterocolitis (pseudomembranous colitis) caused by staphylococci and *Clostridium difficile*. The drug is given intravenously for serious systemic infections caused by staphylococci resistant to other drugs and for streptococcal infections in patients allergic to penicillins.[25] Its half-life is about 6 hours. The drug is eliminated through renal mechanisms, and so dosage must be reduced in persons with renal failure.[15] Weekly administration has been used successfully in patients with end-stage renal failure even when on hemodialysis, because the drug is not cleared by dialysis membranes. Vancomycin is quite irritating to veins and can also cause vestibular toxicity and neutropenia.[25] It must be given slowly intravenously, or it can cause flushing ("red-neck syndrome") and hypotension.[10]

Bacitracin

Bacitracin is a mixture of polypeptides that inhibits the second stage of cell-wall synthesis. It is used only topically for skin infections caused by gram-positive organisms.

MISCELLANEOUS AGENTS FOR TREATMENT OF GRAM-POSITIVE INFECTIONS

Erythromycin

Erythromycin (Erythrocin, others), a *macrolide* antibiotic, is a bacteriostatic organic base. It is used mainly to treat pulmonary infections caused by mycoplasma, *Legionella*, and gram-positive organisms in patients allergic to penicillin.[3] In addition, *Chlamydia* and *Haemophilus* species (such as *H. ducreyi*, chancroid) are effectively treated.

Enteric-coated preparations and erythromycin stearate are well absorbed ($>50\%$); erythromycin usually attains effective blood concentrations of 2 μg/ml or more in an hour or so. The drug diffuses rapidly into tissues and distributes in total body water, though penetration to cerebrospinal fluid is poor. Its excretion is mostly gastrointestinal, with only 5% to 15% eliminated in the urine. Gastrointestinal upset is the most common side effect. Allergic reactions are very rare.

Erythromycin estolate (Ilosone) can be taken with food and can provide longer-lasting therapeutic concentrations than comparable doses of erythromycin base. However, a higher incidence of cholestatic jaundice has been reported for this drug, particularly in pregnant women and other adults, than for other esters of erythromycin, and so caution is necessary.

Lincomycin

Lincomycin (Lincocin) has an antibacterial spectrum similar to that of erythromycin, but it is also effective against *Bacteroides* species. However, with the usual adult dose of 0.5 g every 6 to 8 hours gastrointestinal irritation is sufficient to limit its use.

Clindamycin

Clindamycin (Cleocin) was introduced to replace lincomycin, since its spectrum of activity is similar.[9] Clindamycin can be administered by mouth (150 to 450 mg every 6 hours), intramuscularly, or by intravenous infusion. The drug is bactericidal for gram-positive organisms and bacteriostatic for anaerobic bacilli.[2] Gastrointestinal irritation is less frequent than that with lincomycin but is potentially severe. In addition, neutropenia, eosinophilia, rashes, and elevated hepatic enzymes can develop, especially in those with underlying liver disease.

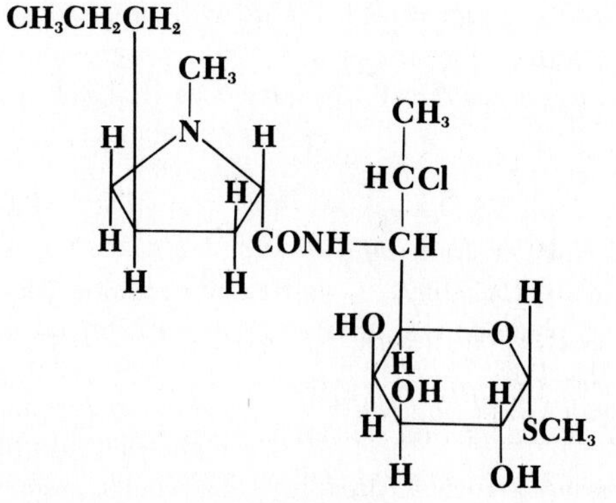

Clindamycin

Pseudomembranous colitis (caused by toxin from *Clostridium difficile*) is a serious complication that limits the usefulness of clindamycin.[1] This compound (or any other antibiotic) should be discontinued in patients who develop diarrhea (more than five stools per day). Pseudomembranous infiltrates can be visualized in the colon, but examination of stools for leukocytes and toxin provide indirect evidence of the condition. If either is present, vancomycin or metronidazole should be administered orally.[29]

METRONIDAZOLE

Metronidazole (Flagyl, others), originally introduced as an oral agent against *Trichomonas* organisms, is also effective in treatment of amebiasis and giardiasis (see Chapter 64).[24] An intravenous form of metronidazole is available for treatment of serious anaerobic bacterial infections (especially *Bacteroides fragilis*).[2] The antimicrobial properties of metronidazole appear to be mediated by a partially reduced intermediate. DNA breakage may be its mechanism of action. The drug diffuses well to all tissues, including the central nervous system. Toxicity includes gastrointestinal disturbances, thrombophlebitis, seizures, peripheral neuropathy, and a disulfiram-like reaction to ethanol. It may be a potential mutagen and carcinogen.

REFERENCES

1. Bartlett JG: Antibiotic-associated pseudomembranous colitis, *Rev Infect Dis* 1:530, 1979.
2. Bartlett JG: Anti-anaerobic antibacterial agents, *Lancet* 2:478, 1982.
3. Brittain DC: Erythromycin, *Med Clin North Am* 71:1147, 1987.
4. Brogden RN, Campoli-Richards DM: Cefixime: a review of its antibacterial activity, pharmacokinetic properties and therapeutic potential, *Drugs* 38:524, 1989.
5. Cuchural GJ Jr, Tally FP, Jacobus NV, et al: Comparative activities of newer β-lactam agents against members of the *Bacteroides fragilis* group, *Antimicrob Agents Chemother* 34:479, 1990.
6. Drusano GL, Schimpff SC, Hewitt WL: The acylampicillins: mezlocillin, piperacillin, and azlocillin, *Rev Infect Dis* 6:13, 1984.
7. Fleming A: On antibacterial action of cultures of penicillium, with special reference to their use in isolation of *B. influenzae*, *Br J Exp Pathol* 10:226, 1929.
8. Goldberg DM: The cephalosporins, *Med Clin North Am* 71:1113, 1987.
9. Klainer AS: Clindamycin, *Med Clin North Am* 71:1169, 1987.
10. Levine JF: Vancomycin: a review, *Med Clin North Am* 71:1135, 1987.
11. Linton AL, Clark WF, Driedger AA, et al: Acute interstitial nephritis due to drugs: review of the literature with a report of nine cases, *Ann Intern Med* 93:735, 1980.
12. Lipman B, Neu HC: Imipenem: a new carbapenem antibiotic, *Med Clin North Am* 72:567, 1988.
13. Luft BJ, Gorevic PD, Halperin JJ, et al: A perspective on the treatment of Lyme borreliosis, *Rev Infect Dis* 11(suppl 6):S1518, 1989.
14. Macfarlane G: *Howard Florey: the making of a great scientist*, Oxford, Eng, 1979, Oxford University Press.
15. Moellering RC Jr, Krogstad DJ, Greenblatt DJ: Vancomycin therapy in patients with impaired renal function: a nomogram for dosage, *Ann Intern Med* 94:343, 1981.
16. Neu HC: Relation of structural properties of beta-lactam antibiotics to antibacterial activity, *Am J Med* 79(suppl 2A):2, 1985.
17. Neu HC: Aztreonam: the first monobactam, *Med Clin North Am* 72:555, 1988.
18. Ohm-Smith MJ, Sweet RL: In vitro activity of cefmetazole, cefotetan, amoxicillin-clavulanic acid, and other antimicrobial agents against anaerobic bacteria from endometrial cultures of women with pelvic infections, *Antimicrob Agents Chemother* 31:1434, 1987.

19. Parry MF: The penicillins, *Med Clin North Am* 71:1093, 1987.

20. Petz LD: Immunologic cross-reactivity between penicillins and cephalosporins: a review, *J Infect Dis* 137(suppl):S74, 1978.

21. Sanders CC: Novel resistance selected by the new expanded-spectrum cephalosporins: a concern, *J Infect Dis* 147:585, 1983.

22. Saxon A: Immediate hypersensitivity reactions to β-lactam antibiotics, *Rev Infect Dis* 5(suppl 2):S368, 1983.

23. Schaad UB, Suter S, Gianella-Borradori A, et al: A comparison of ceftriaxone and cefuroxime for the treatment of bacterial meningitis in children, *N Engl J Med* 322:141,1990.

24. Scully BE: Metronidazole, *Med Clin North Am* 72:613, 1988.

25. Sorrell TC, Packham DR, Shanker S, et al: Vancomycin therapy for methicillin-resistant *Staphylococcus aureus*, *Ann Intern Med* 97:344, 1982.

26. Stratton CW: *Pseudomonas aeruginosa* revisited, *Infect Control Hosp Epidemiol* 11:101, 1990.

27. Sullivan TJ: Antigen-specific desensitization of patients allergic to penicillin, *J Allergy Clin Immunol* 69:500, 1982.

28. Tomasz A: From penicillin-binding proteins to the lysis and death of bacteria: a 1979 view, *Rev Infect Dis* 1:434, 1979.

29. Treatment of *Clostridium difficile* diarrhea, *Med Lett Drugs Ther* 31:94, 1989.

Chapter 59

Antibiotics: aminoglycosides and other drugs used to treat gram-negative infections

PROTEIN-SYNTHESIS INHIBITORS

Certain antibiotics that inhibit protein synthesis are used to treat serious infections caused by many gram-negative bacilli and some gram-positive organisms. However, streptococci, pneumococci, clostridia, anaerobes, and fungi are resistant. Aminoglycosides and tetracyclines inhibit protein synthesis by interfering with the binding of bacterial aminoacyl transfer ribonucleic acids (tRNAs) to the 30 S ribosomal subunit (see Fig. 56-4).

Aminoglycosides

Aminoglycosides (aminocyclitols) are polar cations that are poorly absorbed after oral administration and so are injected intramuscularly or intravenously. The aminoglycosides are not bound to plasma proteins. They have a small volume of distribution but reach tissues well, except for the central nervous system. They are excreted by glomerular filtration. Renal elimination is rapid and plasma half-lives are 2 to 3 hours in patients with normal renal function.

The aminoglycosides are ototoxic and nephrotoxic and may cause neuromuscular blockade. Dose-related ototoxicity manifests itself in vestibular and auditory disturbances caused by damage to hair cells in the cochlea. Whereas streptomycin and neomycin primarily affect vestibular function, kanamycin, gentamicin, and amikacin have relatively greater auditory toxicity. Functional impairment ranges from disturbances in equilibrium and tinnitus to permanent deafness.[13] The risk is greater with decreased renal function because the aminoglycoside accumulates; serum peak and trough concentrations are monitored in an effort to minimize this possibility.[5]

Manifestations of nephrotoxicity, which is usually reversible, range from mild proteinuria to severe azotemia. In patients with preexisting renal dysfunction, adjustment of dosage schedules is mandatory. This can be accomplished by a variety of methods including the use of computer-generated programs.[5]

The neuromuscular blocking action of aminoglycosides may cause apnea, particularly in patients with myasthenia gravis or when large intravenous doses are given rapidly or instilled into the peritoneal cavity. Hypokalemia also predisposes patients to this effect.

Resistance, which develops rapidly to the antibacterial action of streptomycin and more slowly to the other aminoglycosides, can be acquired by induction of enzymes that render the drug inactive (see Fig. 56-6, *D*). This form of resistance is carried by R factors (plasmids) that may also confer resistance to several other nonaminoglycoside antibiotics. The plasmids induce production of enzymes that acetylate or phosphorylate the aminoglycoside. Because these enzymes may be specific for some but not all aminoglycosides, resistance to one aminoglycoside does not necessarily extend to all. For example, *Pseudomonas* may be resistant to gentamicin but susceptible to amikacin or tobramycin.

STREPTOMYCIN

Streptomycin sulfate is used to treat tuberculosis (see Chapter 61) and in combination with penicillin to treat endocarditis caused by streptococcal species, especially *Streptococcus fecalis*. It is also the treatment of choice for tularemia and plague. Resistance may emerge rapidly (induced by R factors), especially when the drug is used alone.

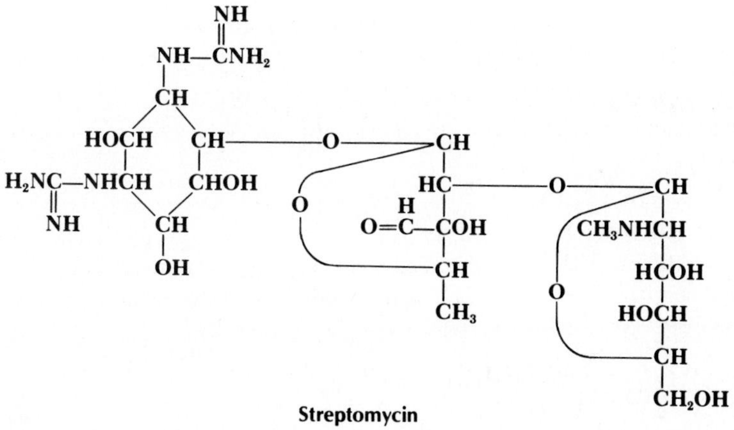

Streptomycin

GENTAMICIN, TOBRAMYCIN, AND NETILMICIN

Gentamicin sulfate (Garamycin, Jenamicin) and tobramycin sulfate (Nebcin) are the most commonly used aminoglycosides. Tobramycin is more effective against *Pseudomonas aeruginosa* and should be used for *Pseudomonas* species known to have lower MICs (minimal inhibitory concentrations). Gentamicin is less expensive and probably has no greater toxicity, especially if serum concentration is monitored closely.[5] Netilmicin sulfate (Netromycin) has similar antimicrobial activity but is reputed to have less ototoxicity.

Gentamicin

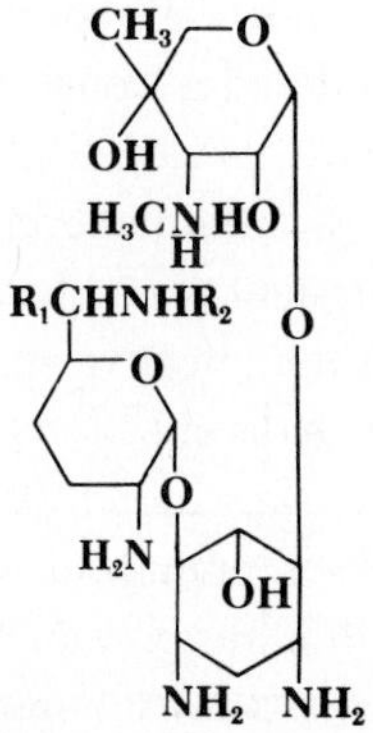

Tobramycin

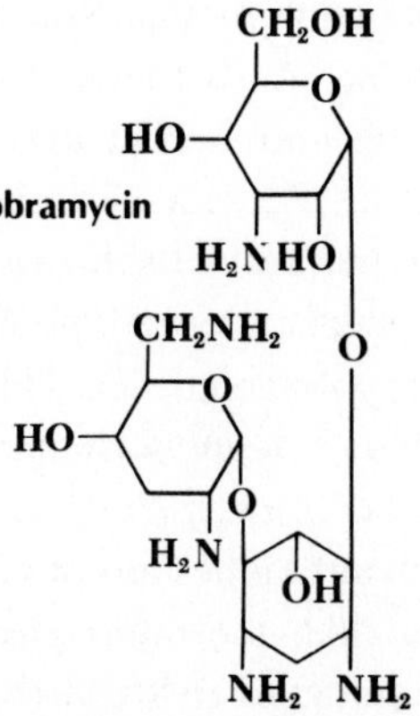

These drugs are used to treat systemic infections caused by susceptible gram-negative bacteria, especially *Pseudomonas*, *Klebsiella*, and *Serratia* species (see Table 59-2). Serum concentrations of these aminoglycosides should be monitored early in therapy and again if the patient's clinical status (especially renal function) changes; trough concentrations predict ototoxicity and nephrotoxicity and should not exceed 2 μg/ml. Peak concentrations between 5 and 7 μg/ml predict clinical efficacy.[12]

Initial dosage of gentamicin and tobramycin for adults with normal renal function is 1.5 mg/kg every 8 hours. Dosage should then be adjusted according to values for peak and trough serum concentrations of the individual patient. One method of doing so is by a computer-assisted Bayesian feedback program.[5,10]

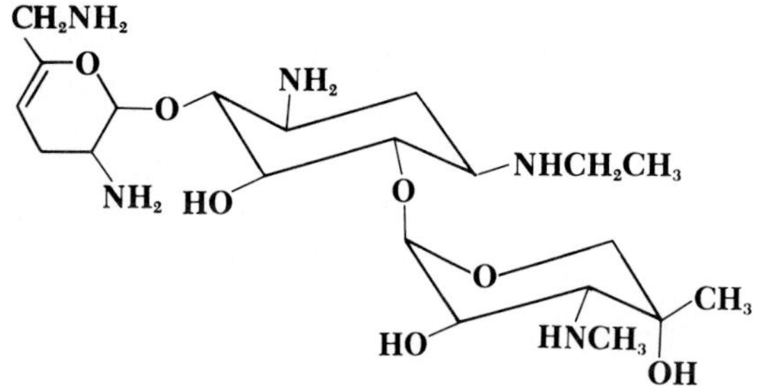

Netilmicin

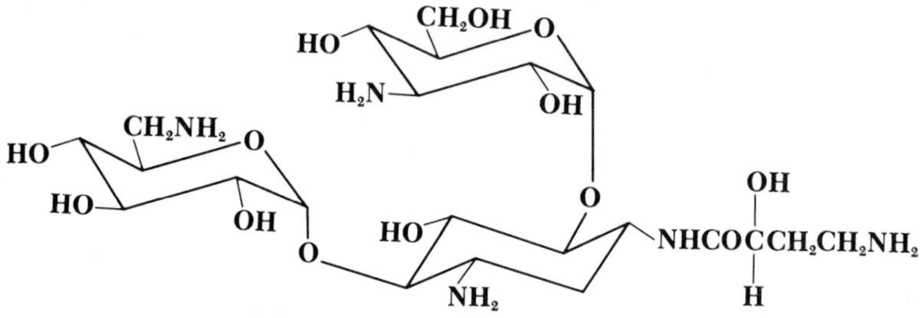

Amikacin

AMIKACIN

Amikacin sulfate (Amikin) is a semisynthetic aminoglycoside with a modification that confers resistance to enzymes that inactivate gentamicin and tobramycin. Resistance of gram-negative bacteria to amikacin rarely develops and remains at a low level. The drug is available in solutions containing 50 and 250 mg/ml. It should be given intramuscularly or intravenously at 7.5 mg/kg every 12 hours (less in renal failure) for a peak serum concentration of 25 to 30 μg/ml and a trough below 5 μg/ml.

SPECTINOMYCIN

Spectinomycin (Trobicin) hydrochloride is an aminocyclitol used as a single 2 g intramuscular injection to treat penicillin-resistant gonorrheal infections or penicillin-allergic patients with gonorrhea. This drug is *not* effective against syphilis. The drug is neither ototoxic nor nephrotoxic and has few side effects.

Tetracyclines

Tetracycline antibiotics are produced by soil organisms. They are broad-spectrum antibiotics that, like the aminoglycosides, inhibit protein synthesis in bacteria by blocking the binding of tRNA to the 30 S ribosomal subunit. However, the bacteriostatic tetracyclines tend to suppress an infection and require phagocytes to completely eradicate bacteria. They are highly effective in treatment of *Mycoplasma pneumoniae*, cholera, rickettsial disease, brucellosis, and nongonococcal urethritis caused by chlamydiae.[8] Tetracycline is used orally in low doses to treat acne. Combination therapy with other agents has limited application, since tetracyclines occasionally interfere with the killing effect of a bactericidal antibiotic, such as penicillin for pneumococcal meningitis.[15]

In addition to the older **tetracycline, chlortetracycline** (Aureomycin), and **oxytetracycline**, several newer derivatives have been introduced (Table 59-1).[8] Of these, **demeclocycline** is rarely, if ever, used as an antibiotic because it can cause severe photosensitization. **Doxycycline** requires less frequent administration than other tetracyclines because of slower elimination and is safe in renal failure. It too may cause phototoxicity. Another slowly excreted member of the family is **minocycline**, which has been touted for infrequent dosing. However, it may cause severe vertigo and nausea, particularly in women.

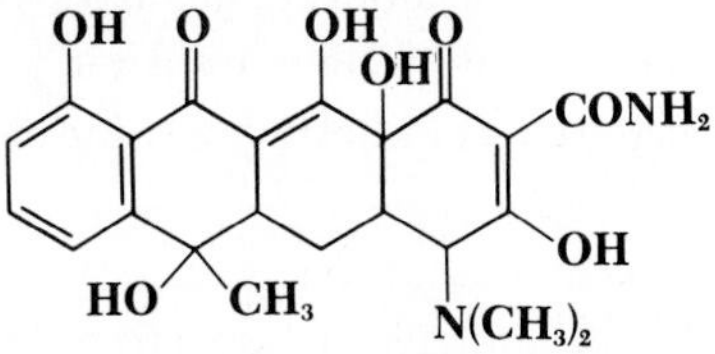

Tetracycline

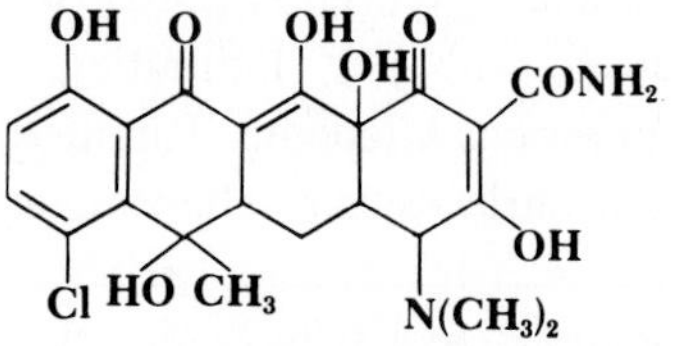

Chlortetracycline

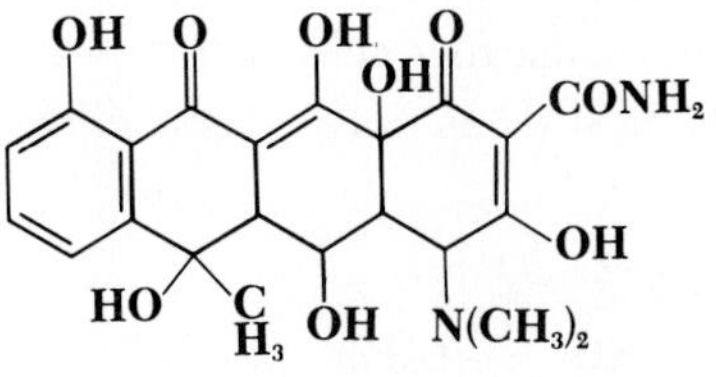

Oxytetracycline

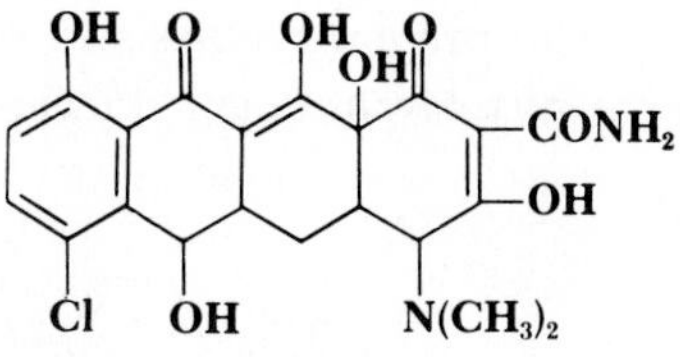

Demeclocycline

PHARMACOKINETICS

Tetracyclines are absorbed rapidly but incompletely from the gastrointestinal tract. Calcium salts and antacids inhibit their absorption; the drug should be taken 30 minutes before meals, and antacids should be avoided for at least an hour afterward.

Tetracycline is widely distributed in most tissues. However, its concentration is low in cerebrospinal fluid, and it is not indicated for meningitis. As a consequence of its chelating properties, tetracycline tends to localize in bones and teeth, where it may be detected by its fluorescence.

ADVERSE EFFECTS

Adverse effects of tetracyclines include nausea, vomiting, enterocolitis, stomatitis, and superinfections. Deposition in developing teeth can cause permanent

TABLE 59-1 Tetracyclines: systemic dosage forms

Tetracycline	Dosage forms (mg)
Demeclocycline hydrochloride (Declomycin)	C: 150; T: 150,300
Doxycycline (Vibramycin, others) hyclate	C,T: 50,100; P: 100,200; S: 50
Methacycline hydrochloride (Rondomycin)	C: 150,300
Minocycline (Minocin)	P: 100
Minocycline (Minocin) hydrochloride	C,T: 50,100; S: 50
Oxytetracycline (Terramycin)	I: 50,125/ml
Oxytetracycline (Terramycin, others) hydrochloride	C: 250
Tetracycline hydrochloride (Acromycin, others)	C: 100-500; P: 100-500; S: 125; T:250,500

C, Capsules; *I,* injection; *P,* powder for injection; *S,* suspension or syrup (per 5 ml); *T;* tablets.

discoloration; hence these agents should be avoided by pregnant women and by children up to 8 years of age. Phototoxicity may occur after administration of demeclocycline and doxycycline. Large intravenous doses of tetracyclines have produced liver damage with fatty infiltration, and so they are no longer used for parenteral therapy of serious infections. Parenteral administration is indicated only for instillation into pleural surfaces as a sclerosing agent.

Chloramphenicol

Chloramphenicol (Chloromycetin) has a broad antibacterial spectrum similar to that of tetracyclines.[8] It has been replaced by cephalosporins as the drug of choice for treatment of typhoid fever or gram-negative meningitis.

Chloramphenicol is a bacteriostatic derivative of nitrobenzene. It binds exclusively to the 50 S ribosomal subunit, thereby interfering with protein synthesis. It also interferes with protein synthesis in human bone marrow cells in tissue culture, an action perhaps relevant to aplastic anemia, its most dangerous adverse effect.

$$O_2N\text{—}C_6H_4\text{—}\underset{|}{\overset{OH}{CH}}\text{—}\underset{|}{\overset{CH_2OH}{CH}}\text{—}NH\text{—}\overset{O}{\overset{\|}{C}}\text{—}CHCl_2$$

Chloramphenicol

An adequate plasma concentration is reached 30 minutes after oral administration; peak concentration occurs in 2 hours. Chloramphenicol is poorly absorbed after intramuscular administration but can be given intravenously.

Toxicity

Chloramphenicol treatment is associated with gastrointestinal disturbances, glossitis, skin rash, and superinfection. Rarely, optic neuritis and encephalopathy may develop with high doses. However, the use of chloramphenicol is severely restricted primarily because of its tendency to produce blood dyscrasias.[4] The frequency of aplastic anemia (1 per 24,000 cases) has led physicians to use other agents. The nitrobenzene moiety may be responsible for the anemia, possibly in those with a genetic predisposition. Chloramphenicol is metabolized chiefly (90%) by conjugation to the monoglucuronide. Elevated plasma concentrations of free drug and metabolites can cause toxicity in older patients with significant hepatic disease.[8] The "gray baby" syndrome (cyanosis and vascular collapse) occurs in premature and newborn infants who lack hepatic glucuronyl transferase, which normally detoxifies the antibiotic by changing it to the inactive glucuronide.

POLYMYXIN B

Polymyxins are basic peptides that act as cationic detergents to cause lysis of the lipoprotein cell membrane. Polymyxin B sulfate (Aerosporin) is particularly active against gram-negative bacteria, but serious nephrotoxicity has limited its internal use. It is employed chiefly to treat local infections: external otitis, eye infections, and skin infections with sensitive organisms. **Colistin sulfate** (Coli-Mycin S) is a very similar compound that can be given parenterally with risks of ototoxicity and nephrotoxicity.

CLINICAL PHARMACOLOGY OF ANTIBACTERIAL AGENTS

Certain generalizations apply to the use of antimicrobial agents for various infections (Table 59-2)[6,9]: (1) Penicillin derivatives remain the treatment of choice for most respiratory tract infections and may be used in combinations for other infections. (2) Cephalosporins are especially effective for patients with hospital-acquired pneumonia and community-acquired gram-negative meningitis and as prophylactic agents.[1,6] (3) Expense should be considered particularly in outpatient therapy, and expensive, albeit broad-spectrum, agents should be avoided except when susceptibility testing shows one to be the only effective agent. (4) Certain drugs fail even when the organism is susceptible to the drug. Some causes of therapeutic failure are listed below:

Incorrect clinical or bacteriologic diagnosis
Improper drug administration or inadequate dosage
Poor patient compliance
Alteration in bacterial flora during drug administration and superinfection with a resistant organism
Infection in a location inaccessible to the drug
Failure to use indicated surgical drainage
Development of drug resistance by mutant forms of the infecting organism
Deficiency in host defenses
Drug toxicity and hypersensitivity

Poor gastrointestinal absorption of antibiotics such as penicillin G may necessitate administration by another route. If certain agents are given with meals, they may lose much of their effectiveness. Cations in antacids and milk reduce absorption of the tetracyclines. Gastrointestinal complications, such as enterocolitis caused by *Clostridium difficile*, may occur in patients who receive various antibiotics and can cause severe electrolyte disturbances or even death.[2]

Pharmacokinetic characteristics are important for selection of antimicrobial agents because maintenance of therapeutic blood and tissue concentrations is usually critical for eradicating infectious agents. For example, aminoglycosides have therapeutic activity only in relation to their concentration in blood. In contrast, the antibiotic effect of a cephalosporin persists after the drug is no longer detectable in the circulation.

TABLE 59-2 Drugs of choice for various infections

Causative agent	Drugs
Gram positive	
Actinomyces	Penicillin or ampicillin; clindamycin
Clostridium	Penicillin, clindamycin
Corynebacterium diphtheriae	Penicillin, erythromycin
*Enterococcus**	Penicillin with gentamicin; vancomycin with gentamicin
Listeria	Ampicillin
Pneumococcus	Penicillin, erythromycin, vancomycin
Staphylococcus aureus (penicillinase producing)	Oxacillin, nafcillin, cloxacillin, vancomycin
Streptococcus pyogenes	Penicillin, erythromycin, cephalosporin
*Streptococcus viridans**	Penicillin with gentamicin; cephalosporin; vancomycin
Gram negative	
Bacteroides	Clindamycin, metronidazole, cefoxitin
Bordetella pertussis	Erythromcyin, trimethoprim-sulfamethoxazole
Brucella	Tetracycline with rifampin
*Enterobacter**	Third-generation cephalosporin, aminoglycoside
*Escherichia coli**	Cephalosporin, ampicillin, trimethoprim-sulfamethoxazole, aminoglycoside
Haemophilus ducreyi	Erythromycin, ceftriaxone
Haemophilus influenzae	Second-generation cephalosporin, ampicillin
*Klebsiella**	Cephalosporin, aminoglycoside
Legionella	Erythomycin, rifampin
Neisseria gonorrhoeae	Ceftriaxone, penicillin, tetracycline, spectinomycin
Neisseria meningitidis	Penicillin, cefotaxime
*Proteus**	Third-generation cephalosporin, aminoglycoside
*Pseudomonas**	Third-generation cephalosporin, aminoglycoside
Salmonella	Ceftriaxone, ampicillin
Shigella	Trimethoprim-sulfamethoxazole, ampicillin, ciprofloxacin
Miscellaneous	
Fusobacterium (Vincent's angina)	Penicillin, clindamycin
Leptospira	Penicillin, tetracycline
Psittacosis (lymphogranuloma group)	Tetracycline, chloramphenicol
Rickettsia	Tetracycline, chloramphenicol
Treponema pallidum	Penicillin, tetracycline

*Susceptibility tests may be essential.

Tissue concentrations are also critical.[3] Some agents (aminoglycosides) are not effective at the pH present in an abscess cavity, whereas others such as metronidazole are just as effective in this environment.

Alterations in microbial flora can occur with antibiotic use, as in development of vaginal candidiasis in patients treated with penicillin or broad-spectrum antibiotics. Usually replacement of normal flora with new organisms (such as pharyngeal flora with gram-negative organisms) is not equivalent to disease. Hence a positive sputum culture is considered important only if accompanied by a new pulmonary infiltrate and fever. Development of resistance in therapy is more likely to occur in immunocompromised patients or in those with certain infections attributable to gram-negative organisms.[18] In general, to treat a leukopenic patient, a β-lactam agent is combined with an aminoglycoside to achieve bactericidal activity and to prevent emergence of resistance to the β-lactam drug.[15] Certain organisms, including *Enterobacter*, *Serratia*, and *Pseudomonas* species, have inducible β-lactamases that limit use of a β-lactam antibiotic alone for serious infections of bone or for bacteremia.[17]

Serious toxicity, particularly drug fever, eruptive skin lesions, and liver disease, may limit use of certain antibiotics. Many agents cause a chemical hepatitis, but they only rarely cause severe hepatic dysfunction. Nevertheless, if disorders of liver function are noted, the drugs should usually be discontinued.

Effectiveness and safety of antibiotic therapy depend on several host factors. Renal and hepatic elimination should be considered (see Appendix B), and dosing intervals may need to be altered for many antibiotics when hepatic or renal function is impaired.[7,11]

Defense mechanisms of the host greatly influence success or failure of any treatment. Debilitating diseases, poor nutrition, or administration of large doses of corticosteroids or other immunosuppressant drugs may affect responses to antibiotic therapy.[18] As mentioned above, many immunocompromised patients can be cured with use of the appropriate agent or agents.[16] Duration of treatment and dosage are important factors, since these patients tend to relapse more easily.

The age of the patient also influences the effectiveness and safety of antibiotic therapy. Infants in the first month of life metabolize or excrete many drugs more slowly; serum concentration should be monitored, and dosage must be adjusted for many antibiotics. Like infants, the elderly or those with hepatic disease may exhibit a reduced capacity to conjugate drugs (such as chloramphenicol) by glucuronidation.

Pregnancy is a contraindication to the use of several antibiotics, including tetracyclines, erythromycin estolate, and various agents that may be teratogenic (metronidazole). Pregnant women are also more sensitive to the hepatotoxicity of tetracyclines.

Liver disease may be aggravated by chloramphenicol, the tetracyclines, and erythromycin. Diminished renal function causes accumulation of aminoglycosides, sulfonamides, some tetracyclines, and most β-lactams. Dosage must be altered for these agents, and, for some, blood concentration should be followed. Computer-assisted dosage schemes are available for many drugs, particularly aminoglycosides and vancomycin.[5,14]

Obstruction or abscess formation can affect the response to antibiotics and make eradication of infection very difficult. Hence surgical drainage should be considered if drug therapy does not produce a favorable response.

Genetic predisposition can affect metabolism or toxicity. Glucose-6-phosphate dehydrogenase deficiency may predispose to hemolytic anemia from antimicrobial drugs such as the sulfonamides and nitrofurantoin. Genetic predisposition also may explain rare but fatal reactions to chloramphenicol.

REFERENCES

1. Antimicrobial prophylaxis in surgery, *Med Lett Drugs Ther* 31:105, 1989.
2. Bartlett JG: Antibiotic-associated pseudomembranous colitis, *Rev Infect Dis* 1:530, 1979.
3. Bergan T, Engeset A, Olszewski W: Does serum protein binding inhibit tissue penetration of antibiotics? *Rev Infect Dis* 9:713, 1987.
4. Best WR: Chloramphenicol-associated blood dyscrasias: a review of cases submitted to the American Medical Association Registry, *JAMA* 201:181, 1967.
5. Burton ME, Brater DC, Chen PS, et al: A Bayesian feedback method of aminoglycoside dosing, *Clin Pharmacol Ther* 37:349, 1985.
6. The choice of antimicrobial drugs, *Med Lett Drugs Ther* 32:41, 1990.
7. Eisenberg JM, Koffer H, Glick HA, et al: What is the cost of nephrotoxicity associated with aminoglycosides? *Ann Intern Med* 107:900, 1987.
8. Francke EL, Neu HC: Chloramphenicol and tetracyclines, *Med Clin North Am* 71:1155, 1987.
9. Guglielmo BJ, Brooks GF: Antimicrobial therapy: cost-benefit considerations, *Drugs* 38:473, 1989.
10. Hassan E, Ober JD: Predicted and measured aminoglycoside pharmacokinetic parameters in critically ill patients, *Antimicrob Agents Chemother* 31:1855, 1987.
11. Manian FA, Stone WJ, Alford RH: Adverse antibiotic effects associated with renal insufficiency, *Rev Infect Dis* 12:236, 1990.
12. Moore RD, Smith CR, Lietman PS: The association of aminoglycoside plasma levels with mortality in patients with gram-negative bacteremia, *J Infect Dis* 149:443,1984.
13. Pancoast SJ: Aminoglycoside antibiotics in clinical use, *Med Clin North Am* 72:581, 1988.
14. Pestotnik SL, Evans RS, Burke JP, et al: Therapeutic antibiotic monitoring: surveillance using a computerized expert system, *Am J Med* 88:43, 1990.
15. Rahal JJ Jr: Antibiotic combinations: the clinical relevance of synergy and antagonism, *Medicine* 57:179, 1978.
16. Rubin RH: Empiric antibacterial therapy in granulocytopenia induced by cancer chemotherapy, *Ann Intern Med* 108:134, 1988.
17. Sanders CC: Novel resistance selected by the new expanded-spectrum cephalosporins: a concern, *J Infect Dis* 147:585, 1983.
18. Wade JC: Antibiotic therapy for the febrile granulocytopenic cancer patient: combination therapy vs. monotherapy, *Rev Infect Dis* 11(suppl 7):S1572, 1989.

Chapter 60

Antiviral agents

Several drugs with proved efficacy are available for therapy of viral infections[14] (Table 60-1). Amantadine has been used for over two decades for prevention and amelioration of influenza A infections. Effective drugs for treating herpes infections have been released; serious infections can now be prevented or treated. Antiretroviral drugs have become available for primary treatment of patients with acquired immunodeficiency syndrome (AIDS).

AMANTADINE

Amantadine hydrochloride (Symmetrel, Symadine) and **rimantadine hydrochloride** (Flumadine) inhibit influenza A virus by preventing uncoating of virus in host cells.[13] In vitro they are effective against both influenza and rubella viruses. Clinically they have value as prophylactic agents for influenza A2 virus infection and, if used within 2 days, for therapy of the early infection.[14,18] Amantadine reduces the duration of clinical illness and diminishes systemic complaints. It also has some therapeutic effect in parkinsonism (see Chapter 30).

Amantadine can produce central nervous system symptoms, including nervousness, difficulty concentrating, insomnia, and, rarely, grand mal seizures. Neurotoxicity is enhanced by concomitant antihistamine and caffeine ingestion. Rimantadine has a lower frequency of central side effects.[7] Dosage of both drugs must be reduced in renal failure.[9] Amantadine is available in 100 mg capsules and as a syrup (50 mg/5 ml), to be taken once or twice daily. Rimantadine is not yet marketed in the United States.

NH_2 $H—C(NH_2)—CH_3$

Amantadine   Rimantadine

RIBAVIRIN

Ribavirin (Virazole) is a nucleoside analog with broad antiviral activity.[14] It is approved in the United States as an aerosol for treatment of respiratory syncytial virus.[3] The drug is administered by means of a small-particle generator at a concen-

TABLE 60-1 Treatment of viral infections[3]

Infection	Antiviral drug	Route of administration	Dosage schedule: Dose	Interval (hours)	Duration (days)
Influenza A	Amantadine	Oral	100 mg	12	3-5
	Rimantadine†	Oral	200 mg	12	5
Respiratory syncytial virus	Ribavirin	Inhalation	0.8 mg/kg/hr	Continuous	3-7
Herpes simplex virus (HSV) conjunctivitis	Vidarabine	Topical	3% ointment	4	10-14
	or idoxuridine	Topical	0.5% ointment	4	10-14
	or trifluridine	Topical	1% solution	2	10-14
HSV encephalitis	Acyclovir	Intravenous	10 mg/kg	8	10
	or vidarabine	Intravenous	15 mg/kg	24	10
HSV mucocutaneous infections*	Acyclovir	Intravenous	5 mg/kg	8	7
		or oral	400 mg	5×/day	7
Genital HSV	Acyclovir	Intravenous	5 mg/kg	8	5
		or oral	200 mg	5×/day	10
		or topical	Thin film	3	7
Herpes zoster	Acyclovir	Oral	800 mg	5×/day	7
Herpes zoster*	Acyclovir	Intravenous	10 mg/kg	8	7
	or vidarabine	Intravenous	15 mg/kg	24	7
Human immunodeficiency (HIV, AIDS) virus*	Zidovudine	Intravenous	1-2 mg/kg	4	Indefinite
		or oral	100 mg	4	Indefinite
Age 3 months to 12 years			180 mg/m^2	6	Indefinite
Cytomegalovrius	Ganciclovir	Intravenous	5 mg/kg	12	14-21

*Immunocompromized.
†Not yet approved by the FDA.

tration of 20 mg/ml and an hourly rate of 0.8 mg/kg.[6] There has been little toxicity with this aerosol. Ribavirin has also been used for infections such as influenza and Lassa fever. Anemia has been reported with oral or intravenous use. The drug is mutagenic, teratogenic, and possibly carcinogenic in experimental animals.

IDOXURIDINE

The initial antiviral drug for herpes infection was idoxuridine (Herplex, Stoxil), an inhibitor of nucleic acid synthesis that is available only for herpes simplex virus (HSV) keratitis, in which it has produced spectacular results. The drug has too much hematologic toxicity for systemic use. More recently introduced agents have better safety margins for therapy of herpetic infections.

VIDARABINE

Vidarabine (adenine arabinoside) inhibits DNA viruses such as HSV and varicella-zoster virus. Its action is poorly understood. Topically, vidarabine is an alternative for treatment of ocular herpes simplex. When administered intravenously, it is efficacious for herpes encephalitis and systemic herpes infections in neonates and immunocompromised patients. However, acyclovir appears more effective in these conditions.[15,17] Vidarabine (Vira-A) is infused over 12 to 24 hours at a daily dosage of 15 mg/kg. It may cause nausea, diarrhea, and, rarely, central nervous system, hematologic, and metabolic effects.

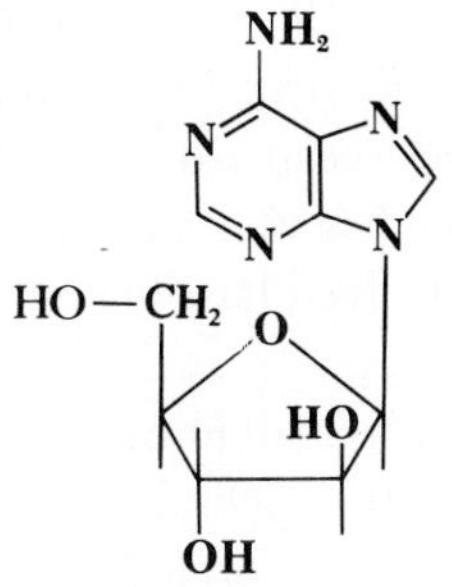

Vidarabine

TRIFLURIDINE

Trifluridine (Viroptic) is a trifluoro analog of thymidine. A solution is instilled into the eye to treat herpes simplex keratitis and keratoconjunctivitis.[3]

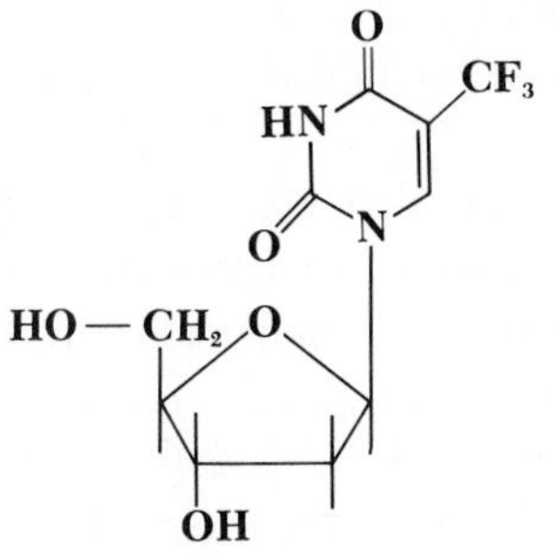

Trifluridine

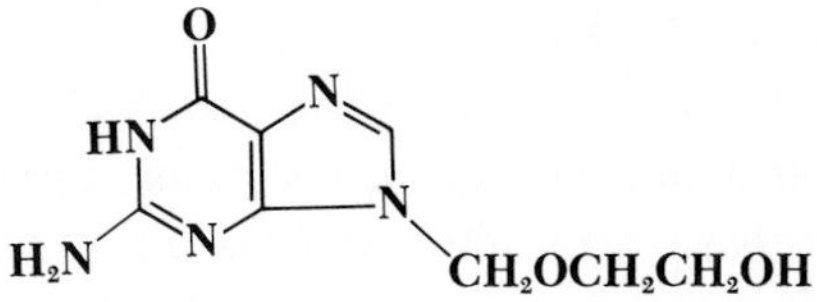

Acyclovir

ACYCLOVIR

Acyclovir (acycloguanosine) is a purine nucleoside analog that is active against herpes viruses. Cells infected with herpes simplex phosphorylate the drug to yield acycloguanosine triphosphate, which preferentially inhibits viral DNA polymerase.[12] This compound is a more potent inhibitor of viral DNA polymerase than of cellular DNA polymerase. *Herpes simplex* virus with altered or absent viral thymidine kinase activity has been isolated from patients receiving multiple courses of acyclovir therapy.[4]

Both topically and orally administered acyclovir (200 mg five times daily) are beneficial in treating primary genital HSV infections; they are less useful for treating recurrence when used after onset of clinical symptoms. Low oral doses (400 mg per day), if given chronically, will prevent recurrence.[1] Intravenous acyclovir is considered the drug of choice for HSV encephalitis.[17] The parenteral drug reduces illness and viral shedding by immunosuppressed patients with mucocutaneous HSV disease. It is also effective for herpes zoster infections and is used particularly in immunocompromised patients.[12] Acyclovir is excreted principally by glomerular filtration, and the dosage must be reduced in patients with renal failure. Adverse responses have included phlebitis at intravenous sites of injection, rash, hematuria, and less frequently central nervous system toxicity with lethargy, confusion, and hallucinations.[12] Reversible renal dysfunction and crystalline nephropathy may also occur.[17] Acyclovir (Zovirax) is available in 200 mg capsules, a suspension of 200 mg in 5 ml, and a 5% ointment. The sodium salt, in 10 ml and 20 ml vials as a powder equivalent to 500 mg and 1 g of acyclovir, respectively, can be dissolved for slow infusion over several hours.

ANTI-HUMAN IMMUNODEFICIENCY VIRUS AGENTS

The advent of AIDS caused by human immunodeficiency virus (HIV) has spurred development of a wide variety of antiviral compounds. Trials with 3′-azido-3′-deoxythymidine (AZT) showed efficacy for AIDS victims with *Pneumocystis carinii* pneumonia (PCP) or for HIV-positive patients with an absolute helper/inducer ($CD4^+$, $T4^+$) T-cell count of less than 200/mm^3 (adults or children). Although commonly referred to in the United States as AZT, the compound has been renamed **zidovudine** (Retrovir).[2] It is available as 100 mg capsules, a syrup with 50 mg/5 ml, and for intravenous infusion (10 mg/ml).

The drug interrupts elongation of DNA chains, making it impossible for the virus to complete DNA synthesis and reproduce. In doses of at least 200 mg every 4 hours, patients with low $CD4^+$ lymphocyte counts had fewer infectious complications than untreated controls, had a transient rise in circulating T4-lymphocytes, and could manifest delayed hypersensitivity.[8] Recently, dosages of 100 mg five times daily significantly reduced the time to onset of PCP in those asymptomatic HIV-positive patients with $CD4^+$ lymphocyte counts <500/mm^2.[16] Serious side effects, such as severe anemia necessitating transfusions, headache, myalgias, and gastrointestinal intolerance, have been observed. The drug may also be carcinogenic. Many other agents, including dideoxyinosine (ddI, didanosine, Videx), dideoxycytidine (ddC), and soluble $CD4^+$, are under investigation.[2]

GANCICLOVIR

Ganciclovir sodium (Cytovene, DHPG) delays DNA replication of the human cytomegalovirus (CMV) agent. The drug is effective in treatment of CMV retinitis, by inducing scarring in active lesions and by preventing progression of the disease in less involved eyes.[11] It may be effective for infections of other organs (gastrointestinal, pulmonary), but too few cases have been studied for efficacy to be proven. Ganciclovir is given intravenously as 1-hour infusions (5 mg/kg) every 12 hours for 14 days; then maintenance therapy of 6 mg/kg is given once daily five times a week to prevent relapse.[3] The principal side effect is leukopenia, but skin rash and mental changes also occur rarely. The drug may interact with imipenem/cilastatin to elicit generalized seizures. Ganciclovir is excreted unchanged in the urine. Because its half-life is increased in patients with renal failure, dosage must be reduced.[5]

INTERFERON

Inducers of endogenous interferon represent a novel approach to antiviral chemotherapy. Interferons are antiviral proteins that exist in multiple molecular forms in different cells where they arise as a consequence of viral infections. They induce enzymes that inhibit synthesis of proteins and degrade viral RNA. Bacteria and their products can also induce formation of interferons by host cells. Alpha interferon, either purified (Alferon N) or recombinant (Intron A, Roferon-A), is marketed for such indications as hairy cell leukemia, genital warts (papilloma virus), and AIDS-related Kaposi's sarcoma.[3] Treatment with 2 to 5 million units of the recombinant preparation daily or twice weekly for 16 to 24 weeks can decrease the pathologic activity of hepatitis B and C viruses.[10] Adverse effects include fever, headache, and myalgia.

REFERENCES

1. Douglas JM, Critchlow C, Benedetti J, et al: A double-blind study of oral acyclovir for suppression of recurrences of genital herpes simplex virus infection, *N Engl J Med* 310:1551, 1984.
2. Drugs for HIV infection, *Med Lett Drugs Ther* 31:11, 1990.
3. Drugs for viral infections, *Med Lett Drugs Ther* 32:73, 1990.
4. Englund JA, Zimmerman ME, Swierkosz EM, et al: Herpes simplex virus resistant to acyclovir: a study in a tertiary care center, *Ann Intern Med* 112:416, 1990.
5. Faulds D, Heel RC: Ganciclovir: a review of its antiviral activity, pharmacokinetic properties and therapeutic efficacy in cytomegalovirus infections, *Drugs* 39:597, 1990.
6. Hall CB, McBride JT, Gala CL, et al: Ribavirin treatment of respiratory syncytial viral infection in infants with underlying cardiopulmonary disease, *JAMA* 254:3047, 1985.
7. Hayden FG, Hoffman HE, Spyker DA: Differences in side effects of amantadine hydrochloride and rimantadine hydrochloride relate to differences in pharmacokinetics, *Antimicrob Agents Chemother* 23:458, 1983.
8. Hirsch MS: Chemotherapy of human immunodeficiency virus infections: current practice and future prospects, *J Infect Dis* 161:845, 1990.
9. Horadam VW, Sharp JG, Smilack JD, et al: Pharmacokinetics of amantadine hydrochloride in subjects with normal and impaired renal function, *Ann Intern Med* 94:454, 1981.
10. Interferon for chronic viral hepatitis, *Med Lett Drugs Ther* 32:1, 1990.
11. Jabs DA, Enger C, Bartlett JG: Cytomegalovirus retinitis and acquired immunodeficiency syndrome, *Arch Ophthalmol* 107:75, 1989.
12. O'Brien JJ, Campoli-Richards DM: Acyclovir: an updated review of its antiviral activity, pharmacokinetic properties and therapeutic efficacy, *Drugs* 37:233, 1989.
13. Oxford JS, Galbraith A: Antiviral activity of amantadine: a review of laboratory and clinical data, *Pharmacol Ther* 11:181, 1980.
14. Reines ED, Gross PA: Antiviral agents, *Med Clin North Am* 72:691, 1988.
15. Shepp DH, Dandliker PS, Meyers JD: Treatment of varicella-zoster virus infection in severely immunocompromised patients: a randomized comparison of acyclovir and vidarabine, *N Engl J Med* 314:208, 1986.
16. Volberding PA, Lagakos SW, Koch MA, et al, the AIDS Clinical Trials Group of the National Institute of Allergy and Infectious Diseases: Zidovudine in asymptomatic human immunodeficiency virus infection: a controlled trial in persons with fewer than 500 CD4-positive cells per cubic millimeter, *N Engl J Med* 322:941, 1990.
17. Whitley RJ, Alford CA, Hirsch MS, et al, the NIAID Collaborative Antiviral Study Group: Vidarabine versus acyclovir therapy in herpes simplex encephalitis, *N Engl J Med* 314:144,1986.
18. Younkin SW, Betts RF, Roth FK, Douglas RG Jr: Reduction in fever and symptoms in young adults with influenza A/Brazil/78 H1N1 infection after treatment with aspirin or amantadine, *Antimicrob Agents Chemother* 23:577, 1983.

Chapter 61

Drugs used to treat mycobacterial infections

FIRST-LINE ANTITUBERCULOSIS DRUGS

Tuberculosis remains a frequently encountered disease. After the advent of effective chemotherapy in the late 1940s, a dramatic decrease occurred in the incidence of pulmonary disease.[8] Systemic forms, such as miliary and bone tuberculosis, have also decreased but remain as frequent in proportion to cases of pulmonary disease as previously. Now both pulmonary and systemic forms are most commonly seen in inner city inhabitants, the elderly, and in patients with AIDS. Tuberculosis must be included in the differential diagnosis of patients with fever of unknown origin, subacute meningitis, or chronic infection at any site.

Appropriate chemotherapy must take into account the slow multiplication of the tubercle bacillus (*Mycobacterium tuberculosis*), its relatively protected intracellular location, and its propensity to become drug resistant, especially during single-drug therapy.[8] Bactericidal activity is accomplished rapidly with combination chemotherapy.[4] The major current problem is failure of compliance,[11] especially among alcoholic patients. In addition, persons from Southeast Asia and Central America are likely to harbor resistant organisms.

The primary agents used in treatment are isoniazid, ethambutol, rifampin, pyrazinamide, and streptomycin.[1,5] Isoniazid and rifampin are highly effective bactericidal agents if used in combination.[3,4] Pyrazinamide is presently recommended as a third drug for the initial 2 months of therapy because it is effective against intracellular organisms.[4] Other compounds are used for secondary treatment of persons with *M. tuberculosis* infections. These alternatives include *p*-aminosalicylic acid, ethionamide, cycloserine, amikacin (see Chapter 59), and capreomycin. Such agents are generally more toxic and slightly less effective, but they may be indicated in selected cases (Table 61-1), especially if the patient has organisms resistant to the primary drugs.

Combinations of drugs are necessary to treat tuberculosis but are not required for prophylaxis. The purpose of combinations is to prevent development of resistant bacilli.

Isoniazid

The effect of isoniazid (INH) on the tubercle bacillus was discovered accidentally during routine screening of intermediates in synthesis of thiosemicarbazones of nicotinamide (a known inhibitor of tubercle bacilli in vitro). Isoniazid (at concentrations of less than 1 μg/ml) kills actively dividing tubercle bacilli and inhibits growth in vitro. The drug presumably inhibits synthesis of mycolic acid. Isoniazid is bactericidal for extracellular populations in body cavities and is also active against intracellular myco-

TABLE 61-1 Drugs for treatment of *Mycobacterium* infections

Drug	Effect	Dosage forms (mg)	Daily dosage	Elimination	Infectious treatment
Primary					
Isoniazid (INH) (Laniazid, Nydrazid)	Cidal	T: 50-300; I: 100/ml; S: 50/5 ml	A: 300 mg Ch: 10-20 mg/kg	Hepatic (metabolism)	*M. tuberculosis, M. kansasii*; included for others but less active
Ethambutol hydrochloride (Myambutol)	Static	T: 100,400	15-25 mg/kg	Renal (excretion)	*M. tuberculosis, M. kansasii*; less active for others; used if isoniazid resistance possible
Rifampin (Rifadin, Rimactane)	Cidal	C: 150,300	A: 600 mg Ch: 10-20 mg/kg	Biliary (excretion)	*M. tuberculosis, M. kansasii, M. leprae*; variable for others
Pyrazinamide	Cidal	T: 500	15-30 mg/kg	Hepatic	Short course, daily or twice weekly, or for 12 months for drug-resistant varieties of *M. tuberculosis*
Streptomycin sulfate	Cidal	I: 400/ml	1 g (to twice weekly)	Renal	*M. tuberculosis*; daily or twice weekly for 3 months (for compliance); not to exceed 120 g
Secondary					
Aminosalicylic sodium (Sodium P.A.S.)	Static	T: 500	12-16 g/d	Renal	Combination therapy in developing countries
Ethionamide (Trecator-SC)	Static	T: 250	0.75-1 g	Hepatic	Retreatment of *M. tuberculosis*; in combination for others
Cycloserine (Seromycin)	Cidal	C: 250	0.75-1 g	Renal	Retreatment of *M. tuberculosis, M. avium/intracellulare* complex, *Nocardia*
Capreomycin sulfate (Capastat)	Static	P: 1000	1 g	Renal	Retreatment of resistant strains
Dapsone	Static	T: 25,100	50-100 mg	Renal	*M. leprae*
Clofazimine (Lamprene)	Cidal	C: 50,100	100-200 mg	Biliary (slow)	*M. leprae, M. avium/intracellulare* complex

Cidal and *static*, Combining forms for "bactericidal" and "bacteriostatic" respectively.
A, Adult; *Ch*, children; *C*, capsule; *I*, injection; *P*, powder for reconstitution; *S*, syrup; *T*, tablet.

bacteria, though it kills them less readily. If used alone for an active infection (usually associated with more than 10^6 bacilli), resistance will develop in a majority of cases within 3 months. Resistance to antitubercular drugs occurs in many regions of the world and is more likely in patients who relapse after previous treatment.[11] Initial therapy is usually started with those drugs to which the organism is likely to be sensitive, such as isoniazid, rifampin, and pyrazinamide. If the patient lives in a geographic region known to have resistant organisms or is being treated after relapse, isoniazid is combined with at least two drugs not previously used, pending susceptibility testing.[5,11]

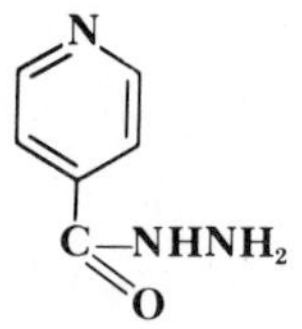

$$\text{4-pyridyl}-C(=O)-NHNH_2$$

Isoniazid

Isoniazid is rapidly absorbed from the gastrointestinal tract, is widely distributed in the body, and penetrates efficiently into the cerebrospinal fluid.[9,10] It is primarily acetylated; metabolites are cleared by the kidney. Persons with slow acetylating ability (an autosomal recessive trait) are subject to hepatotoxicity, particularly if they receive rifampin concomitantly, because of enhanced conversion of isoniazid to hydrazine, a toxic metabolite.[7]

Isoniazid is given to adults in doses of 5 to 10 mg/kg once a day with a maximal dose of 300 mg. Larger doses have been used in tuberculous meningitis but are not necessary. Parenteral administration can be used if patients cannot take oral drug.

Adverse effects of isoniazid include peripheral neuritis, sensory disturbances, hepatic necrosis, arthritic reactions, and hematologic disturbances. Neurotoxicity can be prevented by pyridoxine, which does not affect antimycobacterial activity. The most feared complication is hepatitis. Transaminase elevations are common, but the incidence of significant hepatotoxicity with clinical symptoms increases with age to 2% in persons over 50. Patients should be warned to discontinue the drug if abdominal pain, nausea, or jaundice ensue.

Drug interactions may be significant. Rifampin increases the hepatotoxicity of isoniazid; the drugs must be discontinued by 3% of patients. Isoniazid interferes with metabolism of phenytoin; reduction of phenytoin dosage is usually necessary.

Ethambutol

Ethambutol, though bacteriostatic, is highly effective in combination with other drugs in treatment of tuberculosis.[5] Its mechanism of action is unknown, but it may affect RNA synthesis. Secondary resistance in previously treated patients is low.

The major adverse effect of ethambutol is a dose-dependent optic neuritis. This manifests as loss of visual acuity and alterations in color perception. These responses are reversible and are uncommonly experienced if dosage is limited to a single 15 mg/kg dose each day. Patients receiving ethambutol should be warned to return to their physician if visual impairment occurs; otherwise prospective ophthalmologic testing is not indicated when 15 mg/kg/day is taken. Visual symptoms commonly precede a measurable decrease in visual acuity.[1]

Ethambutol is absorbed rapidly from the gastrointestinal tract and is excreted to a large extent unchanged by the kidney.[9] Consequently, its half-life is prolonged in patients with renal failure; the dosage in this setting should be reduced to 5 to 8 mg/kg. The drug does not normally cross the blood-brain barrier but may do so if the meninges are inflamed.

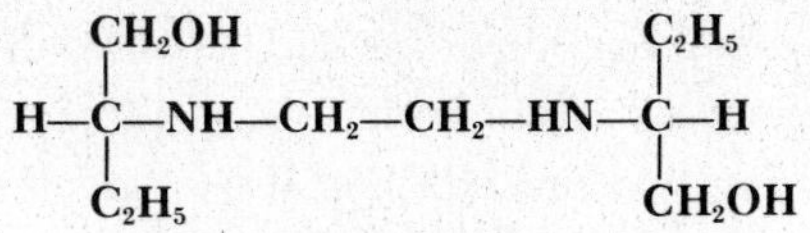

$$
\begin{array}{c}
\quad CH_2OH \qquad\qquad\qquad\qquad\qquad C_2H_5 \\
H{-}C{-}NH{-}CH_2{-}CH_2{-}HN{-}C{-}H \\
\quad C_2H_5 \qquad\qquad\qquad\qquad\qquad CH_2OH
\end{array}
$$

Ethambutol

Rifampin

Rifampin, a semisynthetic derivative of rifamycin B produced by *Streptomyces mediterranei*, is bactericidal for tubercle bacilli.[8] The drug inhibits DNA-dependent RNA polymerase. Oral administration of 600 mg of rifampin produces an effective plasma concentration of 8 μg/ml in less than 2 hours, and antibacterial activity is often still present 10 hours later. Combinations of other drugs with rifampin are now standard therapy for short treatments of pulmonary and extrapulmonary tuberculosis.[3,6,10] Rifampin is also used in combination with antistaphylococcal agents to treat endocarditis and pharyngeal carriage of *Neisseria meningitidis* and *Haemophilus* species.

Resistance to rifampin is increasing, and so it is imperative to use two or more antituberculosis agents concurrently when treating relapse.[11]

Rifampin is absorbed well from the gastrointestinal tract and distributed throughout body fluids, including the cerebrospinal fluid. It is metabolized in the liver and excreted mostly in the bile.[9] Rifampin and its metabolites may stain body fluids (urine, sweat, tears) orange.

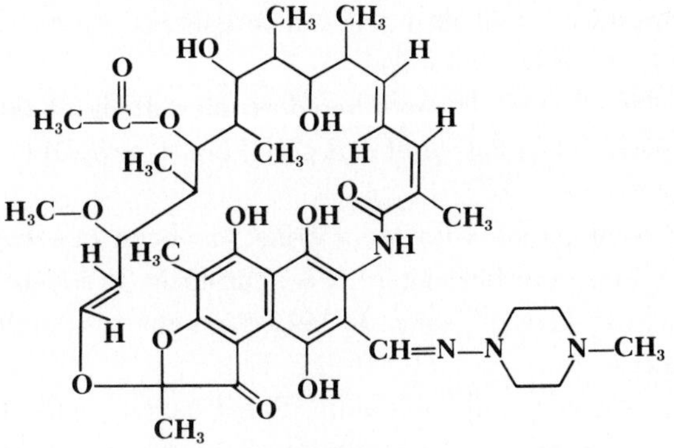

Rifampin

Adverse effects are infrequent (in about 2%) but include hepatotoxicity, abdominal symptoms, leg cramps, and an influenza-like hypersensitivity reaction, especially if the drug is taken intermittently. Drug interactions are numerous because rifampin is a potent inducer of microsomal enzymes (see Chapter 70).

Pyrazinamide

Pyrazinamide (pyrazinoic acid amine), an analog of nicotinamide, is bactericidal at high concentrations for rapidly dividing tubercle bacilli and for organisms in macrophages.[1] Because of this latter activity, it has become a first-line drug for the initial 2 months of therapy when 6-month courses are used.[3,10] The drug is well absorbed and distributes throughout the body. Hepatic damage is infrequent at the recommended dosage of 15 to 30 mg/kg/day. Pyrazinamide can also be given twice weekly (at dosages of 50 to 70 mg/kg). Hyperuricemia, which may lead to gouty arthritis, can occur.

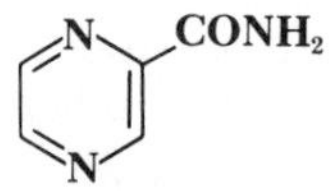

$CONH_2$

Pyrazinamide

Streptomycin

Streptomycin was the first effective drug for treatment of tuberculosis. It must be administered intramuscularly and produces numerous toxic effects, particularly in adults.[5] It is most often used in combination with other drugs to retreat pulmonary infections in patients with organisms known to be resistant. The dose is 7 to 15 mg/kg once daily (20 to 40 mg/kg/day in children, up to 1 g/day) for 4 weeks, or to improve compliance in outpatients the drug can be injected twice weekly. The total amount given to an adult should not exceed 120 g.[1]

SECOND-LINE ANTITUBERCULOSIS DRUGS

Some other compounds are available as alternatives to the aforementioned agents. However, their use should be limited to retreatment of infections proved resistant to the primary agents.

***p*-Aminosalicylic acid** is well absorbed, but compliance is poor due to gastrointestinal disturbances; it is rarely used today.

Ethionamide, like isoniazid, is a pyridine derivative. Its limitation is frequent side effects, especially gastrointestinal upset and peripheral neuropathy, which necessitate its discontinuation.

Cycloserine in combination with other drugs has been effective in treatment of some cases of tuberculosis. Unfortunately, it is neurotoxic. Frequent side effects, such as nausea, vomiting, hypotension, seizures, behavioral changes, and peripheral neuritis, limit its usefulness.

Capreomycin is a polypeptide antibiotic. Renal damage and ototoxicity limit its usefulness. The drug is given parenterally for 2 to 4 months. Since eighth-nerve damage can be severe, hearing tests should be performed prospectively.

DRUGS USED FOR NONTUBERCULOSIS INFECTIONS

Mycobacteria other than *Mycobacterium tuberculosis* may be sensitive to some of the aforementioned agents. *M. kansasii* infections usually respond to isoniazid and rifampin, but *M. avium/intracellulare complex* forms are more difficult to treat. Combinations of four to five drugs, including rifampin, isoniazid, and ethambutol, are employed with ciprofloxacin or amikacin. Recently some success, particularly in patients with AIDS, has been reported with two other substances: rifabutin (a congener of rifampin) and clofazimine. However, these agents are not approved by the FDA for this use, and only clofazimine is available in the United States. *M. fortuitum* and *M. chelonii* (rapid growers) are resistant to the usual antituberculosis drugs but are variably susceptible to amikacin, cefoxitin, trimethoprim-sulfamethoxazole, or ciprofloxacin (susceptibility testing can be performed rather readily to guide the choice of drug).[12] Combination therapy is employed because resistance develops with single-drug therapy.

DRUGS USED IN TREATMENT OF LEPROSY

Chemotherapy of leprosy (Hansens disease), which afflicts 12 to 15 million persons worldwide, has relied on **dapsone** (4,4′-diaminodiphenylsulfone) for over 40 years.[2] This drug has been used in both lepromatous (disseminated) and tuberculoid leprosy (Table 61-1). Unfortunately, single-drug therapy has led to emergence of resistant organisms, and so multidrug therapy with dapsone and rifampin or clofazimine is now standard for lepromatous leprosy.

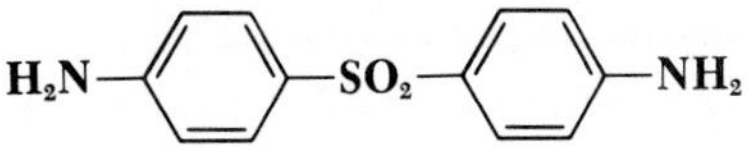

H_2N—C₆H₄—SO_2—C₆H₄—NH_2

Dapsone

Cl, N, $NCH(CH_3)_2$, N, NH, Cl

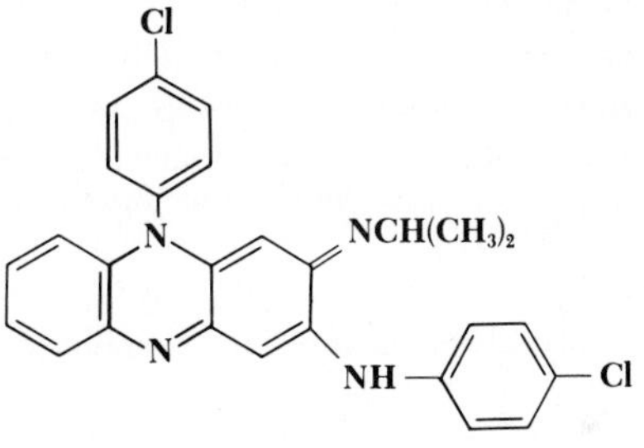

Clofazimine

The precise mechanism of action of dapsone is unknown, but it probably acts like sulfonamides to inhibit bacterial metabolism of *p*-aminobenzoic acid. This mechanism also likely accounts for its efficacy in combination with trimethoprim in *Pneumocystis carinii* infections. The drug is administered once daily, since it has a half-life of 20 to 40 hours. Initially, however, it is given in low doses (one tablet weekly) to minimize adverse reactions. A syndrome of severe skin lesions, hepatomegaly, and psychosis can develop with dapsone therapy.[2] Otherwise its toxicity is similar to that of sulfonamides.

Erythema nodosum of leprosy may be accelerated by the drug, but this reaction is prevented by thalidomide. Thalidomide must be discontinued gradually or reactions will recur, and it must not be used in women of childbearing age because of its teratogenic activity. When thalidomide was marketed in Europe as a hypnotic agent, it caused severe birth defects (phocomelia) in thousands of children.

Antitubercular drugs, including rifampin and ethionamide, kill the bacilli and rapidly decrease the number of organisms. Since relapse can occur with single-drug therapy, treatment is begun with dapsone and rifampin for 6 months. Clofazimine is effective in patients with borderline-lepromatous and lepromatous leprosy and does not induce erythema nodosum of leprosy.[2] It is weakly bactericidal and takes some time to decrease the number of bacilli. Its major side effect is skin discoloration, a red-brown pigmentation particularly at sites of lepromatous involvement; this clears when the drug is discontinued.

REFERENCES

1. American Thoracic Society Statement: Treatment of tuberculosis and tuberculosis infection in adults and children, *Am Rev Respir Dis* 134:355, 1986.
2. Binford CH, Meyers WM, Walsh GP: Leprosy, *JAMA* 247:2283, 1982.
3. Cohn DL, Catlin BJ, Peterson KL, et al: A 62-dose, 6-month therapy for pulmonary and extrapulmonary tuberculosis: a twice-weekly, directly observed, and cost-effective regimen, *Ann Intern Med* 112:407, 1990.
4. Combs DL, O'Brien RJ, Geiter LJ: USPHS Tuberculosis Short-course Chemotherapy Trial 21: effectiveness, toxicity, and acceptability. The report of final results, *Ann Intern Med* 112:397, 1990.
5. Davidson PT: Treating tuberculosis: what drugs, for how long? *Ann Intern Med* 112:393, 1990.
6. Dutt AK, Moers D, Stead WW: Short-course chemotherapy for extrapulmonary tuberculosis: nine years' experience, *Ann Intern Med* 104:7, 1986.
7. Gangadharam PRJ: Isoniazid, rifampin, and hepatotoxicity, *Am Rev Respir Dis* 133:963, 1986.
8. Goldberger MJ: Antituberculosis agents, *Med Clin North Am* 72:661, 1988.
9. Holdiness MR: Clinical pharmacokinetics of the antituberculosis drugs, *Clin Pharmacokinet* 9:511, 1984.
10. Holdiness MR: Management of tuberculosis meningitis, *Drugs* 39:224, 1990.
11. Suwanogool S, Smith SM, Smith LG, Eng R: Drug-resistance encountered in the retreatment of *Mycobacterium tuberculosis* infections, J Chronic Dis 37:925, 1984.
12. Wallace RJ Jr, Bedsole G, Sumter G, et al: Activities of ciprofloxacin and ofloxacin against rapidly growing mycobacteria with demonstration of acquired resistance following single-drug therapy, *Antimicrob Agents Chemother* 34:65, 1990.

Chapter 62

Drugs used to treat fungal infections

A number of agents, given both parenterally and orally, are used to treat deep fungal infections. Because the frequency of certain fungal infections has increased in immunosuppressed patients, these compounds are being administered for both proved and suspected infections. Their significant potential for adverse effects greatly influences the choice of a specific agent for therapy.

NYSTATIN AND AMPHOTERICIN B

Nystatin and amphotericin B (Table 62-1) are *polyene* antibiotics that complex with sterols, principally ergosterol, in fungal membranes.[7] Bacterial membranes are not injured by polyenes. However, mammalian membranes with cholesterol, such as red blood cells, may sustain injury, causing a reutilization type of anemia.

Nystatin is effective topically against *Candida albicans* and some other fungi. It is given orally only for oral candidal infections because its absorption is minimal and its action requires direct contact.

Amphotericin B has been an effective antibiotic against the causative agents of deep-seated mycotic infections,[3,5] such as aspergillosis, mucormycosis, histoplasmosis, cryptococcosis, blastomycosis, coccidioidomycosis, and candidiasis.[2] A total dose of 1 to 2 g is given intravenously over 4 to 8 weeks. Because fever and chills may occur early, test doses of 1 to 5 mg are injected on the first day.[7] If no untoward reaction occurs, a daily dose of 20 to 50 mg (not to exceed 0.5 mg/kg/day) is given over 2 to 5 hours. Adverse reactions include thrombophlebitis at the site of injection, gastrointestinal upset, and renal toxicity. In addition, renal tubular acidosis, hypocalcemia, and K^+ loss can occur. The rise in creatinine concentration in some patients responds to infusion of saline. The drug can enhance the toxicity of agents such as aminoglycosides and pentamidine.[1] Amphotericin B has a long elimination half-life (about 15 days), but plasma concentration rarely exceeds 2 μg/ml. It is available as 50 mg vials that contain 41 mg of deoxycholate. Reconstitution in dextrose in water is necessary because the drug aggregates in saline solution. If a prolonged infusion (24 hours) is given, the preparation must be shielded from light.

TABLE 62-1 Oral and topical dosage forms of antifungal agents

Drug	Tablets or capsules (mg)	Vaginal tablets or suppositories (mg)	Topical preparations*
Polyenes			
Nystatin (Mycostatin, others)	500,000 units	100,000 units	100,000 units
Amphotericin B (Fungizone)			3%
Other antifungal agents used systemically			
Flucytosine (Ancobon)	250,500		
Ketoconazole (Nizoral)	200		2%
Fluconazole (Diflucan)	100-200		
Griseofulvin (Fulvicin, others)	125-500		
Antifungal agents applied topically			
Miconazole nitrate (Monistat, Micatin)		100,200	2%
Clotrimazole (Lotrimin, Mycelex)		100,500	1%
Tolnaftate (Tinactin, others)			1%
Haloprogin (Halotex)			1%
Ciclopirox olamine (Loprox)			1%
Iodochlorhydroxyquin (clioquinol, Vioform, Torofor)			3%
Butoconazole nitrate (Femstat)			2%
Econazole nitrate (Spectazole)			1%
Oxiconazole nitrate (Oxistat)			1%
Sulconazole nitrate (Exelderm)			1%
Terconazole (Terazol 7)			0.4%
Tioconazole (Vagistat)			6.5%
Triacetin (Enzactin, Fungacetin)			25%
Naftifine hydrochloride (Naftin)			1%
Gentian violet			1,2%

*Creams, gels, lotions, ointments, solutions.

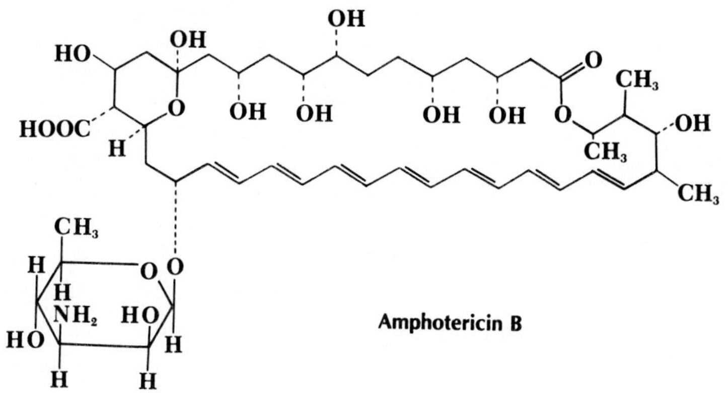

Amphotericin B

OTHER ANTIFUNGAL AGENTS

Certain other antifungal agents are useful for systemic infections (Table 62-1).

Flucytosine is a fluorinated compound administered orally to treat infections caused by *Candida albicans*, especially of the urinary tract or localized infections.[7] For treatment of cryptococcal infections and central nervous system and bone infections caused by *Candida*, the drug is highly effective when combined with amphotericin B. Flucytosine may cause blood dyscrasias, especially leukopenia, hepatic toxicity, and diarrhea.[7] The usual dosage is 100 to 150 mg/kg/day, but serum concentration must be monitored; dosage should be reduced if the concentration exceeds 100 μg/ml.

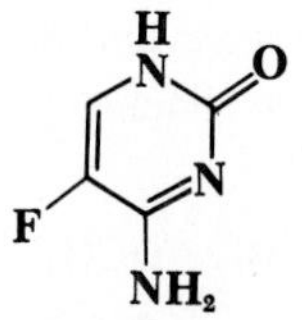

Flucytosine

Ketoconazole is an imidazole derivative that interferes with formation of the fungal plasma membrane sterol. It is very effective for chronic mucocutaneous candidiasis, dermatophytosis, and mild systemic fungal infections, such as histoplasmosis and blastomycosis.[8] The drug is given orally, usually 400 mg/day. Absorption of ketoconazole requires an acidic gastric environment; patients receiving other drugs that increase gastric pH or who are achlorhydric will not adequately absorb the compound. Infrequent toxicity includes gastrointestinal and hepatic manifestations, gynecomastia, and decreased libido. Ketoconazole blunts the adrenal response to ACTH but rarely causes adrenal insufficiency.[8] It inhibits hepatic microsomal drug metabolism and thereby contributes to several drug interactions (see Chapter 70).

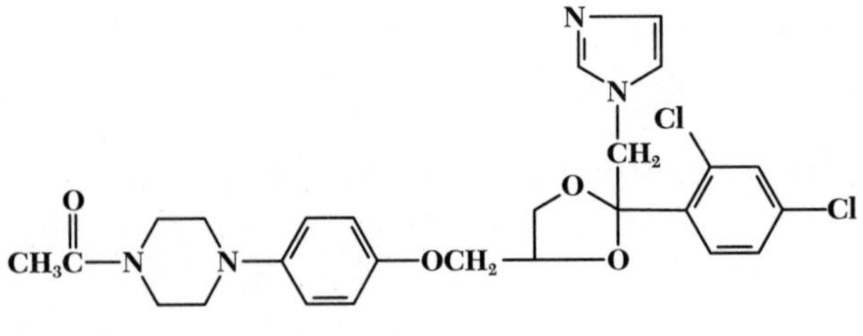

Ketoconazole

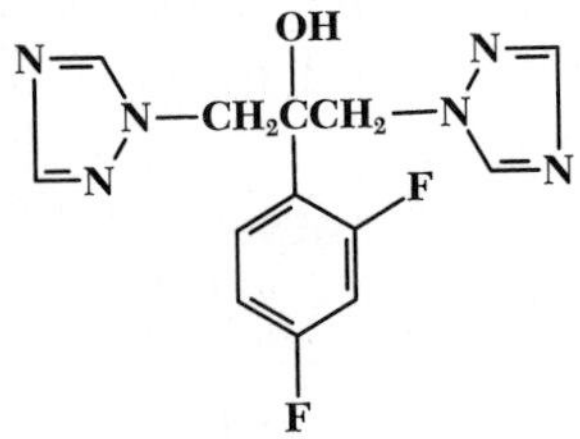

Fluconazole

Fluconazole, a recently introduced imidazole, has greater activity than ketoconazole and penetrates into cerebrospinal fluid.[9] It has been approved for use in severely ill patients with candidal and cryptococcal infections, including cryptococcal meningitis in AIDS patients. In the latter instance, therapy is long-term because relapse after stopping therapy is almost universal. Adverse reactions include hepatitis, gastrointestinal upset, and rarely central nervous system abnormalities. The drug is available for intravenous therapy at an initial dose of 400 mg, followed by 200 mg for serious infections or 100 mg for less serious problems.[4] Fluconazole is excreted and dosage must be reduced in renal failure. Use of the drug in dialysis patients is not established. Awaiting approval is itraconazole; relative to ketoconazole it is effective against more fungi and is absorbed better after oral ingestion.[6,10]

Griseofulvin, produced from a *Penicillium* mold, represents a novel approach to treatment of certain dermatomycoses. When given orally for long periods, griseofulvin is incorporated into the skin, hair, and nails where it exerts fungistatic activity against various species of *Microsporum*, *Trichophyton*, and *Epidermophyton*. Administration for several weeks is necessary for improvement of ringworm. In fungal infections of the nails, treatment may be needed for several months. The most common side effects are gastric discomfort, diarrhea, and headache. Urticaria and skin rash may also occur.

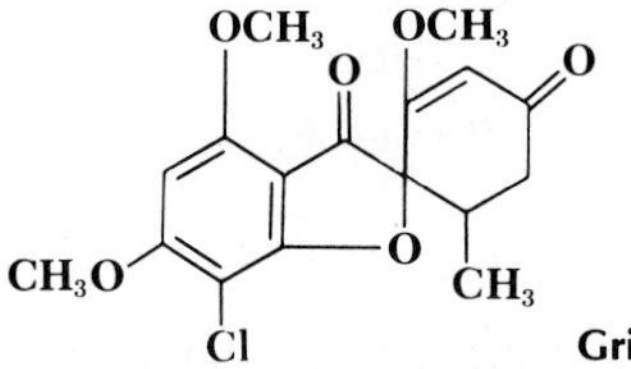

Griseofulvin

Still other antifungal agents have principal use as topical drugs for vaginal or cutaneous mycotic infections (Table 62-1).[2]

Topical preparations of **miconazole**, another imidazole, are available for treatment of dermatophytosis and cutaneous or vaginal candidal infections. The drug has also been used intravenously, on rare occasions, for *C. albicans* infections in patients allergic to amphotericin B and for infections with *Petriellidium boydii*. Miconazole may cause intense pruritus.

Clotrimazole, related structurally to miconazole, is used primarily as a topical fungicide or as vaginal tablets for candidiasis.

Tolnaftate, though effective in epidermophytosis, does not eliminate candidal organisms and is inadequate for fungal infections of the nails, scalp, and soles of the feet.

Undecylenic acid and its zinc salt are topical agents for mild epidermophytosis.

Natamycin (Natacyn), a polyene antibiotic, is used in a 5% ophthalmic suspension for fungal keratitis, blepharitis, and conjunctivitis.

REFERENCES

1. Antoniskis D, Larsen RA: Acute, rapidly progressive renal failure with simultaneous use of amphotericin B and pentamidine, *Antimicrob Agents Chemother* 34:470, 1990.
2. Bodey GP: Topical and systemic antifungal agents, *Med Clin North Am* 72:637, 1988.
3. Cohen J: Antifungal chemotherapy, *Lancet* 2:532, 1982.
4. Fluconazole, *Med Lett Drugs Ther* 32:50, 1990.
5. Gallis HA, Drew RH, Pickard WW: Amphotericin B: 30 years of clinical experience, *Rev Infect Dis* 12:308, 1990.
6. Grant SM, Clissold SP: Itraconazole: a review of its pharmacodynamic and pharmacokinetic properties, and therapeutic use in superficial and systemic mycoses, *Drugs* 37:310, 1989.
7. Medoff G, Kobayashi GS: Strategies in the treatment of systemic fungal infections, *N Engl J Med* 302:145, 1980.
8. National Institute of Allergy and Infectious Diseases Mycoses Study Group: Treatment of blastomycosis and histoplasmosis with ketoconazole: results of a prospective randomized clinical trial, *Ann Intern Med* 103:861, 1985.
9. Robinson PA, Knirsch AK, Joseph JA: Fluconazole for life-threatening fungal infections in patients who cannot be treated with conventional antifungal agents, *Rev Infect Dis* 12(suppl 3):S349, 1990.
10. Tucker RM, Denning DW, Dupont B, Stevens DA: Itraconazole therapy for chronic coccidioidal meningitis, *Ann Intern Med* 112:108, 1990.

Chapter 63

Antiseptics and disinfectants

Antiseptics are drugs that are applied to living tissues to kill or inhibit growth of bacteria. *Disinfectants* are able to kill bacteria when applied to nonliving materials.[5] Related terms are defined as follows:

germicide Anything that destroys bacteria but not necessarily spores.
fungicide Anything that destroys fungi.
sporicide Anything that destroys spores.
sanitizer An agent that reduces the number of bacterial contaminants to a safe level, as may be judged by public health requirements.
preservative An agent or process that, by either chemical or physical means, prevents decomposition.

BRIEF HISTORY

Disinfectants were used long before the discovery of bacteria. The first germicides were deodorants, since foul odors were associated with disease. Chlorinated soda ($NaCl$ and $NaClO$) was used on infected wounds in the nineteenth century and was recommended to purify drinking water, since the soda appeared to diminish bacterial growth. Phenol was used as a deodorant and later as an antiseptic for infected wounds, long before the nature of infections was understood. The use of ethanol as an antiseptic was delayed for many years because Koch (1881) had reported that it did not kill anthrax spores. However, the fact that 70% ethanol has superior germicidal properties was later established by Beyer (1912). Tincture of iodine was introduced into the *United States Pharmacopoeia* in 1830 and was used extensively by the beginning of the Civil War.

Semmelweis, an assistant at the Lying-in Hospital in Vienna, demonstrated the benefits of cleansing the hands with chlorine-containing solutions for prevention of puerperal fever. He noted that the incidence of mortality attributable to puerperal sepsis was lower in women delivered by midwives than in those delivered by medical students (the first case-control study). The students delivered babies after performing autopsies, as noted by Semmelweis because of the odor in the delivery room when the students were present. He suspected that students were carrying "decomposing organic matter" (actually group A streptococci) from the autopsy room to the delivery room. He proved his hypothesis when cleansing of the students' hands reduced fatalities. However, he was ostracized by the medical community, was hospitalized with psychiatric illness, and ultimately committed suicide.

The activity of antiseptics has been standardized by use of the *phenol coefficient*, the ratio of dilutions compared with phenol necessary to kill test organisms in vitro.

TABLE 63-1 Disinfection of medical equipment

Level of disinfection	Germicidal	Sporicidal	Agents
High	Yes	Yes (long exposure)	8% formaldehyde 2% glutaraldehyde
Intermediate	Yes	No	70% ethanol 1% iodine 5000 ppm hypochlorite or iodophor
Low	Yes (not fungicidal or mycobactericidal)	No	75 ppm iodophor 1% phenolic quaternary ammonium compounds

From Simmons BP: Infect Control Urological Care 6:14-25, 1981.

Antiseptics were found to be useless for treating systemic infections, and they are now used only as external agents to prevent growth of bacteria.

ANTISEPTICS AND DISINFECTANTS

The only acceptable disinfectants for initial sterilization of equipment (Table 63-1) are 30-minute exposure to 8% formaldehyde (20% formalin) or 2% alkalinized glutaraldehyde.[5] Organic material, such as blood, exudates, and stool, will totally inactivate other germicides, precluding their use for instrument sterilization.[1] The alkalinized form of glutaraldehyde is as effective as other aqueous forms but less corrosive. These agents, if an adequate contact time of 20 minutes at 20° C is allowed, will kill all bacteria and all viruses, including hepatitis B and HIV.[2] The causative agent of Creutzfeldt-Jakob disease is relatively resistant to formaldehyde, and so instruments used in surgery on possible cases must be autoclaved for 60 minutes at 121° C. Inanimate objects can be treated with 5000 ppm hypochlorite solution.[4]

Alcohol and iodine preparations (iodophors) are commonly used for preoperative preparation of the skin.[3] Ethanol is most bactericidal at 70% concentration by weight and is used in Europe as the standard surgical hand scrub. Tincture of iodine, which stains the skin and is irritating, has been replaced by iodophors such as povidone-iodine (Betadine, others) for routine surgical scrubbing. Iodophors release iodine slowly and are somewhat less irritating to the skin. They rapidly lose activity in the presence of organic matter, such as serum.

Sodium hypochlorite releases chlorine. It is quite effective for cleaning spills and for killing viruses as well as bacteria.

Tetraglycine hydroperiodide (Globaline), and **aluminum hexaurea sulfate triiodide** (Hexadine-S) disinfect water by means of halogen release. Globaline has less activity against ova; Hexadine is the choice of back packers to prevent *Giardia* infection.

The most widely used phenol derivative, **hexachlorophene**, is incorporated into soaps and creams. In a 3% solution, hexachlorophene (pHisoHex) sharply reduces gram-positive bacterial counts on the skin without irritation, but it has been supplanted by iodophors, which have more generalized activity. Hexachlorophene preparations are not safe for newborn infants, because of potential absorption through the skin.

Chlorhexidine gluconate (Hibiclens, Hibistat) is a safe antiseptic comparable to the iodophors, with broad antimicrobial activity. Its major advantage is its prolonged residual action, particularly against regrowth of resident flora.

Surface-active compounds

Surface-active compounds have been popular but are weakly active agents. Their use as disinfectants is limited to soaps for hand washing (if visible surface action is present, people think that more disinfection takes place).

Quaternary ammoniums, such as benzalkonium chloride (Zephiran, others), kill some gram-positive and gram-negative organisms but have little activity against many hospital strains. They should no longer be used in hospitals.

Metal-containing antiseptics

Derivatives of mercury and silver have been widely used as skin antiseptics. They are largely bacteriostatic.

Thimerosal (Mersol, Merthiolate) contains 49% mercury; **merbromin** (Mercurochrome) contains 25% mercury and 20% bromine.

Silver nitrate in 1% solution was traditionally used to prevent ophthalmia neonatorum caused by gonococci but has now been replaced by application of erythromycin to the conjunctival sac of the newborn infant. Silver combined with the sulfonamide sulfadiazine (Silvadene, Flint SSD) is a useful antibacterial cream for burn patients.

Zinc sulfate solution is used in some types of conjunctivitis, and zinc oxide ointment or paste is a traditional remedy in a variety of skin diseases. Calamine lotion contains 8% zinc oxide. Phenolated calamine lotion contains 1% phenol in addition.

Acids

Acids, such as benzoic, salicylic, and undecylenic, have been used for many years as fungistatic agents. Whitfields ointment is a mixture of 6% benzoic acid and 3% salicylic acid used to treat fungal infections of the feet.

OH

Phenol

OH OH
Cl CH$_2$ Cl
Cl Cl
Cl Cl

Hexachlorophene

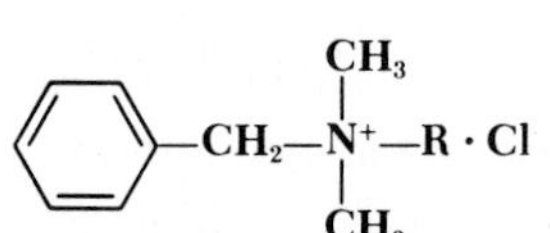

Benzalkonium chloride

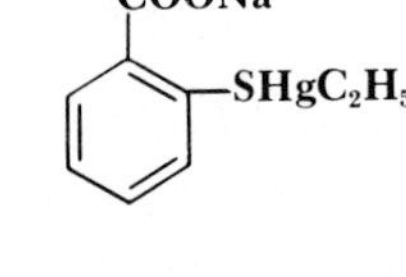

Thimerosal

REFERENCES

1. Ayliffe GAJ: Surgical scrub and skin disinfection, *Infect Control* 5:23, 1984.
2. Gurevich I, Yannelli B, Cunha BA: The disinfectant dilemma revisited, *Infect Control Hosp Epidemiol* 11:96, 1990.
3. Larson EL, Butz AM, Gullette DL, Laughon BA: Alcohol for surgical scrubbing? *Infect Control Hosp Epidemiol* 11:139, 1990.
4. Rutala WA: Draft guideline for selection and use of disinfectants, *Am J Infect Control* 17(Feb):24A, 1989.
5. Simmons BP: Guidelines for hospital environmental control, *Infect Control Urological Care* 6:14, 1981.

Chapter 64

Drugs used to treat amebiasis and other intestinal protozoal infections

Amebiasis is caused by the protozoan *Entamoeba histolytica*. Its clinical presentation can vary from an symptomatic state to dysentery or extraintestinal disease, particularly liver abscess. Antiamebic and other antiprotozoal drugs, which are usually taken for several days, are listed in Table 64-1.

METRONIDAZOLE

Drug therapy of moderate to severe amebiasis is best accomplished by use of metronidazole (Flagyl, others), which is safe, inexpensive, and effective for both intestinal and extraintestinal forms of the disease.[3] The drug also kills *Trichomonas* and *Giardia* (Table 64-1). Metronidazole acts as an artificial electron acceptor after accumulating within the cell as the reduced compound.[5] This diverts electrons from normal pathways of the protozoan. Metronidazole also impairs the ability of DNA to function as a template. Although it is active against cysts and trophozoites, metronidazole is more effective in symptomatic or invasive amebiasis. It is also active in treatment of amebic liver abscess, but complications can occur. These are usually attributable to the size and position of the abscess and not to lack of activity of the drug.[3] Some, however, recommend use of dehydroemetine if there is no dramatic clinical improvement within 72 hours of therapy with metronidazole.[6] Side effects of metronidazole include gastrointestinal symptoms, stomatitis, a disulfiram-like reaction with ethanol, a change in urine color, and, rarely, neuropathy.[5] It should not be used during pregnancy. The drug is taken as tablets containing 250 or 500 mg. A solution is also available for intravenous administration to persons who cannot take oral medication.

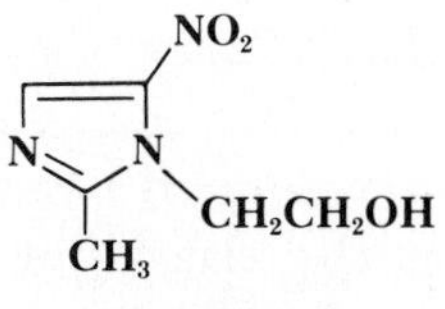

NO_2
N N
CH_2CH_2OH
CH_3

Metronidazole

DEHYDROEMETINE

Although emetine was used for centuries to treat dysentery, toxicity has forced its limitation to treatment of amebiasis.[3] This alkaloid of ipecac is amebicidal in vitro and on trophozoites localized in tissues. Emetine inhibits protein synthesis in the parasites and in host mammalian cells by blocking translocation of peptide chains.[1]

TABLE 64-1 Drugs used to treat amebiasis, other intestinal protozoal infections, and *Trichomonas*

	Drug	Dose (mg)	Interval (hours)	Duration (days)
Amebiasis (*Entamoeba histolytica*)				
Asymptomatic (cyst passers)	Iodoquinol or	650	8	20
	paromomycin or	25-30/kg/d	8	7
	diloxanide furoate*	500	8	10
Symptomatic intestinal disease or hepatic abscess	Metronidazole	750	8	10
	+ iodoquinol	650	8	20
	If no response: dehydroemetine*†	1-1.5/kg	24	≤5
	+ chloroquine phosphate	500	24	14-21
Giardia lamblia	Quinacrine hydrochloride	100	8	5
	Metronidazole‡	250	8	5
	Furazolidone	100	6	7-10
		6/kg§	6	7-10
Balantidium coli	Tetracycline‡	500	6	10
Trichomonas vaginalis	Metronidazole	250‖	8	7

Primary source: Drugs for parasitic infections, Med Lett Drugs Ther 32:23, 1990.
*Available from the Centers for Disease Control, Atlanta, GA 30333 (telephone 404-639-3670; 8:00 AM-4:30 PM EST, Monday through Friday).
†Intramuscular (others oral).
‡Considered investigational for this condition.
§Pediatric dose.
‖Or single 2 g dose.

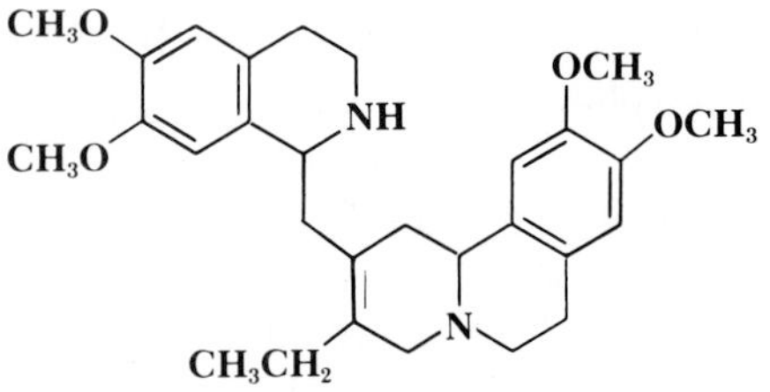

CH_3O, CH_3O, NH, OCH_3, OCH_3, N, CH_3CH_2

Dehydroemetine

Dehydroemetine (Mebadin) is a slightly less toxic moiety. Nevertheless, it is toxic to cardiac and skeletal muscle,[1] and its use is limited to those unable to tolerate metronidazole or to instances of clinical failure.[2,4]

IODOQUINOL

Iodoquinol (diiodohydroxyquin, Yodoxin) is recommended as an intestinal amebicide and for asymptomatic carriers. The related drug iodochlorhydroxyquin caused an epidemic of subacute myelo-optic neuropathy in Japan and is not used in the United States. In rare cases iodoquinol also causes this syndrome, but its most common adverse effects are related to the gastrointestinal tract. Tablets of 210 or 650 mg are available.

The mechanism of action of iodoquinol is not known. It is not well absorbed and so is therapeutic only for intestinal infection. The drug is recommended for additional therapy after metronidazole therapy has been completed.[2]

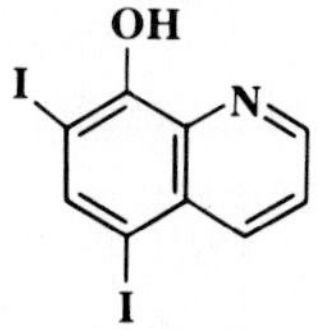

Iodoquinol

CHLOROQUINE

Chloroquine (Aralen) is a well-known antimalarial compound that can be combined with dehydroemetine to treat amebic abscess of the liver.[2] Chloroquine does not affect the intestinal form of *Entamoeba histolytica*.

The oral dosage of chloroquine phosphate is 1 g daily for 2 days, then 500 mg daily for 2 to 3 weeks. Chloroquine hydrochloride (50 mg/ml) is available for intramuscular injection.

MISCELLANEOUS AGENTS

Patients with intestinal amebiasis improve more rapidly when tetracyclines are added to the usual antiamebic regimen. However, tetracyclines alone are not sufficient to effect a cure. Paromomycin (Humatin) and erythromycin are directly amebicidal, whereas tetracyclines modify the bacterial flora to influence amebas indirectly. Paromomycin is an alternative for asymptomatic carriers. Diloxanide furoate (Furamide), an amebicide with minimal side effects, probably should be the drug of choice for asymptomatic intestinal infections.[3] The treatment of *Giardia* infections in children is successfully managed with a suspension of furazolidone (Furoxone).

REFERENCES

1. Balamuth W, Lasslo A: Comparative amoebacidal activity of some compounds related to emetine, *Proc Soc Exp Biol Med* 80:705, 1952.
2. Drugs for parasitic infections, *Med Lett Drugs Ther* 32:23, 1990.
3. Krogstad DJ, Spencer HC Jr, Healy GR, et al: Amebiasis: epidemiologic studies in the United States, 1971-1974, *Ann Intern Med* 88:89, 1978.
4. Mandell WF, Neu HC: Parasitic infections: therapeutic considerations, *Med Clin North Am* 72:669, 1988.
5. Scully BE: Metronidazole, *Med Clin North Am* 72:613, 1988.
6. Thompson JE Jr, Forlenza S, Verma R: Amebic liver abscess: a therapeutic approach, *Rev Infect Dis* 7:171, 1985.

Chapter 65

Drugs used to treat malaria and other extraintestinal protozoal infections

MALARIA

Malaria has been treated for years with derivatives of cinchona bark, from which the alkaloids quinine and quinidine were extracted. Quinine was the standard antimalarial drug until World War II. More effective drugs were synthesized, and new approaches to antimalarial therapy evolved.[5] However, certain strains of the parasite, particularly *Plasmodium falciparum*, have developed resistance to the synthetic drugs.

Classification of antimalarial compounds can be based on their activity in various stages of the life cycle of *Plasmodium* or on their mechanisms of action. Drugs that cure a clinical attack by eliminating the asexual forms are known as *schizonticides*. They include quinine, chloroquine, amodiaquine, mefloquine, and pyrimethamine. Tetracycline and combinations of a sulfonamide with pyrimethamine are effective also and have been combined with quinine for chloroquine-resistant strains.

Radical cure implies the elimination from the body of both the asexual forms and the exoerythrocytic forms of the parasite. Since there are no exoerythrocytic forms of falciparum malaria, the usual schizonticides are sufficient to achieve a radical cure. However, primaquine is necessary for a radical cure in *P. vivax* and *P. ovale* infections.

The cinchona alkaloids and the 4- and 8-aminoquinolines, such as chloroquine and primaquine, had been believed to act by intercalation (insertion between base pairs) into DNA of the parasite to alter the digestion of hemoglobin. Currently, these weak bases are thought to concentrate within intracellular organelles where they alter intracellular transport.[5,9] The antimalarial action of pyrimethamine and sulfonamides, as with bacteria, is to inhibit synthesis of folic acid from *p*-aminobenzoic acid.

Quinine

Quinine, the traditional antimalarial remedy, is combined with other drugs in treatment of chloroquine-resistant *Plasmodium falciparum* (CRPF). The drug is rapidly and nearly completely absorbed. About 20% escapes metabolism by the liver. This portion and the metabolites are excreted in the urine. The half-life of quinine is about 10 hours. If given intravenously to ill patients, some accumulation can occur; dosage reduction is necessary for those who remain severely ill.[9] Quinine sulfate is available in capsules (130 to 325 mg) and tablets (260 and 325 mg). In a patient who cannot tolerate orally administered quinine, the drug may be given as the dihydrochloride (available from the Centers for Disease Control) by slow intravenous infusion. For this purpose 650 mg of quinine is dissolved in 300 ml of saline solution and given over 2 to 4 hours.[9] Blood concentration must be monitored. Alternatively, intravenous administration of 10 mg/kg of quinidine gluconate (an optical isomer of quinine) can be followed by infusion of 0.02 mg/kg/min, alone or with exchange transfusion, to achieve a cure in some cases of severe, complicated malaria.[8] The advantage of quinidine is that measurement of circulating concentration is a routine procedure in clinical laboratories.

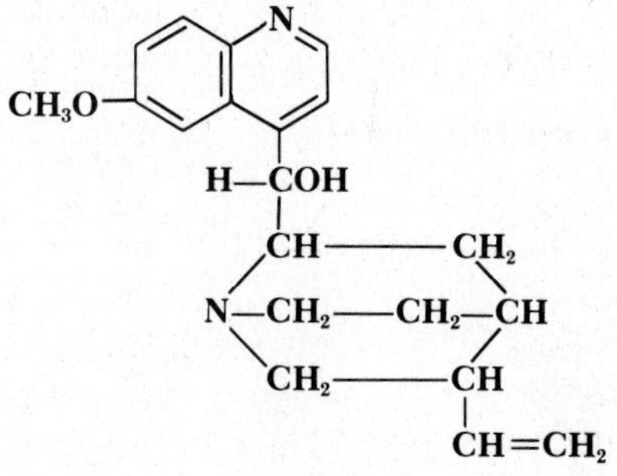

CH_3O N
H—COH
CH—CH$_2$
N—CH$_2$—CH$_2$—CH
CH$_2$—CH
CH=CH$_2$

Quinine

Quinine can produce a variety of toxic effects, including the syndrome *cinchonism*, with nausea, vertigo, tinnitus, and visual disturbances. This symptom complex is associated with blood concentrations above 5 μg/ml. Allergic skin rashes, drug fever, and, rarely, asthmatic attacks have been reported.[9]

Quinine has other uses in medicine. It is given occasionally to relieve leg cramps, in treatment of myotonia congenita, and as a sclerosing agent.

Chloroquine

Chloroquine is a 4-aminoquinoline derivative that underwent extensive testing during World War II, when supplies of quinine were unavailable. Chloroquine became the drug of choice for most forms of malaria.[5]

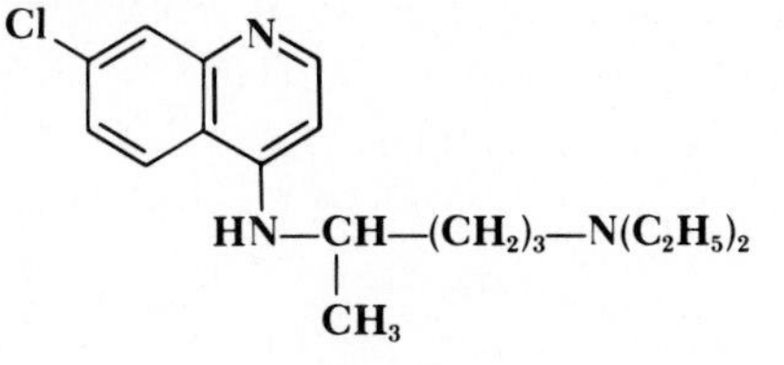

Cl N
HN—CH—$(CH_2)_3$—$N(C_2H_5)_2$
CH_3

Chloroquine

Chloroquine is highly effective against susceptible strains of *Plasmodium* (Table 65-1). It can produce a radical cure in susceptible falciparum malaria but is suppressive only for *P. vivax* and *P. ovale*, since it will not eliminate the exoerythrocytic forms. Thus the drug can terminate clinical attacks very effectively, but relapses occur in vivax malaria.

METABOLISM

Chloroquine is rapidly and almost completely absorbed from the gastrointestinal tract. It is widely distributed throughout the body and is tightly bound to some tissues,

TABLE 65-1 Drugs used to treat extraintestinal protozoal infections

	Drug	Dosage (oral unless specified otherwise)
Malaria (except for chloroquine-resistant *Plasmodium falciparum*)		
Chemoprophylaxis	Chloroquine phosphate	500 mg once weekly (from 2 weeks before until 4 weeks after exposure)
If infection very likely	Primaquine phosphate	15 mg daily for 14 days during last 2 weeks of chloroquine
Treatment	Chloroquine phosphate	1 g, then 500 mg in 6 hours and daily for 2 more days
To prevent relapses	Primaquine phosphate	15 mg daily for 14 days; 45 mg weekly for 8 weeks if G-6-PD deficient
Chloroquine-resistant *P. falciparum (CRPF)*		
Chemoprophylaxis	Mefloquine	250 mg once weekly
Treatment	Quinine sulfate +	650 mg three times daily for 3 days
	pyrimethamine +	25 mg twice daily for 3 days
	sulfadiazine	500 mg four times daily for 5 days
	or	
	Quinine sulfate +	as above
	tetracycline	250 mg four times daily for 7 days
	or	
	Quinine sulfate +	as above
	clindamycin	900 mg three times daily for 3 days
***Pneumocystis carinii* pneumonia (PCP)**		
Treatment	Trimethoprim-sulfamethoxazole	5 mg/kg trimethoprim four times daily, orally or intravenously, for 14 days
	or	
	Pentamidine isethionate	4 mg/kg daily for 14 days intramuscularly or intravenously
Prevention	Trimethoprim-sulfamethoxazole	One double-strength tablet twice daily
	or	
	Pentamidine isethionate	300 mg once monthly as aerosol
Toxoplasmosis	Pyrimethamine +	25 mg daily for 4 weeks
	short-acting sulfonamide	2-6 g daily for 4 weeks
Trypanosomiasis		
Trypanosoma gambiense or *T. rhodesiense*		
Hemolymphatic stage	Suramin*	100-200 mg, then 1 g repeated intravenously on days 1, 3, 7, 14, and 21
	or	
	Pentamidine isethionate	4 mg/kg daily for 10 days
CNS involvement	Melarsoprol*	2 mg/kg daily intravenously for 3 days; after 1 week, 3.6 mg/kg daily for 3 days; repeat in 10-21 days
T. cruzi	Nifurtimox*	8-10 mg/kg daily divided into 4 doses, for 120 days
Leishmanial infections	Sodium stibogluconate*	20 mg/kg daily intravenously or intramuscularly for 20 days (may be repeated)

Primary source: Drugs for parasitic infections, Med Lett Drugs Ther 32:23, 1990.
*Obtain from the Centers for Disease Control, Atlanta, GA 30333 (telephone 404-639-3670), 8:00 AM TO 4:30 PM EST, Monday through Friday).

such as the liver and heart. As a consequence, chloroquine persists in the body for a long time, up to a year after taking a single dose. One half is metabolized by the liver, and the rest is excreted unchanged in urine. Although its elimination half-life is prolonged in severe renal failure, dosage adjustment is rarely necessary.

Chloroquine phosphate (Aralen) is available as 250 and 500 mg tablets (150 and 300 mg base). For treatment a total dose of 2.5 g is given over about 2 days (Table 65-1). Intramuscular chloroquine (40 mg/ml) as the hydrochloride can be given in a dose of 250 mg if necessary for cerebral malaria or severe illness. For chronic suppression of sensitive strains in an endemic area, one 500 mg tablet is taken weekly from 2 weeks before exposure until 4 weeks after leaving.

TOXICITY

The toxicity of antimalarial doses of chloroquine is quite low. Rarely, nausea, dizziness, blurring of vision, headache, diarrhea, and epigastric distress occur. Pruritus of the soles is commonly noted in Africans receiving the drug. It should be given cautiously to persons with liver disease but is safe for pregnant women and nonnursing mothers.

RESISTANCE TO CHLOROQUINE

CRPF is being detected with increasing frequency in South America, Southeast Asia, and Africa. Although chloroquine or quinine therapy may reduce parasitemia, patients relapse within 2 weeks. Drug combinations that include quinine with pyrimethamine and sulfadiazine or with tetracycline or clindamycin have reasonable success (Table 65-1).

Hydroxychloroquine

Hydroxychloroquine sulfate (Plaquenil), another 4-aminoquinoline very similar to chloroquine but without significant advantages over the parent drug, is available in tablets, 200 mg.

Amodiaquin

Amodiaquin is similar to chloroquine in its action, with more potent in vitro activity.[9] It is given by mouth in doses of 0.6 g daily as a suppressive antimalarial or 1.8 g in divided doses the first day, followed by 0.6 g/day for 2 or 3 days for clinical control. Its use has been associated with several cases of agranulocytosis and hepatitis with death in some, and so the Centers for Disease Control has recommended against its use for prophylaxis in malaria.[1]

Amodiaquin

Mefloquine

Mefloquine, a 4-quinolone-methanol compound, is now the chemotherapeutic agent of choice for travel to areas with CRPF.[2] It is a schizonticide in the early asexual blood stages. Oral administration results in peak blood concentration 12 hours later. Mefloquine is an extensively tissue- and protein-bound drug, and its terminal metabolism is very slow (elimination half-life of 6.5 to 30 days).[9] Because the drug may affect fine motor function, it is recommended that airplane pilots not take it. Mild nausea, diarrhea, dizziness, and abdominal pain have also been reported. Mefloquine should be avoided in pregnancy because its safety has not been established. Mefloquine hydrochloride (Lariam) is provided as 250 mg tablets.

Primaquine

Certain 8-aminoquinolines act on the exoerythrocytic stage of malarial parasites. Primaquine is the most effective representative of this group of drugs.

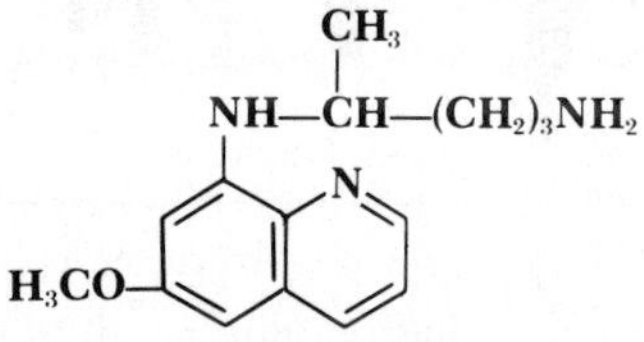

CH_3
$NH—CH—(CH_2)_3NH_2$
N
H_3CO

Primaquine

Primaquine leads to radical cure in *Plasmodium vivax* infections because it acts on hypnozoites of *P. vivax* and *ovale* in the liver.[9] It has limited activity against the asexual forms. Primaquine is given for 14 days in combination with a suppressive agent such as chloroquine to achieve a radical cure of vivax malaria. It is also effective, when combined with clindamycin, against *Pneumocystis carinii*.

Primaquine is rapidly absorbed from the gastrointestinal tract. It is also rapidly metabolized and excreted. Primaquine phosphate is available in tablets, 15 mg base.

Although primaquine is generally well tolerated by Caucasians at the recommended therapeutic dosages, some patients may complain of anorexia, nausea, abdominal cramps, and other vague symptoms. Rarely, there may be depression of bone-marrow activity, with leukopenia and anemia. The drug can cause methemoglobinemia that is aggravated by concomitant use of quinacrine.

Hemolytic anemia can follow primaquine therapy in persons with a genetic deficiency of glucose-6-phosphate dehydrogenase (G-6-PD). In persons of Mediterranean origin with the defect, red blood cells of all ages are hemolyzed, whereas in blacks, usually males, only older red cells are hemolyzed so the anemia is less severe. The level of G-6-PD should be measured in patients in these ethnic groups before the drug is given.[9] Weekly doses of 45 mg can be given for 4 to 6 weeks to persons with a moderate G-6-PD deficiency.

Anti-folate drugs

Pyrimethamine (Daraprim) inhibits the dihydrofolate reductase of malarial parasites. The drug is used in combination with other drugs for treatment of CRPF malaria.

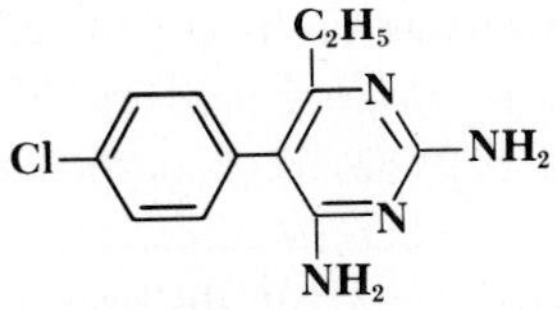

Pyrimethamine

Pyrimethamine appears safe in doses of 25 to 50 mg once or twice a week. Transient megaloblastic anemia has occurred in some persons, perhaps as a result of metabolic antagonism of folic acid or folinic acid. The drug is taken as tablets of 25 mg in combination with sulfonamides for malaria and toxoplasmosis.[4,7] A combination of pyrimethamine with sulfadoxine (Fansidar) has been used to treat presumed exposure to *P. falciparum* for those who have been in an area (Asia, South America) endemic for CRPF. However, because deaths attributable to severe Stevens-Johnson syndrome have been reported, the Centers for Disease Control no longer recommends the drug for prophylaxis.[10]

Trimethoprim (Trimpex, others), a synthetic diaminopyrimidine compound related to pyrimethamine, is also effective treatment for malaria when used in combination with sulfamethoxazole.

Other antimalarial drugs

When combined with quinine, tetracycline, or doxycycline plus clindamycin, is effective in treatment of CRPF.[9] In fact, doxycycline may be effective prophylaxis alone in persons who are intolerant to mefloquine.[10]

TREATMENT OF PNEUMOCYSTIS CARINII *PNEUMONIA*

Trimethoprim-sulfamethoxazole (co-trimoxazole) (see p. 639) has become the treatment of choice for *Pneumocystis carinii* pneumonia (PCP) in patients with AIDS and other immunologic disorders. This combination can be given intravenously at an initial daily dose of 20 mg/kg, divided over four administrations, and continued orally for 14 days. The frequency of allergic skin reactions is increased (to as often as 75%) in patients with AIDS, but some physicians now recommend continued treatment despite the rash.

Intravenous **pentamidine isethionate** (Pentam 300), 4 mg/kg as a single daily dose for 14 days, also achieves success rates of 60% to 80%.[3] This regimen is indicated for those who fail to respond to co-trimoxazole within 7 days or who experience severe adverse reactions to that combination. Pentamidine induces frequent serious side effects, including renal failure, hypoglycemia, hypotension, and hypothermia. Permanent islet cell destruction may cause diabetes mellitus.[3] Dapsone (see p. 679) or a combination of clindamycin with primaquine may be effective alternatives, especially for sulfonamide-allergic or pentamidine-intolerant patients with mild PCP.

Because 85% of all patients with AIDS will develop PCP, preventive therapy with co-trimoxazole (as one double-strength or two single-strength tablets, twice daily) is recommended for all AIDS patients after recovery from PCP and for those with $CD4^+$-lymphocyte counts less than 200/mm^3 (or less than 20%); it is also recommended for all heart transplant patients (dosed twice weekly). For those with serious allergic reactions to co-trimoxazole, aerosolized pentamidine (NebuPent, 300 mg) can be inhaled once monthly via a respiratory delivery device. Although this preventive therapy is effective, relapses of PCP do occur, particularly in the upper lobe.[3]

ANTITRYPANOSOMAL DRUGS

Trypanosomal infections are important diseases in the Southern Hemisphere. Subspecies are responsible for sleeping sickness in tsetse-infested areas of equatorial Africa. Of the three drugs available for routine treatment of human trypanosomiasis, none is well tolerated. **Suramin** (Germanin, others), a nonmetallic dye, is used to treat early cases of both Gambian and Rhodesian forms of the disease.[6] It is given orally first, as a test dose of 0.2 g, to be followed by five 1 g doses intravenously at 3- to 7-day intervals. Renal toxicity is the most severe side effect. **Pentamidine** is also useful in early cases of sleeping sickness.

$$H_2N-\overset{\overset{NH}{\|}}{C}-C_6H_4-OCH_2(CH_2)_3CH_2O-C_6H_4-\overset{\overset{NH}{\|}}{C}-NH_2$$

Pentamidine

Melarsoprol (Arsobal) is an organic compound of arsenic that is effective in treatment of late African trypanosomiasis involvement in the central nervous system.

The drug of choice for Chagas disease is **Nifurtimox** (Lampit).[2] It is effective in 70% to 90% of acute cases but is associated with significant side effects in a majority. The most serious involve the central nervous system, with insomnia, disorientation, and seizures, but the symptoms abate when the drug is discontinued.

LEISHMANIA

Pentavalent antimonials are the drugs of choice for leishmanial infections. Their mechanism of action is unknown. **Sodium stibogluconate** (Pentostam) is given intravenously or intramuscularly (maximum of 800 mg/day).[2] Muscle pain and gastrointestinal side effects occasionally develop. Resistant cases are treated with amphotericin B (see Chapter 62).

REFERENCES

1. Agranulocytosis associated with the use of amodiaquine for malaria prophylaxis, *MMWR* 35:165, 1986.
2. Drugs for parasitic infections, *Med Lett Drugs Ther* 32:23, 1990.
3. Glatt AE, Chirgwin K: *Pneumocystis carinii* pneumonia in human immunodeficiency virus-infected patients, *Arch Intern Med* 150:271, 1990.
4. Krick JA, Remington JS: Toxoplasmosis in the adult: an overview, *N Engl J Med* 298:550, 1978.
5. Krogstad DJ, Herwaldt BL: Chemoprophylaxis and treatment of malaria, *N Engl J Med* 319:1538, 1988.
6. Mandell WF, Neu HC: Parasitic infections: therapeutic considerations, *Med Clin North Am* 72:669, 1988.
7. McCabe RE, Oster S: Current recommendations and future prospects: treatment of toxoplasmosis, *Drugs* 38:973, 1989.
8. Miller KD, Greenberg AE, Campbell CC: Treatment of severe malaria in the United States with a continuous infusion of quinidine gluconate and exchange transfusion, *N Engl J Med* 321:65, 1989.
9. Panisko DM, Keystone JS: Treatment of malaria—1990, *Drugs* 39:160, 1990.
10. Recommendations for the prevention of malaria among travelers, *MMWR* 39(RR-3):1, 1990.

Chapter 66

Anthelmintic drugs

GENERAL CONCEPT

There have been important advances recently in antiparasitic chemotherapy, especially for human intestinal helmintic infections. Newer anthelmintics are safer and are frequently effective in a single course of therapy (Table 66-1). An effective drug for treatment of schistosomiasis, praziquantel, is now available, and the price has been reduced so that mass application at low cost per unit course of treatment is possible.[1] Cost is very important in determining the distribution of anthelmintics[10]; parasites are commonly found in third-world countries that may not be able to purchase expensive medications.

INDIVIDUAL ANTHELMINTICS

Thiabendazole

The first imidazole anthelmintic in general use was thiabendazole. The drug is absorbed rapidly after oral administration, inactivated in the liver by hydroxylation, and excreted as a conjugate in urine and feces.

Thiabendazole has a wide spectrum of anthelmintic activity, but side effects (nausea, chills, vertigo, hypotension, hallucinosis, leukopenia, crystalluria) have limited its use.[4] It remains a first-line drug for strongyloidiasis and an alternative for trichostrongylus, though after a single use many refuse to take the drug again.[5] The drug is ovicidal and larvicidal.

Thiabendazole (Mintezol) is dispensed as chewable tablets (500 mg) and an oral suspension (500 mg/5 ml). The drug is taken twice daily after meals to a maximum of 3 g.

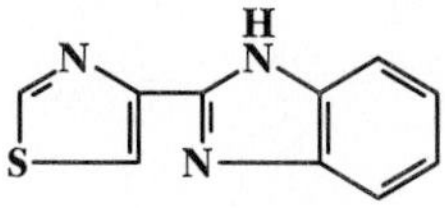

Thiabendazole

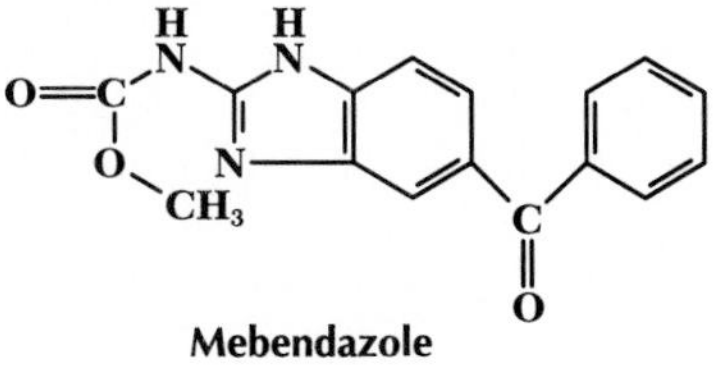

Mebendazole

$CH_3CH_2CH_2S$ ... $NHCOOCH_3$

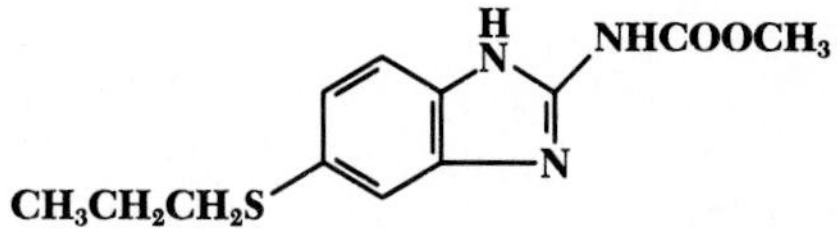

Albendazole

Mebendazole

Mebendazole (Vermox) is one of several thiabendazole congeners that retain a broad spectrum of activity but with fewer untoward reactions. Mebendazole is a first-line drug for *Trichuris*, *Enterobius*, *Ascaris*, and hookworm infections.[2] In most of these the cure rate exceeds 90%. Mebendazole, like thiabendazole, depletes helminth energy stores and disrupts the capacity for cytoskeletal transport by binding to tubulin.[9] The colonic concentration of mebendazole is high because it is poorly absorbed,

TABLE 66-1 Anthelmintic drug applications		
Organism	**Drugs of choice**	**Usual oral adult dose**
Nematodes – intestinal		
Strongyloides stercoralis (threadworm)	Thiabendazole	25 mg/kg twice daily for 2 days
Trichuris trichiura (whipworm)	Mebendazole	100 mg twice daily for 3 days
Enterobius vermicularis (pinworm)	Mebendazole	100 mg single dose, repeat in 2 weeks
	or	
	Pyrantel pamoate	11 mg/kg single dose, repeat in 2 weeks
Ascaris lumbricoides (roundworm)	Mebendazole	100 mg twice daily for 3 days
	or	
	Pyrantel pamoate	11 mg/kg single dose
Necator americanus and *Ancylostoma duodenale* (hookworms)	Mebendazole	100 mg twice daily for 3 days
	or	
	Pyrantel pamoate*	11 mg/kg daily for 3 days
Trichostrongylus species	Pyrantel pamoate*	11 mg/kg single dose
	or	
	Thiabendazole*	25 mg/kg twice in 1 day
Nematodes – extraintestinal		
Wuchereria bancrofti, W. malayi, Loa loa (filariasis)	Diethylcarbamazine	50 mg first day, 150 mg second day, 300 mg third day, then 6 mg/kg/day for 18 days
Onchocerca volvulus	Ivermectin*†	150 μg/kg once, repeated every 6-12 months
Dracunculus medinensis (guinea worm)	Metronidazole*	250 mg three times daily for 10 days
Trichinella spiralis (trichinosis)	Mebendazole* (plus corticosteroids)	200-400 mg three times daily for 3 days, then 400-500 mg three times daily for 10 days
Larva migrans (creeping eruption)	Thiabendazole	25 mg/kg twice daily for 5 days
	or	
	Diethylcarbamazine*	2 mg/kg three times daily for 7-10 days
Trematodes		
Schistosoma haematobium	Praziquantel	20 mg/kg twice in 1 day
S. japonicum, S. mekongi	Praziquantel	20 mg/kg three times in 1 day
S. mansoni	Praziquantel	20 mg/kg twice in 1 day
	or	
	Oxamniquine	15 mg/kg single dose
Clonorchis sinesis (fluke)	Praziquantel	25 mg/kg three times daily for 2 days
Fasciola hepatica (fluke)	Bithionol†	30-50 mg/kg on alternate days for 10 to 15 doses
Cestodes		
Diphyllobothrium latum, Taenia saginata, T. solium, Dipylidium caninum (tapeworms)	Niclosamide	2 g single dose
	or	
	Praziquantel*	10-20 mg/kg single dose
Hymenolepsis nana (dwarf tapeworm)	Praziquantel*	25 mg/kg single dose
	or	
	Niclosamide	2 g first day, then 1 g daily for 6 days
Cysticercus cellulosae	Praziquantel*	50 mg/kg daily for 15 days
	or	
	Albendazole*	5 mg/kg three times daily for 30 days

Primary data from Drugs for parasitic infections, Med Lett Drugs Ther 32:23, 1990.
*Investigational for this indication.
†Available from the Centers for Disease Control, Atlanta, GA 30333 (telephone 404-639-3670, 8:00 AM TO 4:30 PM EST, Monday through Friday).

perhaps accounting for fewer side effects. Since the drug is teratogenic in animals, it should not be given to women who are or may become pregnant.

For most infections, a 100 mg tablet is chewed twice daily for several days. Pinworms can be eradicated with a single dose, but reinfection may necessitate periodic readministration. Filariasis (for which mebendazole is a second-line drug) requires daily therapy for a month.

Albendazole

Albendazole is a new benzimidazole that has been used to treat neurocysticercosis[7] and echinococcosis. It is moderately well absorbed and reaches peak plasma concentration in 2 hours.[4] Its usually mild toxicity includes diarrhea and, rarely, hepatitis; the drug is potentially teratogenic.

Pyrantel

Pyrantel depolarizes and paralyzes worm muscle by persistent nicotinic activation. Intestinal nematodes can then no longer maintain the tone necessary to attach to host tissues and are expelled by host peristalsis.[6]

Because pyrantel is poorly absorbed after oral administration, intestinal parasites are exposed to high concentrations. The small fraction of drug that is absorbed causes minimal side effects (dizziness, headache, rash, fever). Pyrantel pamoate (Antiminth) is marketed as an oral suspension or liquid, 50 mg/ml. It can be given as a single dose with over 90% effectiveness for *Ascaris, Enterobius*, or hookworm infection.

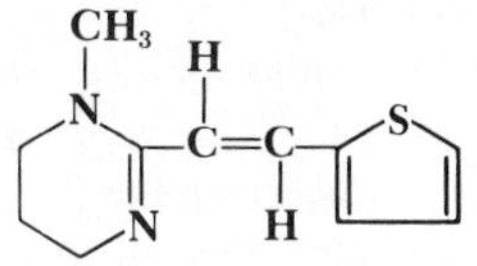

CH_3 H S N C=C N H

Pyrantel

$H_3C—N$ $CH_2—CH_2$ $CH_2—CH_2$ $N—C—N$ O C_2H_5 C_2H_5

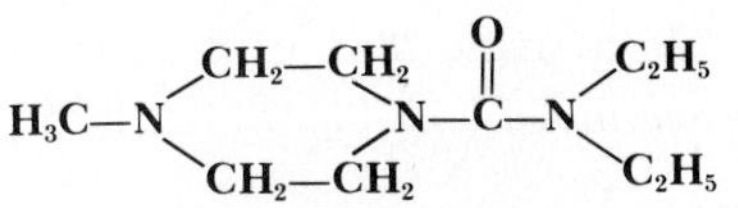

Diethylcarbamazine

Diethylcarbamazine

The drug of choice for some causative agents of filariasis is diethylcarbamazine, a piperazine derivative. Its mode of action is unclear, but it kills microfilariae and may kill adult worms. When the drug was used to kill microfilariae of *Onchocerca volvulus*, violent allergic manifestations occurred. Antihistamines may be helpful. Reversible allergic reactions to the drug itself are less frequent if dosage is increased slowly to the desired level (Table 66-1). Diethylcarbamazine citrate (Hetrazan) is dispensed as 50 mg tablets.

Ivermectin

Ivermectin is a macrocyclic lactone with broad antinematodal activity, particularly for filarioidea and *Onchocerca*. It has a very long half-life and is detectable in tissues for 4 weeks. It is accepted as the best agent against onchocerciasis; a single dose of 150 μg/kg is given every 6 to 12 months with good success.[11] The drug can cause fever, headache, and joint pain. Generally, rash and lymph node tenderness and enlargement occur within 3 days of treatment. Surgical incision of *Onchocerca* nodules before therapy is recommended by some.

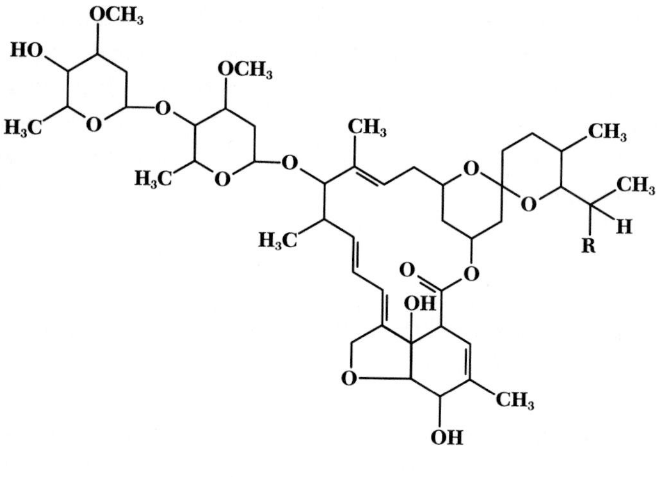

Ivermectin

Niclosamide

Tapeworm infections are treated with niclosamide. The drug inhibits oxidative phosphorylation in the mitochondria of cestodes and kills proximal worm segments and the scolex; these appear in the feces severely damaged.[6] The drug should not be used if there is intestinal obstruction. It is not absorbed by the host, and the incidence of side effects (nausea, abdominal pain, pruritus) is very low.

Niclosamide (Niclocide) is available as 500 mg chewable tablets. Adults and children over 8 take a single dose of 2 g for treatment of *T. saginata, T. solium,* and *Diphyllobothrium latum* (fish tapeworm) infestations.

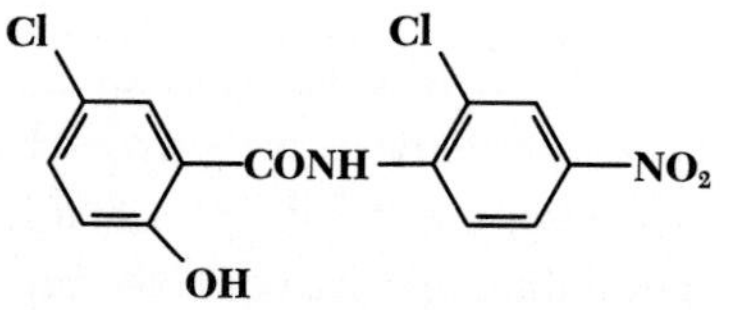

Niclosamide

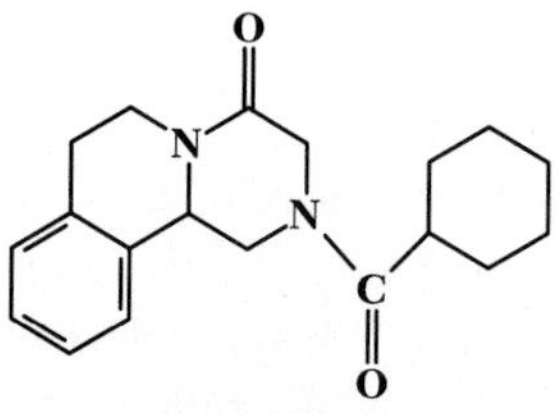

Praziquantel

Praziquantel

Praziquantel has broad anthelmintic activity. It has a better cure rate than niclosamide for *H. nana.* Moreover, praziquantel is particularly effective against the schistosomes that infect humans.[1] It is essential for management of schistosomiasis, one of the more difficult infections to treat, but cost severely limits its use in developing countries.[3]

Praziquantel is readily absorbed from the gut. It is metabolized rapidly by the host but not by the worms, which apparently concentrate the drug. It appears to alter integument permeability to monovalent and divalent cations. In the tapeworm, influx of Ca^{++} is believed responsible for muscular spasticity that dislocates the worm from the intestinal wall. The drug is rapidly absorbed and achieves peak plasma concentration in 1 to 3 hours.[3] Side effects thus far have been mild (sedation, headache, nausea, rash), transient (a few minutes to an hour), and infrequent (less than 5% of patients).[1] Praziquantel (Biltricide), in 600 mg tablets, is given two to three times in 1 day with over 90% effectiveness for all species of schistosomes.[3] It has also been used successfully in treatment of central nervous system cysticercosis, 50 mg/kg divided over three doses daily for 15 days.[4]

OTHER USEFUL ANTHELMINTICS

Piperazine citrate is an alternative therapy for *Ascaris* and *Enterobius* infections. Piperazine is readily absorbed from the intestine and can cause gastrointestinal and allergic reactions.

Metronidazole (Flagyl), used primarily for its amebicidal and trichomonacidal activities (see Chapter 64), also has utility for *Dracunculus* infection.

Oxamniquine (Vansil) is an alternative for infections with *Schistosoma mansoni*, particularly South American strains. In Brazil more than 7 million people have been treated successfully with it.[8] Capsules contain 250 mg of the drug.

Bithionol (Bitin, Lorothidol) has been used for lung and liver flukes but seems to be less effective for liver flukes than is praziquantel. Side effects include photosensitivity and urticaria.

REFERENCES

1. Archer S: The chemotherapy of schistosomiasis, *Annu Rev Pharmacol Toxicol* 25:485, 1985.
2. Drugs for parasitic infections, *Med Lett Drugs Ther* 32:23, 1990.
3. King CH, Mahmoud AAF: Drugs five years later: praziquantel, *Ann Intern Med* 110:290, 1989.
4. Mandell WF, Neu HC: Parasitic infections: therapeutic considerations, *Med Clin North Am* 72:669, 1988.
5. Pelletier LL Jr: Chronic strongyloidiasis in World War II Far East ex-prisoners of war, *Am J Trop Med Hyg* 33:55, 1984.
6. Sheth UK: Mechanisms of anthelmintic action, *Prog Drug Res* 19:147, 1975.
7. Sotelo J, Penagos P, Escobedo F, Del Brutto OH: Short course of albendazole therapy for neurocysticercosis, *Arch Neurol* 45:1130, 1988.
8. Stürchler D: Chemotherapy of human intestinal helminthiases: a review, with particular reference to community treatment, *Adv Pharmacol Chemother* 19:129, 1982.
9. Van den Bossche H, Rochette F, and Hörig C: Mebendazole and related anthelmintics, *Adv Pharmacol Chemother* 19:67, 1982.
10. Wang CC: Current problems in antiparasite chemotherapy, *Trends Biochem Sci* 7:354, 1982.
11. White AT, Newland HS, Taylor HR, et al: Controlled trial and dose-finding study of ivermectin for treatment of onchocerciasis, *J Infect Dis* 156:463, 1987.

Chapter 67

Drugs used in chemotherapy of neoplastic disease

GENERAL CONCEPT

The search for pharmacologic approaches to neoplastic disease has made impressive gains during the past 30 years. Drugs can cure patients having choriocarcinoma, Hodgkins disease, acute lymphatic and myelogenous leukemia, and testicular cancer.[3] In combination with surgery and radiation, drugs have prolonged life in many other forms of cancer, though the quality of life is often impaired.

The current emphasis in cancer chemotherapy is on use of combinations of drugs. Such combinations take into account the phase of the cell cycle affected by each drug and potential synergistic actions in attempts to increase efficacy and decrease emergence of cell resistance. The cell cycle is divided into several phases: G_o, G_1 (gap 1), S (synthesis), G_2, M (mitosis). The resting phase is designated as G_o. In the G_1 phase genes required for replication are activated as cells prepare to enter the S phase. During the S phase there is a pronounced increase in DNA synthesis. The G_2 phase, a period in which DNA repair progresses, is the transition time between DNA synthesis and mitosis (the M phase). Cancer chemotherapeutic agents may be *cell cycle–specific* or *cell cycle–nonspecific*. Resting cells do not respond to cell cycle–specific agents. However, they may respond to alkylating agents or to other drugs that combine directly with DNA.

The lack of specificity of cancer chemotherapeutic agents for malignant cells compared to relatively rapidly but normally proliferating cells such as bone marrow, skin, and intestinal mucosa results in a very narrow margin of safety for these agents. Advances in understanding of drug action, of mechanisms of drug toxicity, of the nature of resistance to the drugs,[1,2,4] and of tumor biology have continually led to changes in dosing and scheduling of certain drugs. For example, continuous infusion of anthracyclines in attempts to decrease cardiotoxicity, continuous infusion of *Vinca* alkaloids to increase cell kill, and low-, moderate-, or high-dose methotrexate (20 to $>20{,}000$ mg/m^2/dose) are all being used or evaluated in current treatment regimens. Because of this constant flux of information, specific dosage and regimens for different diseases are not listed in this chapter. Information as to drug dose and schedule should be obtained by consultation of protocols written to facilitate treatment of the patient.

DEVELOPMENT OF ANTINEOPLASTIC CHEMOTHERAPY

The antineoplastic activity of nitrogen mustards was discovered during World War II as an outgrowth of earlier observations on the leukopenic effect of mustard gas (bis[2-chloroethyl]sulfide). Subsequently, the less toxic nitrogen mustards (bis[2-chloroethyl]amines) and eventually many other alkylating agents were introduced into chemotherapy of neoplastic diseases.

The development of folic acid antagonists and other antimetabolites as potential antitumor agents originated from observations on the role of folic acid in both white cell production and as an "antianemia" factor. It seemed reasonable that compounds structurally related to folic acid could inhibit white cell production, and this was indeed demonstrated. These observations stimulated interest in other metabolic antagonists as possible chemotherapeutic agents, and eventually several purine, pyrimidine, and amino acid antagonists were discovered. Since proliferating cells are the main target for antineoplastic agents, nucleic acid biosynthesis and DNA have been the chief targets of the chemotherapeutic approach to cancer.

CLASSIFICATION

The drugs currently used in management of malignant diseases fall into several categories (Table 67-1). More detailed discussions of their clinical pharmacology and important biochemical reactions can be found elsewhere.[9,12]

The sites and mechanisms of action of various cancer chemotherapeutic agents are indicated in Fig. 67-1.

ALKYLATING AGENTS

The alkylating agents are highly reactive compounds that transfer alkyl groups to important cell constituents by combining with amino, sulfhydryl, carboxyl, and phosphate groups. They are *cell cycle–nonspecific*; they can combine with cells in any phase of their cycle. It is believed that these drugs alkylate DNA, and more specifically guanine, as a primary mechanism of cell kill. This basic action may explain their preferential toxicity for rapidly multiplying cells.

Mechlorethamine (nitrogen mustard) must be injected intravenously because it is highly reactive. More recently, attempts have been made to inject the drug intra-arterially, close to the tumor. Because it disappears very rapidly from the blood, the activity of mechlorethamine lasts only a few minutes.

Mechlorethamine can induce venous thrombosis, severe vomiting, and delayed depression of the bone marrow. In toxic doses it may cause involution of lymphatic tissues and the thymus, ulcerations of gastrointestinal mucosa, convulsions, and death.

The main indication for mechlorethamine is in treatment of Hodgkins disease and lymphomas, but it may also be useful in other malignancies. Other alkylating agents have an advantage over mechlorethamine in that they can be administered orally.

$CH_3N(CH_2CH_2Cl)_2$

Nitrogen mustard

$H_2C(CH_2{-}NH)(CH_2{-}O)\,O{=}P{-}N(CH_2CH_2Cl)_2$

Cyclophosphamide

$CH_3{-}SO_2{-}O{-}(CH_2)_4{-}O{-}SO_2{-}CH_3$

Busulfan

$(ClCH_2{-}CH_2)_2N{-}C_6H_4{-}CH_2{-}CH(NH_2){-}COOH$

Melphalan

TABLE 67-1 Classification of antineoplastic agents

Compound	Abbreviations	Routes of delivery*	Oral dosage forms† (mg)
Alkylating agents			
Mechlorethamine hydrochloride (Mustargen)		IV	
Chlorambucil (Leukeran)		PO	T: 2
Cyclophosphamide (Cytoxan, Neosar)		IV, PO	T: 25,50
Ifosfamide (Ifex)		IV	
Melphalan (Alkeran)		IV, PO	T: 2
Thiotepa	TSPA, TESPA	IV, IT, IM, SC	
Busulfan (Myleran)		PO	T: 2
Carmustine (BiCNU)	BCNU	IV	
Lomustine (CeeNu)	CCNU	PO	C: 10-100
Antimetabolites			
Methotrexate (Folex, Rheumatrex)	MTX	IV, IM, PO, SC, IT	T: 2.5
Mercaptopurine (Purinethol)	6-MP	PO, IV	T: 50
Thioguanine	TG	PO, IV	T: 40
Fluorouracil (Adrucil)	5-FU	IV	
Cytarabine (Cytosar-U)	ARA-C	IV, SC, IT	
Hormones			
Glucocorticoids (prednisone)		PO, IV, IT	
Estrogens (Estinyl, Feminone)		PO	T: 0.25-0.5
Antiestrogen (Nolvadex)		PO	T: 10
Androgens (Halotestin)		PO, IM	T: 2-10
Antibiotics			
Bleomycin sulfate (Blenoxane)	BLM	IV, SC, IM	
Dactinomycin (Cosmegen)	ACT	IV	
Doxorubicin hydrochloride (Adriamycin)	ADR	IV	
Daunorubicin hydrochloride (Cerubidine)	DNR	IV	
Mitoxantrone (Novantrone)	DHAD	IV	
Plicamycin (Mithracin)		IV	
Mitomycin (Mutamycin)	MTC	IV	
Miscellaneous			
Vinblastine sulfate (Velban, others)	VLB	IV	
Vincristine sulfate (Oncovin, Vincasar)	VCR, LCR	IV	
Asparaginase (Elspar)		IV, IM	
Procarbazine hydrochloride (Matulane)	MIH	PO, IV, IM	C: 50
Hydroxyurea (Hydrea)		PO, (IV)	C: 500
Cisplatin (Platinol)	CDDP, DDP	IV	
Dacarbazine (DTIC-Dome)	DTIC, DIC	IV	
Mitotane (Lysodren)	o,p′-DDD	PO	T: 500
Teniposide	VM-26	IV	
Etoposide (VePesid)	VP-16-213	PO, IV	C: 50

**IM*, Intramuscular; *IT*, intrathecal; *IV*, intravenous; *PO*, oral; *SC*, subcutaneous.
†*C*, Capsule; *T*, tablet.

FIG. 67-1 *Mechanism of action of antineoplastic drugs.*

From Goldberg RS, Krakoff I: Hosp Formulary, Oct 1979, p 891. Reprinted from Hospital Formulary, New York, copyright 1980, Harcourt Brace Jovanovich, Inc.

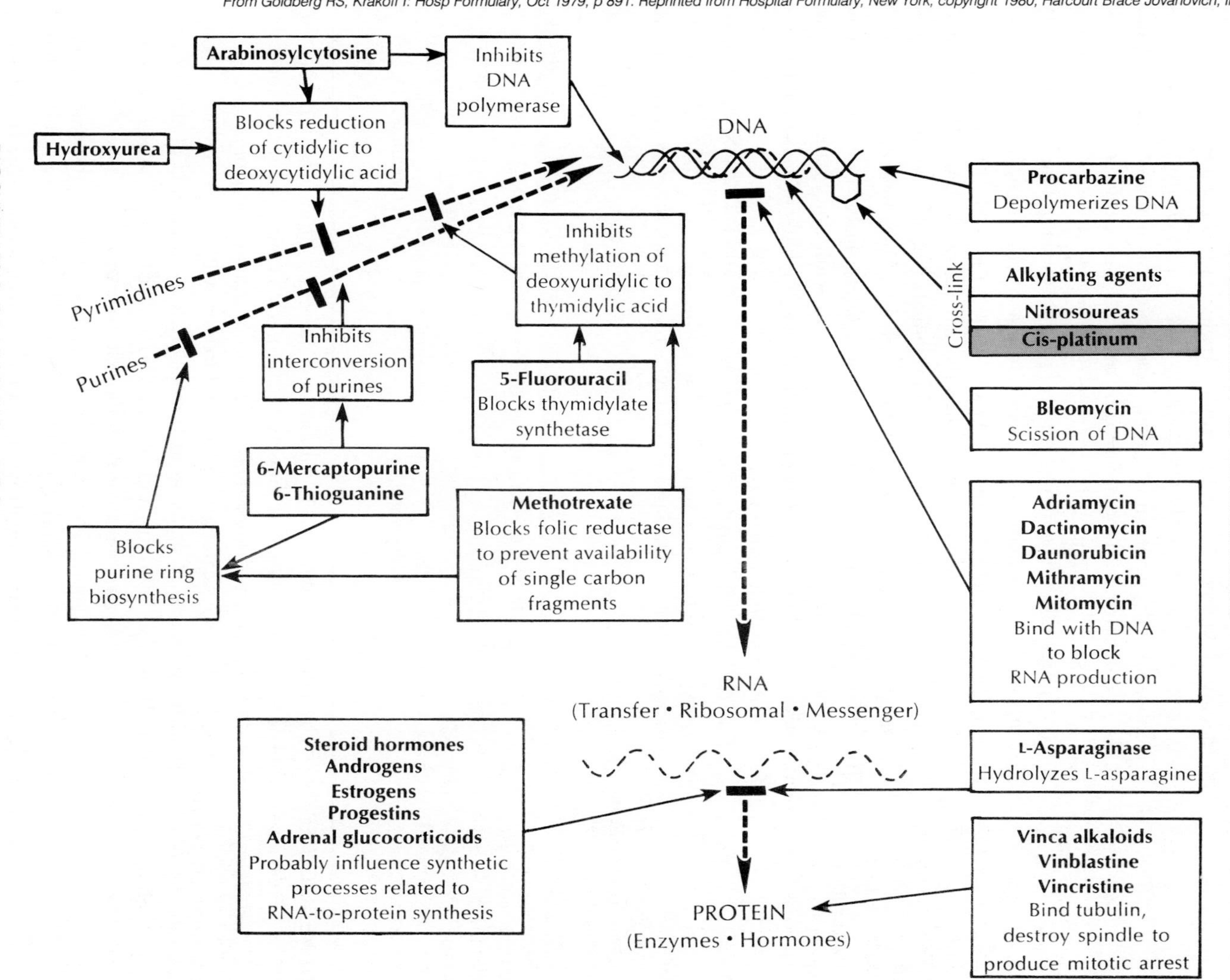

Chlorambucil is used prinicpally in chronic lymphocytic leukemia, Hodgkins disease, multiple myeloma, and macroglobulinemia. **Cyclophosphamide** is a widely used cytotoxic drug, which is metabolically activated in the liver. This drug is generally useful in therapy of lymphomas, acute lymphocytic leukemia in children, multiple myeloma, and many solid tumors. Hemorrhagic cystitis is a characteristic toxic effect of the cyclophosphamide metabolite acrolein. **Ifosfamide**, an analog of cyclophosphamide that is likewise inactive until metabolized by the liver, may prove to have more utility than cyclophosphamide. Attempts to minimize the bladder toxicity of both cyclophosphamide and ifosfamide utilize coadministration of mesna (Mesnex; 2-mercaptoethanesulfonate), a sulfhydryl compound that inactivates acrolein. **Melphalan** (L-sarcolysin) is L-phenylalanine mustard, a derivative of nitrogen mustard. It is used to treat multiple myeloma and some solid tumors, such as those of the ovary, testis, and breast. Occasionally the drug is infused intra-arterially for regional chemotherapy of specific tumors. It is also used in high doses in conjunction with bone marrow reconstitution. **Thiotepa** (triethylenethiophosphoramide) is used parenterally in treatment of carcinoma of the ovary and breast. It can also be given intrathecally for therapy of carcinomatosis. **Busulfan** is used mainly to treat chronic myelocytic leukemia, since it has a somewhat selective action on granulocytes.

Carmustine and **lomustine** are nitrosoureas that alkylate DNA and RNA. Lomustine may have additional actions on DNA synthesis. An important characteristic of the nitrosoureas is their high lipid solubility, which allows them to cross the blood-brain barrier.

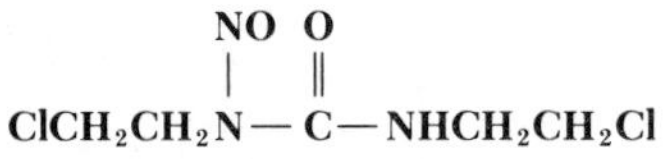

$$ClCH_2CH_2N(NO){-}C(=O){-}NHCH_2CH_2Cl$$

Carmustine

$$ClCH_2CH_2N(NO){-}C(=O){-}N(H)(C_6H_{11})$$

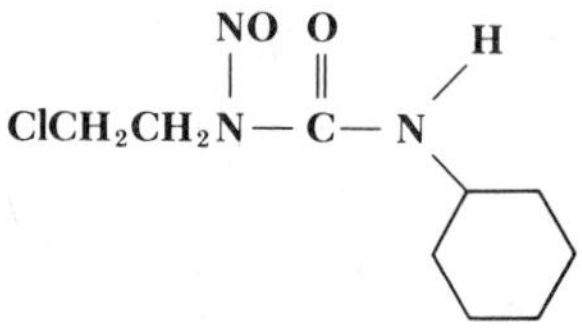

Lomustine

ANTIMETABOLITES

Folic acid antagonists

The folic acid antagonists inhibit nucleic acid synthesis by blocking the enzyme dihydrofolate reductase. **Methotrexate**, formerly known as amethopterin, is effective in treatment of acute leukemias in children and of lymphomas.[6] It is curative in women with choriocarcinoma. In combination with other agents, methotrexate is useful in treatment of many solid tumors, such as carcinoma of the breast, ovary, or colon. It is also used in high doses (>10 g/m^2) with *leucovorin rescue* to treat osteogenic sarcoma. Leucovorin (5-formyltetrahydrofolate) is a reduced folate that bypasses the metabolic block imposed by methotrexate. Methotrexate produces many toxic effects, such as nausea, vomiting, diarrhea, alopecia, aphthous stomatitis, skin rash, and bone-marrow depression. A long-term sequela may be leukoencephalopathy, especially in children treated with cranial radiation or intrathecal methotrexate, or both.

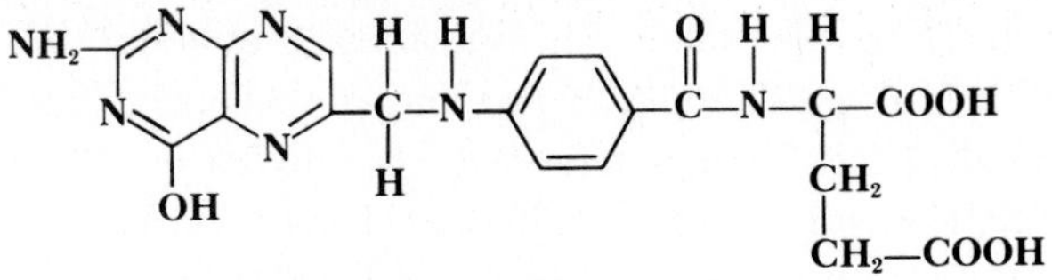

Folic acid (pteroylglutamic acid)

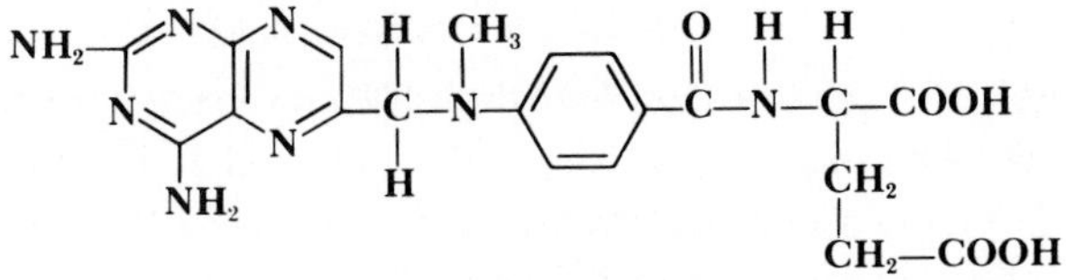

Methotrexate

Purine antagonists

Mercaptopurine, one of the most important purine antagonists, acts by several mechanisms. After metabolism to its ribonucleotide, it competes with enzymes that convert hypoxanthine ribonucleotide (inosinic acid) to adenine and xanthine ribonucleotides. In addition, mercaptopurine is converted to 6-methyl mercaptopurine and its ribonucleotide. This metabolite inhibits the enzyme that synthesizes phosphoribosylamine, which is required for RNA and DNA synthesis. Azathioprine, a precursor of mercaptopurine, is used as an immunosuppressant (see p. 727) and as a remittive agent in rheumatoid arthritis.

Mercaptopurine is effective in therapy of acute lymphocytic[6] and chronic myelocytic leukemias. Its toxic manifestations include bone-marrow depression, gastrointestinal disturbances, and hepatic dysfunction, seen initially as jaundice.

For patients taking allopurinol, a drug that inhibits xanthine oxidase, the dose of mercaptopurine should be decreased.

Thioguanine has essentially the same indications and adverse effects as mercaptopurine. Thioguanine is also metabolized to its ribonucleotide, which enters the pathway of nucleic acid synthesis by substituting for guanine. Thus "fraudulent" polynucleotides that block nucleic acid synthesis are produced.

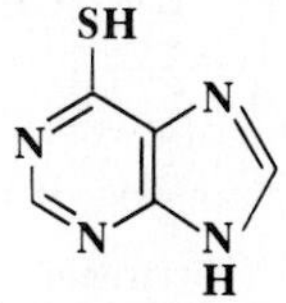

Mercaptopurine

Pyrimidine antagonists

Fluorouracil is a pyrimidine antimetabolite of some usefulness in treatment of carcinoma of the colon, breast, ovary, pancreas, and liver. It is highly toxic and produces hyperpigmentation and photosensitization, as well as the same adverse effects as mercaptopurine. Fluorouracil is available as a solution, 50 mg/ml, for intravenous injection. It is also used topically as solutions or creams (Efudex, Fluoroplex). The solutions contain 1% to 5% fluorouracil, the creams 1% or 5%; the 5% strength is recommended for treatment of superficial basal cell carcinomas.

Fluorouracil is converted to the ribonucleotide 5-fluorouridine monophosphate (5-FUMP), which may be reduced to 5-fluoro-2′-deoxyuridine-5′-phosphate (5-FdUMP). This enzymatic product inhibits thymidylate synthase, which is involved in the production of deoxythymidylate from deoxyuridylic acid. To ensure adequate pools of methylene tetrahydrofolate so that the 5-FdUMP can form a ternary complex with folate and enzyme, protocols now give leucovorin in conjunction with the fluorouracil. Data also indicate that disruption of RNA metabolism by 5-FUMP may be an important mechanism of action of fluorouracil.

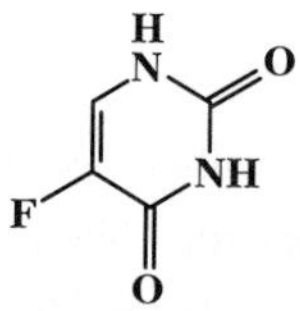

Fluorouracil

Cytarabine (cytosine arabinoside) is a pyrimidine antagonist that differs from deoxycytidine (cytosine deoxyriboside) in that it contains arabinose rather than deoxyribose.[13] It is converted to the nucleotide, which then blocks conversion of cytidine nucleotide to deoxycytidine nucleotide. It also prevents formation of DNA by blocking incorporation of deoxycytidine triphosphate.

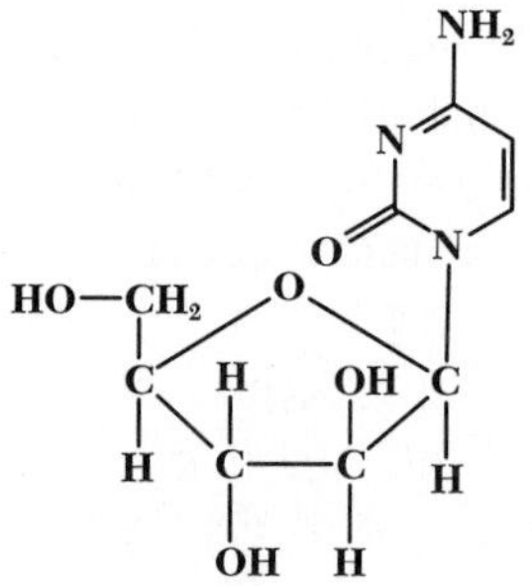

Cytarabine

Cytarabine is not effective after oral administration. It can be given by continuous intravenous infusion or subcutaneously. Cytarabine is used to treat acute lymphocytic and acute myelocytic leukemias. The dose and schedule have ranged from 100 mg/m^2/day for 5 days to 3000 mg/m^2 every 12 hours for 3 days. The drug was once of interest as a possible antiviral agent; however, its margin of safety is too low for this indication.

HORMONAL AGENTS

Steroid hormones, such as estrogens, androgens, and glucocorticoids, are useful in some neoplastic diseases.[7] The estrogens include **diethylstilbestrol diphosphate** (Stilphostrol) and **ethinyl estradiol** (Estinyl, Feminone). Androgens that are widely used, particularly in treatment of carcinoma of the breast, include **testosterone propionate** (Testex) and **fluoxymesterone** (Halotestin, others). The most widely used glucocorticoid is **prednisone**, which is effective in various lymphomas and some other malignancies.

The progestins include **medroxyprogesterone acetate** (Depo-Provera), **hydroxyprogesterone caproate** (Delalutin, others), and **megestrol acetate** (Megace). These progestins are sometimes effective treatment for renal and endometrial carcinomas.

Estrogens, along with castration and other measures, are used to treat prostatic carcinoma. Both androgens and estrogens have been employed in management of advanced mammary carcinoma. The choice depends on the age of the patient. Estrogens are used in women well past the menopause, whereas androgens may be helpful in patients who are still menstruating. The main benefit from such therapy is reduction of pain related to metastatic bone lesions. The rationale for use of estrogens and androgens is the belief that prostatic and mammary carcinomas are to some extent "hormone dependent" with regards to proliferation and differentiation.

Adverse effects of estrogens include gastrointestinal symptoms, hypercalcemia, edema, uterine bleeding, and feminization in males. The adverse effects expected from large doses of androgens in treatment of advanced mammary carcinoma are virilization, edema, and hypercalcemia.

Tamoxifen citrate (Nolvadex), an antiestrogen, competes with estradiol for the estrogen receptor. The drug is not a steroid, but, by competing for the estrogen receptor, it inhibits estrogen-stimulated growth of the tumor. Its main usefulness is in carcinoma of the breast in both postmenopausal and premenopausal women.

ANTIBIOTICS

Bleomycin binds to DNA and has been useful in treatment of squamous cell carcinomas of the head and neck, testicular tumors, and malignant lymphomas.[3] Although bleomycin does not depress the bone marrow, it can cause an unusual toxic manifestation—pulmonary fibrosis, which can be very severe in a small percentage of patients.

Dactinomycin (actinomycin D) combines with DNA and blocks RNA production. It is effective treatment for choriocarcinoma, Wilms' tumor, and testicular carcinoma.[5] The drug causes bone-marrow depression and gastrointestinal toxicity. It may also have a "radiation recall" effect (that is, an increase in toxicity in irradiated tissue).

Doxorubicin (hydroxydaunorubicin) is an anthracycline antibiotic that combines with DNA and is cell cycle–specific; it inhibits the S phase preferentially. Doxorubicin is used to treat lymphomas, leukemia, sarcomas, and neuroblastoma. Mucositis and bone-marrow depression are common acute toxic effects, and a dose-related cardiomyopathy, often fatal, is a late effect. The incidence of the latter toxicity may be increased with concomitant use of chest irradiation or drugs such as cyclophosphamide. Tissue necrosis is severe if extravasation occurs.

Other commonly used anthracyclines include **daunorubicin** and **mitoxantrone**, a recently approved, synthetic agent that does not have the daunosin sugar. Mitoxantrone, like doxorubicin, is cardiotoxic, but it may have use in treatment of breast cancer and leukemia.

Plicamycin (mithramycin) inhibits DNA-dependent RNA synthesis. In addition, the drug affects calcium metabolism, probably by acting on osteoclasts, and it is used to treat the hypercalcemia that occurs with some malignancies. Among numerous toxic effects, thrombocytopenia, bleeding, and gastrointestinal manifestations are most common.

Mitomycin is an alkylating antibiotic that combines with DNA. The drug is used occasionally when other alkylating agents are ineffective. It causes severe bone-marrow depression, gastrointestinal toxicity, and renal toxicity.

MISCELLANEOUS ANTINEOPLASTIC AGENTS

Vincristine and **vinblastine** are alkaloids from the periwinkle plant (*Vinca*). Antineoplastic activity is presumably a consequence of mitotic arrest. Nausea, vomiting, leukopenia, unique neurotoxic effects such as loss of deep tendon reflexes, jaw pain, constipation, seizures, and secretion of inappropriate antidiuretic hormone (SIADH), as well as alopecia, are side effects of *Vinca* alkaloids. Vinblastine is more marrow suppressive than vincristine. *Vinca* alkaloids are very active agents in combination therapy of lymphomas and solid tumors.

L-Asparaginase is an enzyme used to treat leukemia. Apparently some malignant cells require exogenous asparagine, though normal cells synthesize their own. Thus a metabolic difference between normal and neoplastic cells appears to exist for this drug. The discovery of L-asparaginase as an antineoplastic agentresulted from observations on the suppressive effect of guinea pig serum, now known to contain L-asparaginase, on experimental leukemias in vitro. Toxicity includes pancreatitis, hepatitis, bleeding diathesis, and thrombosis. Approximately 10% of patients have a significant allergic reaction to *Escherichia coli* L-asparaginase. A second preparation from *Erwinia* species is available to avoid this problem.

Procarbazine is a synthetic methylhydrazine derivative that finds use in treatment of generalized Hodgkins disease. It causes numerous adverse effects, including gastrointestinal symptoms, bone-marrow depression, a monoamine oxidase inhibitory action, and disulfiram-like reactions.

Hydroxyurea is one of the few agents that has ribonucleotide reductase, a key enzyme in DNA synthesis, as its target. It may be useful in patients with chronic myelocytic leukemia when there is no response to busulfan. Bone-marrow depression is its most serious adverse effect. The drug is available in capsules, and an intravenous form is available for experimental purposes.

The observation that an electric current delivered through platinum electrodes was cytotoxic led to development of **cisplatin** (*cis*-platinum II) as an antineoplastic drug. Platinum functions as an alkylating agent, forming interstrand and intrastrand DNA cross-links. The dose-limiting toxicity is nephrotoxicity, clinically apparent as decreased glomerular filtration rate and salt wasting. Aggressive prehydration seems to decrease this toxicity. Cisplatin also causes a high-frequency hearing loss and is one of the most emetic compounds used in anticancer therapy. It is used to treat sarcomas, testicular carcinomas, and brain tumors.[10] Newer organic platinums, such as carboplatin (Paraplatin), are now available. These compounds may be as beneficial as cisplatin in some patients, but they are still oto- and nephrotoxic. A major advantage of carboplatin is that it is much less emetogenic than cisplatin. For this reason marked hydration is not required, and the drug can be given on an outpatient basis.

Dacarbazine (imidazole carboxamide), though structurally similar to purine precursors, also appears to function as an alkylating agent. It causes severe nausea and vomiting, as well as bone marrow suppression. In addition, a "flulike" syndrome and urticarial rashes have been reported. Dacarbazine is primarily used to treat Hodgkins disease. It also has some activity in therapy of sarcoma, especially in combination with an anthracycline such as doxorubicin.

Mitotane is a synthetic compound related to DDT that has specific toxicity for the adrenal gland. It causes a chemical adrenalectomy.

The epipodophyllotoxins **teniposide** and **etoposide** are derivatives of the mayapple (mandrake). Although related to the podophyllotoxins, these compounds are not tubulin binders (that is, mitotic inhibitors) but interrupt the S and G_2 phases of the cell cycle. They inhibit topoisomerase, a DNA repair enzyme.[11] Etoposide is commercially available. It is especially useful in treatment of lymphomas, leukemia, and testicular

TABLE 67-2 Examples of multiagent protocols*

	Components	Dose (mg/m²)	Days of administration
MOPP	*m*echlorethamine	6	1 and 8
	*O*ncovin (vincristine)	1.4	1 and 8
	*p*rocarbazine	100	1-14
	*p*rednisone	40	1-14
ABVD	*A*driamycin (doxorubicin)	25	1 and 14
	*b*leomycin	10 IU/m²	1 and 14
	*v*inblastine	6	1 and 14
	DTIC	375	1 and 14
CHOP	*c*yclophosphamide	750	1
	*h*ydroxydaunorubicin (= doxorubicin)	50	1
	*O*ncovin (vincristine)	1.4	1
	*p*rednisone	100	1-5
COMLA	*c*yclophosphamide	1500	1
	*O*ncovin (vincristine)	1.4	1, 8, 15
	*m*ethotrexate	120	22, 29, 36, 43, 57, 64, 71
	*l*eucovorin	25†	
	*a*ra-C (cytarabine)	300	Same as methotrexate
VAC (pulse)	*v*incristine	1.5	1 (repeat
	*a*ctinomycin D (dactinomycin)	1.25	1 every
	*c*yclophosphamide	750	1 2 to 3 weeks)

*Modifications and variations of these time-tested regimens, based on empiric or pharmacologic data, may be used.
†Every 6 hours for four doses, 24 hours after methotrexate.

cancer and may be helpful in therapy of brain tumors. Teniposide is primarily used to treat acute leukemia.

CHOICE OF DRUGS IN CANCER CHEMOTHERAPY

In addition to the use of surgery and radiation, various drugs may be beneficial in treating malignancies. In fact, chemotherapy is considered the primary method of treatment in the following conditions: choriocarcinoma, Wilms' tumor, acute and chronic leukemias, disseminated lymphomas, multiple myeloma, and polycythemia vera.[3,8]

As a general rule, the drugs and schedule of choice of these agents for various malignancies are continually in flux as new information is accumulated by cancer chemotherapy study groups performing controlled trials. Several multiagent combinations that have withstood the test of time form the basis for chemotherapy of several types of malignancies. Examples are listed in Table 67-2.

The exponential increase of knowledge about cytokines such as interleukin 2, tumor necrosis factor, and interferons and improved understanding of the cellular biology and biochemistry of empirically proved drugs (for example, anthracyclines, methotrexate, and 6-mercaptopurine) have led to novel therapeutic regimens. Some protocols are designed to be immunoregulatory; others are designed to minimize a drug's toxicity by use of low dosage, constant infusion, and so forth. The clinician should recognize the need to consult with oncologists to obtain the most current information and protocols.

REFERENCES

1. Chan HSL, Thorner PS, Haddad G, Ling V: Immunohistochemical detection of P-glycoprotein: prognostic correlation in soft tissue sarcoma of childhood, *J Clin Oncol* 8:689, 1990.
2. Chatterjee M, Robson CN, Harris AL: Reversal of multidrug resistance by verapamil and modulation by α_1-acid glycoprotein in wild-type and multidrug-resistant Chinese hamster ovary cell lines, *Cancer Res* 50:2818, 1990.
3. DeVita VT Jr, Hellman S, Rosenberg SA, editors: *Cancer: principles and practice of oncology*, ed 2, Philadelphia, 1989, JB Lippincott Co.
4. Endicott JA, Ling V: The biochemistry of P-glycoprotein-mediated multidrug resistance, *Annu Rev Biochem* 58:137, 1989.
5. Frei E III: The clinical use of actinomycin, *Cancer Chemother Rep* 58:49, 1974.
6. Frei E III: Acute leukemia in children: model for the development of scientific methodology for clinical therapeutic research in cancer, *Cancer* 53:2013, 1984.
7. Lippman ME, Eil C: Steroid therapy of cancer. In Chabner BA, editor: *Pharmacologic principles of cancer treatment*, Philadelphia, 1982, WB Saunders, p 132.
8. Pizzo PA, Poplack DG, editors: *Principles and practice of pediatric oncology*, Philadelphia, 1989, JB Lippincott Co.
9. Powis G, Prough RA, editors: *Metabolism and action of anti-cancer drugs*, London, 1987, Taylor & Francis.
10. Rosenberg B: Fundamental studies with cisplatin, *Cancer* 55:2303, 1985.
11. Ross W, Rowe T, Glisson B, et al: Role of topoisomerase II in mediating epipodophyllotoxin-induced DNA cleavage, *Cancer Res* 44:5857, 1984.
12. Schilsky RL, Yarbro JW, Kamen BA: Anticancer drugs. In Williams RL, Brater DC, Mordenti J, editors: *Rational therapeutics: a clinical pharmacologic guide for the health professional*, New York, 1990, Marcel Dekker, Inc, p 611.
13. Valeriote F: Cellular aspects of the action of cytosine arabinoside, *Med Pediatr Oncol* 10(suppl 1):5, 1982.

section eleven

Principles of immunopharmacology

Chapter 68

Principles of immunopharmacology

Basic principles of immunology are involved in the diagnosis, therapy, and prevention of many human diseases. The immune system has an extensive repertoire of antibodies that recognize many natural and synthetic molecules. Immunologic competence enables one to fend off repeated infections with pathogenic organisms, and preventive immunizations are commonplace. The role of immunocompetence in prevention of malignancy is currently of great interest in experimental science, as well as in clinical medicine. The ability of an individual to mount an immune response, however, is also the basis of allergic reactions and autoimmune diseases.

Control of disease by immunologic means has two primary objectives: production of desired immunity and elimination of undesired immune reactions. The first objective is achieved by immunization to selected antigens or by administration of specific antibodies or cytokines; the second is generally achieved through drugs that alter immunity and inflammation. This chapter emphasizes some aspects of immunopharmacology, including immunomodulation, autoimmune disease, and selected mediators of the immune response. Immediate hypersensitivity and allergic reactions are discussed in Chapter 22.

ENHANCEMENT OF THE IMMUNE RESPONSE

Selective enhancement of the immune response is a primary goal in prevention of infectious disease. Identification of specific immune cell populations and their interactions has improved understanding of immunologic defense mechanisms that prevent invasion by bacteria, parasites, or neoplasms.

Immunization

Production of a diverse array of antibodies with varying specificities is an important means of host defense. Immunization elicits antibodies against specific pathogens. The modern science of immunology began in 1796 with Edward Jenner's discovery that immunization with vaccinia (cowpox) prevented development of the more lethal smallpox through the synthesis of antibodies. Since that time development of safe and effective vaccines (a term derived from *vaccinia*) for prevention of infectious diseases has been responsible, in part, for the substantial decline in morbidity and mortality associated with smallpox, rabies, diphtheria, pertussis, tetanus, yellow fever, poliomyelitis, measles, mumps, and rubella. As the incidence of these diseases declined, routine immunizations became primarily the concern of pediatricians. Vaccines against pneumonia, influenza, and hepatitis are frequently used to immunize adults.

Some early vaccines made from live or attenuated organisms caused serious reactions, and their efficacy was questionable. Recombinant DNA technology and peptide

TABLE 68-1 Development of new vaccines

Vaccine	Method	Example
Subunit vaccines	Isolation of polypeptide subunits from infectious agent	Hepatitis B virus
Recombinant vaccines	Synthesis of antigen by recombinant DNA	*Escherichia coli* LT toxin Hepatitis B virus
Recombinant infectious vectors	Genome of infectious agent is inserted into infectious vector	Human sarcoma virus *Shigella* Hepatitis B virus Rabies virus
Synthetic peptides	Synthesis of antigenic sequence or conformational determinants	Cholera toxin Poliomyelitis virus Foot and mouth disease virus

Modified from Steward MW, Howard CR: *Immunol Today* 8:51, 1987.

sequencing and synthesis have been combined to produce new and safer vaccines. Some of these are listed in Table 68-1.

Vaccines against parasitic protozoan and helminthic infections are less successful. Since the response to these organisms probably involves activated T cells and mediators such as γ-interferon, stimulation of a humoral immune response may not suffice. Understanding the mechanisms of gene regulation in parasites may aid in development of better vaccines.

Synthetic vaccines

Synthetic vaccines use chemically synthesized antigens (usually peptides) as the immunizing agent. Design of a vaccine requires identification of pathogen-specific epitopes that are recognized by immunocompetent cells. The success of these vaccines depends on the ability of an antibody to a small peptide to recognize and bind to the same peptide sequence within a larger molecule. T-cell epitopes were recently identified in proteins from various viruses, bacteria, and parasites. T-cell clones in vitro can be used as well to establish that synthetic peptides associate with antigens of the major histocompatibility complex (MHC), a requirement for immunogenicity.[23]

Advantages of synthetic vaccines are twofold. First, because they do not rely on live or attenuated viruses, they are quite safe. Second, antigenic peptides can be synthesized on a large scale. If the sequence of only a few amino acid residues of a viral protein is known, this small peptide can be synthesized and used to immunize against the virus. In practical terms, the amino acid sequence of bacterial or viral proteins can be discerned from the nucleotide sequence of the gene, and many different immunogenic peptides can be synthesized.

Synthetic vaccines have been used to protect animals against foot and mouth disease virus, and it is believed that they can also immunize against tumor antigens. Another application is the long-term prevention of pregnancy. A vaccine against human chorionic gonadotropin (HCG) prevented pregnancy in animals,[30] as did vaccination with a synthetic peptide sequence from a glycoprotein from the zona pellucida.[19] Such results imply that one might be successfully vaccinated against any pathogen if an appropriate peptide sequence can be identified. Unfortunately, many pathogens can so quickly alter their antigens that development of a vaccine is thwarted.

Because clones of specifically primed T lymphocytes are believed to cause autoimmune reactions, vaccination against specific T-cell sequences is currently being explored as one type of therapy for these reactions. Studies in animals with experimental autoimmune encephalitis (EAE) suggest that vaccines against specific subsets of CD4+ T cells arrests the autoimmune response.[8]

Studies with adjuvant-induced arthritis in animals are also encouraging. Administration of T-cell vaccines even after arthritis is established has produced remissions.[8]

ANTIBODIES IN DIAGNOSIS

Antibodies are widely used for diagnostic procedures and also for identification, quantitation, and selection of specific subsets of immune cells. For example, labeled antibodies are used for tissue typing and assays of cell-mediated immunity. The combination of labeled antibodies specific for certain cellular subsets and the techniques of flow cytometry now allows immunologic classification of lymphomas and leukemias.[14] The alarming increase in HIV infection and the acquired immunodeficiency syndrome (AIDS) prompted studies of T-lymphocyte populations; fluoresceinated antibodies to T4 and T8 subsets can quantitate ratios of helper and suppressor cells. Finally, antibodies to tumor-specific antigens have potential for both diagnostic and therapeutic applications. Panels of antibodies facilitate cytologic diagnosis of many different malignancies. Combination of antibodies with radioisotopes for localization of tumors is still experimental but promises to be a valuable diagnostic aid.

ANTIBODIES AS THERAPEUTIC AGENTS

Antibodies that block infectious agents, enhance phagocytosis, or lyse tumor cells are defensive but can be used as therapy for certain diseases. The idea for immunologic treatment originated with Paul Ehrlich, who suggested that toxic antibody molecules could be therapeutic agents. Since Ehrlich's time, significant advances have been made in this direction. Antibodies can lyse malignant tumor cells, direct chemotherapeutic agents, and target radionuclides to specific organs or cells. In addition, monoclonal antibodies to the leukocyte common antigen, CD45, amplify human T-cell responses to mitogens and antigens, including those from HIV. This suggests that antibodies can enhance the immune response of patients with HIV.[12] The use of Fab fragments to treat digitalis toxicity is discussed in Chapter 38.

Immunoglobulins

Immunoglobulin preparations from human blood provide a passive immunity to prevent infection in patients with immune deficiencies, burns, chronic lymphocytic leukemia, or multiple myeloma. They may prevent viral infections such as cytomegalovirus or Kawasaki disease as well.[3] Gamimune N, Sandoglobulin, Gammagard, and Venoglobulin-I are immune globulin preparations for intravenous use.

Immunotoxins

Immunotoxins are formed by linking antibodies to polypeptides that inactivate protein synthesis. The cell-binding antibody directs the toxin to tumor target cells and

Schematic structure of immunotoxin. *FIG. 68-1*

Reproduced, with permission, from Frankel AE, Houston LL, Issell BF, Fathman BF: Annu Rev Med 37:125-142, copyright 1986 by Anuual Reviews Inc.

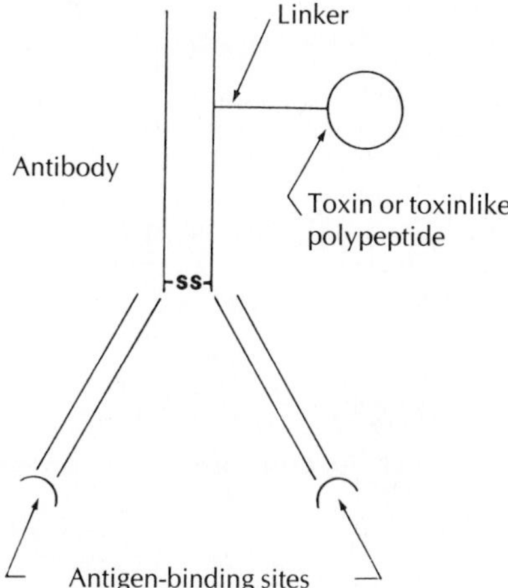

spares normal cells from contact with the chemotherapeutic agent. This approach can be used for tumors of mesenchymal or epithelial origin. Fig. 68-1 shows the general structure of an immunotoxin.

The toxin portion is usually of plant or bacterial origin. Ricin is a plant polypeptide consisting of two chains. The B chain is a lectin that binds to the cell surface; the A chain inhibits protein synthesis. Since immunotherapy requires binding to specific target cells rather than to cell surfaces in general, only the A chain is used to prepare the immunotoxin. Because the A chain is not active outside the cell, it affects only cells that bind it through the antibody portion of the complex. Immunotoxins containing the ricin A chain kill mouse and human tumor cells. Other toxins that can be coupled to antibodies include diphtheria toxin, abrin (a plant-derived toxin), daunorubicin, vinblastine, and methotrexate. Some conjugates are effective at very low concentrations.

Inhibition of protein synthesis requires uptake of the toxin into endosomes and processing within the cell, as indicated in Fig. 68-2.

Although this approach is still experimental, immunotoxins have at least four different clinical applications: T-cell depletion in bone-marrow transplantation, intracavitary treatment of tumors such as ovarian carcinoma or bladder carcinoma, systemic therapy of leukemias and lymphomas, and systemic treatment of refractory metastatic tumors.[10]

Radioimmunotherapy with antibody-linked radionuclides involves a similar approach. Radioimmunotherapy, linking an isotope such as ^{131}I to a tumor-specific antibody, serves to target the tumor and concentrate the radioactivity within it. This approach has been successful in patients with radiosensitive lymphomas, and it may prove particularly valuable for tumors refractive to chemotherapeutic agents.

FIG. 68-2 *According to its antigen specificity, the immunotoxin binds to its antigen and the complex migrates into coated pits on the cell surface. After invagination, a vesicle is formed that becomes acidified and the endosome eventually is processed by the Golgi complex into lysosomes. At some point in this path, immunotoxin escapes and the toxin* (solid circle) *(which may or may not be still linked to the antibody) attacks the ribosome (ricin A chain) or elongation factor 2 (diphtheria toxin).*

Reproduced, with permission, from Frankel AE, Houston LL, Issell BF, Fathman BF: Annu Rev Med 37:125-142, copyright 1986 by Annual Reviews Inc.

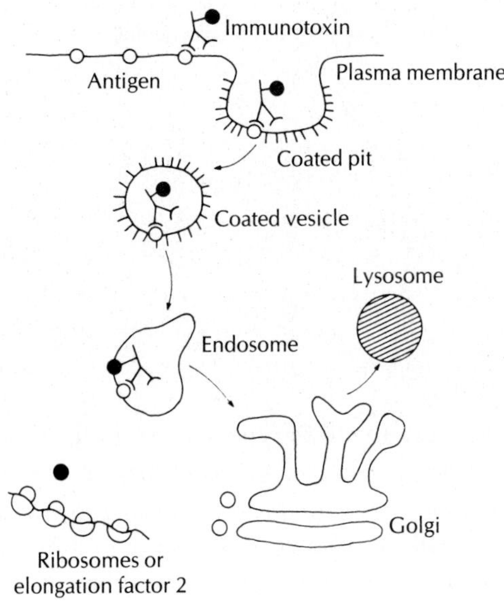

Catalytic antibodies

Catalytic antibodies share functions of both antibodies and enzymes. They are produced by chemical modification of the antigen-binding site and by genetic selection of antibody-producing cells to obtain the desired antigen-binding and catalytic specificities. The resultant antibodies, though not directly lytic for tumor cells, might activate specific cells of the immune system. Antibodies that bind to and hydrolyze specific proteins also have potential as fibrinolytic agents.

Chimeric antibodies

Monoclonal immunotherapy in man is limited because the most easily produced monoclonal antibodies, which are made in mice, are immunogenic in humans. Human hybridoma antibodies have a limited antigen-binding repertoire and are difficult to maintain. Genetically engineered, or chimeric, antibodies that contain features of both mouse and human antibodies circumvent these problems. Combining genes for the constant region of human antibodies with those for mouse variable regions can produce a nonimmunogenic protein that interacts with a wide variety of antigenic determinants. Such antibodies are likely to be used to provide long-term immunity, target specific tumor proteins, remove specific subsets of T cells in transplantation reactions, or modulate components of the coagulation system.[20]

CELLULAR IMMUNOLOGY

T cells recognize foreign antigens in the form of short peptides associated with the major histocompatibility complex (MHC). Competition between peptides for antigen presentation to T lymphocytes can be turned to therapeutic advantage. For example, autoimmune diseases involve activation of self-reactive T cells by autoantigens, which are known to be linked to certain MHC type II markers. These disease-associated MHC molecules have an increased capacity to bind autoantigens and present them to T cells. One possible approach would be to block MHC sites with synthetic peptides. A similar mechanism could apply to allograft rejection.[1]

Peptides bound to MHC types I and II are ligands for T-cell receptors $CD8^+$ and $CD4^+$ with a broad range of specificity. Since each MHC molecule can bind many different peptides, peptides with unrelated sequences could compete for MHC sites. The role of these peptide-recognition sequences in tumor surveillance is currently of great interest. Epitope libraries of bacteriophage vectors are used to screen millions of short peptides for binding to antibodies or immune receptors. Mimetic peptides can be used to block MHC or T-lymphocyte–binding sites in specific disease states.

Tumor immunotherapy

Eradication of tumors by immunologic means has been a long-term goal. However, tumor immunotherapy has fallen far short of its original promise. Initially, the use of antibodies to attack tumors was limited by their impurity and heterogeneity. Later, monoclonal antibodies of defined specificity were used to lyse malignant cells in some types of leukemias and lymphomas.[17] The success of this mechanism depends, however, on recognition of unique tumor antigens and efficient removal of antibody-coated cells by the reticuloendothelial system or by macrophages. Most monoclonal antibodies do not have sufficient specificity, and even highly specific antibodies are unlikely to reduce large tumors.

An alternate approach is the transfer of tumor-specific cultured T cells to provide adoptive immunotherapy. Originally, lymphokine-activated (see *lymphokines*, next section) killer (LAK) cells were used, but these cells can attack both tumor and normal cells. The technique has now been refined to select only tumor-specific cells. These cells, known as tumor-infiltrating lymphocytes (TIL), can be isolated from a tumor, expanded in culture, activated with interleukin-2, and reinfused. The TIL recognize and attack the tumor, without damaging normal cells. The technique works well in animal models, particularly when combined with cytotoxic drugs or cytokines (see next section), and encouraging results were obtained in patients with metastatic melanoma.[25] Some investigators believe that successful adoptive immunotherapy depends upon additional recruitment and activation of host T lymphocytes for tumoricidal activity.[22]

Although still experimental, there is an enormous potential for production of genetically engineered TIL that could be armed with genes for antitumor substances.

CYTOKINES (INTERLEUKINS)

Polypeptide mediators that regulate cellular interactions within the immune system were originally called "interleukins" because it appeared that they were produced by and acted on leukocytes. Because many different cells produce these peptide mediators and they act on both lymphocytic and monocytic cells, the term "cytokine" is more appropriate. *Lymphokine* and *monokine* refer to cytokines from lymphocytes or monocytes respectively.

There are at least 12 interleukins. They are distinct gene products, with molecular weights ranging from approximately 10,000 to 30,000. Amino acid sequences are known for eight human interleukins. These peptides have a wide spectrum of immunologic and nonimmunologic activities. Several share the ability to stimulate cell proliferation, initiate synthesis of new proteins, and enhance production of cellular and humoral mediators of inflammation.[9] Others are important colony-stimulating factors for bone-marrow cells.

Interferons, interleukins, colony-stimulating factors, and macrophage-activating and inhibiting factors are all members of the cytokine family. The cytokine network forms the endocrine arm of the immune system. Individual cytokines are short lived and appear to be regulated by several mechanisms, including binding to autoantibodies and to alpha-2 macroglobulin.

Interleukin-1 (IL-1)

The first two interleukins, IL-1 and IL-2, were originally described as T-cell mitogens. Once the peptides were purified, sequenced, and synthesized, many additional functions were recognized. IL-2 from T lymphocytes was identified as the major thymocyte growth factor, and IL-1, produced by many different types of cells, has many functions, including stimulation of IL-2 production. Effects of IL-1 in vitro are similar to those of tumor-necrosis factor (TNF-α), lymphotoxin, IL-6, and others.[9]

Two forms of IL-1 have been identified by isoelectric focusing; these have only limited homology with respect to peptide sequence, and they appear to have different roles. IL-1β is secreted by activated cells, whereas IL-1α remains associated with the cell.

IL-1 is synthesized primarily by monocytes in response to viruses, bacteria, microbial products, antigens, and inflammatory agents. It is the mediator of fever caused by infection, immunologic reactions, and inflammation, and it evokes an *acute-phase response*. The latter, which entails synthesis of specific acute-phase proteins by the liver and activation of immune cells, involves TNF-α and IL-6 as well.

IL-1 also affects several nonleukocytic target cells. Decreased production of IL-1 or an absence of receptors for IL-1 may play a role in susceptibility to some types of tumors.

Interleukin-2 (IL-2)

IL-2 is a growth factor for helper, suppressor, and cytotoxic T lymphocytes. It is more specific than IL-1 because it acts directly as a growth factor for T lymphocytes, whereas IL-1 activates several components of the systemic acute-phase response.[9] IL-2 is also necessary for activation of all T lymphocytes, regardless of class. IL-2 induces secretion of γ-interferon by T cells, stimulates cytolytic activity of lymphocytes, activates macrophages, and modulates expression of histocompatibility antigens. The human gene for IL-2 has homology with the promoter portion of the human γ-interferon gene and viral enhancer elements. These features might be involved in

FIG. 68-3 *The multiple roles of interleukin-2* (IL-2) *in various immune responses.* Ag, *Antigen;* B-act, *activated B cell;* BCDF, *B-cell differentiation factor;* BCGF, *B-cell growth factor;* γ-IFN, *immune (gamma) interferon;* IL-1, *interleukin-1;* LAK, *lymphocyte-activated killer cell;* MHC, *major histocompatibility complex proteins;* Mϕ, *macrophage;* NK, *natural killer cell;* T-act, *activated T cell;* T-resp, *IL-2 responsive T cell.*

From Robb RJ: Immunol Today 5:203, 1984.

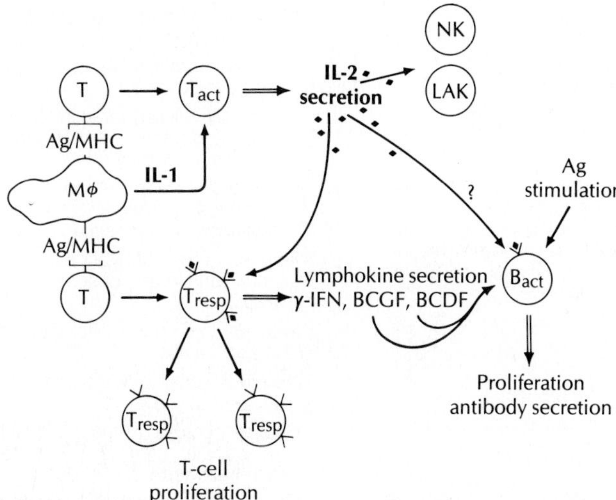

expression of IL-2 during T-cell activation. Some of the relationships between interleukins-1 and -2 and immune cells are shown in Fig. 68-3.

IL-2 enhances the tumoricidal activity of natural killer (NK) cells and also lymphokine-activated killer (LAK) cells, a subpopulation of lymphocytes that can kill tumor cells without prior sensitization of the donor against tumor antigen and without histocompatibility restriction. LAK cells recognize and lyse tumor cells, microorganisms, and cells infected with viruses.[13] The combination of IL-2 and LAK cells appeared promising in trials against certain types of tumors, but the response is variable and often unpredictable.

Some studies indicate that IL-2 can enhance several parameters of immune function in patients with AIDS, but the efficacy of this agent in AIDS or other immunodeficiency syndromes remains to be demonstrated.

IL-2 therapy causes a number of toxic effects. The most common are chills, fever, and diarrhea, but hypotension and various blood dyscrasias have been reported. Patients who received IL-2 immunotherapy developed an acute, but reversible, defect in neutrophil chemotaxis,[15] and in vitro there was also alteration of T-lymphocyte responses.[11]

Other Interleukins

Several other interleukins play a role in growth and differentiation of various cells of the immune system or in activation of inflammatory cells. Table 68-2 lists some of the major activities and sources of lymphokines.

TABLE 68-2 Sources and activities of cytokines

Cytokine	Major sources	Main activities
IL-1	Monocytes/macrophages; NK, endothelial, epithelial cells; fibroblasts; astrocytes	Stimulates T- and B-cell proliferation; induces fever; releases acute-phase proteins, IL-2; stimulates growth of some nonimmune cells
IL-2	Activated T-helper cells	Stimulates T- and B-cell growth; activates killer lymphocytes
IL-3	T-helper, endothelial cells; activated macrophages; fibroblasts	Stimulates proliferation and growth of bone-marrow stem cells
IL-4	T-helper, mast cells	Induces B-cell proliferation, Ia expression, IgG and IgE secretion; enhances antigen-presenting activity
IL-5	T-helper cells	Enhances B-cell proliferation, IgA, IgM, and IgG secretion, IL-2 receptor expression; induces eosinophil differentiation
IL-6	T cells, various subsets	Induces growth of hybridomas; stimulates acute-phase response; synergistic with IL-2 and IL-3
IL-7	Bone-marrow stroma	Induces growth and differentiation of immature B and T cells
IL-8 (NAF)	Macrophages, monocytes	Neutrophil chemotaxis and activation; chemotactic for T cells
TNF	Activated macrophages	Causes necrosis of tumors; T-cell activation; releases IL-1; nonspecific immune enhancement
IFN-γ	T-helper, NK cells	Causes immunoglobulin secretion; antagonizes IL-4; enhances MHC expression; stimulates NK and macrophage activities, release of TNF, expression of macrophage Fc receptor
GM-CSF	Neutrophils; macrophages; bone-marrow blast cells	Growth and differentiation of granulocyte lineages

Adapted from Toder V, Shomer B: Immunol Allergy Clin North Am 10:65, 1990.
GM-CSF, Granulocyte-macrophage colony-stimulating factor; *IFN,* interferon; *IL,* interleukin; *MHC,* major histocompatibility complex; *NAF,* neutrophil-activiating factor; *NK,* natural killer; *TNF,* tumor-necrosis factor.

Tumor-necrosis factor and lymphotoxin

Tumor-necrosis factor (TNF-α), previously known as cachectin, is a major inflammatory mediator produced by macrophages and other cells. It is similar to lymphotoxin, also known as TNF-β, produced by T lymphocytes. Both peptides bind to the same receptor and have similar actions.[4] TNF-α appears important in the host response to invasion by bacteria, viruses, parasites, or tumors, and it may be the primary mediator of endotoxin shock. TNF induces fever both by a direct effect on the hypothalamus and by stimulating synthesis of IL-1. The catabolic effect of TNF on fat metabolism probably causes the cachexia associated with chronic diseases, malignancies, and AIDS.

Despite these deleterious effects, TNF-α is believed to prevent spread of infections by stimulating the acute-phase response, augmenting host resistance, and enhancing phagocytosis of pathogens.[7] It is synergistic with other cytokines in various in vitro systems, and through release and amplification of other cytokines it orchestrates tissue defense against invading microorganisms or tumors. It also has some direct defensive actions. In an experimental model of human prostatic cancer TNF-α was cytotoxic for cancer cell lines but not for prostatic epithelial and stromal cells.[28] Clinical trials in man, however, indicate that its therapeutic margin is too low for TNF to be a useful form of tumor therapy.[4]

Interferons

Interferons (IFN) are important immunoregulatory peptides that were first described as inhibitors of viral replication and later recognized as regulators in the immune system. There are several IFNs that differ with respect to molecular weight and cellular source. α-IFN and β-IFN are produced in leukocytes and fibroblasts, respectively, in response to viral or bacterial infections. Immune interferon, or γ-IFN, is produced by lymphocytes after stimulation by antigens, mitogens, or other lymphokines. Interferons have a broad spectrum of activities: they inhibit replication of viruses, cell division, and various immunologic reactions, they enhance phagocytosis and cytotoxicity of lymphocyte subpopulations, and they modulate B-cell responses.

Reports that interferon has antitumor effects in humans stimulated considerable interest, and intensive effort went into preparations for clinical use. Recombinant interferon was used in clinical studies of acute and chronic viral infections, tumors, and other disorders. Although interferon therapy lessened the severity of viral and bacterial infections in several studies, they have not lived up to expectations as anticancer agents. Combination of IFN with other therapeutic modalities, however, may be effective in certain types of malignancies. A recent trial of γ-IFN in treatment of AIDS was disappointing. Interferon has been used successfully in treatment of chronic hepatitis when other treatment modalities have failed.

Despite initial disappointment when it was assessed in therapeutic trials, γ-IFN is still of great interest because of its role in immunity.[33] IL-2—stimulated production of γ-IFN by NK cells correlates with an increase in cytotoxicity. γ-IFN induces the appearance of new surface markers and receptors associated with differentiation of immune cells. It also enhances expression of MHC antigens that are recognition sites for directed cytotoxicity or replicative signals. γ-IFN plays a pivotal role in antigen processing, and as a maturation factor for B lymphocytes it promotes immunoglobulin synthesis and secretion.[31]

Colony-stimulating factors

Blood cell formation is maintained through growth factors that regulate replication and differentiation of stem cells. IL-3 promotes development of all the hematopoietic lineages. Granulocyte-macrophage colony-stimulating factor (GM-CSF) enhances myelopoiesis in animals and humans, and it activates phagocytosis in neutrophils and macrophages.

Cytokine therapy

Selected recombinant cytokines, singly or in combination, can be used to exploit natural immune defenses or to enhance hematopoietic potential. IL-2 was used successfully to increase cytotoxic lymphocytes, and therapy with this agent initially produced encouraging remissions in certain types of tumors. Unfortunately, elimination of the tumor is rare, and such treatments are expensive and time consuming. Systemic toxicity that accompanies infusion of IL-2 makes it even more undesirable. Targeting to the tumor by means of antibodies might reduce systemic toxicity. Genetically engineered lymphocytes might provide continuous localized delivery of IL-2 or other cytokines to all tumors accessible to the circulation.[26]

Human recombinant interferon is used in combination therapies, notably in combination with zidovudine for treatment of Kaposi's sarcoma. It was combined with cytolytic agents to treat solid tumors and with monoclonal antibodies against lymphomas. Although the results were encouraging in some cases, none of these therapies has proven satisfactory. Results from a recent clinical trial suggest that α-IFN prolongs the response to chemotherapeutic agents and increases survival in patients with multiple myeloma.[18]

Recombinant IL-3 and other colony-stimulating factors are currently being tested in patients with bone-marrow failure. GM-CSF partially reverses neutropenia in patients with AIDS and in patients who are neutropenic as a result of myelosuppressive chemotherapy,[2] and it stimulates myelopoiesis after marrow failure.[32]

IMMUNOSUPPRESSION

A fully responsive immune system is necessary for survival. However, if directed against host tissues, an immune response is potentially harmful. A normal immune response causes rejection of tissue grafts and organ transplants; selective suppression helps to control this unwanted reaction.

Autoimmune disease

Much has been learned about genetically controlled immune responsiveness and about the relationship between tissue antigens and the development of autoimmunity. MHC antigens are involved in inappropriately directed autoimmune responses. Definition of MHC profiles (HLA typing) can identify susceptibilities to various autoimmune diseases, including certain connective tissue and rheumatic diseases. The association of HLA markers is particularly strong for diseases such as ankylosing spondylitis and juvenile-onset rheumatoid arthritis and for diseases that are characterized by chronic inflammatory and aberrant immune reactions, such as myasthenia gravis, insulin-dependent diabetes mellitus, Graves disease, and Addisons disease. Other diseases with specific HLA markers include pemphigus, multiple sclerosis, pernicious anemia, and psoriasis.[27]

Because helper T cells recognize antigen only in association with MHC antigens on the surface of an antigen-presenting cell, the molecular similarity between histocompatibility antigens and those of viruses or bacteria might enable antibodies to the invading microorganism to cross-react with tissues. Another hypothesis is that cell-surface antigens are modified as a result of exposure to microorganisms or toxins or through neoplastic changes. These alterations would then render the host tissue sufficiently antigenic to stimulate an immune response. In addition, there is evidence that Ir (immune response) genes are involved. Thus the pathogenesis could occur at the level of gene expression for control of antibody production.[27]

Control of autoimmune reactions involves reducing the number of lymphoid cells by cytotoxic drugs or irradiation. Unfortunately, this results in generalized immunosuppression. Antibodies or immunotoxins directed against specific T-cell subpopulations promise more selective therapies.

Immunosuppressive drugs

Immunosuppressive therapy of immunologic disease or for the purpose of organ transplantation is relatively nonspecific. It is not directed at the cause of the disease, and it can inhibit normal immune and inflammatory responses as well. Agents such as mercaptopurine, azathioprine, cyclophosphamide, and methotrexate are cytotoxins. They interfere with cell replication and metabolism in various ways, but the result is disruption of normal cell function. Interference with replication of rapidly dividing cells causes several undesirable effects, both acutely (for example, bone-marrow suppression) and long term (for example, an increased incidence of neoplasia). Whether there are additional long-range risks of cytotoxic drugs used to treat autoimmune disease or to prevent organ rejection is not known. Fig. 68-4 compares mechanisms of several immunosuppressive agents.

Glucocorticoids, such as prednisone, have anti-inflammatory as well as immunosuppressive actions. Immune injury activates cells that produce inflammatory mediators; glucocorticoids inhibit production of mediators, such as arachidonate metabolites, that both augment inflammation and activate immune cells. Experiments with lymphocytes in vitro indicate that lipoxygenase products affect proliferative and cytotoxic responses, probably through production of IL-2 or γ-IFN.[24] Corticosteroids may also interfere with production of other cytokines.

Azathioprine (Imuran), a precursor of mercaptopurine, has been used successfully in organ transplantation. It interferes with nucleic acid synthesis in all replicating cells. It first affects the most actively dividing cells, the lymphocytes, to temporarily prevent rejection of the graft. It also inhibits replication of cells in bone marrow and the gastrointestinal tract. Azathioprine in combination with prednisone, which promotes lysis of lymphocytes, provides even greater immune suppression but does not prevent side effects or the increased incidence of secondary infection.[21]

FIG. 68-4

Diagrams show comparison of sites of action of various immunosuppressive agents. Azathioprine inhibits proliferation of effector lymphocytes; prednisone is cytolytic. Since neither is specific for the T lymphocytes most prominently involved in graft rejection, their untoward effects can include bone-marrow suppression and susceptibility to infection. Antilymphocyte globulin adds immunologic attack but will be directed against B- as well as T cells, with consequent infection risks. Only cyclosporin is appropriately specific. By inhibiting production or activity of interleukin-2, it aborts the signal for effector T-cell proliferation.

From Najarian JS: Hosp Pract 17(10):61, 1982; this illustration drawn by Nancy Lou Makris, Wilton, Conn.

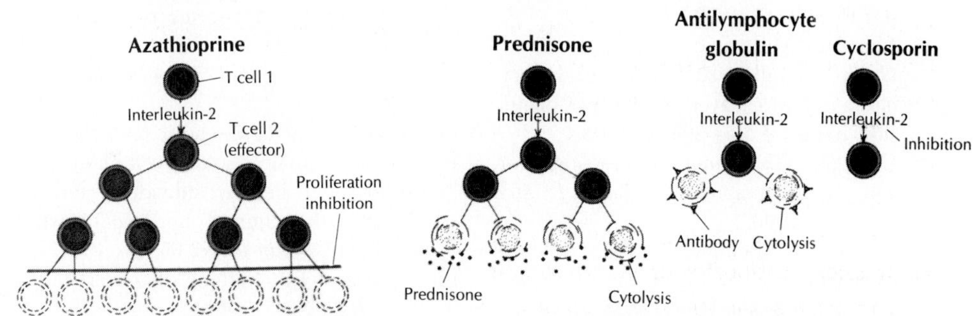

Cyclosporine (Sandimmune), a cyclosporin, is a fungal metabolite that has proved superior to azathioprine in clinical trials of organ transplantation.[5] It is more selective than azathioprine because it primarily affects lymphoid cells and does not cause bone-marrow suppression. Cyclosporine is not directly cytotoxic, but it inhibits activation of lymphocytes before DNA synthesis begins by preventing production of IL-1 and IL-2. This decreases formation of cytotoxic lymphocytes. There is also evidence that cyclosporine interferes with antigen activation of B cells.[29]

A major drawback to use of cyclosporine is nephrotoxicity. Blood concentration must be regulated closely to minimize this adverse effect. The drug can also cause hypertension, hyperkalemia, and impairment of liver function. Combinations of cyclosporine with azathioprine or corticosteroids help to minimize undesirable effects and enhance efficacy in organ transplantation. Administration of misoprostol, a prostaglandin analog, along with cyclosporine and prednisone to renal transplant recipients improved renal function and reduced the incidence of rejection.[6]

PROSPECTS

New technologies in molecular biology and peptide synthesis have expanded the field of immunopharmacology, with development of more selective vaccines, newer therapies for precise and selective control of unwanted or inappropriate immune responses, and "designer" cells that can attack specific types of tumors. Control of HIV infection and its disastrous consequences through manipulation of the immune system remains a viable possibility.

REFERENCES

1. Adorini L, Nagy ZA: Peptide competition for antigen presentation, *Immunol Today* 11:21, 1990.
2. Antman KS, Griffin JD, Elias A, et al: Effect of recombinant human granulocyte-macrophage colony-stimulating factor on chemotherapy-induced myelosuppression, *N Engl J Med* 319:593, 1988.
3. Berkman SA, Lee ML, Gale RP: Clinical uses of intravenous immunoglobulins, *Ann Intern Med* 112:278, 1990.
4. Beutler B: The tumor necrosis factors: cachectin and lymphotoxin, *Hosp Pract* [OFF] 25(2):45, 1990.
5. Canadian Multicentre Transplant Study Group: A randomized clinical trial of cyclosporine in cadaveric renal transplantation, *N Engl J Med* 309:809, 1983.
6. Carpenter CB: Immunosuppression in organ transplantation, *N Engl J Med* 322:1224, 1990.
7. Cerami A, Beutler B: The role of cachectin/TNF in endotoxic shock and cachexia, *Immunol Today* 9:28, 1988.
8. Cohen IR: T-Cell vaccination against autoimmune disease, *Hosp Pract* [OFF] 24(2):53, 1989.
9. Dinarello CA: Interleukin-1 and its biologically related cytokines, *Adv Immunol* 44:153, 1989.
10. Frankel AE, Houston LL, Issell BF, Fathman G: Prospects for immunotoxin therapy in cancer, *Annu Rev Med* 37:125, 1986.
11. Hank JA, Sosman JA, Kohler PC, et al: Depressed in vitro T cell responses concomitant with augmented interleukin-2 responses by lymphocytes from cancer patients following in vivo treatment with interleukin-2, *J Biol Response Mod* 9:5, 1990.
12. Harris PE, Strba-Cechova K, Rubinstein P, et al: Amplification of T cell blastogenic responses in healthy individuals and patients with acquired immunodeficiency syndrome, *J Clin Invest* 85:746, 1990.
13. Heberman RB: Natural killer cells, *Annu Rev Med* 37:347, 1986.

14. Kano K, Ito S, Kitazawa K: Diagnosis and therapy with labeled antibodies, *Immunol Today* 7:95, 1986.

15. Klempner MS, Noring R, Mier JW, Atkins MB: An acquired chemotactic defect in neutrophils from patients receiving interleukin-2 immunotherapy, *N Engl J Med* 322:959, 1990.

16. Larsen CG, Anderson AO, Appella E, et al: The neutrophil-activating protein (NAP-1) is also chemotactic for T lymphocytes, *Science* 243:1464, 1989.

17. Levy R, Miller RA: Biological and clinical implications of lymphocyte hybridomas: tumor therapy with monoclonal antibodies, *Annu Rev Med* 34:107, 1983.

18. Mandelli F, Avvisati G, Amadori S, et al: Maintenance treatment with recombinant interferon alfa-2b in patients with multiple myeloma responding to conventional induction chemotherapy, *N Engl J Med* 322:1430, 1990.

19. Millar SE, Chamow SM, Baur AW, et al: Vaccination with a synthetic zona pellucida peptide produces long-term contraception in female mice, *Science* 246,935, 1989.

20. Morrison SL: Genetically engineered (chimeric) antibodies, *Hosp Pract* [OFF] 24(10):65, 1989.

21. Najarian JS: Immunologic aspects of organ transplantation, *Hosp Pract* 17(10):61, 1982.

22. Parmiani G: An explanation of the variable clinical response to interleukin 2 and LAK cells, *Immunol Today* 11:113, 1990.

23. Pink JRL, Sinigaglia F: Characterizing T-cell epitopes in vaccine candidates, *Immunol Today* 10:408, 1989.

24. Rola-Pleszczynski M: Immunoregulation by leukotrienes and other lipoxygenase metabolites, *Immunol Today* 6:302, 1985.

25. Rosenberg SA, Packard BS, Aebersold PM, et al: Use of tumor-infiltrating lymphocytes and interleukin-2 in the immunotherapy of patients with metastatic melanoma: a preliminary report, *N Engl J Med* 319:1676, 1988.

26. Russell SJ: Lymphokine gene therapy for cancer, *Immunol Today* 11:196, 1990.

27. Schaller JG, Hansen JA: HLA relationships to disease, *Hosp Pract* 16(5):41, 1981.

28. Sherwood ER, Ford TR, Lee C, Kozlowski JM: Therapeutic efficacy of recombinant tumor necrosis factor α in an experimental model of human prostatic carcinoma, *J Biol Response Mod* 9:44, 1990.

29. Shevich EM: Cyclosporine, *Annu Rev Immunol* 3:397, 1985.

30. Stevens VC: Current status of antifertility vaccines using gonadotropin immunogens, *Immunol Today* 7:369, 1986.

31. Trinchieri G, Perussia B: Immune interferon: a pleiotropic lymphokine with multiple effects, *Immunol Today* 6:131, 1985.

32. Vadhan-Raj S, Buescher S, Broxmeyer HE, et al: Stimulation of myelopoiesis in patients with aplastic anemia by recombinant human granulocyte–macrophage colony-stimulating factor, *N Engl J Med* 319:1628, 1988.

33. Vitetta ES, Fernandez-Botran R, Myers CD, Sanders VM: Cellular interactions in the humoral immune response, *Adv Immunol* 45:1, 1989.

section twelve

Poisons and antidotes

Chapter 69

Poisons and antidotes

A poison may be defined as any substance causing death, disease, or injury. Poisons arise from various sources, including bacteria (toxins), industrial pollution, burning of fossil fuels (carbon monoxide), and radionuclides. Drugs also fit the definition of a poison. In fact, the word pharmacology derives from the Greek *phármakon*, which means "drug" or "poison." Poisoning by drugs is usually a matter of degree; a relatively small quantity produces a desired (therapeutic) effect, whereas a large amount is likely to induce untoward or toxic effects.

Toxicology is the science of poisons and poisonings. It encompasses diagnosis, treatment, mechanism of action, and identification of poisons. Persons in this area are clinical, forensic, or industrial toxicologists. Chemical analysis is central to all areas of toxicology, including diagnosis of drug intoxication; recent advances in analytic chemistry have proved invaluable.

Today, and even more in the future, every human will experience some loss of quality of life from environmental poisons: (1) air pollutants, such as auto exhausts, excessive ozone, and smog, (2) food and water contaminated with pesticides, bacteria, viruses, and plasticizers, and (3) buildings with mold in air vents and gases from synthetic building materials.

Since there are more poisons than diseases and almost all medical training is focused on disease, physicians may consider themselves relatively poorly equipped to deal with poisonings. Most areas of the country have access to poison control centers where advice can be sought. Toxicology texts emphasize advanced life support in poisoning cases, but in-home and out-patient care is becoming more and more important. Three goals are particularly important in clinical toxicology: (1) correct diagnosis, (2) assessment of severity, and (3) appropriate initial management.[12]

DIAGNOSIS OF POISONING

Currently, in the United States 10% of all ambulance calls are poison related. Of pediatric admissions 2% to 5% and of adult admissions to medical services 10% to 20% are for toxin ingestions.[5]

The diagnosis of poisoning can be difficult, particularly if the victim is unconscious. The conscious patient may not admit to self-poisoning, and this possibility may not enter the physician's differential diagnosis. A suspicious mind is essential to detect such cases. Intoxication should be suspected when an ill person does not respond to treatment within a reasonable time. Cases of poisoning often mimic the initial signs and symptoms of a disease. In contrast, certain symptoms and pathologic changes are quite characteristic of specific intoxications. The victim's family should be encouraged to produce bottles of medication, particularly empty or partially empty ones, to which the patient had access. Excluding alcohol, fewer than 20 of the 20,000 different pharmaceutic products currently marketed account for 90% of *nonaccidental* toxin ingestions.[5]

POISON CONTROL CENTERS

Poison control centers are an important facet of poison therapeutics. A physician confronted with a case of intoxication can call one of these centers for help in diagnosis and treatment. Initially, three questions must be answered as accurately as possible: (1) what was ingested, inhaled, etc., (2) how much, and (3) when did intoxication occur?[12]

In the United States over 180 million persons in 42 states are served by 70 centers that contribute data to a comprehensive annual report.[14] Extrapolation from this data base indicates that there were more than 2 million poison exposures in this country in 1989, over 90% of which happened in homes. Over 90% of exposures involved intoxication with a single substance; less than 2% involved more than two compounds. Most exposures were accidental; fewer than 10% were intentional. Approximately three-quarters of reported exposures occurred by ingestion, followed in descending frequency by dermal, ophthalmic, inhalation, bites and stings, and parenteral exposures. Of 590 reported deaths the peak number occurred in victims aged 30 to 39.

The types of substances most commonly reported to the poison control centers and those most commonly implicated in death are listed in Tables 69-1 and 69-2, respectively.

TABLE 69-1 Substances most frequently involved in human exposure

Substance	No.	%*
Cleaning substances	160,652	10.2
Analgesics	160,591	10.2
Cosmetics	130,207	8.2
Plants	100,704	6.4
Cough and cold preparations	90,798	5.7
Pesticides (includes rodenticides)	60,045	3.8
Bites/envenomations	58,750	3.7
Hydrocarbons	58,616	3.7
Topicals	56,920	3.6
Foreign bodies	56,356	3.6
Chemicals	53,011	3.4
Sedative/hypnotics/antipsychotics	50,833	3.2
Antimicrobials	50,236	3.2
Food poisoning	48,336	3.1
Alcohols	43,539	2.8
Vitamins	40,922	2.6

From Litovitz TL, Schmitz BF, Bailey KM: Am J Emerg Med 8:394, 1990.
NOTE: Despite a high frequency of involvement, these substances are not necessarily the most toxic, but rather often represent only ready availability.
*Percentages are based on the total number of human exposures rather than the total number of substances.

TABLE 69-2 Categories with largest numbers of deaths

Category	No.	% of all exposures in category
Antidepressants	140	.559
Analgesics	126	.078
Stimulants and street drugs	64	.320
Sedative/hypnotics	78	.153
Cardiovascular drugs	70	.345
Alcohols	53	.122
Gases and fumes	46	.225
Asthma therapies	34	.265
Hydrocarbons	31	.053
Chemicals	27	.051
Cleaning substances	25	.016
Pesticides (including rodenticides)	14	.023

From Litovitz TL, Schmitz BF, Bailey KM: Am J Emerg Med 8:394, 1990.

The relative overall importance of various treatment modalities is indicated by Table 69-3. Clearly, initial decontamination is tremendously important. Ipecac syrup was used in 7% of cases, more often outside a health-care facility in children under 6 years of age. The use of ipecac syrup has been declining since 1985, however, whereas use of activated charcoal has increased. Enhancement of elimination after the poison was absorbed and treatment with specific antidotes were much less commonly reported.

PRINCIPLES OF TREATMENT

General principles in management of poisoning include (1) stabilization of the patient, (2) removal of ingested poison from the stomach, except when contraindicated, or other appropriate forms of decontamination, (3) expeditious evaluation of samples of blood, urine, vomitus, or other body fluids to identify the responsible compound(s), (4) symptomatic and supportive therapy, (5) administration of an antidote for specific intoxications, and (6) measures to hasten removal of absorbed intoxicant from the body.

The importance of emptying the stomach when poisons have been ingested cannot be overemphasized; this mainstay of treatment can be lifesaving in most such intoxications. However, gastric emptying should be avoided when there is potential for seizures, when the airway cannot be protected to prevent aspiration, when the ingested product is corrosive or a petroleum distillate, and when too much time has elapsed since ingestion of the poison. Otherwise, if emesis has not occurred, the conscious patient should be made to vomit, since vomiting is more effective than the most intensive gastric lavage.[1] Many poisons are themselves emetics, but if emesis does not occur spontaneously, it can usually be induced by stimulation of the pharynx with a finger, often after having the victim drink a glass of milk or water, or by emetic drugs. If vomiting cannot be induced, gastric lavage should be performed at once, with particular attention to protecting the airways.

TABLE 69-3 Therapy provided in human exposure cases

Therapy	No.
Initial Decontamination	
Dilution	602,880
Irrigation/washing	293,111
Ipecac syrup	110,800
Activated charcoal	101,525
Cathartic	85,016
Gastric lavage	41,056
Other emetic	3,743
Measures to Enhance Elimination	
Alkalinization (with or without diuresis)	4,526
Hemodialysis	418
Forced diuresis	340
Hemoperfusion (charcoal)	162
Acidification (with or without diuresis)	134
Exchange transfusion	42
Hemoperfusion (resin)	29
Peritoneal dialysis	21
Specific Antidote Administration	
Naloxone	6,082
N-acetylcysteine (oral)	4,972
Atropine	717
Deferoxamine	646
Antivenin/antitoxin	506
Ethanol	440
Hydroxocobalamin	343
Pralidoxime (2-PAM)	275
Physostigmine	246
Dimercaprol (BAL)	205
N-acetylcysteine (IV)	179
FAB fragments	174
Cyanide antidote kit	160
Penicillamine	125
Pyridoxine	113
Methylene blue	93
EDTA	78

From Litovitz TL, Schmitz BF, Bailey KM: Am J Emerg Med 8:394, 1990.

The judicious use of drugs and other therapeutic measures in treating poisonings is of utmost importance. However, overtreatment of the intoxicated patient with large doses of antidote, sedatives, or stimulants can cause more damage than the poison itself.[2]

Emetics

Two drugs used to induce vomiting are syrup of ipecac and apomorphine. For best results fluids should be given before the emetic.

Although its use has declined somewhat, **ipecac syrup** is by far the most widely used emetic.[14] It can be kept at home and is inexpensive and safe. The dose is 15 ml for children over 1 year old and perhaps more for adults; the average time before vomiting is 15 minutes. If necessary, a second 15 ml dose may be administered 20 minutes later. If this fails to evoke emesis, gastric lavage is imperative, since ipecac is an irritant and, when absorbed, a cardiotoxin. Syrup of ipecac should never be given simultaneously with charcoal because charcoal adsorbs the ipecac, thereby preventing its emetic effect. Charcoal can be given after vomiting has stopped.

Subcutaneous injection of **apomorphine hydrochloride** produces emesis within 5 minutes and promotes reflux of the contents of the upper intestinal tract into the stomach. However, prolonged vomiting and, especially in children, the depressant effect of apomorphine can be serious disadvantages, even though naloxone can be given as an antidote. Most toxicologists feel that this emetic should not be used.

ANTIDOTES

Nonsystemic antidotes

Activated charcoal (SuperChar, others) is a black powder. Because the particles are extremely small and contain many pores, the surface area of a gram of the material may exceed 3000 m^2. A compound that is adsorbed to activated charcoal cannot be absorbed from the gastrointestinal tract; its elimination is enhanced and systemic toxicity is minimized. Even after absorption, a substance that returns to the gut via enterohepatic circulation (theophylline, carbamazepine) can be trapped there by charcoal. For those substances to which it binds, activated charcoal tends to be more effective treatment than measures to empty the stomach, although the adsorptive capacity of activated charcoal can be exceeded.[17] A combination of gastric lavage followed by charcoal may be the most beneficial approach in selected cases. Combination of a cathartic with activated charcoal does not appreciably enhance poison removal.

For maximal effectiveness, a highly active preparation of charcoal must be given orally as soon as possible after intoxication. The dose should exceed that of the poison at least tenfold (based on animal studies).[13,17] A suspension containing about 1 g of charcoal per kilogram of body weight is recommended for both adults and children. Administration can be repeated every 4 to 6 hours until the circulating concentration of poison declines to below the toxic range and symptoms abate. In addition to continual trapping of drugs that are excreted in bile, repeated administration minimizes dissociation (desorbing) of the charcoal-toxin complex as it traverses the gut. To expedite treatment, activated charcoal should be kept in homes and at the workplace. Even if it is ineffective, it will seldom harm a conscious patient, and in severe intoxication it may be dangerous to wait until the identity of the poison is known before initiating treatment. Charcoal is not useful after ingestion of caustic alkalis or acids.

Tannic acid forms insoluble salts with many alkaloids and heavy metals. Approximately 30 to 50 g/L of water is an effective concentration. Larger amounts should be avoided because of hepatotoxicity.

Systemic antidotes

In addition to supportive measures and nonsystemic antidotes, several antidotes that act systemically as physiologic, or occasionally pharmacologic, antagonists to specific intoxicants are available. The most important ones are listed in Table 69-4,[3,4] and certain of these that have not been considered elsewhere are discussed below.

DIMERCAPROL

Dimercaprol (2,3-dimercaptopropanol, or BAL) is routinely used to treat mercury, gold, arsenic, and severe lead poisoning. It was developed during World War II as an antidote to vesicant arsenicals that combine with sulfhydryl groups. Dimercaprol is a particularly effective antidote because a pair of adjacent sulfhydryl groups enable it to form a stable ring structure with the metal.

$$\begin{array}{l} CH_2\text{—}SH \\ | \\ CH\text{—}SH \\ | \\ CH_2\text{—}OH \end{array}$$

Dimercaprol

Therapeutic objectives. There are two major objectives in the use of dimercaprol. The first is inactivation of the poison by formation of a complex or a *chelate* (a ringed complex). This prevents combination of the poison with sulfhydryl groups of essential enzymes. The second objective is to promote elimination of the poison from the body; the complex is water soluble at pH 7.5 and is readily excreted. Uncomplexed dimercaprol is metabolized through S-methylation by a microsomal enzyme.

TABLE 69-4 Specific antidotes and their dosages

Drug or toxin	Antidote	Dosage*
Acetaminophen	*N*-Acetylcysteine	*Loading:* 140 mg/kg orally; *oral maintenance:* 70 mg/kg every 4 hours for 17 doses
Anticholinergics	Physostigmine	*Adult*: 1-2 mg; *child*: 0.5 mg; given slowly
Bromide	Sodium chloride	
Carbon monoxide	Oxygen	
Cyanide	Sodium nitrite Sodium thiosulfate	*Adult*: 300 mg; *child:* 10 mg/kg *Adult:* 12.5 g; *child*: 0.3-0.5 g/kg
Ethylene glycol	Ethanol	*Loading:* 1 ml/kg of 95%; *maintenance:* 0.1 ml/kg/hour
Heavy metals	Dimercaprol (BAL), edetate calcium disodium, penicillamine	See text
Isoniazid	Pyridoxine	2 to 5 g slowly
Iron	Deferoxamine	10 to 15 mg/kg/hour for 8 hours
Methanol	Ethanol	Same as for ethylene glycol (above)
Narcotics	Naloxone	*Adult:* 0.4-2 mg; *child:* 0.01-0.1 mg/kg
Nitrites	Methylene blue	1 to 2 ml/kg of 1% solution
Organophosphates	Atropine, pralidoxime	2 mg as needed, 1 g

*Given intravenously unless indicated otherwise

Toxicity and adverse effects. Dimercaprol is potentially dangerous. Side effects include vascular flushing, myalgia, nausea and vomiting, nephrotoxicity, hypotension, pulmonary edema, salivation, lacrimation, and fever. Despite these, dimercaprol has remained in use for over 35 years because it is the most effective antidote for specific metal poisonings.

Contraindications. Dimercaprol is contraindicated in patients with liver disease or severe renal disease and in poisoning by iron, cadmium, or selenium. Dimercaprol forms toxic complexes with the latter metals.

Preparations. Dimercaprol (BAL) is available as a 10% solution (100 mg/ml) in peanut oil. Dosage varies from 2.5 to 3 mg/kg intramuscularly repeated from one to four times a day, depending on the severity of the intoxication.

EDETATE CALCIUM DISODIUM AND EDETATE DISODIUM

Ethylenediaminetetraacetic acid (EDTA) and its salt, edetate disodium, are powerful chelating agents that form a highly stable complex with calcium. Despite the stability of the chelate, calcium is displaced from it by lead, zinc, chromium, copper, cadmium, manganese, and nickel. Edetate calcium disodium is used primarily to treat lead poisoning; it can be combined with dimercaprol to treat severe cases associated with encephalopathy.

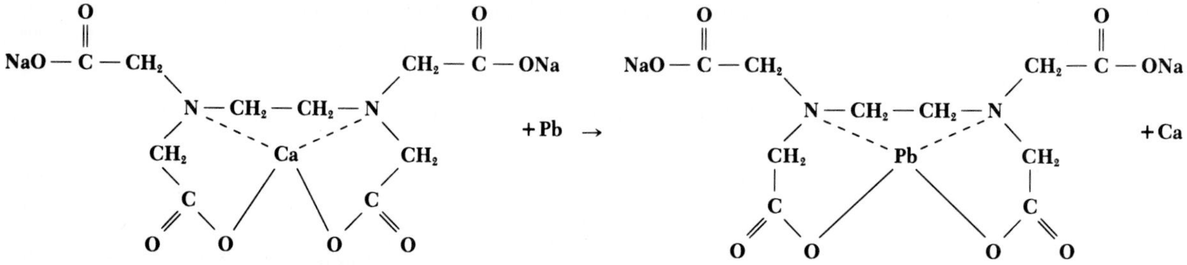

$$\text{Edetate calcium disodium} + Pb \rightarrow \text{Edetate lead disodium} + Ca$$

Edetate calcium disodium **Edetate lead disodium**

The calcium disodium derivative should be used to treat metal intoxications, since the disodium salt will chelate endogenous Ca^{++} to produce hypocalcemia. Recent drug schedules use deep intramuscular injection of edetate. Severe reactions such as fever, headache, vomiting, decreased blood pressure, and histamine-like reactions have been observed with intravenous administration.

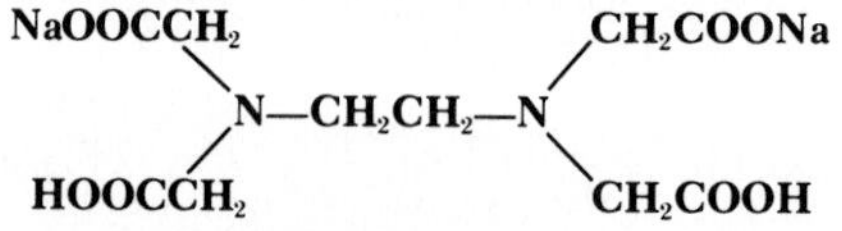

$$(NaOOCCH_2)(HOOCCH_2)N{-}CH_2CH_2{-}N(CH_2COONa)(CH_2COOH)$$

Edetate disodium

Toxicity and adverse effects. The toxicity of edetate is probably caused by binding of essential metal ions. Large doses are nephrotoxic. Edetate is not metabolized; it is excreted by the kidney and is contraindicated in the presence of renal disease.

Preparations. Edetate calcium disodium (Calcium Disodium Versenate) for parenteral use is a 20% solution. To avoid toxic symptoms the total daily dose should not exceed 50 mg/kg of body weight.

Edetate disodium (Endrate, others) is marketed in 20 ml ampules that contain 150 mg/ml. It is used primarily to treat hypercalcemia.

PENICILLAMINE

Therapeutic objectives. Penicillamine and its acetyl derivative, *N*-acetylpenicillamine, chelate copper and other metals such as mercury, lead, and iron. Since other drugs are more effective for the latter metals, penicillamine is employed primarily to remove copper in hepatolenticular degeneration (Wilsons disease). The drug is also of value in treatment of nephrolithiasis associated with cystinuria and in treatment of rheumatoid arthritis.

Toxicity and adverse effects. Adverse effects of penicillamine include acute allergic reactions, leukopenia, eosinophilia, thrombocytopenia, and nephrotoxicity. D-Penicillamine is less toxic and is the preferred form, in contrast to former use of the L or D,L forms.

Penicillamine (Cuprimine, Depen) is marketed as capsules (125 and 250 mg) and tablets (250 mg); 1 to 4 g/day is divided over four doses.

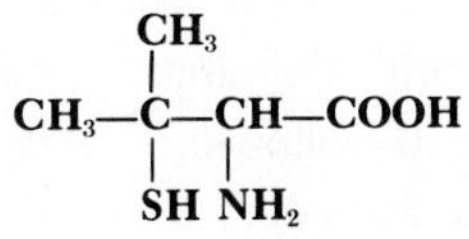

$$CH_3\text{—}C(CH_3)(SH)\text{—}CH(NH_2)\text{—}COOH$$

Penicillamine

DEFEROXAMINE MESYLATE

Deferoxamine is isolated from *Streptomyces pilosus* and has high affinity for ferric iron and low affinity for Ca^{++}. This chelating agent is used to treat acute iron poisoning and chronic iron or aluminum overload. It is metabolized by plasma enzymes and is also excreted unchanged in the urine. The drug is toxic and should be used only if the severity of the poisoning justifies it. Reactions include diarrhea, hypotension, and cataract formation. Deferoxamine (Desferal) mesylate is available in ampules containing 500 mg as powder. The recommended dose in iron poisoning is 1 g, usually intramuscularly but also intravenously, repeated if necessary every 4 to 12 hours. The total dose should not exceed 6 g in 24 hours.

LIFE-SUSTAINING MEASURES

Patients with severe intoxication or underlying systemic disease may require special interventions to enhance drug removal from the body. These include forced diuresis, dialysis, hemoperfusion and filtration, plasmapheresis, exchange transfusion, and drug-specific antibodies.[13]

It is important to stress that such measures are used in only a small fraction of cases (Table 69-3). When deciding whether to institute such an approach, one must consider if it will substantially increase clearance of the poison. In general, if the intervention does not contribute 30% or more to the total clearance of a compound, it is unlikely to be useful. One must also compare the risks of the intervention itself to those of the poison.

Forced diuresis

Forced diuresis[13,19] uses diuretics (usually osmotic or loop diuretics), large volumes of isotonic fluids, or both to speed renal elimination of drugs that are readily reabsorbed from tubular fluid. The normal concentration gradient between drug in the tubular lumen and in plasma, which is produced as water is reabsorbed, favors passive reabsorption. This gradient is reduced when a diuretic diminishes water reabsorption. Likewise, a greater rate of flow within the tubules due to an increased fluid load lowers the gradient and allows less time for passive reabsorption to take place. In addition, alteration of urinary pH can facilitate excretion if it maintains an appreciably greater proportion of lumenal drug in its charged, less readily reabsorbed, form (see p. 50). Sodium bicarbonate is used to alkalinize the urine; because the urine is normally acid, additional acidification is rarely useful (see Table 69-3).

Potential complications of forced diuresis include hyponatremia and hypokalemia, cerebral or pulmonary edema, and systemic acid-base disturbances. It is not used in patients with renal or cardiac failure.

Dialytic therapy

Dialysis also hastens removal of some intoxicants from the circulation. It is expensive and presents some hazards and, therefore, should be limited to specific, serious intoxications. Indications include the following[13]: (1) intoxication with evidence of vital function impairment (deep coma, refractory hypotension, hypothermia); (2) deterioration despite supportive care; (3) possible absorption of a lethal dose or determination of a potentially lethal concentration in blood; (4) intoxication by agents, such as methanol, ethylene glycol, and paraquat, that have delayed effects; (5) impairment of normal excretory function; (6) the presence of diseases, such as chronic obstructive lung disease or heart failure, that increase risk of prolonged coma or development of a life-threatening complication; (7) multi-drug intoxication in which the concentration of no one agent is particularly high, even though the combination may be lethal.

In dialysis a poison passes from blood flowing on one side of a semipermeable membrane down its concentration gradient into a solution (dialysate) on the other side. The peritoneal membrane is the semipermeable membrane in peritoneal dialysis. In hemodialysis, blood passes through an external circuit that comprises the semipermeable membrane. Compounds are poor candidates for dialysis if they are: (1) large molecules, (2) highly lipid soluble, (3) highly bound to plasma proteins, or if they have a volume of distribution greater than 1 to 2 L/kg. Pore size of the usual membranes limits hemodialysis to compounds with molecular weights less than 500 daltons. The other three factors greatly limit the fraction of total drug that is free in the blood and thus available for diffusion from the circulation. The composition, flow rate, volume, and pH of the dialysate can be altered to enhance drug removal.

Peritoneal dialysis

This form of dialysis is rarely used for intoxication (see Table 69-3), even though it is an easy procedure. Hemodialysis is considerably more effective, and forced diuresis may work just as well. Peritoneal dialysis can be used if these other methods are not feasible due to equipment problems or difficulty with vascular access.

HEMODIALYSIS

Catheters for acute hemodialysis can be inserted at the bedside. A single-pass dialysis system, which maintains a maximal concentration gradient across the membrane, is the most efficient. Hemodialysis is useful for salicylate, ethanol, methanol, and ethylene glycol intoxications and for removal of long-acting barbiturates. Short-acting barbiturates are eliminated rapidly enough that dialysis does not add a substantial increment to their clearance. Many potential complications of hemodialysis are related to the procedure itself (infection, local thrombosis, air embolism) or to the need for anticoagulant administration.

Hemoperfusion

In hemoperfusion a substance in blood is exposed to a column containing charcoal or a resin that can adsorb it. Polar compounds tend to be removed better by charcoal. With the resin preparations, in contrast to charcoal, drugs can be eluted by organic solvents for later analysis. Hemoperfusion is more successful than dialysis in removing substances that are relatively large, lipid soluble, or highly bound to plasma proteins.

Hemofiltration

In hemofiltration, a procedure not unlike filtration that normally occurs in renal glomeruli, pressure exerted on one side of a semipermeable membrane forces water and solutes through the membrane to create an ultrafiltrate of plasma, which can be discarded and replaced with another physiologic solution. Certain barbiturates, antibiotics, and digoxin are effectively removed by this procedure. Minimal binding to plasma proteins is required for efficient filtration. Hemofiltration can remove unbound compounds (up to 5,000 daltons) that are too large to pass through dialysis membranes. Unfortunately, hemofiltration is a relatively slow process.

Plasmapheresis

In plasmapheresis a portion of the patient's blood is collected, the plasma is removed, and the red cells are returned in substitute plasma or albumin solution. Usually 3 to 4 L of plasma are replaced in about 3 hours. This approach works well for compounds, such as digitoxin, that have a small volume of distribution but are highly bound to plasma proteins. Plasmapheresis is expensive, and complications may arise from the need for anticoagulation, removal of antibodies, and the hazards of plasma administration.

Exchange transfusion

Unlike plasmapheresis, in exchange transfusion whole blood is replaced. The technique is used to remove methemoglobin, formed by intoxication with aniline dyes, nitrites, and certain other oxidizing agents, and replace it with normal hemoglobin.

Drug-specific antibodies

Specific antidotes are available for only a few types of intoxication (Table 69-4). A recent addition to treatment of drug overdosage is the use of specific Fab fragments to treat digoxin toxicity (see p. 418). Other potential applications of Fab fragments, when they are marketed, include intoxications with tricyclic antidepressants, several antiepileptic compounds, quinidine, and theophylline.

ESSENTIAL FEATURES OF SPECIFIC INTOXICATIONS

Ethylene glycol and diethylene glycol intoxication

Gastric lavage is beneficial early after ingestion of these glycols. Specific treatment is aimed at correcting acidosis with sodium bicarbonate and administration of ethanol to slow conversion of the glycol by alcohol dehydrogenase to its toxic metabolites. Hemodialysis should be used to reduce the body load of ethylene glycol.[10] Calcium gluconate can be administered intravenously with caution if hypocalcemia and muscle spasms result from calcium chelation by the oxalate metabolite. Recent evidence suggests that inhibition of alcohol dehydrogenase by the compound 4-methylpyrazole may be a more effective and safer alternative to use of ethanol in ethylene glycol intoxication,[18] but this compound is not yet available for use.

Diethylene glycol has many industrial uses. Ingestion can cause hepatic and renal failure. In the 1930s its use as a solvent in an elixir of sulfanilamide caused 107 fatalities in 15 states among 353 people taking the preparation. From this catastrophe it was estimated that the oral lethal dose is approximately 1 ml/kg.

Carbon monoxide poisoning

Carbon monoxide[9] is the leading cause of lethal intoxication in the United States. Because it is an odorless and colorless gas that does not irritate air passages, a dangerous state of intoxication can arise before the victim becomes aware of it. Unsuspected sublethal exposure, with flu-like symptoms, is believed to affect several thousand people in this country every year. Smoke and carbon monoxide inhalation from home fires has been estimated responsible for half of all fire-related deaths.

Carbon monoxide competes with and displaces oxygen from ferrous sites on hemoglobin. Environmental exposure in nonsmokers usually produces a carboxyhemoglobin level of less than 2% of total hemoglobin. The level is increased considerably in smokers and can be sufficient to lower the threshold for angina. If exposure is sufficiently severe, tissue hypoxia and acidosis follow.

Symptoms of poisoning include headache, dizziness, nausea, vomiting, loss of muscular control, unconsciousness, and death. Retinal hemorrhages have been observed with subacute poisoning. Carbon monoxide affects the cardiac and respiratory systems by causing hypoxia. Cardiac arrhythmias are common, and myocardial infarction often occurs. The skin becomes cherry red in color when as little as 25% of the hemoglobin is saturated with carbon monoxide. Coma and death can result when about 60% of the hemoglobin is in the form of carboxyhemoglobin; in cardiac patients, lower levels may be fatal.

Oxygen containing 5% to 7% carbon dioxide is used to reverse carbon monoxide poisoning. Carbon dioxide increases ventilatory exchange and also hastens dissociation of carbon monoxide from hemoglobin. Use of two atmospheres of oxygen will speed conversion of carboxyhemoglobin to oxyhemoglobin. Hyperbaric oxygen, the best treatment, reduces the carboxyhemoglobin level by one half in 40 minutes, compared to over 4 hours if room air is breathed.

Cyanide poisoning

Cyanide inhibits cellular respiration by reacting with cytochrome oxidase. Cytotoxic hypoxia results. The minimal lethal dose of cyanide is about 0.5 mg/kg; autopsy data indicate that death predictably occurs at approximately 1.4 mg/kg of body weight.

Symptoms of poisoning, which appear very quickly, include giddiness, headache, palpitations, unconsciousness, convulsions, and death. Diagnosis is usually made by the characteristic odor of bitter almond associated with asphyxia. Prompt treatment with sodium nitrite and thiosulfate can be lifesaving. The rationale for this classic approach to treatment is that cyanide reacts only with iron in the ferric state to form a cytochrome oxidase–cyanide complex. However, methemoglobin competes with cytochrome oxidase for cyanide ion. The concentration gradient favors formation of cyanomethemoglobin, and cytochrome oxidase activity is restored.[20] The objective of therapy is to produce a high concentration (but not more than 30%) of methemoglobin ($HbFe^{+++}$) by intravenous administration of nitrite.

$$HbFe^{++} + NaNO_2 \rightleftarrows HbFe^{+++}$$

Actual detoxification is finally achieved by injection of thiosulfate, which reacts with cyanide to form thiocyanate (SCN^-). Thiocyanate is then excreted in the urine. More than one such set of treatments may be necessary.

$$Na_2S_2O_3 + CN^- \rightleftarrows SCN^- + Na_2SO_3$$

Some investigators question the use of nitrates to treat cyanide intoxication,[7] partially on the basis of evidence that methemoglobin formation, relative to tissue cyanide uptake, may be too slow to be of value. They propose combining hemodialysis and intravenous infusion of sodium thiosulfate with supportive measures that include gastric lavage followed by activated charcoal and administration of oxygen. Hemodialysis is believed to help (1) by removing extracellular cyanide, particularly if it is still being absorbed; (2) by correcting the lactic acidosis that is common to cyanide toxicity; and (3) by hastening removal of the thiocyanate end-product.

ENVIRONMENTAL POISONING

Environmental contaminants are a concomitant of modern life. For example, albeit an extreme one, in Canada some totally self-contained houses were built in which no one could live because of gases released from synthetic materials. Similarly, persons hypersensitive to formaldehyde have been forced to move to new locations to avoid this chemical released from insulation. Air ducts in buildings can be sources of bacteria or molds that cause toxic reactions. These areas should be explored when other sources of poisons cannot be identified.

Heavy metal poisoning

Various metals may produce vastly different symptoms, but a common characteristic is their tendency to accumulate and produce chronic as well as acute poisoning.

Lead poisoning was recognized in colonial times, and in 1723 Massachusetts passed a law preventing distillation of rum and liquors in retorts or pipes containing lead. In 1975 the Centers for Disease Control reported that more than 28,000 young children suffered from excessive lead absorption. Ingestion is unsafe if it exceeds 0.5 mg/day; 3 months of daily ingestion at this rate is required to reach dangerous concentrations. A few small chips of old paint may contain more than 100 mg of lead.

The half-life of lead in blood and soft tissue is about 15 days; in bone it is about 15 years. Over 90% of total body lead is in bone. Chelating agents remove lead from blood and soft tissue but will not remove lead tightly bound to bone.

Most lead enters through the gastrointestinal tract and lungs. Daily adult consumption of lead is about 300 μg but absorption is only 10%. Children, on the other hand, absorb about half of the lead they ingest.[6] Lead concentrations are also many times higher in children compared to adults because children breathe closer to the ground where lead-particle densities are higher. This coupled with a more permeable blood-brain barrier makes children much more susceptible to lead poisoning. Analysis of bones demonstrates over a hundredfold increase in the average total-body lead burden of children compared to unexposed ancestors. As new data are obtained, the level of lead believed to have no effect on children is continually revised downward.

Early symptoms of lead poisoning include anorexia, apathy, irritability, and perhaps sporadic vomiting. Neurocognitive impairment manifests as diminished intelligence, attention deficits, behavior problems, and EEG alterations.[16] After the early symptoms, acute encephalopathy characterized by ataxia, persistent vomiting, lethargy, stupor, convulsions, and coma may rapidly ensue. Twenty-five percent of children who survive encephalopathy suffer permanent brain damage. Organic lead produces symptoms predominantly of the central nervous system, whereas inorganic lead poisoning is accompanied by disturbances in hemoglobin synthesis.

The primary screening procedure for lead toxicity is the free erythrocyte protoporphyrin (FEP) test. It is used to detect metabolic evidence of toxicity. Measurements of urinary δ-aminolevulinic acid and coproprophyrin III are also useful for assessing lead poisoning. The toxic concentration of lead in whole blood is above 0.5 μg/ml, whereas a concentration of FEP above 1.1 μg/ml is consistent with lead intoxication. Urine lead concentrations above 0.2 μg/ml, urine coproporphyrin concentrations higher than 0.8 μg/ml, and urinary δ-aminolevulinic acid concentrations higher than 19 μg/ml indicate dangerous amounts of lead absorption.

In patients with encephalopathy, chelation therapy is started with dimercaprol and edetate calcium disodium for 5 to 7 days, depending on severity. Seizures should be controlled with a benzodiazepine. If the patient is symptomatic but without encephalopathy, dimercaprol may be omitted. Patients should be separated from the source of lead, since edetate calcium disodium increases absorption of lead from the intestine.

Mercury contaminates the atmosphere from burning fossil fuels and enters the food chain through fish exposed to contaminated water. The latter cycle was illustrated by the tragic deaths of those eating mercury-contaminated fish from Minamata Bay in Japan; mercury wastes from insecticide manufacture were poured into the bay from industrial plants. Another deplorable event was the death of 459 victims in Iraq who ate bread prepared from wheat treated with a methylmercury fungicide.

The approximate lethal dose of $HgCl_2$ is 1 g, and symptoms of mercury poisoning are first observed at a whole blood concentration of 1 μg/ml. The half-life of methyl mercury is 65 days; therefore repeated exposure leads to accumulation. Methyl mercury is a subtle, difficult to detect, long-lasting poison that easily enters the central nervous system. Symptoms of chronic mercury poisoning most frequently involve the central nervous system and include tremor and psychotic behavior. Other symptoms include gingivitis, stomatitis, excessive salivation, dermatitis, anorexia, anemia, and weight loss. Acute poisoning produces gastroenteritis with severe abdominal pain and bloody diarrhea. Proteinuria may occur. Anuria and uremia are common.

Depending on the molar ratio of antidote to poison, dimercaprol forms either a chelate or a complex with mercury. The complex is water soluble at pH 7.5, binds mercury more tightly than the chelate does, and is rapidly excreted.

H_2C-S, $HC-S$ (both S bound to Hg), CH_2OH

Mercury chelate

$CH_2-S-Hg-S-CH_2$; $HC-SH$ $\quad$ $HS-CH$; CH_2OH $\quad$ CH_2OH

Mercury complex

Thallium was used to a greater extent than arsenic for poisoning in antiquity. Acute poisoning is currently caused by rodenticides and depilatory preparations. Cases of chronic industrial poisoning have resulted from contact with metal alloys, jewelry, optical lenses, thermometers, and pigment manufacture. Manifestations of poisoning, mainly gastrointestinal or central, include hematemesis, bloody diarrhea, tremor, choreiform movements, ataxia, convulsions, cyanosis, and death. Among the most lethal of metal poisons, thallium exhibits a high incidence of long-term neurologic sequelae. The average acute lethal dose of thallium sulfate is about 1 g.

Diagnosis is delayed if it depends only on the alopecia that occurs about 3 weeks after exposure. Hair loss is complete, including hair in the axillary and pubic regions. Black pigmentation around hair roots can be seen as early as 3 days after exposure. Lunule stripes develop as a result of transient disturbances in nail growth. Pronounced tachycardia appears 1 to 4 weeks after initial exposure.

To treat acute intoxication, gastric lavage or emesis should be instituted promptly. Activated charcoal is given twice daily for 5 days along with potassium chloride daily for 5 to 10 days. Dimercaprol is used in maximum doses.

Soluble **gold** salts have been given intramuscularly to treat rheumatoid arthritis (see p. 371) for over half a century. Dermatitis and stomatitis with fever are the most common manifestations of acute toxicity. Gold also causes nephritis with albuminuria, gastritis, colitis, and hepatitis. Other organ systems affected are the hematopoietic system, where gold may produce agranulocytosis or aplastic anemia, and the respiratory system, where it rarely initiates a pneumonitis characterized by diffuse interstitial inflammation, fibrosis, and lymphocyte and plasma cell infiltration. Dimercaprol is an effective antidote when given early. Penicillamine, as an oral chelating agent, is also reported to be effective.

Arsenic, a protoplasmic poison, is found in herbicides, fungicides, and pesticides. Fortunately, its emetic effect can be lifesaving. Other toxic effects are erosion of the gastrointestinal tract, intense diarrhea, and anuria. Inhalation of arsine gas rapidly causes hemolysis and jaundice; the released hemoglobin blocks renal tubules. Arsenic can induce encephalopathy even though it enters the brain slowly and central levels remain relatively low.

Dimercaprol is the antidote of choice, since organic and inorganic trivalent arsenicals have a high affinity for adjacent thiol groups with formation of stable five-membered rings:

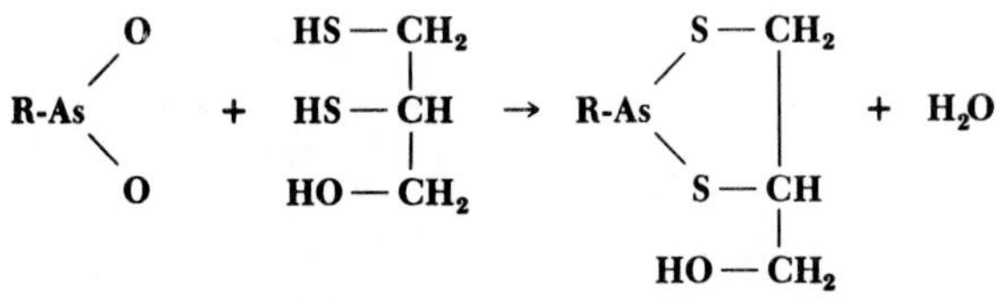

```
       O        HS—CH2               S—CH2
      /            |                /    |
R-As      +     HS—CH    →    R-As       |     +  H2O
      \            |                \    |
       O        HO—CH2               S—CH
                                         |
                                     HO—CH2
Trivalent arsenical   BAL        BAL-arsenic complex
```

Ferrous **iron**, such as that supplied in dietary supplements, can be fatal to children. Symptoms include vomiting, gastrointestinal erosions, hemorrhage, cyanosis, coma, and respiratory depression. Acidosis and shock require prompt treatment. Gastric lavage must be instituted, or emesis can be induced if it hasn't already occurred. Chelation with injectable deferoxamine is appropriate if the amount of iron in serum exceeds the transferrin iron-binding capacity.[15] Whole bowel irrigation, the production of diarrhea by oral or nasogastric introduction of a large amount of polyethylene glycol-electrolyte solution, is a potential new approach to minimizing iron absorption.[15]

Aluminum compounds are widely distributed in nature. Despite an oral intake of 10 to 100 mg daily, little aluminum is absorbed. Absorption may be excessive, however, in uremic patients maintained on long-term hemodialysis who receive aluminum-containing antacids to decrease phosphate absorption. A few such patients develop a peculiar neurologic syndrome characterized by speech and motor abnormalities, personality changes, dementia, and psychosis, and some have died. Osteomalacia also occurs. Inhalation of fumes containing Al_20_3 causes lung damage with shortness of breath, cyanosis, substernal pain, and often spontaneous pneumothorax (Shavers disease).

Insecticides

Although pesticides are designed to kill insects and other pests, they can also kill humans. The organochlorine compounds are central nervous system stimulants that cause convulsions. They are absorbed through the skin as well as from the gastrointestinal tract.

The **cyclodiene** insecticides (for example, dieldrin and chlordane) cause seizures along with tremor, nausea, vomiting, and ataxia. Endrin is the most toxic compound in this group.

The **chlorinated ethane derivatives** are related to DDT. DDT has been largely replaced by methoxychlor, a less toxic but less effective insecticide. Sudden death from ventricular fibrillation has occurred after ingestion of these substances, caused by sensitization of the myocardium to endogenous catecholamines. In DDT poisoning, death may also result from respiratory failure secondary to medullary paralysis.

These compounds tend to accumulate in fat and induce the microsomal enzyme system.[3]

The **chlorocyclohexanes** are represented by benzene hexachloride and its γ isomer, lindane, which is used to treat pediculosis. They can induce severe convulsions as well as pulmonary edema, liver and kidney damage, and agranulocytosis. Like DDT, these substances can sensitize the myocardium. Renal and hepatic damage caused by organochlorine compounds are managed the same as when induced by other causes.

Other types of insecticides are thiocyanates, phosphate esters, organophosphate compounds (anticholinesterases), fluorides, and botanicals such as nicotine, pyrethrins, and rotenoids. For symptoms and treatment of organophosphate poisoning refer to Chapter 14.

Rodenticides

In contrast to insecticides, rodenticides are designed to kill animals that have essentially the same biochemical pathways as humans. These agents include (1) anticoagulants such as coumarins and indandiones; (2) heavy metals such as arsenicals, thallium, copper, and lead salts; (3) botanicals such as squill and strychnine; and (4) miscellaneous substances such as fluoroacetate, phosphorous, and zinc phosphide. The treatment for rodenticide poisoning depends on the poison because the substances vary in composition and actions.

Solvents

A significant number of poisonings occur from solvents used at home and in industrial settings. Lipid solvents readily cross cellular membranes. The brain is a major target organ where solvents have depressant or convulsant actions depending on the molecule. In general, aliphatic hydrocarbons induce coma; reflexes are weak or absent. Aromatic solvents tend to cause motor unrest, tremors, jactitations, and hyperactive reflexes. Chronic exposure may cause chronic neurotoxic symptoms.[8] Intentional solvent sniffing is a major form of abuse (see Chapter 34).

Toluene in many ways exemplifies the typical solvent; it is extensively used in industrial and in some household products. Toluene is the primary intoxicant in glue-sniffing. Although it replaces the more dangerous benzene as a household solvent,[11] it is a psychotropic and neurotoxic agent. Neurologic symptoms are its most frequent effects. Toluene can cause sudden death, addictive-like behavior, renal abnormalities, hepatic and hematologic illness, and an acute brain syndrome with EEG changes, visual hallucinations, confusion, and seizures. Since it accumulates in bone narrow and is only slowly eliminated, toluene exposure can also cause blood dyscrasias.

The distribution of toluene into tissues is faster after inhalation than after ingestion. Exercise enhances uptake of inhaled toluene, largely by increasing respiration and cardiac output.

Toluene is sometimes contaminated with benzene. For example, industrial-grade toluene contains as much as 25% benzene. Toluene combinations with other solvents are more toxic than would be predicted on the basis of additive toxic actions of each component alone.

REFERENCES

1. Arena JM: Poisoning, *Emerg Med* 8(4):171, 1976.
2. Arena JM: *Poisoning: toxicology, symptoms, treatments*, ed 4, Springfield, Ill, 1979, Charles C Thomas, Publisher.
3. Bayer MJ, Rumack BH: *Poisoning and overdose*, Rockville, Md, 1983, Aspen Systems Corp.
4. Bryson PD: *Comprehensive review in toxicology*, Rockville, Md, 1986, Aspen Systems Corp.
5. Goldfrank LR: Overview: general management and diagnostic tools. In Goldfrank LR, Flomenbaum NE, Lewin NA, Weisman RS, Howland MA, editors: *Goldfrank's toxicologic emergencies*, ed 4, Norwalk, Conn, 1990, Appleton & Lange, p 3.
6. Goldfrank LR, Osborn H, Hartnett L: Lead. In Goldfrank LR, Flomenbaum NE, Lewin NA, Weisman RS, Howland MA, editors: *Goldfrank's toxicologic emergencies*, ed 4, Norwalk, Conn, 1990, Appleton & Lange, p 627.
7. Gonzales J, Sabatini S: Cyanide poisoning: pathophysiology and current approaches to therapy, *Int J Artif Organs* 12:347, 1989.
8. Gregersen P: Neurotoxic effects of organic solvents in exposed workers: two controlled follow-up studies after 5.5 and 10.6 years, *Am J Ind Med* 14:681, 1988.
9. Ilano AL, Raffin TA: Management of carbon monoxide poisoning, *Chest* 97:165, 1990.
10. Jacobsen D, McMartin KE: Methanol and ethylene glycol poisonings: mechanism of toxicity, clinical course, diagnosis and treatment, *Med Toxicol* 1:309, 1986.
11. Klaassen CD, Amdur MO, Doull J: *Casarett and Doull's toxicology: the basic science of poisons*, ed 3, New York, 1986, Macmillan Publishing Co.
12. Lewander WJ, Lacouture PG: Office management of acute pediatric poisonings, *Pediatr Emerg Care* 5:262, 1989.
13. Li PKT, Lai KN: Active therapeutic approaches to drug intoxication, *Adverse Drug React Acute Poisoning Rev* 2:55, 1988.
14. Litovitz TL, Schmitz BF, Bailey KM: 1989 Annual report of the American Association of Poison Control Centers National Data Collection System, *Am J Emerg Med* 8:394, 1990.
15. Mann KV, Picciotti MA, Spevack TA, Durbin DR: Management of acute iron overdose, *Clin Pharm* 8:428, 1989.
16. Needleman HL: The persistent threat of lead: medical and sociological issues, *Curr Probl Pediatr* 18:703, 1988.
17. Neuvonen PJ, Olkkola KT: Oral activated charcoal in the treatment of intoxications: role of single and repeated doses, *Med Toxicol* 3:33, 1988.
18. Porter GA: The treatment of ethylene glycol poisoning simplified, *N Engl J Med* 319:109, 1988.
19. Winchester JF: Poisoning: is the role of the nephrologist diminishing? *Am J Kidney Dis* 13:171, 1989.
20. Vennesland B, Castric PA, Conn EE, et al: Cyanide metabolism, *Fed Proc* 41:2639, 1982.

section thirteen

Drug interactions

Chapter 70

Drug interactions

When several drugs are administered concurrently, they may influence each other favorably or unfavorably. Drug interactions may be of great clinical importance when the margin of safety of one or more of the drugs is small. The interactions present as either an enhanced or diminished drug effect. Enhanced drug effects may manifest themselves as idiosyncratic responses that can occasionally have dire consequences. Some estimate that up to 10% of all hospitalizations (particularly in elderly patients) are due to drug interactions, many, if not most, of which are avoidable. The clinically significant drug interactions can be minimized by avoidance of combinations of drugs known to be incompatible, according to current pharmacologic literature and tables such as those presented in this chapter. Ultimately, however, it is the physician's familiarity with the clinical literature and understanding of the mechanisms underlying drug interactions that are most likely to prevent their occurrence.

MECHANISMS UNDERLYING ADVERSE EFFECTS OF DRUG INTERACTIONS

Adverse drug interactions may be divided into *pharmacokinetic* and *pharmacodynamic* interactions.[1,2,4,5] The pharmacokinetic interactions may be at the level of (1) absorption, (2) distribution, (3) metabolism, or (4) excretion. Pharmacodynamic interactions influence the response to a drug once it reaches its site of action and may occur at the receptor site, may alter response by changing the physiologic milieu, and so forth.

Intestinal absorption

Drug interactions involving absorption are presented in Table 70-1. Important examples include calcium-, magnesium- or aluminum-containing antacids that interfere with absorption of tetracycline, which forms a chelate with the metals. Antacids containing aluminum also interfere with phosphate absorption. Carbonates and phytates (cereals) prevent absorption of iron. Cholestyramine and colestipol (bile acid–binding resins) may interfere with absorption of many drugs, particularly warfarin and digitalis glycosides.

Antacids may also influence drug absorption by pH-related changes in the lipid-soluble, nonionized fraction of weak acids in the gastrointestinal tract. Recall from p. 34 that the nonionized moiety is much better absorbed from the stomach (as opposed to the small intestine where pH-dependent lipid solubility appears to play a lesser role). Because of this, antacids would be expected to diminish gastric absorption of weak acids. Absorption from the small intestine would not be affected. In addition, some drugs such as ketoconazole require an acidic environment to dissolve and then to

TABLE 70-1 Drug interactions at sites of absorption

Proposed mechanism	Drug affected	Drug causing effect	Results of interaction
Formation of complexes, chelation, adsorption	Atenolol	Antacids	Decreased absorption
	Bishydroxycoumarin	Antacids	Increased absorption
	Captopril	Antacids	Decreased absorption
	Carbamazepine	Activated charcoal	Decreased absorption, increased elimination
	Cephalexin	Cholestyramine	Decreased absorption
	Chlorothiazide	Cholestyramine	Decreased absorption
	Chlorpromazine	Antacids	Decreased absorption
	Ciprofloxacin (and other quinolone antibiotics)	Al^{+++}- or Mg^{++}-containing antacids, including sucralfate	Decreased absorption
	Diflunisal	Antacids	Decreased absorption
	Digitoxin	Cholestyramine	Decreased absorption, increased elimination
	Digoxin	Activated charcoal, antacids, cholestyramine, kaolin-pectin	Decreased absorption
	Isoniazid	Antacids	Decreased absorption
	Methyldopa	Oral iron	Decreased absorption
	Penicillamine	Antacids	Decreased absorption
	Phenobarbital	Activated charcoal	Decreased absorption, increased elimination
	Phenylbutazone	Cholestyramine	Decreased absorption
	Phenytoin	Activated charcoal	Decreased absorption
	Piroxicam	Activated charcoal	Increased elimination
	Propranolol	Antacids, cholestyramine	Decreased absorption
	Quinine	Activated charcoal	Increased elimination
	Ranitidine	Antacids	Decreased absorption
	Tenoxicam	Cholestyramine	Increased elimination
	Tetracyclines	Antacids	Decreased absorption
	Theophylline	Activated charcoal	Decreased absorption, increased elimination
	Thyroxine	Cholestyramine	Decreased absorption
	Tolbutamide	Activated charcoal	Decreased absorption
	Valproate	Activated charcoal	Decreased absorption
	Warfarin	Cholestyramine	Decreased absorption, increased elimination
Alteration in gastric pH	Cimetidine	Antacids	Decreased absorption
	Ketoconazole	Antacids, histamine H_2-antagonists, omeprazole	Decreased absorption
	Tetracyclines	Cimetidine, sodium bicarbonate	Decreased absorption

Continued.

TABLE 70-1 Drug interactions at sites of absorption—cont'd

Proposed mechanism	Drug affected	Drug causing effect	Results of interaction
Alteration in gastric motility			
Increase	Acetaminophen	Metoclopramide	Increased rate of absorption
	Chlorothiazide	Metoclopramide	Increased rate of absorption
	Cimetidine	Metoclopramide	Decreased absorption
	Digoxin	Metoclopramide	Decreased absorption
	Ethanol	Metoclopramide	Increased rate of absorption
	Lithium	Metoclopramide	Increased rate of absorption
Decrease	Acetaminophen	Opioid analgesics, propantheline	Decreased rate of absorption
	Benzodiazepines	Antacids	Decreased rate of absorption
	Bishydroxycoumarin	Amitriptyline	Increased absorption
	Chlorothiazide	Propantheline	Decreased rate of absorption
	Digoxin	Propantheline	Increased absorption
	Ethanol	Propantheline	Decreased rate of absorption
	Isoniazid	Antacids	Decreased rate of absoprtion
	Lithium ion	Propantheline	Decreased rate of absorption
	Phenytoin	Antacids	Decreased rate of absorption
	Propranolol	Antacids	Decreased rate of absorption
Effects on gastrointestinal mucosa	Aminoglycoside antibiotics	Ethanol	Increased absorption caused by mucosal damage
	Digoxin	Neomycin, sulfasalazine	Decreased absorption
	Furosemide	Phenytoin	Decreased absorption
Effects on gastrointestinal flora	Digoxin	Broad-spectrum antibiotics	Increased absorption
Alteration of gut or first-pass hepatic metabolism			
Induction	Cyclosporine	Carbamazepine, phenobarbital, rifampin, phenytoin	Decreased absorption
Inhibition	Cyclosporine	Erythromycin, ketoconazole	Increased absorption
	Mercaptopurine	Allopurinol, methotrexate	Increased absorption
	Felodipine, imipramine, labetalol, lidocaine, metoprolol, nisoldipine, propranolol, verapamil	Cimetidine	Increased absorption

be absorbed; antacids or other drugs that reduce gastric acidity can prevent their absorption.

Other gastrointestinal drug interactions may be of clinical significance. Antibiotics that alter the bacterial flora in the intestine can decrease formation of vitamin K and thus increase the anticoagulant action of the coumarins. Similarly, in about 10% of patients gut bacteria metabolize digoxin, decreasing its availability. Certain antibiotics can eliminate the responsible flora and thereby increase the bioavailability of digoxin. Some drugs, such as phenytoin and triamterene, inhibit an intestinal conjugase that breaks down the polyglutamate portion of naturally occurring folic acid and, by this mechanism, can cause megaloblastic anemia.

Direct chemical interactions occur not only in the gastrointestinal tract but also when drugs are mixed for intravenous infusions. For example, carbenicillin and other ureidopenicillins inactivate aminoglycosides if mixed for intravenous infusion.

Distribution

Many drugs are bound to plasma proteins to varying degrees, and the bound fraction fails to exert pharmacologic actions. For example, two antibiotics having the same potency in a protein-free culture medium will have different clinical effectiveness if their affinities for plasma proteins differ greatly. The most important adverse drug interactions caused by displacement from plasma proteins occur with the coumarin anticoagulants (Table 70-2). Although in general the increase in concentration of free drug is expected to be transient, in many instances the displacer inhibits drug metabolism as well. For example, phenylbutazone displaces warfarin from its binding sites and also inhibits its metabolism and may thereby cause bleeding.

Displacement of tolbutamide from plasma binding by dicumarol can result in severe hypoglycemia. Chloral hydrate transiently increases the anticoagulant action of warfarin because its metabolite, trichloroacetic acid, competes with the anticoagulant for plasma protein binding.

Metabolism or biotransformation

Inhibition of the metabolism of one drug by another is a well-established mechanism of enhanced drug effect (Table 70-3). By their enzyme-inhibiting action, the anticholinesterases enhance the effects of acetylcholine, succinylcholine, and some other choline esters. Allopurinol inhibits xanthine oxidase and thus increases plasma

TABLE 70-2 Drug interactions caused by displacement from plasma protein-binding sites

Drug displaced	Causative agents
Coumarin anticoagulants	Chloral hydrate, clofibrate, diazoxide, ethacrynic acid, mefenamic acid, nalidixic acid, phenytoin, NSAIDs including salicylate
Diazepam	Heparin, valproic acid
Phenytoin	NSAIDs including salicylate, tolbutamide, valproic acid
Tolbutamide	Phenylbutazone, salicylates, dicumarol
Valproic acid	Salicylate

TABLE 70-3 Examples of drugs that inhibit hepatic metabolism of other drugs

Drug causing inhibition	Drugs inhibited
Acetaminophen	Fenoldopam (competition for sulfation)
Amiodarone	Digoxin, flecainide, metoprolol, phenytoin, procainamide, quinidine, warfarin
Bishydroxycoumarin	Tolbutamide
Calcium-channel blockers: verapamil > diltiazem; no effect, dihydropyridines	Carbamazepine, cyclosporine, metoprolol, propranolol, quinidine, theophylline
Chloramphenicol	Carbamazepine, chlorpropamide, oral anticoagulants, phenobarbital, phenytoin, tolbutamide
Chlorpromazine	Phenytoin, propranolol
Cimetidine = etintidine (negligible effect of famotidine, nizatidine, ranitidine, roxatidine)	Benzodiazepines, carbamazepine, chloroquine, desipramine, 5-fluorouracil, imipramine, lidocaine, meperidine, metoprolol, metronidazole, moricizine, nifedipine, pentoxifylline, phenytoin, piroxicam, propranolol, quinidine, theophylline, urapidil, verapamil
Disulfiram	Benzodiazepines, phenytoin, theophylline, warfarin
Erythromycin	Alfentanil, bromocriptine, carbamazepine, cyclosporine, theophylline
Ethanol (acute ingestion)	Diazepam, meprobamate, pentobarbital, phenytoin, tolbutamide, warfarin
Flecainide (inhibition of P-450 IID6)	Propranolol
Fluconazole	Chlorpropamide, glipizide, glyburide, phenytoin, tolbutamide
Fluoxetine	Diazepam
Isoniazid	Carbamazepine, haloperidol, phenytoin
Ketoconazole	Chlordiazepoxide, cyclosporine, methylprednisolone, prednisolone, terfenadine
Methylphenidate	Phenobarbital, phenytoin, primidone
Omeprazole	Diazepam, phenytoin
Oral contraceptives	Alprazolam, caffeine, chlordiazepoxide, cyclosporine, diazepam, imipramine, nitrazepam, oral anticoagulants, prednisolone, theophylline
Oxyphenbutazone	Phenytoin, tolbutamide, warfarin
Phenylbutazone	Phenytoin, tolbutamide, warfarin
Probenecid	Zidovudine (AZT, decreased glucuronidation)
Propafenone	Metoprolol, warfarin
Propoxyphene	Carbamazepine, doxepin, phenytoin
Propranolol	Diazepam, flecainide, lidocaine, nifedipine, nisoldipine
Quinidine (specifically inhibits P-450 IID6)	Desipramine, imipramine, propafenone, propranolol
Quinolone antibiotics: enoxacin > ciprofloxacin = pefloxacin; no effect, ofloxacin and norfloxacin	Caffeine, theophylline, inactive enantiomer of warfarin (so no effect on hemostasis)
Sulfonamides	Carbamazepine, phenytoin, tolbutamide, warfarin
Tamoxifen	Warfarin
Ticlopidine	Theophylline
Valproic acid	Epoxide hydrolase for carbamazepine-10, 11-epoxide, the active metabolite of carbamazepine

concentrations of mercaptopurine and azathioprine. Monoamine oxidase inhibitors have caused severe reactions by preventing destruction of catecholamines in the body. Cimetidine and some quinolone antibiotics halve the clearance of some drugs with narrow therapeutic margins, such as warfarin and theophylline. In some instances a drug may diminish hepatic blood flow and inhibit drug metabolism by that mechanism. In this way β-adrenergic receptor blocking agents raise lidocaine concentrations.

Many drugs can accelerate their own metabolism and also that of other drugs by induction of hepatic microsomal enzymes (Table 70-4). Phenobarbital accelerates metabolism of hydrocortisone, estrogens, androgens, progesterone, and many other agents. Phenobarbital combined with phenytoin greatly increases the clearance of quinidine, probably as a consequence of enzyme induction. Other agents that induce hepatic metabolism include glutethimide, phenytoin, rifampin, and chlorinated hydrocarbon insecticides, such as DDT.

Enzyme induction decreases the effectiveness of certain other drugs and may have life-threatening consequences if the inducer is discontinued without changing the dosage of the second drug. For example, if phenobarbital is suddenly discontinued without lowering the dosage of a coumarin anticoagulant, severe hemorrhagic episodes may develop.

TABLE 70-4 Examples of drugs that induce hepatic metabolism of other drugs

Inducing agent	Drug induced
Carbamazepine	Cyclosporine, haloperidol, oral anticoagulants, phenytoin, valproic acid
Cigarette smoking	Theophylline
Ethanol (chronic, before hepatic impairment)	Meprobamate, oral anticoagulants, pentobarbital, phenytoin, tolbutamide
Glutethimide	Oral anticoagulants
Griseofulvin	Oral anticoagulants
Isoniazid	Acetaminophen (increasing formation of toxic metabolite)
Moricizine	Theophylline
Oral contraceptives	Glucuronidation of acetaminophen, clofibrate, diflunisal, morphine, salicylate, temazepam
Phenobarbital	Chloramphenicol, chlorpromazine, cimetidine, cyclosporine, digitoxin, disopyramide, griseofulvin, oral anticoagulants, oral contraceptives, phenylbutazone, phenytoin, theophylline, verapamil
Phenytoin	Carbamazepine, clonazepam, cyclosporine, diazepam, digitoxin, doxycycline, glucocorticoids, methadone, oral anticoagulants, oral contraceptives, pancuronium, quinidine, theophylline, valproic acid
Rifampin	Chloramphenicol, cyclosporine, diazepam, digitoxin, digoxin, fluconazole, glucocorticoids, haloperidol, oral anticoagulants, oral contraceptives, quinidine, theophylline, tolbutamide
Vigabatrin	Phenytoin

Renal excretion

There are several examples of drug interactions resulting from an influence on renal tubular excretion of drugs. The best is the inhibition of penicillin secretion by probenecid. A variety of organic acids and organic bases (Table 70-5) can compete with each other for renal secretion.

Acidification of the urine after oral administration of ammonium chloride or alkalinization with sodium bicarbonate may have a demonstrable effect on renal clearance of several drugs, but the quantitative importance is not great except in phenobarbital or salicylate intoxication. The excretion of amphetamine is greatly decreased in a relatively alkaline urine. However, since the urine is normally acidic, this phenomenon becomes important only in unusual circumstances.

Another important renal drug interaction involves interruption of secretion of digoxin by quinidine, amiodarone, verapamil, spironolactone, or cyclosporine.[3] These drugs reduce distal tubular secretion of digoxin, thus increasing digoxin concentration in the plasma. In addition, quinidine decreases the volume of distribution of digoxin, probably by reducing the binding of digoxin in muscle.

Pharmacodynamic interactions

Numerous pharmacodynamic interactions take place at the receptor level. Innumerable synergisms and antagonisms discussed throughout the text are examples of pharmacodynamic interactions. Representative examples are also presented in Table 70-6. These interactions may be at the same receptor or at different receptors.

TABLE 70-5 Agents actively secreted by the proximal renal tubules

Organic acids	Organic bases
Acetazolamide	Acecainide (*N*-acetylprocainamide)
p-Aminohippurate	Amantadine
Captopril	Amiloride
Cephalosporins (most)	Cimetidine
Ciprofloxacin	Ethambutol
Dyphylline	Flecainide
Heparin	Mecamylamine
"Loop" diuretics	Mepacrine
Methotrexate	Metformin
Nonsteroidal anti-inflammatory agents that form acyl-glucuronide metabolites (carprofen, diflunisal, indomethacin, ketoprofen)	*N*-Methylnicotinamide
	Procainamide
	Pseudoephedrine
	Tetraethylammonium
Penicillins	Triamterene
Probenecid	Trimethoprim
Salicylates	
Sulfonamides	
Sulfonylureas	
Thiazide diuretics	

Significance of adverse drug reactions

Some drug interactions among those listed in Tables 70-1 to 70-6 may be life threatening, whereas others are relatively less important and require only a simple adjustment in the dosage. A major determinant of the seriousness of an interaction is the therapeutic margin of the drugs involved. With anticoagulants, anticonvulsants, oral hypoglycemic drugs, digitalis, and antiarrhythmic agents, the margin of safety is not great, and relatively small changes in plasma concentration resulting from drug interactions can have catastrophic results. On the other hand, drugs with large margins of safety do not cause serious problems as a consequence of drug interactions. This principle should be kept in mind when one is examining tables of drug interactions.

TABLE 70-6 Examples of pharmacodynamic drug interactions

Drug or condition altering response	Drug with altered response	Comments
Amiodarone	β-Blockers, calcium antagonists	Increased cardiac toxicity
	Anesthetics	α-Blockade enhances hypotensive effect
Acidemia	Sympathomimetics	Decreased effect
Aminoglycoside antibiotics	Neuromuscular blockers	Increased effect
β-Adrenergic receptor antagonists	Clonidine	Blood pressure overshoot during withdrawal
Chlorpromazine	Captopril	Hypotension, especially postural
Digitalis	β-Blockers	Profound bradycardia
Diuretics	Antihypertensives	Increased effect
Guanidinium antihypertensives	Directly acting α-receptor agonists	Increased effect
HMG CoA-reductase inhibitors (lovastatin)	Fibric acid derivatives (clofibrate, gemfibrozil)	Myopathy, rhabdomyolysis
Hypercalcemia	Cardiac glycosides	Increased toxicity
Inhibitors of prostaglandin synthesis	Captopril	Decreased effect
	Lithium ion	Increased renal reabsorption, increased plasma concentration
	"Loop" diuretics	Predominately decreased effect
	Propranolol	Decreased antihypertensive effect
Magnesium depletion	Cardiac glycosides	Increased toxicity
Methyldopa	Haloperidol	Dementia
Phenytoin	Lithium ion	Increased effect
Potassium depletion	Cardiac glycosides	Increased toxicity
Reserpine	Indirectly acting α-receptor agonists	Decreased effect
Tricyclic antidepressants	Directly and indirectly acting α-receptor agonists	Increased effect
	Guanidinium antihypertensives	Decreased effect
	Clonidine	Decreased effect

REFERENCES

1. Hansten PD: *Drug interactions*, ed 5, Philadelphia, 1985, Lea & Febiger.
2. McInnes GT, Brodie MJ: Drug interactions that matter: a critical reappraisal, *Drugs* 36:83, 1988.
3. Rodin SM, Johnson BF: Pharmacokinetic interactions with digoxin, *Clin Pharmacokinet* 15:227, 1988.
4. Tatro DS, Olin BR, Hebel SK, editors: *Drug interaction facts*, ed 2, St Louis, 1990, JB Lippincott Co.
5. Vasko MR, Brater DC: Drug interactions. In Chernow B, editor: *The pharmacologic approach to the critically ill patient*, ed 2, Baltimore, 1988, Williams & Wilkins, p 21.

section fourteen

Prescription writing and drug compendia

Chapter 71

Prescription writing and drug compendia

PRESCRIPTION WRITING

A prescription is a written order given by a physician to a pharmacist.[2] In addition to the Prescription writing and drug compendianame of the patient and that of the physician, the prescription should contain the name or names of the drugs ordered and their quantities, instructions to the pharmacist, and directions to the patient.

Prescription writing has changed in modern medicine as a result of several developments. Most preparations today are compounded by pharmaceutical companies, and the pharmacist's current roles in most cases are dispensing and advising patients as to precautions they should take, potential drug interactions, and adverse reactions. Also, the practice of writing long, complicated prescriptions containing many active ingredients, adjuvants, correctives, and various vehicles has been abandoned in favor of pure compounds. Even when combinations of several active ingredients are desirable, they are still provided by pharmaceutical companies. Although convenient, the custom of prescribing trademarked mixtures has the disadvantage that the physician may be so accustomed to prescribing a mixture of drugs by a trade name that he becomes uncertain about the individual components, some of which may be unnecessary or undesirable in a given case. Physicians should be cautious to avoid this pitfall.

A drug may be prescribed by its official name, which is listed in the *United States Pharmacopoeia* (*USP*), by its nonproprietary (often called "generic") name or *United States Adopted Name* (*USAN*), or by a manufacturer's trade name.[1] The designation USAN has been coined for generic or nonproprietary names adopted by the American Medical Association–United States Pharmacopoeia Nomenclature Committee in cooperation with the respective manufacturers. Adoption of USAN names does not imply endorsement by these organizations.

There is considerable advantage to prescribing drugs by their official or nonproprietary names. This often allows the pharmacist to dispense a more economical product than a trademarked preparation of one company (so-called generic substitution). It also reduces the expense of each pharmacy's maintaining a multiplicity of very similar preparations, a saving that could ultimately benefit the patient. Whether there is a cost in terms of decreased drug efficacy or increased toxicity is unclear. The outcome of this debate should be of great interest in medical economics.

On the other hand, the physician may have reasons for prescribing one manufacturer's product. This is often the only way to be certain that the preparation given to the patient will be what is intended, not only in its active ingredients but even to the point of its appearance and taste.

Approval of a generic formulation by the Food and Drug Administration (FDA) requires demonstration of "bioequivalence." This has been defined in regulatory terms as the generic drug's absorption differing no more than a defined percentage (from 20% to 30% depending on the therapeutic margin of the drug) from the brand-name product. This means, for example, that a product may have from 80% to 120% absorption compared to the standard. If an individual manufacturer's product is consistent in this regard, substitution of a generic formulation for the brand-name product may cause no problems. However, if a patient's pharmacy switches from a product with 80% absorption to one with 120% of the bioavailability of the standard or vice versa, problems could conceivably ensue. Physicians and patients should be alert to this potential.

Parts of a prescription

Traditionally a prescription is written in a certain order and consists of four basic parts:

1. *Superscription.* This is simply *Rx*, the abbreviation for *recipe*, meaning "take thou," the imperative of *recipere*.
2. *Inscription.* This indicates the ingredients and their amounts. If a prescription contains several ingredients in a mixture, it is customary to write them in the following order: (1) the basis, or principal ingredient, (2) the adjuvant, which may contribute to the action of the basis, and (3) the corrective, which may eliminate some undesirable property of the active drug or the vehicle, which is the substance used for dilution. Today this part of the prescription is usually simply the drug name, preferably nonproprietary.
3. *Subscription.* This contains directions for dispensing. Often it consists only of *M.*, the abbreviation for *misce*, meaning "mix (thou)." This section rarely appears today.
4. *Signature.* This is often abbreviated as *Sig.* and contains the directions to the patient, such as "Take one teaspoonful three times a day before meals." It is also helpful to include the indication for the medication, for example, "for ulcers." Whenever possible, instructions of a general nature, such as "take as directed," should be avoided, since the patient may misunderstand or forget oral directions given by the physician.

In addition to these basic parts of a prescription, it should have the patient's name and the physician's signature, followed by the prescriber's degree. The current trend is that the physician may sign his or her name in one of two places to designate whether generic substitution is permitted. Some state laws require that if substitution is to be *prohibited*, the physician must actually write "dispense as written" or a similar phrase.

Modern trends in prescription writing

The parts of the prescription described in the previous paragraphs represent a tradition that is undergoing considerable change. Latin, even in the form of abbreviations, is not necessary. Its main purpose in the past was to conceal from the patient the nature (and often worthlessness) of a drug. At the present time, prescriptions are written in English. Even such abbreviations as *M.* or *Sig.* may be avoided. It is also advisable to avoid the use of the decimal point and to state the number of milligrams in a dose instead of using the decimal fraction of a gram.

Much confusion results when the name of a drug is not included on the label so that a patient knows only its physical characteristics, for example, a green tablet. A critical component of good practice is that the physician be cognizant of all drugs that a patient is taking. Accordingly, physicians should ask the pharmacist to name the drug on the label, indicating their wish by checking an appropriate box on the prescription form. They also indicate in another area the number of allowable refills.

Prescriptions and the Federal Controlled Substances Act

Prescriptions for drugs with abuse potential are regulated by the Federal Drug Enforcement Administration (DEA). The drugs controlled by the act are placed in five categories, or schedules (Table 71-1).

All prescriptions for controlled drugs (schedules II to V) must contain the full name and address of the patient, full name, address, and DEA number of the prescribing doctor, signature of the prescribing doctor, and date. Prescriptions for schedule II drugs are not refillable. Schedules III and IV drugs may be refilled up to five times within 6 months of initial issuance if so authorized by the prescribing physician. Prescriptions for schedule V drugs may be refilled as authorized by the prescribing physician.

Typical prescription

John Doe, M.D.
555 Medical Arts Building
City
Telephone: 361-4282

Name David Smith — *Date* May 9, 1992

Address 201 Hall St. — *Age* 42

Tetracycline, 250 mg capsules
Dispense twenty
Label: Take one capsule four times a day for 5 days

Signature:

Refills ________ *Dispense as written* ________

DEA No. ________ *Substitution permitted* ________

DRUG COMPENDIA

Authoritative information on drugs can be found in the *United States Pharmacopoeia* as well as in many textbooks of pharmacology. The *United States Pharmacopoeia* was first published in 1820 and became official in 1906, when it was so designated by the first Food and Drug Act. The *United States Pharmacopoeia* is revised by physicians, pharmacists, and medical scientists who are elected by delegates to the United States Pharmacopoeial Convention. The delegates originate from schools of medicine and pharmacy, from medical and pharmaceutical societies, and from some departments of the government. Its current official position is based on the Federal Food, Drug,

TABLE 71-1 Criteria for scheduling drugs

	Schedule I	Schedule II	Schedule III	Schedule IV	Schedule V
Potential for abuse	+ + + +	+ + + +	+ + +	+ +	+
Accepted medical use in U.S.	None	Yes, with severe restrictions	Yes	Yes	Yes
Potential dependence					
Psychologic	+ + + +	+ + + +	+ + +	+ +	+
Physical	+ + + +	+ + + +	+ +	+ +	+
Examples	Heroin LSD Marijuana MDA Methaqualone Phencyclidine	Amphetamine Cocaine Codeine Dronabinol Methadone Morphine Pentobarbital Phenmetrazine	Codeine combinations Glutethimide Phendimetrazine	Diazepam Flurazepam Pentazocine Phentermine Propoxyphene*	Antitussive preparations with codeine Buprenorphine Diphenoxylate combinations

LSD, Lysergic acid diethylamide; *MDA,* 3,4-methylenedioxyamphetamine.
*Bulk chemical in Schedule II.

and Cosmetic Act of 1938, which recognizes it as an "official compendium." The *United States Pharmacopoeia* is published every 5 years. For a drug to be included there must be good evidence for its therapeutic merit or its pharmaceutical necessity.

AMA Drug Evaluations is a valuable source of information, published about every 3 years, on most drugs that are available in the United States. It is particularly useful in describing currently accepted therapeutic practices and available preparations.

If physicians could limit their use of drugs to those that are listed in the *United States Pharmacopoeia* or those that have been recommended by *AMA Drug Evaluations*, they would be protected against unfounded claims or the power of advertising. When a new drug represents a therapeutic advance, physicians may be unable to wait for such authoritative reviews. They must often rely on written or verbal statements of recognized experts in the field. In any case, they should not depend solely on advertising literature or drug circulars and package inserts (including the *Physicians' Desk Reference*, or *PDR*).

REFERENCES

1. Cutting W: A note on names, Clin Pharmacol Ther 4:569, 1963.
2. Friend DG: Principles and practices of prescription writing, Clin Pharmacol Ther 6:411, 1965.

Appendixes

Appendix A

Drug concentrations in blood

The concentration of drugs in the blood is of interest in clinical medicine and medicolegal situations. The tabular presentation of drug concentrations in the blood on pp. 767 to 772 is intended as a source of information and as a guide to the available literature. It should be recognized that the figures given are often based on a few cases and are subject to change as more information accumulates. Furthermore, the significance of blood concentrations depends on numerous factors, and the tables should be consulted with full recognition of the role of modifying influences.

IMPORTANCE OF DRUG CONCENTRATIONS IN SERUM

The determination of drug concentrations in serum is not important when the pharmacologic effects of the drug can easily be monitored. For example, in the use of coumarin anticoagulants or antihypertensive agents the effects of the drugs (assessed as prothrombin time or blood pressure, respectively) provide a good indication of adequacy of serum concentrations and dosage. On the other hand, there are drugs such as anticonvulsants that are used prophylactically and provide therapeutic problems in the absence of knowledge of their serum concentrations. Studies have demonstrated that the correlation of serum concentration of these drugs with response is closer than the correlation of dose to response.[1,2] The determination of concentrations in the serum is also useful for revealing noncompliance with the physician's instructions.

The relationship between serum concentration and a drug's effects is complicated by numerous factors such as (1) tolerance, (2) drug interactions, (3) the underlying disease, (4) protein binding, and (5) active metabolites. The first three factors in modifying the relationship between concentration and effect are easily understood. The importance of the latter two is not always appreciated.

The role of protein binding is illustrated by the following problem.

PROBLEM A. *The therapeutic concentration of phenytoin is 20 mg/L. It is about 95% bound to plasma albumin. In the case of uremia, hypoalbuminemia, or the presence of other drugs that displace phenytoin from its binding sites, the bound fraction can decrease to 90%. What will be the effect on the free drug fraction and the potential toxicity of phenytoin? If the total phenytoin concentration in the plasma is reported to be 20 mg/L, the free fraction will now be 2 mg/L, which is twice the concentration with normal albumin binding and could be toxic.*[3]

The complicating effect of active metabolites is demonstrated in the case of procainamide. This drug is metabolized to *N*-acetylprocainamide, which also has antiarrhythmic activity. Hence the serum concentration of procainamide alone may not reflect the overall antiarrhythmic effect.

DEFINITION OF BLOOD CONCENTRATIONS

therapeutic blood concentration The concentration of drug in blood, serum, or plasma after therapeutically effective dosage in humans. The values in Table A-1 are generally those reported with oral administration of the drug. Only agents for which monitoring is clinically necessary or at least useful are included.

toxic blood concentration The concentration of drug in blood, serum, or plasma that is associated with serious toxic symptoms in humans (Table A-2).

lethal blood concentration The concentration of drug in blood, serum, or plasma that has been reported to cause death or is so far above therapeutic or merely toxic concentrations that it would be expected to cause death in humans (Table A-2).

• • •

The following tables give the therapeutic, toxic, and lethal blood concentrations of a large number of drugs.

TABLE A-1 Therapeutic drug concentrations (μg/ml)*

	Peak	Steady state average	Trough
Antiarrhythmics			
N-Acetylprocainamide		10-25	
Amiodarone		1-2.5	
Bretylium		0.5-3	
Cibenzoline		0.2-0.4	
Disopyramide		2-6	
Flecainide		0.2-1	
Lidocaine		1.5-6	
Mexiletine		0.7-2	
Moricizine		0.5-1	
Procainamide		4-12	
Propafenone		0.5-3	
Quinidine		2-6	
Sotalol		4	
Tocainide		3-12	
Antibiotics			
Amikacin	20-25		<5
Chloramphenicol		10-20	
Gentamicin	5-8		<2
Kanamycin	20-25		<5
Netilmicin	5-8		<2
Tobramycin	5-8		<2
Vancomycin	20-25		<5
Antiepileptic agents			
Carbamazepine		6-12	
Clonazepam		0.013-0.072	

*Ranges may vary among different laboratories because of different assay methods.

Continued.

TABLE A-1 Therapeutic drug concentrations (μg/ml) – cont'd

	Peak	Steady state average	Trough
Ethosuximide		40-100	
Methsuximide		10-40	
Phenobarbital		15-35	
Phenytoin		10-20	
Primidone		6-12	
Valproate		50-100	
Psychotherapeutic agents			
Amitriptyline		0.12-0.25	
Chlordiazepoxide		0.5-5	
Chlorpromazine		0.05-0.3	
Clomipramine		0.1-0.25	
Desipramine		0.1-0.25	
Diazepam		0.1-0.25	
Imipramine		0.15-0.75	
Haloperidol		0.004-0.025	
Lithium ion		0.5-1.5 mEq/L	
Nortriptyline		0.025-0.2	
Protriptyline		0.07-0.17	
Miscellaneous			
Aspirin (salicylate)			
Antipyretic, analgesic		20-100	
Anti-inflammatory		100-250	
Cyclosporin A (cyclosporine)		0.2-0.4	
Digitoxin		0.01-0.03	
Digoxin		0.0008-0.002	
Theophylline		10-20	

TABLE A-2 Toxic and lethal blood concentrations*

Compound	Toxic concentrations (mg/L)†	Lethal concentrations (mg/L)
Acetaminophen	30-300	>160
Acetone	200-300	550
Alprazolam	0.12-0.39	
Aminophylline	>20	50-250
Amitriptyline	0.5-3.4	2-20
Amobarbital	8-21	13-96
Amoxapine	>0.2	>0.6
Amphetamine	>0.1	0.5-41
Arsenic	1	9-15
Atropine		0.2
Barbital	60-80	>100
Benzene	>0	0.94
Benztropine	0.05	0.7
Boron (boric acid)	40	50
Bromide	500-1500	2000
Brompheniramine	>0.05	>1
Caffeine	>40	79-181
Carbamazepine	20-60	
Carbon monoxide	15%-35% (saturation of hemoglobin)	50%
Carbon tetrachloride	20-50	100-200
Carisoprodol	>30	>100
Chloral hydrate (see trichloroethanol)		
Chlordane	0.0025	1.7-4
Chlordiazepoxide	5-60	>20
Chloroform	60-182	390
Chlorpromazine	>0.5	3-35
Chlorpropamide	200-750	
Chlorprothixene	>0.2	
Chloroquine	>0.6	3-16
Clonazepam	>0.6	
Cocaine	0.9	1-20
Codeine	0.5	1.4-5.6
Copper	5.4	2.5-63
Cyanide	0.1-2.2	>5
Cyclizine	0.76	15
Desipramine	>0.5	5-20
Dextromethorphan		>3
Diazepam	>5	>20
Diazinon	>0	200

Sources: Winek CL: *Drug & chemical blood-level data 1989,* Pittsburgh, Pa, 1988, Fisher Scientific. Garriott JC: *Interpretation of 119 drug concentrations in blood,* San Antonio. 1990, Bexar County Medical Examiner's Office. *Garriott JC: Interpretation of chemical concentrations in blood,* San Antonio, 1990, Bexar County Medical Examiner's Office.

*The values listed are mostly derived from actual blood assays. The upper range of toxic concentrations may be greater than the listed lethal concentrations because of variation in individual sensitivity or intervening therapy, or both.

†The current convention of toxicologists is to express concentrations as mg/L, which is the same as μg/ml and parts per million.

Continued.

TABLE A-2 Toxic and lethal blood concentrations—cont'd

Compound	Toxic concentrations (mg/L)	Lethal concentrations (mg/L)
Dicumarol	>22	
Dicyclomine	>0.5	
Dieldrin	0.15-0.3	
Digitoxin		0.32
DIgoxin	0.0021	0.015
Diphenhydramine	>1	>8
Disopyramide	3	>20
Doxepin	>0.14	0.7-29
Ethanol (see ethyl alcohol)		
Ethosuximide	150	250
Ethyl alcohol	800-1000 (legal)	>3500
Ethyl ether	90	1400-1890
Ethylene glycol	>0	2000-4000
Fenfluramine	0.2-0.9	6-15
Fentanyl	0.02	0.02
Fluoride		2
Flurazepam	0.2	0.5-4
Glutethimide	5-78	10-100
Haloperidol	0.01	
Halothane		200
Hydrocodone		0.6
Hydrogen sulfide		0.92
Hydromorphone	0.02	0.02-1.2
Hydroxyzine		20
Ibuprofen	>100	
Imipramine	0.5-1.5	1-7
Iron	6	20-50
Isoniazid	20	70
Lead		1.1-3.5
Lidocaine	8	6-33
Lindane	0.02	0.2
Lithium	13.9	13.9-34.7
Lorazepam	0.3-0.6	
Loxapine	0.1	1
Lysergide (LSD)	0.001-0.004	
Magnesium	90-130	
Maprotiline	0.45-0.8	2-13
Meperidine	5	8-20 (oral) 1-8 (i.v.)
Mepivacaine	10	50
Meprobamate	60-120	100-300
Mercury (inorganic)	0.18-0.62	0.4-22
Mercury (organic)	>0.2	>0.6
Mesoridazine		>2
Methadone	0.1	0.1-1.8

TABLE A-2 Toxic and lethal blood concentrations—cont'd

Compound	Toxic concentrations (mg/L)	Lethal concentrations (mg/L)
Methamphetamine	0.1	2
Methanol	200	400
Methapyrilene		4.4-30
Methaqualone	2-12	5-42
Methohexital		100
Methylphenidate	0.8	2.3
Methyprylon	17	50
Metoprolol	>10	
Mexiletine	2	2
Morphine	0.2	0.2
Nicotine	10	5-52
Nortriptyline	0.5	10
Orphenadrine	2	4-75
Oxalate		10
Oxazepam	2	
Oxycodone	0.2	5
Paraldehyde	200-400	>480
Paraquat	8.5	35
Pentazocine	0.5	1-5
Pentobarbital	>5	10-169
Phenacetin	>30	100
Phencyclidine	0.09-0.22	0.3-25
Phenmetrazine	0.5	0.5-5
Phenobarbital	40-60	65-116
Phentermine	0.2	1
Phenylbutazone	100	400
Phenytoin	20-50	94
Primidone	50-80	100
Procainamide	10	>20
Procaine	>21	
Prochlorperazine	>1	5
Procyclidine		0.4-7.8
Promazine	>1	>5
Propoxyphene	0.3-0.6	1-17
Propranolol	2	4-29
Protriptyline	0.5-2	>1
Quinidine	9-28	30-50
Quinine	6	12
Salicylate	150-300	>500
Secobarbital	>3	5-52
Strychnine	2	2.8-12
Thallium	>1	0.5-11
Theophylline	20	50-250
Thiopental	>7	11-26
Thioridazine	2.4	4-13

Continued.

TABLE A-2 Toxic and lethal blood concentrations—cont'd

Compound	Toxic concentrations (mg/L)	Lethal concentrations (mg/L)
Thiothixene	1-2	3-12
Tolbutamide		600
Toluene	>0.5	10
Trazodone		15-28
Trichloroethanol	>50	100-640
Trifluoperazine	1.2-3	3-8
Trimethobenzamide	>10	
Trimipramine		>5
Tripelennamine		10
Valproic acid	200	
Verapamil		4

REFERENCES

1. Choonara IA, Rane A: Therapeutic drug-monitoring of anticonvulsants: state of the art, Clin Pharmacokinet 18:318, 1990.
2. Perry PJ, Pfohl BM, Holstad SG: The relationship between antidepressant response and tricyclic antidepressant plasma concentrations: a retrospective analysis of the literature using logistic regression analysis, Clin Pharmacokinet 13:381, 1987.
3. Reidenberg MM, Odar-Cederlöf I, von Bahr C, et al: Protein binding of diphenylhydantoin and desmethylimipramine in plasma from patients with poor renal function, N Engl J Med 285:264, 1971.

Appendix B

Pharmacokinetic characteristics of drugs

Values in this table are derived from multiple publications in the literature. They apply to adults and should be applied to children with caution if at all. When discrepant results were reported from different laboratories, a decision was made as to which methodology (assay, study design, and so on) was likely to be the most accurate. The ranges reflect those reported among the multiple sources reviewed. Drugs in development and available in countries other than the United States are included in anticipation of future availability.

Class / Drug	Bioavail-ability (%)	Renal elimi-nation (%)	Protein bound (%)	V_d (L/kg)	Elimination half-life (hours)	Clearance (ml/min/kg)	Effect of diseases: ESRD V_d	ESRD Cl	Cirrhosis V_d	Cirrhosis Cl	Other
Analgesics and antagonists											
Acetaminophen	75-85	0	Negligible	0.8-1.4	2-4	5	No Δ	No Δ			
Buprenorphine	30	0		2.8	2-3	20					
Butorphanol		<5	80	7	2.5-3	43					
Codeine	80			3.5-6	4	15	7.3	No Δ			
Dezocine		<1		11-12	2.2-2.8	50				31	
Hydromorphone	50	6		2.9	2.4	15					
Meperidine	56	5-7	60-80	4.2-5.2	3-7	7.5-12	No Δ	No Δ	No Δ	8	Bioavailability ↑ to 87% in cirrhosis
Meptazinol	9		27	5	2	30					
Methadone	80-90	4	60-90	3.6	20-30	1.4-2.1					
Morphine	25-50	10	35	2-4	1.7-4.5	8-27	No Δ	No Δ	No Δ	11	Bioavailability ↑ to 100% in cirrhosis
Nalbuphine	10	<7		4.3-7	2.2-3.7	22					Bioavailability ↑ to 45% in the elderly
Naltrexone	5-60	8	20	16	3-10	18-22					
Pentazocine	18	<5		5-7	3-5	17-20			No Δ	10	Bioavailability ↑ to 70% in cirrhosis
Propoxyphene	40	0	80	16	8-24	14	No Δ	No Δ			Toxic metabolite eliminated by kidney
Anesthetics (and other agents used primarily in anesthetic practice)											
Alcuronium		80-85	40	0.28-0.36	3-3.5	1.3-1.4		0.5			
Alfentanil		<1	88-95	0.3-1	1.5-2	4.4-6.5		No Δ		1.6	
Aminopyridine	95	90		3.2	3.9	9.3					
Atracurium		0	82	0.15-0.18	0.3-0.4	5.5-6.1					Metabolized by plasma esterases
Bupivacaine				1	2.7	8.3					
Etidocaine				1.9	2.7	16					
Etomidate		2	75	2-4.5	4-5.5	11.6-25					
Fazadinium		0	17	0.18-0.23	1	1.9-2.3					
Fentanyl		6-8	79-87	2-5	2.5-3.5	5.7-12.7					
Gallamine		85-100	30-70	0.21-0.24	2.3-2.7	1.2-1.6		0.2-0.3			

Ketamine		2-3		1.8-3.1	2.2-3.5	14-19					
Lofentanil			92								
Mepivacaine				1.2	1.9	11					
Metocurine		45-60	70	0.42-0.57	3.5-5.8	1.2-1.8		↓			
Minaxolone				1.6-2.2	0.75	17-25					
Pancuronium		30-40	70-85	0.15-0.38	1.7-2.2	1.1-2.1	No Δ	0.3			
Propofol		<1		3-14	3-6.5	19-33					
Sufentanil		1-2	92	1.7-5.2	2.5	10-21					
Thiopental		<1	84	1.9	10	3.2	No Δ	No Δ			
Tubocurarine		40-60	30-50	0.22-0.39	0.5-4	1.8-2.7	No Δ	↓			
Vecuronium		25	30	0.19-0.27	0.4-1.3	3-6.4				2.7	
Antianxiety agents, sedatives, and hypnotics											
Adinazolam				3.7	3.8	12					
Alprazolam	80-90	20	70	1-1.5	10-20	0.6-1.6					
Barbital		80			2.4-3.3						
Bromazepam			72	1.4	10-15	0.8					
Brotizolam	70		89-95	0.7	3.6-8	1.5-2.5					
Buspirone	1-13	<1	95	5.3	2-8	45	No Δ			↓	Bioavailability probably ↑ in cirrhosis
Chloral hydrate			70-80	0.6	4-10	1					
Chlordiazepoxide	100	0	94-97	0.3-0.6	6-25	0.25-0.54				0.15	
Clobazam		0	90	0.9-1.5	17-50	0.35-0.65					
Clomethiazole	10	<3	64	4.4	4.8	16.4				10	Bioavailability ↑ to 100% in cirrhosis
Chlorazepate		0		0.33	2	1.8					
Clotiazepam		0	99	2.5	9-10	3-4			1.6	2.5	
Desmethyl-diazepam	50		98	0.45	60	0.1					
Diazepam	100	0	98	1-2	20-70	0.25-0.54					
Estazolam					17						
Ethchlorvynol		0		3.5	19-32	1.7-2					
Flumazenil	16-28	<1	40	0.6-1.6	0.7-1.3	10-17			No Δ	10	Bioavailability ↑ to 65% in cirrhosis
Flunitrazepam	85	0	80	3.3	15-25	3.5					
Flurazepam			97	22	50-100	4.5					

CHF, Congestive heart failure; *Cl*, clearance; Cl_{Cr}, creatinine clearance; *COPD*, chronic obstructive pulmonary disease; *ESRD*, end-stage renal disease; K_m, Michaelis-Menten constant; V_d, volume of distribution.

Continued.

Class / Drug	Bioavailability (%)	Renal elimination (%)	Protein bound (%)	V_d (L/kg)	Elimination half-life (hours)	Clearance (ml/min/kg)	Effect of diseases: ESRD V_d	ESRD Cl	Cirrhosis V_d	Cirrhosis Cl	Other
Glutethimide		< 2	50	2.7	5-22	2.3					
Hexobarbital	> 90	< 1	50	1.2	3.5	3.9					
Loprazolam	70		80	4	7-8						
Lorazepam	93	0	90-93	0.7-1.6	10-20	0.7-1.2					
Lormetazepam	70-80	0			9-15	2.6-4.3					
Medazepam					1-2						
Meprobamate		10	Negligible		6-17						
Methaqualone		0	70-90	6	20-60	1.7					
Methohexital		< 1		2.2-5.2	3.9-8	11					
Midazolam	40-50	< 1	94-97	0.8-1.5	1.5-5.1	4-9				3.3	Bioavailability ↑ to 75% in cirrhosis
Nitrazepam	80	0	87	1.6-2.6	20-48	0.85-1.2					
Oxazepam	> 90	0	98	0.6-2	4-13	0.9-2					
Paraldehyde		0			3.5-10						
Pentobarbital			50-65	1.2	20-25	0.5-0.6					
Phenobarbital	100	20	50	0.9	24-140	0.1					
Prazepam		0		14	1.3	140					
Quazepam		0	> 95	5	27-41						
Temazepam	> 80	0	96-98	0.8-1.5	7-17	1-2					
Triazolam	100	0	80-90	0.7-1.7	2-4.5	3-9					
Zolpidem	70	< 1	92	0.54	1.5-2.4	4-3				↓	
Zopiclone	80	4-5	45	1.4	5	3.3					
Anticholinergics and cholinergics											
Atropine				2.7	4.1	7.6					
Cisapride	40-50	< 1	98	2.4	7-10						
Edrophonium				1.1	1.8	9.6					
Metoclopramide	60-75	80	40	2-3.4	2.5-5	8-11	No Δ	2-4			
Neostigmine	10-20	67	Negligible	0.9	1.3	8.4		1.7			
Pirenzepine	21-33	50	12	1.3-3.4	11-14	2.8-3.6	No Δ	1.4			
Pyridostigmine	10-20	80-90		1.5	1.9	9		2			
Anticoagulants, antifibrinolytics, and antiplatelet agents											
Dipyridamole	45		99	2.4	12	2-4					
Epsilon-aminocaproic acid		70-86		0.39	4.9	2.7		↓			

Streptokinase				0.016	1-1.5	0.15				
Sulfinpyrazone	100	25-50	>95	0.06	2.2-2.7	0.28				
Sulotroban		50-60			0.7-3	10		↓		
Ticlopidine	80-90	2	98		24-33					
TPA				0.1	0.5	9.8				
Tranexamic acid		90			1.5			1/8 normal		
Warfarin	100	0	99	0.14	35-45	0.045	No Δ	No Δ	No Δ	No Δ
Antidepressants, antipsychotics, and antimanic agents										
Amitriptyline	48	<2	95	14	16	12.5				
Amoxapine		0			8					
Bromperidol	50	<1	90		24					
Bupropion		0		40	7.5-19	57				
Chlorpromazine	40	0	95	20	30	8.5				
Clomipramine		1-3	95	7-20	34-36	5.5				
Clozapine	27			2	10	2.5				
Desipramine	40-50	18	90	20-60	15-60	10-30				
Dothiepin	30	<1		11-78	14-24	23-63				
Doxepin	13-45	0		9-33	8-25	14				
Fluoxetine		2-5	94	20-40	2.2-4 days	10			No Δ	4.2
Flupentixol	50			12-14	26-36	5.3				
Fluphenazine			99		16					
Fluvoxamine		0	77		15					
Haloperidol	60-65	<1	92	14-21	10-22	12				
Imipramine	30-75	18	95	20-40	16-20	8-17				
Lithium ion	100	100	0	0.67	8-41	0.35		↓		
Lofepramine	10		>99			163				
Maprotiline	37-67			15-28	20-60					
Medifoxamine	21	<1		3.9	3	15				
Mianserin	30-75		90	16	10-40	8.7				
Nortriptyline	50-80	0	95	20-30	15-56					
Perphenazine			92		9.4					
Protriptyline	80-90		90-95	20-55	55-200	3.6				
Rolipram	74			0.5	8.4	6.1				
Sulpiride		100	0	1	6	2	No Δ	0.6		
Tranylcypromine				2.7	2.4	14				
Trazodone	70-90	<1	90-95	0.9-1.3	4.7-6.3	2.3-2.8				

CHF, Congestive heart failure; *Cl*, clearance; Cl_{Cr}, creatinine clearance; *COPD*, chronic obstructive pulmonary disease; *ESRD*, end-stage renal disease; K_m, Michaelis-Menten constant; V_d, volume of distribution.

Continued.

Class / Drug	Bioavailability (%)	Renal elimination (%)	Protein bound (%)	V_d (L/kg)	Elimination half-life (hours)	Clearance (ml/min/kg)	Effect of diseases: ESRD V_d	ESRD Cl	Cirrhosis V_d	Cirrhosis Cl	Other
Trimipramine	41		95	31	23	16					
Antiepileptics											
Carbamazepine	70	2-3	75	1	4-6	0.9					Undergoes autoinduction
Clonazepam	98	0	86	3.2	24	1.6					
Ethosuximide		17-40	Negligible	0.7	35-55	0.17					
Lamotrigine		<7	40-60	1.2	24	0.4					
Phenytoin	100	2	90	0.6	24						V_{max} = 8.4 mg/kg/d; K_m = 8.5 mg/L
Primidone	90-95	40	19	0.6	5-15	0.85-1.7					
Valproate	100	3-7	90	0.19	6-15	0.15					Clearance 1/3 normal in elderly
Vigabatrin		50-65	0	0.8	5-7.4	1.7					
Antihistamines											
Astemizole		0	97		20 days						
Azelastine	80	<5	78-88		25						
Brompheniramine				11.7	25	6					
Cetirizine		60		0.5	7.4	0.7	No Δ	↓			
Chlorpheniramine	34	20		5.9-11.7	14-24	1.4-4.7					
Cimetidine	60	50-70	20	1.3	1-5	8-10	No Δ	3	0.6	No Δ	Bioavailability ↑ to 75% in cirrhosis
Diphenhydramine	40-60	2	78	3.3-6.8	3.4-9.3	8.6-18.6				6	
Doxylamine					10	3.2-3.7					
Etintidine		35-40		2	1.2-1.6	15					
Famotidine	37-45	65-80	15-22	0.8-1.4	2.5-4	5.6-6.4	No Δ	1	No Δ	No Δ	
Flunarizine	85	0	99	43-78	17-18 days						
Hydroxyzine		0		16-19.5	14-20	9.8-16.5			23	No Δ	
Methapyrilene	14	<2		3.9	1.6	28					
Nizatidine	100	54-65	28-35	0.8-1.3	1.3-1.6	10-11	No Δ	2.3			
Orphenadrine	95	8			16						
Oxatomide		<1	91		20						

Promethazine	25	< 1	93	13.5	12	16					
Ranitidine	50	80	15	1.2-1.8	1.5-2.5	9-10		2.5			Bioavailability ↑ to 70% in cirrhosis
Roxatidine	> 95	55-60	6-7	3.2	6	5	2	1.3			
Terfenadine			97		16-23						
Tripelennamine				10	3-4.5	32					
Tripolidine					5						
Anti-inflammatory agents											
Alclofenac		10-50	> 99	0.1	1.5-2.5						
Auranofin		50			70-80 days						
Azapropazone		60	> 99	0.15	10-15	0.14		0.05		0.03	
Carprofen		3-12	98		13-27						
Diclofenac		< 1	> 99	0.12-0.17	1-2	3.7					
Diflunisal		8	> 99	0.1-0.13	5-20	0.11				0.05	
Etodolac		0	95	0.4	6-7						
Fenbufen		4	> 98	2-4	10						
Fenclofenac				0.2-0.25	20-38						
Fenoprofen		30	> 99	0.1	2-3	0.6-1.3					
Flufenamic acid		< 1	> 90		9						
Flurbiprofen		< 15	99	0.1	3-5	0.3					
Ibuprofen		1	99	0.15-0.17	2-2.5	0.75					
Indomethacin		30	> 90	0.12	6	1-2					
Isoxicam					10-54						
Ketoprofen		< 1	99	0.11	1.5-4	0.6-1.7					
Ketorolac		5-10	> 99	0.17-0.25	4-6	0.35-0.62		No Δ			
Meclofenamic acid		2-4	> 99		3						
Mefenamic acid		< 6			3-4						
Nabumetone		< 1	> 99	0.11	24	0.06					
Naproxen		< 1	99	0.1	12-15	0.07					
Oxaprozin	100	< 1	> 99	0.15-0.25	50-60	0.04	↓	No Δ	No Δ	No Δ	
Oxyphenbutazone		< 2	99		27-64						
Penicillamine	40-70	40	80	1.5-3		10.7					
Phenylbutazone		1	99	0.17	50-100	0.02					

CHF, Congestive heart failure; *Cl*, clearance; Cl_{Cr}, creatinine clearance; *COPD*, chronic obstructive pulmonary disease; *ESRD*, end-stage renal disease; K_m, Michaelis-Menten constant; V_d, volume of distribution.

Continued.

Class Drug	Bioavail-ability (%)	Renal elimi-nation (%)	Protein bound (%)	V_d (L/kg)	Elimination half-life (hours)	Clearance (ml/min/kg)	Effect of diseases: ESRD V_d	ESRD Cl	Cirrhosis V_d	Cirrhosis Cl	Other
Piroxicam		10	>99	0.12-0.15	45-55	0.04-0.05					
Pirprofen			>99	0.11-0.17	6-7	0.28					
Proquazone	6-8	0	>98	0.15	0.6-1.3	9.5					
Salicylates (low dose)	70	Dependent on urine pH	80-90	0.15	2-3	0.8					Dose-dependent elimination
Salicylates (high dose)			↓	↑	15-30	0.2					
Sulindac sulfide		7	95		16						
Tenoxicam		0	>99	0.15	60-75	0.02-0.06					
Tiaprofenic acid		60	98	0.4-1	1.5-2.5	0.6-1.4					
Tolfenamic acid		<8	>99	0.16	2.5	2.2					
Tolmetin		15	>99	0.10-0.14	1-1.5	1.8					
Antiparkinson agents											
Bromocriptine	6		90-96		3	13					
Carbidopa	40-70	30			2.1						
Levodopa	33-63	0		0.9-1.6	0.8-1.7	23					
Antispasticity agents											
Baclofen	100	70-80	30	0.84	3-7	2.6		↓			
Dantrolene	70	0			8						
Antiulcer agents											
Misoprostol			85		1.5						
Omeprazole	35-60	0	95	0.3-0.4	0.5-1.5	7-8.6					
Bronchodilators											
Albuterol (salbutamol)	43-50	50-64	7	2-2.5	2.4-4	7-8	0.8	2.5			
Dyphylline		85	<3	0.8	1.8-2.3	4.8		↓			
Enprophylline		90	47	0.5-0.6	1.6	3-4					
Ipratropium	3-7			4.6	1.6	31					
Isoproterenol	25	40			0.05						
Metaproterenol	10		10	7.6	2-6	14					
Prenalterol	27	60	<5	3.4	2	21					

Terbutaline	10-20	55-60	15-25	0.9-1.5	3-20	3.8					
Theophylline	95	0	55	0.4-0.7	4-12	1			No Δ	0.7	Clearance is about half normal in COPD and in CHF
Cardiovascular agents											
Antianginal agents											
Amlodipine	52-88		93-97	21.4	34-48	7-14					
Diltiazem	30-40	<5	80-85	2-8	3.5-5	14-20		No Δ			
Felodipine	10-25	<1	99	8-12	10-25	12-24	No Δ	No Δ	5.6	7	Bioavailability doubles in CHF
Isosorbide dinitrate	30	0	30	1.4	1	32		No Δ			
Isradipine	15-20	0	97	1.6-2.9	2-5	10.5				↓	Bioavailability doubles in cirrhosis
Nicardipine	6-30	<1	>90	0.6-0.9	3.5-5	7-17		No Δ		↓	
Nifedipine	40-50	<1	92-98	0.8	3.5-4	6-15				3	Bioavailability doubles in cirrhosis
Nimodipine	5-13		98	0.9-2.3	1-6	14				↓	
Nisoldipine	4	0	>99	1.6-4.1	10-15	8-16		No Δ	6.4	7	Bioavailability ↑ to 15% in cirrhosis
Nitrendipine	11-16	<1	98	2-6	8-12	19		No Δ		↓	Bioavailability may ↑ in cirrhosis
Nitroglycerin	36	<1		3	3 min	300-1000					
Verapamil	34	3-4	90	5-6	3-5	14-20			3	5	Bioavailability doubles in cirrhosis
Antiarrhythmic agents											
Acecainide (*N*-Acetyl-procainamide)	80-90	60-85	10	1.2-1.6	6-10	2-3.1	No Δ				$Cl = 0.34 + 0.024\ Cl_{Cr}$
Amiodarone	22-86	0	96	70	25-50 days	2					
Aprindine	75	2		4	50	1					
Bretylium	25	100	8-10	5.0	6-11	10	No Δ	2			
Cibenzoline	85-100	50-60	55	4.0	6-15	9-15	No Δ	2.5			
Disopyramide	65-85	40-60	50-70	0.6	4-10	1.5-2	No Δ	↓		2.5	Clearance is about 1/3 normal in CHF
Encainide	30-85	0	80	3.8-5.7	0.5-4	25	↓	15	No Δ	17	All activity resides in metabolites
Flecainide	90-95	30-50	40	5.5-7.3	7	16	No Δ	5	No Δ	4	

CHF, Congestive heart failure; *Cl*, clearance; Cl_{Cr}, creatinine clearance; *COPD*, chronic obstructive pulmonary disease; *ESRD*, end-stage renal disease; K_m, Michaelis-Menten constant; V_d, volume of distribution.

Continued.

Class / Drug	Bioavailability (%)	Renal elimination (%)	Protein bound (%)	V_d (L/kg)	Elimination half-life (hours)	Clearance (ml/min/kg)	Effect of diseases: ESRD V_d	ESRD Cl	Cirrhosis V_d	Cirrhosis Cl	Other
Lidocaine	30	5	50-70	1.6	1.8	10	No Δ	No Δ	2.4	6	Volume of distribution and clearance are 1/2 normal in CHF; bioavailability ↑ to 90% in cirrhosis
Lorcainide	Dose-dependent	<3	85	6.5	7-8	14-21		No Δ		12	Clearance is about 1/3 normal in CHF
Mexiletine	90	30-55	50-60	5.9	8-12	6.3-8.3		No Δ	No Δ	2.3	
Moricizine					9						
Pirmenol	80-90	25	85	1.5	6-18	2.9					
Procainamide	75-85	50-70	15	2.4	2.6-3.5	8.6-9.8		↓			
Propafenone	5-12	<1	77-89	2.5-4.4	2-5	11		No Δ		↓	
Quinidine	70	15-40	70-95	2-3.5	5-12	2.5-5		No Δ			Both volume of distribution and clearance are 1/2 normal in CHF
Sotalol	100	60-75	54	0.7-1.5	5-8	1.5-2.1					$Cl = 0.27 + 0.018\ Cl_{Cr}$
Tocainide	90-100	40	50	2.2	12-14	2-2.5	No Δ	0.5-1.3			
Antihypertensives											
Acebutolol	20-60	15-30	11-19	1.2	3-4	8.8					Active metabolite is eliminated by the kidney
Alprenolol	15	<1	85		2-3						
Amosulalol	100	35		0.75	2.8	1.9					
Atenolol	45-55	75-85	<5	1.2	6-9	1.3-2.1	No Δ				$Cl = 0.047 + 0.0107\ Cl_{Cr}$
Benazepril		85	96		11	0.04		↓			
Betaxolol	80-90	15	55	4.9-9.8	14-22	4.7		No Δ			
Bevantolol	60	<10	>95	1.5	1.5-2			No Δ			
Bisoprolol	90	50	30	2.9	9-12	1.8-3.4	No Δ		No Δ		$Cl = 1.36 + 0.014\ Cl_{Cr}$
Captopril	60-70	80	20-30	0.7-0.8	1.9-2.2	12-13.3		1.5-2			
Carteolol	85	65	15	4	3-7	10		↓			
Cilazapril	45-75	90	24	0.3	36-49	1.8-4.1					$Cl = 0.61 + 0.026\ Cl_{Cr}$
Clonidine	75-100	40-70	20-30	2-4	7-18	3-5		↓			
Delapril					1.2			↓			
Diazoxide	85-90	20	>90	0.18	15-30	0.1	No Δ	No Δ			
Doxazosin	60-70	1	98-99	1	18-20	1.2-2.2		No Δ			
Enalapril	40	100	50		5	6.7		↓			

Esmolol		0	56	2-3.5	7-9 min	170-285					
Fosinopril	25-29		95	0.14	3.7	0.6		↓			
Guanabenz		<1	90	5	4.3	9			↓	2	
Guanadrel		40	20	10	4	41	No Δ				$Cl = 0.42 + 0.337\ Cl_{Cr}$
Guanfacine	60-100	24-37	64	3.9-6.5	12-23	2.6-5.2		No Δ			
Hydralazine	10-35	<10		6-8	0.7-1	75-140		No Δ			
Indoramin	24-31	<10	92	7.4-7.7	4-5.5	20			9.5	12	
Ketanserin	50	<4	94	5-10	6-14	6-10			4.7	4.6	
Labetalol	11-86	<5	50	5.6	3-3.5	21	No Δ	No Δ			Bioavailability doubles in cirrhosis
Lisinopril	25-30	100	0	1.8	13	0.7		↓			
Medroxalol	30	8		16	11	16					
Mepindolol	80	<1	50-60		3			No Δ			
Methyldopa	25-30	50-65	<15	0.5-0.6	1.3-1.8	3.3-5.7		↓			
Metoprolol	50	5-10	12	4.9	2.5-5	10-20		No Δ	No Δ	9	Bioavailability ↑ to 85% in cirrhosis
Minoxidil	95	12-20	0	2.6-5	3-4	20					$Cl = 4.87 + 0.18\ Cl_{Cr}$
Moxonidine		60-70	8	3	2.1	12-15	2.4	4.8			
Nadolol	30-50	60-75	20-30	1.5	14-24	1-3					$Cl = 0.025 + 0.0087\ Cl_{Cr}$
Nitroprusside		0									Thiocyanate metabolite (toxic) is eliminated by the kidney
Oxprenolol	20-60	2-5	80		1.3-1.5						
Penbutolol	95	4-6	>95		22						
Pentopril		40			2						
Perindopril	19	60-70	10-18		31	1.2-2.3				No Δ	Bioavailability ↑ to 30% in cirrhosis
Pinacidil	60	4-10	65	3.4	1.5-3	9.5			2.6	4.9	
Pindolol	75	36-39	57	2.1	3-4	6.9-7.7		No Δ		No Δ	
Prazosin	50-70	<10	90-95	0.57	2.5-4.5	2.4-3.3		No Δ			
Propranolol	36	0	99	4-4.5	2.5-5	12	No Δ	No Δ	↑	8	Bioavailability doubles in cirrhosis
Quinapril					1.8-3.4	1.8-3.3					$Cl = 0.022\ Cl_{Cr} - 0.15$
Ramipril			56		11	5.7		1.6		No Δ	
Rilmenidene	100	64	<10	4.5	8-9	6.6	No Δ		No Δ		$Cl = 1.06 + 0.048\ Cl_{Cr}$
Terazosin	90	10-15	90-94	0.25-0.43	10-18	1.1					
Timolol	50-60	15	10	1.7	2.7	7.7					
Trimazosin	63				2.9	0.9					
Urapidil	63-80	10-15	75-80	0.4-0.8	1.8-4	1.8-3.8				↓	

CHF, Congestive heart failure; *Cl*, clearance; Cl_{Cr}, creatinine clearance; *COPD*, chronic obstructive pulmonary disease; *ESRD*, end-stage renal disease; K_m, Michaelis-Menten constant; V_d, volume of distribution.

Continued.

Class / Drug	Bioavail-ability (%)	Renal elimi-nation (%)	Protein bound (%)	V_d (L/kg)	Elimination half-life (hours)	Clearance (ml/min/kg)	Effect of diseases: ESRD V_d	ESRD Cl	Cirrhosis V_d	Cirrhosis Cl	Other
Blood lipid-lowering agents											
Bezafibrate	100	35-40	95	0.24-0.35	2.1	1.4					$Cl = 0.14 + 0.015\ Cl_{Cr}$
Ciprofibrate		7			81			↓			
Clofibrate	95	40-70	92-97	0.14	15-17.5	0.1		0.05		↓	
Fenofibrate		0	>99		20-27			↓			
Gemfibrozil	100		97-99		7.6			No Δ			
Lovastatin	<5	0	>95		1.1-1.7	4.3-7.8		No Δ			
Pravastatin	18	47	45	0.9	0.8-3.2	13.5					
Probucol	2-8	<2			23-47 days						
Simvastatin	<5	<1	>95								
Cardiac inotropes											
Amrinone	90	10-40	35-50	1.4	2-4.4	3.9-8.8					Both V_d and clearance are about 1/2 normal in CHF
Digitoxin	95	33	90	0.73	6-8 days	0.05	No Δ	No Δ			
Digoxin	75	70-80	25	3.9	42	1.8	↓				$Cl = 0.33 + 0.0126\ Cl_{Cr}$
Enoximone	45-70	<1	85	4.2	6.2	9.6					
Milrinone	90	80-85		0.32-0.56	0.8-0.9	4.3-6.2					$Cl = 0.036\ Cl_{Cr} - 0.24$
Xamoterol	5	60-70	3	1.1-2	8-16	3			No Δ	↓	
Chemotherapeutic agents											
Antibacterials											
Aminocyclitols											
Spectinomycin		75	0	0.15-0.24	1.6	1	No Δ	↓			
Aminoglycosides											
All	0	100	0	0.25	2-3	1.2	No Δ				$Cl = 0.04 + 0.01\ Cl_{Cr}$
Carbapenems											
Clavulanic acid		27-32		0.35	1-1.5	2-5					
Imipenem	0	60-70	20	0.23-0.42	1	3.5		↓			

Cephalosporins											
Cefaclor	50	50-60	25	0.36	0.7-0.8	5.5		↓			
Cefadroxil	85	90-95	16	0.3	1.3	2.5		↓			
Cefamandole		>95	74	0.19	0.5-1.5	2.8		↓			
Cefatrizine	40	80	60-65	0.3	1	3.2					
Cefazolin	90	80-100	85	0.14	1.6-2.3	1	↑				$Cl = 0.06 + 0.0056\ Cl_{Cr}$
Cefepime		80	16	0.25	0.3	1.6	No Δ				$Cl = 0.014 + 0.0124\ Cl_{Cr}$
Cefetamet	40-50	>90	22	0.29-0.35	2.1-2.4	1.7-2	No Δ	0.2			
Cefixime	40-52	40	63	0.1	3-5	1.0-2.4	↓				$Cl = 0.82 + 0.013\ Cl_{Cr}$
Cefmenoxime		80	43-75	0.17	1	2.8	No Δ				$Cl = 0.29 + 0.02\ Cl_{Cr}$
Cefmetazole		85		0.16	1.3	1.8	No Δ				$Cl = 0.0041 + 0.017\ Cl_{Cr}$
Cefonicid		82-96	98	0.1	3-5	0.3	No Δ				$Cl = 0.02 + 0.003\ Cl_{Cr}$
Cefoperazone		25	90	0.17	1.6-2.4	1.1	No Δ	No Δ		↓	
Ceforanide		80-82	80-82	0.14-0.17	2.5-3	0.7-1	No Δ				$Cl = 0.074 + 0.086\ Cl_{Cr}$
Cefotaxime		50-60	20-40	0.28-0.48	1-1.5	3.6-4.5	No Δ			2.7	$Cl = 1.2 + 0.025\ Cl_{Cr}$
Cefotetan		80	80-90	0.12	3	0.46		0.04			
Cefotiam		50-70	40	0.34	0.9-1.6	4.2-6.4		3.2			Dose-dependent elimination
Cefoxitin		80	74	0.27	0.7	4.7					$Cl = 0.05\ Cl_{Cr} - 0.19$
Cefpiramide		22	96	0.1	4.5	0.27					
Cefroxadine	90	80-96	10	0.35	0.9-1.1	4.1	No Δ				$Cl = 0.034\ Cl_{Cr}$
Cefsulodin		50	25-35	0.26	1.6	2					$Cl = 0.362 + 0.01\ Cl_{Cr}$
Ceftazidime		70-80	17	0.25	1.5-3	1.7	No Δ				$Cl = 0.15 + 0.016\ Cl_{Cr}$
Ceftizoxime		90-100	30	0.23-0.35	1.4	1.9-2.5	No Δ				$Cl = 0.007 + 0.0157\ Cl_{Cr}$
Ceftriaxone		40-65	83-96	0.16	6-9	0.15-0.3		No Δ	↓	↓	
Cefuroxime	30-40	95-100	33-50	0.2	1.2	1.5-2.1					$Cl = 0.28 + 0.013\ Cl_{Cr}$
Cephacetrile	95	>90	25-35	0.37	1-1.5	3.4		↓			
Cephalexin	95	90-96	15	0.33	0.9-1.2	3.6		↓			
Cephalothin		50-80	65-70	0.32	0.4-0.6	8.2		↓			
Cephapirin		50	60	0.22	0.6-0.7	4.3		↓			
Cephradine	>90	80-95	14	0.32	0.7-0.8	5.3		↓			
Chloramphenicol and thiamphenicol											
Chloramphenicol	75-90	5-10	25-50	0.5-0.8	3-5	2.5-3.2			No Δ	0.7-2.1	
Thiamphenicol		60-90	<10		2-3			↓			

CHF, Congestive heart failure; *Cl*, clearance; Cl_{Cr}, creatinine clearance; *COPD*, chronic obstructive pulmonary disease; *ESRD*, end-stage renal disease; K_m, Michaelis-Menten constant; V_d, volume of distribution.

Continued.

Class / Drug	Bioavail-ability (%)	Renal elimi-nation (%)	Protein bound (%)	V_d (L/kg)	Elimination half-life (hours)	Clearance (ml/min/kg)	Effect of diseases: ESRD V_d	ESRD Cl	Cirrhosis V_d	Cirrhosis Cl	Other
Macrolide antibiotics											
Azithromycin	40	15		23	41	10.5					
Clindamycin	85	10-15	60-90	0.66	2.5-3.5	2.1-3.5		No Δ	No Δ	1.7	
Erythromycin	10-80	10-15	70-85	0.78	1.1-2	6.9	↑	No Δ		6	
Josamycin		<20	15		0.9-2					↓	
Lincomycin		5-15	70	0.54	4.7-5.6	1.2		↓			
Roxithromycin		50	96	0.4	10-13	0.6	No Δ	0.3			
Monobactams											
Aztreonam	<1	65	50-60	0.2	1.7	1-2	No Δ	0.35	No Δ	0.8	
Carumonam		70-90	18	0.18	1.5	1.5					Cl = 0.123 + 0.0134 Cl_{Cr}
Moxalactam		60-80	50-60	0.28	2-4	1.7	No Δ				Cl = 0.14 + 0.016 Cl_{Cr}
Nitroimidazole											
Ornidazole		<4	5-10	0.86	14	0.7			No Δ	0.5	
Penicillins											
Amdinocillin (Mecillinam)		50-70	5-10	0.5	1	3-6					Cl = 0.97 + 0.027 Cl_{Cr}
Amoxicillin	95	50-70	17	0.66	0.9-2.3	6.5		↓			
Ampicillin	60	90	18	0.3	0.8-1.5	2.7					Cl = 0.21 + 0.025 Cl_{Cr}
Azlocillin		65	30	0.18	0.8	2.6	No Δ	↓			
Carbenicillin		80	50	0.13	1	1.5					Cl = 0.15 + 0.0097 Cl_{Cr}
Cloxacillin	40	75	95	0.1	0.5	2.2		No Δ			
Dicloxacillin	50-85	60	96	0.09	0.7	1.6		No Δ			
Methicillin		85-90	30-50	0.45	0.5-0.85	6.1		↓			
Mezlocillin		60-70	16-42	0.14	1	4	No Δ			1.8	Cl = 0.97 + 0.03 Cl_{Cr}
Nafcillin	35	25	90	0.35	1-2	7.5		No Δ			
Oxacillin	35	45	92	0.3	0.5	6.1		No Δ			
Penicillin		90-100	50-65	0.23	0.5	5.3					Cl = 0.51 + 0.048 Cl_{Cr}
Piperacillin		53-73	21	0.18-0.22	1	2.6	No Δ	0.7			
Temocillin		85	85	0.15-0.24	5-6	0.35		0.15			
Ticarcillin		85-90	45-65	0.21	1.2-1.5	1.9		↓			

Polymyxins											
Colistin		60-75	50	0.47	3-4.5	1.4		↓			
Polymyxin B		60-90			3-6			↓			
Quinolones											
Ciprofloxacin	60-85	60-70	20-30	2.2-5	3-6.5	5.5-10.5	No Δ		No Δ	No Δ	Cl = 3.15 + 0.047 Cl_{Cr}
Enoxacin	87-98	45-70	20-25	1.6-4.4	3.1-7.4	2.3-6.7	No Δ				Cl = 1.26 + 0.044 Cl_{Cr}
Fleroxacin	100	60-70	23	1.3	11-14	1.2	No Δ				Cl = 0.37 + 0.0067 Cl_{Cr}
Norfloxacin	30-40	30-40	10-15		3.5-6.5			↓			
Ofloxacin	95-100	70-100	20-30	1.1-1.6	5-7.5	3.3-4.1	No Δ	0.8			
Pefloxacin	90-100	9	20-30	1.5-1.9	7.5-11	1.7-2.1	No Δ	No Δ	No Δ	0.6	
Sulfonamides											
Sulfadiazine	100	66	55	0.3	7.5-9	0.5					
Sulfamethox-azole	100	20-30	65	0.25	9-11	0.32		↓			
Sulfasalazine	<20	10-20	50	0.26	6-14	0.6-2.1					
Sulfisoxazole	95	50-55	90	0.16	5.5-6	0.32		↓			
Trimethoprim	100	50	70	2.1	8-11	2.2		↓			
Tetracyclines											
Doxycycline	90-95	30-40	80-90	0.75-1.9	15-25	0.53		No Δ			
Minocycline	95-100	8-12	70-80	1.1-1.6	12-18			No Δ			
Tetracycline	80	60	65	1.5	6	1.7		↓			
Urinary bacterio-static											
Cinoxacin		60	65-70	0.25	1-1.5	2.3	No Δ	↓			
Vancomycin											
Teicoplanin		75-100	90	0.5-1	30-130	0.19	No Δ				Cl = 0.063 + 0.00093 Cl_{Cr}
Vancomycin		90-100	30	0.47-0.9	6-11	0.9-1.2					Cl = 0.04 + 0.0075 Cl_{Cr}
Antifungals											
Amphotericin B		3	95	4	15 days	0.43		No Δ			
Fluconazole	>90	80	11	0.9	25-30	0.34	No Δ	0.09			
Flucytosine	85	80-90	3-4	0.7	3-5.5	2					Cl = 0.011 Cl_{Cr}
Itraconazole	40-100	0	>99		35	4-5	No Δ	No Δ			
Ketoconazole		<1	99	1.25	4-7.5	3		No Δ			
Miconazole	0	0	98	21	24	10	↓	No Δ			

CHF, Congestive heart failure; *Cl*, clearance; Cl_{Cr}, creatinine clearance; *COPD*, chronic obstructive pulmonary disease; *ESRD*, end-stage renal disease; K_m, Michaelis-Menten constant; V_d, volume of distribution.

Continued.

Class / Drug	Bioavail-ability (%)	Renal elimi-nation (%)	Protein bound (%)	V_d (L/kg)	Elimination half-life (hours)	Clearance (ml/min/kg)	Effect of diseases: ESRD V_d	ESRD Cl	Cirrhosis V_d	Cirrhosis Cl	Other
Antimalarials											
Chlorguanide		50			6-12						
Chloroquine	80-90	55	55	150-250	6-10 days	10-12					
Halofantrine		0		100-570	1.3-6.6 days	2.5-19					
Hydroxychloroquine		25			44 days						
Mefloquine		0	98	13-41	6.5-35 days	0.26-1.2					
Primaquine	75	4		3	7.6	5					
Proquanil		50			6-12						
Pyrimethamine		<1	85	2.3-2.9	35-175	0.25-0.4					
Quinine		20	90	1.8	8.5-11	9.2		No Δ			
Antineoplastics and antimetabolites											
Adriamycin					14						
Azathioprine (mercaptopurine)	60	<2	20	0.55	1	11					
Bleomycin		60		0.3	9	0.38		↓			
Busulfan		0.5-3	3-15	1	2.5-3.4	4.5					
Carboplatin		50-75	15-24	0.23-0.28	6	1.1-2.1					$Cl = 0.52 + 0.013\ Cl_{Cr}$
Carmustine (BCNU)				3.3	1.5	56					
Chlorambucil				0.86	1	0.55					
Cisplatin		27-45	>90	0.5	0.3-0.5	17		↓			
Cyclophosphamide	60-90	10-15	60	0.62	4-7.5	0.8-1.1		No Δ			Clearance of active metabolites is decreased in renal disease
Cytarabine		6		2.6	0.5-3.3			No Δ			
Doxorubicin	5	<15	80-85	22	36	4					
Etoposide	25-75	20-60	94	0.2-0.5	4-8	0.37-0.86		0.3			
Fluorouracil	50-80	<5	10	0.25	0.1	33					
Melphalan	25-90	12	90	0.6-0.75	1.1-1.4	5.2					
Methotrexate	24-70	80-90	45-50	0.76	8-12	1.5-2.1		↓			

Mitomycin-C				0.5	0.7	3.4			
Mitoxantrone		<7	>95	15.5	37	4.7			↓
Tamoxifen	25-50	0			7 days				
Teniposide		4-14	99	0.2-0.7	6-10	0.2-0.4			
Trimetrexate				0.6-0.8	12-15	0.4			
Vinblastine			75	24	1-1.5	10.6			
Vincristine		12	75	8.6	1-2.5	1.8			
Antiparasitics and anthelmintics									
Levamisole	60-70	<6		1.6	3.6-5.6	4.3			
Mebendazole	22	0		1.2	1.1	15.1			↓
Metronidazole	100	6	10	0.8-1	8	0.7-1.3	No Δ	No Δ	0.25
Ornidazole	>90	<5	10-15	0.7	10-14	0.7		No Δ	0.4
Oxamniquine	50	2			2.2				
Pentamidine		100	3					↓	
Praziquantel	5-7				1-1.5				↓
Suramin			>99	0.5	44-54 days	0.005			
Tinidazole	100	25	12-20	0.6-0.8	12-17	0.6	No Δ	No Δ	
Antituberculosis and antileprosy agents									
p-Aminosalicylic acid		40-60	50-70	0.24	0.7	4		↓	
Capreomycin			50						
Clofazimine	70	<1			2-3 months				
Cycloserine (terizidone)		50			8-12				
Dapsone	70-80	5-15	70-90	1.2-1.5	10-30	0.6			
Ethambutol	75-80	80	20-30	2.3	3	8.6		↓	
Ethionamide	100	<1	24		2				
Isoniazid		5-25	0	0.6	0.7-6.5	2.5-7		No Δ	
Pyrazinamide		<1		0.7	7.4-9.6	0.9			
Rifampin		<10	90	1	3.5	3.5			
Thiacetazone		15	30		12				
Viomycin			85						

CHF, Congestive heart failure; *Cl*, clearance; Cl_{Cr}, creatinine clearance; *COPD*, chronic obstructive pulmonary disease; *ESRD*, end-stage renal disease; K_m, Michaelis-Menten constant; V_d, volume of distribution.

Continued.

Class / Drug	Bioavail-ability (%)	Renal elimi-nation (%)	Protein bound (%)	V_d (L/kg)	Elimination half-life (hours)	Clearance (ml/min/kg)	Effect of diseases: ESRD V_d	ESRD Cl	Cirrhosis V_d	Cirrhosis Cl	Other
Antiviral agents											
Acyclovir	15-30	75-80	9-22	0.7	2-3	4.2					Cl = 0.41 + 0.05 Cl_{Cr}
Amantadine	100	100	0	5.1-6.6	12	4.9		↓			
2′,3′-Dideoxy-inosine (ddI)	38	36		1	0.5	17					
Foscarnet	17	80		1.3	90	2.2-3.1					
Ganciclovir (DHPG)	4-7	99	1-2	0.47-0.64	2.5-4	3					Cl = 0.03 Cl_{Cr}
Ribavirin	45	24	0	8.7	35	3.8					
Rimantadine		10-16		19-25	24-33	9				No Δ	
Vidarabine		40-60			3.5	2		↓			
Zidovudine (AZT)	42-81	10-20	15	1.4	1-1.5	22		No Δ	No Δ	6.6	
Dermatologic agents											
Etretinate	40		98	3	80-100 days						
Isotretinoin	25	0	>99		10-30	5					
Methoxsalen		0	90	0.9-8.9	0.6-2.4	10.2-157					
Diuretics											
Acetazolamide					13						
Amiloride		50	40		17-26			↓			
Bendroflumethi-azide	90			1-1.5	2.5-5	4.3		↓			
Benzthiazide	100				10						
Bumetanide	80-90	50		0.15	1	2-3.5		↓			
Chlorothiazide	30-50			1	15-25	4.3		↓			
Chlorthalidone	65				24-55			↓			
Clopamide					8-12						
Furosemide	40-60	50		0.15	1-1.5	1.5-3		↓			
Hydrochlorothi-azide	65-75			2-5	3-10	4.6		↓			
Hydroflumethiazide	75			5	6-10	6.4		↓			
Indapamide	93			1.6	6-15			↓			
Mannitol		80	0	0.5	1.2	7		0.03			

Polythiazide					25			↓		
Triamterene	55	7	60	3	2-5	14		↓		Metabolite accounts for most of activity
Trichlormethiazide					1-4	3.4		↓		
Drugs of abuse										
Amphetamine			20	3.5-4.6						
Cocaine	70-100	<1	45	2-2.7	0.8-1.2	23-35				
Nicotine	30	10	5-20							
Phencyclidine	50-90	9-10	60-70	6.2	7-51	5.4				
Δ^9-Tetrahydro-cannabinol	4-24		95	7.1	57					
Hypoglycemic agents										
Acarbose	0.5-1.7	1.7	15	0.32	2.8	143				
Acetohexamide		Minor			1-1.3					Active metabolite is eliminated by the kidney
Chlorpropamide	>90	47	88-96	0.1-0.3	24-48	0.03		↓		
Glibornuride			95	0.25	5-12					
Gliclazide		<20	85-95	0.24	8-11	0.19				
Glipizide	80-100	5-7	97	0.13-0.36	3-7	0.4-0.6				
Glyburide	45	50	99	0.16-0.3	1.4-2.9	0.9-1.1				
Phenformin		54	12-20	5-10	5-15					
Tolazamide		7			4-7					
Tolbutamide	95	0	95-97	0.1-0.15	4-6	0.28		No Δ	0.14	
Hypouricemic agents and colchicine										
Allopurinol	67	30	<5		2-8					Active metabolite is eliminated by the kidney
Colchicine		5-17	31	2.2	19	1.3		↓		
Probenecid	100	<2	85-95	0.15	5-8	0.25-0.4				
Miscellaneous agents										
Acetylcysteine	6-10	30		0.34	2.3	3.5				
Aminoglutethimide		35-50	20-25	1.1	9-16	0.8-1		↓		
Clodronate	1-2	70-90	36	0.25	1.8-2.3	1.7		↓		
Cyclosporine	<5-80	<1	96-99	3.5-7.4	3-16	6-10	No Δ	No Δ	2.5	

CHF, Congestive heart failure; *Cl,* clearance; *Cl_{Cr}*, creatinine clearance; *COPD,* chronic obstructive pulmonary disease; *ESRD,* **end-stage renal disease;** K_m, **Michaelis-Menten constant;** V_d, volume of distribution.

Continued.

Class / Drug	Bioavailability (%)	Renal elimination (%)	Protein bound (%)	V_d (L/kg)	Elimination half-life (hours)	Clearance (ml/min/kg)	Effect of diseases: ESRD		Cirrhosis		Other
							V_d	Cl	V_d	Cl	
Dihydroergotamine mesylate	9	11		15	14	25					
Disulfiram					7						
Domperidone	15	1	92	5.7	7.5-16	7-10		No Δ			
Edetate (EDTA)				0.05-0.23	2-3	0.8	No Δ				$Cl = 0.102 + 0.0077\ Cl_{Cr}$
Epoetin (Erythropoietin)	31	<5		0.02-0.11	8-10	0.03-0.08					
Iloprost	16	0			0.5	24					
Nabilone	96				2	0.7					
Pentoxifylline	20	0	0	2.4-4.2	0.8	19			No Δ	↓	Bioavailability doubles in cirrhosis
Tolrestat			99		10						
Steroids											
Betamethasone	70	5	65	1.4	5.5	3					
Budesonide	11	0	88	4.3	2	20					
Dexamethasone	50-80	8	70	0.8-1	3-4	2.8-3.5					
Methylprednisolone	80	<10	40-60	1.2-1.5	1.9-6	4-8					
Prednisone	98	34		2.2	2.5-3.5	10				↓	$Cl = 3.8 + 0.036\ Cl_{Cr}$
Triamcinolone				1.4-2.1	1.4	11-16					
Sympathomimetics and other drugs affecting the sympathetic nervous system											
Caffeine		0.5-1.5	15-30	0.54-0.7	4-5	1.3-1.5				0.2	
Dobutamine				0.2	2.5 min	60					
Dopexamine					7	36					
Ibopamine		<1			0.75					↓	
Ritodrine	30		35	29	15	23					
Thyroid and antithyroid drugs											
Methimazole	95	7	0	0.6	3-6	1.4		No Δ			
Propylthiouracil	75	<10	80	0.3-0.4	1-2	3.9					
Thyroxine					6 days						
Triiodothyronine					1 day						

CHF, Congestive heart failure; *Cl*, clearance; Cl_{Cr}, creatinine clearance; *COPD*, chronic obstructive pulmonary disease; *ESRD*, end-stage renal disease; K_m, Michaelis-Menten constant; V_d, volume of distribution.

Index

H

N

S

W

X

Y

Z